R. Korinthenberg
(Hrsg.)

Aktuelle Neuropädiatrie 2002

Peter-Emil-Becker-Lecture 2002
Wissenschaftspreis der Gesellschaft für Neuropädiatrie 2002
Kontroversen in der Neuropädiatrie: Pro und Contra
Pädiatrische Neurophysiologie
Funktionelle Bildgebung – Eine Erweiterung der neurophysiologischen Untersuchungstechniken
Pathophysiologie und Behandlung der Infantilen Zerebralparese
Neuropharmakologie
Neuromuskuläre Erkrankungen
Therapie mit Immunglobulinen bei neurologischen Erkrankungen im Kindesalter
Stoffwechselleiden und Genetik
Neurologie in Neonatologie und Intensivmedizin
Epilepsie 1: prächirurgische Befunde und chirurgische Behandlung
Epilepsie 2: Pathophysiologie, Verlauf, Differentialdiagnose
Epilepsie 3: medikamentose und diatetische Behandlung
Verschiedenes
Stellungnahmen der Gesellschaft für Neuropädiatrie zu Therapieverfahren

Novartis Pharma Verlag
Nürnberg 2003

Prof. Dr. med. R. Korinthenberg

Klinik für Neuropädiatrie und Muskelerkrankungen
Zentrum für Kinderheilkunde und Jugendmedizin
Universitätsklinikum Freiburg
Mathildenstraße 1
D-79106 Freiburg

ISSN 0721-6106
ISBN 3-933185-59-9 Novartis Pharma Verlag, Nürnberg

Die Deutsche Bibliothek – CIP-Einheitsaufnahme

Satz: Fotosatz H. Strütt & D. Rünzi, 79650 Schopfheim
Druck: Freimund-Druckerei, 91564 Neuendettelsau

Vorwort

Vom 4. bis 7. April 2002 fand in Freiburg die 28. Jahrestagung der Gesellschaft für Neuropädiatrie statt. Das Programm umfasste wissenschaftliche Sitzungen und Fortbildungsveranstaltungen, die sämtlich auf das Interesse einer großen Zahl von Teilnehmern trafen. Vor allem auch in den Hauptsitzungen wurde versucht, neue wissenschaftliche Methoden und Grundlagenwissen aufzuarbeiten und für die praktische Arbeit im klinischen Alltag verwertbar zu machen.

Im vorliegenden Kongressband konnten neben den Referaten der P.E. Becker- und Wissenschafts-Preisträger fast alle Hauptvorträge und eine große Zahl der wissenschaftlichen Beiträge Aufnahme finden. Die Redner der »Pro und Kontra«-Sitzung waren aufgefordert worden, wissenschaftliche Argumente zu noch umstrittenen Vorgehensweisen gegeneinander zu stellen. Es resultierte eine hochinteressante Veranstaltung, die die Diskussionskultur in der Gesellschaft gefördert hat. Zusammen mit den Beiträgen des Vorsymposiums der Arbeitsgemeinschaften »Pädiatrische Neurophysiologie« und »Frühe Hirnläsionen« ist es gelungen, relevante Manuskripte zur Pathophysiologie der Cerebralparesen zusammenzustellen und mit den Beiträgen der Sitzung zur Therapie der ICP zu kombinieren. Unter dem Kapitel »Neuromuskuläre Erkrankungen« findet sich die Zusammenstellung von Referaten, welchen den aktuellen Stand der Therapieforschung auch in dieser Krankheitsgruppe sehr umfassend darstellen. Großen Raum nehmen auch die epileptologischen Themen ein, mit den Schwerpunkten Chirurgie, diätetische Behandlung und neue Medikamente. Schließlich finden sich in der Rubrik »Verschiedenes« zahlreiche Beiträge, die dem Leser für seinen neuropädiatrischen Alltag nützlich sein mögen.

Das Buch soll für die Leser, die an dem Kongress in Freiburg teilnehmen konnten, eine brauchbare Erinnerungshilfe sein. Für die Kolleginnen und Kollegen, die nicht nach Freiburg kommen konnten, möge es einen Einblick in die abgehandelten Themen geben.

Freiburg, den 1. Juli 2002

Prof. Dr. Rudolf Korinthenberg

Inhaltsverzeichnis

4. Pädiatrische Neurophysiologie

5. Funktionelle Bildgebung – Eine Erweiterung der neurophysiologischen Untersuchungstechniken

6. Pathophysiologie und Behandlung der Infantilen Zerebralparese

9. Therapie mit Immunglobulinen bei neurologischen Erkrankungen im Kindesalter

10. Stoffwechselleiden und Genetik

11. Neurologie in Neonatologie und Intensivmedizin

12. Epilepsie 1: prächirurgische Befunde und chirurgische Behandlung

14. Epilepsie 3: medikamentöse und diätetische Behandlung

15. Verschiedenes

Autoren- und Sachwortverzeichnis

1. Peter-Emil-Becker-Lecture 2002

Laudatio Jean Aicardi
Emil Becker Prize Awardee 2002

I. Krägeloh-Mann

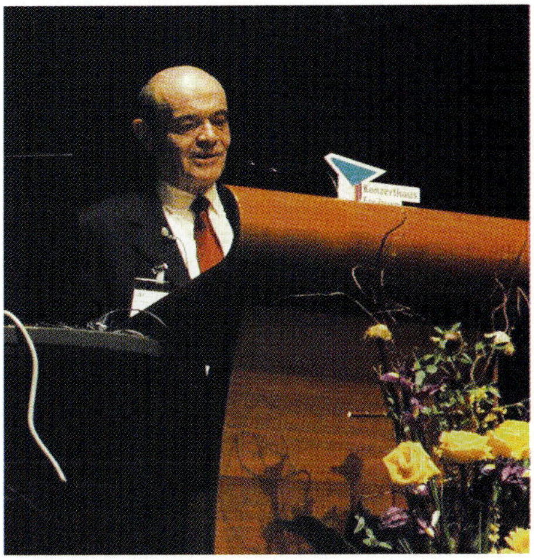

Jean Aicardi was born in Paris in 1926. He got his school and university education in Paris and became MD in 1955. He then went to Havard Medical school as a Research Fellow where he worked with Ronnie Byers.

Back in France, he was first in Hopital Des Enfants Malades, then from 64 to 79 in St. Vincent de Paul, one of the first departments of Child Neurology in Europe, then back again Aux Enfants Malades until 91.

In 1969, he became chief investigator, in 1986 research director at the national institute of health and medical research (INSERM).

After having retired in Paris he was appointed honorary professor of Child Neurology at the Institute of Child Health, University of London and Honorary Consultant at Great Ormond Street. He is there still part of the year, since 2 years he is also Honorary Consultant at Hopital Robert Debré in Paris.

Jean Aicardi went very early beyond national borders, his international activities are very vast. He was visiting professor in Cincinnati, Sydney, Sherbrooke, Buenos Aires, Melbourne, Vancouver, Tokyo, Edinburgh, Barcelona, Brisbane, Miami, Riyadh.

He got and gets regularly invited for major lectures all over the world.

He is member in 19 national and international societies, honorary member of the Gesellschaft für Neuropädiatrie since 1989. He is chief-editor of »Epileptic Disorders« and editor in 8 mainly international journals , the second – and the first non-french – was Neuropediatrics, where he was invited to join the editorial board in 1979.

His huge publicationlist reveals an eminent epileptologist, just to mention his book »Epilepsy in Children«. But this is far from being his only interest. He is one of the rare child neurologists covering the whole field. Just to mention that several syndromes carry his name. This explains why he could write his book »Diseases of the Nervous System in Childhood« almost alone, a book, which has won highest appreciation by a large readership.

The Society of Child Neurology in German speaking countries has elected Jean Aicardi as this year' P.E. Becker lecturer due to his merits as an eminent researcher and outstanding child neurologist and teacher.

Disorders of cortical development. Their diagnosis and some remarks on the relationships between imaging, structure and paroxysmal dysfunction

J. Aicardi, MD, FRCP

With the development of modern neuroimaging techniques cortical development disorders (CDDs), formerly a narrowly specialized chapter of neuropathology, have grown to be one of the major issues in child neurology.

The term CDDs seems more comprehensive than those of neuronal migration disorders as other mechanisms than migration are clearly in cause in many cases of cortical dysplasias (which is used ambiguously to designate either a specific form of cortical disorganization or as a general term of all CDDs) or that of malformations of cortical development, as malformations are the result of abnormal development which is abnormal but not »malformed«.

Although the clinical, imaging, neurophysiological, etiologic and therapeutic aspects of CDDs have been extensively reviewed (Dobyns and Truwit 1995, Raymond et al 1995, Barkovich et al 1996, Guerrini et al 1996, Kuzniecky and Barkovich 2001), they still raise many unanswered questions as to their mechanisms of formation and of interference with normal cortical functions especially epilepsy.

This paper will discuss briefly the diagnosis of CDDs, the relationships between imaging and pathological findings and the possible mechanisms of epilepsy, the most common clinical manifestation of CDDs. The discussion will mainly deal with focal CDDs because of their diagnostic difficulties and of the problems posed by their surgical therapy. The controversial issue of the classifications of the CDDs (Barkovich et al 1996, Sarnat and Flores-Sarnat 2001) will not be dealt with. Only a simple topographic classification separating diffuse, unilateral, focal and multifocal CDDs, will be used as it is essential in the approach of the clinical and, especially the treatment problems.

Diagnosis of Cortical Development Disorders

The diagnosis of CDDs has become really practical with the development of modern neuroimaging and, especially, that of MRI, the major tool which is being constantly improved both in its resolution and by the introduction of new methods such as diffusion-weighed MR, quantitative MR and functional MRI (fMRI). Other techniques, especially PET (Chugani ete al 1993) and, to a lesser extent, SPECT, are also used to confirm the presence or nature of some lesions or, in some cases, to demonstrate a lesion that is not evidenced by MRI. Functional MRI may become an important tool as it can localize some critical functions such as motricity or language therefore helping to predict the likely effects of resection.

The primary basis for a diagnosis of CDDs is represented by clinical symptoms or signs even though it is well recognized that some CDDs can remain asymptomatic for long periods or even for the whole life (Chevassus-au-Louis et al 1999). Epilepsy, neurological deficits, mental retardation or learning disorders in this order are the major presenting manifestations. Given the high frequency of CDDs as a cause of epilepsy (up to 25% of children with intractable seizures (Kuzniecky et al 1993) and the fact that the clinical spectrum of epilepsy associated with malformations of the cerebral cortex is very broad, any epilepsy that is not idiopathic could be related with underlying cortical dysplasia and these should be suspected in all patients with cryptogenic or symptomatic epilepsy not explained by antecedents or by physical findings. The clinical diagnosis may be considerably helped by the presence of clinical findings, e.g. cutaneous abnormalities, associated malformations etc. and, in some cases, even the likely type of CDD can be strongly suspected (e.g. the bilateral perisylvian syndrome). However, although most of the severe forms of childhood epilepsy are caused by CDDs, this is not an absolute rule, as relatively benign and remitting epilepies may also be observed (Dravet al 1996).

Relatively minor neuropsychological problems, e.g. dyslexia, may have a relation with dysplastic cortical areas, found at autopsy in a few cases, but the role of these lesions in the symptomatology remains uncertain and such disturbances do not constitute an indication to systematically look for CDDs.

The diagnosis is usually relatively easy in those frequent cases in which clearcut MRI abnormalities are found. A more difficult issue is raised when no definitely abnormal MR image is found, even with high-resolution MR, in patients with resistant epilepsy for whom epilepsy surgery may be considered despite normality of MRI. In some such cases, a diagnosis of CDD may be suggested by other techniques such as PET (Chugani 1993). The EEG is sometimes highly suggestive of CDD, especially in diffuse lesions such as lissencephaly or pachygyria, by showing diffuse high amplitude fast rhythms or a slow spike-wave pattern. In some focal CDDs, especially in Taylor type cortical dysplasia, almost continuous or prolonged focal discharges of repetitive rhythmical spikes or low amplitude fast rhythms, are recorded over the malformed area and are characteristic. In most cases, however, the EEG is nonspecific and does not even necessarily localize the lesions (Boyd et al 2001). In some cases, a diagnosis of CDD can be confirmed only by pathological study of the cortex resected on an electrophysiological basis despite its normal macroscopic appearance (Sisodiya 2000). However, interpretation of histological appearance is often difficult. In a recent pathologic study of 327 cortical samples from patients with intractable epilepsy, 51 were difficult to interpret or showed 'nonspecific signs' (Pasquier et al 2002). This heterogeneous group included cases of microdysgenesis (Menke and Veith 1992) whose clinical significance remains disputed (Lyon and Gastaut 1985). Recent work suggests that, at least in some of these cases, microdysgenesis is a pathological entity with clinical relevance and may have possible cytological links with other variants of cortical dysplasia (Thom et al 200). In some such cases, resection of the abnormal area has resulted in control of epilepsy.

Another circumstance of diagnosis is in the prenatal period especially for women who had borne a previous child with one of the cortical malformations known to be genetically transmitted. Although ultrasonography can detect only extensive focal CDDs and at a late stage, the development of intrauterine MR may improve this situation.

Relationship of neuroimaging and structure

Most CDDs are recognizable on MRI scans when several sequences, including fluid attenated inversion-recovery sequences (FLAIR), thin cuts and 3D acquisition with reformatting are used (Barkovich 1996).

Diffuse, unilateral and some multifocal forms have specific or very suggestive imaging features (Dobyns and Truwit 1995) and multiple subtypes have been described (Kato et al 1999, Hanefeld 1999, Ross et al 2001).

Focal CDDs (often simply referred to as cortical dysplasias) generally appear as areas of thickened cortex with blurred gray/white interface with a variable signal, often increased in T2 sequences, small number of sulci and sometimes a rippled surface.

Very small dysplastic areas may be difficult to find and require special techniques such as surface rendering, curvilinear reconstruction or quantitative MR. However some dysplasias remain undetectable even with the best techniques and with the help of diffusion MR or PET. The latter may not correspond to the anatomical lesion.

Even when the lesions are visible, they do not necessarily correspond exactly to the epileptogenic zone. The major arguments for correspondence of the visible lesion with the epileptogenic zone is drawn from the fact that removal of the macroscopic lesion is often associated with significant control of the seizures (Palmini et al 1991). However, this is not a constant experience and cases are on record of persistence of seizures after apparently complete resection or, conversely, good control after only partial removal (Munari et al 2000). Moreover, determining whether resection of a cortical dysplasia has been complete can be very difficult as the limits between normal and dysplastic tissue may be blurred and few cases have been completely examined from this point of view. It seems that a zone of »penumbra« may surround the core of the lesion (Andermann 2000).

Sisodiya et al (1998) analyzed quantitatively the MRI scans of 18 patients with cortical dysplasia and compared them with those of 30 neurologically normal control subjects, examining the regional distribution of gray and subcortical matter volumes using statitical parametric analysis Fifteen of the 18 patients demonstrated abnormalities of this distribution beyond the margins of the visualized lesions and 9 of 10 patients with unilateral dysplastic lesions had volumetric abnormality in the contralateral hemisphere. The histological features were not studied outside the clearly dysplastic area removed therapeutically. Such abnormal volume distribution could represent either additional, less marked, dysplastic lesions or, perhaps, represent changes secondary to altered connectivity and remodeling of local circuitry. The possible contribution of the more diffuse abnormalties to epileptogenesis remained speculative, but these findings are intriguing and might account in part for the greater difficulties of control in cases of dysplasia than in those with other epileptogenic lesions. Not infrequently, electrocorticography or depth electrode studies show that the origin of seizure discharges lies outside the visible dysplastic area.

Thus, understanding of relations between imaging and structure is not complete. Moreover, imaging is not specific for the type of lesion and may be similar with lesions of different histopathology and epileptogenicity (see below). Occasionally, however, it may be possible to suspect the presence of Taylor type dysplasia on images, e.g. when increased signal is present on T2-weighted images but this seems unreliable.

Relationship between CDDs and Epilepsy

Not all CDDs are associated with epilepsy. However, seizures are the most common clinical manifestation and CDDs are found in 20 to 60% of the brains of persons with apparently cryptogenic refractory epilepsy as against 1% in control brains. By MRI, 8 to 14% of children with refractory epilepsy have CDDs (Li et al 1995, Steffenburg et al 1998). Although such figures are clearly biassed as cases of epilepsy are more likely to receive MRI or to be represented in autopsy studies, the association is confirmed by the results of resection which suggest that about 50 to 60% of patients in whom an apparently complete removal could be achieved are rendered seizure-free after a 2-year follow-up (Sisodiya 2000) and by the observation that the best predictor of a good outcome is the completeness of resection of the macroscopically defined dysplastic area (Palmini et al 1991). The role of CDDs is also confirmed by the good correspondence between EEG abnormalities and MRI and/or operative demonstration of dysplasia. However, interictal surface EEG is far from demonstrating a close correlation between paroxysmal abnormalities and the location of focal CDDs. EEG spiking is often more diffuse and multilobar, or even generalized, thus potentially misleading. Palmini et al recorded on electrocorticography, in some of their patients, apparently »ictal« continuous epileptogenic discharges from the surface of CDD cortex and, in some cases, from surrounding cortex that appeared normal on inspection but was subsequently proven histologically to harbor CDD. Completeness of resection of the cortex generating these discharges was correlated with a significantly better outcome. Other investigators (Mattia et al 1995, Kothare et al 1998) also adduced evidence demonstrating that CDD may have intrinsic epileptogenicity. However, paroxysmal discharges are absent in many cases, even though they have also been recorded from different areas including subcortical heterotopias (Dubeau et al 1995, Munari et al 1996) and their disappearance following surgery did not predict a seizure-free outcome in 9 of 12 patients of Palmini et al. Similarly, cases are on record for which resections away from the visualized dysplastic area under corticographic or stereo-electroencephalographic guidance led to a 80%–100% reduction in seizure frequency in some patients (Leblanc et al 1991, Landy et al 1992, Munari et al 2000). In some cases with bilateral dysplastic areas, leaving in place the lesion in one hemisphere, shown by electrocorticography or stereo-electroencephalography not to generate spiking, could result in satisfactory control (Munari et al 2000). It seems reasonable to conclude that the evidence that epileptogenesis is associated with CDDs is good but not absolute and this has a bearing upon therapeutic decisions.

Intrinsic epileptogenicity of CDDs in some cases is supported by pathological and experimental data.

Several investigators (Ferrer 1992, Spreafico et al 1998) have demonstrated specific histopathologic changes in human tissue from CDDs. Studies aimed at characterizing the fine circuitry in resected malformed regions have indicated a potential excitation/inhibition imbalance. This was suggested by the distribution and structure of subtypes of nonpyramidal inhibitory interneurons in dysplasia, reminiscent of that reported in nonmalformed cortex rendered epileptic (Spreafico et al 1998). Excessive expression of glutamate receptors has also been reported in human dysplastic cortex (review in Chevassus-au-Louis et al 1999). This is consistent with decreased inhibition and/or increased excitation and may contribute to its intrinsic excitability. Fine studies at cell level are currently attempting to precise the neurotansmitters used by abnormal cells and their possible role in hyperexcitability (Crino et al 2001).

Changes observed in animals with genetic or experimentally induced cortical development disorders also support hyperexcitability of malformed areas. Spontaneous seizures occur in genetic models of cortical malformations but not in experimentally-induced dysplasias. However, the possibility of spontaneous minimal seizures in these models is not excluded as detection of such events may not be possible without continuous EEG-recording.

In vitro increase in seizure susceptibility is present in hippocampal slices of rats treated with methylazoxymethanol (MAM) an agent that induces cortical malformations. This is shown by the occurrence of spontaneous and evoked epileptiform activity in response to subconvulsive changes in extracellular potassium concentration. Furthermore, in MAM treated rats, a majority of CA1 pyramidal neurons function as »burster« spiking neurons that respond to stimulation with a stereotyped burst of action potentials, and small heterotopic neurons clusters in the same area are capable of generating synchronized epileptiform discharges in the absence of synaptic input, thus sugggesting their epileptogenic propensity (Chevasus-au-Louis 1999). In the freeze-model of CDD, there is an increase in NMDA-mediated excitation and a concurrent decrease of glutamatergic input onto inhibitory interneurons thus resulting in a decrease of inhibition (Luhman et al 1998).

Thus, the hyperexcitability and the epileptogenic potential of human and experimental CDDs seems to be reasonably established.

However, the precise manner in which epilepsy is generated remains very imperfectly known. One point of particular importance is to determine what are the exact relations between the dysplastic areas, as defined by MRI and/or gross inspection, and the epileptogenic zone (EZ) as this is clearly important for practical surgical decisions.

As already indicated, the congruence of CDD and EZ is far from perfect. Evidence for foci distant from the CDD is frequent and multifocality is possible. Origin of ictal discharge outside the dysplastic area has been noted. This may be explained by inhomogeneity of the lesions with only part of them reaching an epileptogenic threshhold or by the presence of a milder degree of lesions grossly undetectable around the visible CDD or at a distance from it. Another possible explanation may be that the presence of a malformation is somehow associated with more diffuse hyperexcitability in the non-malformed cortex. Such distal abnormalities may become worse when the dysplastic area is removed. Experimental studies of the freeze model that results in a microgyric lesion show that epileptiform responses to subconvulsive stimulation of the white matter are present in cortical regions adjacent to the microgyrus whereas the microgyrus itself is not the focus of abnormal seizure discharges (Hablitz and DeFazio 1998). These can persist even when the microgyrus is dissected out of the slice. An anatomic substrate for this hyperexcitability could be the excess of glutamatergic projections that has been described in the area bordering the microgyrus. These fibers are probably thalamic afferent fibers rerouted because of the absence of their normal target in the microgyrus (Chevassus-au-Louis et al 1999). The profound reorganization of cortical networks around CDDs due to rerouting, sprouting and other synaptic changes may well account for the hyperexcitability that exists in the vicinity of dysplastic lesions.

Recent data show that distant synaptic communications may exist between some malformations and other cortical areas. These may account for distant diffusion of epileptogenesis. A possible example in humans could be periventricular heterotopias, in which the origin of seizures from the heterotopias themselves has been demonstrated, whereas the EEG abnormalities often recorded from the temporal cortex (pathologically normal) have been shown not to be the cause of the seizures: removal of the spiking temporal cortex dos not control the epilepsy (Dubeau et al 1995).

There is thus evidence that CDDs may have distant consequences on the apparently normal cortex and that CDDs might act as the leading point of more or less widely distributed epileptogenic circuits, also termed *distributed epileptogenesis* (Sisodiya 2000). Such circuits might be the source of persistent auras following resection od CDDs or even of recurrences, after some time has allowed restoration of parts sufficient to sustain autonomous epileptic activity.

Other widespread changes in excitability and/or of structure have also been described both in animal models such as persistence of transient projections normally eliminated during development or long-term survival of the normally transient Cajal-Retzius cells. The frequent presence of hippocampal lesions in association with ipsilateral CDDs (dual pathology) could be an example of a similar phenomenon in humans.

The complexity of relations between epilepsy and lesion is a strong incitation to a complete investigation of the likely mechanisms in each individual case, rather than the use of a standardized surgical therapy. Moreover, there are indications that the different types of CDD probably do not have the same degree of epileptogenicity and this has also a bearing on therapy.

Variable epileptogenicity of different types of CDD

Although there is no strict relation between types of CDD and type and severity of epilepsy, some correlations are worth mentioning.

Most of the diffuse CDDs are associated with severe epilepsies with generalized (especially infantile spasms) but also with focal seizures. However, children with type II lissencephaly rarely have epilepsy as a prominent feature. Bilateral periventricular heterotopias are often associated with generalized epilepsy. However, temporal lobe seizures are often present and may wrongly suggest a limbic origin to the seizures.

Focal CDDs are of special interest because of the possibility of surgical treatment in some cases. Taylor type focal cortical dysplasia appears to be highly epileptogenic. This is probably the result of the intrsinsic epileptogenicity of this malformation. Non-Taylor types are usually less severe. Polymicrogyria is probably less epileptogenic than Taylor type dysplasia, although it may be the cause of intractable seizures. Unilateral polymicrogyria involving the major part of the cortex of one hemisphere can be associated with a remarkable syndrome that features focal motor seizures resembling those of idiopathic focal epilepsies and an EEG aspect of continuous spike-wave complexes during sleep or electrical status epilepticus of slow sleep (CSWS or ESES). The epilepsy in this syndrome is relatively benign and may remit spontaneously, although cognitive deterioration often occurs during the period of CSWS (Guerrini et al 1996, Caraballo et al 1999).

The epilepsy in schizencephaly and in the bilateral perisylvian syndrome is probably related to the presence of polymicrogyria. In schizencephaly, epilepsy may be relatively benign. In the series of Granata's et al, only 57% of the patients had seizures and these were controlled with drug treatment in half the cases. There may thus be close relationships between histology and epileptogenesis.

Conclusion

Although neuroimaging is the most important clue to the diagnosis of CDDs and to determination of the extent and limits of lesions, it is not always sufficient, especially when surgical treatment of epilepsy is considered, as there is no absolute correspondence between data from MR imaging, pathological extent of lesions and definition of the epileptogenic zone. Any discrepancy between data from clinical, imaging and EEG (especially ictal) studies requires additional investigations that may include PET or SPECT or spectrographic MR in order to better define the abnormal cortical areas. Often, invasive methods especially intracranial recording (corticography or depth electrodes) are necessary and simple lesionectomy should be used only when all data are consistent.

The mechanisms of epileptogenesis also require further studies to try to clarify the relationships between pathology and the origin and diffusion of the discharges.

The heterogeneity of CDDs should be further investigated especially with respect to their epileptogenic propensity so that appropriate therapeutic methods are selected for individual cases.

References

1. Andermann F (2000). The cortical dysplasias and epilepsy: where have we been, where are we and where are we going ? In: Spreafico R, Avanzini G, Andermann F, eds: *Abnormal Cortical Development and Epilepsy,* London, John Libbey, pp.3–19.
2. Barkovich AJ, Kuzniecky RI, Dobyns WB et al (1996). A classification scheme for malformations of cortical development. *Neuropediatrics,* 27:59–63.
3. Boyd SG, Dan B (2001). Cerebral dysplasias: review from a neurophysiological perspective. *Neuropediatrics,* 32,279–285.
4. Caraballo R, Cerosimo R, Fejerman N (1999). A particular type of epilepsy in children with congenital hemiparesis associated with unilateral polymicrogyria. *Epilepsia,* 40:865–871.
5. Chevassus-au-Louis N, Baraban SC, Gaïarsa JL, Ben-Ari Y (1999). Congenital malformations and epilepsy: new insights from animal models. *Epilepsia,* 40:811–821.
6. Chugani HT, Shewmon DA, Shields WD et al (1993). Surgery for intractable infantile spasms: neuroimaging perspectives. *Epilepsia,* 34:764–771.
7. Crino PB, Duhaime AC, Baltuch C, White R (2001). Differential expression of glutamate and GABA-A receptor mRNA in cortical dysplasia. *Neurology,* 56:906–913.
8. Dobyns WB, Truwit CL (1995). Lissencephaly and other malformations of cortical development: 1995 update. *Neuropediatrics,* 26:132–149.
9. Dravet C, Guerrini R, Mancini J et al (1996). Different outcomes of epilepsy due to cortical dysplastic lesions. In: Guerrini R et al, eds. *Dysplasias of Cerebral Cortex and Epilepsy.* Philadelphia, Lippincott-Raven, pp. 323–328.
10. Dubeau F, Tampieri D, Lee N et al (1995). Periventricular and subcortical nodular heterotopia. A study of 33 patients. *Brain,* 118:1273–1287.
11. Dubeau F, Li LM, Bastos A et al (2000). Periventricular nodular heterotopia: further delineation of the clinical syndromes. In: Spreafico R et al, eds. *Abnormal Cortical Development and Epilepsy.* London, John Libbey, pp.203–217.
12. Duncan JS (1997). Imaging and epilepsy. *Brain,* 120:339–377.
13. Ferrer I, Pineda M, Tallada M et al (1992). Abnormal local-circuits neurons in epilepsia partialis continua associated with focal cortical dysplasia. *Acta Neuropathol,* 83:647–652.
14. Ferrer I, Alcantara S, Zujer MI, Cisnos C (1993). Structure and pathogenesis of cortical nodules induced by prenatal X-irradiation: an autoradiographic and Golgi study. *Acta Neuropathol,* 85:205–212.
15. Granata T, D'Incerti L, Ferri L et al (2000). Schizencephaly: clinical and genetic findings in a case series. In: Spriafico R, Avanzini G, Andermann F, eds. *Abnormal Cortical Development and Epilepsy.* London, John Libbey, pp.181–190.
16. Guerrini R, Dravet C, Bureau M et al (1996). Diffuse and localized dysplasia of cerebral cortex: clinical presentation, outcome and proposal for a morphologic MRI classification based on a study of 90 patients. In: Guerrini R, Andermann F, Canapicchi R, Roger J, Zifkin BG, Pfanner P, eds. *Dysplasias of Cerebral Cortex and Epilepsy.* Philadelphia, Lippincott-Raven, pp. 65–73.
17. Hablitz JJ, DeFazio T (1998). Excitability changes in freeze-induced cortical microgyria. *Epilepsy Res,* 32, 78–82.
18. Hanefeld F (1999). Oligogyric microcephaly. *Neuropediatrics,* 30:102–103.
19. Kato M, Tagikawa N, Yamada S et al (1999). Diffuse pachygyria with cerebellar hypoplasia: a milder form of microlissencephaly or a new genetic syndrome. *Ann Neurol,* 46:660–663.

20. Kothare SV, Vaulandingham K, Armon C et al (1998). Seizures onset from periventricular nodular heterotopias: depth electrode study. *Neurology,* 51:1723–1727.
21. Kuzniecky R, Murro A, King D et al (1993). Magnetic resonance imaging in childhood intractable partial epilepsies: pathologic correlations. *Neurology,* 43:681–687.
22. Kuzniecky R, Barkovich A (2001). Malformations of cortical development and epilepsy. *Brain Dev,* 23–2–11.
23. Landy HJ, Ramsey RE, Ajmone-Marsan et al (1992). Temporal lobectomy for seizures associated with unilateral schizencephaly. *Surg Neurol,* 37,477–481.
24. Leblanc R, Tampieri D, Robitaille Y et al (1991). Surgical treatment of intractable epilepsy associated with schizencephaly. *Neurosurgery,* 29:421–429.
25. Li LM, Dubeau F, Andermann F et al (1997). Periventricular nodular heterotopia and intractable temporal lobe epilepsy: poor outcome after temporal lobe resection. *Ann Neurol,* 41;662–668.
26. Luhman HJ, Raabe K (1996). Characterization of neuronal migration disorders in neocortical structures: I. Expression of epileptiform actvity in an animal model. *Epilepsy Res,* 26:67–74.
27. Lyon G, Gastaut H, (1985). Considerations on the significance attributed to unusual cerebral histological findings recently described in 8 patients with generalized epilepsy. *Epilepsia,* 26;365–367.
28. Mattia D, Olivier A, Avoli M (1995). Seizure-like discharges recorded in human dysplastic cortex maintained in vitro. *Neurology,* 45:1391–1395.
29. Meencke HJ, Veith G (1992). Migration disturbances in epilepsy. In: Engel J Jr et al, eds. *Molecular Biology of Epilepsy.* Amsterdam, Elsevier, pp.31–40.
30. Munari C. Francione S, Kahane P et al (1996). Usefulness of stereo-EEG investigations in partial epilepsy associated with cortical dysplastic lesions and gray matter heterotopia. In: Guerrini R et al, eds. *Dysplasias of Cerebral Cortex and Epilepsy.* London, John Libbey, pp. 383–394.
31. Munari C, Minotti L, Tassi L. et al (2000). Surgical management of severe partial epilepsy symptomatic of neuronal migration disorders : physiopathological considerations and perspectives of research. In : Spreafico R et al, eds. *Abnormal Cortical Development and Epilepsy.* London, John Libbey, pp.303–318.
32. Palmini A, Andermann F, Olivier A et al (1991). Focal neuronal migration disorders and intractable epilepsy: a study of 30 patients. *Ann Neurol,* 30:741–749.
33. Palmini A, Gambardella A, Andermann F et al (1995). Intrinsic epileptogenicity of human dysplastic cortex as suggested by corticography and surgical results. *Ann Neurol* 37:476–487.
34. Pasquier B, Péoc'h M, Fabre-Bocquentin B et al (2002) Surgical pathology of drug-resistant partial epilepsy. A 10-year experience with a series of 327 consecutive resections. *Epileptic Dis* 4: 99–119
35. Raymond AA, Fish DR, Sisodiya SM et al (1995). Abnormalities of gyration, heterotopia, tuberous sclerosis, focal cortical dysplasia, microdysgenesis and dysgenesis of the archicortex in epilepsy. *Brain,* 118 :629–660.
36. Ross ME, Swanson E, Dobyns WB (2001). Lissencephaly and cerebellar hyposplasia (LCH): a heterogeneous group of cortical malformations. *Neuropediatrics,* 32:256–263.
37. Sarnat HB, Flores-Sarnat L (2001). A new classification of malformations of the nervous system: an integration of morphological and molecular genetic criteria as patterns of genetic expression. *Eur J Paediatr Neurol,* 5:57–64/
38. Sisodiya SM, Free SL, Stevens J et al (1995). Widespread cerebral structural changes in patients with cortical dysgenesis and epilepsy. *Brain,* 118:1039–1050.
39. Sisodiya SM (2000). Surgery for malformations of cortical development. *Brain,* 123: 1039–1050.
40. Spreafico R, Pasquier B, Minotti L et al (1998). Immunocytochemical investigation on dysplastic human tissue from epileptic patients. *Epilepsy Res,* 32:34–48.
41. Steffenburg U, Hedström A, Lindroth A et al (1998). Intractable epilepsy in a population-based series of mentally retarded children. *Epilepsia,* 39:767–775.
42. Thom M, Moran NF, Plant GT et al (1999). Cortical dysplasia with angiodysgenesis and chronic inflammation in multifocal partial epilepsy. *Neurology* 52: 654–657.

2. Wissenschaftspreis der Gesellschaft für Neuropädiatrie 2002

Glutarazidurie Typ I: Basismechanismen und modulierende Faktoren des neuronalen Zelluntergangs

S. Kölker

Zusammenfassung

Die Glutarazidurie Typ I ist biochemisch durch die Akkumulation organischer Säuren, insbesondere Glutarsäure und 3-Hydroxyglutarsäure (3-OH-GA), charakterisiert. Klinisch ist der Erkrankungsverlauf durch das Auftreten einer akuten Enzephalopathie während des Säuglings- und frühen Kleinkindalters charakterisiert, die häufig zu einer bilateralen Schädigung des Striatums führt.

Es konnte in neuronalen Zellkulturen und *in vivo* gezeigt werden, dass insbesondere 3-OH-GA an der Neuropathogenese der Erkrankung beteiligt ist. 3-OH-GA induziert einen als exzitotoxischen Zelluntergang beschriebenen Mechanismus, der über die vermehrte Aktivierung von ionotropen Glutamatrezeptoren, insbesondere *N*-Methyl-D-Aspartat-Rezeptoren, vermittelt wird. Eine vermehrte Produktion reaktiver Sauerstoffspezies ist hierbei ebenfalls von Bedeutung. Basierend auf diesen Ergebnissen wurde postuliert, dass die postnatalen zerebralen Reifungsprozesse – insbesondere im glutamatergen System – ein Zeitfenster für die Entwicklung einer akuten Enzephalopathie markieren.

Es ist klinisch bedeutsam, dass sich die akute Enzephalopathie charakteristischerweise im Rahmen einer fieberhaften Infektionserkrankung manifestiert. In Analogie hierzu wurde *in vitro* nachgewiesen, dass die 3-OH-GA-induzierte Zellschädigung durch eine Kombination der inflammatorischen Zytokine Interleukin-1β und Interferon-γ potenziert wird. Mechanistisch spielen hierbei die Expression der induziblen NO-Synthase (iNOS) und eine vermehrte NO-Produktion eine Rolle. Somit konnte erstmals die Bedeutung eines neuroimmunologischen Ansatzpunktes für die Pathogenese der Glutarazidurie Typ I aufgezeigt werden.

Einleitung

Die Glutarazidurie Typ I (GA-I, Synonym: Glutaryl-CoA-Dehydrogenase-Defizienz; McKusick 231670) ist eine neurometabolische Erkrankung, die durch die autosomal-rezessiv vererbte Defizienz des mitochondrialen Enzyms Glutaryl-CoA-Dehydrogenase (EC 1.3.99.7) verursacht wird. Sie ist biochemisch durch eine Akkumulation organischer Säuren, insbesondere Glutarsäure und 3-OH-GA charakterisiert. Von klinischer Seite wird der Erkrankungsverlauf unbehandelter Kinder durch die Entwicklung einer akuten Enzephalopathie, deren Manifestationsmaximum zwischen dem 6. und 12. (–18.) Lebensmonat liegt, kompliziert (2, 6). Charakteristische Folge dieser krisenhaften metabolischen Entgleisung ist eine akute striatale Destruktion mit daraus resultierender dyston-dyskinetischer Bewegungsstörung (6). In der Zwischenzeit konnte gezeigt werden, dass vor allem 3-OH-GA das Potential besitzt, einen exzitotoxischen Mechanismus zu induzieren. Von Relevanz ist hierbei eine Aktivierung von *N*-Methyl-D-Aspartat (NMDA)-Rezeptoren und eine Beeinträchtigung des intrazellulären Energiestoffwechsels (7, 12).

Dieser Mechanismus allein betrachtet kann jedoch sicherlich nur einen Teil der komplexen Neuropathogenese der Erkrankung erklären. Die vorliegende Arbeit diskutiert die Bedeutung inflammatorischer Zytokine als modulierende Faktoren.

Methoden

Zellkulturen

Gemischte neuronale (80%)/gliale (20%) Primärkulturen aus dem Hippokampus neonataler Ratten (P1) wurden für 12 Tage kultiviert (9). Zur Abklärung der beteiligten Pathomechanismen wurden ionotrope Glutamatrezeptorantagonisten (MK-801, D-AP5, CNQX), Superoxiddismutase, Katalase sowie NO-Synthase-Inhibitoren (Aminoguanidin, L-NAME) verwendet. Zur *in vitro*-Simulation der NO-Effekte wurde ein NO-Donor (SNAP) eingesetzt. Die Zellvitalität wurde mittels Trypanblaufärbung und LDH-Release bestimmt.

Intrastriatale Injektion von 3-Hydroxyglutarsäure

Die Toxizität von 3-OH-GA wurde in adulten Ratten nach intrastriataler Applikation (AP: 0 mm, ML: 3,0 mm, V: 4,0 mm von der Dura) anhand von Kresylviolett-gefärbten Schnittpräparaten untersucht.

iNOS-Induktion und Nitrit-Messung

Zur Etablierung eines Induktionsmodells für iNOS durch inflammatorische Zytokine (IL-1β, IFN-γ) wurden neben den hippokampalen auch astrozytäre Primärkulturen aus Rattencortex verwendet (11). Die iNOS-Expression wurde auf Proteinebene (Western blot, Immunfärbung), die NO-Produktion wurde indirekt mittels Nitritmessung (Griess-Reagenz) bestimmt.

Ergebnisse

Charakterisierung der Neurotoxizität von 3-Hydroxyglutarsäure in vitro und in vivo

Die hippokampalen Primärkulturen der Ratte zeigten während der Kultivierungsdauer eine zunehmende Empfindlichkeit gegenüber Glutamat, NMDA und 3-OH-GA. Der 12. Kulturtag wurde – bei maximaler Differenz zwischen Kontroll- und induzierter Schädigung – als optimaler Zeitpunkt für die folgenden Experimente bestimmt. Abbildung 1 zeigt im Vergleich die durch NMDA, Glutamat und 3-OH-GA induzierte Zellschädigung und den neuroprotektiven Effekt

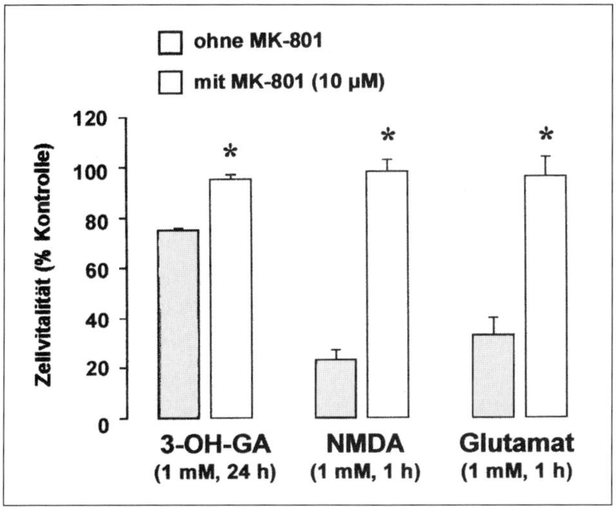

Abb. 1: Neurotoxizität von 3-OH-GA, NMDA und Glutamat (je 1 mM) in hippokampalen Kulturen der Ratte (12. Kulturtag). 3-OH-GA wurde 24 h lang, NMDA und Glutamat je 1 h lang inkubiert. Die Zellvitalität wurde 24 h nach Beginn der Inkubation mittels Trypanblaufärbung ermittelt. Eine Koinkubation mit dem NMDA-Rezeptorantagonisten MK-801 wirkte neuroprotektiv. Die Kontrolle wurde auf 100% normalisiert. *p < 0,001 ohne vs mit MK-801 (Student's t-Test).

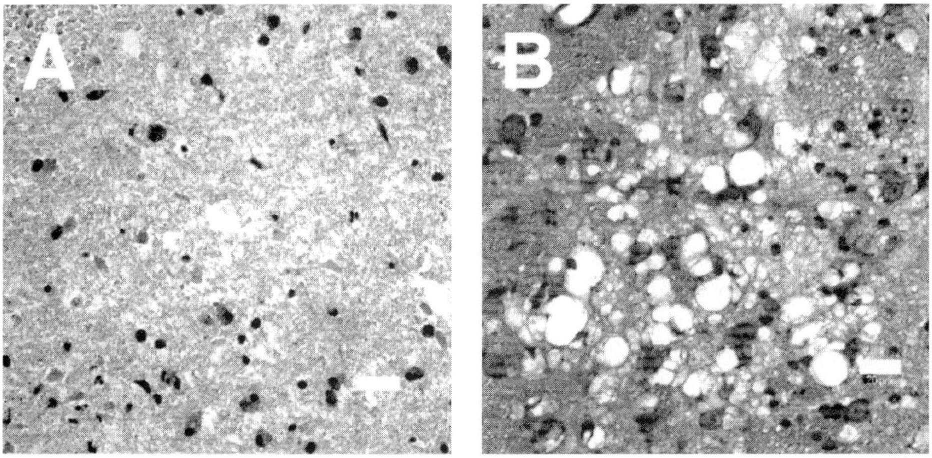

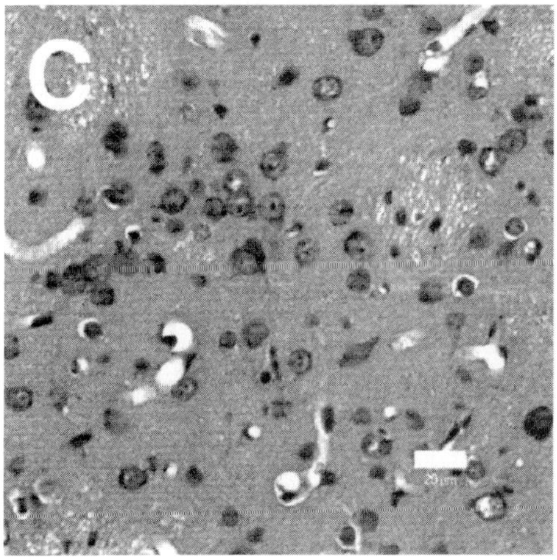

Abb. 2: Neurotoxizität von 3-OH-GA nach intrastriataler Injektion in adulten Ratten. Die Abbildung zeigt Kresylviolett-gefärbte Koronarschnitte des Striatums (auf Bregmalevel), die 24 h nach Applikation von 6 µmol 3-OH-GA (A, B) oder 6 µmol NaCl (C) angefertigt wurden. 3-OH-GA verursachte eine striatale Läsion mit deutlicher Reduktion der Zelldichte (A) und einer Vakuolenbildung (B). Somit ergaben sich deutliche histologische Ähnlichkeiten mit striatalen Läsionen, wie sie *post mortem* bei Kindern mit GA-I gefunden wurden, die im Rahmen einer akuten Enzephalopathie verstorben sind. Skalierung: 20 µm.

des NMDA-Rezeptorantagonisten MK-801. Grundlage der steigenden Empfindlichkeit gegenüber einer exzitotoxischen Schädigung ist u. a. eine zunehmende Expression von NMDA-Rezeptoren auf Nervenzellen während der Kulturdauer. Die Relevanz einer NMDA-Rezeptor-vermittelten Zellschädigung nach 3-OH-GA-Exposition wurden durch intrastriatale Injektion von 3-OH-GA in adulten Ratten bestätigt. Die ipsilateral erzeugten Läsionen wiesen eine deutliche Verminderung der Zelldichte (Abb. 2A) und z.T. eine Vakuolisierung auf (Abb. 2B). Abbildung 2C zeigt im Vergleich dazu die Histologie derselben Region in einem NaCl-behandelten Kontrollgehirn. Eine NMDA-Rezeptorblockade durch MK-801 zeigte auch in diesem Modell eine neuroprotektive Wirkung, wohingegen der AMPA-Rezeptorantagonist DNQX die 3-OH-GA-induzierte Läsion nicht beeinflusste (de Mello et al., 2001).

Die Aktivierung von rekombinanten Glutamat-Rezeptoren durch 3-OH-GA wurde weiterhin in HEK293-Zellen untersucht. 3-OH-GA (1 mM) induzierte hierbei Ströme (24 ± 6 pA; $n = 6$) in NR1/NR2A-exprimierenden Zellen, aber nicht in rekombinanten AMPA-Rezeptoren. An unterschiedlichen Modellen konnte somit gezeigt werden, dass bei der 3-OH-GA-induzierten neuronalen Zellschädigung exzitotoxische Mechanismen und insbesondere eine Aktivierung von NMDA-Rezeptoren (aber nicht von AMPA-Rezeptoren) von Bedeutung sind.

Inflammatorische Zytokine als modulierende Faktoren

Es ist bekannt, dass IL-1β und IFN-γ die zerebrale Expression von iNOS in Astrozyten und Mikroglia induzieren und eine exzitotoxische Zellschädigung verstärken können (5). Um den Effekt dieser beiden Zytokine auf die Neurotoxizität von 3-OH-GA untersuchen zu können, wurde zunächst ein standardisiertes Induktionsmodell für iNOS in astroglialen Kulturen etabliert. Eine

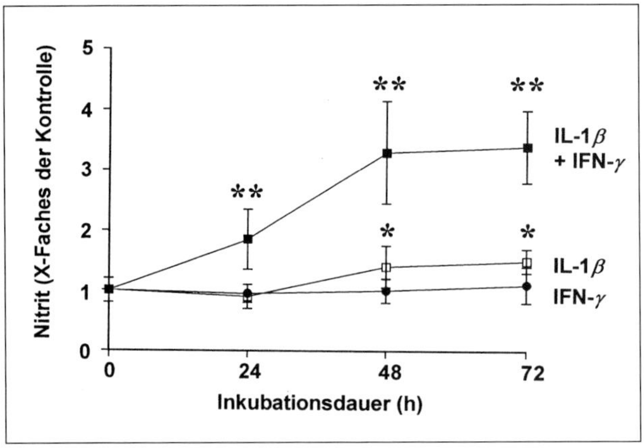

Abb. 3: Zeitabhängige Wirkung von IL-1β und IFN-γ auf die Nitritkonzentration in kortikalen, astroglialen Kulturen der Ratte. Die NO-Produktion wurde indirekt über die Messung des Oxidationsprodukts Nitrit bestimmt (spektrophotometrische Messung nach Zugabe des Griess-Reagenzes). Die Nitritkonzentration im Kulturmedium wurde auf das Gesamtprotein der kultivierten Astrozyten normiert und als X-Faches des Kontrollniveaus dargestellt. Die Kombination von IL-1β und IFN-γ wies einen synergistischen Effekt auf, der nach 48–72 h ein Maximum erreichte. *$p < 0{,}05$; **$p < 0{,}001$* vs 0 h (ANOVA mit *post hoc* Scheffés Test).

Kombination beider Zytokine induzierte eine vermehrte NO-Produktion, die zeitabhängig anstieg (Maximum: 48–72 h *post incubationem).* Dahingegen stimulierten IL-1β und IFN-γ allein die NO-Produktion kaum bzw. nicht (Abb. 3). Parallel zur steigenden NO-Produktion wurde eine Zunahme des iNOS-Proteins mittels Western blot nachgewiesen (9). Vergleichbare Ergebnisse fanden sich nach einer Stimulation der hippokampalen Primärkulturen mit den genannten Zytokinen. IL-1β (200 U/ml) und/oder IFN-γ (500 U/ml) hatten nach einer Inkubation von 48 h folgenden Einfluss auf die NO-Produktion (x-Faches des Kontrollniveaus): IL-1β (1,5-fache Steigerung), IFN-γ (1,6-fache Steigerung), IL-1β + IFN-γ (2,7-fache Steigerung). Durch eine Immunfärbung des astrozytären Markerproteins GFAP und iNOS konnte gezeigt werden, dass iNOS spezifisch in Astrozyten exprimiert wurde (Abb. 4).

Die dargestellten Zytokinbehandlungen selbst hatten in den hippokampalen Primärkulturen keinen Einfluss auf die Zellvitalität. Jedoch wurde die 3-OH-GA-induzierte Zellschädigung durch die kombinierte Vorbehandlung mit IL-1β und

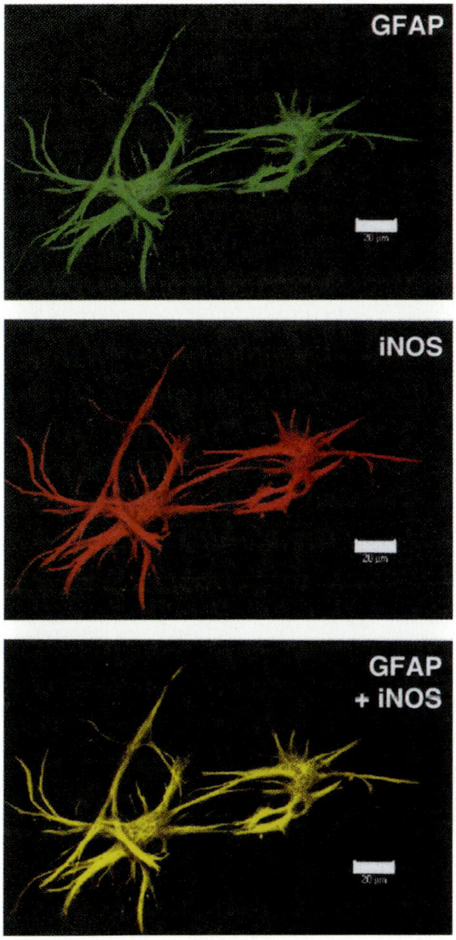

Abb. 4: Astrozytäre Expression von iNOS nach Zytokinbehandlung in hippokampalen Kulturen der Ratte. Die hippokampalen Kulturen (20% Astrozyten, 80% Neurone) wurden beginnend am 10. Kulturtag 48 h lang mit IL-1β (200 U/ml) und IFN-γ (500 U/ml) behandelt. Eine Doppelimmunfärbung gegen das astrozytäre Markerprotein GFAP und iNOS wurde am 12. Kulturtag nach Methanolfixation durchgeführt. Die zytokinbehandelten Astrozyten zeigten sowohl eine Expression von GFAP *(oben,* grün) als auch von iNOS *(Mitte,* rot) in der konfokale Laserscanningmikroskopie. Eine Kolokalisation von GFAP und iNOS *(unten,* gelb) bestätigte die spezifische iNOS-Expression in Astrozyten. In nicht-behandelten Astrozyten konnte eine GFAP- aber keine iNOS-Expression nachgewiesen werden (nicht dargestellt). Skalierung: 20 µm.

Tab. 1: Protektiver Effekt von NOS-Inhibitoren und Superoxiddismutase/Katalase auf die basale und zytokin-potenzierte Neurotoxizität von 3-Hydroxyglutarsäure.

Substanz (-en) *(Konzentration, Inkubationszeit)*	**Zellvitalität** *(%Kontrolle; Mittelwert ± SD)*
Kontrolle[#]	100 ± 5
3-OH-GA (1 mM, 24 h)	75 ± 5 *
+ Aminoguanidin (100 µM, 24 h)[a]	72 ± 9 *
+ L-NAME (100 µM, 24 h)[a]	62 ± 10 *
+ Superoxiddismutase/Katalase (je 50 U/ml, 24 h)[a]	98 ± 10 †
3-OH-GA (1 mM, 24 h) + IL-1β (200 U/ml)[b] + IFN-γ (500 U/ml)[b]	50 ± 5 *,†,‡
+ Aminoguanidin (100 µM, 24 h)	79 ± 9 *,‡
+ L-NAME (100 µM, 24 h)	79 ± 8 *,‡
+ Superoxiddismutase/Katalase (je 50 U/ml, 24 h)	95 ± 7 ‡

[#] Die Kontrolle wurde auf 100% normalisiert.
[a] Aminoguanidin, L-NAME und Superoxiddismutase/Katalase hatten bei den verwendeten Konzentrationen keinen Effekt auf die Zellvitalität.
[b] Vorbehandlung (48 h) vor der Behandlung mit 3-OH-GA
* $p < 0{,}05$ vs Kontrolle, † $p < 0{,}05$ vs 3-OH-GA, ‡ $p < 0{,}05$ vs 3-OH-GA + IL-1β/IFN-γ (ANOVA mit *post hoc* Scheffés Test).

IFN-γ deutlich gesteigert (Tab. 1). Der potenzierende Effekt auf den 3-OH-GA-induzierten Zelluntergang war für diese Zytokinkombination spezifisch und konnte nicht durch IL-1β (73 ± 7% der Kontrolle) oder IFN-γ (74 ± 8% der Kontrolle) alleine erzielt werden.

Um die zugrundeliegenden Mechanismen der zytokinstimulierten Potenzierung zu differenzieren, wurde zunächst untersucht, ob der NO-Donor SNAP (0,5–500 µM) die Wirkung von 3-OH-GA (1 mM) potenzierte. Tatsächlich steigerte SNAP konzentrationsabhängig die 3-OH-GA-induzierte Zellschädigung, wodurch sich ein weiterer Hinweis für die Bedeutung von NO in diesem Scenario ergab (nicht dargestellt). Der iNOS-spezifische Inhibitor Aminoguanidin (100 µM) sowie der unselektive NOS-Inhibitor L-NAME (100 µM) verhinderten den durch IL-1β und IFN-γ induzierten NO-Anstieg. Beide NOS-Inhibitoren hemmten ausschließlich den Anteil der zytokin-getriggerten Potenzierung der 3-OH-GA-Schädigung, nicht aber die durch 3-OH-GA *per se* induzierte Schädigung (Tab. 1). Somit kommt iNOS als Quelle der vermehrten NO-Produktion nach Zytokinvorbehandlung in Betracht. Es ist bekannt, dass eine vermehrte NMDA-Rezeptor-Stimulation die Produktion von Superoxidanionradikalen fördert (10). Eine vermehrte Generierung reaktiver Sauerstoffspezies wurde nach 3-OH-GA-Exposition in neuronalen Kulturen nachgewiesen (8). Superoxidanionradikale bilden mit NO rasch das starke Neurotoxin Peroxynitrit (3). Die Bildung von Peroxynitrit wird als wesentliche Voraussetzung der NO-Toxizität angesehen (1). Es wurde daher untersucht, ob Superoxiddismutase und Katalase (je 50 U/ml), die eine Umwandlung von Superoxidanionradikalen zu H_2O und O_2 katalysieren, die 3-OH-GA-induzierte Zellschädigung beeinflussen können. Tatsächlich hemmten Superoxiddismutase/Katalase die 3-OH-GA-induzierte Schädigung und verhinderten ebenfalls eine Potenzierung durch inflammatorische Zytokine (Tab. 1).

Diskussion

Die bisherigen Studien zeigten, dass 3-OH-GA als endogenes Neurotoxin wirksam ist und über eine NMDA-Rezeptoraktivierung (direkt und indirekt) exzitotoxische Mechanismen initiiert (7, 8, 12). Da die NMDA-Rezeptorexpression, -zusammensetzung und -verteilung während der Gehirnentwicklung deutlich variiert, kann postuliert werden, dass das Zeitfenster der akuten Enzephalopathie mit den ontogenetischen Veränderungen im glutamatergen System zusammenhängt. Die hierbei involvierten Faktoren sind bislang jedoch erst unzureichend charakterisiert.

Die dargestellten Ergebnisse erweitern das bisherige Konzept, indem sie neuroimmunologische Aspekte berücksichtigen. Die Präzipitation der akuten Enzephalopathie im Rahmen fieberhafter Infekte muss vor diesem Hintergrund neu interpretiert werden (6). Die bisherigen Überlegungen basierten auf der Annahme der Verstärkung einer mitochondrialen Dysfunktion unter katabolen Bedingungen (6, 12). Kaum Beachtung hingegen fanden inflammatorische Zytokine im pathogenetischen Geschehen der GA-I, obwohl bereits früher gezeigt werden konnte, dass IL-1β und IFN-γ selektiv einen NMDA-Rezeptor-vermittelten Zelluntergang verstärken (5). Diesen Mechanismus konnten wir nun in unserem Modell ebenfalls für 3-OH-GA verifizieren. Für den aufgezeigten Potenzierungseffekt sind mehrere Teilmechanismen notwendig: (1) NMDA-Rezeptorstimulation, (2) Generierung von Superoxidanionradikalen und (3) NO-Produktion. Hieraus ergeben sich unterschiedliche Angriffspunkte für die Entwicklung neuroprotektiver Strategien. Die Übertragbarkeit und funktionelle Bedeutung der in unterschiedlichen Modellsystemen generierten Vorstellungen ist derzeit noch nicht zu beurteilen. Alternative Mechanismen, wie z.B. die IFN-γ-induzible Produktion des NMDA-Rezeptoragonisten Chinolinsäure, bedürfen einer systematischen Erforschung.

Danksagung

Die vorliegende Studie wurde durch ein Forschungsstipendium der DFG (KO 2010/1-1) gefördert. Für die mannigfaltige Unterstützung bei der Realisation des Projekts bedanke ich mich herzlich bei (in alphabetischer Reihenfolge): Priv.-Doz. Dr. B. Ahlemeyer, Prof. Dr. C. F. de Mello, Prof. Dr. G. F. Hoffmann, Dr. F. Hörster, Dr. R. Hühne, Priv.-Doz. Dr. G. Köhr, Prof. Dr. Dr. J. Krieglstein, Priv.-Doz. Dr. E. Mayatepek, Dr. J. G. Okun, V. Pawlak, Prof. Dr. P. Seeburg, Prof. Dr. M. Wajner

Literatur

1. Beckman JS, Koppenol WH (1996) Nitric oxide, superoxide, and peroxynitrite: the good, the bad, and the ugly. Am J Physiol 27: C1427–C1437.
2. Bjugstad KB, Goodman SI, Freed CR (1998) Age at symptom onset predicts severity of motor impairment and clinical outcome of glutaric aciduria type 1. J Pediatr 137: 681–686.
3 Dawson TM, Gonzalez-Zulueta M, Kusel J, Dawson VL (1998) Nitric oxide: diverse actions in the central and peripheral nervous system. Neuroscientist 4: 96–112.
4. De Mello CF, Kölker S, Ahlemeyer B, de Souza FR, Fighera MR, Mayatepek E, Krieglstein J, Hoffmann GF, Wajner M (2001) Intrastriatal administration of 3-hydroxyglutaric acid induces convulsions and striatal lesions in rats. Brain Res 916: 70–75.
5. Hewett SJ, Csernansky CA, Choi DW (1994) Selective potentiation of NMDA-induced neuronal injury following induction of astrocytic iNOS. Neuron 13: 487–494.
6. Hoffmann GF, Athanassopoulos S, Burlina AB, Duran M, deKlerck JBC, Lehnert W, Leonard JV, Monavari AA, Müller E, Muntau AC, Naughten ER, Plecko-Starting B, Superti-Furga A, Zschocke J, Christensen E (1996) Clinical course, early diagnosis, treatment, and prevention of disease in glutaryl-CoA dehydrogenase deficiency. Neuropediatrics 27: 115–123.
7. Kölker S, Ahlemeyer B, Krieglstein J, Hoffmann GF (2000) Maturation-dependent neurotoxicity of 3-hydroxyglutaric and glutaric acids in vitro: a new pathophysiologic approach to glutaryl-CoA dehydrogenase deficiency. Pediatr Res 47: 495–503.
8. Kölker S, Ahlemeyer B, Krieglstein J, Hoffmann GF (2001) Contribution of reactive oxygen species to 3-hydroxyglutarate neurotoxicity in primary neuronal cultures from chick embryo telencephalons. Pediatr Res 50: 76–82.
9. Kölker S, Ahlemeyer B, Hühne R, Mayatepek E, Krieglstein J, Hoffmann GF (2001) Potentiation of 3-hydroxyglutarate neurotoxicity following induction of astrocytic iNOS in neonatal rat hippocampal cultures. Eur J Neurosci 13: 2115–2122.
10. Lafon-Cazal M, Pietri S, Culcasi M, Bockaert J (1993) NMDA-dependent superoxide production and neurotoxicity. Nature 364: 535–537.
11. McCarthy KD, DeVellis J (1980) Preparation of separate astroglial and oligodendroglial cell cultures from rat cerebral tissue. J Cell Biol 85: 890–902.
12. Ullrich K, Flott-Rahmel B, Schluff P, Musshoff U, Das A, Lücke T, Steinfeld R, Christensen E, Jakobs C, Ludolph A, Neu A, Röper R (1999) Glutaric aciduria type I: Pathomechanism of neurodegeneration. J Inherit Metab Dis 22: 392–403.

3. Kontroversen in der Neuropädiatrie: Pro und Contra

Therapie der Kraniopharyngiome – Konservatives Vorgehen

C.B. Ostertag, M. Trippel, R. Unsöld, P.C. Warnke

Zusammenfassung

Bei Kraniopharyngeomen im Kindes- und Jugendalter wird eine Therapie bevorzugt, die sich darauf beschränkt, den chirurgischen Eingriff so klein wie möglich zu halten, und eine fraktionierte Strahlentherapie folgen zu lassen. Bei ausgedehnten Tumoren mit Kompression bzw. Infiltration des Hypothalamus und des Chiasmas, wo mit postoperativen ophthalmologischen und/oder endokrinologischen Ausfällen zu rechnen ist, und wo eine völlige Resektion von vornherein nicht möglich erscheint, sollte ein stereotaktisches Vorgehen bevorzugt werden, d.h. die Sicherung der histologischen Diagnose durch eine Biopsie sowie, bei Vorhandensein einer zystischen Komponente, die Entlastung der Zyste durch eine Aspiration und evtl. Zystoventrikulostomie. Dem sollte eine fraktionierte Strahlentherapie (kleinvolumige Konformationsbestrahlung) folgen. Die mikrochirurgische Resektion ist u.E. nur gerechtfertigt bei begründeter Aussicht auf Radikalität und bei dokumentierter minimaler Morbidität. Diese Therapieoption wird im wesentlichen für intraselläre und transsphenoidal anzugehende Kraniopharyngeome in Frage kommen. Selbst aus neurochirurgischer Sicht wird das aggressive Vorgehen mittlerweile kritisch bewertet.

Einleitung

Kraniopharyngiome sind, auch im Kindes- und Jugendalter, seltene Tumoren (0,5 bis 1,0 Fall / 1Million Einwohner/Jahr), die solide/zystisch/verkalkend wachsen, dabei die suprasellären Strukturen (z.B. Chiasma, Hypothalamus, Boden des 3. Ventrikels) verdrängen und/oder infiltrieren. Histomorphologisch sind Kraniopharyngiome gutartige Tumore, deren Wachstum nichtlinear, langsam, gelegentlich schubweise verläuft. Sowohl der natürliche Verlauf als auch therapeutische Maßnahmen können durch eine hohe Morbidität gekennzeichnet sein.

Über die beste Therapiemethode, d.h. zwischen aggressiver und konservativer chirurgischer Therapie, wird seit 40 Jahren unverändert heftig, teilweise emotional, gestritten. Manche Neurochirurgen betrachten diesen Tumor als eine persönliche Herausforderung (2). »Optimum treatment in childhood consists in making every effort to effect a total excision« (13,17,28). Die radikale Entfernung ist jedoch nur in einen kleinen Prozentsatz möglich und selten ohne, z.T. erhebliche, zusätzliche Morbidität zu erreichen. Hiervon ausgenommen sind intraselläre, infradiaphragmatische und kleine supraselläre, nicht-infiltrative Kraniopharyngiome (1, 8, 11).

»The best treatment is conservative surgery and postoperative radiation therapy« (12,15). Für das chirurgisch konservative Vorgehen steht an erster Stelle die rasche Druckentlastung von Hypothalamus, Chiasma und eines eventuellen Hydrozephalus. Wir bevorzugen die stereotaktische Punktion von Zysten bzw. die Aspiration eines Zysteninhaltes. Auf diesem Wege kann auch die Diagnose durch Mikroskopieren des Zysteninhaltes (Cholesterinkristalle) und durch eine Gewebsentnahme aus der Zystenwand (Nachweis von differenziertem Epithel) rasch geklärt werden. Falls notwendig, kann auch eine Teilresektion erfolgen (»limited surgery«). Durch dieses schrittweise Vorgehen wird erreicht, dass sich Funktionen erholen können, keine zusätzlichen funktionellen Ausfälle erzeugt werden und dass Zeit gewonnenen wird für die sorgfältige Planung einer kleinvolumigen Strahlentherapie.

Die *stereotaktische Punktion* erfolgt bei Kindern in Intubationsnarkose, bei Jugendlichen in Lokalanästhesie. Eine optimierte Planung des Zuganges erfolgt durch Bildfusion (CT/MR). Über ein sorgfältig geplantes Bohrloch wird eine Führungssonde mit einem Durchmesser von ein bis zwei Millimetern bis in die Zyste(n) eingeführt, der Zysteninhalt aspiriert und, nach Spülung, entleert. Gelegentlich erfolgt eine innere Drainage durch Einlage eines Reservoirkatheters. Durch eine Gewebsentnahme aus der Zystenwand gelingt es meist auch, die histologische Diagnose zu sichern. Der Eingriff selbst dauert 60 bis 90 Minuten und erfordert einen stationären Aufenthalt von drei bis vier Tagen.

Obwohl es sich um einen gutartige Tumore handelt, sind Kraniopharyngiome strahlenempfindlich, d.h., es besteht eine Differenz hinsichtlich der Strahlenempfindlichkeit zwischen normalem Gehirn und Tumor. Die *stereotaktische kleinvolumige Radiotherapie* verbindet die Vorteile der Fraktionierung mit einer fokalen Dosisapplikationen. Voraussetzung ist eine sorgfältige Darstellung und Definition des Zielvolumens. Die stereotaktische Bestrahlung erfordert eine Fixierung des Kopfes, d. h., sie wird in sorgfältiger Maskentechnik oder mit Hilfe eines stereotaktischen Rahmens durchgeführt. Auf ein möglichst kleines Volumen wird eine Herddosis von 50 bis 60 Gy mit 1,8 bis 2 Gy täglich appliziert (3, 12, 21). Durch mehrere Studien bei kindlichen Patienten mit Kraniopharyngiomen, z.T. mit einer Nachbeobachtungszeit von > 20 Jahren, ist sowohl die Wirksamkeit der Bestrahlung als auch die Rate an strahlenbedingten Nebenwirkungen bekannt. Es herrscht Übereinstimmung darüber, dass die partielle Entfernung eines Kraniopharyngioms nur dann gerechtfertigt ist, wenn eine Strahlentherapie, gegebenenfalls nach einem zeitlichen Intervall, folgt. Es ist jedoch auch sicher, dass selbst eine Strahlentherapie mit sehr kleinen Feldern für das kindliche Gehirn nicht folgenlos ist, und, wenn unumgänglich, möglichst bis zu einem Lebensalter von fünf bis sechs Jahren hinausgeschoben werden soll (4). Über das sehr seltene Vorkommen von Zweittumoren im Niedrig- Dosisbereich nach Bestrahlung eines Kraniopharyngioms ist berichtet worden (16).

Eigene Erfahrungen

Die Ergebnisse der konservativen chirurgischen Therapie mit nachfolgender Strahlentherapie sind in mehreren Serien sehr gut belegt mit z. T. langer Nachbeobachtungszeit (3, 6, 7, 10, 12, 14, 15, 19, 21, 22, 25). In einer Serie von 185 Patienten mit Kraniopharyngiomen (Freiburg 1972 bis 2002) wurden ausschließlich stereotaktische Methoden angewendet (bildgestützte Zugangsplanung und -optimierung, Bohrlochtrepanation, Punktion, Aspiration, innere Drainage, Gewebsentnahme). In dieser Serie fanden sich 70 Patienten im Jugend- oder Kindesalter (≤ 20 Jahre). Eine retrospektive Analyse von 45 Patienten im Kindesalter (1984 bis 1999) mit einem medianen Alter von 9 ± 3,7 Jahre, männlich/weiblich 24/21 Patienten, liegt vor. Vorangegangene Behandlung vor dem stereotaktischen Eingriff: Shuntanlage 10 Patienten, Teilresektion 15 Patienten. Bei 37 Patienten erfolgte eine stereotaktische Zystenentleerung, bei 8 Patienten nur eine Biopsie und bei 16 Patienten eine innere Drainage (Ventrikulozystostomie). Es wurde keine perioperative Letalität und keine permanente Morbidität verzeichenet. Nach diesen operativen Maßnahmen erfolgte, nach unterschiedlichen Wartezeiten bei 31 Patienten eine kleinvolumige stereotaktische Strahlentherapie. Diese Patienten wurden 10,5 ± 5,3 Jahre (Median) nachbeobachtet. Der kindliche Performance Status war bei der letzten Beobachtung signifikant verbessert (präoperativ 76 ± 13, letzte Nachbeobachtung 89 ± 10, $p = 0.0005$). Während der Beobachtung sind 3 Patienten verstorben (2 Patienten durch Progression, eine Patientin durch Shunt-Komplikationen. Die 5/10 Jahresüberlebensrate betrug 96/93 Prozent. Das 5/10 Jahre-progressionsfreie Überleben lag bei 82/80 Prozent. Bei 27 Patienten bestand präoperativ eine Visus/Gesichtsfeld-Einschränkung, die postoperativ bei 24 Patienten gebessert, bei 18 Patienten unverändert und bei drei Patienten passager verschlechtert war. Der endokrinologische Befund war bei 42 Patienten unverändert, eine Substitution eines Diabetes insipidus war bei drei Patienten nach dem Eingriff erforderlich (9).

Andere Therapieoptionen

Andere Therapiemodalitäten sind die *stereotaktische Radiochirurgie,* die *stereotaktische intrakavitäre Bestrahlung* durch Radioisotope und die *intrakavitäre Chemotherapie.* Die stereotaktische Radiochirurgie beinhaltet eine einzeitig applizierte, fokussierte Dosis, unter Umständen mit multiplen Isozentren. Kritische Strukturen sind auch hier Chiasma und Hypothalamus. Mehrere Autoren berichten über eine Tumorkontrolle von über 80% bei einer Morbidität von < 10 Prozent (5, 26). Die stereotaktische Instillation radioaktiver Isotope wie Yttrium-90, Rhenium-186 und Phosphor-32, d.h. von Beta strahlenden kolloidalen Lösungen in Kraniopharyngiom Zysten wird seit mehreren Jahren angewandt. Sie führt zur einer Zystenreduktion in ca. 80 Prozent. Eine Morbidität über 12 Prozent machen diese Methode jedoch risikoreich. Durch die Betastrahlung werden Anteile des Kraniopharyngioms außerhalb der Zystenwand nicht erreicht. Die in den meisten Fällen notwendige Strahlentherapie lässt sich durch die intrakavitäre Bestrahlung nicht ersetzen (27). Die Anwendung einer intrakavitären Chemotherapie, z. B. mit Bleomycin, ist noch problematischer. Neben einer hohen Morbidität durch direkte Schädigung des Chiasmas oder in der Zystenwand verlaufender Gefäße sind hier auch vereinzelte Todesfälle beschrieben worden (24). Wir wenden diese zuletzt genannten Methoden in Freiburg nicht an. Auch die stereotaktische interstitielle Bestrahlung durch Einlage von Jod-125 Seeds kommt nur in Ausnahmefällen in Betracht.

Diskussion und Therapieempfehlung

In einer Meta-Analyse hat A. Raimondi, einer der großen Pioniere der pädiatrischen Neurochirurgie, eindringlich darauf hingewiesen, dass auch durch das moderne Instrumentarium des Neurochirurgen der nicht-entfernbare Tumor nicht entfernbarer wird. Die Schwierigkeit, den Tumor chirurgisch komplett und ohne Morbidität zu entfernen, ist ein Charakteristikum des Tumors, und ist nicht unbedingt auf das Geschick des Chirurgen zurückzuführen. Zweifellos ist jedoch die Routine für jeden Operateur von größter Wichtigkeit (23). Der ungetrübte Optimismus mancher aggressiver Operateure ist vor dem Hintergrund der Erfolge der modernen Strahlentherapie nicht länger gerechtfertigt (20). Aufgrund der bislang vorliegenden Daten und unter Berücksichtigung eigener retrospektiver Analysen kommen wir zu folgender Therapieempfehlung: Kraniotomie und mikrochirurgische Resektion erscheinen nur gerechtfertigt bei begründeter Aussicht auf komplette Entfernung und bei dokumentierter Routine, d. h. minimaler Morbidität des behandelnden Zentrums. Diese Therapieoption wird im wesentlichen bei infradiaphragmatischen und transphenoidal zu operierenden Kraniopharyngiomen infrage kommen. Bei ausgedehnten Tumoren mit hypothalamischer Kompression bzw. Infiltration, nicht zu erwartender vollständiger Entfernung und zu erwartenden postoperativen ophthalmologischen und/oder endokrininologischen Ausfällen sollte das konservative Vorgehen bevorzugt werden. Der ersten Behandlungsmaßnahme kommt eine entscheidende Bedeutung zu.

Bei der Seltenheit des Kraniopharyngioms (ca. 80 Patienten pro Jahr in Deutschland) macht es keinen Sinn, diese Patienten gleichmäßig im Lande zu verteilen und zu behandeln. Nur durch eine Konzentration in wenigen Behandlungszentren, die alle diagnostischen, operativen und strahlentherapeutischen Optionen haben, können kindliche Kraniopharyngiome optimal behandelt werden (18). Neuropädiatrische, ophthalmologische, endokrinologische und neurochirurgische Expertise sind Voraussetzung. Alle weltweit bislang vorgelegten klinischen Daten sind retrospektive Analysen, zumeist mit geringem Fallzahlen, kurzen Beobachtungszeiten und unvollständiger ophthalmologischer und endokrininologischer Verlaufsdokumentation. Es ist dringend notwendig, mit prospektiven, »kontrollierten« Studien zu beginnen, damit unnötige Eingriffe bzw. Therapiefolgen vermieden werden.

Literatur

1. Abe T, Lüdecke DK.Transnasal surgery for infradiaphragmatic craniopharyngiomas in pediatric patients. Neurosurgery. 1999 May;44(5):957–64
2. Amacher AL. Craniopharyngioma: the controversy regarding radiotherapy. Childs Brain. 1980;6(2):57–64.
3. Becker G, Kortmann RD, Skalej M, Bamberg M.The role of radiotherapy in the treatment of craniopharyngioma--indications, results, side effects. Front Radiat Ther Oncol. 1999;33:100–13.
4. Brada M, Thomas DG. Craniopharyngioma revisited. Int J Radiat Oncol Biol Phys. 1993 Sep 30;27(2):471–5.
5. Chiou SM, Lunsford LD, Niranjan A, Kondziolka D, Flickinger JC.Stereotactic radiosurgery of residual or recurrent craniopharyngioma, after surgery, with or without radiation therapy. Neuro-oncol. 2001 Jul;3(3):159–66.
6. Danoff BF, Cowchock FS, Kramer S.Childhood craniopharyngioma: survival, local control, endocrine and neurologic function following radiotherapy. Int J Radiat Oncol Biol Phys. 1983 Feb;9(2):171–5
7. De Vile CJ, Grant DB, Kendall BE, Neville BG, Stanhope R, Watkins KE, Hayward RD.Management of childhood craniopharyngioma: can the morbidity of radical surgery be predicted? J Neurosurg. 1996 Jul;85(1):73–81
8. Fahlbusch R, Honegger J, Paulus W, Huk W, Buchfelder M.Surgical treatment of craniopharyngiomas: experience with 168 patients. J Neurosurg. 1999 Feb;90(2):237–50
9. Guthoff R: Ophthalmologische und endokrinologische Befunde bei primär mikrochirurgisch und bei stereotaktisch-radiotherapeutisch behandelten Patienten mit Kraniopharyngiomen. Dissertation, Medizinische Fakultät, Freiburg i.Br. 2000
10. Habrand JL, Ganry O, Couanet D, Rouxel V, Levy-Piedbois C, Pierre-Kahn A, Kalifa C. The role of radiation therapy in the management of craniopharyngioma: a 25-year experience and review of the literature. Int J Radiat Oncol Biol Phys. 1999 May 1;44(2):255–63.
11. Hayward R.The present and future management of childhood craniopharyngioma. Childs Nerv Syst. 1999 Nov;15(11–12):764–9.
12. Hetelekidis S, Barnes PD, Tao ML, Fischer EG, Schneider L, Scott RM, Tarbell NJ. 20-year experience in childhood craniopharyngioma. Int J Radiat Oncol Biol Phys. 1993 Sep 30;27(2):189–95.
13. Hoffman HJ: Surgical management of craniopharyngioma. Pediatr Neurosurg 1994 21(suppl1), 44–49,
14. Isaac MA, Hahn SS, Kim JA, Bogart JA, Chung CT: Management of craniopharyngioma. Cancer J 2001 Nov-Dec;7(6):516–20
15. Kramer S (1976) Craniopharangioma: The best treatment is conservative surgery and postoperative radiation therapy. In: Morley TP (edit) Current controversies in neurosurgery. WB Saunders, Philadelphia
16. Kranzinger M, Jones N, Rittinger O, Pilz P, Piotrowski WP, Manzl M, Galvan G, Kogelnik HD.Malignant glioma as a secondary malignant neoplasm after radiation therapy for craniopharyngioma: report of a case and review of reported cases. Onkologie. 2001 Feb;24(1):66–72.
17. Matson DD, Crigler JF Jr.Management of craniopharyngioma in childhood. J Neurosurg. 1969 Apr;30(4):377–90.
18. Muller HL, Bueb K, Bartels U, Roth C, Harz K, Graf N, Korinthenberg R, Bettendorf M, Kuhl J, Gutjahr P, Sorensen N, Calaminus G.Obesity after childhood craniopharyngioma – German multicenter study on pre-operative risk factors and quality of life. Klin Padiatr. 2001 Jul-Aug;213(4):244–9.
19. Raimondi AJ, Rougerie J.A critical review of personal experiences with craniopharyngioma: clinical history, surgical technique and operative results. 1983. Pediatr Neurosurg. 1994;21(2):134–50;
20. Raimondi AJ (1993) Craniopharyngioma: complications and treatment failures weaken case for aggressive surgery. Crit Rev Neurosurg 3:7–24

21. Rajan B, Ashley S, Gorman C, Jose CC, Horwich A, Bloom HJ, Marsh H, Brada M. Craniopharyngioma – a long-term results following limited surgery and radiotherapy. Radiother Oncol. 1993 Jan;26(1):1–10
22. Regine WF, Kramer S.Pediatric craniopharyngiomas: long term results of combined treatment with surgery and radiation. Int J Radiat Oncol Biol Phys. 1992;24(4):611–7
23. Sanford RA.Craniopharyngioma: results of survey of the American Society of Pediatric Neurosurgery. Pediatr Neurosurg. 1994;21 Suppl 1:39–43.
24. Savas A, Erdem A, Tun K, Kanpolat Y.Fatal toxic effect of bleomycin on brain tissue after intracystic chemotherapy for a craniopharyngioma: case report. Neurosurgery. 2000 Jan;46(1):213–6;
25. Scott RM, Hetelekidis S, Barnes PD, Goumnerova L, Tarbell NJ. Surgery, radiation, and combination therapy in the treatment of childhood craniopharyngioma – a 20-year experience. Pediatr Neurosurg. 1994;21 Suppl 1:75–81.
26. Sims E, Doughty D, Macaulay E, Royle N, Wraith C, Darlison R, Plowman PN.Stereotactically delivered cranial radiation therapy: a ten-year experience of linac-based radiosurgery in the UK. Clin Oncol (R Coll Radiol). 1999;11(5):303–20
27. Voges J, Sturm V, Lehrke R, Treuer H, Gauss C, Berthold F.Cystic craniopharyngioma: long-term results after intracavitary irradiation with stereotactically applied colloidal beta-emitting radioactive sources. Neurosurgery. 1997 Feb;40(2):263–9
28. Yasargil MG, Curcic M, Kis M, Siegenthaler G, Teddy PJ, Roth P.Total removal of craniopharyngiomas. Approaches and long-term results in 144 patients. J Neurosurg. 1990 Jul;73(1):3–11.

Chemotherapie – Standard in der Behandlung von Kindern mit Hirntumoren!

J. Kühl

Zusammenfassung

Aufgrund der Ergebnisse prospektiv randomisierter Studien kann festgestellt werden, dass die zytostatische Chemotherapie einen sicheren Platz in der Behandlung von allen Kindern mit einem Medulloblastom und analog einem supratentoriell lokalisierten PNET hat. Dies gilt auch für Kinder mit einem sezernierenden Keimzelltumor. Bei Kindern mit einem anaplastischen Ependymom, dessen Prognose mit alleiniger Bestrahlung sehr schlecht war, ist es derzeit nicht vertretbar, auf eine zusätzliche Chemotherapie zu verzichten, wenngleich noch randomisierte Studien fehlen. Auch die schlechte Prognose von Kindern mit Gliomen hoher Malignität WHO° III/IV zwingt gerade unter Berücksichtigung aktueller Ergebnisse der HIT-Studien zusätzlich Chemotherapie einzusetzen. Zur Schonung von kleinen Kindern mit einem progressiven Gliom niedriger Malignität WHO° I/II eignet sich eine milde Chemotherapie im Rahmen kontrollierter Studien, um die Strahlentherapie in ein höheres Alter hinauszuzögern. Somit ist die Chemotherapie mittlerweile bei einem breiten Spektrum von Hirntumoren im Kindesalter indiziert.

Einleitung

In der Pädiatrischen Onkologie konnte in den letzten 20 Jahren die Prognose von Kindern mit Krebserkrankungen durch den systematischen Einsatz der zytostatischen Chemotherapie dramatisch verbessert werden. Die Einführung der Chemotherapie bei Kindern mit Hirntumoren verlief dagegen zögerlich. Aktuelle Studien konnten jedoch zeigen, dass die Chemotherapie mittlerweile zum Standard auch bei der Behandlung von Kindern mit Hirntumoren gehört und nur noch bei wenigen Entitäten experimenteller Natur ist.

Medulloblastom

Der häufigste maligne Hirntumor im Kindesalter ist das Medulloblastom. Es handelt sich dabei wie bei den meisten Krebserkrankungen im Kindesalter um einen embryonalen, speziell um einen primitiv neuroektodermalen Tumor (PNET). Der PNET reagiert auf Chemotherapie ebenso sensibel wie andere embryonale Tumoren. Da in malignen Hirntumoren wie dem Medulloblastom die Blut-Tumor-Schranke nicht intakt ist, konnten in Phase II-Studien mit Kombinationsregimen, die Cyclophosphamid oder Cisplatin enthielten, Responseraten von 60–70% erzielt werden (Kühl 1988).

Die Arbeitsgruppe für Hirntumoren der Gesellschaft für Pädiatrische Onkologie und Hämatologie (GPOH) entschloss sich 1988 gemeinsam u.a. mit der Gesellschaft für Neuropädiatrie die Wirksamkeit einer intensiven Sandwich-Chemotherapie, die aus Procarbazin, Ifosfamid, Etoposid, hochdosiertem Methotrexat, Cisplatin und Cytarabin bestand, bei Kindern ab einem Alter von drei Jahren zu untersuchen. Mit dieser postoperativen Chemotherapie konnte bei 67% der Patienten, die einen Resttumor und/oder solide ZNS-Metastasen hatten, ein Response, d.h. eine komplette oder partielle (> 50%) Rückbildung erzielt werden (Kühl et al. 1993). Wir konnten sogar zeigen, dass Patienten, die durch die Chemotherapie in komplette Remission kamen, eine annähernd so gute progressions-freie Überlebensrate *(PFÜ)* erreichten, wie Patienten ohne Resttumor und ohne Metastasen. Nach einem kompletten Response betrug die 5-Jahre PFÜ 57%; dagegen nach einem weniger als kompletten Response nur 20% (Kühl et al. 1998). Dieses Ergebnis stützte die Hypothese, dass die nachfolgende Bestrahlung dann in höherem Maße kurativ sein kann, wenn es gelingt, die postoperative Tumorzellmasse durch eine neoadjuvante Chemotherapie um einen ca. 2 log Zellkill zu reduzieren.

In den ersten internationalen prospektiv randomisierten Phase III Studien der 70er Jahre wurde die Effektivität der Kombinationen von CCNU und Vincristin von der SIOP[1] und CCG[2] bzw. MOPP (Mustargen, Vincristin, Procarbazin und Prednison) von der POG[3] untersucht (Tait et al. 1990, Evans et al. 1990, Krischer et al. 1991). Die 5-Jahre ereignis- bzw. rezidiv-freie Überlebensrate *(EFÜ/RFÜ)* lagen im jeweiligen Chemotherapiearm der drei Studien tendenziell höher: SIOP 56% vs. 42%, CCG 59% vs. 50% und POG 68% vs. 57%. Diese Ergebnisse ließen vermuten, dass eine adjuvante Chemotherapie bei Kindern mit einem Medulloblastom sinnvoll ist. Von der Chemotherapie profitierten am meisten Kinder mit einem bereits initial hohen Rezidivrisiko, d.h. mit fortgeschrittenem Tumorstadium(T3/4), mit initialer Metastasierung, nach inkompletter Resektion des Tumors und mit niedrigem Alter. Besonders drastisch fiel der Unterschied aus in der Studie CCG-942 bei Kindern mit fortgeschrittener Tumorerkrankung und Metastasen mit einem 5-Jahre EFS von 46% nach Bestrahlung und Chemotherapie gegen 0% nach alleiniger Bestrahlung (Evans et al. 1990).

Um die Effektivität der adjuvanten Chemotherapie mit CCNU und Vincristin zu verstärken, wurde diese Kombination durch Cisplatin ergänzt. In Philadelphia wurde mit dieser 3-fach Kombination bei Kindern mit Hochrisiko-Medulloblastom eine 5-Jahre PFÜ von 85% erzielt (Packer et al. 1991). Kinder mit Standardrisiko, die keine Chemotherapie erhielten, hatten mit nur 52% eine wesentlich schlechtere Überlebensrate. Daher erhielten in einer Folgestudie (CCG-9892) Kinder mit Standardrisiko, d.h. ohne Metastasen im Alter von 3–10 Jahren, diese Erhaltungschemotherapie mit CCNU, Cisplatin und VCR. Die PFÜ lag nach 5 Jahren mit 79% erstaunlich hoch, obwohl zur Schonung des Gehirns

[1)] International Society of Paediatric Oncology
[2)] Childrens Cancer Group
[3)] Pediatric Oncology Group

der jungen Patienten die kranio-spinale Bestrahlungsdosis auf 23,4 Gy reduziert worden war (Packer et al. 1999). Wie wichtig die Reduktion der kranio-spinalen Bestrahlungsdosis ist, haben die Ergebnisse einer CCG/POG-Studie gezeigt, in der die neuro-kognitiven Folgen einer kranio-spinalen Bestrahlung mit 36 Gy gegen 23,4 Gy verglichen wurden (Mulhern et al. 1998). Kinder, die eine reduzierte Dosis erhalten hatten, erreichten bei der neuropsychologischen Testung einen signifikant höheren »Full Scale«-IQ, im Vergleich zu den konventionell bestrahlten Kindern. Dies galt besonders für Kinder unter 9 Jahren (IQ 85 vs. 70), aber auch für ältere Kinder (IQ 92 vs. 83). Diese Studie musste allerdings abgebrochen werden, da im reduzierten Bestrahlungsarm gehäuft Rezidive auftraten, was mit dem völligen Verzicht auf Chemotherapie in dieser Studie erklärt werden konnte (Deutsch et al. 1996). In unserer Studie HIT'88/'89, in der alle Kinder eine intensive postoperative Chemotherapie erhielten, war die PFÜ von Patienten ohne Metastasen, die weniger als 30 Gy kranio-spinal erhielten, nicht schlechter als die PFÜ der Patienten, die mit mehr als 30 Gy bestrahlt wurden. Die Chemotherapie war offensichtlich in der Lage, eine Häufung von Rezidiven bei Patienten, die eine reduzierte kranio-spinale Bestrahlungsdosis erhielten, zu verhindern.

Die Frage, ob bei Standardrisikopatienten ohne Metastasen die Prognose durch eine zusätzliche Chemotherapie deutlich verbessert werden kann, wurde in der 3. Medulloblastomstudie der SIOP (PNET-3) prospektiv randomisiert untersucht. Im Standardarm erhielten die Kinder nur eine postoperative Bestrahlung und im experimentellen Arm zusätzlich eine postoperative Chemotherapie mit Carboplatin, VP16 und Vincristin sowie Cyclophosphamid, VP16 und VCR, die unserem HIT-SKK Protokoll nachempfunden war, allerdings kein Methotrexat enthielt (Taylor et al. 2001). Die Studie konnte eindeutig einen signifikanten Vorteil der Sandwich-Chemotherapie im Vergleich zur alleinigen postoperativen Bestrahlung zeigen mit einer EFÜ von 72% vs. 59% nach 5 Jahren. Bei Kindern ohne Metastasen und ohne Resttumor war der Unterschied besonders deutlich. Somit steht endlich fest, dass auch Kinder mit Standardrisiko-Medulloblastom von einer Chemotherapie profitieren, was lange von Radioonkologen bestritten worden war.

In unserer prospektiv randomisierten Therapiestudie HIT'91 hatten wir in Deutschland und Österreich bereits parallel zur PNET-3 Studie untersucht, ob die HIT-Sandwich-Chemotherapie, die in einer variierten Form ohne MTX in PNET-3 so erfolgreich war, der Erhaltungs-Chemotherapie mit Cisplatin, CCNU und Vincristin, die in Philadelphia so erfolgreich eingesetzt worden war, bei Kindern ohne Metastasen überlegen ist (Kühl 1998). In dieser Studie war entgegen unserer Erwartung die adjuvante Erhaltungs-Chemotherapie der HIT-Sandwich-Chemotherapie deutlich überlegen (Kortmann, Kühl et al. 2000). Mit einer PFÜ von 78% konnte bei Kindern ohne solide ZNS-Metastasen (Chang Stadium M0/1) mit der Erhaltungs-Chemotherapie ein annähernd gleich hohes Niveau wie in den amerikanischen Studien erzielt werden. Dieses Ergebnis ist um so erstaunlicher, als es in einer multizentrischen Studie, an der sich 69 Kliniken in Deutschland, Österreich und der Schweiz beteiligen, erreicht wurde. Damit kann die adjuvante Chemotherapie mit Cisplatin, CCNU und Vincristin nach Operation und Bestrahlung derzeit als der »Golden Standard« bei Kindern über 3 Jahren angesehen werden.

Bei Kindern unter 3 Jahren verhält sich das Medulloblastom wesentlich aggressiver als bei älteren Kindern und Jugendlichen. Dies ist wahrscheinlich auf molekularbiologischer Ebene determiniert. So konnte bei jüngeren Kindern, die bereits initial klinisch manifeste Metastasen hatten, häufiger eine Amplifikation des c-myc Onkogens nachgewiesen werden (Scheurlen et al. 1998). Frühe Rezidive sind Ausdruck dieser Aggressivität. In einer Chemotherapiestudie der CCG lag die PFÜ von Kindern unter 3 Jahren nur noch bei 32% nach 5 Jahren (Zeltzer et al. 1999). Die Bestrahlung des Gehirns, das bei kleinen Kindern noch nicht vollständig ausgereift ist, führte zu neuro-kognitiven und neuro-endokrinologischen Funktionsstörungen, die ihre Lebensqualität erheblich beeinträchtigte (Chapman et al. 1995, Hoppe-Hirsch et al. 1995).

In unserer Studie HIT-SKK'92 erhielten alle Kinder unter 3 Jahren mit einem Medulloblastom postoperativ drei modifizierte HIT-Zyklen sowie Methotrexat, das intraventrikulär über eine Rickham-Kapsel oder ein Ommaya-Reservoir gegeben wurde (Kühl 1997). Mit diesem innovativen Therapieelement sollte die kraniospinale Bestrahlung ersetzt und die Sanierung eines okkulten Befalls des Liquorraumes erzielt werden. Kinder, die am Ende der Chemotherapie in kompletter Remission waren, wurden nicht mehr bestrahlt. Auch für uns überraschend konnte mit diesem experimentellen Therapieansatz knapp die Hälfte der 45 behandelten Kinder geheilt werden. Die PFÜ lagen nach 4 Jahren bei 77% für Kinder ohne einen Resttumor, bei 42% für Kinder mit einem Resttumor und bei 27% für Kinder mit Metastasen eines Stadiums M2/3 (Kühl et al. 1999). Von 19 im ersten Ansatz geheilten Kindern (ohne Stadium M2/3) waren 16 nicht bestrahlt worden. Dieses Ergebnis widerspricht dem Dogma, dass Kinder mit Medulloblastom ohne Bestrahlung nicht geheilt werden können! Neurospychologische Untersuchungen der behandelten Kinder konnten zeigen, dass sich der Verzicht auf die Bestrahlung günstig auf die neuro-kognitive Leistungsfähigkeit ausgewirkt hatte (Ottensmeier, Kühl 1999). Die Lebensqualität der geheilten Kinder hat sich auch dadurch verbessert, dass die Kinder nicht unter den anderen Nebenwirkungen der Bestrahlung, wie z.B. neuro-endokrinologischen Störungen zu leiden haben.

Mit zunehmend verbesserter Kontrolle der Erkrankung innerhalb der kranio-spinalen Achse scheint die relative Inzidenz an Metastasen außerhalb des Zentralnervensystems zuzunehmen. So traten in einer Serie aus Boston bei 9 von 50 Kindern, die nur bestrahlt wurden, Metastasen außerhalb des ZNS (Knochenmetastasen) auf, dagegen bei keinem der 39 Kinder, die zusätzlich eine Chemotherapie erhielten (Tarbel et al. 1991). Daher lag die PFÜ nach 5 Jahren deutlich höher (72% vs. 55%) bei Kindern, die zusätzlich zur Bestrahlung mit einer Chemotherapie behandelt wurden.

Zusammenfassend spielt somit die Chemotherapie eine sehr wichtige Rolle in der modernen Behandlung von Kindern mit einem Medulloblastom. Bei Kindern ohne Metastasen soll eine hohe Heilungsrate bei geringen Spätfolgen durch die Reduktion der Strahlentherapie erreicht werden. Bei Kindern mit Metastasen soll die bisher noch unbefriedigende Prognose verbessert werden. Bei Kindern unter 4 Jahren soll die Chemotherapie die Bestrahlung ersetzen. Bei allen Patienten soll dadurch das Auftreten von systemischen Metastasen außerhalb des ZNS verhindert werden.

Primitiv Neuroektodermaler Tumor (PNET)

Supratentoriell gelegene PNET sprechen ebenso gut auf Chemotherapie an, wie Medulloblastome. In älteren Zusammenstellungen lag die Überlebensrate dennoch unter 20%, wobei auffiel, dass nur die Kinder überlebten, die sowohl Strahlen- als auch Chemotherapie erhielten (Dirks et al. 1996). In den HIT-Studien lag das PFÜ mit 55% nach 4 Jahren im Erhaltungschemotherapiearm HIT'91 jedoch deutlich über den historischen Daten, aber niedriger als beim Medulloblastom.

Ependymom

Im Vergleich zum Medulloblastom ist das Ependymom ein weniger chemotherapiesensibler Tumor. In einer konsekutiven Studie am Royal Marsden Hospital mit einem renomierten strahlentherapeutischen Institut konnte gezeigt werden, dass Kinder, die eine Erhaltungs-Chemotherapie mit CCNU und Vincristin erhielten, mit einer 10-Jahres Überlebensrate von 54% (vs. 34%) besser abschnitten, als Kinder, die zuvor nur postoperativ nachbestrahlt wurden (Bloom et al. 1990). Andere Studien waren bisher nicht in der Lage, den zusätzlichen Benefit der Chemotherapie zu belegen. Dies lag vor allem daran, dass in diesen Studien nicht zwischen einem Ependymom niedriger vs. hoher Malignität unterschieden wurde. Aber nur beim hochmalignen anaplastischen Ependymom WHO°III ist überhaupt mit einem Effekt der Chemotherapie zu rechnen.

In einer aktuellen retrospektiven Untersuchung konnte gezeigt werden, dass Kinder mit einem anaplastischen Ependymom WHO° III mit einer 5-Jahre EFS von unter 20% eine sehr viel schlechtere Prognose hatten als Kindern mit einem Ependymom WHO° II (Horn et al. 1999). Dagegen lag die PFÜ von Kindern mit ausschließlich anaplastischen Ependymomen, die im Rahmen der HIT-Studien zusätzlich zur Bestrahlung alle auch eine Chemotherapie erhielten, nach 5 Jahren über 40% (Timmermann et al. 2000). Dieses Ergebnis war deutlich besser als die bisherigen Erfahrungen mit alleiniger postoperativer Strahlentherapie. Mit der Kombination von hyperfraktionierter Bestrahlung mit lokaler Dosissteigerung und intensiver Chemotherapie wurde in einer oligozentrischen Studie eine 5-Jahres PFÜ von 74% erzielt, wobei ein vergleichsweise hoher Anteil an anaplastischen Ependymomen vorlag (Needle et al. 1997).

Gliom hoher Malignität

Hochmaligne Gliome wie das anaplastische Astrozytom WHO° III und das Glioblastoma multiforme WHO° IV sind weniger chemotherapiesensibel als das Medulloblastom. Dennoch konnte in einer alten Studie der CCG (-943) in den 70er Jahren gezeigt werden, dass die PFÜ von Kindern, die eine adjuvante Chemotherapie mit CCNU und Vincristin erhielten, mit 46% (vs. 18%) signifikant höher lag, als die von Kindern, die postoperativ nur bestrahlt wurden

(Sposto et al. 1989). In der Folgestudie wurde untersucht, ob eine Sandwichchemotherapie nach dem »8in1«-Protokoll der adjuvanten Chemotherapie mit CCNU und Vincristin überlegen sein könnte. Der Unterschied war jedoch nicht signifikant. Das erreichte Niveau von 33% bzw. 26% lag immer noch höher als im reinen Strahlentherapiearm der vorausgegangenen Studie (Finlay et al. 1995).

In unserer Studie HIT'91 wurde bei Kindern mit malignen Gliomen (ohne Ponsgliome), die eine Sandwich-Chemotherapie erhielten, ein exzellentes Ergebnis mit einer Überlebensrate von ca. 60% nach 5 Jahren erzielt (Wolff et al. 2002). Bei Kindern, deren Tumor zu mehr als 90% reseziert werden konnte, lag die Überlebensrate sogar bei ca. 80%. Neue chemotherapeutische Ansätze werden derzeit untersucht um die Prognose von Kindern mit einem wenig oder nicht resektablen Tumor bzw. mit einem Ponsgliom zu verbessern. Dies erfolgt im Rahmen der HIT-GBM-Studien, deren Strategie vorsieht, alle 2 Jahre sequentiell das Therapiekonzept zu ändern und neue innovative Therapieansätze, wie z.B. Immuntherapie oder Differenzierungstherapie zu prüfen. In der aktuellen Studie HIT-GBM-C wird derzeit u.a. eine synchrone Radio-Chemotherapie durchgeführt, die bereits in der Vorstudie zu besseren Responseraten führte als früher die alleinige Strahlentherapie. Insbesondere bei Kindern mit Ponsgliomen wurden erfreuliche Verbesserungen des klinischen Beschwerdebildes aber vereinzelt auch nahezu komplette Remissionen im MRT erzielt, die allerdings nicht dauerhaft anhielten.

Benignes Gliom WHO°I und Gliom von niedriger Malignität WHO°II

Lange Zeit hielt man Tumoren von niedriger Malignität oder gar benigne Tumoren für chemotherapieresistent. Dies galt besonders für die Hirntumoren. Da sich aber auch benigne und niedrigmaligne Astrozytome dann klinisch bösartig verhalten, wenn sie nicht reseziert werden können, kamen diese Kinder ins Blickfeld der Onkologen. Insbesondere bei jüngeren Kindern, denen eine Bestrahlung wegen der neuro-psychologischen und neuro-endokrinologischen Spätfolgen sowie dem Zweitmalignomrisiko nach Strahlentherapie nicht zugemutet werden sollte, wurde die Wirksamkeit von Zytostatika untersucht. Erste Ergebnisse amerikanischer Studien hatten gezeigt, dass eine milde Chemotherapie in der Lage war bei jungen Kindern eine Tumorprogression aufzuhalten, was wichtig ist z.B. bei Kindern mit einem dienzephalen Syndrom oder um bei Kindern mit einem Optikus-/Chiasmagliom den drohenden Visusverlust aufzuhalten. Bei einigen Kindern gelang es sogar den Tumor zur Rückbildung zu bringen (Schmandt, Packer 2000).

In der ersten HIT-LGG-Studie, die eingebettet war in eine internationale SIOP-Studie, wurde der Wert einer Chemotherapie bei Kindern mit einem benignen oder niedrigmalignen Gliom untersucht. Kinder, deren Tumor nicht reseziert werden konnte, der progredient wuchs und/oder eine ernste Symptomatik wie z.B. das dienzephale Syndrom verursachte, erhielten eine Chemotherapie mit Carboplatin und Vincristin, wenn sie jünger als 5 Jahre waren. Die Responserate (CR, PR und SD) lag bei 95%. Der Wert der Chemotherapie wurde auch daran gemessen, wie lange eine Strahlentherapie hinausgezögert werden konnte, und ob einigen Kindern eine Bestrahlung erspart werden konnte. Von den Kindern, die primär Chemotherapie erhielten, mussten tatsächlich 78 von 84 Kindern nach 3 Jahren immer noch nicht bestrahlt werden (Gnekow et al. 2000). Dies hatte für diese Kinder den Vorteil, dass die Bestrahlung in ein Alter hinausgeschoben werden kann, in welchem die Spätfolgen der Bestrahlung weniger gravierend sind. Von den nicht-bestrahlten Kindern hatten ca. 20% einen Progress, der erneut chemotherapeutisch oder wegen einer infausten Tumorsituation nicht mehr behandelt wurde.

Literatur

1. Bloom HJG, Glees J, Bell J (1990) The treatment and long-term prognosis of children with intracranial tumors: a study of 610 cases, 1950–1981. Int J Radiat Oncol Biol Phys 18: 723–45
2. Chapman CA, Waber DP, Bernstein HJ, Pomeroy SL, La Vally B, Sallan SE, Tarbell N (1995) Neurobehavioral and neurologic outcome in long-term survivors of posterior fossa brain tumors: role of age and perioperative factors. J Child Neurol 10: 209–12
3. Deutsch M, Thomas PRM, Krischer J, Boyett JM, Albright L et al. (1996) Results of a prospective randomized trial comparing standard dose neuraxis irradiation (3600 cGy /20) with reduced dose neuraxis irradiation (2340 cGy /13) in patients with low-stage medulloblastoma. Pediatr Neurosurg 24: 167–77
4. Dirks PB, Harris L, Hoffman HJ, Humphreys RP, Drake JM, Rutka JT (1996) Supratentorial primitive neuroectodermal tumors in children. J. Neurooncol. 29: 75–84, 1996
5. Evans AE, Jenkin RDT, Sposto R, Ortega JA, Wilson CB, Wara W, Ertel IJ, Kramer S, Chang CH, Leikin SL, Hammond GD (1990) The treatment of medulloblastoma : results of a prospective randomized trial of radiation therapy with and without CCNU, vincristine and prednisone. J Neurosurg 72: 572– 82
6. Finlay JL. Boyett JM, Yates AJ, Milstein JM, Geyer JR, Bertolone SJ, McGuire P, Cherlow JM, Tefft M, Turski PA, Wara WM, Edwards M, Sutton LN, Berger MS, Epstein F, Ayers G, Allen JC, and Packer RJ (1995) Randomized phase III trial in childhood high-grade astrocytoma comparing vincristine, lomustine, and prednisone with eight-drugs-in1-day regimen. J Clin Oncol 13: 112–23
7. Gnekow AK, Kaatsch P, Kortmann R, Wiestler OD (2000) HIT-LGG: Effektivität von Carboplatin-Vincristin bei progredienten Gliomen niedrigen Malignitätsgrades im Kindesalter – Zwischenbericht. Klin Pediatr 212: 177–84
8. Hoppe-Hirsch E, Brunet L, Laroussinie F et al. (1995) Intellectual outcome in children with malignant tumors of the posterior fossa: influence of the field of irradiation and quality of surgery. Child's Nerv Syst 11: 340–6
9. Horn B, Heideman R, Geyer R, Pollack I, Packer R, Goldwein J, Tomita T, Schomberg P, Ater J, Luchtman-Jones L, Rivlin K, Lamborn K, Prados M, Bollen A, Berger M, Dahl G, McNeil E, Patterson K, Shaw D, Kubalik M, and Russo C (1999) A multi-institutional retrospective study of intracranial ependymoma in children: identification of risk factors. J Pediatr Hematol Oncol 21: 203–11
10. Kortmann RD, Kühl J, Timmermann B, Mittler U, Urban C, Budach V, Richter E, Willich N, Flentje M, Berthold F, Slavc I, Wolff J, Meisner, C, Wiestler O, Sörensen N, Warmuth-Metz M, Bamberg M (2000) Postoperative neoadjuvant chemotherapy before radiotherapy as compared to immediate radiotherapy followed by maintenance chemotherapy in the treatment of medulloblastoma in childhood: HIT'91. Int J Radiat Oncol Biol Phys 46: 269–79
11. Krischer JP, Ragab AH, Kun L, Kim TH, Laurent JP, Boyett JM, Cornell CJ, Link M, Luthy AR, Camitta B (1991) Nitrogen mustard, vincristine, procarbazine and prednisone as adjuvant chemo-therapy in the treatment of medulloblastoma. J Neurosurg74: 905–9
12. Kühl J (1988) Chemotherapie bei Hirntumoren im Kindesalter. Literaturübersicht und Pilotprotokoll. Klin Pädiatr 100: 214–20

13. Kühl J, Berthold F, Bode U, Bucsky P, Graf N, Gnekow A, Maass E, Bamberg M, Kaatsch P, Kleihues P, Rating P, Riehm H, Sörensen N (1993) Preradiation chemotherapy of children with poor-prognosis medulloblastoma. Am J Pediatr Hematol Oncol 15, Suppl A: 67–71
14. Kühl J (1997) Delayed or no radiation therapy after postoperative chemotherapy in children less than 3 years of age with medulloblastoma. In: Kühl J (Hrsg.) Ergebnisse der Pädiatrischen Neuro-Onkologie III. Im Selbstverlag, Würzburg
15. Kühl J, Müller HL, Berthold F, Kortmann RD, Deinlein F, Maaß E, Graf N, Gnekow A, Scheurlen W, Göbel U, Wolf J, Bamberg M, Kaatsch P, Kleihues P, Rating D, Sörensen N, Wiestler OD (1998) Pre-radiation chemotherapy of children and young adults with malignant brain tumors: results of the German pilot trial HIT '88/'89. Klin Pädiatr 210: 227–33
16. Kühl J (1998) Modern treatment strategies in medulloblastoma. Child's Nerv Syst 14: 2–5
17. Kühl J, Bode U, Deinlein F, Ottensmeier H, Wahrmuth-Metz M et al. (1999) Cure of infants with medulloblastoma (M0/M1-stage) by postoperative chemotherapy only. Med Pediatr Oncol 33: 169 (O-107)
18. Mulhern RK, Kepner JL, Thomas PR, Armstrong FD, Friedman HS, Kun LE (1998) Neuropsychologic functioning of survivors of choldhood medulloblastoma randomized to receive conven-tional or reduced-dose craniospinal irradiation: A pediatric oncology group study. J Clin Oncol 16: 1723–8
19. Needle MN, Goldwein JW, Grass J, Cnaan A, Bergman I, Molloy P, Sutton L, Zhao H, Garvin JH, Philips PC (1997) Adjuvante chemotherapy for the treatment of intracranial ependymoma of childhood. Cancer 80: 341–7
20. Ottensmeier H, Kühl J (1999) Pilotstudien HIT-SKK'87 und '92: Zwischenergebnisse der neuropsychologischen Begleitstudie bei Kindern mit Medulloblastom. Monatsschr Kinderheilkd 147: 988
21. Packer RJ, Sutton LN, Goldwein JW, Perilongo G, Bunin G, Ryan J, Cohen BH, D'Angio G, Kramer ED, Zimmerman RA, Rorke LB, Evans AE, Schut L (1991) Improved survival with the use of adjuvant chemotherapy in the treatment of medulloblastoma. J Neurosurg 74: 433–40
22. Packer RJ, Goldwein J, Nicholson HS, Vezina LG, Allen JC, Ris MD, Muraszko K, Rorke LB, Wara W, Cohen BH, Boyett JM (1999) Treatment of children with medulloblastomas with reduced-dose craniospinal radiation therapy and adjuvant chemotherapy: A children's cancer group study. J Clin Oncol 17: 2127–36
23. Scheurlen WG, Schwabe GC, Joos S, Mollenhauer J, Sörensen N, Kühl J (1998) Molecular analysis of childhood PNET defines markers associated with poor outcome. J Clin Oncol 16: 2478–24
24. Schmandt SM, Packer RJ (2000) Treatment of low-grade pediatric glioma. Curr Opin Oncol 12: 194–8
25. Sposto R, Ertel IJ, Jenkin RDT, Boesel CP, Venes JL, Ortega JA, Evans AE, Wara W and Hammond D (1989) The effectiveness of chemotherapy for treatment of high grade astrocytoma in children: results of a randomized trial from the CCSG. J Neuro-Oncol 7: 165–77
26. Tait DM, Thornton-Jones H, Bloom HJG, Lemerle J, Morris-Jones P (1990) Adjuvant chemotherapy for medulloblastoma: The first multi-centre control trial of the International Society of Paediatric Oncology (SIOP I). Eur J Cancer 26: 464–9
27. Tarbell NJ, Loeffler JS, Silver B, Lynch E, Lavally BL, Kupsky WJ, Scott RM, Sallan SE (1991) The change in patterns of relapse in medulloblastoma. Cancer 68: 1600–04
28. Taylor RE, Bailey CC, Lucraft H, Robinson K, Weston C, Lashford LS (2001) Results of a randomised study of pre-radiotherapy chemotherapy (Carboplatin, Vincristine, Cyclophosphamide, Etoposide) with radiotherapy alone in Chang stage M0/M1 medulloblastoma (SIOP/UKCCSG PNET-3). Med Pediatr Oncol 37: 191 (O114)
29. Timmermann B, Kortmann RD, Kühl J et al. (2000) Combined postoperative irradiation and chemo-therapy for anaplastic ependymomas in childhood: Results of the German prospective trials HIT '88/89 and HIT'91. Int J Radiat Oncol Biol Phys 46: 287–95
30. Zeltzer PM, Boyett JM, Finlay JF, Albright AL et al. (1999) Metastasis stage, adjuvant treatment and residual treatment are prognostic factors for medulloblastomas in children: conclusions from the children's cancer group 921 randomized phase III study. J Clin Oncol 17: 832–45

Chemotherapie bereits Standard in der Behandlung von Hirntumoren? – Kontra – Kontroversen in der Neuropädiatrie – Pro und Kontra

R.-D. Kortmann, B. Timmermann, J. Scheiderbauer, E. Dannenmann-Stern, E. Rex, M. Bamberg

Zusammenfassung

Operation gefolgt von Bestrahlung stellt unverändert die Standardtherapie bei Hirntumoren im Kindesalter dar. Nach den bisherigen Erfahrungen kann die Chemotherapie eine Bestrahlung nicht ersetzen. Die seit ca. 3 Jahrzehnten intensiv untersuchten chemotherapeutischen Protokolle haben nach anfangs hochgesetzten Erwartungen nur in wenigen Ausnahmesituationen einen gesicherten Stellenwert erhalten. Es konnte zwar eine Wirkung der chemotherapeutischen Agenzien innerhalb von Phase II-Protokollen gesehen werden, ein zusätzlicher Überlebensvorteil konnte jedoch nur in wenigen Fällen bewiesen werden. Gemessen an den heutigen gültigen Grundanforderungen an klinische Studien im Sinne der sogenannten »Evidence Based Medicine« hat die zusätzliche Chemotherapie einen gesicherten Stellenwert beim Medulloblastoma mit hohen Risikofaktoren und bei nicht seminomatösen intrakraniellen Keimzelltumoren. Bei allen anderen Hirntumoren im Kindesalter ist sie ungesichert. Eine Behandlung außerhalb klinischer Studien sollte daher nicht erfolgen.

Einleitung

Hirntumoren im Kindesalter repräsentieren etwa 20% aller pädiatrischen malignen Neoplasien. Durch Fortschritte und Optimierung in den neurochirurgischen Operationsverfahren ist es in den letzten Jahren zunehmend möglich geworden, intrakranielle Tumoren makroskopisch vollständig zu entfernen. Während die Bestrahlung nach der Operation die wichtigste Therapie bei der kurativen Behandlung von Hirntumoren im Kindesalter darstellt, wird der Einsatz einer zusätzlichen Chemotherapie kontrovers diskutiert. Seit etwa 30 Jahren werden chemotherapeutische Protokolle eingesetzt, um die Prognose zu verbessern oder die Strahlentherapie in Dosierung und Ausdehnung der Therapiefelder zu reduzieren. Bis heute ist die Frage eines therapeutischen Gewinnes jedoch in vielen Fällen ungeklärt, gleichzeitig wird dem zusätzlichen Nebenwirkungspotential der Chemotherapie zu wenig Beachtung geschenkt.

Die Interpretation des Stellenwertes einer zusätzlichen Chemotherapie wird häufig dadurch erschwert, dass erfolgversprechende Erfahrungen aus Phase II-Studien in Therapiestandards überführt werden, ohne dass sie innerhalb von Phase III-Studien auf ihren therapeutischen Vorteil überprüft wurden. Einzelne

Tumorerkrankungen entziehen sich jedoch aufgrund geringer Inzidenz sinnvoller Phase III Studien, so dass spezielle biometrische Analyseverfahren gefordert sind.

Vor diesem Hintergrund müssen aktuelle chemotherapeutische Protokolle vor den Gesichtspunkten »Toxizitäten« und »Kosten« daher kritisch gesehen werden, so dass derzeit Behandlungen außerhalb prospektiver kontrollierter Studien als ethisch und ökonomisch fragwürdig anzusehen sind.

Design klinischer Studien

Die Etablierung von Therapiestandards erfordert klar definierte und standardisierte klinische Studien mit adäquaten biometrischen Vorgaben, Analysen und standardisierten Qualitätskontrollen, um eine Reproduzierbarkeit der gewonnenen klinischen Ergebnisse zu erreichen. Biometrisch abgesicherte Daten, die in Phase II-Studien gewonnen wurden müssen in Folge innerhalb prospektiver kontrollierter Phase III-Studien mit bisherigen etablierten Therapiestandards verglichen und die Überlegenheit bewiesen werden (»Evidence Based Medicine«). Erst dann kann von einem neuen, gesicherten Therapiestandard gesprochen werden. Die Erfüllung dieser Grundanforderungen ist heute Voraussetzung, um eine innovative Therapie in die reguläre Praxis zu überführen. Vor diesem Hintergrund werden im Folgenden die bisher gewonnenen klinischen Erfahrungen mit zusätzlicher Chemotherapie bei Hirntumoren im Kindesalter analysiert.

Medulloblastom

In der Therapie der strahlenempfindlichen Medulloblastome stellt die Radiatio des gesamten Liquorraumes die wesentlichste postoperative Therapiemaßnahme dar. Heute können mit der Kombination aus Operation und Bestrahlung 5-Jahres-Überlebensraten zwischen 60 und 80% und nach 10 Jahren zwischen 40 bis 60% erzielt werden (Bailey et al. 1995, Bamberg et al. 1980, Berry et al. 1981, Evans et al. 1990). Die Qualität der Strahlenbehandlung ist mit dem therapeutischen Ergebnis eng verbunden (Tab. 1). Das hohe Qualitätsniveau hat in den letzten Jahren wahrscheinlich maßgeblich dazu beigetragen, die Überlebenszeiten anzuheben (Kortmann et al., 1999). So konnte in der HIT '91 Studie eine 3 Jahre rückfallfreie Überlebenszeit für Kinder mit niedrigem Risikoprofil von 72% erreicht werden (Kortmann et al., 2000).

Gesamtdosen von 35 bis 36 Gy im Bereich der Neuroachse gelten als Standard. Eine Dosisreduktion auf 23,4 Gy scheint nach retrospektiven Analysen möglich zu sein, wenn keine Risikofaktoren vorliegen (Brand et al. 1987, Halberg et al. 1991). Die amerikanische Pilotstudie von Packer erreichte für das Patientenkollektiv mit Standard Risiko ein 5-Jahre rückfallfreies Überleben von 79%. Die Ergebnisse wurden jedoch bei einem hochselektionierten Patientenkollektiv erzielt. In den größeren, multizentrischen Studie der CCSG- und SIOP (SIOP II-Studie) war jedoch eine Dosisreduktion mit einer erhöhten Rückfallrate und einer reduzierten Überlebenszeit verbunden (Bailey et al. 1995, Thomas et al., 2000). Die randomisierte Studie der CCSG (36 versus 23,4 Gy) zeigte eine unver-

Tab. 1: Der Einfluß der Qualität der Bestrahlung beim Medulloblastom auf das therapeutische Ergebnis

Autor/ Studie	**Pat.**	**»niedrige Qualität«**	**»hohe Qualität«**	**Überleben**	**Signifikanzen**
Packer et al., 1991	108	RT 1975–82 n = 67	RT 1983–89 n = 41	5 Jahre ÜL 49% vs.82% 5-J-PFÜ	Signifikant P = 0.004
Graben-bauer et al., 1996	40	RT vor 1980	RT nach 1980	5 Jahre ÜL 64% versus 80%	Signifikant p = 0.02
Miralbell, et al.1997	77	36 inadäquate Helmfelder	41 adäquate Helmfelder	5 Jahre progr.-freies ÜL 94% versus 72%	Signifikant p = 0.016
Carrie et al., 1999	169	Ger. Abw.: 67 (40%) Grß Abw.: 53 (31%), Hiervon : 36 eine grß Abw. 11 zwei grß Abw. 6 drei grß Abw.	49 (29%)	3 J. Rückfallrate 33% : alle Patienten 23% : korr. Therapie 17% : eine grß Abw. 67% : zwei grß Abw. 78% : drei grß Abw.	Signifikant. p = 0.04
Packer et al., 1999	63	Abweichungen 20	Keine Abweich. 43	5 Jahre progr.-freies ÜL 81% vs. 70%	Nicht signif. p = 0.42

CSA : kraniospinale Achse, RT : Radiotherapie, ÜL : Überleben, PFÜ : progressionsfreies Überleben, Ger. Abw. . geringe Abweichungen, Grß. Abw. . Große Abweichungen

tretbar hohe Rezidivrate außerhalb der hinteren Schädelgrube die zum frühzeitigen Abbruch der Studie führte (Thomas et al., 2000). Hyperfraktionierte Bestrahlungskonzepte unter Einschluss lokaler Dosiseskalationen scheinen ausschlaggebend für eine weitere Anhebung der Überlebenszeiten zu sein (Allen et al., 1996 Prados et al., 1993, 1999). Dieses innovative Konzept wird in der aktuellen Studie HIT 2000 innerhalb eines Phase III Protokolles prospektiv untersucht.

Chemotherapie

In den bisherigen, publizierten Phase-III-Studien profitierten nur Kinder mit einem hohen Rezidivrisiko, d.h. mit fortgeschrittenem Tumorstadium (T3/4), mit initialer Metastasierung, nach einer unvollständigen Resektion des Tumors und mit einem niedrigem Alter von einer zusätzlichen Chemotherapie (Tait et al., 1990, Bailey et al. 1995, Evans et al. 1990, Krischer et al. 1991, Tarbell et al. 1991) (Tab. 2).

Mit der Kombination Cisplatin, CCNU und Vincristin wurde bei Kindern mit »high risk« Medulloblastom ein progressionsfreies Überleben von 85% nach 5 und 9 Jahren erzielt (Packer et al. 1994). Für »standard risk« Kindern ist die Stellung der zusätzlichen Chemotherapie jedoch unklar. In der prospektiven Studie der CCG (9792) wurde dasselbe Protokoll für Kinder mit »standard risk« eingesetzt und zeigte eine progressionsfreie Überlebensrate nach 5 Jahren von 79%, ohne dass jedoch die Wirksamkeit im Rahmen einer Phase III - Studie bisher bewiesen wurde (Packer et al. 1999). Die korrespondierenden 3 Jahre progressionsfreien Überlebensraten lagen in der HIT '91 Studie bei 78%, wobei

Tab. 2: Medulloblastom : Effizienz einer zusätzlichen Chemotherapie/retrospektive Analyse (Y), randomisierte Studien (X) : Alleinige Strahlentherapie versus Chemotherapie in Komb. mit Strahlentherapie

Autor	Pat.-Zahl, alleinige RT	Pat.-Zahl, RT und Chx.	Überleben ohne Chx.	Überleben mit Chx.	Signifikanz
Tarbell [Y] 1991	50	39	5-J-rez.-fr. ÜL : 55,0%, keine Diff high/low risk	5-J-rez.-fr. ÜL: 72%, keine Diff high/low risk	keine
Tait [X], 1990 (SIOP I)	low risk: 56 high risk: 81	low risk: 57 high risk: 82	5-J-rez.-fr. ÜL: nicht anal. 5-J-rez.-fr. ÜL: 38%	5-J-rez.-fr. ÜL: nicht anal. 5-J-rez.-fr. ÜL: 55%	signifikant
Evans [X], 1990 (CCSG)	118	115	5-J-ereig..-fr. ÜL: 50%	5-J-ereig..-fr. ÜL: 59%	keine, jedoch Vorteil d. Chx bei high risk Pat.
Krischer et al., 1991	35	36	5 J. ereignisfrei: 57% 5 J. Gesamt-ÜL: 56,1	5 J. ereignisfrei: 68% 5 J. Gesamt- ÜL: 73,6%	P = 0.18 P = 0.07
Bailey [X], 1995 (SIOP II)	low risk: 110 high risk: 71	low risk: 114 high risk: 62	5-J-rez.-fr. ÜL: 64,7% 5-J-rez.-fr. ÜL: 51,0%	5-J-rez.-fr. ÜL: 58,9% 5-J-rez.-fr. ÜL: 53,0%	keine keine

das hohe Qualitätsniveau der Bestrahlung maßgeblich das gute Ergebnis erreichen konnte (Kortmann et al., 2000).

Supratentorieller PNET

Die stPNET sind mit ca. 2–3% aller Hirntumoren im Kindesalter sehr selten. Sie entstehen überwiegend in den Großhirnhemisphären oder der Pinealisregion (Pinealoblastom). Die Kinder sind etwas jünger und das lokale Wachstumsverhalten ist aggressiver als beim Medulloblastom. Die Therapie orientierte sich in der Regel an den Protokollen für das Medulloblastom. Dennoch lagen die Überlebensraten nach kombinierter Strahlen- und Chemotherapie um 20–30% niedriger als beim Medulloblastom (Cohen et al. 1996). Phase III Studien liegen nicht vor, so dass über den Stellenwert einer zusätzlichen Chemotherapie keine gesicherten Daten vorliegen. Lokale strahlentherapeutische Dosiseskalationen stehen offenbar im Vordergrund, um die lokale Tumorkontrolle zu verbessern. Nach den Ergebnissen einer Pilotserie von Halperin (Halperin et al. 1993) und Marymont (Marymont et al. 1996) konnte in vielen Fällen durch eine hyperfraktionierte Bestrahlung eine anhaltende, komplette Remission bei jedoch geringen Patientenzahlen erreicht werden, so dass dieses radiotherapeutische Konzept in der HIT 2000 Studie prospektiv untersucht wird.

Ependymome

Die Einführung der Strahlentherapie in die Behandlung der Ependymome konnte die Ergebnisse entscheidend verbessern (Rousseau et al. 1994). Mit einer

Tab. 3: Überlebenszeiten bei Ependymomen WHO Gr. II und III.

Autor (Zeitraum)	Patienten/ Tumorsitz	Histologie	Therapie	Überleben
Nazar et al, 1990 (1970–87)	35 k. Ang. zum Tumorsitz	Mitoti. Index I–III I: 12 Pat, II: 12 Pat., III: 11 Pat.	CSA / Tumorgebiet, keine näheren Ang., Tumordos. > 45 Gy,	5 Jahre gesamt: 44,6% I: 69,3%, II: 1,8%, III 0%
Goldwein et al., 1990 (1970–1988)	51 infratentoriell: 33 supratentoriell: 18	WHO Gr. II: 38 WHO Gr. III:13	CSA, Ganzhirn, Tumorregion 50 Gy, (0–61 Gy)	5 Jahre progr.-frei: 30%, gesamt: 46% < 45 Gy: 18% > 45 Gy: 51% 29/30 Rückfälle lokal
Grabenbauer et al., 1991 (1978–1991)	31 infratentoriell: 17 supratentoriell: 9	WHO Gr. II: 23 WHO Gr. III: 8	CSA: 13 Pat (21–57 Gy) Nur Ganzhirn: 3 Nur Tumorregion: 12 (42–72 Gy) Chx. 6 Pat.	5 Jahre progr.-frei: 42% gesamt: 54%, < 54 Gy: 50%, > 54 Gy: 58% 8/13 Rückfälle nur lokal, kein Unterschied RT lokal oder CSA
Vanyutsel, et al., 1992 (1952–88)	93 infratentoriell: 53 supratentoriell: 40	WHO Gr.I/II: 41 WHO Gr.III/IV: 49	CSA: 60 Pat. Ganzhirn/Tumor: 33 Pt. CSA: 20–35 Gy Tumor 45–55 Gy	5 Jahre progr.-frei: 41%, gesamt: 52% WHO Gr. I/II: 60%, WHOGr. III/IV:26%, p < 0,005 Kompl. Res.: 58%, Inkompl. Res.: 36% , p < 0,05
Rousseau et al., 1994 (1975–89)	80 infratentoriell: 63 supratentoriell: 13	WHO Gr. II: 54 WHO Gr. III: 18 PNET mit Ependym.: 8	Tumorregion (21,3–55,8Gy): 28 Pat. Ganzh. / CSA (30–40 Gy): 37 Pat. 33 Pat Chx.: CCNU,VCR	5 Jahre progr.-frei: 38%, gesamt: 56% Kompl. Res.: 75%, Inkompl. Res.: 41% < 50 Gy: 51%, > 50 Gy: 69%
Evans et al., 1996 (CCG 942) (1975–81)	Phase III Nur RT: 14 (A) RT + Chx.: 22 (B)	WHO Gr. II: 29 WHO Gr. III: 6 Intermed.: 1	CSA:35-40 Gy, boost 50–55 Gy CCNU, VCR, Predinson	10 Jahre progr.-frei: A: 35% ,B: 40% p: n.s. 10 Jahre gesamt: A: 29%, B: 40% p: n.s.
Needle et al., 1997	19 infratentoriell: 11 supratentoriell: 8.	WHO Gr. II: 10 WHO Gr. III: 9 10/19 inkompl. Res.	16 Pat: RT hfx 2x1,0 Gy, 65–72 Gy 14 Pat. Nur Tumorgebiet) Carbopl., VCR, Ifosf., Etop.	5 Jahre progr.-frei: 74% 5 Jahre gesamt: 79%
Timmermann et al., 2000 (HIT 88/89 und 91)	55 infratentoriell: 29 supratentoriell: 26	Nur WHO Gr. III	40 Pat. . RT Neuroachse (5 Pat. mit M1-3) 35,2 Gy / 54 Gy (Tumor) 13 Pat. RT Tumoregion Chx. Nach HIT Protokoll	3 Jahre progr.-frei Kompl. Res.: 83,3% Inkompl. Res.: 38,5% P: 0,0043 CSA: 56,3% RT Tumorregion: 92,3% P: n.s. 20 / 25 Rückfällen lokal

kompletten Resektion und Nachbestrahlung wurden progressionsfreie Überlebenszeiten zwischen 60% und 75% nach 5 Jahren und zwischen 50% und 60% nach 10 Jahren erzielt (Tab. 3).

Als wesentlicher prognostischer Faktor muss das Ausmaß der Resektion angesehen werden. In den Studien HIT '88/89 und '91 betrug das 3 Jahre progressionsfreie Überleben nach kompletter Resektion 83,3% und bei Resttumor 38,5% (Timmermann et al. 2000). Das Risiko für eine leptomeningealen Ansiedlung wird unter 15% geschätzt (Goldwein et al. 1991). So traten auch in den Studien HIT '88/89 und HIT '91 bei 25 Kindern mit Rückfall in 20 Fällen ausschließlich lokale Rezidive auf und bei weiteren 2 Kindern in Verbindung mit Metastasen. Nur drei Kinder erlitten trotz spinaler Bestrahlung eine reine Metastasierung ohne Lokalrezidiv (Timmermann et al. 2000). Nach heutigem Kenntnisstand scheint ein Verzicht auf eine Bestrahlung des gesamten Liquorraumes bei fehlender Tumoraussaat zum Zeitpunkt der Diagnose möglich zu sein.

Die hyperfraktionierte Bestrahlung mit lokaler Dosiseskalation scheint nach neueren Erfahrungen mit einer verbesserten lokalen Tumorkontrolle verbunden zu sein. In einer Phase II Studie mit 19 Kindern, von den 9 einen anaplastischen Tumor aufwiesen, wurde nach inkompletter Tumorresektion eine hyperfraktionierte Bestrahlung mit 2 x tgl. 1,0 Gy bis zu 72 Gy gefolgt von einer Chemotherapie durchgeführt (Needle et al., 1997). Es konnte ein progressionsfreies Überleben von 74% nach 5 Jahren erzielt werden. In der POG-8132-Studie mit überwiegend Grad-II-Tumoren erreichten Kinder mit inkomplett resezierten Tumoren nach vorläufigen Ergebnissen ein progressionsfreies Überleben nach 3 Jahren von ca. 70% (Kovnar et al. 1996). Im Vergleich dazu erbrachte eine konventionelle Strahlentherapie weniger als 50% (Goldwein et al., 1990, Timmermann et al., 2000). In der Studie HIT 2000 wurde die lokale Dosiseskalation mit Hyperfraktionierung als strahlentherapeutische Frage eingeführt.

Chemotherapie

Die zusätzliche Chemotherapie besitzt nach aktuellem Kenntnisstand keinen gesicherten Stellenwert. Die Erfahrungen des Royal Marsden Hospital mit adjuvanter Chemotherapie (CCNU, Vincristin), nach der die Überlebenswahrscheinlichkeit nach 10 Jahren mit 54% signifikant höher im Vergleich zu 34% nach alleiniger Bestrahlung (Bloom et al. 1990) war, konnte in der CCG-Studie nicht bestätigt werden. Die progressionsfreie Überlebensrate von 22 Kindern nach 10 Jahren betrug 35% bei einem Gesamtüberleben von 39%, ohne dass ein Unterschied im Vergleich zu 14 Kindern ohne Chemotherapie gesehen werden konnte (Evans et al. 1996). Ein Problem in der Bewertung der Chemotherapie besteht darin, dass der Anteil an anaplastischen Ependymomen in den einzelnen Studien sehr gering ist, jedoch nur bei der anaplastischen Variante ein signifikanter Effekt zu erwarten ist. In der oben erwähnten Studie von Needle wurde eine Chemotherapie nach hyperfraktionierter Bestrahlung durchgeführt. Der Stellenwert dieser zusätzlichen Behandlung ist zwar vielversprechend, bleibt aber in diesem Behandlungskonzept bisher ungeklärt.

Niedrigmalignes Astrozytom (WHO Grad I/II)

Diese Untergruppe umfasst eine Vielzahl histologischer Subtypen an unterschiedlichen anatomischen Lokalisationen und ist häufig mit der Neurofibromatose Recklinghausen verbunden (Alvord et al. 1988, Bloom et al. 1990). Die

Tab. 4: Überlebenszeiten nach Behandlung (Operation, Bestrahlung, Chemotherapie) von niedrig malignen Gliomen im Kindesalter

Autoren	Pat.	Behandlung	Überleben Progr.-frei	Überleben Gesamt	Nachbeob.-Zeit
Montgomery et al., 1997, 1962–75	16	RT 3.5 Gy–65.0 Gy	k.A.	5/10 Jahre: 80% 12/16 Pat. leben	1–14 Jahre mittel 6,3 Jahre
Horwich et al., 1985, 1951–81	29	RT: 45–50 Gy ED: 1,8–2,0 Gy	5 Jahre 100% 10 Jahre 90%	5 Jahre 100% 10 Jahre 93%	1–30 Jahre median: 10 Jahre
Wong et al., 1987 1953–84	36	RT: 24 Pat. RT bei Progr. 12 Pat.. 35–61 Gy, ED 1,5 - 2,0 Gy	10 Jahre 55%	10 Jahre 87%	7 Mon. - 33,4 Jahre mittel 9,4 Jahre
Kovalic et al., 1990 1956–1986	33	OP+RT: 22 Pat. Nur RT: 11 Pat. 37,86–61 Gy ED: 0,76–2,0 Gy	5 Jahre 85% 10 Jahre 75% 15 Jahre 75%	5 Jahre 94% 10 Jahre 81% 15 Jahre 74%	2–31 Jahre Mittel: 12,3 Jahre
Pierce et al., 1990 1971–86	24	Nur RT 45–56,6 Gy ED 1,8–2,0 Gy	6 Jahre 88%	6 Jahre 100%	24 Mon.–17 Jahre median 6 Jahre
Bataini et al., 1991 1970–1986	57	Nur RT 40–60 Gy ED 1,45–2,15 Gy	5 Jahre 89,5% 10 Jahre 82,0%	5 Jahre 83,5% 10 Jahre 83,5%	2,5–16,5 Jahre Mittel 7,5 Jahre
Jenkin et al., 1993 1958–90	87	RT (a): 38 Pat. Beob (b): 49 Pat..	A b 5 J. 80%/64% 10 J. 73%/64% 15 J. 65%/64%	a b 5 J. 94%/95% 10 J. 79%/92% 15 J. 69%/80%	K. A.
Fisher et al., 1998 1963–1995	19	RT (Makr. Tumor) Median 54 Gy ED 1,8 Gy	10 Jahre: 68%	10 Jahre: 80%	K. A.
Grabenbauer et al., 2000, 1975–1997	25	Nur RT 45–60 Gy ED 1,6–2,0 Gy	10 Jahre: 69%	10 Jahre: 94%	1,5–23,0 Jahre Mittel: 9 Jahre
Kortmann et al., 2000 / SIOP / GPOH 1992–1999	96	RT bei Progredienz 81 Pat: 54 Gy ED 1,8 Gy 15 P.: Brachyth.: 60 Gy	3 Jahre: 87,1%	3 Jahre: 95,7%	0–96 Monatc Mittel 19,4 Mon
Petronio et al., 1991 1983–89	19	Chemotherapie VCR, CCNU, Act.-D, BCNU, 5-FU u.a.	4 Jahre: 60%	100 im Nachbeob.-Zeitraum	6,6–303 Wochen median 79 Wochen
Packer et al., 1997 1989 - 93	78	Chemotherapie Carboplatin / VCR	2 Jahre: 75% 3 Jahre: 68%	97% im Nachbeob.-Zeitraum	18 Mon.–6 Jahre Median: 30 Mon.
Walker et al., 2000 / SIOP / GPOH 1992–99	132	Chemotherapie bei Progredienz Carboplatin / VCR	3 Jahre: 48,7%	3 Jahre: 88,7%	K. A.

klinische Symptomatik hängt in erster Linie von Sitz und Wachstumstendenz der Tumoren ab. Nach totaler Exzision folgt gewöhnlich keine adjuvante Nachbehandlung. Der positive Effekt der Bestrahlung auf Visus und Tumorkontrolle ist seit Jahrzehnten bekannt. Die niedrig malignen Astrozytome im Kindesalter zeigen eine deutlich günstigere Prognose gegenüber den Erwachsenen, die mit einer geringeren Neigung zur Entdifferenzierung erklärt wird (Dirks et al. 1994). Die 5 bis 10 Jahre progressionsfreien Überlebensraten liegen in den meisten retrospektiven Analysen zwischen 70 und 90% (Tab. 4). In teilweise über 90% der Fälle erreicht die Bestrahlung eine Kontrolle der Visusfunktion (Tab. 5). Es besteht derzeit Konsensus, dass bei Kindern eine postoperative Strahlenbehandlung indiziert ist, wenn eine Tumorprogression im CT/MRT erkennbar ist oder klinisch neurologische Symptome zunehmen bzw. der Visusverlust droht (Listernick et al. 1997).

In der prospektiven internationalen kooperativen Studie (SIOP Low Grade Glioma) wurde bei Kindern ab dem 5. Lebensjahr mit progredientem Tumorwachstum eine Strahlentherapie der erweiterten Tumorregion bis 54 Gy Zielvolumendosis durchgeführt. Nach einer Interimanalyse bei 96 Patienten konnte eine Ansprechrate von 93,3% erreicht werden. Die progressionsfreien und Gesamtüberlebensraten lagen bei 87,1% bzw 95,7% bei einem Nachbeobachtungszeitraum von median 19,4 Monaten, so dass die Bestrahlung innerhalb dieses Behandlungsansatzes als effektiv gelten muß (Kortmann et al. 2000).

Tab. 5: Visus nach Bestrahlung von niedrig malignen Gliomen der Mittellinie (Gliome der Sehbahn) im Kindesalter

Autor	Patienten	Gesamtdosis (GD) Einzeldosis (ED)	Besser	Stabil	Schlechter
Horwich et al., 1985	23	GD 45–50 Gy ED 1,8–2,0 Gy	Sehschärfe (23) 10 (43%) Gesichtsfeld (23) 4 (18%)	 11 (48%) 19 (82%)	 2 (9%) /
Flickinger et al., 1988	22	GD 38–56,86 Gy ED 1,4–2,0 Gy	2 (9%)	14 (77%)	3 (14%)
Wong et al., 1987	17	GD 35–61 Gy ED 1,5–2,0 Gy	6 (35%)	9 (53%)	2 (12%)
Pierce et al., 1990	23	GD 45–56,6 Gy ED 1,8–2,0 Gy	23 (30%)	14 (61%)	2 (9%)
Bataini et al., 1991	44	GD 40–60 Gy ED 1,45–2,15 Gy	Sehschärfe 25 (57%) Gesichtsfeld 19 (61%)	 16 (36%) 11 (35%)	 3 (7%) 1 (3%)
Erkal et al., 1997	13	GD 40–60 Gy ED 1,8–2,0 Gy	9 (34%)	14 (54%)	3 (12%)
Grabenbauer et al., 2000	25	GD 45–60 Gy ED	Sehschärfe (25) 9 (36%) Gesichtsfeld (20) 3 (15%)	 13 (52%) 16 (80%)	 3 (12%) 1 (5%)

Chemotherapie

Zur Reduktion therapieinduzierter Spätfolgen, wurde in Phase II-Studien das Ansprechen niedrigmaligner Gliome auf Zytostatika untersucht (Janss et al. 1995, Packer et al. 1997, Petronio et al. 1991). In einer retrospektiven Analyse an 32 Kindern, die unterhalb des 5. Lebensjahres eine initiale Chemotherapie mit Vincristin und Actinomycin D erhielten, konnte bei 17 Kindern die Bestrahlung im Mittel um 40 Monate hinausgezogert werden (Janss et al. 1995). Bei Kindern unter 5 Jahren konnte ein Protokoll bestehend aus Carboplatin und Vincristin eine 5 Jahre progressionsfreie Überlebensrate von 74% erreichen (Packer et al. 1997). Derzeit wird in der o.g. internationalen Studie der SIOP die Effektivität dieser Chemotherapie untersucht. Vorläufige Ergebnisse bei 132 Patienten konnten die amerikanischen Ergebnisse nicht bestätigen, die 3 Jahre progressionsfreien Überlebensrate lag nur bei 48,7% bei einem Gesamtüberleben von 88,7% (Walker et al., 2000). Die mittlere Verzögerung bis zum Beginn der Strahlentherapie lag bei 21 Monaten. Die anschließende, in ihrer Effizienz bewiesene Bestrahlung konnte in der Mehrheit ein erneutes Ansprechen erreichen mit einem progressionsfreien Überleben von 91,3% bzw. einem Gesamtüberleben von 100% bei 23 Patienten (Kortmann et al. 2000). Der Einsatz der Chemotherapie muss daher sehr kritisch gesehen werden. Die in ihrer Effizienz unbewiesene Chemotherapie verursacht potentiell ein höheres Risiko für irreversible neurologische Schäden, vor allem Blindheit, zumal in den bisherigen Studien der Einfluss auf die Visusfunktion nicht systematisch untersucht wurde.

Hochmalignes Astrozytom/Glioblastom (WHO Grad III/IV)

Das Therapiekonzept entspricht dem Vorgehen bei malignen Gliomen im Erwachsenenalter. Nach dem operativen Eingriff folgt die Bestrahlung der erweiterten Tumorregion mit Dosierungen zwischen 54 und 60 Gy. Unverändert gelten auch bei Kindern die Daten für Erwachsene von Walker aus dem Jahre 1978, nach denen die postoperative Strahlentherapie eine mediane Überlebenszeit von etwa 10 bis 12 Monaten erreicht. Nach der deutschen HIT 91-Studie zeigen WHO III-Gliome eine deutlich bessere Prognose. Acht von 19 Patienten mit Grad III-Tumoren überlebten 8 Jahre im Vergleich zu 1 von 12 Patienten mit Glioblastom (Kühl et al., 1998). Einen wesentlichen prognostischen Faktor stellt das Alter bei Diagnosestellung dar. Das mediane Überleben lag bei etwa einem Jahr bei Patienten über dem 8. Lebensjahr und bei fast 2 Jahren bei Patienten jünger als 8 Jahre (Kühl et al. 1998).

Chemotherapie (Tab. 6)

Die CCSG (Children Cancer Study Group) untersuchte innerhalb zweier randomisierten Studien den Stellenwert einer zusätzlichen Chemotherapie (Finlay et al. 1995, Sposto et al. 1989). Bei Grad 3 und Grad 4 Tumoren wurde eine Verbesserung des 5-Jahre ereignisfreien Überleben von 18% ohne Chemotherapie auf 46% mit CCNU, Vincristin und Prednison erreicht (Sposto et al. 1989). In der Folgestudie fiel das Ergebnis deutlich schlechter aus mit einem 3-

Tab. 6: Neuere klinische Studien zur Untersuchung der Wirksamkeit einer zusätzlichen Systemtherapie bei hochmalignen Gliomen

Autor	Pat. n	Behandlung	Histologien	Überleben
Sposto et al., 1989 (CCG)	58	Phase III Studie RT versus RT + CCNU, VCR, Prednison	Hochmaligne Gliome	5 Jahre ereignisfrei Nur RT: 18% RT + Chx.: 46%
Finlay et al., 1995 (CCG)	85 87	Phase III - Studie RT anschl. CCNU VCR Pred »8 in 1« anschl. RT	Hochmaligne Gliome	5 Jahre progr.-frei: 33%, Gesamt: 36%. Kein Unterschied zwischen Th.-armen
Geyer et al., 1995	39 (< 24 Mon.)	»8 in 1«, »verzögerte« Bestrahlung	Astrocytom WHO Gr. III Glioblastom	3 Jahre progr.-frei Alle Pat.: 36% WHO Gr. III: 44% WHO Gr. IV: 0%
Finlay et al., 1996	18	Hochdosis-Chemotherapie und autologe KMT / Rezidive	Hochmaligne Gliome	16% therapiebed. Todesfälle 5 von 18 (28) leben nach 39–59 Monaten
Graham et al., 1997	12	Hochdosischemotherapie und autologe KMT (Primärtherapie und Rezidiv)	»Gliale Tumoren« 6 Primärtherapie 6 Therapie bei Rückfall	Überleben: 2 von 12
Bouffet et al., 1997	22	Etoposid, Thiotepa, autologe KMT (neu diagn., Rezidiv)	Hochmaligne Gliome	15% leben nach 54–65 Monaten
Heideman et al., 1997	41	Chemotherapie vor Bestrahlung	Astrozytom WHO Gr. III: 13 Glioblastom: 25 Oligodendrogliom III 3	3 Jahre progr.-frei: 18% 3 Jahre gesamt: 35%
Wolff et al., 2001	22	Trophosphamid/Etoposid Simultan zur Bestrahlung (54 Gy)	Glioblastom	Med. Überl.: 12 Mon. (Kontroll-Gr. ohne RT: 12 Mon.)
Wolff et al., 2002	52	HIT '91 Prot. + RT 54 Gy 22 Pat.: Erhaltungschx. 30 Pat.: »Sandwich«-Chx.	Astrozytom WHO Gr. III: 25 Glioblastom: 27	Med. ÜL Kompl. Res: 5,2 Jahre Inkompl. Res. 1,2 Jahre P < 0,0005

KMT: Knochenmarktransplantation, CCG: Childrens Cancer Group

Jahre progressionsfreien Überleben bei anaplastischen Astrozytomen von 29% und bei Glioblastomen von 20% und liegt damit in Bereichen, der auch durch eine alleinige Bestrahlung erreicht wird (Finlay et al., 1995). Aktuellere Protokolle mit Stammzell- oder Knochemarktransplantation sind zum Teil sehr toxisch und haben keinen Durchbruch erzielt.

Nach der deutschen HIT-Studie '88/89 erreichten 57% der Patienten mit WHO Grad III Gliomen die 3-Jahresgrenze, jedoch keiner mit Glioblastom (Kühl et al. 1998). In der Folgestudie HIT '91 erreichte jedoch eine Chemotherapie vor Bestrahlung bei Kindern mit komplett resezierten Tumoren ein deutlich besseres Ergebnis. 11 von 15 Kindern blieben nach 5 Jahren rezidivfrei, hierunter jedoch etliche Kinder mit WHO Grad III Tumoren (Wolff et al., 2002). Die GPOH verfolgt eine Strategie mit sequentiellen Phase II Protokollen (HIT-GBM). Hierbei wurde Trophosphamid sowie eine Immuntherapie nach Strahlentherapie untersucht (HIT-GBM-A) bzw. ein radio-/chemotherapeutischer Behandlungsansatz mit Cisplatin, Ifosfamid und Etoposid (HIT-GBM-B). Nach aktueller Auswertung lag die mediane Überlebenszeit für 20 Patienten jedoch nur bei 12 Monaten und unterschied sich nicht von historischen Kontrollgruppen nach alleiniger postoperativer Bestrahlung (HIT – GBM A) (Wolff et al., 2001). In der aktuellen HIT-GBM C Studie wird der radiochemotherapeutische Ansatz fortgesetzt und durch eine nachfolgende Chemotherapie ergänzt.

Hirnstamm-Gliom

Die Behandlung der Wahl stellt die Strahlentherapie dar. Bei konventioneller Fraktionierung resultiert eine 5-Jahres-Überlebenszeit von 0–45% (Albright et al. 1986, Freeman et al. 1988, Freeman et al. 1986, Halperin et al. 1989). Die Prognose von Patienten mit Tumoren im Bereich des Mittelhirns und des Thalamus ist mit einer 5-Jahres-Überlebensrate zwischen 67 und 73% deutlich besser. Vor dem Hintergrund eines rasch proliferierenden Tumorgewebes wurden zu Beginn der 80er Jahre von der POG (Pediatric Oncology Group) und CCG (Childrens Cancer Group) Hyperfraktionierungsschemata in eskalierenden Dosierungen untersucht (Tab. 7). Eine Besserung der klinischen Symptome war unabhängig vom Dosiskonzept festzustellen und lag zwischen 71% und 80%. Allerdings stieg das Risiko für radiotherapieinduzierte Nekrosen im Tumorgebiet und die Notwendigkeit einer Steroideinnahme in den hohen Dosisleveln an. Die intensiven Bemühungen auch unter Einsatz einer zusätzliche Chemotherapie, die Überlebenszeiten zu verbessern, waren enttäuschend. Die medianen Überlebenszeiten lagen bei ca. 9 bis 11 Monaten. Diese negativen Erfahrungen konnten in der HIT-GBM A Studie bei 20 Kindern bestätigt werden. Die mediane Überlebenszeit lag bei 8 Monaten (Wolff et al., 1996). Neuere Ansätze mit Temozolomide, Thiotepa, Topotecan oder Antiöstrogenen waren ebenfalls enttäuschend, so dass innovative, experimentelle Therapieansätze gefordert sind (Heideman et al. 1993, Blaney et al. 1996, Estlin et al. 1998, Broniscer et al. 2000). Hirnstammgliome werden derzeit innerhalb des HIT GBM Konzeptes prospektiv untersucht.

Als Standard gilt die alleinige Bestrahlung der Tumorregion mit einem Sicherheitssaum. Die konventionelle Fraktionierung bis 54 Gy bei einer Fraktionierung von 1,8–2,0 Gy gilt weltweit als Standard.

Intrakranielle Keimzelltumoren

Überwiegend sind die Tumoren mittelliniennah in der Pinealisregion, seltener »ektopisch« supraselIär oder im dritten Ventrikel lokalisiert und können sich subependymal entlang der Seitenventrikel nach ventral sowie in Richtung des 4. Ventrikels ausbreiten. Überwiegend finden sich reine Germinome die histogenetisch den germinalen Tumoren von Hoden und Ovar entsprechen. Seltener kommen Cho-rio- und embryonale Karzinome oder Dottersack-

Tab. 7: Phase I/II und III-Studien zur hyperfraktionierten Strahlentherapie von Hirnstammgliome, teilweise in Kombination mit simultaner, zusätzlicher Chemotherapie

Autor	Patienten	Dosiskonzept	Überleben
Freeman et al., 1988 (POG)	38	2 x 1,1 Gy, 66,0 Gy	Pogressionsfrei / median: 6,5 Monate Gesamt / median: 11 Monate
Freeman et al., 1991 (POG)	57	2 x 1,17 Gy, 70,2 Gy	Pogressionsfrei / median: 6 Monate Gesamt / median: 10 Monate Steroidpflicht > 3 Mon: 9%
Freeman et al., 1993 (POG)	41	2 x 1,26 Gy, 75,6 Gy	Pogressionsfrei / median: 7 Monate Gesamt / median: 10 Monate Steroidpflicht > 3 Mon: 61%
Packer et al., 1987 (CCG)	16	2 x 1,2 Gy, 64,8 Gy	Pogressionsfrei / median: 7 Monate Gesamt / median: 9 Monate
Packer et al., 1993 (CCG)	53	2 x 1,0 Gy, 72,0 Gy	Gesamt 1 Jahr 38% 2 Jahre 14%. 3 Jahre 8%
Packer et al., 1994 (CCG)	66	2 x 1,16 Gy, 78,0 Gy	Gesamt 1 Jahr 35% 2 Jahre k.a. 3 Jahre 6% Steroidpflicht: 50%
Shrieve et al., 1992	41	2 x 1,0 Gy, 66–78 Gy	Gesamt / median: 72 Wochen Keine Dosisabhängigkeit
Lewis et al., 1997	28	Hyperfraktioniert – akzeleriert 2 x 1,8 Gy 48,6 / 50,4 Gy	Gesamt / median: 8,5 Monate
Kretschmar et al., 1993	35	2 x 1,1 Gy, 66,0 Gy Vor RT 4 Kurse Cisplatin/ Cyclophophamid	Kompl. Remission: 0 Part. Remission 3 (8,6%) »stable disease«: 23 (65,7%) Progredienz: 9 (25,7%) Medianes Überleben: 8 Monate
Packer et al., 1996 (CCG)	32	2 x 1,16 Gy, 72,0 Gy + beta Interferon	Pogressionsfrei / median: 5 Monate Gesamt / median: 9 Monate
Walter et al., 1998	9	2 x 1,17 Gy, 70,2 Gy + simultan Carboplatin	8 von 9 Pat. nach median 44 Wochen verstorben
Mandell et al., 1999 POG Phase III	66 64	1x 1,8 Gy / 54 Gy (I) 2 x 1,17 Gy, 70,2 Gy (II) + simultan Cisplatin (I + II)	I Pogressionsfrei / median: 6 Monate Gesamt / median: 9 Monate II Pogressionsfrei / median: 5 Monate Gesamt / median: 8 Monate
Allen et al., 1999	34	2 x 1,0 Gy, 72,0 Gy + simultan Carboplatin	Pogressionsfrei / median: 8 Monate Gesamt / median: 12 Monate

POG: Pediatric Oncology Group, CCG: Childrens Cancer Group, ZVD Zielvolumendosis

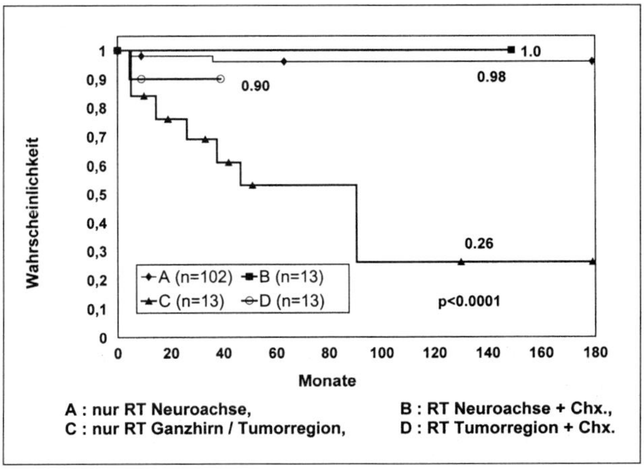

Abb. 1: Rückfallfreie Überlebenszeiten in Abhängigkeit vom Therapiekonzept bei reinen intrakraniellen Germinomen. Ergebnisse der MAKEI/SIOP-Studien (Kortmann et al, 2001)

Tumoren (Yolk sac) vor, die ebenso wie die Germinome in ihrer reinen Form oder kombiniert als gemischte Keimzelltumoren auftreten können (Bjornsson et al. 1985).

Wesentlicher Bestandteil der Diagnose zur Differenzierung intrakranieller Keimzelltumoren ist der Nachweis von Tumormarkern in Serum und Liquor (β-HCG, AFP). Hiernach wird in sogenannte sezernierende bzw. nicht sezernierende Keimzelltumoren unterschieden. Besonders wichtig ist die Bestimmung der Tumormarker, da bei positivem Markernachweis die Behandlung mit einer Chemotherapie begonnen wird.

Das Therapiekonzept bei intrakraniellen Keimzelltumoren orientiert sich an den langjährigen günstigen Ergebnissen der interdisziplinären Deutschen MAKEI-Studie der Gesellschaft für Pädriatische Onkologie und Hämatologie zusammen mit der APRO.

Germinome

Therapiestandard ist die alleinige Bestrahlung der Neuroachse. Hierdurch kann eine Tumorkontrolle innerhalb des ZNS in nahezu 100% der Fälle erreicht werden (Tab. 8, Abb. 1). Einschränkungen der Zielvolumina sind mit einem erhöhten Rückfallrisiko verbunden (Bamberg et al., 1999, Kortmann et al., 2001). Die schrittweise Dosisreduktion in den MAKEI/SIOP Protokollen wurde nicht von Einbußen begleitet, so dass heute eine Gesamtdosis von 30 bzw. 45 Gy als Standard gilt. Eine aktuelle Vorauswertung der SIOP CNS GCT Studie zeigt, dass 24 bzw. 40 Gy ebenfalls auszureichen scheinen (Kortmann et al., 2001).

Andere Arbeitsgruppen empfehlen eine kombinierte Behandlung bestehend aus einer intensiven Chemotherapie gefolgt von einer lokal erweiterten Bestrahlung (Bouffet et al. 1999) (Tab. 8). Die bisherigen Daten bei einer kombinierten Chemo- und Strahlentherapie der erweiterten Tumorregion sind jedoch widersprüchlich (Bouffet et al. 1999, Cefalo et al. 1995). Die Rate von Feldrandrezidiven betrug in der Untersuchungsserie der italienischen Arbeitsgruppe 71% (Bouffet et al. 1999). In prospektiven Studie der SFOP (Societe francaise

Tab. 8: Überlebensraten nach alleiniger Bestrahlung, kombinierter Chemo/Radiotherapie und alleiniger Chemotherapie bei Behandlung reiner Germinome

Autor	Patienten	Therapie nach Biopsie/Resektion	Ergebnis (RFS)(5 Jahre)	
Shibamoto et al., 1988	24	RT nur Tumor	87%	
	40	RT CSA	91%	
	9	RT Ganzhirn	78%	
	8	RT Spinal +Ventrikel	88%	
Allen et al., 1987	11	Chx + RT CSA	91%	
Wolden et al., 1995	24	Ventrikel/Ganzhirn /Tumor Gy	95%	
Bamberg et al., 1999	11	RT CSA 36 Gy+Tu 14 Gy	100%	
	49	RT CSA 30 Gy+Tu 15 Gy	88,8%	
Bouffet et al., 1999	44	Chx. + RT Tumor	98% (3Jahre)	
Balmaceda et al., 1996	45	Nur Chx.	50%	
Haddock et al., 1997	48	12 RT CSA/Tumor	**5-Jahre**	**10-Jahre**
		11 RT Ganzhirn/Tumor	94%	94%
		24 RT Ventrikel	94%	94%
			29%	0%
Kitamura et al., 1999	13	Chx. / RT Tumor: 24 Gy	100%	
Aoyama et al., 1998	41	a) 23 RT CSA/Tumor	**10-Jahre**	
		b) 10 RT Ganzhirn/Tumor	a) 90%	
		c) 8 RT Tumor	b) 76%	
			c) 22%	
Hardenbergh et al., 1997	40	30 RT CSA/Tumor	100%	
		10 RT Ganzhirn/Tumor	100%	
Cefalo et al., 1995	7	Chx. / RT Tumorregion	5 Rückfälle (Ventrikelsystem)	
Kortmann et al., 2001	155	a) 102 RT CSA	a) 99,5% (ZNS)	
		b) 53 RT Ganzhirn + Chx,	b) 71,7% (ZNS)	
		CSI + Chx, RT Tumor + Chx		
		nur Op. (Chx)		

CSA: craniospinale Achse, Chx.: Chemotherapie, RT: Radiotherapie

d'oncologie pediatrique) lagen in 7% der Fälle Rezidive außerhalb der primären Tumorregion und intrakraniell vor (Cefalo et al. 1995).

Die alleinige, intensive Chemotherapie ist mit einer zu hohen Rückfallrate (22 von 42 Patienten zeigten ein Rezidiv) und mit einer unvertretbaren Akuttoxizität verbunden (4 therapiebedingte Todesfälle) (Balmaceda et al. 1996).

Nichtseminomatöse Keimzelltumoren (»Sezernierende Keimzelltumore«)

Sezernierende Keimzelltumoren werden primär einer Chemotherapie zugeführt gefolgt von einer möglichen Operation zur Entfernung des Resttumors, der meist nur noch nekrotisches oder teratomatöses Gewebe enthält. Anschließend folgt die Strahlentherapie. Die 2-Jahres-Überlebensraten (krankheitsfrei) konnten durch kombinierte Behandlung (Chemotherapie/Strahlenbehandlung des Liquorraumes) von nur 6% (Operation/Strahlenbehandlung) auf über 80% gesteigert werden (Calaminus et al. 1994, 1997) (Tab. 9).

Tab. 9: Überlebensraten nach Behandlung nicht seminomatöser Keimzelltumoren

Autor	Therapie nach Biopsie/Resektion	Patienten	5 Jahre rückfallfr. Überleben
Allen et al., 1987	Vinblastin, Bleomycin, Cyclophosphamid, Cisplatin CSA: 35 Gy + Tu 20 Gy	4	50%
Itoyama et al., 1990	Cisplatin, Etoposid, Vinblastin 50–55Gy Ganzhirn CSA: 25 Gy	4	50%
Balmaceda et al., 1996	Carboplatin, Bleomycin, Etoposid	26	50%
Calaminus et al., 1997	Cisplatin, Etoposid, Ifosfamid (4 Kurse) CSA 30 Gy + Tu 24 Gy	19	81%
Robertson et al., 1997	Cisplatin/Etoposid + RT CSA bzw. Ganzhirn, bzw. Tumorgebiet 50,4–55,8 Gy	18	67% (4 Jahre)
Calaminus et al., 1998	Cisplatin, Etoposid, Bleomycin Ifosfamid, Vinblastin CSA 30 Gy + Tu 20 Gy	27	58%
Baranzelli et al., 1998	Vinblastin, Bleomycin, Carbo Etoposid, Ifosfamid	18	33%

Auch hier wird gegenwärtig in ausländischen Arbeitsgruppen bei sezernierenden Keimzelltumoren nach kompletter Resektion und fehlender Liquoraussaat eine lokal erweiterte Bestrahlung in Kombination mit einer Chemotherapie überprüft (Flamant et al. 1990). Die alleinige Chemotherapie ist zwar hocheffektiv hinsichtlich der Ansprechraten, jedoch gleichzeitig mit einem hohen Rückfallrisikoverbunden (Balmaceda et al. 1996). In dem o.g. das SIOP-CNS-GCT 96 Protokoll wird derzeit bei sezernierenden Keimzelltumoren mit fehlender leptomeningealer Metastasierung eine Chemotherapie mit 4 Kursen PEI gefolgt von einer Bestrahlung der Tumorregion untersucht. Bei nachgewiesener Metastasierung innerhalb des ZNS erfolgt eine Bestrahlung des gesamten Liquorraumes.

Zusammenfassung

Operation gefolgt von Bestrahlung stellt unverändert die Standardtherapie bei Hirntumoren im Kindesalter dar. Die zusätzliche Chemotherapie konnte bei den strahlensensiblen Medulloblastomen im Rahmen von Phase III-Studien nur bei metastatischer Erkrankung einen gesicherten Überlebensvorteil zeigen. Die derzeit von der pädiatrischen Onkologie favorisierte zusätzliche Erhaltungschemotherapie bei niedrigen Risikofaktoren wird zwar als Standard angesehen, der mögliche Vorteil wurde jedoch nie innerhalb einer randomisierten Phase III-Studie überprüft. Die ausgezeichnete 5-Jahre-Überlebensrate von 79% wird jedoch offenbar maßgeblich durch die Fortschritte bei strahlentherapeutischen

Techniken und durch verbesserte neurochirurgische Vorgehensweisen erreicht. Beim Ependymom steht die lokale Tumorkontrolle im Vordergrund. Zusätzliche Chemotherapien konnten in der Phase III-Studie der CCG keinen gesicherten Vorteil zeigen. Auch in übrigen Phase II-Protokollen ist der Stellenwert umstritten. Im Vordergrund stehen Maßnahmen zur Verbesserung der lokalen Tumorkontrolle mittels strahlentherapeutischer Verfahren (Hyperfraktionierungen), die aktuell in prospektiven Studien weltweit untersucht werden. Bei der Behandlung niedrigmaligner Gliome im Kindesalter steht die Kontrolle neurologischer Funktionen im Vordergrund. Der Therapiestandard besteht aus einer Operation gefolgt von einer Bestrahlung bei progredienter Erkrankung. Die Bestrahlung von Gliomen der Sehbahn erreicht in einem hohen Maße eine Verbesserung bzw. Stabilisierung der Visusfunktion. Die Rolle der Chemotherapie innerhalb des Gesamtbehandlungskonzeptes unterliegt aktuell prospektiven Studien. Unbekannt ist bisher der Einfluss auf neurologische Funktionen, so dass ein Einsatz außerhalb kontrollierter Studien derzeit nicht vertretbar ist. Auch bei den hochmalignen Gliomen und Hirnstammgliomen stehen Operation und Bestrahlung im Vordergrund. Die zusätzliche Chemotherapie konnte keinen Durchbruch erreichen. Vergleichende Protokolle mit beschränkten Patientenzahlen zeigten keinen gesicherten Überlebensvorteil, wobei die Interpretation der Resultate häufig durch unterschiedliche Anteile von WHO Grad III- und IV-Tumoren erschwert wird. Die seltenen intrakraniellen Keimzelltumoren werden vorwiegend von den strahlensensiblen Germinomen gestellt. Die alleinige Bestrahlung mit reduzierten Dosiskonzepten erreicht eine nahezu 100%ige Heilungsrate. Einschränkungen der Zielvolumina kombiniert mit einer Chemotherapie sind mit einem erhöhten Rückfallrisiko verbunden. Alleinige chemotherapeutische Protokolle sind bei Rückfallraten von bis zu 50% unvertretbar, so dass insgesamt die zusätzliche Chemotherapie bzw. alleinige Chemotherapie keinen gesicherten Stellenwert besitzt. Lediglich bei den nicht seminomatösen Keimzelltumoren konnte die zusätzliche Chemotherapie eine durchgreifende Verbesserung der Prognose von 6% langfristigem Überleben nach alleiniger Bestrahlung gegenüber 86% nach kombinierter Therapie erzielen.

Literatur

1. Albright AL, Gutkehlch AN, Packer RJ, Price RA, Rourke LB: Prognostic factors in pediatric brain stem gliomas. J. Neurosurg. 65 (1986) 751–755
2. Allen J, Siffert J, Donahue B, Nirenberg A, Jakacki R, Robertson P, DaRosso R, Thoron L, Rosovsky M, Pinto R: A phase I/II study of carboplatin combined with hyperfractionated radiotherapy for brainstem gliomas. Cancer 86 (1999) 1064–1069
3. Allen JC, Donahue B, DaRosso R, Nierenberg A: Hyperfractionated craniospinal radiotherapy and adjuvant chemotherapy for children with newly diagnosed medulloblastoma and other primitive neuroectodermal tumors. Int. J. Radiat. Oncol. Biol. Phys. 30 (1996) 1155–1161
4. Allen JC, Kim JH, Packer RJ: Neoadjuvant chemotherapy for newly diagnosed germ-cell tumors of the central nervous system. J. Neurosurg. 67(1), (1987 Jul) 65–70
5. Alvord EC, Jr., Lofton S: Gliomas of the optic nerve or chiasm. Outcome by patients' age, tumor site, and treatment. J. Neurosurg. 68 (1988) 85–98

6. Aoyama H, Shirato H, Kakuto Y, Inakoshi H, Nishio M, Yoshida H, Hareyama M, Yanagisawa T, Watarai J, Miyasaka K: Pathologically-proven intracranial germinoma treated with radiation therapy. Radiother-Oncol. 47(2), (1998 May) 201–205
7. Bailey CC, Gnekow A, Wellek S, Jones M, Round C, Brown J, Phillips A, Neidhardt MK: Prospective randomised trial of chemotherapy given before radiotherapy in childhood medulloblastoma. International Society of Pediatric Oncology (SIOP) and the (German) Society of Pediatric Oncology (GPO): SIOP II. Med. Ped. Oncol. 25 (1995) 166–178
8. Balmaceda C, Heller G, Rosenblum M, Diez B, Villablanca JG, Kellie S, Maher P, Vlamis V, Walker RW, Leibel S, Finlay JL: Chemotherapy without irradiation – a novel approach for newly diagnosed CNS germ cell tumors: results of an international cooperative trial. The First International Central Nervous System Germ Cell Tumor Study. J. Clin. Oncol. 14 (1996) 2908–2915
9. Bamberg M, Kortmann RD, Calaminus G, Becker G, Meisner C, Harms D, Gobel U: Radiation therapy for intracranial germinoma: results of the German cooperative prospective trials MAKEI 83/86/89. J. Clin. Oncol. 17 (1999) 2585–2592
10. Bamberg M, Schmitt G, Quast U: Therapie und Prognose des Medulloblastoms, Fortschritte durch neuartige Bestrahlungstechniken. Strahlentherapie 156 (1980) 1–17
11. Baranzelli MC, Patte C, Bouffet E, Portas M, Mechinaud-Lacroix F, Sariban E, Roche H, Kalifa C: An attempt to treat pediatric intracranial alphaFP and betaHCG secreting germ cell tumors with chemotherapy alone. SFOP experience with 18 cases. Societe Francaise d'Oncologie Pediatrique. J. Neurooncol. 37(3), (1998 May) 229–239
12. Bataini JP, Delanian S, Ponvert D: Chiasmal gliomas: results of irradiation management in 57 patients and review of literature. Int. J. Radiat. Oncol. Biol. Phys. 21 (1991) 615–623
13. Berry MP, Jenkin RD, Keen CW, Nair BD, Simpson WJ: Radiation treatment for medulloblastoma. A 21-year review. J. Neurosurg. 55 (1981) 43–51
14. Bjornsson J, Scheithauer BW, Okazaki H, Leech RW: Intracranial germ cell tumors: pathobiological and immunohistochemical aspects of 70 cases. J. Neuropathol. Exp. Neurol. 44 (1985) 32–46
15. Blaney SM, Phillips PC, Packer RJ, Heideman RL, Berg SL, Adamson PC, Allen JC, Sallan SE, Jakacki RI, Lange BJ, Reaman GH, Horowitz ME, Poplack DG, Balis FM: Phase II evaluation of topotecan for pediatric central nervous system tumors. Cancer 78 (1996) 527–531
16. Bloom HJ, Glees J, Bell J, Ashley SE, Gorman C: The treatment and long-term prognosis of children with intracranial tumors: a study of 610 cases, 1950–1981 (published erratum appears in Int J. Radiat. Oncol. Biol. Phys. 1990 Sep;19(3): 829). Int. J. Radiat. Oncol. Biol. Phys. 18 (1990) 723–745
17. Bouffet E, Baranzelli MC, Patte C, Portas M, Edan C, Chastagner P, Mechinaud Lacroix F, Kalifa C: Combined treatment modality for intracranial germinomas: results of a multicentre SFOP experience. Societe Francaise d'Oncologie Pediatrique. Br. J. Cancer 79 (1999) 1199–1204
18. Bouffet E, Mottolese C, Jouvet A, Philip I, Frappaz D, Carrie C, Brunat Mentigny M: Etoposide and thiotepa followed by ABMT (autologous bone marrow transplantation) in children and young adults with high-grade gliomas. Eur. J. Cancer 33 (1997) 91–95
19. Brand WN, Schneider PA, Tokars RP: Long-term results of a pilot study of low dose cranial-spinal irradiation for cerebellar medulloblastoma. Int. J. Radiat. Oncol. Biol. Phys. 13 (1987) 1641–1645
20. Broniscer A, Leite CC, Lanchote VL, Machado TM, Cristofani LM: Radiation therapy and high-dose tamoxifen in the treatment of patients with diffuse brainstem gliomas: results of a Brazilian cooperative study. Brainstem Glioma Cooperative Group. J. Clin. Oncol. 18 (2000) 1246–1253
21. Calaminus G, Andreussi L, Garre ML, Kortmann RD, Schober R, Gobel U: Secreting germ cell tumors of the central nervous system (CNS). First results of the cooperative German/Italian pilot study (CNS sGCT). Klein. Padiatr. 209 (1997) 222–227
22. Calaminus G, Bamberg M, Baranzelli MC, Benoit Y, di Montezemolo LC, Fossati Bellani F, Jurgens H, Kuhl HJ, Lenard HG, Curto ML: Intracranial germ cell tumors: a comprehensive update of the European data. Neuropediatrics 25 (1994) 26–32

23. Calaminus G, Garre ML, Kortmann RD, Mann JR, Göbel U: CNS germcell tumors in children. Results of the German MAKEI '89 protocols and SOIP CNS GCT 93P/96 study. Germ Cell Tumors IV eds.: Jones WG, Appleyard I, Harnden P, Joffe JK, John Libbey & Co Ltd., (1998) 247–254
24. Carrie C, Hoffstetter S, Gomez F, Moncho V, Doz F, Alapetite C, Murraciole X, Maire JP, Benhassel M, Chapet S, Quetin P, Kolodie H, Lagrange JL, Cuillere JC, Habrand JL: Impact of targeting deviations on outcome in medulloblastoma: study of the French Society of Pediatric Oncology (SFOP). Int. J. Radiat. Oncol. Biol. Phys. 45 (1999) 435–439
25. Cefalo G, Gianni MC, Lombardi F, Balzarini L, Fossati-Bellani F: Intracranial germinoma: does a cisplatinum-based chemotherapeutic regimen permit to avoid whole CNS irradiation. Med. Ped. Oncol. 25 (1995) 303
26. Cohen BH, Packer RJ: Chemotherapy for medulloblastomas and primitive neuroectodermal tumors. J. Neurooncol. 29 (1996) 55–68
27. Dirks PB, Jay V, Becker LE, Drake JM, Humphreys RP, Hoffman HJ, Rutka JT: Development of anaplastic changes in low-grade astrocytomas of childhood. Neurosurgery 34 (1994) 68–78
28. Erkal HS, Serin M, Cakmak A: Management of optic pathway and chiasmatic-hypothalamic gliomas in children with radiation therapy. Radiother. Oncol. 45 (1997) 11–15
29. Estlin EJ, Lashford L, Ablett S, Price L, Gowing R, Gholkar A, Kohler J, Lewis IJ, Morland B, Pinkerton CR, Stevens MC, Mott M, Stevens R, Newell DR, Walker D, Dicks Mireaux C, McDowell H, Reidenberg P, Statkevich P, Marco A, Batra V, Dugan M, Pearson AD: Phase I study of temozolomide in paediatric patients with advanced cancer. United Kingdom Children's Cancer Study Group. Br. J. Cancer 78 (1998) 652–661
30. Evans AE, Anderson JR, Lefkowitz Boudreaux IB, Finlay JL: Adjuvant chemotherapy of childhood posterior fossa ependymoma: cranio-spinal irradiation with or without adjuvant CCNU, vincristine, and prednisone: a Childrens Cancer Group study. Med Pediatr. Oncol. 27 (1996) 8–14
31. Evans AE, Jenkin RDT, Sposto R, Ortega JA, Wilson CB, Wara W, Ertel IJ, Kramer S, Chang CH, Leikin SL, Hammond GD: The treatment of medulloblastoma: results of a prospective randomized trial of radiation therapy with and without CCNU, vincristine and prednisone. J. Neurosurg. 72 (1990) 572–582
32. Finlay JL, Boyett JM, Yates AJ, Wisoff JH, Milstein JM, Geyer JR, Bertolone SJ, McGuire P, Cherlow JM, Tefft M: Randomized phase III trial in childhood high-grade astrocytoma comparing vincristine, lomustine, and prednisone with the eight-drugs-in-1-day regimen. Childrens Cancer Group. J. Clin. Oncol. 13 (1995) 112–123.
33. Finlay JL, Goldman S, Wong MC, Cairo M, Garvin J, August C, Cohen BH, Stanley P, Zimmerman RA, Bostrom B, Geyer JR, Harris RE, Sanders J, Yates AJ, Boyett JM, Packer RJ: Pilot study of high-dose thiotepa and etoposide with autologous bone marrow rescue in children and young adults with recurrent CNS tumors. The Children's Cancer Group. J. Clin. Oncol. 14 (1996) 2495–2503
34. Fisher BJ, Bauman GS, Leighton CE, Stitt L, Cairncross JG, Macdonald DR: Low-grade gliomas in children: tumor volume response to radiation. J. Neurosurg. 88 (1998) 969–974
35. Flickinger JC, Torres C, Deutsch M: Management of low-grade gliomas of the optic nerve and chiasm. Cancer 61 (1988) 635–642
36. Freeman CR, Krischer J, Sanford RA, Burger PC, Cohen M, Norris D: Hyperfractionated radiotherapy in brain stem tumors: results of a Pediatric Oncology Group study. Int. J. Radiat. Oncol. Biol. Phys. 15 (1988) 311–318
37. Freeman CR, Krischer J, Sanford RA, Cohen ME, Burger PC, Kun L, Halperin EC, Crocker I, Wharam M: Hyperfractionated radiation therapy in brain stem tumors. Results of treatment at the 7020 cGy dose level of Pediatric Oncology Group study #8495. Cancer 68 (1991) 474–481
38. Freeman CR, Krischer JP, Sanford RA, Cohen ME, Burger PC, Del Carpio R, Halperin EC, Munoz L, Friedmann HS, Kun LE: Final Results of a Study of Escalating Doses of Hyperfractionated Radiotherapy in Brain Stem Tumors in Children: A Pediatric Oncology Group Study. Int. J. Radiat. Oncol. Biol. Phys. 27 (1993) 197–206

39. Freeman CR, Suissa S: Brainstem tumors in children: results of a survey of 62 patients treated with radiotherapy. Int. J. Radiat. Oncol. Biol. Phys. 12 (1986) 1823–1828
40. Geyer JR, Zeltzer PM, Boyett JM, Rorke LB, Stanley P, Albright AL, Wisoff JH, Milstein JM, Allen JC, Finlay JL: Survival of infants with primitive neuroectodermal tumors or malignant ependymomas of the CNS treated with eight drugs in 1 day: a report from the Childrens Cancer Group. J. Clin. Oncol. 12 (1994) 1607–1615
41. Goldwein JW, Corn BW, Finlay JL, Packer RJ, Rorke LB, Schut L: Is craniospinal irradiation required to cure children with malignant (anaplastic) intracranial ependymomas? Cancer 67 (1991) 2766–2771
42. Goldwein JW, Leahy JM, Packer RJ, Sutton LN, Curran WJ, Rorke LB, Schut L, Littman PS, D'Angio GJ: Intracranial ependymomas in children Int. J. Radiat. Oncol. Biol. Phys. 19 (1990) 1497–1502
43. Grabenbauer G, Schuchardt U, Buchfelder M, Rödel C, Gusek Ǵ, Marx M, Doerr H, Fahlbusch R, Huk W, Wenzel D, Sauer R: Radiation therapy of optico-hypothalamic gliomas (OHG) radiographic response, vision and late toxicity. Radiother. Oncol. 54 (2000) 239–245
44. Grabenbauer GG, Barta B, Erhardt J, Buchfelder M, Thierauf P, Beck JD, Sauer R: (Prognostic factors and results after the combined surgical and radiotherapy treatment of ependymomas). Strahlenther. Onkol. 168 (1992) 679–685
45. Grabenbauer GG, Beck JD, Erhardt J, Seegenschmidt MH, Seyer H, Thierauf P, Sauer R: Postoperative radiotherapy of medulloblastoma: Impact of radiation quality on treatment outcome. Am J. Clin. Oncol. 19 (1996) 73–77
46. Graham ML, Herndon JE, Casey JR, Chaffee S, Ciocci GH, Krischer JP, Kurtzberg J, Laughlin MJ, Longee DC, Olson JF, Paleologus N, Pennington CN, Friedman HS: High-dose chemotherapy with autologous stem-cell rescue in patients with recurrent and high-risk pediatric brain tumors. J. Clin. Oncol. 15 (1997) 1814–1823
47. Haddock MG, Schild SE, Scheithauer BW, Schomberg PJ: Radiation therapy for histologically confirmed primary central nervous system germinoma. Int. J. Radiat. Oncol. Biol. Phys. 38(5), (1997 Jul 15) 915–923
48. Halberg FE, Wara WM, Fippin LF, Edwards MS, Levin VA, Davis RL, Prados MB, Wilson CB: Low-dose craniospinal radiation therapy for medulloblastoma. Int. J. Radiat. Oncol. Biol. Phys. 20 (1991) 651–654
49. Halperin EC, Friedman HS, Schold SC, Jr., Fuchs HE, Oakes WJ, Hockenberger B, Burger PC: Surgery, hyperfractionated craniospinal irradiation, and adjuvant chemotherapy in the management of supratentorial embryonal neuroepithelial neoplasms in children. Surg. Neurol. 40 (1993) 278–283
50. Halperin EC, Wehn SM, Scott JW, Djang W, Oakes WJ, Friedmann HS: Selection of management strategy for pediatric brainstem tumors. Med. Pediatr. Oncol. 17 (1989) 116–125
51. Hardenbergh PH, Golden J, Billet A: Intracranial germinoma: the case for lower dose radiation therapy. Int. J. Radiat. Oncol. Biol. Phys. 39 (1997) 419–426
52. Heideman RL, Kuttesch J, Jr., Gajjar AJ, Walter AW, Jenkins JJ, Li Y, Sanford RA, Kun LE: Supratentorial malignant gliomas in childhood: a single institution perspective. Cancer 80 (1997) 497–504
53. Heideman RL, Packer RJ, Reaman GH, Allen JC, Lange B, Horowitz ME, Steinberg SM, Gillespie A, Kovnar EH, Balis FM: A phase II evaluation of thiotepa in pediatric central nervous system malignancies. Cancer 72 (1993) 271–275
54. Horwich A, Bloom HJ: Optic gliomas: radiation therapy and prognosis. Int. J. Radiat. Oncol. Biol. Phys. 11 (1985) 1067–1079
55. Itoyama Y, Kochi M, Yamamoto H, Kuratsu J, Uemura S, Ushio Y: Clinical study of intracranial nongerminomatous germ cell tumors producing alpha-fetoprotein. Neurosurgery. 1990 Sep; 27(3): 454–60, J. Neurosurg. 82(4), (1995 Apr) 523–529
56. Janss AJ, Grundy R, Cnaan A, Savino PJ, Packer RJ, Zackai EH, Goldwein JW, Sutton LN, Radcliffe J, Molloy PT: Optic pathway and hypothalamic/chiasmatic gliomas in children younger than age 5 years with a 6-year follow-up. Cancer 75 (1995) 1051–1059

57. Jenkin D, Angyalfi S, Becker L, Berry M, Buncic R, Chan H, Doherty M, Drake J, Greenberg M, Hendrick B: Optic glioma in children: surveillance, resection, or irradiation? Int. J. Radiat. Oncol. Biol. Phys. 25 (1993) 215–225
58. Kitamura K, Shirato H, Sawamura Y, Suzuki K, Ikeda J, Miyasaka K: Preirradiation evaluation and technical assessment of involved-field radiotherapy using computed tomographic (CT) simulation and neoadjuvant chemotherapy for intracranial germinoma. Int. J. Radiat. Oncol. Biol. Phys. 43(4), (1999 Mar 1) 783–788
59. Kortmann RD, Calaminus G, Timmermann B, Göbel U, Bamberg M: Reine intrakranielle Germinome: Bedeutung von Zielvolumen und Bestrahlungsdosis – Analyse der Studien MAKEI '83/'86/'89/SIOP CNS GCT 96., Klinische Pädiatrie 149 (2001) 426 (Abstract)
60. Kortmann RD, Kuhl J, Timmermann B, Mittler U, Urban C, Budach V, Richter E, Willich N, Flentje M, Berthold F, Slavc I, Wolff J, Meisner C, Wiestler O, Sorensen N, Warmuth Metz M, Bamberg M: Postoperative neoadjuvant chemotherapy before radiotherapy as compared to immediate radiotherapy followed by maintenance chemotherapy in the treatment of medulloblastoma in childhood: results of the German prospective randomized trial HIT '91. Int. J. Radiat. Oncol. Biol. Phys. 46 (2000) 269–279
61. Kortmann RD, Timmermann B, Kuhl J, Willich N, Flentje P, Meisner C, Bamberg M: HIT '91 (Prospective, co-operative study for the treatment of malignant brain tumors in childhood): Accuracy and acute toxicity of the irradiation of the craniospinal axis – Results of the quality assurance program. Strahlentherapie und Onkologie 175 (1999) 162–169
62. Kortmann RD, Zanetti I, Mueller S, Taylor RE, Scarlello G, Perilongo G, Walker DA, Gnekow AK, Garre ML: Radiotherapy in low grade glioma : an interim analysis of the SIOP low grade glioma study. IXth Symposium Pediatric Neuro-Oncology (Abstractband) (2000)
63. Kovalic JJ, Grigsby PW, Shepard MJ, Fineberg BB, Thomas PR: Radiation therapy for gliomas of the optic nerve and chiasm. Int. J. Radiat. Oncol. Biol. Phys. 18 (1990) 927–932
64. Kovnar EH: Hyperfractionated irradiation for childhood ependymoma: early results of a phase III Pediatric Oncology Group Study. VIIth Symposium Pediatric Neuro-Oncology (Abstractband) (1996)
65. Kreth FW, Faist M, Warnke PC, Rossner R, Volk B, Ostertag CB: Interstitial radiosurgery of low-grade gliomas. J. Neurosurg. 82 (1995) 418–429
66. Kretschmer CS, Tarbell NJ, Barnes PD, Krischer JP, Burger PC, Kun L: Pre-irradiation chemotherapy and hyperfractionated radiation therapy 66 Gy for children with brain stem tumors. A phase II study of the Pediatric Oncology Group, Protocol 8833. Cancer 72 (1993) 1404–1413
67. Krischer JP, Ragab AH, Kun L, Kim TH, Laurent JP, Boyett JM, Cornell CJ, Link M, Luthy AR, Camitta B: Nitrogen mustard, vincristine, procarbazine, and prednisone as adjuvant chemotherapy in the treatment of medulloblastoma. A Pediatric Oncology Group study. J. Neurosurg. 74 (1991) 905–909
68. Kühl J, Müller HL, Kortmann RDB, L., Deinlein F, Maa E, Graf N, Gnekow A, Scheurlen W, Göbel U, Wolff JEA, Bamberg M, Kaatsch P, Kleihues P, Rating D, Wiestler ODT, D.M. Preirradiation chemotherapy of children and young adults with malignant brain tumours: results of the German pilot trial HIT '88/'89. Klein. Pädiatr. 210 (1998) 227–233
69. Lewis J, Lucraft H, Gholkar A: UKCCSG study of accelerated radiotherapy for pediatric brain stem gliomas. United Kingdom Childhood Cancer Study Group. Int. J. Radiat. Oncol. Biol. Phys. 38 (1997) 925–929
70. Listernick R, Louis DN, Packer RJ, Gutmann DH: Optic pathway gliomas in children with neurofibromatosis 1: consensus statement from the NF1 Optic Pathway Glioma Task Force. Ann. Neurol. 41 (1997) 143–149
71. Mandell LR, Kadota R, Freeman C, Douglass EC, Fontanesi J, Cohen ME, Kovnar E, Burger P, Sanford RA, Kepner J, Friedman H, Kun LE: There is no role for hyperfractionated radiotherapy in the management of children with newly diagnosed diffuse intrinsic brainstem tumors: results of a Pediatric Oncology Group phase III trial comparing conventional vs. hyperfractionated radiotherapy Int. J. Radiat. Oncol. Biol. Phys. 43 (1999) 959–964
72. Marymont MH, Geohas J, Tomita T, Strauss L, Brand WN, Mittal BB: Hyperfractionated craniospinal radiation in medulloblastoma. Pediatr. Neurosurg. 24 (1996) 178–184

73. Miralbell R, Bleher A, Huguenin P, Ries G, Kann R, Mirimanoff RO, Notter M, Nouet P, Bieri S, Thum P, Toussi H: Pediatric medulloblastoma: radiation treatment technique and patterns of failure. Int. J. Radiat. Oncol. Biol. Phys. 37 (1997) 523–529
74. Montgomery AB, Griffin T, Parker RG, Gerdes AJ: Optic nerve glioma: the role of radiation therapy. Cancer 40 (1977) 2079–2080
75. Nazar GB, Hoffman HJ, Becker LE, Jenkin D, Humphreys RP, Hendrick EB: Infratentorial ependymomas in childhood: prognostic factors and treatment. J. Neuro-surg. 72 (1990) 408–417
76. Needle MN, Goldwein JW, Grass J, Cnaan A, Bergman I, Molloy P, Sutton L, Zhao HQ, Garvin JH, Phillips PC: Adjuvant chemotherapy for the treatment of intracranial ependymoma of childhood. Cancer 80 (1997) 341–347
77. Packer RJ, Ater J, Allen J, Phillips P, Geyer R, Nicholson HS, Jakacki R, Kurczynski E, Needle M, Finlay J, Reaman G, Boyett JM: Carboplatin and vincristine chemotherapy for children with newly diagnosed progressive low-grade gliomas. J. Neurosurg. 86 (1997) 747–754
78. Packer RJ, Boyett JM, Zimmerman RA, Albright AL, Kaplan AM, Rorke LB, Selch MT, Cherlow JM, Finlay JL, Wara WM: Outcome of children with brain stem gliomas after treatment with 7800 cGy of hyperfractionated radiotherapy. A Childrens Cancer Group Phase I/II Trial. Cancer 74 (1994) 1827–1834
79. Packer RJ, Boyett JM, Zimmermann RA, Rorke LB, Kaplan AM, Albright AL, Selch MT, Finlay JL: Hyperfractionated radiation therapy (72Gy) for Children with brain stem gliomas: a Children's Cancer Group Phase I/II Trial. Cancer 72 (1993) 1414–1421
80. Packer RJ, Goldwein HS, Nicholson LG, Vezina JC, Allen MD, Ris K: Treatment of children with medulloblastomas with reduced-dose craniospinal radiation therapy and adjuvant chemotherapy : A children's cancer group study. J. Clin. Oncol. 17 (1999) 2127–2136
81. Packer RJ, Littman PA, Sposto RM, D'Angio G, Priest JR, Heideman RL, Bruce DA, Nelson DF: Results of a pilot study of hyperfractionated radiation therapy for children with brain stem gliomas. Int. J. Radiat. Oncol. Biol. Phys. 13 (1987) 1647–1651
82. Packer RJ, Prados M, Phillips P, Nicholson HS, Boyett JM, Goldwein J, Rorke LB, Needle MN, Sutton L, Zimmerman RA, Fitz CR, Vezina LG, Etcubanas E, Wallenberg JC, Reaman G, Wara W: Treatment of children with newly diagnosed brain stem gliomas with intravenous recombinant beta-interferon and hyperfractionated radiation therapy: a childrens cancer group phase I/II study. Cancer 77 (1996) 2150–2156
83. Packer RJ, Sutton LN, Goldwein JW, Perilongo G, Bunin G, Ryan J, Cohen BH, D'Angio G, Kramer ED, Zimmerman RA: Improved survival with the use of adjuvant chemotherapy in the treatment of medulloblastoma. J. Neurosurg. 74 (1991) 433–440
84. Packer RJ, Sutton LN, Elterman R, Lange B, Goldwein J, Nicholson HS, Mulne L, Boyett J, D'Angio G, Wechsler-Jentzsch K: Outcome for children with medulloblastoma treated with radiation and cisplatin, CCNU, and vincristine chemotherapy. J. Neurosurg. 81(5), (1994 Nov) 690–698
85. Petronio J, Edwards MS, Prados M, Freyberger S, Rabbitt J, Silver P, Levin VA: Management of chiasmal and hypothalamic gliomas of infancy and childhood with chemotherapy. J. Neurosurg. 74 (1991) 701–708
86. Pierce SM, Barnes PD, Loeffler JS, McGinn C, Tarbell NJ: Definitive radiation therapy in the management of symptomatic patients with optic glioma. Survival and long-term effects. Cancer 65 (1990) 45–52
87. Prados MD, Edwards MSB, Chang SM, Russo C, Davis R, Rabbitt J, Page M, Lamborn K, Wara WM: Hyperfractionated craniospinal radiation therapy for primitive neuroectodermal tumors: Results of a phase II study. Int. J. Radiat. Oncol. Biol. Phys. 43 (1999) 279–285
88. Prados MD, Wara WM, Edwards MHB, Cogen PH: Hyperfractioned craniospinal radiation for primitive neuroectodermal tumors; early results of a pilot study. Int. J. Radiat. Oncol. Biol. Phys. 28 (1993) 431–438
89. Robertson PL, DaRosso RC, Allen JC: Improved prognosis of intracranial non-germinoma germ cell tumors with multimodality therapy. J. Neurooncol. 32(1), (1997 Mar) 71–80
90. Rousseau P, Habrand JL, Sarrazin D, Kalifa C, Terrier Lacombe MJ, Rekacewicz C, Rey A: Treatment of intracranial ependymomas of children: review of a 15-year experience. Int. J. Radiat. Oncol. Biol. Phys. 28 (1994) 381–386

91. Shibamoto Y, Abe M, Yamashita J: Treatment results of intracranial germinoma as a function of the irradiated volume. Int. J. Radiat. Oncol. Biol. Phys. 15 (1988) 285–290
92. Shrieve DC, Wara WM, Edwards MS, Sneed PK, Prados MD, Cogen PH, Larson DA, Levin VA: Hyperfractionated radiation therapy for gliomas of the brainstem in children and in adults. Int. J. Radiat. Oncol. Biol. Phys. 24 (1992) 599–610
93. Sposto R, Ertel IJ, Jenkin RD, Boesel CP, Venes JL, Ortega JA, Evans AE, Wara W, Hammond D: The effectiveness of chemotherapy for treatment of high grade astrocytoma in children: results of a randomized trial. A report from the Childrens Cancer Study Group. J. Neurooncol. 7 (1989) 165–177
94. Tait DM, Thornton-Jones H, Bloom HJG: Adjuvant chemotherapy for medulloblastoma: The first multi-centre control trial of the International Society of Pediatric Oncology (SIOP I). Eur. J. Cancer 26 (1990) 464–469
95. Tarbell NJ, Loeffler JS, Silver B, Lynch E, Lavally BL, Kupsky WJ, Scott RM, Sallan SE: The change in patterns of relapse in medulloblastoma. Cancer 68 (1991) 1600–1604
96. Thomas PR, Deutsch M, Kepner JL, Boyett JM, Krischer J, Aronin P, Albright L, Allen JC, Packer RJ, Linggood R, Mulhern R, Stehbens JA, Langston J, Stanley P, Duffner P, Rorke L, Cherlow J, Friedman HS, Finlay JL, Vietti TJ, Kun LE: Low-stage medulloblastoma: final analysis of trial comparing standard-dose with reduced-dose neuraxis irradiation. J. Clin. Oncol. 18(16), (2000 Aug) 3004–3011
97. Timmermann B, Kortmann RD, Kuhl J, Meisner C, Slavc I, Pietsch T, Bamberg M: Combined postoperative irradiation and chemotherapy for anaplastic ependymomas in childhood: results of the German prospective trials HIT 88/89 and HIT 91 Int. J. Radiat. Oncol. Biol. Phys. 46 (2000) 287–295
98. Vanuytsel LJ, Bessell EM, Ashley SE, Bloom HJ, Brada M: Intracranial ependymoma: long-term results of a policy of surgery and radiotherapy. Int. J. Radiat. Oncol. Biol. Phys. 23 (1992) 313–319
99. Walker DA, Taylor RE, Perilongo G, Zanetti I, Gnekow AK: Vincristine (VCR) carboplatin (CBDCA) in low grade glioma: an interim report of the international consortium on low grade glioma (ICLGG). IXth Symposium Pediatric Neuro Oncology 2000; (Abstractband)
100. Walter AW, Gajjar A, Ochs JS, Langston JW, Sanford RA, Kun LE, Heideman R: Carboplatin and etoposide with hyperfractionated radiotherapy in children with newly diagnosed diffuse pontine gliomas: a phase I/II study. Med. Pediatr. Oncol. 30 (1998) 28–33
101. Wolden SL, Wara WM, Larson DA, Prados MD, Edwards MS, Sneed PK: Radiation therapy for primary intracranial germ-cell tumors. Int. J. Radiat. Oncol. Biol. Phys. 32(4), (1995 Jul 15) 943–949
102. Wolff JEA, Scheurlen W, Kühl J: HIT-GBM: Clinical multicenter study for glioblastoma in childhood and infancy. Med. Pediatr. Oncol. 27 (1996) 587
103. Wolff JE, Molenkamp G, Westphal S, Pietsch T, Gnekow A, Kortmann RD, Kuehl J: Oral trofosfamide and etoposide in pediatric patients with glioblastoma multiforme. Cancer 89(10), (2000 Nov 15) 2131–2137
104. Wolff JEA, Gnekow AK, Kortmann RD, Pietsch T, Urban C, Graf N, Kühl J: Preradiation Chemotherapy for Pediatric Patients with High-Grade Glioma. Cancer (2002) 264–271
105. Wong JY, Uhl V, Wara WM, Sheline GE: Optic gliomas. A reanalysis of the University of California, San Francisco experience. Cancer 60 (1987) 1847–1855

Antikoagulation nach akutem Hirnschlag im Kindesalter

M. Steinlin, J. Pavlovic

Ein juveniler Hirninfarkt ist meist ein unerwartetes und sehr erschreckendes Ereignis. Eine sofortige und erfolgreiche Therapie zur Verbesserung des weiteren Verlaufes ist von allen Betroffenen gewünscht und gefordert. Im Verlaufe der letzten 20 Jahre hat sich die Betreuung des Erwachsenen nach einem akuten ischämischen Hirninfarkt stark verändert. Bei Kindern besteht jedoch auf Grund mangelnder pädiatrischer Daten noch immer eine große Unsicherheit betreffend die Indikationen der verschiedenen Therapien. Unsere Entscheidungen basieren größtenteils auf den Daten, die bei Erwachsenen nach einem akuten Hirnschlag erhoben wurden.

Der Vorteil einer akuten thrombolytischen Therapie im Kindesalter ist noch nicht nachgewiesen worden. In der Cochrane Review von Wardlaw et al. (1) betreffend Thrombolysetherapie beim Erwachsenen zeigte sich bei einer akuten Thrombolyse (innert 4–6 Stunden nach dem Ereignis) eine gesteigerte Frühmortalität um 68/1000 Patienten, eine gesteigerte Gesamtmortalität um 36/1000 Patienten sowie eine Zunahme der symptomatischen Blutungen um 70/1000 Patienten. Trotz diesen negativen Effekten in der Akut- und Subakutphase kann im Langzeitverlauf durch die Thrombolysetherapie die Gesamtmortalität und -morbidität um 44/1000 Patienten vermindert werden. Somit kann gesagt werden, dass bei den Überlebenden diejenigen Patienten, welche Thrombolyse erhalten haben gegenüber den Unbehandelten bezüglich Morbidität deutlich profitieren. Wird berücksichtigt, dass sowohl Mortalität als auch Morbidität bei den Kindern gegenüber den Erwachsenen geringer ist und dass Kinder andere ätiologische Hintergründe für das Auftreten eines Schlaganfalles haben, so muss die Indikation zur Thrombolyse im Kindesalter sehr kritisch, sorgfältig und auch restriktiv gestellt werden. Ein besseres Wissen über Mortalität und insbesondere über das Ausmaß der Morbidität sowie auch ausreichende Erfahrungen betreffend Thrombolyse im Kindesalter sind notwendig, um den schwierigen Entscheid einer Thrombolyse treffen zu können.

In der Akutphase des juvenilen Hirninfarktes stellt sich meist die Frage der Antikoagulation versus Therapie mit Plättchenaggregationshemmern. Auch hier gibt es verschiedene Cochrane Reviews, welche sich mit diesem Entscheid bei Erwachsenenpatienten befasst haben. Gubitz et al. (2) analysierten Arbeiten, welche den Effekt auf Mortalität und Morbidität bei Therapien mit unfraktioniertem und low molecular weight Heparin, Heparinoiden, oraler Antikoagulation sowie Thrombininhibitoren untersuchten. Dabei konnte gezeigt werden, dass keine der Therapien Mortalität und Morbidität beeinflussten. Zwar konnte bei 9/1000 Patienten eine wiederholte Ischämie verhütet werden, dagegen trat aber bei 9/1000 Patienten eine akute, symptomatische intrakranielle Blutung auf.

Bei 4/1000 Patienten konnte eine pulmonale Embolie verhindert werden, hingegen trat bei 9/1000 Patienten eine große extrakranielle Blutung auf. Interessanterweise fanden die Autoren keinen signifikanten Unterschied zwischen den verschiedenen Antikoagulantientherapien, insbesondere konnte kein Vorteil des moderneren low molecular weight Heparin gegenüber den anderen Antikoagulantien gefunden werden. In einer zweiten Cochrane Review analysierten Gubitz et al. (3) auch den Einsatz von Thrombocytenaggregationshemmern bereits während der Akutphase, das heißt innerhalb der ersten 14 Tage nach dem Ereignis. Dabei haben die beiden großen Studien CAST (4) und IST (5) 98% der Patienten für diese Metaanalyse beigetragen. Bei beiden Studien wurde Aspirin in einer Dosis von160–300 mg/Tag innerhalb der ersten 48 Stunden nach dem Ereignis verabreicht. Hier konnte eine deutliche Verbesserung von Mortalität und Morbidität sowie auch der vollständigen Erholung der Patienten gezeigt werden. Es konnten gegenüber der Antikoagulation zwar nur sieben wiederholte Ischämien/1000 Patienten verhindert werden, es kam aber auch nur zu zwei intrakraniellen Blutungen/1000 Patienten. Thrombocytenaggregation hatte keinen Einfluss auf das Auftreten von tiefen Beinvenenthrombosen, jedoch konnte eine Lungenembolie / 1000 Patienten verhütet werden. Im Langzeitverlauf traten pro 1000 Patienten 10 mehr auf, welche sich vollständig erholten und 13 mehr, welche ein selbstständiges Leben führen konnten. Somit ist in der Akutphase des ischämischen Schlaganfalles bei Erwachsenen die Thrombocytenaggregation die Therapie der ersten Wahl. Unter Berücksichtigung der risikoarmen und auch billigen Therapie sollte diese Maßnahme auch bei den Kindern eingesetzt werden. Sicherlich kann dem entgegengehalten werden, dass diese Resultate fast ausschließlich bei Ischämien im Rahmen von Arteriosklerosen erhoben wurden. Solange jedoch bei anderen Ätiologien keine bessere Akuttherapie nachgewiesen worden ist, ist der Einsatz von potentiell meist auch gefährlicheren und teureren Therapien außerhalb von Studien nicht gerechtfertigt.

Auch bei Erwachsenen wurden einzelne Indikationen der Therapien speziell berücksichtigt. Als häufige Indikation zur Heparinisierung gefolgt von Langzeitantikoagulation von 3–6 Monaten wird die arterielle Dissektion betrachtet. Interessanterweise konnte bei einer Cochrane Review von 2001 keine randomisierte oder Vergleichstudie zu diesem Thema gefunden werden. Lyrer und Engelter (6) fanden in verschiedenen Studien Daten von 359 Patienten, welche eine arterielle Dissektion erlitten hatten. Die verschiedenen Therapieformen und ihr Effekt auf Mortalität und Morbidität sind hier zusammengefasst:

	N	**Mortalität**	**Morbidität**
Tc-aggreagation	98	2%	20%
Antikoagulation	188	1.5%	11%
Operation	85	9%	11%
Nihil	88	22%	47%

Unter Berücksichtigung, dass es sich hier um sehr uneinheitliche Studien mit verschiedensten Studiendesigns gehandelt hat, muss die Schlussfolgerung gezogen werden, dass bis heute keine sichere Evidenz für einen positiven Effekt irgendeiner Therapie nachgewiesen werden konnte. Unter Berücksichtigung des tendenziell verbesserten Outcomes nach einer Therapie im Vergleich zu keiner Therapie schlagen die Autoren den Einsatz des risikoarmen und billigen Aspirins auch bei Ischämien auf Grund einer arteriellen Dissektion vor. Heparin ist der Thrombocytenaggregation dann unterlegen, wenn eine mögliche Blutung unter Therapie als sehr gefährlich betrachtet werden muss. Dies gilt besonders dann, wenn eine volumenmäßig sehr große Ischämie vorhanden ist, oder aber wenn sich die Dissektion des Gefäßes intrakraniell befindet und bei einer möglichen Blutung an der Stelle der Dissektion eine Subarachnoidalblutung auftreten würde.

Ein Drittel der Kinder mit akutem Hirnschlag leidet gleichzeitig auch an kardialen Problemen, welche nur teilweise bei Auftreten des Hirnschlages bereits bekannt sind. Auch hier können wieder verschiedene Cochrane Reviews gefunden werden, welche sich beim Erwachsenen mit den verschiedenen Aspekten der Therapie nach Auftreten eines Hirnschlages als Folge des kardialen Grundproblems beschäftigen (7, 8). Dabei zeigt sich, dass bei Patienten mit Thromboembolien bei Vorhofflimmern die Antikoagulation das Thromboembolierisiko deutlich vermindert. Hingegen konnte kein Effekt der Antikoagulation oder Thrombocytenaggregation bei Patienten mit Thromboembolien bei Herzproblemen im Sinusrythmus gezeigt werden.

Allein bei Infarkten auf Grund einer Sinusvenenthrombose scheint die Antikoagulation die Therapie der ersten Wahl zu sein. Allerdings gibt es dazu keine größeren Studien und auch keine Cochrane Review. Einhauptl et al. 1991 (9) und Levine et al. bereits 1988 (10) zeigten, dass bei symptomatischen Sinusvenenthrombosen durch eine Antikoagulation nicht nur Mortalität und Morbidität gesenkt werden konnten, sondern dass auch eine raschere Erholung unter der Therapie mit Heparin aufgetreten ist.

Aus diesen Ausführungen ist ersichtlich, dass in der Akutphase des cerebralen Schlaganfalles im Erwachsenenalter die Indikation zur Antikoagulation nur selten gegeben ist. Es ist somit auch nicht erstaunlich, dass in der Langzeitbehandlung zur Verhütung eines Rezidivs die Thrombocytenaggregation, primär mit Acetylsalicylsäure, an erster Stelle steht (11). Dies ist die einzige Indikation, welche in einer kleineren Studie auch bei Kindern durchgeführt worden ist. Strater et al. (12) konnten zeigen, dass die Heparin- verglichen mit Acetylsalicylsäuretherapie bei Kindern nach Schlaganfall betreffend Wiederauftreten eines zweiten Schlaganfalles keinen Vorteil beinhaltet.

Es ist für unsere Entscheidungen im Alltag wichtig, dass wir uns bewusst sind, dass Studien zur Therapie des Schlaganfalles bei Kindern noch fehlen, in den meisten Studien wurden sie sogar ausgeschlossen. Wir wissen von den bereits bestehenden Arbeiten über den akuten cerebrovaskulären Insult im Kindesalter, dass Kinder eine bessere Prognose, sowohl betreffend Mortalität, Morbidität als auch Rezidivgefahr haben (13, 14). Nichtsdestotrotz zeigen Kinder nach einem akuten Schlaganfall signifikante, für das weitere Leben belastende Spätfolgen. Neurologisch am häufigsten ist eine bleibende Hemisymptomatik. Bedeutend sind aber insbesondere die neuropsychologischen Folgeprobleme, welche diese

Kinder in ihrer Schulkarriere, Berufsausbildung und später auch Berufsausübung beeinträchtigen können. Wir wissen, dass bei Kindern eine Arteriosklerose sehr selten ist, bei den meisten ist der akute Schlaganfall ein »multiple risk factor« Problem. Wichtig für die Ursache des Schlaganfalles sind vor allem infektiöse und parainfektiöse Reaktionen sowie auch (meist hereditäre) Hyperkoagulopathien. Es ist unbekannt, wieweit die verschiedenen Ätiologien einen Therapieeffekt beeinflussen können. Haben Kinder mit hereditären Koagulopathien möglicherweise einen größeren Nutzen von der Antikoagulation? Gibt es noch andere solche genetischen Dispositionen, welche allenfalls die Therapieindikationen beeinflussen könnten? Sprechen die kindlichen Gefäße und das kindliche Gehirn anders auf Heparin an als Erwachsene?

Solange wir diese Fragen noch nicht beantwortet haben, müssen wir uns bewusst sein, dass die Antikoagulation eine risikoreiche Therapie ist und deshalb sorgfältig indiziert werden sollte. Ich bin überzeugt, dass wir vorläufig folgende Regeln noch einhalten sollten:

Thrombolyse im Kindesalter ist nur sehr kritisch, sorgfältig und restriktiv zu indizieren.

Die Antikoagulation ist nur in wenigen Spezialfällen indiziert.

Die Thrombocytenaggregation sollte so rasch als möglich nach dem Ereignis der cerebralen Ischämie eingesetzt werden.

Sorgfältige Untersuchungen der verschiedenen Risikofaktoren sind indiziert, um gezielt das Wiederholungsrisiko vermindern zu können.

Längerfristig sollten Studien zur Evaluation von Kindern mit akut ischämischen Insulten durchgeführt werden, insbesondere auch mit der Frage, ob es Kinder mit einem höheren Risiko der Mortalität und Morbidität gibt, und ob allenfalls dieses Risiko spezifisch angegangen werden kann. Bei Erwachsenen konnte gezeigt werden, dass das Vorliegen einer Mutation im Apolipoprotein E Gen einen positiven Effekt auf die Erholung nach einer cerebralen Ischämie hat (15). Ähnliche Hinweise finden sich für Kinder in einer Arbeit von Mercuri et al. (16), die zeigt, dass Neugeborene mit einer akuten cerbrovaskulären Ischämie eine deutlich schlechtere weitere Entwicklung zeigen, wenn gleichzeitig das Vorliegen einer hereditären Koagulopathie gefunden werden konnte. Daneben sollten auch Multizenterstudien betreffend Effekte der verschiedenen Therapien initiiert werden. Nur so können wir die wichtige Frage der Therapie auch für Kinder nach einem Schlaganfall adäquat beantworten.

Literatur

1. Wardlaw JM, delZoppo G, Yamaguchi T: Thrombolyses for acute ischaemic stroke. (Cochrane Review). In: The Cochrane Library, Issue 4, 2001. Oxford: Update Software
2. Gubitz G, Counsell C, Sanderock P, Signorini D : Anticoagulation for acute ischaemic stroke (Cochrane Review). In: The Cochrane Library, Issue 4, 2001. Oxford: Update Software
3. Gubitz G, Sanderock P, Counsell C: Antiplatelet therapy for acute ischaemic stroke (Cochrane review). In: The Cochrane Library, Issue 4, 2001. Oxford: Update Software
4. CAST (Chinese acute stroke trial) Collaborative group. A randomised placebo-controlled trial of early aspirin use in 20'000 patients with acute ischaemic stroke. Lancet 1997;349:1641–1649
5. IST (International stroke trial collaborative group. The international stroke trial): A randomised trial of aspirin, subcutaneous heparin, both, or neither among 19435 patients with acute stroke. Lancet 1997;349:1569–1581
6. Lyrer P and Engelter S. Antithrombotic drugs for carotid artery dissection. (Cochrane review). In: The Cochrane Library, Issue 4, 2001. Oxford: Update Software
7. Koudstaal PJ: Anticoagulation versus antiplatelet therapy for preventing stroke in patients with nonrheumatic atrial fibrillation and a history of stroke or transient ischaemic attacks. (Cochrane review). In: The Cochrane Library, Issue 4, 2001. Oxford: Update Software
8. Lipp GYP, Gibbs CR: Antiplatelet agents versus control or anticoagulation for heart failure in sinusrythmus. (Cochrane review). In: The CochraneLlibrary, Issue 4, 2001. Oxford: Update Software
9. Einhauptl KM, Villringer A, Meister W, Mehlraein S, Garner C, Pellkofer M, Haberl RL, Pfister HW, Schmiedek P: Heparin treatment in sinus venous thrombosis. Lancet 1991; 338: 597–600
10. Levine SR, Twyman RE, Gilman S: The role of anticoagulation in cavernous sinus thrombosis. Neurology 1988; 38: 517–522
11. Algra A, De Schryver ELLM, van Gijn J, Kapelle LJ, Koudstaal PJ: Oral anticoagulation versus antiplatelet therapy for preventing vascular events after transient ischaemic attack or minor stroke of presumed arterial origin (Cochrane review). In: The Cochrane Library, Issue 2, 2002. Oxford: Update Software.
12. Strater R, Kurnik K, Heller C, Schobess R, Luigs P, Nowak Gottl U: Aspirin versus low-dose low-molecular-weight heparin : Antithrombotic therapy in paediatric ischemic stroke patients : a prospective follow-up study. Stroke 2001; 32: 2554–8
13. DeSchryver ELLM, Kapelle LJ, Jennekens-Schinkel A, Peters BAC: Prognosis of ischemic stroke in childhood: a long-term follow-up study. Dev Med Child Neurol 2000;15:316–324
14. Ganesan V, Hogan A, Shack N et al: Outcome after ischaemic stroke in childhood. Dev Med Child Neurol 2000;42:455–461
15. MCarron MO, Muir KW, Weir CJ, Dyker AG, Bone I, Nicoll JA, Lees KR: The apolipoprotein E epsilon4 allele and outcome in cerebrovascular disease. Stroke 1998; 29:1882–7
16. Mercuri E, Cowan F, Gupte G, Manning R, Laffan M, Rutherford M, Edwards AD, Dubowitz L, Roberts I. Pediatrics 2001; 107: 1400–1404

4. Pädiatrische Neurophysiologie

Somatosensibel evozierte Potentiale – Chancen und Grenzen der Methode in der Neuropädiatrie

R. Boor

Zusammenfassung

Somatosensibel evozierte Potentiale (SEP) ermöglichen eine objektive Beurteilung der Funktion peripherer Nerven und somatosensibler Bahnen des zentralen Nervensystems. Nach Stimulation des N. medianus werden bei Kindern die Nahfeldpotentiale N9 (Generator im Plexus brachialis), N13a (Hinterhorn des unteren Halsmarks), N13b (kranio-zervikaler Übergang), N20 (Kortex) sowie die Fernfeldpotentiale P13 (kranio-zervikaler Übergang) und P14 (Lemniscus medialis) klinisch verwendet. Nach Stimulation des N. tibialis werden die Nahfeldpotentiale N8 (peripherer Nerv), N22 (Hinterhorn des lumbosakralen Rückenmarks), P40 (Kortex) sowie das Fernfeldpotential P30 (Lemniscus medialis) abgeleitet. Die SEP ermöglichen eine Stufendiagnostik des somatosensorischen Systems. Sie werden eingesetzt bei Erkrankungen des peripheren Nervenssystems, bei Störungen im Bereich der Cauda equina, des Rückenmarks und des kranio-spinalen Übergangs, bei Läsionen lemniskaler und thalamokortikaler Bahnen sowie bei Schädigungen der Hirnrinde. Die lemniskale Antwort P14 lässt sich erst ab einem Alter von 4 Jahren sicher ableiten. Die kortikalen Reizantworten werden bei jungen Kindern stark durch die Vigilanz beeinflusst. Unter Berücksichtigung dieser Besonderheiten und Einflussfaktoren liefern die SEP bei Kindern verlässliche Ergebnisse.

Einleitung

Nach elektrischer Stimulation eines gemischten Nervens kommt es zum Auftreten somatosensibel evozierter Potentiale (SEP). Gerade bei Kindern sind die SEP für die klinische Beurteilung des somatosensorischen Systems unverzichtbar. Säuglinge, Kleinkinder sowie retardierte Kinder müssen jedoch meist im medikamentös induzierten Schlaf untersucht werden, was die kortikalen SEP-Komponenten stark beeinflussen kann (Fagan et al. 1987). Hier bietet sich die Verwendung subkortikal generierter Potentiale an. Normwerte somatosensibel evozierter Potentiale nach Reizung des N. medianus sowie des N. tibialis im Kindesalter sind publiziert (Boor et al. 1998a, Boor et al. 1998b, Boor und Goebel 2000, George und Taylor 1991, Taylor und Fagan 1988, Taylor et al. 1996).

Nach Reizung des N. medianus werden folgende Nahfeld-Potentiale abgeleitet: Die Komponente N9 wird im Plexus brachialis generiert; die N11 repräsentiert den präsynaptischen Impuls im Hinterstrang; bei der N13a handelt es sich um ein postsynaptisches Potential aus dem Hinterhorn des kaudalen Halsmarks;

die N13b wird in der Nähe des Foramen magnum generiert und die N20 in der Area 3b des primären somatosensorischen Kortex. Zusätzlich lassen sich folgende Fernfeld-Potentiale ableiten: Die P13 stellt präsynaptische Aktivität aus dem Bereich des kranio-zervikalen Übergangs dar. Die P14 wird im Lemniscus medialis generiert. Die N18 hat einen medullären Generator. Aufgrund der Variabilität der N18 und der Schwierigkeit, diese Komponente exakt zu messen, ist ihr klinischer Wert bei Kindern jedoch noch unklar. Die Potentiale N9, N13a, N13b, P13 und N20 sind bei gesunden Kindern regelmäßig abgrenzbar. Das Fernfeldpotential P14 ist erst bei Kindern im Alten von über 4 Jahren verlässlich ableitbar (Boor et al. 1998a, Boor und Goebel 2000).

Nach Reizung des N. tibialis werden die Potentiale N8 (peripherer Nerv in der Kniekehle), N20 (Cauda equina), N22 (postsynaptisches Potential aus dem Hinterhorn des unteren Lumbal- und oberen Sakralmarks) abgeleitet. Das Fernfeldpotential P30 hat einen lemniskalen Generator und das Nahfeldpotential P40 stammt aus dem Fußareal des primären somato-sensorischen Kortex.

Methodik

Der N. medianus wird am Handgelenk mit monophasischen elektrischen Rechteckimpulsen von 0.2 ms knapp oberhalb der motorischen Reizschwelle gereizt. Der N. tibialis wird am Innenknöchel stimuliert. 500 Antworten werden mit einer Zeitachse von 50 ms (Medianus-SEP) bzw. 100 ms (Tibialis-SEP) gemittelt. Zum Nachweis der Reproduzierbarkeit werden mindestens 2 gemittelte Kurven übereinandergelagert. Kinder mit einem Entwicklungsalter von unter 4–5 Jahren werden mit Chloralhydrat sediert.

Die Ableitelektroden (Silber-Elektroden auf der Haut, Impedanz unter 5 kOhm) für die Medianus-SEP befinden sich über der linken oder rechten Fossa supraclavicularis (Erb'scher Punkt, EP1 und EP2), über dem Dornfortsatz des siebten und zweiten Halswirbels (cv7 und cv2), auf der frontalen Kopfhaut (Fz) sowie links und rechts zentroparietal jeweils 2 cm hinter C3 oder C4 (C3' und C4'). Eine Elektrode über dem kontralateralen Erb'schen Punkt dient als nonzephale Referenz. Die »Ohrreferenz« wird am ipsilateralen Ohrläppchen (A1, A2) aufgeklebt. Vergleichbare Ergebnisse liefert eine Referenz am Mastoid. Die vordere Halsreferenz befindet sich über der Fossa jugularis (jug). Die Ableitpunkte für die Tibialis-SEP befinden sich in den Kniekehlen (Pf1, Pf2), über den Dornfortsätzen des fünften (L5) und des ersten (L1) Lendenwirbels sowie über der Zentralregion (Cz', 2 cm hinter Cz). Als Referenzelektroden dienen der Beckenkamm (IC), das Ohrläppchen oder Mastoid (A1, A2) sowie Fz. Potentiale negativer Polarität werden in den Abbildungen mit einem Ausschlag nach oben dargestellt. Die Abbildungen 1 und 2 zeigen Beispiele normaler Medianus- und Tibialis-SEP sowie die verwendeten Montagen.

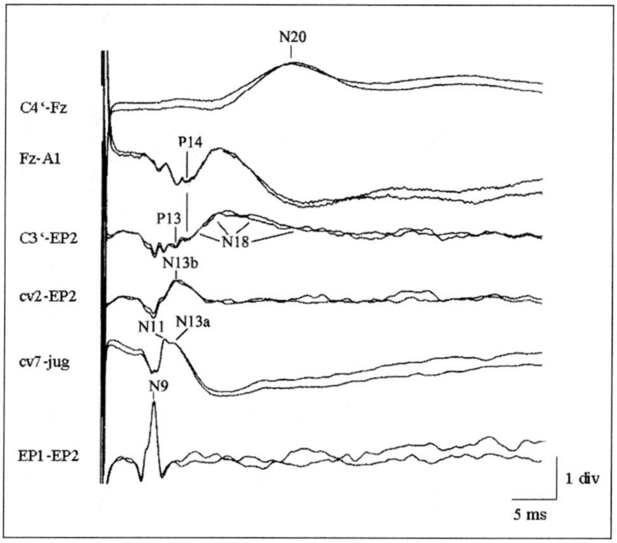

Abb. 1: Normale Medianus-SEP im medikamentös induzierten Schlaf bei einem 45 Monate alten Kind. Man erkennt die Nahfeld-Potentiale N9, N11, N13a, N13b, N20 sowie die Fernfeldpotentiale P13, P14 und N18. Amplituden: 1 div, 2 µV in Kanal 2; 1 div, 5 µV in den übrigen Kanälen.

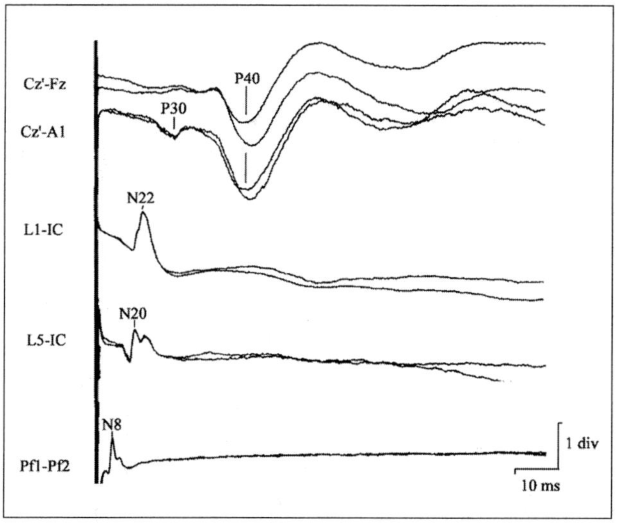

Abb. 2: Normale Tibialis-SEP im medikamentös induzierten Schlaf bei einem 19 Monate alten Kleinkind. Man erkennt die Nahfeldpotentiale N8, N20, N22, P40 sowie das Fernfeldpotential P30. Amplituden: 1 div, 2 µV in den Kanälen 1–3; 1 div, 5 µV in Kanal 4; 1 div, 10 µV in Kanal 5.

Anwendungsbeispiele und Grenzen der SEP

Nahfeld- und Fernfeld-SEP nach Reizung des N. medianus sowie des N. tibialis lassen sich bei Kindern aller Altersstufen verlässlich ableiten. Die SEP ermöglichen eine Stufendiagnostik des somatosensorischen Systems. Die Komponenten N9 nach Stimulation des N. medianus und N8 nach Stimulation des N. tibialis sowie die Interpeaklatenzen (IPL) N9-N13a und N8-N22 geben Hinweise auf die Funktion der peripheren Nerven oder der Plexus (Abb. 3). Die Komponenten N11 (Medianus) und N20 (Tibialis) sowie die zugehörigen IPL N9-N11, N8-N20 sind zur Beurteilung der proximalen Nerven sowie der Plexus ebenfalls einsetz-

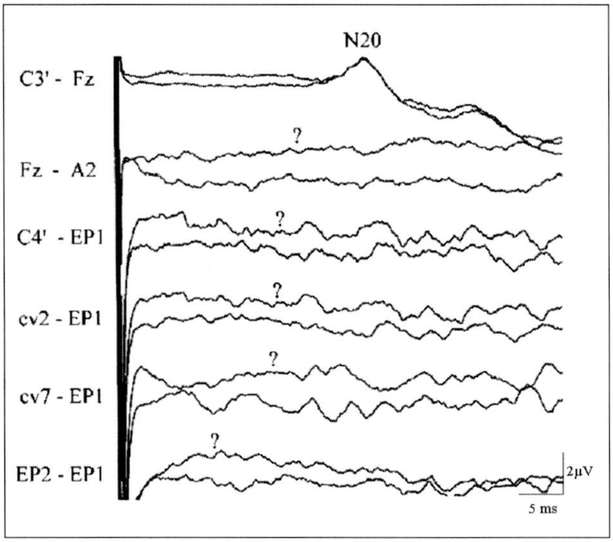

Abb. 3: Medianus-SEP bei Guillain-Barré Syndrom im Alter von 4 Jahren, wach. Es fehlen die peripheren, spinalen sowie die subkortikal generierten Komponenten. Lediglich die kortikale N20 ist mit verzögerter Latenz nachweisbar.

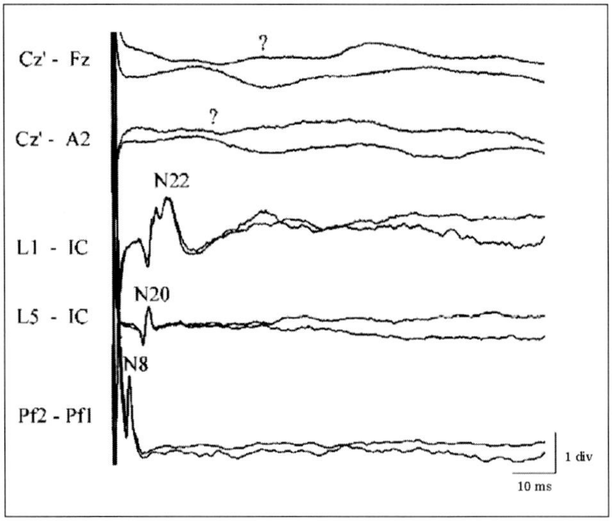

Abb. 4: Tibialis-SEP bei Morbus Pelizaeus-Merzbacher im Alter von 23 Monaten, Schlaf. Die peripheren und spinalen Komponenten sind normal dargestellt; es fehlen die lemniskale Komponente P30 sowie die kortikalen Potentiale. Amplituden: 1 div, 2 µV in den Kanälen 1–4; 1div, 10 µV in Kanal 5.

bar. Deren Aussagekraft ist jedoch dadurch eingeschränkt, dass sie nicht bei allen gesunden Probanden abgeleitet werden können (Boor et al. 1998a, Boor et al. 1998b, Boor und Goebel 2000). Die postsynaptisch generierten spinalen Potentiale N13a (Medianus) und N22 (Tibialis) weisen – bei normalen peripheren Antworten – auf eine Schädigung des Myelons hin. Pathologische subkortikale Komponenten P13 und N13b (Medianus) zeigen bei unauffälligen peripheren und spinalen Komponenten eine Funktionsstörung des Hinterstrangs an. Ähnlich kann die lemniskal generierte P30 (Tibialis) verwendet werden. Ab einem Alter von 4 Jahren lässt sich bei Kindern – ähnlich wie bei Erwachsenen – die lemniskale Komponente P14 nach Armnervenstimulation verwerten (Boor et al. 1998,

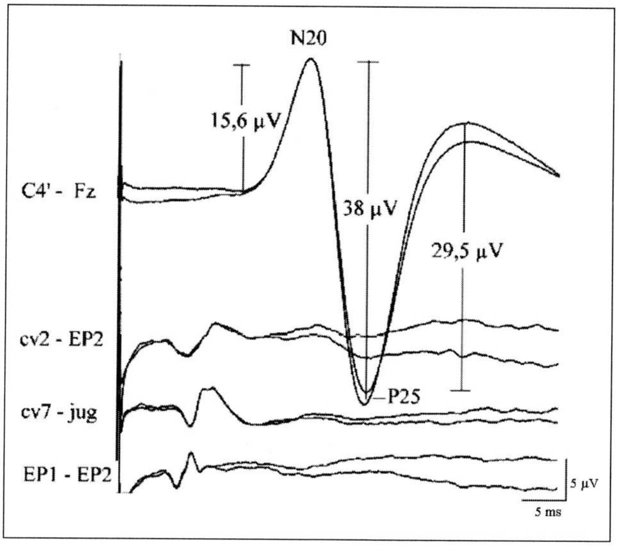

Abb. 5: Spätinfantile neuronale Ceroidlipofuscinose, 10 Jahre, wach: kortikale Riesenpotentiale.

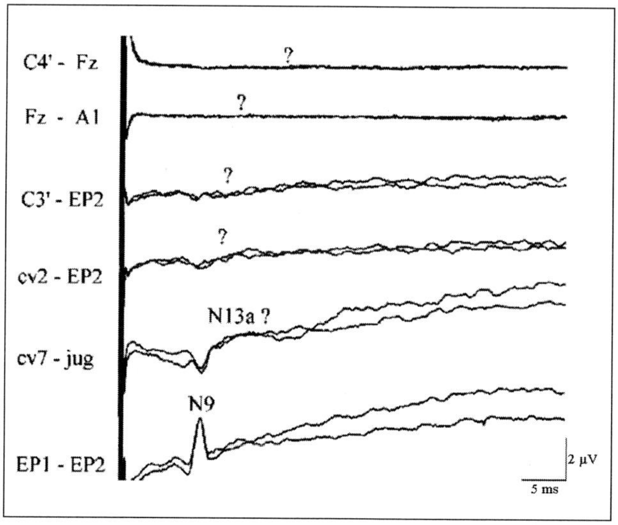

Abb. 6: Hirntod, 14 Jahre: Es fehlen alle Komponenten, welche intrakraniell oder am kranio-zervikalen Übergang generiert werden. Auch die zervikale Antwort N13a ist auffallend breit und nur schwer abgrenzbar.

Boor und Goebel 2000). Mit den SEP lassen sich auch suklinische Läsionen der Hinterstränge erkennen, und die Methode weist eine hohe Sensitivität bei der Erkennung einer zervikalen Myelopathie bei Patienten mit Achondroplasie und Mucopolysaccharidosen auf (Boor et al. 1999, Boor et al. 2000).

Die zentralen Leitzeiten N13a-N20 bzw. N22-P40 weisen auf Funktionsstörungen der zentralen Bahnen hin, wie sie beispielsweise bei Leukodystrophien vorkommen (Abb. 4). Kortikale Riesenpotentiale zeigen eine erhöhte Erregbarkeit des somatosensorischen Kortex an (Abb. 5). Die kortikalen Medianus-SEP sind ein wichtiger prognostischer Indikator bei Patienten im Koma (Abb. 6).

Die Erfahrungen mit der dargestellten SEP-Stufendiagnostik bei Früh- und Neugeborenen sind bislang gering. Leider ist das Fernfeld-Potential P14 bei vielen jüngeren Kindern nicht ableitbar und erst bei älteren Kindern und Erwachsenen klinisch verwertbar. Nach Beinnervenstimulation ist zu beachten, dass die Tibialis-SEP die sakralen Segmente S3–S5 nicht erfassen. Vorsicht ist bei einer Schädigung der Bahnen durch Kompression geboten, da die kortikalen Potentiale infolge der synaptischen Verstärkung und Synchronisation unauffällig sein können. Hier hilft die zusätzliche Ableitung der peripheren, spinalen und subkortikalen Potentiale, die oberhalb der Läsion präsynaptisch generiert werden. Viele jüngere Kinder werden im medikamentös induzierten Schlaf untersucht, welcher die kortikalen Komponenten beeinflusst. Dann ist bereits die Beurteilung der frühen kortikalen Antworten schwierig. Deshalb verwenden wir spätere kortikale Komponenten nicht zur klinischen Diagnostik.

Schlussfolgerung

Die beschriebene SEP-Technik ist klinisch verlässlich anwendbar. Die vorgestellte Stufendiagnostik erlaubt die Identifizierung und topische Zuordnung von Schädigungen des somatosen-sorischen Systems. Im Kindesalter sind die subkortikalen Komponenten P13 und N13b, die in der Umgebung des kraniozervikalen Übergangs generiert werden, zuverlässig ableitbar. Dabei stellt das Fernfeldpotential P13 die wertvollste Komponente zur Beurteilung der Hinterstrangfunktion dar. Gerade bei jungen Kindern, bei denen die klinische Beurteilbarkeit des somatosensiblen Systems oft eingeschränkt ist, sind die SEP von großer klinischer Relevanz.

Literatur

1. Boor R, Goebel B, Taylor MJ (1998a) Subcortical somatosensory evoked potentials after median nerve stimulation in children. Eur J Paediatr Neurol 2: 137–143.
2. Boor R, Goebel B, Doepp M, Taylor MJ (1998b) Somatosensory evoked potentials after posterior tibial nerve stimulation – normative data in children. Eur J Paediatr Neurol 2: 145–152.
3. Boor R, Fricke G, Brühl K, Spranger J (1999) Abnormal subcortical somatosensory evoked potentials indicate high cervical myelopathy in achondroplasia. Eur J Pediatr 158: 662–667.
4. Boor R, Goebel B (2000) Maturation of nearfield and farfield somatosensory evoked potentials after median nerve stimulation in children under four years of age. Clin Neurophysiol 111: 1070–1081.
5. Boor R, Miebach E, Brühl K, Beck M (2000) Abnormal somatosensory evoked potentials indicate compressive myelopathy in mucopolysaccharidosis. Neuropediatrics 31: 122–127
6. Fagan ER, Taylor MJ, Logan WJ (1987) Somatosensory evoked potentials: Part I. A review of neural generators and special considerations in pediatrics. Pediatr Neurol 3: 189–196.
7. George SR, Taylor MJ (1991) Somatosensory evoked potentials in neonates and infants: developmental and normative data. Electroencephalogr Clin Neurophysiol 80: 94–102.
8. Taylor MJ, Fagan ER (1988) SEP to median nerve stimulation: normative data for paediatrics. Electroencephalogr Clin Neurophysiol 71: 323–330.
9. Taylor MJ, Boor R, Ekert PG (1996) Preterm maturation of the somatosensory evoked potential. Electroencephalogr Clin Neurophysiol 100: 448–452.

Transkranielle Magnetstimulation (TMS): Chancen und Grenzen in der Neuropädiatrie

V. Mall

Zusammenfassung

Die TMS gilt als Standard für die Untersuchung der corticospinalen Bahn in der Erwachsenenneurologie und findet zunehmend Anwendung in der Neuropädiatrie. Durch den Einsatz verschiedener Stimulations- und Ableitetechniken gelingt die differenzierte Darstellung funktioneller Eigenschaften des corticospinalen Systems. Die Bestimmung der Zentralmotorischen Latenz durch die Einzelpulsstimulation gilt als »Golden Standard« in der klinischen Routine und kann bei Kindern ohne wesentliche Modifikationen durchgeführt werden. Die Zentralmotorische Latenz dient als Parameter für die Integrität der schnellen corticospinalen Bahn. Die Triple Stimulation stellt eine Weiterentwicklung der Methode zur Erhöhung der Sensitivität für zentrale Leitungsblöcke dar. Durch die Kombination mit peripheren elektrischen Stimuli wird die Amplitudenvariabilität der motorisch evozierten Potentiale reduziert. Die Bestimmung der Amplitude nach Triple Stimulation wird somit zu einem hochsensitiven Parameter für Störungen der Integrität der schnellen corticopsinalen Bahn. Der motorische Cortex kann mit Hilfe der Bestimmung der motorischen Schwelle untersucht werden. Die Exzitabilität nach Single Pulse Stimulation ist ein Parameter, der durch die Regulierung von Na^{+}- und K^{+}-Kanälen beeinflusst wird. Im Gegensatz hierzu wird die Fazilitierung und Inhibierung eines motorisch evozierten Potentiales durch einen vorangegangenen konditionierenden Stimulus hierdurch nicht beeinflusst. Mit der Paired Pulse Technik lassen sich vielmehr GABAerge intracorticale Interneurone abbilden, denen eine wesentliche Bedeutung in der Regulierung neuronaler Plastizität zugeschrieben wird.

Einleitung

Die TMS gilt als Standard für die Untersuchung der corticospinalen Bahn in der Erwachsenenneurologie und findet zunehmend Anwendung in der Neuropädiatric (Heinen et al., 1998; Heinen et al., 1999; Fietzek et al., 2000; Eyre et al., 2000; Müller et al., 1991). Als schmerzfreie und für die Routine schnell durchführbare Methode ist sie für den Einsatz bei Kindern geradezu prädistiniert. Durch den Einsatz verschiedener Stimulations- und Ableitetechniken gelingt die differenzierte Darstellung verschiedener funktioneller Eigenschaften des corticospinalen Systems (Abb. 1). Im folgenden soll auf die Untersuchung der corticospinalen Bahn und des motorischen Cortex eingegangen werden.

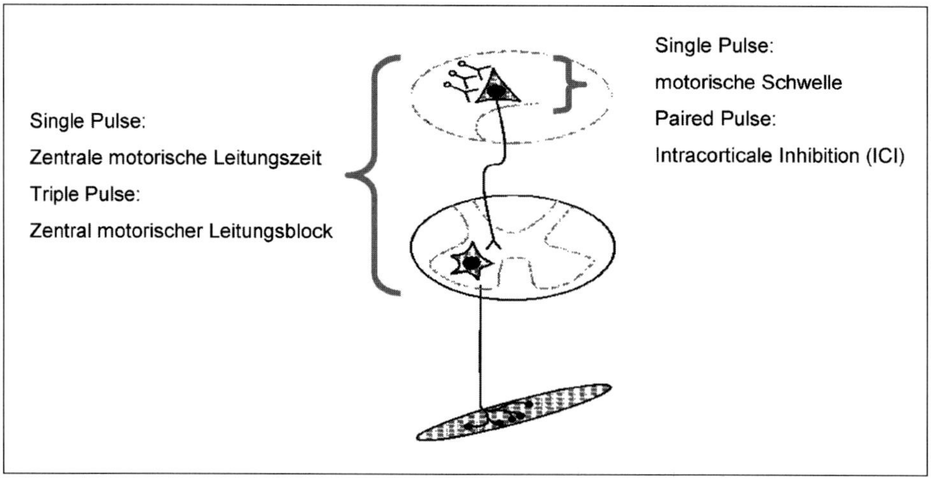

Abb. 1: Schematisch vereinfachte Darstellung des corticospinalen Systems. Mit der TMS lassen sich durch die im Text aufgeführten Untersuchungsmethoden Eigenschaften des motorischen Cortex und der corticospinalen Bahn darstellen.

Die Untersuchung der corticospinalen Bahn in der klinischen Routine: Bestimmung der zentralen motorischen Leitungszeit (ZML) mit der Single Pulse TMS

Die Einzelpulsstimulation und die Bestimmung der ZML gilt als »Golden Standard« der TMS in der klinischen Routine (Abb. 2). Die Untersuchungszeit kann für die klinische Routine auf 15–20 Minuten beschränkt werden. Stimulationsort (Rundspule: Vertex) und Stimulationsintensität (bei Kindern unter 10 Jahren in der Regel 100% der Stimulatorleistung) sind unkritisch. Damit ist die Stimulation transkraniell ebenso wie von peripher (Stimulationsort zur oberen Extremität: C7, zur unteren Extremität L5, Stimulationsintensität: 25–45%) auch bei unruhigen Patienten gut durchführbar. Die Literaturangaben bez. der Normwerte zeigen leichte Differenzen, spätestens ab dem 7. Lebensjahr dürfen Erwachsenen-gleiche Werte angenommen werden; vor dem 5. Lebensjahr sind alterspezifische Normwerte anzuwenden. Zu beachten ist bei der Ableitung zur unteren Extremität, dass bei ca. 10% der gesunden Probanden unter 10 Jahren keine Potentiale ableitbar sind. Fehlende motorische Potentiale an der unteren Extremität in dieser Altersklasse können also nicht als pathologisch gewertet werden. Zusammenfassend handelt es sich bei der Single Pulse TMS zur Bestimmung der ZML um eine Methode, die ohne größere Modifikationen bei Kindern unkompliziert eingesetzt werden kann.

Die Untersuchung der corticospinalen Bahn bei besonderen Fragestellungen: Darstellung zentraler Leitungsblöcke mit der Triple Stimulation

Leitungsblöcke lassen sich prinzipiell besser mit der Amplitude als mit der Leitungszeit abbilden und korrelieren in hohem Maß mit der klinischen Beein-

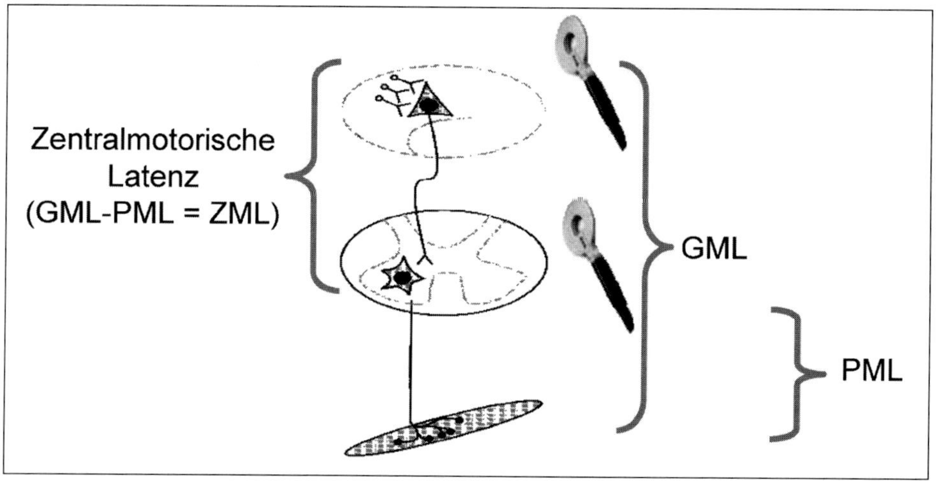

Abb. 2: Die Bestimmung der zentralen motorischen Leitungszeit (ZML) durch Subtraktion der peripheren motorischen Leitungszeit (PML, Stimulation mit der Magnetspule über C7 bzw. L5) von der gesamtmotorischen Leitungszeit (GML, transkranielle Stimulation mit der Magnetspule über dem Vertex).

trächtigung. Diese Grundregel der klinischen Neurophysiologie stellt eine Einschränkung der Aussagekraft der konventionellen Single Pulse TMS dar. Auf Grund zentraler Desynchronisationsphänomene übersteigt die Varianz der Amplitude nach zentraler Stimulation die nach peripherer Stimulation um ein Vielfaches. Gering bis mittel stark ausgeprägte Leitungsblöcke können so unter Umständen durch die konventionelle Single Pulse TMS nicht erkannt werden. Die Triple Puls Stimulation kombiniert die transkranielle magnetische Stimulation mit 2 peripheren elektrischen Stimuli (Magistris et al., 1998). Es kommt hierdurch zur Eliminierung der Effekte, die bei der Single Pulse TMS durch die zentrale Desynchronisation verursacht werden. Die Variabilität der Amplitude wird durch diese Stimulationstechnik minimiert. Die über dem Zielmuskel abgeleitete Amplitude korreliert mit der Anzahl der erregten alpha-Motoneurone. Bei einer intakten corticospinalen Bahn werden 100% der alpha-Motoneurone, die den Zielmuskel innervieren, erregt. Bereits ein zentraler Leitungsblock, der zu einer ausbleibenden Erregung von 5–10% der alpha-Motoneurone führt, wird durch eine signifikante Amplitudenreduktion erkannt. Hierdurch konnte die Sensitivität für zentrale Leitungsblöcke gegenüber der Single Pulse TMS signifikant erhöht werden (Magistris et al., 1999). Auch die Korrelation zwischen dem TMS-Untersuchungsergebnis und der klinischen Beeinträchtigung konnte durch die Triple Stimulation signifikant gesteigert werden. Diese Vorteile werden mit einer Reihe erheblicher Nachteile erkauft. Die Untersuchung ist durch ihre periphere elektrische (supramaximale) Erb-Stimulation ausgesprochen schmerzhaft. Diese Stimulationsart ist beim erwachsenen Patienten nur in Ausnahmefällen möglich, bei Kindern grundsätzlich undenkbar. Wird die Erb-Stimulation durch eine Oberarmstimulation ersetzt, kann die Schmerzhaftigkeit der Untersuchung auf ein Minimum reduziert werden. In eigenen Untersuchungen an 15 erwachsenen Probanden konnten wir die Methode für diese Stimulationsart

	Erwachsene	Kinder
Stimulationsorte peripher	Erb	Oberarm
Untersuchungszeit	30 Min.	30 Min.
Compliance	sehr schmerzhaft	tolerabel

Abb. 3: Pädiatrische Modifikationen zur Durchführung der Triple Stimulation (TST). Die schmerzhafte Stimulation über Erb wird durch die Stimulation am Oberarm ersetzt. Die Untersuchung wird damit für den Patienten gut tolerierbar, erfordert jedoch bei gleich langer Untersuchungsdauer und bezüglich Artefakten störanfälligen Stimulationsorten weiterhin ein hohes Maß an Kooperation.

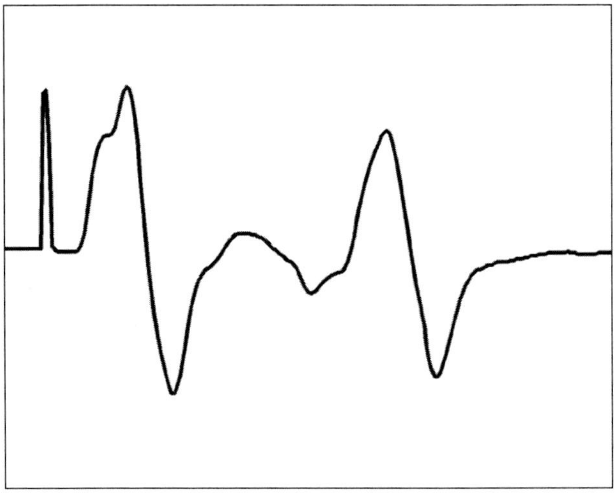

Abb. 4: Darstellung der Ableitungen eines erwachsenen Probanden. Der erste negative Peak (nach oben zeigend) ist das Ergebnis einer rein peripheren supramaximalen Stimulation. Der zweite negative Peak korreliert zur Anzahl der nach zentraler Stimulation erregten alpha-Motoneurone, die bei intakter corticospinaler Bahn 100% beträgt. Die Amplitude nach peripherer Stimulation (erster Peak) gilt somit als Kontrolle für die Amplitude des 2. Peaks, die beim Gesunden maximal 15% kleiner sein darf.

validieren (s. Abb. 3, 4). Erste Untersuchungen bei Jugendlichen sind erfolgversprechend. Zusammenfassend handelt es sich bei der Triple Stimulation um eine Methode die erheblicher Modifikationen bedarf, um bei Jugendlichen eingesetzt zu werden. Sie verlangt auch dann noch ein hohes Maß an Kooperation, so dass sie speziellen klinischen und wissenschaftlichen Fragestellungen vorbehalten bleibt.

Die Untersuchung der cortikalen Erregbarkeit: Die Bestimmung der motorischen Schwelle mit der Single Pulse TMS

Während die Bestimmung der motorischen Schwelle in der klinischen Routine wünschenswert, aber nicht zwingend ist, gilt sie bei der wissenschaftlichen Anwendung der TMS als Standard, da die Stimulationsintensität gemäß internationaler Konventionen grundsätzlich von der motorischen Schwelle abgeleitet wird. Die motorische Schwelle ist das Maß für die Erregbarkeit des motorischen Cortex durch einen transkraniellen magnetischen Stimulus und zeigt große inter-individuelle Unterschiede. Sie zeigt ein stetiges Abfallen vom Kindes- bis zum Erwachsenenalter. Sie lässt sich durch pharmakologische Substanzen wie Lamotrigin beeinflussen, was auf einen Na^+- und K^+- Kanal vermittelten Mechanismus schließen läßt. Die Bestimmung kann mit der Rundspule durchgeführt werden und ist auch am unruhigen Patienten in relativ kurzer Zeit (5–10 Minuten) durchführbar. Die Bestimmung der motorischen Schwelle stellt somit ein unkompliziertes Verfahren dar, mit der die Exzitabilität des motorischen Cortex untersucht werden kann.

Die Untersuchung der intracorticalen Inhibition: Die Paired Pulse Technik

Wird dem Teststimulus (der transkranielle magnetische Stimulus, der ein motorisch evoziertes Potential auslöst) ein unterschwelliger Stimulus (der somit kein motorisches Potential auslöst) vorangestellt, wird die Größe der Amplitude des (durch den Teststimulus ausgelösten) motorischen Potentials beeinflusst. Beträgt das Interstimulusintervall unter 5 ms kommt es zu einer Verkleinerung der Amplitude, zwischen 5 und 12 ms zu einer Vergrößerung. Aufgrund Varianz der Amplituden bei der TMS wird die Amplitudengröße aus mehreren Stimuli gemittelt, die Kombination der Paired Pulse-Technik mit der Triple Stimulationstechnik bringt diesbezüglich keinen signifikanten Vorteil (Mall et al., 2001). Der Amplitudenquotient nach konditionierter (mit vorherigem unterschwelligen Stimulus) und unkonditionierter (ohne vorherigem Stimulus) gilt als Maß für die Inhibition bzw. Fazilitierung. Auch dieser Mechanismus lässt sich pharmakologisch beeinflussen. So führt Lorazepam zu einer Verstärkung der Inhibition woraus auf einen vorwiegend GABAerg vermittelten intracorticalen Wirkmechanismus geschlossen werden kann. GABAergen intracorticalen Interneuronen werden regulative Eigenschaften bezüglich der neuronalen Plastizität zugeschrieben. Die Regulation neuronaler Plastizität konnte an Erwachsenen in Lernexperimenten gezeigt werden (Ziemann et al., 2001). Die durch Lernvorgänge induzierte neuronale Plastizität wird durch eine Verstärkung der GABAergen Inhibition reduziert, durch eine Reduktion GABAerger Inhibition verstärkt.

Die Anwendung der Methode bedarf der Adaptation der Methode an pädiatrische Rahmenbedingungen (s. Abb. 5). Wir konnten nachweisen, dass Kinder eine wesentlich geringere intracorticale Inhibition aufweisen als Erwachsene (s. Abb. 6), was für einen Maturationsprozess intracorticaler GABAerger Regelkreise spricht. Quantitative und qualitative Veränderungen der $GABA_A$-Rezeptoren konnten durch histologische Untersuchungen und in PET-Studien gefunden werden (Brooks-Kayal, Pritchett, 1993; Chugani et al., 2001). Auch wenn eine Metaanalyse der Studien auf Grund der unterschiedlichen Altersgruppen nicht möglich ist, wird die Hypothese der Reifung der intracorticalen GABAergen Regelkreise hierdurch gestärkt. Über die klinischen Implikationen kann hier nur spekuliert werden. Eine größere Häufigkeit zerebraler Krampfanfälle im Kindesalter ist bekannt, eine mögliche Ursache könnte die leichtere

	Erwachsene	Kinder
Spule	fokal	nicht fokal
Interstimulus-intervalle	5-8	1
Untersuchungszeit	45 Min.	15 Min.
Impulszahl pro Intervall	4	12

Abb. 5: Pädiatrische Modifikation zur Durchführung der Paired Pulse Technik. Durch die Reduzierung der Untersuchung auf ein Interstimulusintervall kann die Untersuchungzeit signifikant verkürzt werden und auch bei Kindern ab 6 Jahre durchgeführt werden.

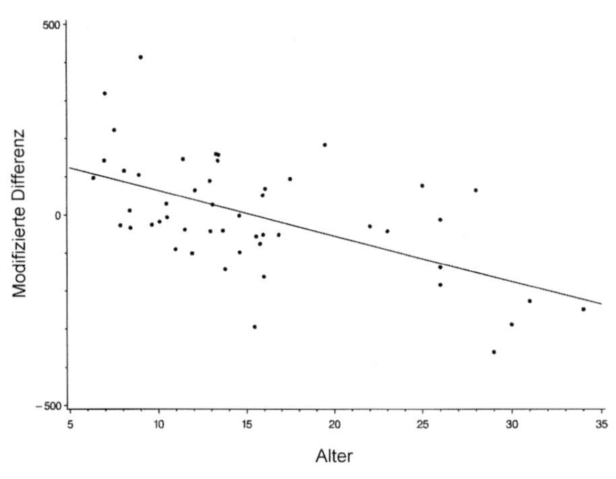

Abb. 6: Darstellung der Ergebnisse nach Paired Pulse Stimulation. Die modifizierte Differenz (modDIFF = Alter –0.4 x Amplitude (nach unkonditionierter Stimulation)) dient als mathematisches Modell zur Darstellung des linearen Zusammenhangs zwischen Alter und intracorticaler Inhibition. Ein niedriger Wert entspricht einer hohen Inhibition, ein hoher Wert einer geringen Inhibition.

Erregungsausbreitung aufgrund einer verminderten intracorticalen Inhibition darstellen. Des weiteren könnte eine verminderte intracorticale Inhibition im Kindesalter zu einer erhöhten neuronalen Plastizität beitragen und somit motorische Lernvorgänge unterstützen.

Literatur

1. Brooks-Kayal AR, Pritchett DB (1993) Developmental changes in human gamma-aminobutyric acidA receptor subunit composition. *Annals of Neurology,* **34**, 687–693.
2. Chugani DC, Muzik O, Juhasz C, Janisse JJ, Ager J, Chugani HT (2001) Postnatal maturation of human $GABA_A$-receptors measured with positron emission tomography. *Annals of Neurology,* **49**, 618–626.
3. Eyre JA, Miller S, Clowry GJ, Conway EA, Watts C (2000) Functional corticospinal projections are established prenatally in the human foetus permitting involvement in the development of spinal motor centres. *Brain,* **123**, 51–64.

4. Fietzek UM, Heinen F, Berweck S, Maute S, Hufschmidt A, Schulte-Mönting J, et al (2000) Development of the corticospinal system and hand motor function: central conduction times and motor performance tests. *Developmental Medicine & Child Neurology,* **42**, 220–227.
5. Heinen F, Glocker FX, Fietzek UM, Meyer B-U, Lücking CH, Korinthenberg R (1998) Absence of transcallosal inhibition following focal magnetic stimulation in pre-school children. *Annals of Neurology,* **43**, 608–612.
6. Heinen F, Kirschner J, Fietzek UM, Glocker FX, Mall V, Korinthenberg R (1999) Absence of transcallosal inhibition in adolescents with diplegic cerebral palsy. *Muscle & Nerve,* **22**, 255–257.
7. Müller K, Hömberg V, Lenard H-G (1991) Magnetic stimulation of motor cortex and nerve roots in children. Maturation of cortico-motoneuronal projections. *Electroencephalography and clinical Neurophysiology,* **81**, 63–70.
8. Magistris MR, Rösler KM, Truffert A, Landis T, Hess CW (1999) A clinical study of motor evoked potentials using a triple stimulation technique. *Brain,* **122**, 265–279.
9. Magistris MR, Rösler KM, Truffert A, Myers JP (1998) Transcranial stimulation excites virtually all motor neurons supplying the target muscle. A demonstration and a method improving the study of motor evoked potentials. *Brain,* **121**, 437–450.
10. Mall V, Glocker FX, Fietzek UM, Heinen F, Berweck S, Korinthenberg R, et al (2001) Inhibitory conditioning stimulus in transcranial magnetic stimulation reduces the number of excited spinal motor neurons. *Clinical Neurophysiology,* **112**, 1810–1813.
11. Ziemann U, Muellbacher W, Hallett M, Cohen LG (2001) Modulation of practice-dependent plasticity in human motor cortex. *Brain,* **124**, 1171–1181.

Ipsilaterale corticomotoneuronale Verbindungen bei Patienten mit frühkindlichen Hirnschädigungen: Relevanz für die Handmotorik

A. Schulze-Bonhage, A. Chatzikonstantinou, C.E. Elger

Zusammenfassung

Mit Hilfe fokaler transcranieller Magnetstimulation wurden plastische Veränderungen corticospinaler Projektionen bei Epilepsiepatienten mit frühkindlichen Hirnschädigungen untersucht. Funktionelle ipsilaterale corticomotoneuronale Verbindungen wurden signifkant häufiger nachgewiesen bei prä- und perinatalen Schädigungen des Motorcortex im Vergleich zu postnatalen Läsionen. Der Nachweis solcher ipsilateraler pyramidaler Projektionen korrelierte nicht mit der Güte der residuellen Handmotorik.

Schädigungen des Motorcortex werden in der Regel besser funktionell kompensiert, wenn sie sehr früh entstehen. Bereits 1866 von Vulpian als klinische Beobachtung erwähnt, wurde diese Auffassung später basierend auf Ablationsexperimenten als sog. »Kennard-Doktrin« bekannt (1, 2). Insbesondere bei ausgedehnten Läsionen, die weite Areale des primären Motorcortex miteinbeziehen, wird als ein möglicher Mechanismus einer besseren Regeneration früher Läsionen eine strukturelle Reorganisation des motorischen Cortex der intakten Hemisphäre mit Neuausbildung oder aber fehlender selektiver Elimination ipsilateraler Projektionen zu spinalen Motoneuronen angesehen, die aufgrund der kontralateralen corticalen Läsion ihrer normalen Afferenzen beraubt sind (3, 4).

Für den Erhalt einer distalen Feinmotorik, insbesondere der relativ unabhängigen Bewegungen der Finger, werden corticomotoneuronale Verbindungen des Tractus corticospinalis für unverzichtbar gehalten (5). Normalerweise lassen sich bei Stimulation des Motorcortex und Registrierung über distalen Handmuskeln nur von der kontralateralen Hemisphäre motorische Potentiale auslösen (6). Stimulationsexperimente bei Patienten mit ausgedehnten frühkindlichen Hirnschädigungen erbrachten in einigen Fällen den Nachweis ipsilateraler corticospinale Projektionen (4). Es wurde daraufhin postuliert, dass diese die Grundlage einer besseren funktionellen Restitution motorischer Funktionen darstellen (z.B. 7). In der vorliegenden Studie wurde untersucht, (a) ob bei frühen unilateralen Schädigungen des Motorcortex ipsilaterale corticomotoneuronale Projektionen des primären Motorcortex der intakten Hemisphäre zu Handmuskeln häufiger nachweisbar sind als bei späten Läsionen und (b) ob ihr Nachweis korreliert mit einer relativ besser erhaltenen Integrität der Handmotorik.

Patienten und Methodik

36 konsekutive Epilepsiepatienten mit Schädigungen motorischer corticaler Areale wurden mit Hilfe fokaler transcranieller Magnetstimulation untersucht. Die Stimulation erfolgte mit Hilfe eines Magstim 200-Magnetstimulators und einer fokalen 8-förmigen planen Spule. Diese wurde unilateral über dem motorischen Cortex der intakten Hemisphäre in einem Winkel von 45 Grad zur Linie Cz-Tragus positioniert, motorisch evozierte Potentiale (MEP) wurden bilateral mit Hilfe von Oberflächenelektroden über den Mm. interossei dorsales I registriert. Die Präsenz ipsilateraler corticomotoneuronaler Projektionsbahnen wurde anhand der Registrierung ipsilateraler MEP mit annähernd gleicher Latenz wie zur kontralateralen Seite bestimmt (vgl. Abb. 1).

Die Präsenz ipsilateraler MEP wurde korreliert zur Qualität der residuellen Handmotorik. Hierzu wurden die Patienten klassifiziert in solche mit einem Mindestkraftgrad von 3/5 (nach MRC) bei einer Fingerbewegung und in solche, die keine Bewegungen der Fingermotorik gegen die Schwerkraft ausführen konnten. Die statistische Auswertung der Korrelation ipsilateraler MEP kurzer Latenz zum Auftreten der Läsion des Motorcortex bei pränatalen und postnatalen Schädigungen erfolgte mit Hilfe des Chi^2-Tests.

Ergebnisse

Ipsilaterale MEP kurzer Latenz waren nachweisbar bei 18/36 der untersuchten Patienten (vgl. Abb. 2). Sie traten signifikant häufiger auf bei pränataler Schädigung des Motorcortex als bei postnataler Schädigung und waren in keinem Falle bei einem Alter von mehr als 1,5 Jahren bei Ausbildung der Läsion nach-

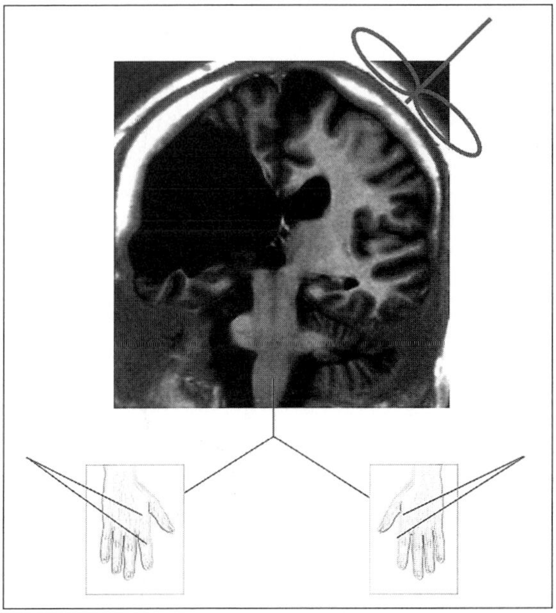

Abb. 1: Schema der Versuchsanordnung. Fokale transcranielle Magnetstimulation des primären Motorcortex der gesunden Hemisphäre mit bilateraler Registrierung motorisch evozierter Potentiale mit Hilfe von Oberflächenelektroden über den Mm. interossei dorsales I.

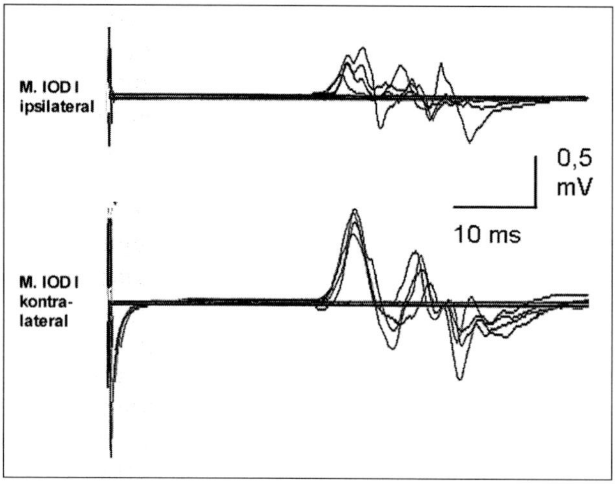

Abb. 2: Beispiel einer MEP-Registrierung mit ipsilateralen (oben) und kontralateralen (unten) MEP gleicher Latenz über den Mm. interossei dorsales I bei fokaler transcranieller Magnetstimulation über dem handmotorischen Areal der intakten Hemisphäre bei einem Patienten mit unilateraler pränataler Schädigung.

weisbar (Abb. 3). Die Amplituden der ipsilateral evozierten MEP waren signifikant niedriger als der kontralateralen.

Der Nachweis der ipsilateralen corticomotoneuronalen Verbindungen zeigte keine Korrelation zu dem Grad der Parese der Handmotorik.

Schlussfolgerung

Mit Hilfe fokaler transcranieller Magnetstimulation ließen sich bei einem Teil der untersuchten Patienten ipsilaterale cortico-motoneuronale Projektionen ausgehend von der intakten Hemisphäre nachweisen. Ihr Vorhandensein vorwiegend bei pränatalen Schädigungen des motorischen Cortex ist Ausdruck einer Reorganisation des corticospinalen Systems, die bei frühem Auftreten einer Schädigung (i.d.R. pränatal) zu einer strukturellen Reorganisation führt. Mögliche Ursachen für den Nachweis solcher ipsilateralen pyramidalen Bahnen können eine fehlende Elimination ontogenetisch primär bilateral angelegten Projektionssysteme oder ein collaterales Sprouting von Motoneuronen des primären Motorcortex der intakten Seite induziert durch eine Deafferenzierung der kontralateral zur Läsionsseite gelegenen spinalen Motoneurone sein (»branching«).

Die Untersuchung der residuellen Handmotorik der paretischen Seite zeigte jedoch, dass die Präsenz solcher solcher funktionell nachgewiesenen corticomotoneuronalen Verbindungen nicht hinreichend ist für die Integrität der Handmotorik. Eine Korrelation zur Qualität der Handmotorik ließ sich nicht nachweisen. Insbesondere fehlte eine Korrelation nicht nur bei Patienten mit mäßig ausgedehnten Läsionen, bei denen zusätzliche Einflüsse corticospinaler Projektionen von der Läsionsseite von funktioneller Relevanz sein und die funktionelle Bewertung des Einflusses ipsilateraler Projektionen erschweren können, sondern auch bei zur Behandlung einer pharmakorefraktären Epilepsie hemisphärekto-

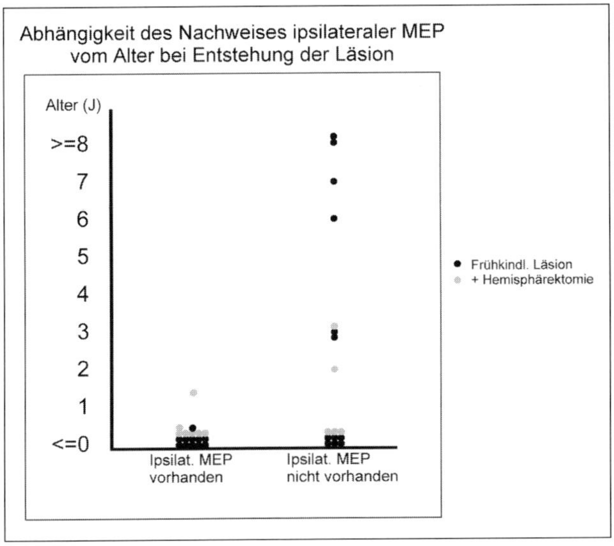

Abb. 3: Abhängigkeit der Präsenz ipsilateraler MEP bei fokaler transcranieller Magnetstimulation über dem intakten Motorcortex vom Alter des Patienten bei Auftreten der Läsion in Jahren. Ipsilaterale corticomotoneuronale Projektionen waren in der untersuchten Patientengruppe nur bei Schädigung des kontralateralen Motorcortex bis zu einem maximalen Alter von 1,5 Jahren nachweisbar.

mierten Patienten, bei denen ein Beitrag erhaltener Projektionsbahnen vom contralateralen Motorcortex ausgeschlossen werden kann.

Die fehlende funktionelle Effizienz der nachgewiesenen plastischen Veränderungen des corticospinalen Systems bei früher Schädigung stellt in Frage, ob die nachgewiesene Form corticaler Reorganisation eine sinnvolle Adaptation darstellt (vgl. hierzu (9)). Die gegenüber kontralateral geminderten Amplituden der MEP (vgl. Abb. 3) erscheinen allein nicht ausreichend, um die stark beeinträchtigte Motorik zu erklären. Es erscheint eher, dass ipsilaterale Projektionssysteme eine differenzierte Handmotorik mit unabhängigen und ausreichend kraftvollen Fingerbewegungen nicht tragen können (vgl. 10, 11). Eine mögliche Ursache für die funktionell unbefriedigende Regeneration könnte eine defiziente Ansteuerung der vom primär motorischen Cortex ausgehenden Efferenzen durch übergeordnete, prämotorische Zentren sein.

Literatur

1. Vulpian A. Lecons sur la physiologie générale et comparée du système nerveux. Paris, Baillière, vi, 1866, pp. 920 ff.
2. Kennard MA. Relation of age to motor impairment in man and in subhuman primates. Arch Neurol Psychiatr 1940; 44: 377–397
3. Barth TM, Stanfield BB. The recovery of forelimb-placing behaviour in rats with neonatal unilateral cortical damage involves the remaining hemisphere. J Neurosci 1990; 10: 3449–3459
4. Carr LJ, Harrrison LM, Evans AL, Stephens JA. Patterns of central motor reorganization in hemiplegic cerebral palsy. Brain 1993; 116: 1223–1247
5. Lawrence DG, Hopkins DA. The development of motor control in the rhesus monkey: evidence concerning the role of corticomotoneuronal connections. Brain 1976; 99: 235–254

6. Schulze-Bonhage A, Cichon BM, Ferbert A. Cortical representation of proximal and distal arm muscles as assessed by focal transcranial magnetic stimulation. Electromyogr clin Neurophysiol 1998; 38: 81–86
7. Hömberg V, Stephan KM, Netz J. Transcranial stimulation of motor cortex in upper motor neuron syndrom: its relation to the motor deficit. Electroenceph clin Neurophysiol 1992; 81: 377–388
8. Benecke R, Meyer B.-U., Freund H.-J. Reorganisation of descending motor pathways in patients after hemispherectomy and severe hemispheric lesions demonstrated by magnetic brain stimulation. Exp Brain Res 1991; 83: 419–426
9. Turton A, Lemon RN. The contribution of fast corticospinal input to the voluntary activation of proximal muscles in normal subjects and in stroke patients. Exp Brain Res 1999; 129: 559–572
10. Passingham R, Perry H, Wilkinson F. Failure to develop a precision grip in monkeys with unilateral neocortical lesions made in infancy. Brain Res 1978; 145: 410–414
11. Wiesendanger M. The pyramidal tract: its structure and function. In: Towe A, Luschei E (eds.) Handbook of Behavioral Neurobiology Vol. 5, pp. 401–491. Plenum, NY, 1981

Transkranielle Magnetstimulation bei Kindern nach schwerem Schädel-Hirn-Trauma: Funktion und Regeneration der kortikospinalen Bahnen

A.C. Binder, U.S. Maisch, U. Ziemann, H.J. Böhles, M. Kieslich

Zusammenfassung

Die transkranielle Magnetstimulation (TMS) ist eine nicht invasive Methode zur Darstellung der Funktion der kortikospinalen Bahnen. Wir untersuchten 8 Kinder, die im frühen Kindesalter ein schweres SHT erlitten haben und stellten fest, dass sowohl die kortiko-muskuläre Latenz als auch die zentral motorische Überleitungszeit (CMCT) auf der geschädigten Körperhälfte verlängert war. Besonders die motorische Schwelle über dem geschädigten Motorcortex zeigte sich noch Jahre nach dem Ereignis gegenüber der gesunden Körperseite erniedrigt.

Diese Ergebnisse demonstrieren, dass die transkranielle Magnetstimulation mit hoher Sensitivität Defizite im motorischen System nachweist. Besonders die erniedrigte motorische Schwelle legt die Schlussfolgerung nahe, dass das kindliche Gehirn bei einer Schädigung in der vulnerablen Phase wesentlich mehr Plastizität und Potential zur Regeneration besitzt als der Erwachsene, um das entstandene Defizit auszugleichen.

Einleitung

Die transkranielle Magnetstimulation (TMS) ist eine relativ neue Methode zur nicht invasiven und schmerzfreien Reizung des motorischen Cortex (M1)(1). Seit 1986 findet die transkranielle Magnetstimulation des motorischen Systems routinemäßig Anwendung in der Erwachsenen Neurologie und etablierte sich als eine wenig schmerzhafte und rasch durchführbare »bedsite« Methode in der klinisch-neurophysiologischen Diagnostik. Koh und Eyre veröffentlichten 1988 erstmals Ergebnisse über die transkranielle Magnetstimulation bei Kindern. Allgemein dient die transkranielle Magnetstimulation zur Erfassung von Läsionen im Bereich des Motorcortex und des kortikospinalen Traktes.

Wir untersuchten mit Hilfe der TMS die Funktion und Reorganisation des motorischen Cortex und des kortikospinalen Traktes bei Kindern nach schwerem Schädel-Hirn-Trauma.

Methodik

8 Patienten im Alter von 10 bis 18 Jahren mit Schädel-Hirn-Trauma im frühen Kindesalter wurden im Rahmen der Studie klinisch-neurologisch untersucht und

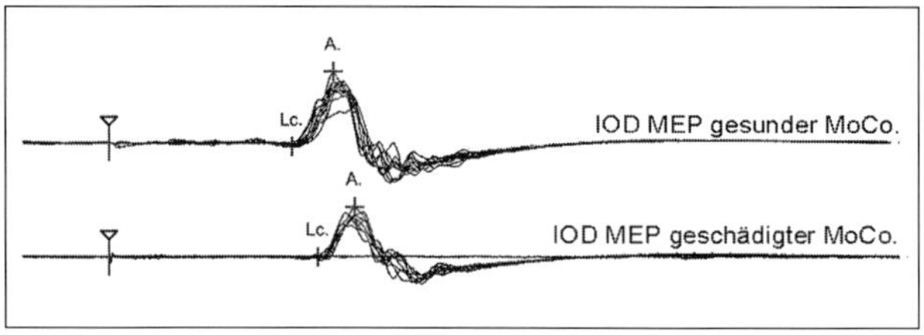

Abb. 1: Aufzeichnung motorisch evozierter Potentiale des Handareals.

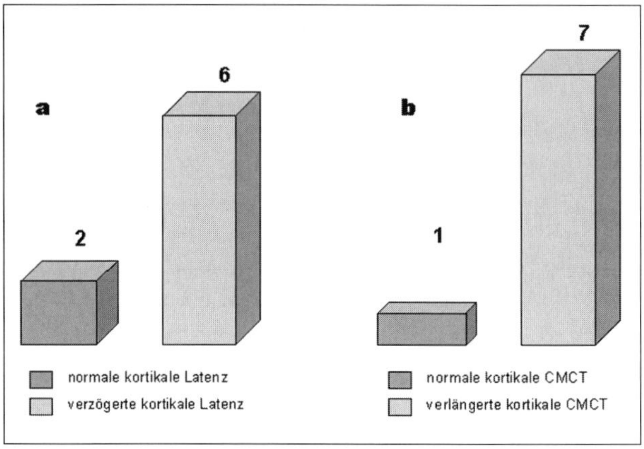

Abb. 2: Verhalten von kortikaler Latenz (a) und CMCT (b) des IOD bei Stimulation über dem geschädigten MoCo von n = 8 Kindern.

im Anschluss eine transkranielle Magnetstimulation des Motorcortex und der Spinalwurzeln durchgeführt. Gereizt wurde mittels einer 8ter Spule, mit der eine fokale Stimulation des motorischen Cortex möglich ist. Die Ableitung der so ausgelösten motorisch evozierten Potentiale (MEP) erfolgte am vorinnervierten m. interosseus dorsalis I (IOD) und m. tibialis anterior (TIB). Die MEPs wurden bezüglich kortikaler und spinaler Latenz, Amplitude, zentral motorischer Überleitungszeit (CMCT) und motorischer Schwelle analysiert. Die kortikale und spinale Latenz bezeichnen den zeitlichen Abstand zwischen der Reizung des Motorcortex bzw. des Spinalmarks bis zum Erscheinen des MEP am Zielmuskel. Die CMCT beschreibt die Zeit, die die Erregung benötigt um vom motorischen Cortex zum α-Motorneuron zu gelangen. Die minimalste Reizstärke mit der ein MEP über 50 µV ausgelöst wird und mindestens einmal reproduzierbar ist, ist per definitionem die motorische Schwelle. Diese Parameter, erhoben über dem gesunden Motorcortex, wurden von uns mit den Ergebnissen des geschädigten Motorcortex verglichen.

Ergebnisse

Die Analyse der kortiko-muskulären Latenz zeigte im Seitenvergleich in 6 von insgesamt 8 Patienten eine eindeutig verzögerte Latenz über dem geschädigten motorischen Cortex bei Ableitung vom m. interosseus dorsalis I (s. Abb. 1 u. 2a). Bei wiederholter Stimulation des geschädigten Motorcortex und Ableitung

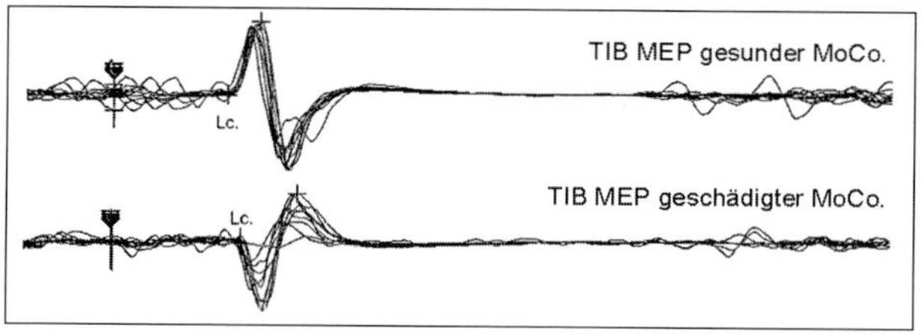

Abb. 3: Aufzeichnung motorisch evozierter Potentiale des Beinareals.

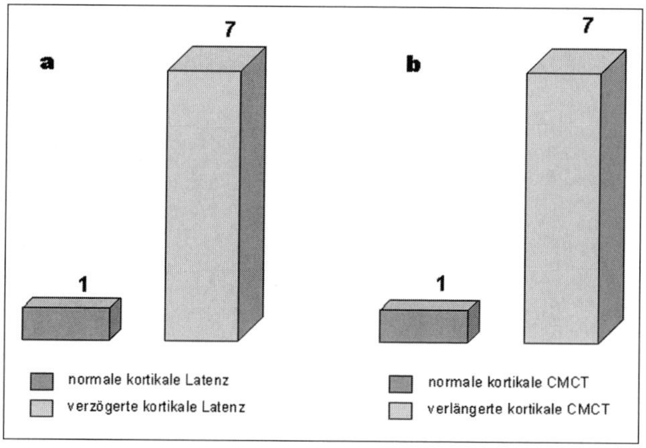

Abb. 4: Verhalten von kortikaler Latenz (a) und CMCT (b) des TIB bei Stimulation über dem geschädigten Motorcortex von n = 8 Kindern.

der MEPs vom m. tibialis anterior zeigte sich die Latenz im Seitenvergleich bei 7 von 8 Patienten verzögert (s. Abb. 3 u. 4a).

Die CMCT des Hand- und des Beinareals stellte sich in 7 von 8 Patienten bei Reizung des geschädigten motorischen Cortex ebenfalls verlängert dar (s. Abb. 2b u.4b).

Insbesondere fand sich bei Ableitung vom m. tibialis anterior in 5 von 8 Patienten eine Senkung der motorischen Schwelle bei Reizung der geschädigten Hemisphäre (s. Abb. 5).

Es zeigten sich bei allen Kindern keine auffallenden Seitendifferenzen zwischen gesundem und geschädigtem motorischen Cortex bei Analyse der Amplitude und der spinalen Latenz.

In der klinisch-neurologischen Untersuchung zeigten 4 Patienten einen komplett unauffälligen neurologischen Status ohne Hinweis auf ein neurologisches Defizit und 4 Patienten minimalste Zeichen einer nur diskreten oder latenten Hemiparese. Alle Patienten mit einem unauffälligen neurologischen Status befanden sich unter denjenigen Kindern, die deutliche Veränderungen der TMS-Parameter auf der geschädigten Körperseite aufwiesen.

Diskussion

Betrachtet man die erhaltenen Parameter in ihrer Gesamtheit, legen diese Ergebnisse die Schlussfolgerung nahe, dass im Kindesalter im Gegensatz zu

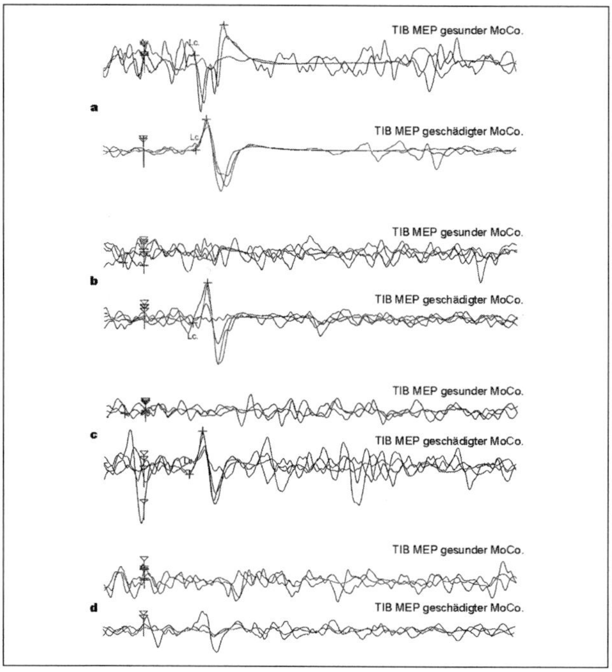

Abb. 5: Aufzeichnung mittels unterschiedlicher Reizstärke ermittelter motorisch evozierter Potentiale zur Bestimmung der motorischen Schwelle:
a) Reizstärke von 70%
b) Reizstärke von 60%
c) Reizstärke von 50%
d) Reizstärke von 45%

Erwachsenen noch Jahre nach einer akuten cerebralen Schädigung im Rahmen eines schweren Schädel-Hirn-Traumas eine Reorganisation der motorischen kortiko-neuronalen Bahnen stattfindet (2). Erkennbar durch die heute, 5–10 Jahre nach dem akuten Ereignis, noch erniedrigte motorische Schwelle über dem geschädigten motorischen Cortexareal.

Des weiteren ist die transkranielle Magnetstimulation in der Lage eine Änderung der motorischen Repräsentation des defizienten motorischen Systems während der motorischen Regenerationsphase nachzuweisen (3, 4).

Selbst bei Patienten ohne oder mit nur sehr diskreten klinischen Zeichen auf ein neurologisches Defizit kann die transkranielle Magnetstimulation deutliche Hinweise auf einen Integritätsverlust des motorischen Cortex und des kortikospinalen Traktes geben.

Literatur

1. Ziemann U (2001) Transkranielle Magnetstimulation: Neue Einsatzmöglichkeiten zur Messung kortikospinaler Erregbarkeit. Akt neurol 28:249–264
2. Transversa R et all. (2000 Sep) Neurophysiological follow-up of motor cortical output in stroke patients. Clin Neurophysiol 111(9):1695–703
3. Trompetto C et all. (2000 Oct) Motor recovery follwing stroke: a transcranial magnetic stimulation study. Clin Neurophysiol 111(10):1860–7
4. Ziemann U (2000) Transcranial magnetic stimulation: Its current role in the evaluation of patients post-stroke. Neurology Report Vol.24 No.3:82–93

Klinische und wissenschaftliche Anwendungen der Magnetoenzephalographie (MEG) im Kindesalter

T. Bast, A. Rupp, A. Seitz, M. Scherg, D. Rating

Zusammenfassung

In der Pädiatrie nimmt das MEG eine Außenseiterstellung innerhalb der Methoden der Hirnfunktionsdiagnostik ein, da die Messung von Magnetfeldern, die durch die intrazellulären Ströme der kortikalen Neurone entstehen, technisch aufwendig und daher nicht überall verfügbar ist. Der Vorteil des MEG gegenüber dem EEG besteht vor allem in dem deutlich geringeren Einfluss der elektrischen Eigenschaften des Volumenleiters auf die Analyse und Lokalisation äquivalenter Stromdipole. Im MEG kommen nahezu ausschließlich tangentiale Quellen zur Darstellung; im EEG hingegen dominieren radiale Aktivitäten. Das MEG ist dem EEG daher in der Detektion tangentialer (fissuraler) Aktivität, z.B. in der Zentralregion oder Sylvischen Fissur, überlegen. Bei rein radialen Quellen kann dem MEG hingegen wesentliche Information entgehen. Aufgrund dieser komplementären Abbildungseigenschaften hirnelektrischer Aktivität ist die simultane Ableitung von EEG und MEG sinnvoll.

Das MEG wird bevorzugt in der neurophysiologischen Forschung zur Analyse von Perzeption und kortikaler Verarbeitung (z.B. visuell oder akustisch) eingesetzt. Hierbei ergänzt das MEG wegen seiner wesentlich höheren zeitlichen Auflösung bis zu mehreren kHz die Ergebnisse der funktionellen MRT, die im Vergleich ein höheres räumliches Auflösungsvermögen besitzt.

Ein Schwerpunkt der epileptologischen MEG-Forschung liegt im Bereich der benignen Partialepilepsien. Daneben wird das MEG im Rahmen der prächirurgischen Epilepsiediagnostik als ergänzende nicht-invasive Methode zur Identifikation irritativer Zonen (Spikelokalisation) und funktioneller Areale (evozierte Felder) angewendet. Hierbei kann das MEG Informationen zur intrinsischen Epileptogenität einer Läsion, z.B. bei kortikaler Malformation, beitragen. Bei einigen unserer Patienten mit symptomatischen Partialepilepsien lag die Rate an detektierten Spikes höher als im EEG, z.B. bei fronto- oder temporobasaler irritativer Zone oder im Schlaf (wegen Überlagerung des EEG-Signals durch physiologische Schlafveränderungen mit radialer Orientierung).

Das MEG liefert, vor allem kombiniert mit dem Oberflächen-EEG, als nicht-invasive Methode zusätzliche Informationen in der epileptologischen und neurophysiologisch-funktionellen Diagnostik.

Physikalische und technische Grundlagen

Jeder elektrische Strom erzeugt gemäß dem Biot-Savart-Gesetz ein Magnetfeld das senkrecht zum entsprechenden elektrischen Potentialfeld steht. Dies gilt auch für die sehr kleinen (50–500 fT) Magnetfelder, die durch intraneuronale elektrische Ströme erzeugt werden. Bei der Magnetoenzephalographie (MEG) handelt es sich um die berührungsfreie Messung dieser Magnetfeldänderungen. Wie für das EEG gilt, dass die einzelne Zelle kein detektierbares Signal erzeugt. Gemessen wird die Summe der elektromagnetischen Signale von Zellen mit gleicher Orientierung zum selben Zeitpunkt. Diese Bedingung wird intrakortikal überwiegend durch die Pyramidenzellen erfüllt und zum Signal tragen überwiegend exzitatorische postsynaptische Potentiale bei.

David Cohen gelang es erstmals 1968 mit hochempfindlichen Spulen den menschlichen Alpha-Rhythmus zu messen (3). 1972 setzte er erstmals supraleitende Detektoren ein (4). Da die zu messenden Magnetfelder wesentlich kleiner als die Störfelder der Laborumgebung (d.h. aller technischen Geräte) sind, muss eine Messung in magnetisch abgeschirmten Kabinen erfolgen (Abb. 1). MEG Messungen sind hoch anfällig für jede Art technischer und biologischer elektrischer Artefakte. Durch die Entwicklung der SQUIDS (Supraconducting Quantum Interference Devices) konnten Vielkanal-Ganzkopf-MEG-Geräte mit niedrigem Rauschniveau eingeführt werden. Für die im folgenden angeführten Beispiele erfolgte die Messung mit einem 122-Kanal Ganzkopf-Gradiometer (Neuromag-122®, Abb. 1 [Salmelin 1993]).

Für die Messung der neuronal entstehenden Magnetfelder gelten folgende Besonderheiten:

1. Die Größe des Magnetfeldes nimmt mit dem Abstand im Quadrat ab. Dies erlaubt dem MEG lediglich eine Aussage bis zu einer intrakraniellen Tiefe von ca. 5 cm.

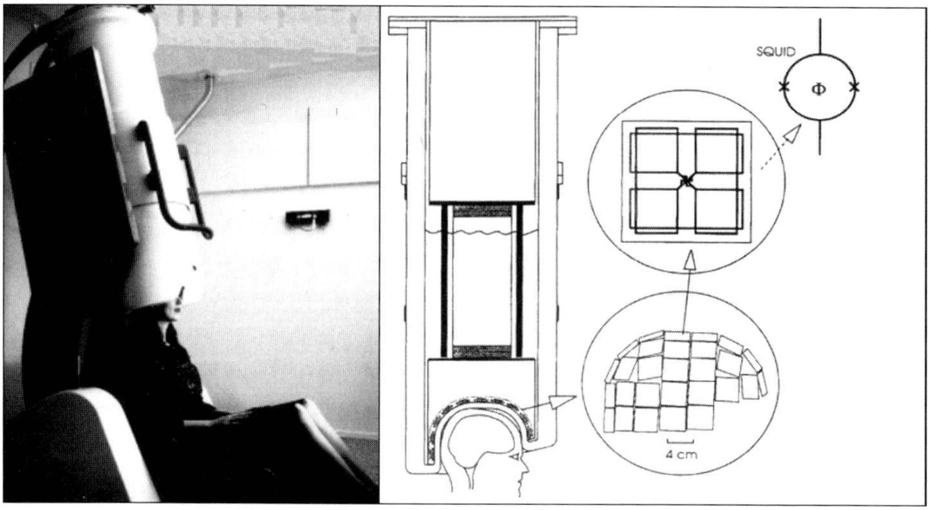

Abb. 1: Neuromag-122® Ganzkopf-Gradiometer und Abschirmkammer (Salmelin 1993)

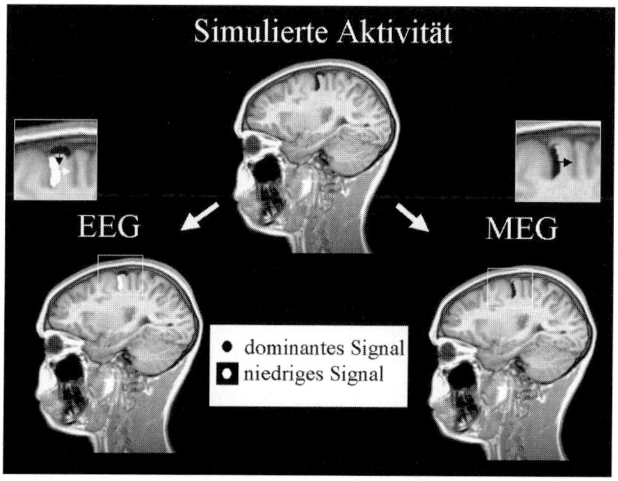

Abb. 2: Simulation kortikaler Aktivität und resultierender Signale in EEG und MEG
Oben: angenommen wird eine Aktivierung eins Gyrus an der Oberfläche (radiale Neurone) und in der Fissur (tangentiale Neurone).
Unten: Das EEG Signal (links) wird dominiert durch die oberflächlichen, radialen Neurone. Das MEG (rechts) erfasst ausschließlich Aktivitäten der fissuralen, tangentialen Neurone.
Die vergrößerten Ausschnitte zeigen das resultierende Dipolmodell.

2. Die Magnetfelder werden nicht durch die Volumenleitereigenschaften der den Kortex umgebenden Gewebe beeinflusst. Dies bedingt den größten Vorteil des MEG gegenüber dem EEG: Für die 3-dimensionale Berechnung eines äquivalenten Stromdipols (»Dipollokalisation«) spielt das zu Grunde liegende Kopfmodell eine entscheidende Rolle, wenn es sich um EEG Messungen handelt. Realistische Kopfmodelle minimieren hierbei den Fehler durch Verzerrung der elektrischen Fernpotentiale, können ihn aber nicht wirklich individuell vermeiden. Gerade für den kindlichen Schädel ist wenig über die elektrischen Eigenschaften der Umgebungsgewebe bekannt. Für die MEG Quellenlokalisation reichen in der Regel einfache Kopfmodelle aus.
Die im folgenden demonstrierten Befunde wurden auf der Grundlage eines elipsoiden Kopfmodelles mit multipler Quellenanalyse erstellt (BESA2000®). Die Überlagerung mit individuellen 3D-T1-MRT Datensätzen erfolgte mit BrainVoyager® (BrainInnovation, R. Göbel, Maastricht).
3. Das MEG erfasst nahezu ausschließlich Aktivitäten, die durch tangential zur Kopfoberfläche fließende elektrische Ströme entstehen. Rein radial orientierte elektrische Quellen erzeugen keinen messbaren magnetischen Gradienten an der Kopfoberfläche und entgehen dem MEG komplett. Für den Kortex gilt vereinfacht: im MEG stellen sich ausschließlich die Aktivitäten der fissuralen Neurone dar, da deren Dendriten tangential zur Kopfoberfläche verlaufen (ca. 2/3 aller Pyramidenzellen liegen in den Fissuren). Im EEG überwiegen dagegen die Aktivitäten der oberflächlichen, radial orientierten Neurone an der Oberkante der Gyri. Die tieferen, tangentialen Aktivitäten tragen zwar ebenfalls zum EEG Signal bei, werden jedoch nicht unerheblich von den radialen Aktivitäten überlagert. Abbildung 2 zeigt eine 2-dimensionale Simulation. Da EEG und MEG quasi teilkomplementäre Informationen liefern empfiehlt sich die simultane Messung mit beiden Methoden.
4. Während die EEG Elektroden auf der Kopfhaut befestigt sind, kann sich der Kopf frei im DEWAR (Kryostat, s. Abb. 1) des MEG bewegen. Zu Beginn

einer Messung wird die Kopfposition bestimmt. Diese darf während einer Messung nicht verändert werden, was eine gewisse Kooperationsfähigkeit des Patienten voraussetzt. Wir selbst konnten in der Regel Kinder ab einem Alter von sechs Jahren untersuchen. Bei Patienten mit Bewegungsunruhe gelingt häufig eine Ableitung im Schlaf.

Im Vergleich von MEG und EEG ergeben sich die in Tabelle 1 aufgeführten Unterschiede.

Tab. 1: Vergleich von EEG und MEG

EEG	MEG
Allgemeines	
Begrenzte Kanalzahl (32–64)	Hohe Kanalzahl (bis über 300)
Überall verfügbar	Begrenzt verfügbar
»Günstig«	»Teuer«
Auch bei unkooperativen Patienten einsetzbar	Wegen Bewegungsanfälligkeit nur bei kooperativen Patienten oder im Schlaf
Technik und biophysikalische Aspekte	
Signalentstehung durch Potentialdifferenzen durch Ströme im Volumenleiter	Signalentstehung durch Magnetfeldänderungen durch intrazelluläre Ströme in Neuronen
Niedrigeres Signal-zu-Rausch Verhältnis	Höheres Signal-zu-Rausch Verhältnis
Bei Frequenzen von 1–40 Hz ca. 10 : 1	Bei Frequenzen von 1–40 Hz ca. 4 : 1
	Abbildungstiefe bis ca. 5 cm
Dipollokalisation/ Quellenanalyse stark abhängig vom Kopfmodell (Volumenleitung)	Dipollokalisation/ Quellenanalyse wenig abhängig vom Kopfmodell
Signal wird dominiert durch oberflächliche, radial orientierte Neurone. Die Aktivität fissuraler, tangentialer Neurone wird ebenfalls, allerdings überlagert abgebildet.	Zum Signal tragen nahezu ausschließlich fissurale, tangential orientierte Neurone bei (2/3 aller Pyramidenzellen).

Klinische und wissenschaftliche Anwendungen des MEG

Untersuchung ereigniskorrelierter Aktivitäten

Im Bereich der Neurowissenschaften wird das MEG überwiegend zur Analyse von Perzeption und kortikaler Verarbeitung durch die Untersuchung ereigniskorrelierter Veränderungen eingesetzt.

In der Grundlagenforschung trägt das MEG unter anderem Informationen zur Psychoakustik (21, 23), zum visuellen System (16, 24, 29) und zur Analyse von Schmerzverarbeitung bei (27).

Bei der Analyse der Perzeption und der kortikalen Verarbeitung überschneiden sich die Fragestellungen der MEG basierten Forschung mit denen des fMRT. Während das fMRT eine höhere lokalisatorische Aussagekraft hat, ist die zeitliche Auflösung des MEG (und auch des EEG) ungleich höher, so dass die elektrophysiologischen Methoden für alle Prozesse mit rascher kortikaler Ver-

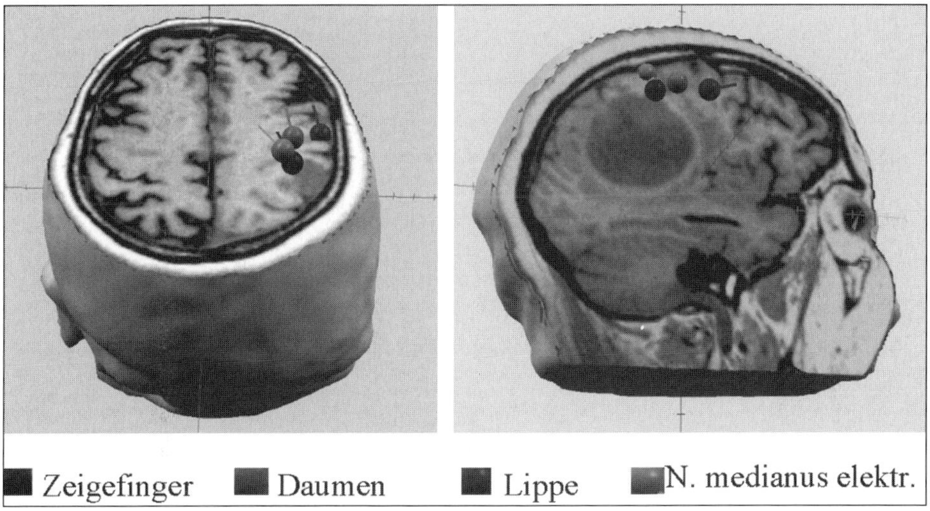

Abb. 3: Dipollokalisation somatosensibel evozierter Felder bei einem Tumorpatienten mittels taktiler Stimulation der kontralateralen Finger und elektrischer Medianusstimulation (Dr. Kai Druen, Sektion Biomagnetismus, Abteilung Neurologie der Universitätsklinik Heidelberg).

arbeitung und Propagation von Interesse sind. Für die zukünftige Forschung zeichnet sich ab, dass es sinnvoll sein kann, für das fMRT und das MEG die selben Paradigmen zu verwenden, um eine maximale Information zu erhalten (»fMRT: wo liegt das Zentrum einer Aktivierung?, MEG: welchen zeitlichen Verlauf nimmt die Aktivierung?«).

Bei Kindern liegen deutlich weniger Untersuchungen vor, z.B. zur Entwicklung der Somatosensibililtät (5), zu Plastizität von Sensibilität und Sprachkortex (22) oder auch Veränderungen des auditorischen Kortex bei Dyslexie (8).

Die Untersuchung ereigniskorrelierter Aktivitäten bietet auch Anwendungsmöglichkeiten in der klinischen Praxis: So kann die Zentralregion im Rahmen einer prächirurgischen Abklärung durch die Lokalisation somatosensibel oder motorisch evozierter Felder identifiziert werden (11, 15) (Abb. 3). Auch eine Lateralisation und Lokalisation der Sprachfunktion ist möglich (1, 2, 25).

Epilepsiediagnostik

Im Bereich der Epilepsiediagnostik kann das MEG immer dann hilfreich sein, wenn es sich um die Analyse tangentialer Aktivitäten handelt (s.o.). Einen besonderen Nutzen lässt das MEG hierbei für Aktivitäten erwarten, die sich in Fissuren (auch mesial im Interhemisphärenspalt) oder an der Hirnbasis (fronto- oder temporobasal) abspielen. In Einzelfällen konnten wir für diese Lokalisationen die Überlegenheit des MEG gegenüber dem EEG, was die Anzahl detektierter Spikes betrifft, demonstrieren (Abb. 4).

Im Bereich der pädiatrischen Epileptologie liegen zahlreiche Berichte zu Untersuchungen bei idiopathischen fokalen Epilepsien vor. In der Regel geht es um eine Analyse der klassischen, tangential orientierten rolandischen Sharp-

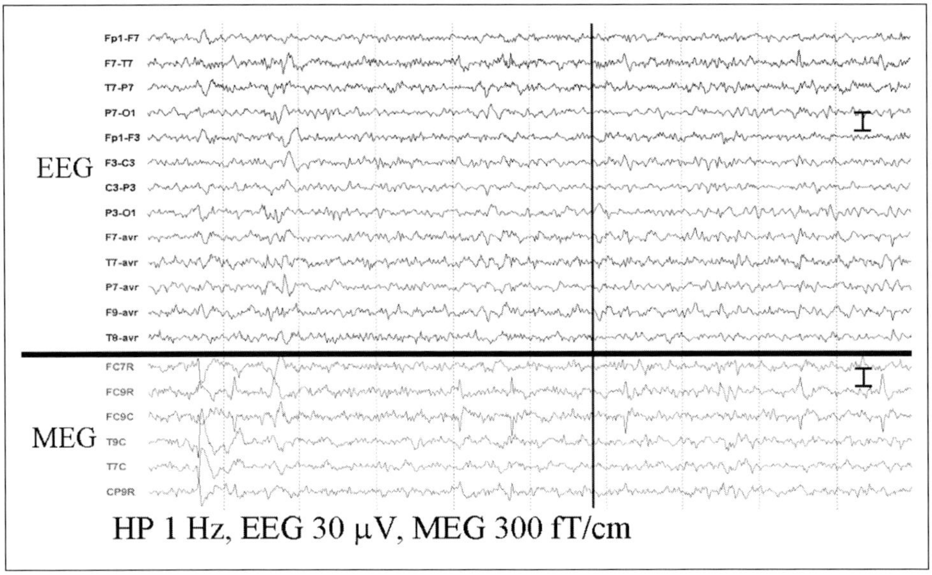

Abb. 4: Simultanes EEG und MEG bei einem Patienten mit Temporallappenepilepsie links. Die Spikes sind im MEG wesentlich deutlicher dargestellt. Dies liegt an der tangentialen Orientierung bei temporobasalen Spikes.

waves (14) mit dem Versuch, neuropsychologische Phänomene mit Lokalisation und Aufbau dieser Sharp-waves in Verbindung zu setzen (10, 30, 31). Neben den typischen Rolandoepilepsien sind auch die atypischen Formen, insbesondere das Landau-Kleffner-Syndrom, von Interesse für den MEG Einsatz (20, 26). Paetau et al. gelang es mit Hilfe des MEG nachzuweisen, dass sich bei Patienten mit Landau-Kleffner-Syndrom Spikes durch akustische Reize provozieren lassen (18). Ähnliche Untersuchungen gibt es zu den taktil evozierten Riesenpotentialen bei Rolandoepilepsien (12, 13). Bei einem eigenen Patienten konnten wir durch Stimulation des Daumens und (wenn auch weniger deutlich) des Zeigefingers der kontralateralen Hand Sharp-waves provozieren die sich von den spontanen Sharp-waves hinsichtlich der Lokalisation und des Aufbaus nicht unterschieden (Abb. 5). Interessant war hierbei die deutliche Somatotopie: die Stimulation des kleinen Fingers und der Lippe führte lediglich zu physiologischen evozierten Aktivitäten.

Bei Erwachsenen ließ sich zeigen, dass die MEG Quellenlokalisation als ergänzende nicht-invasive Methode im Rahmen einer prächirurgischen Abklärung hilfreich ist. So formulierten Stefan et al. bereits sehr früh, dass es ein Ziel der MEG Analyse sein kann, das Ausmaß und die Anzahl invasiver diagnostischer Prozeduren zu reduzieren (28). So kann z.B. die Lokalisation einer irritativen Zone (interiktale Spikes) in Bezug zu einer sichtbaren Läsion mit Hilfe des MEG eingehend untersucht werden (Abb. 5 und 6).

Auch bei Kindern liegen zwischenzeitlich positive Resultate bei Vergleich von MEG Quellenlokalisation und invasiver Diagnostik (15, 17) und gerade auch in der Korrelation zum OP-Outcome (15, 19) vor.

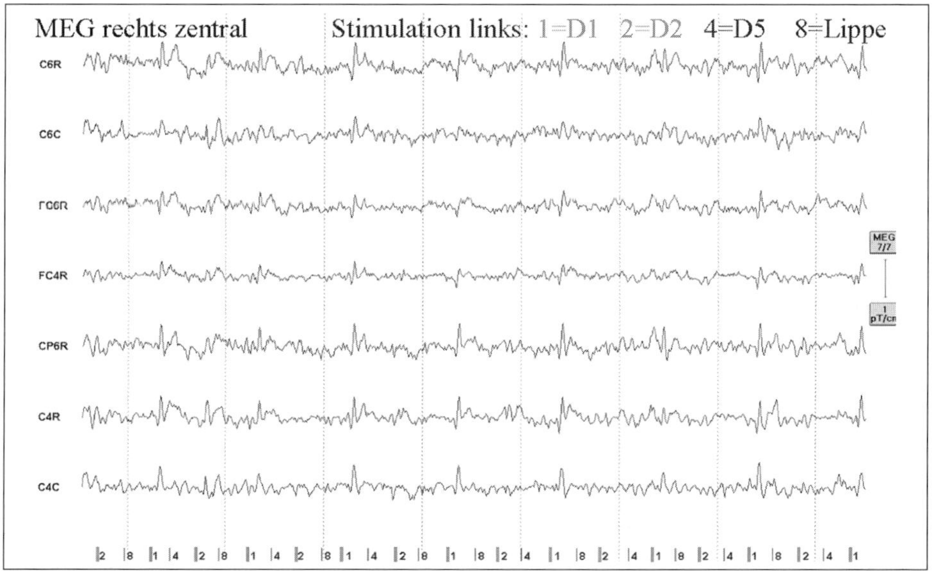

Abb. 5: 8jähriger Patient mit BECTS (spontane SW rechts zentrotemporal). MEG Ableitung mit taktiler Stimulation der Finger und Lippe links. Beachte: Auf Trigger 1 (Daumen links) erfolgt jeweils ein »Riesenpotential«.

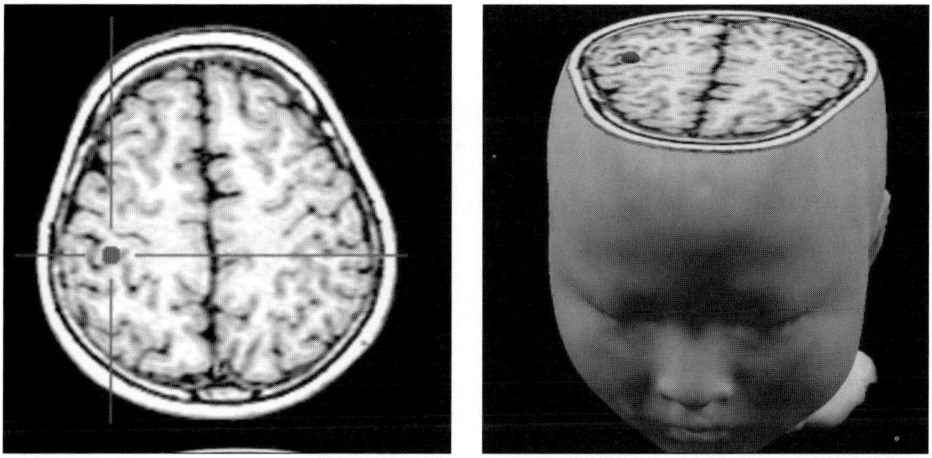

Abb. 6: 8jähriger Patient mit BECTS. Die Quellenlokalisation von 250 gemittelten Somatosensibel evozierten Felder zeigt einen Ursprung im Handareal postzentral. Die multiple Quellenlokalisation zeigt, dass sich die evozierten Felder räumlich und zeitlich genau wie die spontanen Sharp-Waves verhalten, so dass es sich um getriggerte Sharp-Waves handelt.

Auch jenseits der Epilepsiechirurgie rückt das MEG in das Interesse, da es gerade im Kindesalter als nicht-invasive Methode die Möglichkeit zusätzlicher Information bietet. Selbst Kinder mit West-Syndrom wurden jüngst mittels MEG untersucht, wenngleich die Ergebnisse bei 14 Patienten recht diffuse, bilaterale Ergebnisse erbrachten (7).

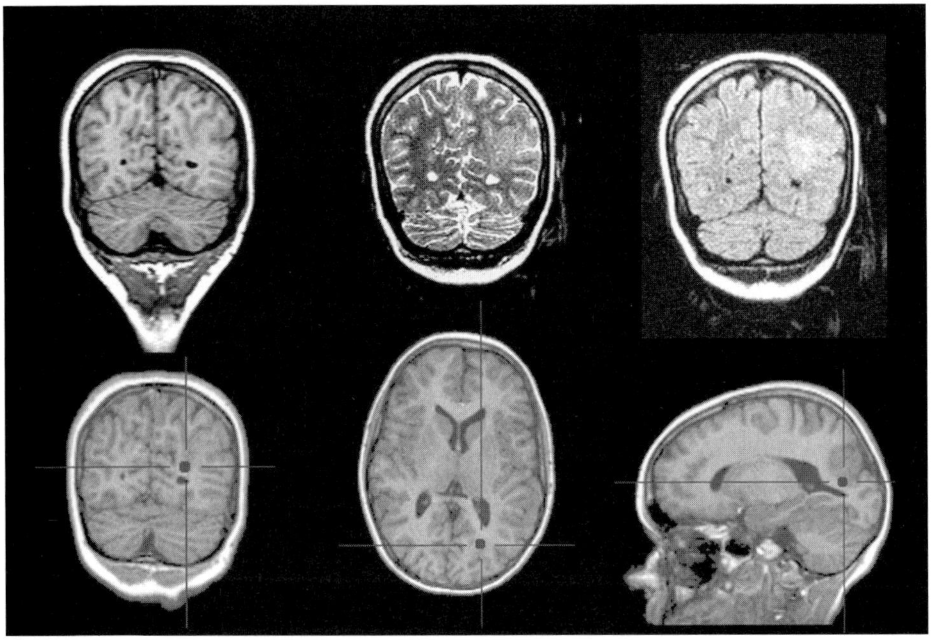

Abb. 7: CR, w, 14,5 Jahre: Fokale kortikale Dysplasie links okzipital. T1, T2 und Flair gewichtete MRT. Quellenlokalisation des Onsets von 21 gemittelten MEG Spikes innerhalb der sichtbaren Läsion.

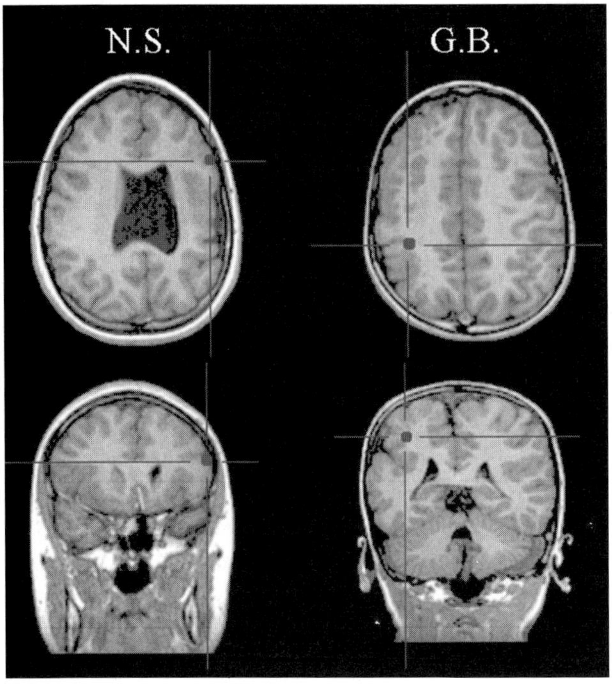

Abb. 8: Links: NS, w, 12,5 Jahre: Polymikrogyrie. Quellenlokalisation von 41 gemittelten MEG Spikes. Onset im vorderen Übergangsbereich der Läsion.
Rechts: GB, m, 7,5 Jahre: Polymikrogyrie. Quellenlokalisation von 27 gemittelten MEG Spikes. Spikeonset in der hinteren Übergangszone.

Schlussfolgerung

Das MEG bietet sich als Methode immer dann an, wenn es um die zeitliche und räumliche Analyse rascher kortikaler Prozesse mit Beteiligung tangential orientierter Neurone geht. In der Neuropsychologie gilt dies insbesondere für die Untersuchung psychoakustischer Phänomene (Heschl Gyrus). Für die Epileptologie sind die typischen und atypischen idiopathischen fokalen Epilepsien von besonderen Interesse. Das MEG liefert als nicht-invasive Methode im Rahmen der prächirurgischen Lokalisationsdiagnostik bedeutende zusätzliche Informationen.

Literatur

1. Breier JI, Simos PG, Wheless JW, Constantinou JE, Baumgartner JE, Venkataraman V, Papanicolaou AC (2001) Language dominance in children as determined by magnetic source imaging and the intracarotid amobarbital procedure: a comparison. J Child Neurol 16:124–130
2. Castillo EM, Simos PG, Venkataraman V, Breier JI, Wheless JW, Papanicolaou AC (2001) Mapping of expressive language cortex using magnetic source imaging. Neurocase 7: 419–422
3. Cohen D (1968) Magnetoencephalography: Evidence of magnetic fields produced by alpha-rhythm currents. Science, 161: 784–786
4. Cohen D (1972) Magnetoencephalography: Detection of the brain´s electrical activity with a superconduction magnetometer. Science, 175: 664–666
5. Gondo K, Tobimatsu S, Kira R, Tokunaga Y, Yamamoto T, Hara T (2001) A magnetoencephalographic study on development of the somatosensory cortex in infants. Neuroreport 12: 3227–3231
6. Gutschalk A, Patterson RD, Rupp A, Uppenkamp S, Scherg M (2002) Sustained magnetic fields reveal separate sites for sound level and temporal regularity in human auditory cortex. Neuroimage 15: 207–216
7. Hattori H, Yamano T, Tsutada T, Tsuyuguchi N, Kawawaki H, Shimogawara M (2001) Magnetoencephalography in the detection of focal lesions in West syndrome. Brain Dev 23: 528–532
8. Heim S, Eulitz C, Kaufmann J, Fuchter I, Pantev C, Lamprecht-Dinnesen A, Matulat P, Scheer P, Borstel M, Elbert T (2000) Atypical organisation of the auditory cortex in dyslexia as revealed by MEG. Neuropsychologia 38:1749–1759
9. Hoechstetter K, Rupp A, Stancak A, Meinck HM, Stippich C, Berg P, Scherg M (2001) Interaction of tactile input in the human primary and secondary somatosensory cortex – a magnetoencephalographic study. Neuroimage 14: 759–767
10. Kamada K, Moller M, Saguer M, Kassubek J, Kaltenhauser M, Kober H, Uberall M, Lauffer H, Wenzel D, Vieth J (1998) Localization analysis of neuronal activities in benign rolandic epilepsy using magnetoencephalography. J Neurol Sci 154: 164–172
11. Kober H, Nimsky C, Moller M, Hastreiter P, Fahlbusch R, Ganslandt O (2001) Correlation of sensorimotor activation with functional magnetic resonance imaging and magnetoencephalography in presurgical functional imaging: a spatial analysis. Neuroimage 14: 1214–1228
12. Kubota M, Takeshita K, Sakakihara Y, Yanagisawa M (2000) Magnetoencephalographic study of giant somatosensory evoked responses in patients with rolandic epilepsy. J Child Neurol 15: 370–379
13. Minami T, Gondo K, Yanai S, Yamamoto T, Tasaki K, Ueda K (1995) Rolandic discharges and somatosensory evoked potentials in benign childhood partial epilepsy: magnetoencephalographical study. Psychiatry Clin 49: 227–228

14. Minami T, Gondo K, Yamamoto T, Yanai S, Tasaki K, Ueda K (1996) Magnetoencephalographic analysis of rolandic discharges in benign childhood epilepsy. Ann Neurol 39: 326–334
15. Minassian BA, Otsubo H, Weiss S, Elliott I, Rutka JT, Snead OC (1999) Magnetoencephalographic localization in pediatric epilepsy surgery: comparison with invasive intracranial electroencephalography. Ann Neurol 46: 627–633
16. Ohtani Y, Okamura S, Shibasaki T, Arakawa A, Yoshida Y, Toyama K, Ejima Y (2001) Magnetic responses of human visual cortex to illusory contours. Neurosci Lett 321: 173–176
17. Otsubo H, Ochi A, Elliott I, Chuang SH, Rutka JT, Jay V, Aung M, Sobel DF, Snead OC (2001) MEG predicts epileptic zone in lesional extrahippocampal epilepsy: 12 pediatric surgery cases. Epilepsia 42:1523–1530
18. Paetau R (1994) Sounds triggers spikes in the Landau-Kleffner syndrome. J Clin Neurophysiol. 11: 231–241
19. Paetau R, Hamalainen M, Hari R, Kajola M, Karhu J, Larsen TA, Lindahl E, Salonen O (1994) Magnetoencephalographic evaluation of children and adolescents with intractable epilepsy. Epilepsia 35: 275–284
20. Paetau R, Granstrom ML, Blomstedt G, Jousmaki V, Korkman M, Liukkonen E (1999) Magnetoencephalography in presurgical evaluation of children with the Landau-Kleffner syndrome. Epilepsia 40: 326–335
21. Pantev C, Lutkenhoner B (2000) Magnetoencephalographic studies of functional organization and plasticity of the human auditory cortex. J Clin Neurophysiol 17: 130–142
22. Papanicolaou AC, Simos PG, Breier JI, Wheless JW, Mancias P, Baumgartner JE, Maggio WW, Gormley W, Constantinou JE, Butler II J (2001) Brain plasticity for sensory and linguistic functions: a functional imaging study using magnetoencephalography with children and young adults. Child Neurol 16: 241–252
23. Rupp A, Hack S, Gutschalk A, Schneider P, Picton TW, Stippich C, Scherg M (2000) Fast temporal interactions in human auditory cortex. Neuroreport 27: 3731–3736
24. Schroeder CE, Mehta AD, Givre SJ (1998) A spatiotemporal profile of visual system activation revealed by current source density analysis in the awake macaque. Cereb Cortex 8: 575–592
25. Simos PG, Papanicolaou AC, Breier JI, Wheless JW, Constantinou JE, Gormley WB, Maggio WW (1999) Localization of language-specific cortex by using magnetic source imaging and electrical stimulation mapping. J Neurosurg 91: 787–796
26. Sobel DF, Aung M, Otsubo H, Smith MC (2000) Magnetoencephalography in children with Landau-Kleffner syndrome and acquired epileptic aphasia. AJNR 21:301–307
27. Soros P, Knecht S, Bantel C, Imai T, Wusten R, Pantev C, Lutkenhoner B, Burkle H, Henningsen H (2001) Functional reorganization of the human primary somatosensory cortex after acute pain demonstrated by magnetoencephalography. Neurosci Lett 298:195–198
28. Stefan H, Schneider S, Feistel H, Pawlik G, Schuler P, Abraham Fuchs K, Schlegel T, Neubauer U, Huk WJ (1992) Ictal and interictal activity in partial epilepsy recorded with multichannel magnetoelectroencephalography: correlation of electroencephalography/electrocorticography, magnetic resonance imaging, single photon emission computed zomography, and positron emission tomography findings. Epilepsia 33: 874–887
29. Taylor MJ, George N, Ducorps A (2001) Magnetoencephalographic evidence of early processing of direction of gaze in humans. Neurosci Lett 316: 173–177
30. van der Meij W, Huiskamp GJ, Rutlen GJ, Wieneke GH, van Huffelen AC, van Nieuwenhuizen O (2001) The existence of two sources in rolandic epilepsy: confirmation with high resolution EEG, MEG and fMRI. Brain Topogr 13:275–282
31. Yoshinaga H, Amano R, Oka E, Ohtahara S (1992) Dipole tracing in childhood epilepsy with special reference to rolandic epilepsy. Brain Topogr. 4: 193–199

5. Funktionelle Bildgebung – Eine Erweiterung der neurophysiologischen Untersuchungstechniken

PET und SPECT – Methodische Grundlagen und Aktivierungsstudien bei Akinese, Dystonie, Botulinumtoxin-Therapie und Tiefenhirnstimulation

A.O. Ceballos-Baumann, H. Boecker

Zusammenfassung

Die Positronenemissionstomographie (PET) und die Single-Photonen-Emissionstomographie (SPECT) stellen zwei Bildgebungsmodalitäten dar, mit denen weitgehend nicht-invasiv Hirnfunktionen *in vivo* untersucht und lokalisiert werden können. In der Neuropädiatrie ist die häufigste klinische Indikation für funktionelle Bildgebung die Epilepsie, daneben die Neuroonkologie. SPECT und PET Studien wurden ferner bei verschiedenen pädiatrischen Krankheiten wie der Dystonie, der Anorexia Nervosa, dem Autismus, dem Gilles de la Tourette Syndrom und dem Aufmerksamkeits-Defizit-Hyperaktivitäts-Syndrom durchgeführt. Der wissenschaftliche Einsatz von PET und SPECT in der Neuropädiatrie ist mit vielschichtigen wissenschaftlichen, methodischen und ethischen Herausforderungen verbunden. Beispielsweise ist die Dynamik der Hirnentwicklung und -Reifung bei der Interpretation der Ergebnisse von wesentlicher Bedeutung. Gut geplante Studien erlauben die Überprüfung von *a priori* Hypothesen, die auf dezidierten Krankheitsmodellen basieren. In dieser Übersicht soll das Hauptaugenmerk auf dem wissenschaftlichen Einsatz der PET und SPECT liegen. Nach einer Einführung in die Möglichkeiten und Probleme dieser bildgebenden Methoden in der Neuropädiatrie werden als Beispiele für das Studiendesign funktionell bildgebender Untersuchungen Aktivierungsstudien zu Bewegungsstörungen wie der Dystonie und bei Patienten mit Tiefenhirnstimulation vorgestellt.

Einleitung

Die nuklearmedizinischen Untersuchungsmethoden stellen einen wichtigen Beitrag dar zur Diagnose, zum Staging und zur Verlaufskontrolle unterschiedlicher Erkrankungen des Zentralnervensystems (ZNS) im Kindesalters. Dabei lassen sich mit der Positronenemissionstomographie (PET) und der Single Photonen Emissions Tomographie (SPECT) quasi nicht-invasiv Hirnfunktionen (z.B. cerebraler Blutfluss, Rezeptorbindung etc.) *in vivo* untersuchen und lokalisieren. Während die PET als emissions-tomographisches Verfahren auf einer Applikation kurzlebiger Positronen-emittierender Isotope beruht wird bei der SPECT durch rotierende Gamma-Kameras die Aktivitätsverteilung von Gammastrahlen im Gehirn gemessen.

Im folgenden sollen die methodischen Grundlagen der PET und SPECT Bildgebung zusammengefasst werden und schwerpunktmäßig Untersuchungen bei Parkinson- und Dystonie Patienten behandelt werden um so pathophysiologisch relevante Aspekte bei Patienten mit Bewegungsstörungen herauszustellen. Neben vielfältigen Studien bei erwachsenen Patienten, auf die in der nachfolgenden Übersicht anhand einiger Beispiele der Autoren detaillierter eingegangen werden soll, wird auch auf die in jüngerer Zeit zunehmenden Publikationen zu SPECT und PET bei Bewegungsstörungen speziell bei Kindern verwiesen, z.B. bei Phenytoin induzierte Choreoathetose (Saito et al., 2001), bei paroxysmaler kinesigener Dyskinesie (Shirane et al., 2001), Aufmerksamkeitsdefizit-Hyperaktivitäts-Syndrom und Parkinson-Syndrom bei Juveniler Zeroidlipofuszinose (Aberg et al., 2000) (Übersicht zu hyperkinetischen Syndromen: (Overmeyer und Taylor, 2000)).

Grundlagen von SPECT und PET

Die ersten Messungen zur Erforschung des Hirnstoffwechsels *in vivo* wurden in den 40iger Jahren mit Isotopen durchgeführt. Die sogenannte Stickstoffoxid-Methode erlaubte die Messung des hemispheralen Hirnblutflusses. In Kombination mit arteriellen und venösen Messungen von Glukose und Sauerstoff ließ sich der globale zerebrale Metabolismus quantifizieren. Das Bestreben, regionale anstatt globale Metabolismus- und Perfusions-Daten zu erheben, führte zur Entwicklung der Hirnszintigraphie. Diese Technik beruht auf der externen Detektion radioaktiver Isotope, welche sich nach parenteraler Verabreichung lokal in pathologischem und gesunden Gewebe verteilen. Der Einsatz der zerebralen Szintigraphie in der funktionellen Hirndiagnostik wurde durch die Entwicklung der computerisierten transversalen axialen Tomographie im Jahr 1973 – mit ihrer ungleich höheren räumlichen Auflösung – in der klinischen Routine weitgehend abgelöst. Bei dieser Technik tastet ein Röntgenstrahl den Kopf aus zahlreichen Winkeln, wodurch das Strahlenintensitätsprofil dreidimensional registriert wird. Die räumliche Verteilung der Absorptionswerte kann somit als Serie axialer Schnittbilder präsentiert werden. Diese Art der dreidimensionalen Datenverarbeitung ist seither Grundlage weiterer Bildgebungsmodalitäten wie SPECT, PET und der Kernspintomographie.

Single-Photonen-Emissions-Tomographie (SPECT)

Da es bei der konventionellen planaren Szintigraphie zu Überlagerungen aus verschiedenen Bildebenen kommt, hat sich die SPECT mit 360° um den Patienten rotierenden Gamma-Kameras für dreidimensionale Hirnuntersuchungen etabliert. Hierbei wird die Aktivitätsverteilung in ausgewählten Objektschichten des Gehirns gemessen, wobei nach jedem Winkelschritt eine zweidimensionale Projektion des Objektes aufgenommen wird. Aus allen Projektionen lässt sich ein Satz von parallelen Schichten rekonstruieren, wodurch sich Schnittbilder in beliebigen Schnittebenen darstellen lassen. So wird eine genauere topographische Zuordnung innerhalb des Gehirns ermöglicht. Neben dem einzelnen rotierenden Messkopf sind neuerdings Systeme mit multiplen rotierenden Messköpfen auf dem Markt, wodurch eine höhere räumliche Auflösung ohne Verlust an Ausbeute erreicht wird.

Positronen-Emissions-Tomographie (PET)

Die PET kombiniert die Technik der Detektion von Isotopen mit Bildrekonstruktionsmethoden, die initial für die computerisierte Röntgenstrahltomographie (CT) entwickelt wurden. Die PET misst die regionale Konzentration von Positronen-emittierenden Radionukliden im Körper und darüber Veränderungen von regionalem Hirnblutfluss, Metabolismus sowie biochemischen Parametern. PET-Untersuchungen werden durchgeführt, indem entweder intravenös oder als Gas zur Inhalation, ein Tracer gekoppelt mit einem Positronenemitter (z.B. ^{15}O, ^{11}C, und ^{13}N) verabreicht wird. Wenn inkorporiert, verursachen diese Isotope von Elementen, die natürlich vorkommen, keine Störung physiologischer Vorgänge. Nach Verabreichung solcher Tracer lassen sich Patienten oder Probanden in der PET-Kamera untersuchen. Mit den sogenannten Sinogrammen als initialen Rohdaten können nach aufwendiger Datenaufarbeitung tomographische Bilder der regionalen zerebralen Tracer-Aufnahme erstellt werden, welche die Grundlage weiterer spezifischer Analysen bilden. Die Genauigkeit des endgültigen Bilder hängt von der Auflösung des Scanners und der adäquaten Aufbereitung der Rohdaten ab. Die meisten Korrekturen geschehen im Hinblick auf Streustrahlung, zufällige Koinzidenzen und Abschwächung im Gesichtsfeld des Tomographen.

Voraussetzung für die PET ist die Produktion Positronen-emittierender Nuklide durch ein Zyklotron. Insbesondere ^{15}O-markierte Bluflusstracer sind sehr kurzlebig. Daher muss ein Zyklotron in direkter Nachbarschaft zu einer PET-

Kamera lokalisiert sein. Im Zyklotron werden Gase in einem elektrischen Feld ionisiert. Protonen aus dieser Ionenquelle werden über ein Radiofrequenzfeld entlang einer durch statische magnetische Felder vorgegebenen zirkulären Bahn beschleunigt. Schließlich wird der Ionenstrahl elektrostatisch abgelenkt und zur Bombardierung eines Zieles zur Schaffung von Positronenstrahlern verwendet. Der in den vorliegenden Studien verwendete Positronenstrahler ^{15}O wird durch Bestrahlung von $^{14}N_2$ durch Deuteronen geschaffen. Die Positronenstrahler zerfallen durch Emission eines Positrons und eines Neutrinos in ein stabiles Nuklid. Der Elektroneneinfang spielt bei den leichten Elementen keine oder nur eine vernachlässigbare Rolle. Das Neutrino geht keine Wechselwirkung ein. Der Messung zugänglich ist nicht der eigentlich gesuchte Ort des Positronenquelle, sondern der Ort der Positronenvernichtung. Das Positron fliegt im wasseräquivalenten Weichteilgewebe ca. 2 mm, bis es abgebremst wird und schließlich zusammen mit einem Elektron ein wasserstoffähnliches System, das Positronium bildet, das sich gleich selbst vernichtet. Bei der Massenumwandlung (Positronenvernichtung) werden gemäß der Einstein'schen Beziehung $E=mc^2$ zwei Photone von je 511 keV unter 180° zueinander emittiert. Kleine Veränderungen in diesem Winkel hängen von der kinetischen Energie des Positrons zur Zeit der Vernichtung ab. Dieser Winkel ist eine intrinsische Eigenschaft des emittierenden Isotops. Diese Winkelschwankung in der Größenordnung von ± 0,5° führt zu einer weiteren Unsicherheit in der Ortsbestimmung von ebenfalls 1–2 mm.

Es ist die simultane Emission der zwei Photone, die es erlaubt, die Quantität und den Ort der Positronenvernichtung zu berechnen. Ein Ring von Detektoren ist in die PET-Kamera eingelassen. Gegenüberliegende Detektoren sind miteinander verschaltet, so dass das nahezu simultane Eintreffen von Gammaquanten auf gegenüberliegenden Detektoren als ein Koinzidenz-Ereignis registriert wird. Wenn die Vernichtung außerhalb eines Feldes zwischen zwei Detektoren geschieht, dann wird das Ereignis nicht registriert.

Strahlendosis bei SPECT und PET

Die nuklearmedizinische *in vivo* Diagnostik mit PET und SPECT, bei der offene radioaktive Stoffe appliziert werden, ist mit einer Strahlenexposition für den Patienten verbunden. Dabei werden in der klinischen Routinediagnostik effektive Dosen von einigen mSv erreicht, was in der Größenordnung der normalen bis ca. dreifachen jährlichen natürlichen Strahlenexposition liegt. Bei Kindern werden – im Vergleich zu Erwachsenenuntersuchungen – niedrigere, an die jeweilige Körperoberfläche angepasste Strahlendosen verwandt (Vergleiche Richtlinien der »Paediatric Task Group« der EANM).

Richtlinien für PET und SPECT Untersuchungen bei Kindern in Deutschland

Während nach der Strahlenschutzverordnung von 1989 Untersuchungen zu wissenschaftlichen Zwecken bei Probanden < 18 Jahren kontraindiziert waren (i.e. Geschäftsfähigkeit des Probanden Vorraussetzung für Einwilligung, entsprechend § 41, (6) 1.), besteht nach der Neufassuung der Strahlenschutzverordnung von 2001 eine Novellierung der diesbezüglich entscheidenden Kriterien. So sind neuerdings an »geschäftsunfähigen und beschränkt geschäftsfähigen Probanden« Anwendungen radioaktiver Stoffe oder ionisierender Strahlung zulässig, wenn 1. »Das Forschungsziel nicht anders erreicht werden kann«, 2. »Die Anwendung gleichzeitig zur Untersuchung oder Behandlung des Probanden angezeigt ist« und 3. »der gesetzliche Vertreter oder der Betreuer seine Einwilligung abgegeben hat, nachdem er von dem das Forschungsvorhaben leitenden Arzt über Wesen, Bedeutung, Tragweite und Risiken aufgeklärt worden ist.« (weitere Details siehe § 88 (3), (Strahlenschutzverordnung 2001).

Anwendungen der PET und SPECT erfordern, dass das untersuchte Kind während der Datenakquision (ca. 30–60 Minuten) still liegt. Dies ist erst ab einem Alter möglich, in dem eine Einsicht in die entsprechenden Erfordernisse der Untersuchung gewährleistet ist. Häufig ist i.R. solcher Untersuchung eine individuell angepasste Sedation (entspr. »Society of Nuclear Medicine Procedure Guideline for Pediatric Sedation in Nuclear Medicine«) erforderlich. Aus diesem Umstand resultiert, dass Hirnaktivierungsstudien bei Kindern mit Sedation nur eingeschränkt möglich sind.

Grundlagen von Hirnaktivierungsstudien

Aktivierungsstudien mit PET registrieren und lokalisieren Veränderungen des regionalen zerebralen Blutfluss (rCBF), welche einem bestimmten Verhalten oder physiologischen Prozess zugeordnet werden können. Aktivierungsstudien beruhen entsprechend auf statistischen Vergleichen des rCBF während definierter experimenteller Zustände des Hirns und ermöglichen so die bildliche Darstellung normaler und pathologischer Hirnfunktion während motorischer, sensorischer und kognitiver Leistungen. Die damit verbundenen Durchblutungsänderungen werden als Index synaptischer Aktivität verstanden, da der rCBF sehr eng mit der zugrundeliegenden neuronalen, insbesondere der synaptischen Aktivität, korreliert (Raichle et al., 1983).

SPECT und PET Studien bei Bewegungsstörungen

Einführung

Anfang der 90iger Jahre wurde begonnen, mit Hirnaktivierungsstudien die Pathophysiologie von hypo- und hyperkinetischen Bewegungsstörungen zu erforschen. Hierbei hat insbesondere die PET dazu beigetragen, das Konzept der Basalganglien-Thalamokortikalen Regelkreisen zu erhärten (Abb. 1). Die funktionelle Auflösung moderner PET-Scanner liegt zwischen 4–8 mm, abhängig davon ob individuelle oder Gruppen-gemittelte Untersuchungen durchgeführt werden. Die Auflösung ist adäquat, um Blutflussveränderungen im Nucleus lentiformis und Caudatum-Kopf zu unterscheiden, lässt hingegen leider nicht eine

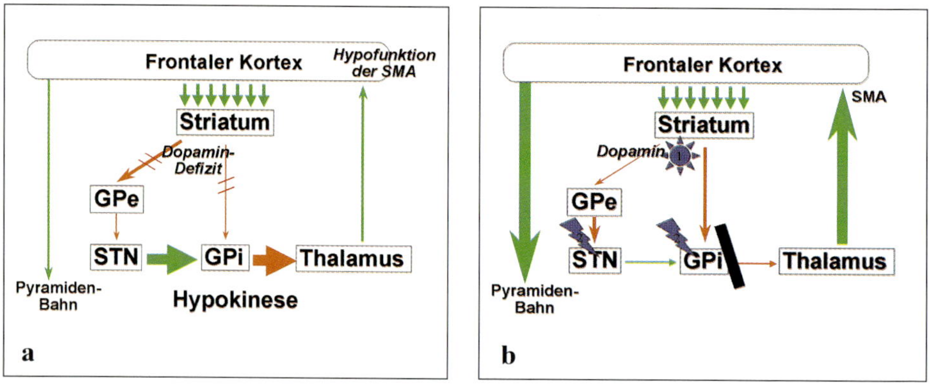

Abb. 1a, b: Basalganglien-thalamokortikaler Regelkreis am Beispiel der Hypokinese und ihrer Modifikation durch stereotaktische Verfahren und Dopaminsubstituion.

In diesem Schema am Modell der Hypokinese bei Morbus Parkinson bildet der Globus pallidus internus (GPi) die Output-Station der Basalganglien. Dopamin- D2-Rezeptor-kontrollierte striatale GABA-Neurone projizieren in das äußere Pallidumglied und erreichen als »indirekte Projektion« über den Globus pallidus externus (GPe) und Nucleus subthalamicus (STN) das innere Pallidumglied (GPI), während Dopamin-D1-Rezeptor-kontrollierte striatale GABA-Neurone direkt in das innere Pallidumglied projizieren.
Der striatale Dopaminmangel bei Morbus Parkinson führt zu einer Aktivitätszunahme der indirekten Projektion zum GPi. Dies wiederum bedingt eine Enthemmung des Nucleus subthalamicus (STN) mit überaktiven exzitatorischen (grün) Projektionen zum GPI, dessen resultierende Aktivitätssteigerung zu einer übermäßiger Hemmung (rot) thalamokortikaler Projektionen, damit zu einer Hypofunktion der SMA und Hypokinese führt. An dem »gestörten« Regelkreis lassen sich die Zielpunkte invasiver Verfahren erklären: Dopaminsubstitution, chronische Hochfrequenzstimulation im N. subthalamicus (STN) bez. Globus pallidus internus (GPi), posteroventrale Pallidotomie (Balken).

sichere funktionelle Differenzierung von Putamen, Pallidum und Nucleus subthalamicus zu. Die seit kurzem verfügbare vollkommen nichtinvasive funktionelle Magnetresonanztomographie (fMRT) ist trotz immanenter Vorteile (insbesondere keine Radioaktivität, ferner bessere räumliche und zeitliche Auflösung) gerade bei bewegungsgestörten Patienten – im Vergleich zur PET – mit praktischen Problemen verbunden. Das liegt in erster Linie am eingeengten geschlossen MRT System im Gegensatz zum offenen PET-Scanner, der Lautstärke während der Untersuchungen und der hohen Empfindlichkeit der fMRT für Bewegungsartefakte. Bisher finden sich lediglich vereinzelte fMRT Untersuchungen bei Bewegungsstörungen in der Literatur (Haslinger et al., 2001b; Sabatini et al., 2000). Wir konnten die fMRT mit Erfolg bei hypokinetischen Parkinson-Patienten einsetzen (Haslinger et al., 2001b), sehen allerdings große Schwierigkeiten bei ausgeprägten Hyperkinesen. Allerdings ist bei der breiten Verfügbarkeit der fMRT und der raschen Entwicklung spezifischer fMRT Software- und Hardware mit einem zukünftig geringeren Einsatz der PET Technik bei Aktivierungsstudien zu rechnen. Für bestimmte Fragestellungen – wie beispielsweise die Evaluierung von implantierten tiefen Hirnstimulationsystemen und Hyperkinesen mit Beteiligung kranialer oder zervikaler Regionen – wird allerdings die PET voraussichtlich die Methode der Wahl bleiben.

Akinese – Morbus Parkinson

Hypofunktion im Basalganglien-thalamokortikalen Regelkreis bei Akinese

Mit PET Aktivierungsstudien lassen sich die funktionellen Effekte der Dopaminverarmung in den Basalganglien und im Kortex zu studieren. Laut Lehrmeinung zu den Basalganglienverbindungen stellen die wichtigsten Efferenzen des Striatums – über Zwischenschaltungen im Globus pallidus und Thalamus – der prämotorische frontale Kortex, insbesondere die supplementär motorische Area (SMA), sowie der präfrontale Kortex dar (Alexander und Crutcher, 1990). Entsprechend lässt sich ableiten, dass Dopaminverarmung zu einer Deafferentierung dieser kortikalen Areale führt. Playford et al. (Playford et al., 1992) untersuchten diese Hypothese indem sie die Zunahme der regionalen Hirndurchblutung bei Parkinson-Patienten während der Durchführung freigewählter Bewegungen eines »joysticks« analysierten. Die Patienten waren zwar im Mittel etwa 15–20% langsamer in ihren Bewegungen, konnten diese aber vollständig durchführen. Sie zeigten eine verminderte Aktivierung im kontralateralen Ncl. lentiformis, in der SMA, im anterioren Cingulum und im dorsolateralen präfrontalen Kortex im Vergleich zu altersabgestimmten Kontrollpersonen. Dieselben Aktivierungsdefizite im Vergleich zur Ruhekondition wurden auch bei der Durchführung von sequentiellen Fingerbewegungen gezeigt (Samuel et al., 1997a). Sie waren besonders ausgeprägt, wenn die Fingerbewegungen mit beiden Händen ausgeführt wurden. Neu war hierbei, dass Parkinson-Patienten – im Vergleich zu den Kontrollpersonen – eine Überaktivität im parietalen Kortex bei bestehender Unteraktivität in der SMA und im dorsolateralen präfrontalen Kortex (DLPFC) aufwiesen. Diese parietale Überaktivität wird als ein funktioneller Bypass-Mechanismus (über cerebelläre-parietale Projektionen) interpretiert, mit dem Parkinson-Patienten das striato-frontale Defizit kompensieren.

Pharmakologische Beeinflussung des Basalganglien-thalamokortikalen Regelkreises

Die funktionelle Reafferentierung der entkoppelten frontalen Assoziationsfelder nach Dopaminergika wurde unter simultaner parenteraler Apomorphin-Gabe (D1-und D2 Dopaminagonist) mit dem »joystick«-Paradigma während frei gewählter Bewegungen untersucht (Jenkins et al., 1992). Die Linderung der Akinesie ging mit einer signifikanten Zunahme des regionalen Hirnblutflusses in der SMA und im DLPFC einher. Diese Ergebnisse sind in Einklang mit Befunden aus SPECT Studien, in denen ebenfalls eine Zunahme der Durchblutung in der SMA mit ^{133}Xe als rCBF-Tracer nach Apomorphin und L-Dopa bei Parkinson-Patienten beschrieben wird (Rascol et al., 1992; Rascol et al., 1994). Vor kurzem konnten diese Befunde der durch Dopaminergika reversiblen Hypoaktivität mesial frontaler Rindenfelder in einer ereigniskorrelierten fMRT repliziert und erweitert werden (Haslinger et al., 2001a).

Stereotaktische Modifikation des Basalganglien-thalamokortikalen Regelkreises

Die Einführung der Tiefenhirnstimulation hat zu einer Renaissance der Stereotaxie bei Bewegungssstörungen geführt. Neben der Therapie der Parkinson-Akinese (2001; Limousin et al., 1995), verschiedener Tremor-Formen (Alesch et al., 1995) wird sie zunehmend auch bei jugendlichen Patienten mit generalisierter Dystonie eingesetzt, insbesondere bei der klassischen Torsionsdystonie mit dem DYT1 Gen (Coubes et al., 2000). $H_2^{15}O$-PET Untersuchungen stellen praktisch die einzige *in vivo* Methode dar, um die Effekte der elektrischen Hirnstimulation auf weitverteilte neuronale Systeme zu untersuchen, mit dereinzigartigen Möglichkeit zerebrale Konnektivität und ihre Modulation zu erforschen. Der rCBF kann wiederholt während aufgabenspezifischer Aktivierungen bei gleichzeitiger Änderung der Stimulationsparameter in einer einzigen PET-Untersuchung gemessen werden. Die fMRT kann hingegen z. Zt. ausschließlich unmittelbar postoperativ, solange die Elektroden über einen externen nicht-implantierten Impulsgeber stimuliert werden können, unter großen Sicherheitsvorkehrungen eingesetzt werden.

Stereotaktische Verfahren wurden mit PET-Aktivierungstudien zunächst bei Patienten vor und nach posteroventrolateraler Pallidotomie untersucht (Ceballos-Baumann et al., 1994; Grafton et al., 1995; Samuel et al., 1997b). Die Rationale für diese Intervention besteht in der Unterbrechung des exzessiven inhibitorischen Outputs aus den Basalganglien als Folge der Dopaminverarmung. Klinisch gesehen zielt die Pallidotomie auf eine Linderung von L-Dopa-Dyskinesien, Akinesie und Rigor. Die untersuchten Patienten führten zur Aktivierung wieder das »joystick«-Paradigma durch. Eingeschränkte Aktivierung wurde vor der Operation in der SMA, dem lateral prämotorischen Kortex und dem DLPFC beobachtet, die nach dem Eingriff entsprechend der Besserung der Akinesie sistierte (Abb. 2). Diese Ergebnisse unterstreichen das Konzept, dass die Pallidotomie zum größten Teil über eine Reduktion der inhibitorischen pallidothalamischen Projektionen wirkt (siehe Abb. 1).

Die tiefe Hirnstimulation wurde im Ncl. subthalamicus (STN) und Globus pallidus internus (GPI) bei Parkinson-Patienten (Ceballos-Baumann et al., 1999; Davis et al., 1997; Limousin et al., 1997) und im Ncl. ventralis intermedius (VIM) des Thalamus bei Patienten mit Parkinson-Tremor (Deiber et al., 1993) und essentiellem Tremor untersucht (Ceballos-Baumann et al., 2001). In Analogie zu den Befunden bei der Pallidotomie konnte gezeigt werden, dass die Besserung der Akinese bei Morbus Parkinson auf eine Zunahme der bewegungsabhängigen Aktivierung prämotorischer und supplementär-motorischer Areale bei STN und GPI Stimulation zurückzuführen ist. Ein Patient mit generalisierter Dystonie wurde während ein- und ausgeschalteter Gpi Stimulation untersucht (Kumar et al., 1999): Das Einschalten des Stimulators führte zu einem Nachlassen der Dystonie und einer Minderung der bewegungsassozierten Aktivierung im prämotorischen und präfrontalen Cortex.

Bei der tiefen Hirnstimulation im VIM-Kern konnten die von Hassler postulierten kortikalen Projektionsgebiete des VIM-Thalamus bildgeberisch dargestellt werden: Tiefe Hirnstimulation im VIM-Thalamus-Kern führte zu einer Deaktivierung der rechtsseitigen retroinsulären Area (parietoinsulärer vesti-

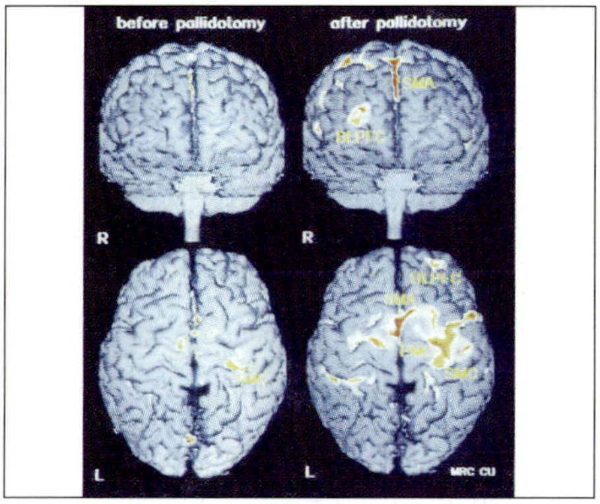

Abb. 2: PET-Aktivierungsbilder eines Parkinson-Patienten vor (links) und nach (rechts) posteroventraler Pallidotomie. Aktivierungsbedingte Zunahmen des regionalen Blutflusses als Index für synaptische Aktivität während frei gewählter Bewegungen mit der zur Pallidotomie kontralateralen Seite Arm sind auf die kortikale Oberfläche des individuellen NMR projiziert. Die orange-gelben Gebiete zeigen Voxels bis zur einer Tiefe von 10, die statistisch signifikant über der Schwelle von Omnibus $p < 0.001$ liegen. Man beachte den Unterschied im Aktivierungsmuster nach der Pallidotomie mit ausgedehnterer Aktivierung im lateral prämotorischen Kortex (PMC), in der supplementär motorischen area (SMA) und im dorsolateralen präfrontalen Kortex (DLPFC) während der Patient auditorisch getriggerte »joystick« Bewegungen in frei gewählte Richtungen ausführt.

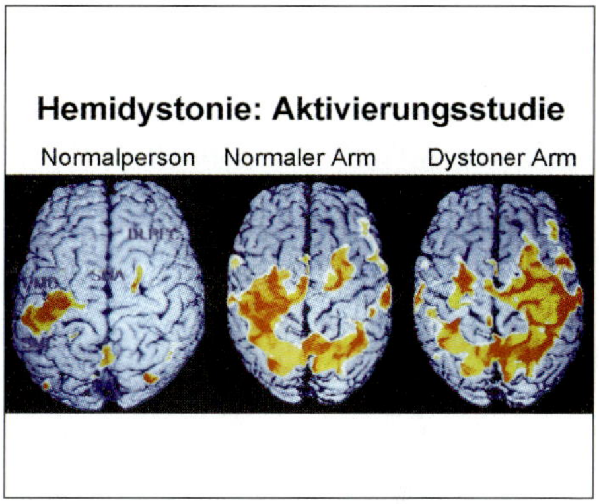

Abb. 3: PET-Aktivierungsbilder eines 20 jährigen Patienten mit einer Hemidystonie aufgrund einer posterolateralen thalamischen Läsion (Mitte und rechts) und einer gesunden Kontrollperson (links). Aktivierungsbedingte Zunahmen des regionalen Blutflusses als Index für synaptische Aktivität während frei gewählter Bewegungen mit dem »normalen« Arm und dem dystonen Arm sind auf die kortikalen Oberflächen des individuellen NMR projiziert. Man beachte den Unterschied im Aktivierungsmuster mit ausgedehnterer Aktivierung des lateralen prämotorischen Kortex (PMC), der supplementär motorischen Area (SMA), der parietalen Assoziationsrinde, des sensomotorischen Kortex (SMC) und des dorsal präfrontalen Kortex (DLPFC), während der Patient Bewegungen mit dem dystonen Arm durchführt. Die Aktivierungsfläche ist ebenfalls erhöht, wenn der Patient die Aufgabe mit dem »normalen« Arm durchführt, verglichen mit einer Kontrollperson, die dieselbe Aufgabe ausübt.

bulärer Kortex), wodurch das häufige Problem des Schwindels VIM stimulierter Patienten erklärbar wird. Die Aktivierung des motorischen Kortex bei effektiver VIM-Stimulation ist mit dem tremorlytischen Effekt assoziert und muss offenbar spezifisch für die VIM-Stimulation sein, da sie weder nach Thalamotomien im VIM (Boecker et al., 1997) noch nach Läsionen im Thalamus bei Hemidystonie (Ceballos-Baumann et al., 1995a) beobachtet wurde. Die mit dem gewünschten tremorlytischen Effekt der VIM-Stimulation einhergehende Aktivierung im motorischen Kortex wurde mit systematischen Veränderungen der Stimulationsparameter Frequenz und Amplitude während rCBF-PET Messungen näher untersucht. Dabei wurden in vivo regional differentielle Effekte der Stimulationsparameter Amplitude und Frequenz bei VIM Stimulation dargestellt. Sie bestätigen die Hypothese der Tiefenhirnstimulation im VIM-Thalamus als aktivem Prozess, welcher zu gesteigerter, am ehesten inhibitorischer, synaptischer Aktität führt (Ceballos-Baumann et al., 2001; Haslinger et al., 2001a).

In einer Studie zur Stimulation des Nucleus subthalamicus (STN) wurde die Interaktion zwischen diesem motorischen Kern und dem kognitiven Schaltkreis zum anterioren Zingulum direkt nachgewiesen (Schroeder et al., in press). Parkinson-Patienten wurden mit einer Reaktions-Konflikt-Aufgabe (Stroop-Aufgabe) unter ein- und ausgeschalteter STN-Stimulation untersucht. Während sich die motorische Symptomatik verbesserte, kam es bei eingeschalteter Stimulation zu einer signifikanten Verschlechterung in den Reaktionszeiten bei Konflikt (Interferenz). Dies war mit einer Aktivierungsabnahme im ventralen Striatum und anterioren Cingulum (ACC), als wesentliche Strukturen des anterior cingulären striatofrontalen Regelkreises, assoziiert. Die Ergebnisse bestätigen die aus tierexperimentellen Untersuchungen erwachsene Hypothese einer integrativen Funktion des STN zwischen Motorik und Kognition und untersteichen die Bedeutung nicht-motorischer Verbindungen des STN. Über die Störung dieser Verbindungen können unerwünschte kognitive Wirkungen der STN-Stimulation bei Parkinson-Patienten erklärt werden. Diese Ergebnisse entsprechen den gegensätzlichen Voraussagen des von Marsden und Obeso geprägten Konzeptes des »Paradoxons der stereotaktischen Chirurgie« (Ausschalten einer physiologischen wichtigen Struktur führt zu einer klinischen Besserung). Das motorische System, entkoppelt von Efferenzen und Afferenzen zum STN, funktioniert weiter bei routinierten, vorhersehbaren und automatisierten Bewegungen, da sie unter STN-Stimulation durch Fazilitierung frontaler Funktionen verbessert werden. Bei neuen und unerwarteten Situationen, die nicht-automatisierte Reaktionen erfordern, führt hingegen die Störung des anterior cingulären frontostriatalen Regelkreises zu Inflexibilität mentaler und motorischer Reaktionen.

Hyperkinese – Dystonie

Dystonie

Die oftmals bizarren Phänomene und das im Gegensatz zum Morbus Parkinson bisher fehlende pathoanatomische Korrelat der idiopathischen Dystonien hat Neurologen und Psychiater lange Zeit mit einer wenig fruchtbaren Kontroverse um Organizität versus Psychogenie beschäftigt. Neuropathologische, neurochemische Untersuchungen und strukturelle Bildgebung haben bei den idiopathischen Dystonien bisher keine spezifischen Befunde erbracht. Mittels funktioneller Bildgebung wurde aber in den letzten Jahren ein erheblicher Erkenntnisgewinn generiert.

Dystonie: 18-Fluoro-Deoxy-Glukose-Untersuchungen (^{18}F-FDG-PET)

Vor der Ära der Aktivierungsstudien haben Untersuchungen des Glukose-Metabolismus mit ^{18}F-FDG-PET bei idiopathischer Dystonie in Ruhe längere Zeit widersprüchliche Ergebnisse geliefert. Es wurde ein normaler (Otsuka et al., 1992), erhöhter (Chase et al., 1988) und erniedrigter (Karbe et al., 1992) Stoffwechsel beschrieben. Bei zervikaler Dystonie wurde über einen normalen Metabolismus allerdings mit Verlust des normalen Verhältnisses zwischen Basalganglien und Thalamus berichtet (Stoessl et al., 1986). In jüngerer Zeit wurde wiederum ein erhöhter Metabolismus im Ncl. lentiformis bei Patienten mit zervikaler Dystonie (Galardi et al., 1996; Magyar-Lehmann et al., 1997) und mit idiopathischer Torsionsdystonie ITD (Eidelberg et al., 1995) gemessen. Bei der ITD-Studie fand sich der relative Hypermetabolismus neben dem Ncl. lentiformis auch im prämotorischen Kortex. In einer weiterführenden ^{18}F-FDG-Untersuchung bei asymptomatischen und symptomatischen DYT1 Gen-Trägern, einem Gen mit einer etwa 30% Pänetranz für die idiopathische Torsionsdystonie, wurden zwei Muster einer metabolischen regionalen Kovarianz beschrieben (Eidelberg et al., 1998): erhöhte metabolische Aktivität im Ncl. lentiformis, Cerebellum und SMA bei Gen-Trägern ohne und solchen mit nur aktionsinduzierten Symptomen; hingegen gesteigerter Metabolismus im Thalamus, Mittelhirn und Cerebellum bei Patienten mit Dystoniezeichen in Ruhe. Die widersprüchlichen Ergebnisse liegen bei den älteren Studien teilweise an heterogenen Patientenkollektiven, sicherlich aber auch an der Schwierigkeit, mit ^{18}F-FDG eine dynamische Motorikstörung mit den durch ^{18}F-FDG bedingten langen Datenakquisitionszeiten zu erfassen. Aktivierungstudien mit Messung des regionalen cerebralen Blutflusses (rCBF) mit PET, eventuell mit fMRT, stellen im Vergleich zu ^{18}F-FDG-Studien eine versatilere Möglichkeit dar, Dystonie *in vivo* zu untersuchen, da Messungen unter verschiedenen Funktionszuständen möglich sind.

Dystonie: Sensorisches System

Tempel und Perlmutter (Tempel und Perlmutter, 1990) wandten Aktivierungsstudien als erste an, um die Integrität der zentralen somatosensorischen Verbindungen bei Patienten mit idiopathischer Torsionsdystonie und Schreibkrampf zu untersuchen. Sie benützten vibrotaktile Stimulation, um den sensomotorischen Kortex (SMC) zu aktivieren und untersuchten die resultierende Zunahme des rCBF. Dystone Patienten wiesen eine reduzierte Zunahme der Durchblutung in dem kontralateralen SMC während vibrotaktiler Stimulation auf. Die Autoren interpretierten die Hypoaktivität des SMC in dem Sinne, dass der SMC bei Dystonie einer exzessiven Hemmung aus den Basalganglien ausgesetzt ist. In einer Nachanalyse ihrer vibrotaktilen Stimulation bei einer Untergruppe von sechs Schreibkrampfpatienten (Tempel und Perlmutter, 1993) wurde zusätzlich zum SMC auch in der kaudalen SMA eine erniedrigte rCBF-Antwort gefunden. Kürzlich hat die gleiche Arbeitsgruppe bei Patienten mit Blepharospasmus ohne Handdystonie wiederum eine ähnliche Minderaktiverung im SMC bei Anwendung von vibrotaktiler Stimulation im Gesicht beschrieben (Feiwell et al., 1999).

Dystonie: Motorisches System

Die Tatsache, dass bei den meisten Patienten mit sekundärer Dystonie strukturelle Veränderungen in den Basalganglien oder im Thalamus gefunden werden (Burton et al., 1984; Lee et al., 1994; Pettigrew und Jankovic, 1985), führte zur Hypothese, dass Dystonien auf abnorme Efferenzen aus dem Globus pallidus oder Thalamus in prämotorische und motorische Projektionsfelder zurückzuführen sind. Läsionsmodelle bei nicht-menschlichen Primaten weisen als

Substrat der Dystonie ebenfalls auf eine Enthemmung thalamokortikaler Projektionen hin. Damit ergaben sich folgende Fragen und Hypothesen, die sich mit PET-Aktivierungsparadigmen untersuchen lassen, die planerische und exekutive Komponenten der Motorik testen:

1. Ist das Aktivierungsmuster bei idiopathischer Torsionsdystonie (ITD) im Vergleich zu Gesunden verändert und ist die Hypothese korrekt, dass die ITD mit einer Überaktivität thalamokortikaler Projektionen vergesellschaftet ist?
2. Zeigen Patienten mit idiopathischer Dystonie und erworbener Hemidystonie nach Läsionen in den Basalganglien oder Thalamus unterschiedliche Aktivierungsmuster?
3. Wird ein abnormes zentrales Aktivierungsmuster bei idiopathischer Dystonie durch eine peripher ansetzende Botulinum-Toxin-Therapie beeinflusst?

Um diese Fragestellungen zu bearbeiten, wurden folgende Paradigmen durchgeführt und mit den Aktivierungseffekten von Kontrollpersonen verglichen:

1. rCBF Messung bei Patienten mit ITD und Kontrollpersonen in Ruhe und während einfacher, frei gewählter Armbewegungen mit der dominanten Hand als aktivierende Bedingung.
2. Messung des rCBF bei Patienten mit erworbener Hemidystonie (EHD) in Ruhe und während einfacher, frei gewählter Armbewegungen mit dem dystonen Arm und mit der nicht betroffenen Seite.
3. Messung des rCBF bei Patienten mit Schreibkrampf (SK), einer idiopathischen Handdystonie, in Ruhe und während stereotypen Schreibens vor und nach effektiver Behandlung mit Botulinum-Toxin (BOTX) in einer erneuten Untersuchung sowie bei Kontrollpersonen.

Gemeinsam mit den ITD-Patienten zeigten die Patienten mit erworbener Dystonie eine gesteigerte Aktivierung in rostralen prämotorischen und dorsolateral präfrontalen Feldern. Hingegen wurde im Vergleich zu den ITD-Patienten bei Patienten mit erworbener Dystonie ebenfalls eine bewegungsabhängige Überaktivität und keine Unteraktivität im exekutiven motorischen Kortex (kaudale SMA und primärmotorischer Kortex) gefunden. Überaktivität frontaler Assoziationsfelder stellt demnach ein gemeinsames pathophysiologisches Substrat dystoner Syndrome dar, während die Hypofunktion des motorischen exekutiven Kortex bei der idiopathischen Variante auftritt. Dieser differentielle Befund spiegelt am ehesten die Tatsache wider, dass die erworbene Dystonie auf unterbrechende Läsionen der Regelkreise zwischen Basalganglien, Thalamus und frontalem Kortex zurückzuführen ist, und dass bei der idiopathischen Torsionsdystonie die zugrundeliegende Pathologie sowohl die Basalganglien als auch den motorischen Kortex betrifft (Ceballos-Baumann et al., 1995a; Ceballos-Baumann et al., 1995b). Um die Anomalie bei idiopathischer Dystonie im exekutiven motorischen Kortex näher definieren zu können, wurde ein Paradigma gewählt, das keine Entscheidungen erfordert und motorisch exekutive Funktionen betont: Dystonie wurde bei Schreibkrampf-Patienten durch eine automatische und früherlernte Aufgabe, nämlich kontinuierliches stereotypes Schreiben ausgelöst und vor einer zweiten Untersuchung durch lokalisierte Injektionen mit Botulinum-Toxin in die dystonen Muskeln gelindert. Das Schreibparadigma erwies sich als außerordentlich aktivierend und die bewegungsabhängige Hypofunktion des primären motorischen Kortex bei den Schreibkrampf-Patienten kam statistisch noch deutlicher hervor als bei den idiopathischen Torsionsdystonie-Patienten während frei gewählter Bewegungen. Ähnlich wie die idiopathische Torsionsdystonie und erworbene Hemidystonie war der Schreibkrampf mit einer Überaktivität in frontalen Assoziationsgebieten vergesellschaftet. Die therapeutischen Effekte der Botulinum-Toxin Injektionen waren bei den Schreibkrampf-Patienten mit einer zusätzlichen Überaktivität in der parietalen Assoziationsrinde vergesellschaftet (Ceballos-Baumann und Brooks, 1998; Ceballos-Baumann et al., 1997). Die eingeschränkte Aktivierung des primären motorischen Kortex wurde allerdings durch eine effektive Botulinum-Toxin Therapie nicht verändert. Das impliziert, dass die bewegungsabhängige Hypofunktion des exekutiven motorischen Kortex eine direkte Konsequenz der Pathologie bei idiopathischer Dystonie darstellt und nicht sekundär, etwa durch Kokontraktion bedingt wird.

Alle Befunde zusammen lassen für die idiopathische (primäre) Dystonie folgende Schlüsse zu:

1. Bewegungsabhängige Überaktivität des prämotorischen Kortex ist ein gemeinsames kennzeichnendes Phänomen dystoner Syndrome unterschiedlicher Ätiologie.
2. Hypofunktion des motorischen Kortex stellt eine konsistente Anomalie nur bei primärer Dystonie und nicht bei sekundärer Dystonie dar.

In Verbindung mit einer elektrophysiologisch nachgewiesenen bewegungsabhängigen erhöhten kortikalen Exzitabilität (Ikoma et al., 1996; Rona et al., 1998) können Mechanismen wie eine defekte kortikale interneuronale Hemmung als Erklärung für die bewegungsabhängige Hypofunktion des motorischen Kortex postuliert werden. Diese lässt sich, wic kürzlich bei Patienten mit aktionsinduzierter Handdystonie gezeigt, mittels der repetitiven transkraniellen repetitiven magnetischen Stimulation modulieren und eröffnet ein experimentellen Weg, die kortikale Dysfunktion bei primärer Dystonie therapeutisch anzugehen (Siebner et al., 1999). Die bewegungsassozierte Minderaktivierung des motorischen Kortex während des Schreibens und anhaltender Handkontraktion konnte in einer weiteren PET Studie bei Schreibkrampf-Patienten bestätigt werden (Ibañez et al., 1999). Diese Autoren interpretierten die Ergebnisse ebenfalls im Sinne eines Verlusts an kortikaler Inhibition während der Generierung von motorischen Befehlen.

Kortikale Reorganisation nach Botulinum-Toxin Therapie

In der oben schon erwähnten Aktivierungsstudie bei Schreibkrampfpatienten konnte durch den Vergleich der Aktivierungsmuster vor und nach Therapie der Nachweis einer BOTOX-induzierten kortikalen Reorganisation erbracht werden, die offenbar die weiter bestehende Minderaktivierung des motorischen Kortex kompensiert. In der Tat wurde beim Vergleich der Schreibkrampf-Gruppe vor und nach BOTOX-Injektionen eine verstärkte Aktivierung in prämotorischen Feldern, im primär sensorischen Kortex, im posterioren (A7) und inferioren paritalen Kortex (A40) gefunden. Die posterioren und inferioren parietalen Rindenfelder repräsentieren sekundäre sensorische Assoziationsfelder. Ihre Überaktivität könnte die Folge von Veränderungen nach Reorganisation in den primären sensorischen Zentren sein, die wiederum zu den höheren sensorischen Assoziationszentren projezieren. Beim Vergleich der Aktivierungseffekte vor und nach BOTOX in der Schreibkrampf-Gruppe zeigte sich außerdem, dass im Frontalhirn eine vermehrte Aktivierung in prämotorischen Feldern, speziell in der kaudalen SMA, zu verzeichnen war. Kaudale prämotorische Felder haben direkte kortikospinale Projektionen (Dum und Strick, 1991) und können direkt durch die BOTOX-induzierte Entkoppelung von Vorderhornzellen betroffen werden. Hier wird jedoch postuliert, dass die BOTOX-induzierte Überaktivität von prämotorischen Feldern sekundär in Folge der Enthemmung im parietalen Bereich entsteht, da diese parietalen Felder direkte Efferenzen zum prämotorischen Kortex aufweisen (Pandya und Seltzer, 1982). Eine alternative Erklärung der kortikalen Reorganisation mit prämotorischer und parietaler Überaktivität nach BOTOX-Behandlung kann eine Veränderung in der Bewegungsstrategie sein. Zusammengefasst ergeben sich die Erklärungen, dass die Veränderungen eine direkte Konsequenz der von BOTOX-induzierten Entkoppelung von Vorderhornzellen oder einer Veränderung in der Bewegungsstrategie nach Behandlung sind. Für die erste dieser beiden Erklärungen spricht, dass die exzessive Aktivierung im parietalen Kortex der kortikalen Plastizität in einer PET-Untersuchung nach Denervierung bei Patienten nach traumatischer Armamputation entspricht (Kew et al., 1994).

Literatur

1. (2001). Deep-brain stimulation of the subthalamic nucleus or the pars interna of the globus pallidus in Parkinson's disease. N Engl J Med 345: 956–63.
2. Aberg L, Liewendahl K, Nikkinen P, Autti T, Rinne JO, Santavuori P (2000). Decreased striatal dopamine transporter density in JNCL patients with parkinsonian symptoms. Neurology 54: 1069–74.
3. Alesch F, Pinter MM, Helscher RJ, Fertl L, Benabid AL, Koos WT (1995). Stimulation of the ventral intermediate thalamic nucleus in tremor dominated Parkinson's disease and essential tremor. Acta Neurochir Wien 136: 75–81.
4. Alexander GE, Crutcher MD (1990). Functional architecture of basal ganglia circuits: neural substrates of parallel processing. Trends Neurosci 13: 266–71.
5. Boecker H, Wills A, Ceballos-Baumann A, Thomas DGT, Marsden CD, Brooks DJ (1997). Stereotactic thalamotomy in tremor dominant Parkinson's disease: a H215O PET study of motor activation. Ann Neurol 41: 108–111.
6. Burton K, Farrell K, Li D, Calne DB (1984). Lesions of the putamen and dystonia: CT and magnetic resonance imaging. Neurology 34: 962–965.
7. Ceballos-Baumann AO, Boecker H, Bartenstein P, von Falkenhayn I, Riescher H, Conrad B, Moringlane JR, Alesch F (1999). A positron emission tomographic study of subthalamic

nucleus stimulation in Parkinson disease: enhanced movement-related activity of motor-association cortex and decreased motor cortex resting activity. Arch Neurol 56: 997–1003.
8. Ceballos-Baumann AO, Boecker H, Fogel W, Alesch F, Bartenstein P, Conrad B, Diederich N, von Falkenhayn I, Moringlane JR, Schwaiger M, Tronnier VM (2001). Thalamic stimulation for essential tremor activates motor and deactivates vestibular cortex. Neurology 56: 1347–54.
9. Ceballos-Baumann AO, Brooks DJ (1998). Activation PET scanning in dystonia. Adv Neurol 78: 135–152.
10. Ceballos-Baumann AO, Obeso JA, Vitek JL, Delong MR, Bakay R, Linazasoro G, Brooks DJ (1994). Restoration of thalamocortical activity following posteroventral pallidotomy in Parkinson's disease. Lancet 344: 814–814.
11. Ceballos-Baumann AO, Passingham RE, Marsden CD, Brooks DJ (1995a). Motor reorganisation in acquired hemidystonia: a PET activation study. Ann Neurol 37: 746–757.
12. Ceballos-Baumann AO, Passingham RE, Warner T, Playford ED, Marsden CD, Brooks DJ (1995b). Overactivity of prefrontal and underactivity of motor cortical areas in idiopathic dystonia: a PET activation study. Ann Neurol 37: 363–372.
13. Ceballos-Baumann AO, Sheean G, Passingham RE, Marsden CD, Brooks DJ (1997). Botulinum toxin does not reverse the cortical dysfunction associated with writer's cramp: a PET study. Brain 120: 571–582.
14. Chase TN, Tamminga CA, Burrows H (1988). Positron emission tomographic studies of regional cerebral glucose metabolism in idiopathic dystonia. Adv Neurol 50: 237–241.
15. Coubes P, Roubertie A, Vayssiere N, Hemm S, Echenne B (2000). Treatment of DYT1-generalised dystonia by stimulation of the internal globus pallidus. Lancet 355: 2220–1.
16. Davis KD, Taub E, Houle S, Lang AE, Dostrovsky JO, Tasker RR, Lozano AM (1997). Globus pallidus stimulation activates the cortical motor system during alleviation of parkinsonian symptoms (see comments). Nat Med 3: 671–674.
17. Deiber MP, Pollak P, Passingham R, Landais P, Gervason C, Cinotti L, Friston K, Frackowiak R, Mauguiere F, Benabid AL (1993). Thalamic stimulation and suppression of parkinsonian tremor. Evidence of a cerebellar deactivation using positron emission tomography. Brain 116: 267–79.
18. Dum RP, Strick PL (1991). The origin of corticospinal projections from the premotor areas in the frontal lobe. J Neurosci 11: 667–689.
19. Eidelberg D, Moeller JR, Antonini A, Kazumata K, Nakamura T, Dhawan V, Spetsieris P, deLeon D, Bressman SB, Fahn S (1998). Functional brain networks in DYT1 dystonia (see comments). Ann Neurol 44: 303–12.
20. Eidelberg D, Moeller JR, Ishikawa T, Dhawan V, Spetsieris P, Przedborski S, Fahn S (1995). The metabolic topography of idiopathic torsion dystonia. Brain 118: 1473–84.
21. Feiwell RJ, Black KJ, McGee-Minnich LA, Snyder AZ, MacLeod AM, Perlmutter JS (1999). Diminished regional cerebral blood flow response to vibration in patients with blepharospasm. Neurology 52: 291–7.
22. Galardi G, Perani D, Grassi F, Bressi S, Amadio S, Antoni M, Comi GC, Canal N, Fazio F (1996). Basal ganglia and thalamo-cortical hypermetabolism in patients with spasmodic torticollis. Acta Neurol Scand 94: 172–6.
23. Grafton ST, Waters C, Sutton J, Lew MF, Couldwell W (1995). Pallidotomy increases activity of motor association cortex in Parkinson's disease: a positron emission tomographic study. Ann Neurol 37: 776–783.
24. Haslinger B, Boecker H, Buechel C, Vesper T, Bartenstein P, Conrad B, Schwaiger M, Ceballos-Baumann AO (2001a). Linear and nonlinear increases of rCBF associated with variations of deep brain stimulation amplitude (abstract). Neuroimage 6: 1182.
25. Haslinger B, Erhard P, Kampfe N, Boecker H, Rummeny E, Schwaiger M, Conrad B, Ceballos-Baumann AO (2001b). Event Related Functional Magnetic Resonance Imaging in Parkinson's Disease Before and After Levodopa. Brain 124: 558–570.
26. Ibañez V, Sadato N, Karp B, Deiber MP, Hallett M (1999). Deficient activation of the motor cortical network in patients with writer's cramp. Neurology 53: 96–105.
27. Ikoma K, Samii A, Mercuri B, Wassermann EM, Hallett M (1996). Abnormal cortical motor excitability in dystonia. Neurology 46: 1371–6.

28. Jenkins IH, Fernandez W, Playford ED, Lees AJ, Frackowiak RS, Passingham RE, Brooks DJ (1992). Impaired activation of the supplementary motor area in Parkinson's disease is reversed when akinesia is treated with apomorphine. Ann Neurol 32: 749–57.
29. Karbe H, Holthoff VA, Rudolf J, Herholz K, Heiss WD (1992). Positron emission tomography demonstrates frontal cortex and basal ganglia hypometabolism in dystonia. Neurology 42: 1540–4.
30. Kew JJM, Ridding MC, Rothwell JC, Passingham RE, Leigh PN, Sooraikumaran SS, Frackowiak RSJ, Brooks DJ (1994). Reorganisation of cortical blood flow and transcranial magnetic stimulation maps in human subjects after upper limb amputation. J Neurophysiol: 2517–2524.
31. Kumar R, Dagher A, Hutchison WD, Lang AE, Lozano AM (1999). Globus pallidus deep brain stimulation for generalized dystonia: clinical and PET investigation. Neurology 53: 871–4.
32. Lee MS, Rinne JO, Ceballos-Baumann A, Thompson PD, Marsden CD (1994). Dystonia following head trauma. Neurology 44: 1374–1378.
33. Limousin P, Greene J, Pollak P, Rothwell J, Benabid AL, Frackowiak R (1997). Changes in cerebral activity pattern due to subthalamic nucleus or internal pallidum stimulation in Parkinson's disease. Ann Neurol 42: 283–91.
34. Limousin P, Pollack P, Benazzouz A, Hoffmann D, Le Bas JF, Brousolle E, Perret JE, Benabid AL (1995). Effect on parkinsonian signs and symptoms of bilateral subthalamic nucleus stimulation. Lancet: 91–95.
35. Magyar-Lehmann S, Antonini A, Roelcke U, Maguire RP, Missimer J, Meyer M, Leenders KL (1997). Cerebral glucose metabolism in patients with spasmodic torticollis. Mov Disord 12: 704–8.
36. Otsuka M, Ichiya Y, Shima F, Kuwabara Y, Sasaki M, Fukumura T, Kato M, Masuda K, Goto I (1992). Increased striatal 18F-dopa uptake and normal glucose metabolism in idiopathic dystonia syndrome. J Neurol Sci 111: 195–199.
37. Overmeyer S, Taylor E (2000). Neuroimaging in hyperkinetic children and adults: an overview. Pediatr Rehabil 4: 57–70.
38. Pandya DN, Seltzer B (1982). Intrinsic connections and architectonics of posterior parietal cortex in the rhesus monkey. J Comp Neurol 204: 196–210.
39. Pettigrew LC, Jankovic J (1985). Hemidystonia: a report of 22 patients and a review of the literature. J Neurol Neurosurg Psychiatry 48: 650–657.
40. Playford ED, Jenkins IH, Passingham RE, Nutt J, Frackowiak RS, Brooks DJ (1992). Impaired mesial frontal and putamen activation in Parkinson's disease: a positron emission tomography study. Ann Neurol 32: 151–161.
41. Raichle ME, Martin WR, Herscovitch P, Mintun MA, Markham J (1983). Brain blood flow measured with intravenous H2(15)O. II. Implementation and validation. J Nucl Med 24: 790–8.
42. Rascol O, Sabatini U, Chollet F, Celsis P, Montastruc JL, Marc VJP, Rascol A (1992). Supplementary and primary sensory motor area activity in Parkinson's disease: Regional cerebral blood flow changes during finger movements and effects of apomorphine. Arch Neurol 49: 144–148.
43. Rascol O, Sabatini U, Chollet F, Fabre N, Senard JM, Montastruc JL, Celsis P, Marc VJ, Rascol A (1994). Normal activation of the supplementary motor area in patients with Parkinson's disease undergoing long-term treatment with levodopa. J Neurol Neurosurg Psychiatry 57: 567–571.
44. Rona S, Berardelli A, Vacca L, Inghilleri M, Manfredi M (1998). Alterations of motor cortical inhibition in patients with dystonia. Mov Disord 13: 118–24.
45. Sabatini U, Boulanouar K, Fabre N, Martin F, Carel C, Colonnese C, Bozzao L, Berry I, Montastruc JL, Chollet F, Rascol O (2000). Cortical motor reorganization in akinetic patients with Parkinson's disease: a functional MRI study. Brain 123: 394–403.
46. Saito Y, Oguni H, Awaya Y, Hayashi K, Osawa M (2001). Phenytoin-induced choreoathetosis in patients with severe myoclonic epilepsy in infancy. Neuropediatrics 32: 231–5.

47. Samuel M, Ceballos-Baumann AO, Blin J, Uema T, Boecker H, Krams M, Passingham RE, Brooks DJ (1997a). Evidence for lateral premotor and parietal overactivity in Parkinson's disease during sequential and bimanual movements: a PET study. Brain 120: 963–76.
48. Samuel M, Ceballos-Baumann AO, Turjanski N, Boecker H, Holmes AP, Obeso JA, DeLong MR, Bakay R, Vitek JL, Thomas DGT, Quinn NP, Brooks DJ (1997b). Pallidotomy in Parkinson's disease increases SMA and prefrontal activation during performance of volitional movements: an H215O PET study. Brain 120: 963–976.
49. Schroeder U, Kühler A, Haslinger B, Erhard P, Tronnier VU, Fogel W, Lange KW, Boecker H, Ceballos-Baumann AO (2002). Subthalamic nucleus stimulation affects striato-anterior cingulate cortex circuit in a response conflict task: a PET study. Brain 125: 995–2004.
50. Shirane S, Sasaki M, Kogure D, Matsuda H, Hashimoto T (2001). Increased ictal perfusion of the thalamus in paroxysmal kinesigenic dyskinesia. J Neurol Neurosurg Psychiatry 71: 408–10.
51. Siebner HR, Tormos JM, Ceballos-Baumann AO, Auer C, Catala MD, Conrad B, Pascual-Leone A (1999). Low-frequency repetitive transcranial magnetic stimulation of the motor cortex in writer's cramp (In Process Citation). Neurology 52: 529–37.
52. Stoessl AJ, Martin WR, Clark C, Adam MJ, Ammann W, Beckman JH, Bergstrom M, Harrop R, Rogers JG, Ruth TJ, et al (1986). PET studies of cerebral glucose metabolism in idiopathic torticollis. Neurology 36: 653–7.
53. Tempel LW, Perlmutter JS (1990). Abnormal vibration-induced cerebral blood flow responses in idiopathic dystonia. Brain 113: 691–707.
54. Tempel LW, Perlmutter JS (1993). Abnormal cortical responses in patients with writer's cramp (published erratum appears in Neurology 1994; 44: 2411). Neurology 43: 2252–7.

Funktionelle Magnetresonanztomographie

J. Hennig

Zusammenfassung

Die funktionelle Magnetresonanztomographie bietet die Möglichkeit der detaillierten Beobachtung und Untersuchung der funktionellen Entwicklung des Gehirns. In Ergänzung der morphologischen Entwicklungsvorgänge bietet sie damit die Möglichkeit einer völlig neuen Einsicht der Entwicklungsvorgänge gerade beim Kleinkind. Die Nichtinvasivität des Verfahrens erlaubt dabei hochdetaillierte Untersuchungen auch subtiler Veränderungen durch longitudinale Studien. Klinische Anwendungen liegen zum einen in der objektiven Diagnose sensorischer Verarbeitungsstörungen sowie in der prächirurgischen Operationsplanung.

Neue Techniken der Bildgebung, die in den letzten 20 Jahren entwickelt wurden, haben zu einer dramatischen Verbesserung unseres Verständnisses der Reifung des menschlichen Gehirns geführt. Während vor Einführung dieser Techniken Autopsien und Läsionsstudien die einzige Grundlage zur Verfolgung der Entwicklungsvorgänge vom Gehirn darstellten, ist es mit Techniken wie Ultraschall, Magnetresonanztomographie, Computertomographie (CT), Positrons-Emissions-Tomographie (PET) und Single-Photon-Emission-Tomographie (SPECT) nunmehr möglich, diese Vorgänge im Detail am lebenden Patienten zu untersuchen. Vor allem die Kernspintomographie hat dabei aufgrund ihrer Nichtinvasivität und der damit gebotenen Möglichkeiten auch longitudinale Beobachtungen an Individuen durchzuführen sowie ihren hervorragenden Kontrast für relevante Strukturen insbesondere bei der Marktreifung ganz erheblich zu einer Verbesserung unseres Verständnisses beigetragen (siehe hierzu (1)).

Seit einigen Jahren wurde durch die Entdeckung des BOLD-Kontrastes durch Ogawa (2) die Möglichkeit geschaffen, neben der anatomischen morphologischen Bildgebung auch eine Darstellung der Lokalisation kortikaler Aktivierung zu erlangen. Mit Hilfe dieser fMRT (funktionelle Magnetresonanztomographie) genannten Technik gelingt es, durch gezielte Stimulationsaufgaben aktivierte Areale objektiv zu bestimmen. Die fMRT am Erwachsenen hat in den letzten Jahren einen wahren Siegeszug vor allem im Bereich der kognitiven Neurowissenschaften angetreten und wird verstärkt auch in der neurochirurgischen Operationsplanung eingesetzt. Erste Ergebnisse an Kleinkindern und Kindern belegen, dass diese Technik in der Lage ist, über die morphologische Entwicklung hinaus auch die funktionelle Entwicklung des Gehirns darzustellen (3). Gerade für die Beobachtung von Entwicklungsprozessen, welche sich in einem frühen Lebensstadium abspielen, hat die funktionelle MRT dadurch einen völlig neuen Einblick in die funktionelle Hirnentwicklung gegeben. Im Folgenden soll zunächst kurz die zugrunde liegende Technik dargestellt werden, folgen einige Anwendungsbeispiele der fMRT in der Neuropädiatrie.

fMRT Methode

Eine direkte Beobachtung neuronaler Vorgange wie sie mittels EEG und MEG durchgeführt wird, ist kernspintomographisch derzeit nicht möglich. Der fMRT liegt vielmehr die Beobachtung zugrunde, dass ein neuronaler Reiz eine hämodynamische Antwort nach sich zieht, welche sich durch entsprechende Messmethoden beobachten und darstellen lässt. Die Grundlage dieses BOLD-Kontrastes liegt dabei in der Tatsache, dass neuronale Aktivierung ein Energie verbrauchender Prozess ist und daher jede lokale Steigerung der neuronalen Aktivität durch ein entsprechendes Stimulationsparadigma zu einer Erhöhung des Sauerstoffverbrauchs führt. Durch die Arbeiten von Fox und Raichle (4) ist es seit vielen Jahren bekannt, dass das Gehirn diesen erhöhten lokalen Energiebedarf durch eine unmittelbar und regional begrenzte Erhöhung des regionalen Blutflusses (rCBF) begegnet. Diese Erhöhung der arteriellen Blutzufuhr führt durch Ausdehnung der postkapillären Venolen zu einer Erhöhung des regionalen Blutvolumens (rCBV) (Abb. 1). Zumindest beim Erwachsenen wird dabei der erhöhte Sauerstoffbedarf durch eine überproportional erhöhte Zufuhr

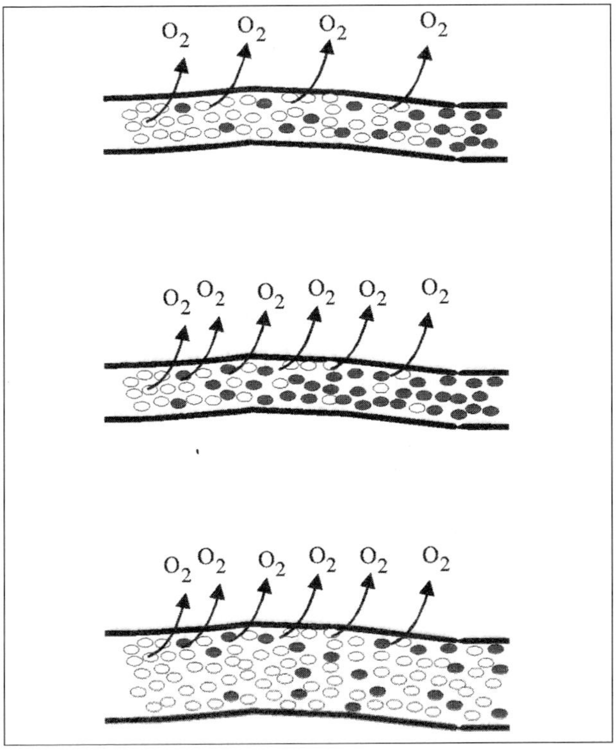

Abb. 1: Schematische Darstellung der hämodynamischen Antwort auf eine neuronale Aktivierung:
(oben) in Ruhe wird aus arteriellem Blut mit oxygeniertem Hämoglobin (weisse Kreise) Sauerstoff extrahiert, im venösen Blut ergibt sich eine Anreicherung von deoxygeniertem Hämoglobin (schwarze Kreise).
(Mitte) bei Aktivierung steigt der Sauerstoffverbrauch an, mehr Sauerstoff wird extrahiert.
(unten) das Gefässsystem reagiert mit einer Erhöhung des regionalen Blutflusses (rCBF), durch die elastische Expansi on der Venen kommt es auch zu einer Erhöhung des regionalen Blutvolumens (rCBV). Infolge der überproportionalen Erhöhung von rCBF und rCBV nimmt der Anteil an oxygeniertem Blut im aktivierten Volumen trotz erhöhtem Sauerstoffverbrauch zu.

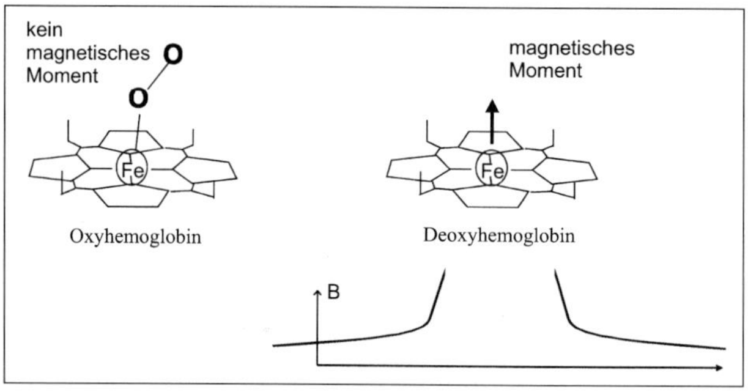

Abb. 2: Oxygeniertes Hämoglobin (links) besitzt nur ein schwaches magnetisches Moment, Deoxyhämoglobin ist dahingegen stark magnetisch. Durch die Wechselwirkung dieses lokalen Magnetfeldes mit dem äußeren Feld B kommt es in der unmittelbaren mikroskopischen Umgebung zu einem sogenannten Suszeptibilitätseffekt, welcher zu einer Signalauslöschung in der Umgebung venösen Blutes führt.

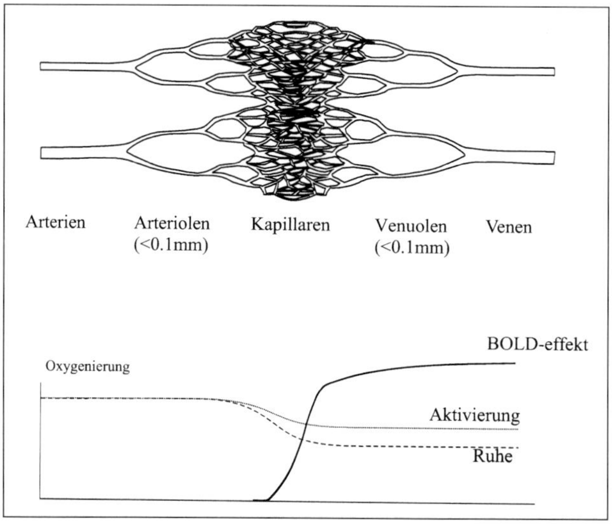

Abb. 3: Schematische Darstellung der Gefäßversorgung im Parenchym. Die Extraktion von Sauerstoff erfolgt ausschließlich über die Kapillaren. Durch die rel. Erhöhung der lokalen Sauerstoffkonzentration bei Aktivierung kommt es zu einer Signalerhöhung vor allem im postkapillären venösen Bett.

sauerstoffhaltigen arteriellen Blutes hypokompensiert, so dass in der Gesamtbilanz die Konzentration des oxygenierten Blutes (HbO) zunimmt. Diese Verschiebung von einer erhöhten Konzentration von Oxyhämoglobin ist nun kernspintomographisch dadurch beobachtbar, dass Oxyhämoglobin und Desoxyhämoglobin in ihren magnetischen Eigenschaften starke Unterschiede aufweisen. So besitzt Desoxyhämoglobin aufgrund des freien Elektronpaars am Eisenkern ein sehr starkes magnetisches Moment, welches sich makroskopisch durch eine Änderung des lokalen Magnetfeldes in der unmittelbaren Umgebung der blutführenden Gefäße bemerkbar macht. Oxyhämoglobin besitzt dahingegen ein sehr viel schwächeres magnetisches Moment und beeinflusst die Umgebung entsprechend wesentlich schwächer. Durch sogenannte suszeptibiltätsempfindliche Messsequenzen wie das Echo-Planar-Imaging (EPI) lässt sich die Verschiebung von Desoxyhämoglobin nach Oxyhämoglobin durch eine Signalerhöhung beobachten (5). Zu Beachten ist hierbei, dass die Sauerstoffextraktion praktisch ausschließlich im Kapillarbett stattfindet und der größte Anteil des bei Aktivierung stärker oxygenierten Blutvolumens in den postkapillären Vennolen stromabwärts vom aktivierten Kortex auftritt (Abb. 3). Der BOLD-Effekt ist also systematisch nach stromabwärts verschoben, wobei aufgrund der räumlichen Nähe der postkapillären Vennolen zum Kapillarbett von typischerweise 100 mm dieser Effekt bei der üblichen Ortsauflösung von ca. 1 bis 4 mm keine Rolle spielt.

Da eine absolute Beurteilung des Aktivierungszustandes in einer Einzelmessung zumindest derzeit praktisch nicht möglich ist, erfolgt die Messung bei der fMRT typischerweise durch Alternierung einer Kontrollbedingung (im allgemeinen Ruhe Bedingung) und der eigentlichen Aktivierungsbedingung. Die Reizdarbietung kann dabei in Abhängigkeit von dem Untersuchungsparadigma entweder durch einen kurzen Einzelreiz (sogenanntes Single Event Paradigma) oder bei geeignetem Aktivierungsparadigma als Blockparadigma über einen längeren Zeitraum stattfinden. Zur Verbesserung der statistischen Auswertung wird dabei die Aktivierungs- und Kontrollbedingung mehrfach alterniert. Aufgrund der langen Zeitkonstanten der hämodynamischen Antwort, liegt die zeitliche Auflösung für die Beobachtung einer Aktivierung in der fMRT, in der in mehrere Sekunden die zeitlich detaillierten Messungen wie sie im EEG oder MEG durchgeführt werden, ist somit mit dieser Technik nicht möglich. Demgegenüber bietet die fMRT allerdings die sehr viel genauere Ortsauflösung, welche mit in Verbindung mit der gleichzeitigen Aufnahme eines entsprechend hochaufgelösten anatomischen Datensatzes zu einer sehr genauen neuroanatomischen Lokalisation der aktivierten Areale führt.

fMRT: Anwendung bei Kindern

Anwendungsgebiete der fMRT bei Kindern sind zum einen wie schon erwähnt der Einsatz zur Beobachtung der funktionellen Entwicklung, wobei hierbei vor allem das visuelle System im Zentrum des derzeitigen Interesses steht. Dies ist vor allem dadurch begründet, dass zum einen das visuelle System sich mittels fMRT sehr gut untersuchen lässt, zum anderen gerade die funktionelle Entwicklung der visuellen Areale in einer sehr frühen Phase beim Kleinkind abläuft, in welcher sich durch fehlende Möglichkeit einer aktiven Kommunikation andere Untersuchungstechniken nur schwer und indirekt einsetzen lassen. Vor einem Ansatz der fMRT zur Untersuchung neuronaler Vorgänge ist hierbei natürlich als erstes abzuklären, inwieweit der im vorigen Kapitel geschilderte BOLD-Kontrast und die zugrunde liegende Kopplung zwischen neuronaler Aktivität und hämodynamischer Antwort bereits im frühkindlichen Gehirn realisiert ist. Neben der strukturellen Entwicklung der Markscheiden ist bereits aus früheren Untersuchungen bekannt, dass das frühkindliche Gehirn gegenüber dem Erwachsenen aufgrund der aktiven strukturellen Umbauvorgängen einen erhöhten Energieumsatz aufweißt, welches sich auch in einem um 30% oder mehr höheren rCBF widerspiegelt. Die Grundvoraussetzungen und Ruhebedingungen sind daher im kindlichen Gehirn gegenüber Erwachsenen deutlich unterschieden, so dass ein Prozedere für BOLD-Effekt durch eine weitere überproportionale Steigerung des RCBF nicht notwendigerweise erwartet werden kann. So wurde in Studien von Meek (6) und Martin (7) in der Tat bei Kleinkindern bei visueller Stimulation eine signifikante Signalerniedrigung statt der gewohnten Signalerhöhung beobachtet. Ein störender Faktor muss bei der Interpretation dieser Ergebnisse allerdings beachtet werden, dass die Untersuchungen bei Kleinkindern obligatorisch unter Sättigung durchgeführt wurden. In weiteren Studien gelang es Joeri (8) und Martin (9) allerdings nachzuweisen, dass Pentobarbital auch bei Erwachsenen zu einer Erniedrigung des BOLD-Effektes in Einzelfällen sogar zu einer Umkehr führt. Dieses sättigungsabhängige Effekt war allerdings bei Kindern wesentlich geringer. Vor allem konnte auch gezeigt werden, dass bei Sättigung mit Halotan, welches im Gegensatz zu Pentobarbital zu einer Erhöhung des RCBF führt, die selben Aktivierungsmuster auftraten, so dass davon ausgegangen werden kann, dass zumindest bei Kleinkindern in den ersten 6 Monaten keine Überkompensierung des regional erhöhten Sauerstoffbedarfs stattfindet und daher ein negativer BOLD-Effekt erwartet werden kann. Bezüglich der Lokalisierung der Hirnaktivierung bei Stimulation mittels eines Schachbrettreizes ist bei Kleinkindern eine starke Verlagerung nach Anterior im kalzarinischen Sulcus zu beobachten, ein Areal, welches neuroanatomisch wahrscheinlich zum extrastriatären Kortex der visuellen Area V2 zugeordnet werden kann. Neben dieser Aktivierung in V2 konnte Martin auch subkortikale Aktivierung im Thalamus beobachten. Diese Aktivierung, welche ausschließlich bei Kleinkindern auftritt, wird nach Interpretation der Autoren dem »secondary visual passway« zugeordnet. Dieser Verarbeitungsweg, welcher aufgrund der Neuroanatomie postuliert wird und für nicht bewußtes Sehen zuständig ist, wird bei Erwachsenen vor allem in der unbewußten Wahrnehmung bei Blinden in Verbindung gebracht (10).

Durch Übertragung von Reizparadigmen etwa zum Farbsehen, zum Kontrastsehen und zur Bewegungswahrnehmung auf die Gegebenheiten der Untersuchungen bei Kleinkindern und Kindern ist es inzwischen möglich, die funktionelle Entwicklung der kortikalen Areale und der unterschiedlichen kortikalen Verarbeitungsschritte im Detail nachzuvollziehen. Es fehlen derzeit allerdings noch statistisch ausreichend abgestützte Untersuchungen um über die derzeit vorliegenden Machbarkeitsstudien hinaus bereits Aussagen zur funktionellen Entwicklung des visuellen Systems beim Kleinkind vornehmen zu können.

Klinische Anwendungen und Ausblick

Fest etablierte und mit ausreichenden Patientenzahlen belegte klinische Anwendungen sind derzeit noch in Entwicklung. Untersucht wird dabei zum einen – wie beim Erwachsenen – der Einsatz der fMRT in der neurochirurgischen Operationsplanung zur Detektion eloquenter Areale, was gerade bei Kleinkindern in Anbetracht der entwicklungsbedingten Plastizität anhand anatomischer Landmarken nicht ohne weiteres möglich ist. Weitere klinische Anwendungen liegen im Einsatz zu Messung kortikaler Aktivierung bei sensorischer Stimulation (vor allem auditorisch) zum Nachweis entsprechender Defizite bei Kleinkindern.

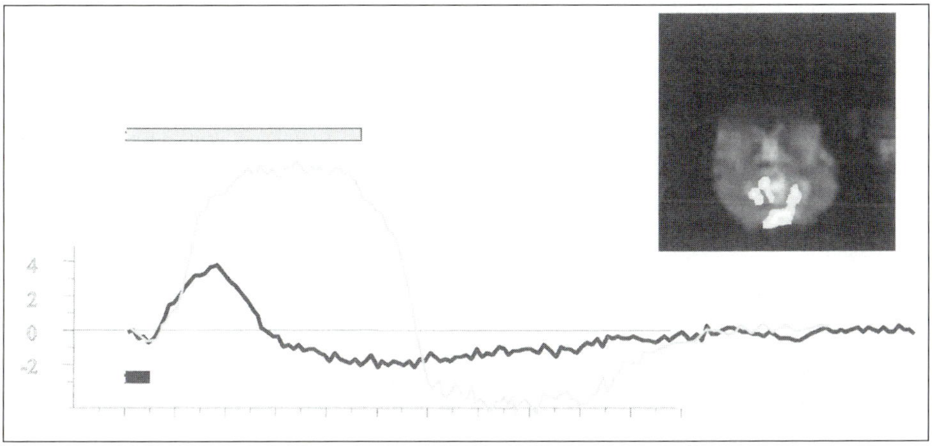

Abb. 4: Typische BOLD-Signale bei kurzer Stimulation (schwarze Linie, sogenanntes single-event design) und bei andauernder Stimulation in einem Block-design. Die single-event response zeigt eine bessere zeitliche Auflösung, im Blockdesign ist dahingegen der Gesamteffekt stärker.

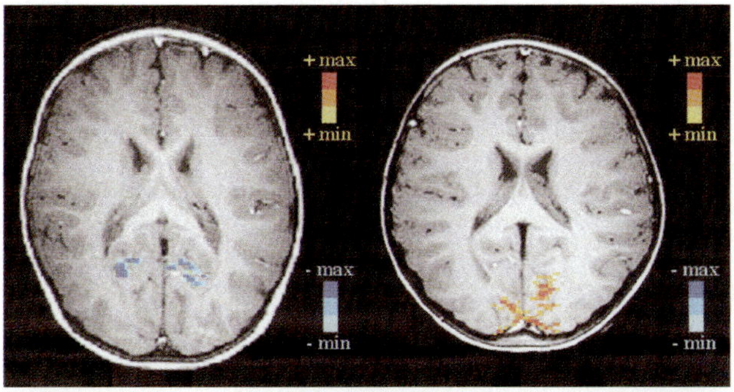

Abb. 5: Kortikale Aktivierung bei einem Kleinkind (2 Jahre, links) im Vergleich zu einem 8-Jährigen (rechts). Die aktivierten Areale beim Kleinkind sind nach vorne verlagert, die BOLD-Antwort ist negativ (blau) im Vergleich zum positiven Effekt (rot) bei Älteren (von E. Martin, Kinderspital Zürich).

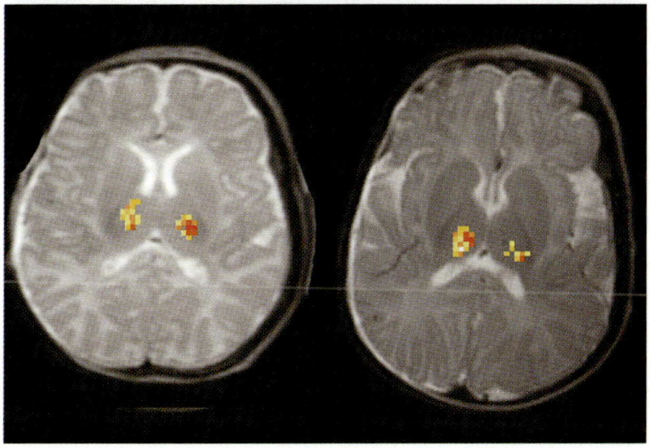

Abb. 6: Subkortikale Aktivierung bei visueller Stimulation, wie sie nur bei Kleinkindern (links: 3 Monate; rechts: 5 Monate) beobachtet wird (von E. Martin, Kinderspital Zürich).

Literatur

1. Valk J, van der Knaap MS (1995) Magnetic Resonance of Myelin, Myelination, & Myelin Disorders Springer-Verlag New York
2. Ogawa S, Tank D, Menon R, et al (1992) Intrinsic signal changes accompanying sensory stimulation: Functional brain mapping with magnetic resonance imaging. Proc Natl Acad Sci 89: 5951
3. Martin E, Marcar VL (2001) Functional MR imaging in pediatrics. Magn Reson Imaging Clin N Am 9-1: 231–245
4. Fox P, Raichle M (1986) Focal physiological uncoupling of cerebral blood flow and oxidative metabolism during somatosensory stimulation in human subjects. Proc Natl Acad Sci 83: 1140
5. Kwong K, Belliveau J, Chesler D, et al (1992) Dynamic magnetic resonance imaging of human brain activity during primary sensory stimulation. Proc Natl Acad Sci 89: 5675
6. Meek JH, Firbank M, Elwell CE, et al (1998) Regional hemodynamic responses to visual stimulation in awake infants. Pediatr Res 43: 840
7. Martin E, Thiel T, Joeri P, et al (1999) Visual processing in infants and children studied using functional MRI. Pediatr Res 46: 135
8. Joeri P, Huisman T, Loenneker T, et al (1996) Reproducibility of fMRI and effects of pentobarbital sedation on cortical activation during visual stimulation. Neuroimage 3: 280
9. Martin E, Thiel T, Joeri P, et al (2000) The effect of pentobarbital on visual processing in man. Hum Brain Mapp 10: 132
10. Sahraie A, Weiskrantz L, Barbur JL, et al (1997) Pattern of neuronal activity associated with conscious and unconscious processing of visual signals. Proc Natl Acad Sci 94: 9406

Rechtshemisphärische Sprachorganisation im fMRT und neuropsychologische Profile bei Patienten mit kongenitalen linksseitigen Hirnläsionen

K. Lidzba, M. Staudt, W. Grodd, I. Krägeloh-Mann

Zusammenfassung

Patienten mit angeborenen Läsionen der linken Hemisphäre (LH) und durch fMRT nachgewiesene rechtshemisphärische (RH) Sprachdominanz wurden mit Kontrollpersonen verglichen bezüglich der exakten Topographie der Hirnaktivierung bei Sprachproduktion sowie bezüglich kognitiver Fähigkeiten.

Die Patienten aktivierten bei einer Sprachproduktionsaufgabe RH Areale homolog zu den klassischen LH Spracharealen. Bezüglich der Sprachleistung gab es zwischen den beiden Gruppen keine Unterschiede.

Abkürzungen

AI = Asymmetrie-Index, GIQ = Gesamt-IQ, HIQ = Handlungs-IQ, LH = Linke Hemisphäre/linkshemisphärisch, MW = Mittelwert, RH = Rechte Hemisphäre/rechtshemisphärisch, SA = Standardabweichung , TE = Echozeit, TR = Repetitionszeit, VIQ = Verbal-IQ

Einleitung

Läsionen von sprachrelevanten Strukturen in der linken Hemisphäre (LH) führen bei Erwachsenen häufig zu permanenten Aphasien. Entstehen solche Läsionen jedoch in der Prä- oder Perinatalperiode, können die betroffenen Kinder in der Regel eine rechtshemisphärische (RH) Sprachorganisation entwickeln bei (weitgehend) intakten verbalen Fertigkeiten (Vargha-Khadem et al., 1994).

Eine RH Sprachorganisation wurde bei solchen Kindern nachgewiesen u.a. mit Hilfe des Wada-Tests (Rasmussen & Milner, 1977; Rey et al., 1988; Satz et al., 1988; Woods, et al., 1988) und mit fMRT (Hertz-Pannier et al., 1997; Staudt et al., 2001). Die genaue kortikale Topographie der atypisch in der RH organisierten Sprachfunktion wurde bislang jedoch noch nicht untersucht.

Die Befunde zu RH Sprachorganisation nach frühen LH Läsionen führten zu einer lebhaften Diskussion über eine mögliche Äquipotenz beider Hemisphären versus eine Prädisposition der LH für Sprachfunktionen.

In der hier beschriebenen Studie sollte zum einen die topographische Organisation von Sprachfunktionen in der RH untersucht werden (Staudt et al., 2002)

und zum anderen die Auswirkungen einer solchen atypischen Sprachorganisation auf die Sprachfunktion.

Topographie

Patienten und Kontrollen

Fünf junge Erwachsene zwischen 18 und 25 Jahren (drei Frauen) mit angeborener rechtsseitiger Hemiparese (Tabelle 1) aufgrund von linksseitigen periventrikulären Läsionen (Abb. 1). Alle Patienten sprechen deutsch als

Tab. 1: Demographische und klinische Daten, Asymmetrie-Indices des Planum temporale (PT) aller Patienten

Patient	Geschl.	Alter (Jahre)	Einschränkung Handmotorik*	Gestationsalter (Wochen)	Asymmetrie des PT
TK	m	18	3	39	−0.18
UE	w	21	1	41	−0.33
HT	m	22	2	33	−0.29
KC	w	24	2	39	−0.67
MJ	w	25	2	36	−0.40

* Einteilung der handmotorischen Einschränkung mit Hilfe der sequenziellen Finger-oppositions-Aufgabe: 1 = keine signifikante Einschränkung, 2 = deutliche Verlangsamung oder unvollständige Ausführung, 3 = unabhängige Fingerbewegungen sind unmöglich (Staudt et al., 2000).

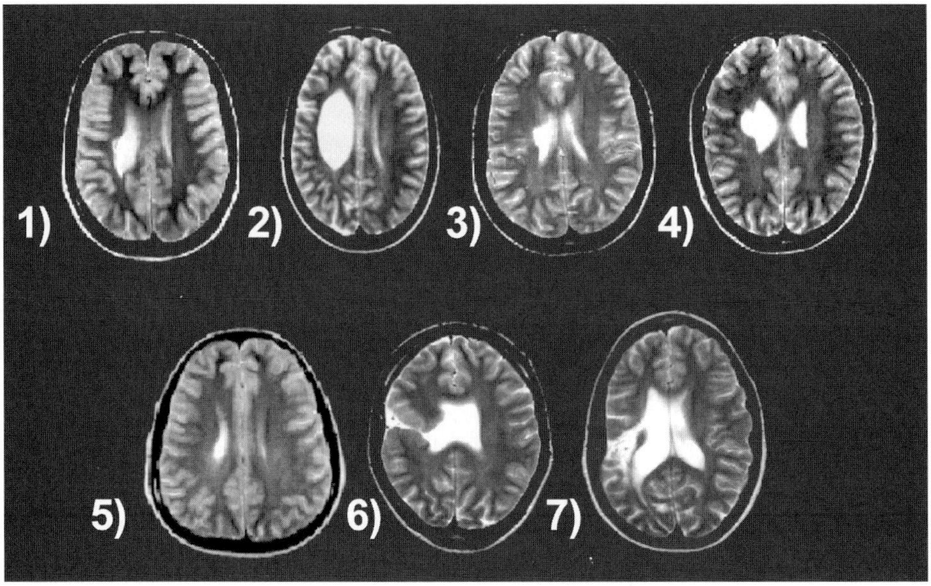

Abb. 1: Axiale Protonendichte-MR Aufnahmen der Patientengruppe. 1)–5) Patienten mit linksseitigen periventrikulären Läsionen; 6) Patient mit linksseitiger Schizencephalie; 7) Patientin mit linksseitigem kortiko-subkortikalen Infarkt. Studie I (Topographie): Patienten 1)–5); Studie II (Psychologie): Patienten 1)–7).

Muttersprache und haben eine reguläre Schullaufbahn absolviert.

Bei einer stillen Wortproduktionsaufgabe zeigten alle Patienten im fMRT eine ausgedehntere Aktivierung in der rechten als in der linken Hemisphäre.

Die Prä- und Perinatal-Anamnese war bei zwei Patienten unauffällig; zwei Patienten waren Frühgeborene (33. und 36. SSW); ein Patient wurde bei pathologischem CTG zum Termin durch Kaiserschnitt geboren. Keiner der Patienten litt an Epilepsie.

Bei keinem der Patienten bestand eine familiäre Disposition für Linkshändigkeit oder eine atypische Asymmetrie des Planum temporale, welche als Marker für eine angeborene RH Sprachorganisation gelten (Hecaen et al., 1981; Habib et al., 1995).

Fünf gesunde Rechtshänder zwischen 19 und 23 Jahren (drei Frauen) dienten als Kontrollgruppe.

Methode

Alle MRT-Messungen wurden mit einem 1,5 Tesla Siemens Vision Scanner durchgeführt.

Strukturelle Bilder: axiale dual spin-echo Schichten (TR 4800 ms, TE 14 und 85 ms, Auflösung 2 x 2 x 4 mm^3) und T1-gewichteter 3D Datensatz (128 lückenlose Sagittalschnitte, TR 9,7 ms, TE 4 ms, Auflösung 1,5 x 1 x 1 mm^3).

Funktionelle Daten: Ganzhirn-Multischicht Echoplanarbildgebung (EPI) (vgl. Klose et al., 1999: 27 Axialschnitte, TR 8 s, TE 84 ms, 4 mm Schichtendicke, 1 mm gap, horizontale Auflösung 2 x 2 mm^2).

Block-Design mit 4 Epochen Ruhe und 4 Epochen Wortproduktion im Wechsel (je Epoche 6 Aufnahmen des gesamten Gehirns; insgesamt 48 Aufnahmen). Zwischen den einzelnen Bildakquisitionen (je 4,87 sek.) gab es jeweils eine kurze Pause von 3,13 sek., die zur Instruktion des Probanden genutzt wurde (neuer Anfangsbuchstabe für die Wortproduktionsaufgabe oder »Pause!« in der Ruhebedingung).

Wortproduktionsaufgabe: Es waren »Wörterketten« mit vorgegebenem Anfangsbuchstaben zu produzieren. Jedes Wort sollte mit dem Endbuchstaben des vorhergehenden Wortes anfangen (Beisp.: **B**anan**e**-**E**lefan**t**-**T**omat**e**...). Als einzige Einschränkung sollten Wiederholungen von Wörtern vermieden werden.

Datananalyse: Die Vorverarbeitung und statistische Analyse der funktionellen Daten wurden mit Hilfe von SPM99 (Statistical Parametric Mapping, Wellcome Department of Cognitive Neurology, University College London) durchgeführt. Nach der Vorverarbeitung der Datensätze gingen wir in folgenden vier Schritten vor:

I. Berechnung von Aktivierungskarten für jeden Patienten einzeln ($p < 0,05$ auf Voxel-Ebene, korrigiert für Mehrfachvergleiche). Nach Auszählung der aktivierten Voxel in jeder Hemisphäre Berechnung eines Asymmetrie-Index (AI) mit AI = (R-L) / (R+L). Negative Werte stehen damit für mehr aktivierte Voxel in der linken Hemisphäre.

II. Erstellung von gruppenspezifischen Aktivierungskarten in einer »fixed-effect« Analyse (auch hier $p < 0,05$, korr.)

III. Vergleich der beiden Gruppen in einer »random-effect« Analyse, um Bereiche zu identifizieren, die in einer der beiden Gruppen signifikant höhere Aktivierung zeigen ($p < 0{,}01$ auf Voxel-Ebene, korr. nur auf Cluster-Ebene mit $p < 0{,}05$).

IV. Direkter Vergleich zwischen der jeweiligen dominanten Hemisphäre (rechts bei Patienten vs. links bei Kontrollen) und der jeweiligen nichtdominanten Hemisphäre (links bei Patienten und rechts bei Kontrollen) nach Spiegelung des funktionellen Datensatzes der Kontrollpersonen in x-Richtung (dadurch Projektion der LH Aktivierung auf die RH).

Ergebnisse

Wie erwartet, wies die Kontrollgruppe eine starke Asymmetrie zur LH hin auf (mittlerer AI = –0,97; SA = 0,06). Die rechtsseitige Asymmetrie bei den Patienten war dagegen weniger stark: mittlerer AI = +0,69; SA = 0,25.

Fixed-effect Analyse

Abbildung 2 zeigt die Gruppen-Aktivierungskarten bei Patienten und Kontrollen.

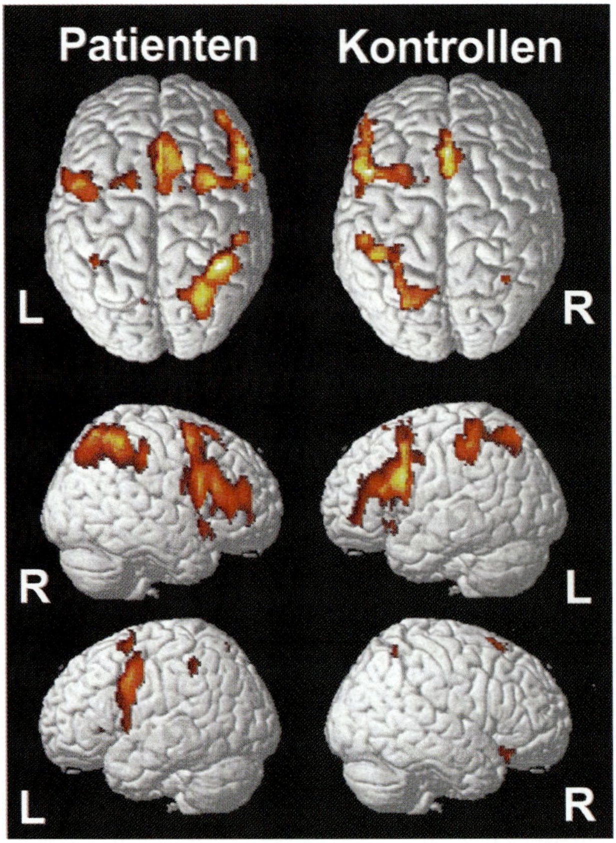

Abb. 2: »Fixed-effect« Analyse für Patienten (links) and Kontrollen (rechts), mit ($p < 0.05$) Aktivierungs-Schwelle auf Voxel-Ebene, korrigiert für Mehrfachvergleiche. Aktivierungskarten sind dem SPM99 single-subject template überlagert.

Beide Gruppen wiesen das globale Maximum im Gyrus frontalis inferior auf (BA 44, »Broca-Areal« bzw. »Broca-Analogon« bei den Patienten). Von hier aus dehnte sich die Aktivierung in posteriorer und dorsaler Richtung in den prämotorischen Cortex aus (BA 6), nach anterior in präfrontale Areale (BA 45, 46, 10) und in ventraler Richtung in das Operculum und die Insula.

Weitere große Cluster liegen im Parietallappen dorsal (BA 7) und ventral (BA 40) des Sulcus intraparietalis, sowie im fronto-mesialen Cortex (BA 6, 32).

Entsprechend der geringeren Lateralität in der Patientengruppe konnten nur hier weitere Aktivierungscluster in der nicht dominanten LH gefunden werden. Diese lagen im Gyrus frontalis inferior (BA 6,44) und im Bereich des Sulcus intraparietalis (BA 7,40).

Random-effect Analyse

Die Random-effect Analyse der RH zeigte einige kleine Areale in der RH auf, die bei den Patienten stärker aktiviert waren, als die korrespondierenden LH Areale der Kontrollgruppe. Nach Korrektur für Mehrfachvergleiche blieb jedoch keine dieser Aktivierungen statistisch signifikant (weder auf Voxel- noch auf Cluster-Ebene; jeweils $p > 0{,}4$ korrigiert). Auch im umgekehrten Vergleich (größere LH Aktivierung bei den Kontrollen als in der RH der Patienten) überstand keine Aktivierung die Korrektur für Mehrfachvergleiche (jeweils $p > 0{,}97$ korrigiert).

Psychologie

Patienten und Kontrollen

Sieben junge Erwachsene zwischen 18 und 25 Jahren (vier Frauen) mit kongenitalen Schädigungen der LH und RH Sprachdominanz im fMRT. Fünf der Patienten sind bereits in Teil I beschrieben, zwei weitere Patienten litten je an einer linksseitigen Schizenzephalie und einem pränatalen linksseitigen kortiko-subkortikalen Infarkt (Abb. 1).

Sieben gesunde Rechtshänder (angeglichen in Alter, Geschlecht und Bildungsniveau) dienten als Kontrollprobanden.

Methoden

Alle Teilnehmer wurden dem Hamburg-Wechsler Intelligenztest für Erwachsene (HAWIE-R; Tewes, 1991) unterzogen. Es lassen sich ein Gesamt-IQ (GIQ), ein Verbal-IQ (VIQ) sowie ein Handlungs-IQ (HIQ) berechnen.

Zusätzlich wurden drei verschiedene Wortflüssigkeitsaufgaben durchgeführt: »Wörterkette« (beschrieben in Teil I), Kategorien (jeweils 1 Minute lang *Tiere, Obstsorten* und *Gemüsesorten* aufzählen) und Anfangsbuchstaben (jeweils 1 Minute lang Wörter mit den Anfangsbuchstaben *F, A* und *S* aufzählen, nicht erlaubt sind Namen oder Zahlwörter). Pro Aufgabe wurde die Anzahl der insgesamt produzierten Wörter berechnet.

Ergebnisse

Zwischen Patienten- und Kontrollgruppe ergeben sich keine signifikanten Unterschiede in den Aufgaben zur Wortflüssigkeit *(Wörterkette: 64,0 ± 14,0 vs. 72,7 ± 15,1; p > 0,3; Kategorien: 52,9 ± 15,5 vs. 60,0 ± 11,8; p > 0,2; Anfangsbuchstaben: 44,7 ± 9,2 vs. 44,2 ± 7,2; p > 0,9. Student t-Test, jeweils MW und SA bei Patienten vs. Kontrollen).*

Zwischen Patienten- und Kontrollgruppe zeigten sich keine signifikanten Unterschiede im mittleren Gesamt-IQ oder im mittleren Verbal-IQ *(GIQ: 104,7 ± 14,3 vs. 115,1 ± 9,0; p = 0,13; VIQ: 108,14 ± 16,2 vs. 112,43 ± 10,2; p > 0,5. Student t-Test, jeweils MW und SA bei Patienten vs. Kontrollen).*

Ein signifikanter Unterschied zeigt sich jedoch zwischen Patienten und Kontrollen beim Handlungs-IQ *(HIQ: 98,3 ± 14,2 vs. 112,7 ± 6,6; p < 0,05. Student t-Test).* Die mittlere Differenz VIQ minus HIQ beträgt in der Patientengruppe *9,9 ± 15,1;* in der Kontrollgruppe *–0,43 ± 9,8 (p = 0,16; Student t-Test).*

Diskussion

Die von uns untersuchten Patienten zeigten eine RH Sprachorganisation nach prä- und perinatalen Schädigungen der LH. Die fMRT-Aktivierungsmuster dieser Patienten bei einer stillen Sprachproduktionsaufgabe sind erstaunlich symmetrisch zu denen von gesunden Rechtshändern. Beide Gruppen zeigen Aktivierungen in inferio-lateralen und mesialen Teilen des Frontallappens, sowie in der Umgebung des Sulcus intraparietalis der jeweils dominanten Hemisphäre.

Der Gruppenvergleich zeigt auf Voxelebene keine signifikanten Unterschiede der Aktivierungsmuster der jeweils dominanten Hemisphäre.

Dies kann als Hinweis dafür gesehen werden, dass nach frühen LH Hirnschädigungen RH Areale rekrutiert werden, die *homolog* zu den LH Sprachарealen gesunder Rechtshänder sind.

Die möglichen Auswirkungen früher unilateraler Läsionen auf kognitive Funktionen werden lebhaft diskutiert (z.B. Vargha-Kahdem et al., 1994; Eisele & Aram, 1995). Dem sich entwickelnden Gehirn wird von allen Studien zugebilligt, bestimmte Läsionen besser verarbeiten zu können als das reife Gehirn. Dennoch besteht nur wenig Einigkeit darüber, wie schwer und wie spezifisch die Defizite sind, die zurückbleiben.

Anhand der hier untersuchten Patienten konnten auch wir zeigen, dass die RH prinzipiell in der Lage ist, Sprachfunktionen zu kontrollieren. Patienten und Kontrollen unterscheiden sich nicht signifikant im Verbal-IQ oder in der Wortflüssigkeit. Über subtilere Sprachleistungen, wie sie z.B. von Reilly et al. (1998) untersucht wurden, kann hier jedoch keine Aussage gemacht werden.

Auffällig ist dennoch, dass die Gruppe der Patienten bei annähernd gleichem Verbal-IQ signifikant schlechtere Leistungen als die Kontrollpersonen im Handlungsteil des HAWIE-R zeigten. Defizite in visuo-spatialen und damit originär rechtshemisphärischen Funktionen nach frühen LH Läsionen wurden schon in den 70er Jahren von Teuber und auch danach immer wieder gefunden (Strauss et al., 1990; Helmstädter et al., 1994; Mariotti et al., 1998). Teuber (1974) prägte den

Begriff des »Crowding«: Die atypische Organisation von Sprachfunktionen in der RH führe dort zu einem Mangel an neuronalem Substrat, wodurch die ursprünglichen RH Funktionen beeinträchtigt würden.

Die Ergebnisse der fMRT zeigt nun, dass trotz der angenommenen Rivalität zwischen Sprach- und visuo-spatialen Funktionen um neuronales Substrat in der RH die Sprachfunktion in zu den klassischen Spracharealen korrespondierenden Hirnarealen lokalisiert zu sein scheint. Dieser Befund unterstützt Spekulationen über die funktionelle Überlegenheit von Sprache gegenüber anderen kognitiven Funktionen, wie sie z.B. von Mariotti et al. (1998) angestellt wurden.

Es sind weitere Studien geplant, um das topographische Schicksal originär RH Funktionen, wie visuell-räumliches Denken oder Sprachprosodie (Wildgruber et al, im Druck), nach RH Sprach(re-)organisation weiter zu verfolgen.

Literatur

1. Eisele J, Aram D (1995) Lexical and grammatical development in children with early hemisphere damage: A cross-sectional view from birth to adolescence. In: Fletcher P, MacWhinney B. (Herausg.) The Handbook of Child Language. Basil Blackwell, Oxford
2. Habib M., Robichon F., Levrier O., Khalil R., Salamon G. (1995) Diverging asymmetries of temporo-parietal cortical areas: a reappraisal of Geschwind/Galaburda theory. Brain Lang. 48: 238–258
3. Hecaen H., De Agostini M., Monzon-Montes A. (1981) Cerebral organization in left-handers. Brain Lang. 12: 261–284.
4. Helmstädter C, Kurthen M., Linke D.B., Elger C.E. (1994) Right hemisphere restitution of language and memory functions in right hemisphere language-dominant patients with left temporal lobe epilepsy. Brain 117: 729–737.
5. Hertz-Pannier L., Gaillard W.D., Mott S.H., Cuenod C.A., Bookheimer S.Y., Weinstein S., Conry J., Papero P.H., Schiff S.J., LeBihan D., Theodore W.H. (1997) Noninvasive assessment of language dominance in children and adolescents with functional MRI: a preliminary study. Neurology 48: 1003–1012
6. Klose U., Erb M., Wildgruber D., Müller E., Grodd W. (1999) Improvement of the acquisition of a large amount of MR images on a conventional whole body system. Magn. Reson. Imaging 17: 471–474
7. Mariotti P., Iuvone L., Torrioni M.G., Silveri M.C. (1998) Linguistic and non-linguistic abilities in a patient with early left hemispherectomy. Neuropsychologia 36: 1303–1312
8. Rasmussen T., Milner B. (1977) The role of early left-brain injury in determining lateralization of cerebral speech functions. Ann. N. Y. Acad. Sci. 299: 355–369.
9. Reilly J., Bates E., Marchman V.(1998) Narrative discourse in children with early focal brain injury. Brain Lang. 61: 335–375
10. Rey M., Dellatolas G., Bancaud J., Talairach J. (1988) Hemispheric lateralization of motor and speech functions after early brain lesion: study of 73 epileptic patients with intracarotid amytal test. Neuropsychologia 26: 167–172
11. Satz P., Strauss E., Wada J., Orsini D.L. (1988) Some correlates of intra- and interhemispheric speech organization after left focal brain injury. Neuropsychologia 26: 345–350
12. Staudt M., Grodd W., Niemann G., Wildgruber D., Erb M., Krägeloh-Mann I. (2001) Early left periventricular brain lesions induce right hemispheric organization of speech. Neurology 57: 122–125
13. Staudt M., Lidzba K., Grodd W., Wildgruber D., Erb M., Krägeloh-Mann I. (2002) Right-Hemispheric Organization of Language Following Early Left-Sided Brain Lesions: Functional MRI Topography. NeuroImage im Druck

14. Staudt M, Niemann G., Grodd W., Krägeloh-Mann I. (2000) The pyramidal tract in congenital hemiparesis: relationship between morphology and function in periventricular lesions. Neuropediatrics 31: 257–264
15. Strauss E., Satz P., Wada J. (1990) An examination of the crowding hypothesis in epileptic patients who have undergone the carotid amytal test. Neuropsychologia 28: 1221–1227
16. Teuber H.L. (1974) Why two brains? In: The Neurosciences: Third Study Program. Schmitt F.O., Worden F. G. (Herausg.). MIT Press, Cambridge.
17. Tewes U. (1991) Hamburg-Wechsler Intelligenztest für Erwachsene. Revision 1991. Verlag Hans Huber, Bern
18. Vargha-Khadem F., Isaacs E., Muter V. (1994) A review of cognitive outcome after unilateral lesions sustained during childhood. J. Child Neurol. 9 (Suppl): 267–273
19. Wildgruber D., Pihan H., Ackermann H., Erb M., Grodd W. (2002) Dynamic brain activation during processing of emotional intonation: influence of acoustic parameters, emotional valence, and sex. NeuroImage, im Druck
20. Woods R.P., Dodrill C.B., Ojemann G.A. (1988) Brain injury, handedness, and speech lateralization in a series of amobarbital studies. Ann. Neurol. 23: 510–518

Motorisches fMRI bei Kindern: Prächirurgisches Mapping der Handrepräsentation

M. Staudt, W. Grodd, M. Erb, H. Holthausen, K. Strobl, I. Krägeloh-Mann

Einleitung

Motorische fMRI-Experimente erfordern eine aktive Mitarbeit des Patienten und sind deshalb bei Kindern, insbesondere solchen mit mentaler Retardierung, schwieriger durchzuführen als bei kooperativen Erwachsenen.

Wir stellen hier ein Messprotokoll vor, das den Anforderungen dieses Kollektivs angepasst ist, und berichten über vorläufige Ergebnisse der Anwendung bei pädiatrischen epilepsie-chirurgischen Patienten.

Patienten und Kontrollen

Bislang wurden 10 Patienten (Alter: 6–22 Jahre) mit fokalen Epilepsien vor (möglicher) epilepsiechirurgischer Intervention untersucht. Bei den zugrundeliegenden Läsionen handelte es sich um Malformationen (n = 6), prä- oder perinatal erworbene Infarkte im Versorgungsgebiet der A. cerebri media (n = 2) und um Defekte nach Schädel-Hirn-Traumen (n = 2), die im Alter von 2 Monaten bzw. 3 Jahren eingetreten waren. Als Kontrollen dienten 4 gesunde Kinder im Alter von 5–9 Jahren.

Fragestellung

Ziel der Untersuchungen war die Identifikation der kortikalen motorischen Handrepräsentation, was bei Patienten mit frühen Läsionen aus zwei Gründen nicht allein anhand anatomischer Kriterien geschehen kann: Einmal wegen der Möglichkeit einer abgelaufenen Reorganisation, zum anderen bei Zerstörung oder Veränderung der normalen anatomischen Landmarken durch die Läsionen bzw. Fehlbildungen. Hier bietet sich die fMRI zur Darstellung kortikaler Aktivierung während einfacher Handbewegungen an.

Messprotokoll

Technische Angaben

1,5 Tesla Siemens SONATA; EchoPlanarImaging (EPI) mit 27 axialen Schichten, TE 37 ms; »Block Design« mit 8 Epochen von Handbewegung im Wechsel mit 8 Epochen von Ruhe, Epochenlänge: je 30 s, damit Gesamtlänge der

Messung: 8 min. Auswertung mit SPM99, Aktivierungsschwelle $p < 0,05$ (korrigiert) auf Voxel-Level.

»Pädiatrische« Modifikationen

Alle Messungen erfolgten mit Anwesenheit des Untersuchers sowie eines Elternteils im Messraum. Als Aktivierungsbedingung wurde repetitives Drücken der Hand des Untersuchers gewählt, was gegenüber Öffnen/Schließen der leeren Hand zwei Vorteile aufweist: Zum einen wird über den direkten Körperkontakt ängstlichen Kindern Sicherheit vermittelt, zum anderen wird die Kooperation des Patienten vom Untersucher unmittelbar erfahren, so dass er ggf. korrigierend eingreifen kann. Schließlich wurde nach jedem Scan (Dauer 2,4 s) eine Pause von 3,6 s ohne Messlärm eingeführt, in der zu dem Kind gesprochen werden kann. In jeder dieser Pausen, also alle 6 s, wird das jeweilige Kommando (»Drücken!« oder »Pause!«) gegeben, zusätzlich kann das Kind durch kurze Anweisungen korrigiert oder ermuntert werden. Um diese Kommunikation zu ermöglichen, muss ohne Gehörschutz für das Kind gemessen werden, was die Auswahl nicht allzu lauter Sequenzen erforderlich macht.

Ergebnisse

Mit der geschilderten Methodik wurde in allen 14 untersuchten Fällen eine kortikale Aktivierung motorischer Areale nachgewiesen (Beispiel siehe Abb. 1).

In der Patientengruppe wurden zwei verschiedene Konstellationen beobachtet:

Bei drei Patienten mit Malformationen unter Einschluss der Zentralregion, die deutliche Hemiparesen aufwiesen (handmotorische Behinderung Grad 2–3,

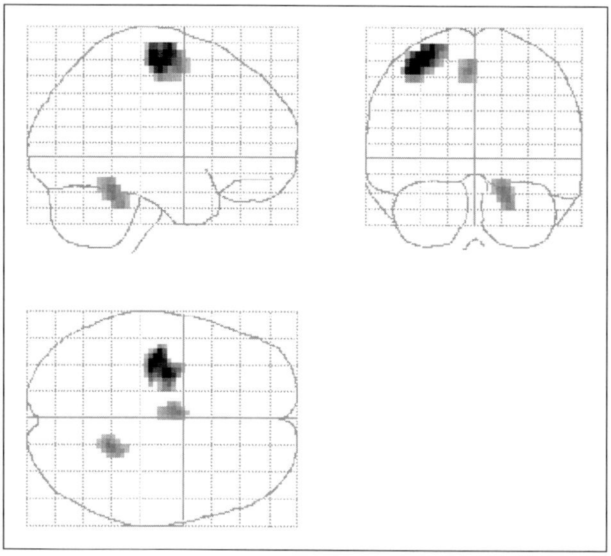

Abb. 1: fMRT bei repetitivem Greifen der rechten Hand von einem gesunden 5-jährigen Kontrollkind. SPM99, $p < 0,05$ korrigiert. Maximum intensity projection (»glass brain«) mit Ansichten in sagittaler (links oben), koronarer (rechts) und axialer Projektion (unten).
Gut erkennbar sind die kräftige Aktivierung des kontralateralen sensomotorischen Kortex, des supplementär-motorischen Areals sowie des ipsilateralen Cerebellum.

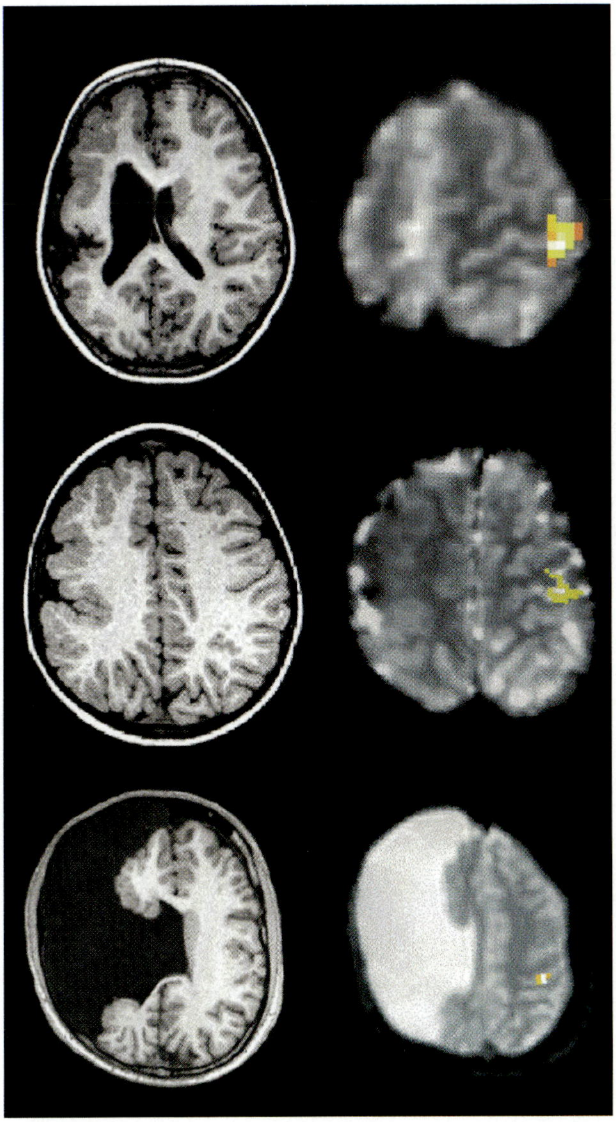

Abb. 2: Drei Patienten mit ausgedehnten Malformationen einer Hemisphäre (links: axiale T1-gewichtete MRT-Schichten) und fMRT-Aktivierung in der intakten Hemisphäre bei Bewegung der paretischen Hand, überlagert auf EPI-Schichten (rechts). SPM99, $p < 0{,}05$.

vgl. Beitrag »Kortikale Reorganisation bei Patienten mit Zerebralparese«), fanden wir während Bewegung der paretischen Hand überschwellige fMRI-Aktivierung immer nur in der Zentralregion der intakten Hemisphäre. Diese abnorme, reorganisierte Repräsentation der paretischen Hand in der ipsilateralen, intakten Hemisphäre wurde bei allen drei Patienten auch durch den Nachweis von schnell-leitenden kortiko-spinalen Projektionen aus der intakten Hemisphäre zu beiden Händen durch transkranielle Magnetstimulation (TMS) bestätigt. Klinisch fielen diese Patienten auch durch deutliche Spiegelbewegungen auf (= Mitbewegungen der jeweils anderen Hand bei willkürlichen unimanuellen Bewegungen), was als Folge der gemeinsamen Repräsentation beider Hände in der Zentralregion der intakten Hemisphäre interpretiert werden kann.

Bei den übrigen Patienten (n = 7) fanden wir fMRI-Aktivierung bei Bewegung der zur Läsion kontralateralen Hand immer in der Zentralregion der geschädigten Hemisphäre. Damit ergab sich in diesen Fällen kein Hinweis auf Reorganisation, weder inter- noch intrahemisphäriell, auch wenn die oft hochepileptogenen Malformationen oder Defekte bis unmittelbar an die Zentralregion heranreichten.

Schlussfolgerungen

1. Bei Wahl geeigneter Messbedingungen werden motorische fMRI-Untersuchungen auch bei weniger kooperationsfähigen Kindern möglich.
2. Eine Reorganisation der primär-motorischen Handrepräsentation sahen wir hier nur bei Malformationen, die die Zentralregion umfassten. Die Funktionsübernahme erfolgte stets durch die Zentralregion der intakten Hemisphäre, war funktionell unvollständig und ging mit deutlichen Spiegelbewegungen einher.

Bedeutung der diffusionsgewichteten Bildgebung (DWI) in der Früherkennung von diffusen axonalen Verletzungen (DAI) bei kindlichen Hirnverletzungen

M. Kieslich, S. Weidauer, W. Schneider, R. Gerlach, S. Vlaho, V. Boda, M. Wesendahl, H. Boehles

Zusammenfassung

Diffuse axonale Verletzungen (DAI) entstehen durch Scherverletzungen der Axone und ihrer versorgenden Mikrogefäße im Rahmen von Akzelerations-Dezelerations-Verletzungen des Gehirns. Prädilektionsorte sind der Hirnstamm, die parasagittale weiße Substanz, das Corpus callosum sowie die Grenzbezirke der kortikalen grauen und weißen Substanz. Im Rahmen der initialen posttraumatischen Computertomographie (CT) und konventionellen Magnetresonanztomographie (MRT) mit T1- und T2-Wichtung lassen sich DAI oft nicht, bzw. erst ab einer gewissen Größe der Läsionen oder bei kombinierten petechialen Einblutungen, darstellen. Erst nach Wochen und Monaten bilden sich kleine narbige Läsionen aus. Die diffusionsgewichteten MRT-Sequenzen (DWI) sind sehr sensitiv für ischämische Läsionen und zytotoxische Ödeme. Letztere sind typisch für die Frühphase nach Axonrupturen. Die Untersuchung zeigt, dass die DWI bereits in der posttraumatischen Frühphase sensitiv für diffuse axonale Verletzungen (DAI) ist und somit hilft, Kinder mit erhöhtem Risiko für posttraumatische Residualzustände zu erkennen und entsprechende Therapie- und Rehabilitationsentscheidungen zu modifizieren.

Einleitung

Diffuse axonale Verletzungen (DAI) entstehen durch Scherverletzungen der Axone und ihrer versorgenden Mikrogefäße im Rahmen von Akzelerations-Dezelerations-Verletzungen des Gehirns, vorwiegend im Rahmen von Schädel-Hirn-Verletzungen, die mit einer im Winkel zur Sagittalebene wirkenden erhöhten Beschleunigung einhergehen. Hierbei kann es durch Abscherung kleiner Gefäße zu petechialen Blutungen aber vor allem zur Schädigung des axonalen Zytoskeletts mit reaktivem zytotoxischem Ödem kommen. Eine Maximalform der DAI finden sich beim abusiven Schütteltrauma (»Shaken Infant Syndrom«), bei dem es durch Schütteln des Kindes zu intracavitären Rotationsbewegungen des Gehirns kommt, welche ausgeprägte großflächige Hirnläsionen mit multiplen petechialen Einblutungen durch zusätzliche intraparenchymatöse Gefäßrupturen zur Folge haben (4).

Im Rahmen der initialen posttraumatischen Computertomographie (CT) und konventionellen Magnetresonanztomographie (MRT) mit T1- und T2-Wichtung lassen sich DAI oft nicht, bzw. erst ab einer gewissen Größe der Lasionen oder bei kombinierten petechialen Einblutungen, darstellen. Im weiteren Akutverlauf kann eventuell ein Hirnödem auftreten. Erst nach Wochen und Monaten bilden sich multiple kleine narbenartige Läsionen, möglicherweise mit begleitender Hirnatrophie, aus.

Grundlage der diffusionsgewichteten Bildgebung (DWI) ist die extra- und intrazellulär unterschiedliche Diffusion von Wassermolekülen in Neuronen und Glia. Eine DWI-Signalerhöhung ergibt sich aufgrund einer umschriebenen Abnahme der Diffusion, welche Folge der Abnahme des Extrazellulärraumes und Zunahme der räumlich relativ begrenzteren Diffusion innerhalb der Zelle ist. Die diffusionsgewichteten MRT-Sequenzen sind sehr sensitiv für ischämische Läsionen, zum Beispiel bei Hirninfarkten, aber auch für zytotoxische Ödeme, wie sie zum Beispiel nach einem Status epileptikus aber auch im Rahmen von axonalen Scherverletzungen auftreten können (2, 9, 10).

Ziel der folgenden Untersuchung war es, die Sensitivität der diffusionsgewichteten Bildgebung (DWI) bezüglich der Früherkennung von DAI, insbesondere ohne assoziierten petechialen Einblutungen, zu untersuchen.

Methodik und Patientengut

Sieben pädiatrische Patienten mit Hirnverletzungen wurden innerhalb der ersten neun posttraumatischen Tage kernspintomographisch untersucht. Die traumatischen Läsionen wurden nach Form und Lage charakterisiert, die klinischen Befunde analysiert und der posttraumatische Residualzustand mittels der Glasgow Outcome Scale evaluiert. Neben der initialen CT erfolgten bei allen Patienten kernspintomographische Untersuchungen mit einem Siemens Vision 1,5 T MR-System. Das standardisierte Untersuchungsprotokoll beinhaltete T1-, T2-, FLAIR- (fluid attenuated inversion recovery) und T2*-Sequenzen. Zusätzlich wurden triplanare DWI- (diffusion-weighted imaging) Sequenzen akquiriert.

Ergebnisse

Bei den 7 Patienten handelte es sich um 5 Mädchen und 2 Jungen im Alter zwischen 1 und 15 Jahren (mittleres Alter 11 Jahre). In 3 Fällen handelte es sich um Verkehrsunfälle mit hoher Geschwindigkeit (»high velocity accidents«), in 4 um Stürze aus bis zu 5 Meter Höhe (»crush injuries«). Die initialen Glasgow Coma Scales (GCS) lagen zwischen 5 und 15 Punkten. Die initial durchgeführten CT's zeigten bei 6 Kindern Schädelfrakturen, bei 4 Kindern epidurale, bei 3 subdurale und bei 1 zusätzlich eine subarachnoidale und intraparenchymale Blutung mit Ventrikeleinbruch. Die initiale neurologische Symptomatik reichte von isolierten Cephalgien, Erbrechen, sekundärer Eintrübung und Ataxie über ein hirnorganisches Psychosyndrom bis hin zu einem akuten Mittelhirnsyndrom.

Die kernspintomographischen Untersuchungen erfolgten zwischen dem 2. und 9. posttraumatischen Tag (Mittelwert 6,7 Tage). Zwei Patienten mit initial guten GCS-Werten von 12 und 13 Punkten wiesen ausgedehnte Diffusionsstörungen ohne petechiale Parenchymeinlutungen auf. Patient 1 mit bis dahin unzureichend erklärtem hirnorganischen Psychosyndrom zeigte als morphologisches Korrelat eine pontine DWI-Läsion. Patient 5 zeigte ausgedehnte DWI-Läsionen der rechtshemisphärischen periventrikulären weißen Substanz. Bei Kontroll-MRT-Untersuchungen 5 bzw. 6 Monate später waren diese Läsionen nicht mehr nachweisbar, bei Patient 1 resultierte neben einem kognitiven Defektzustand eine pontine T2-Läsion. Patient 6 wies eine ausgeprägte Diffusionsstörung des Splenium corporis callosi sowie eine ponto-mesencephale DWI-Läsion auf. Beide Läsionen waren mit Einblutungen assoziiert.

Dieser Befund ging mit einem prolongiertem Koma sowie einem resultierenden ausgeprägten hirnorganischen Psychosyndrom mit Verlangsamung und IQ-Verlust im Sinne einer schweren fremdabhängigen Behinderung einher. Patient 4 zeigte eine isolierte kleine links frontale Scherverletzung mit petechialer Einblutung. Drei Patienten wiesen keine DWI-Läsionen auf.

Die Nachbeobachtungszeit betrug zwischen 3,5 und 10 Monaten (Mittelwert 7 Monate). Fünf Patienten zeigten eine völlige Erholung, 2 eine schwere Behinderung. Hierbei handelte es sich um die beiden Patienten mit pontinen Läsionen (Tab. 1).

Tab. 1: Deskriptive Patientendaten

Patienten	**1**	**2**	**3**	**4**	**5**	**6**	**7**
Alter (Jahre)	15,08	10,83	10	16,08	1,25	11,92	11,58
Unfallmechanism.	Verkehrs-unfall	Sturz (3 m)	Sturz (5m)	Verkehrs-unfall	Sturz (2 m)	Verkehrs-unfall	Sturz (2 m)
Initiale CT	SDH Fronto-Basisfrakt.	EDH Kalotten-fraktur	SDH EDH Basisfrakt. Kalotten-fraktur	Hirnödem Orbitafrakt.	EDH Kalotten-fraktur	SDH SAB/IVH Kalotten-fraktur	EDH Kalotten-fraktur
GCS	12	14	11	5	13	5	15
Symptomatik	Psycho-Syndrom Ataxie	Erbrechen	Eintrübung	Psycho-Syndrom	vermehrte Müdigkeit	Psycho-Syndrom Mittelhirn-syndrom	Cephalgie
MRT-Latenz (Tg.)	6	9	8	6	2	7	9
DWI-Läsionen	pontin	–	–	li frontale Mikroblutung	re hemisph. weiße Substanz	Corp. call. pontin mesenceph.	–
DAI-Schweregrad	III°			I°	I°	III°	
Follow-up (Mon.)	5	7	8	3,5	6	10	9
Outcome	mäßige Behinderg.	völlige Erholung	völlige Erholung	völlige Erholung	völlige Erholung	schwere Behinderg.	völlige Erholung

Diskussion

Prädilektionsorte diffus axonaler Verletzungen sind der Hirnstamm, die parasagittale weiße Substanz, das Corpus callosum, die Basalganglien sowie die Grenzbezirke der kortikalen grauen und weißen Substanz. DAI können, müssen aber nicht, mit petechialen hirnparenchymatösen Einblutungen einhergehen.

Histologisch imponieren ödematöse Bezirke mit Myelinverlust auf dem Boden einer Entzündungsreaktion der rupturierten Axone, welche mit einer Silberfärbung und immunozytochemisch mit Antikörpern gegen Beta-Amyloid Precursor Protein (β-APP) dargestellt werden können. Morphologisch typisch sind ballonförmige Auftreibungen der proximalen Axonstümpfe (»axon balloons« or »retraction balls«) 3 bis 4 Tage nach dem Trauma. Nach 2 bis 3 Wochen verschwinden diese und es entsteht regeneratives gliales Narbengewebe mit Substanzverlust und Waller'scher Degeneration (1, 3).

Adams et al. teilte die DAI im Rahmen einer Postmortem-Studie in 3 Schweregrade ein. Grad 1 weist lichtmikroskopische Veränderungen in der weißen Substanz auf, Grad II zeigt zusätzlich eine fokale makroskopische Läsion im Corpus callosum und Grad III zusätzliche makroskopische Läsionen im rostralen Hirnstamm. Der Schweregrad der DAI korrelierte mit dem Schweregrad der posttraumatischen Vigilanzstörung und der Prognose (1). Hierfür spricht auch das schlechte Outcome der o. g. Patienten 1 und 6.

Klinisch können DAI mit hirnorganischen Pychosyndromen (siehe Patient 1), schweren Vigilanzstörungen bis hin zu prolongierten Komazuständen (siehe Patient 6) einhergehen, aber sie können auch klinisch relativ stumm, zum Beispiel im Rahmen von einer Commotio-Symptomatik (siehe Patient 5), vorliegen (8). Prognostisch bedeutsam sind sie, da sie gehäuft mit kognitiven Defektzuständen einhergehen und auch Ursache eines persistierenden vegetativen Zustandes sein können (12).

Aufgrund der Sensitivität der DWI gegenüber zytotoxischen Ödemen, wie sie im Rahmen von diffusen axonalen Verletzungen vorkommen, ergibt sich die Frage nach der DAI-Früherkennung in der posttraumatischen Akutphase. Bislang gibt es wenig Literatur zur DWI in der Frühphase von Schädel-Hirn-Traumen (SHT), insbesondere bei Kindern. Liu et al berichtete von 9 Erwachsenen Patienten mit pathologischen DWI-Befunden 1 bis 18 Tage nach dem SHT (7). Su et al berichtet von 89% DWI Läsionen bei 20 Kindern mit non-akzidentellen Verletzungen. Die DWI Läsionen imponierten viel extensiver als in den korrespondierenden T1/T2-Wichtungen, bzw. waren in denen gar nicht nachweisbar. Der Schweregrad korrelierte signifikant mit dem Outcome (10).

DAI kommen wahrscheinlich häufiger vor, als sie diagnostiziert werden. Insbesondere leichtere Formen werden häufig nicht erkannt. Paterakis et al. fanden in einer Kohorte von 33 Patienten mit unauffälligen CT-Befunden bei 24 (73%) DAI-Läsionen während der ersten 48 posttraumatischen Stunden (8). Auch können sie, wie bei Patient 5, klinisch stumm und reversibel sein. Takayama et al. berichteten von einem 24-jährigen Patienten mit reversiblen und klinisch asymptomatischen Corpus callosum DWI-Befund am 12. posttraumatischen Tag (11).

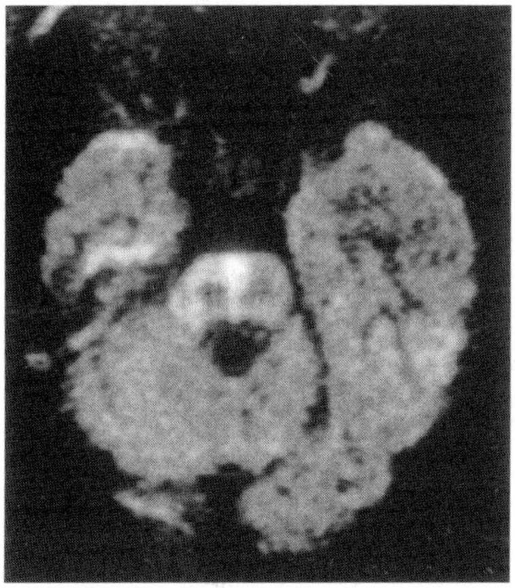

Abb. 1: Pontine DWI-Läsion (Patient 1).

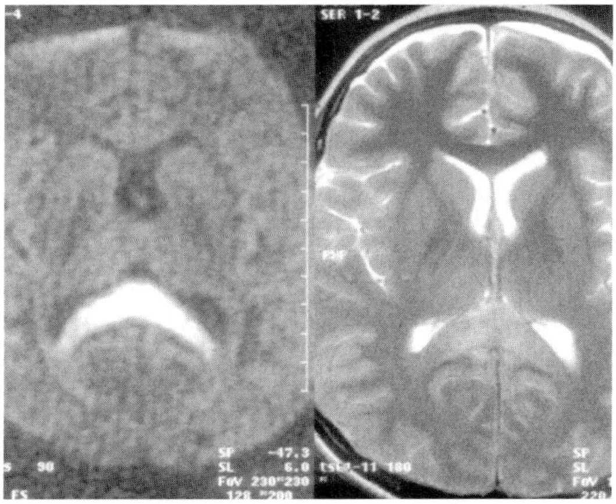

Abb. 2: DWI-Läsion im Splenium corporis callosi mit korrespondierendem diskreten Befund in der T2-Sequenz (Patient 6).

Eine mögliche Alternative zur frühen Erfassung von DAI stellt die Iodine-123 Single-Photon Emission CT (SPECT), mit ihrer Möglichkeit den reduzierten Blutfluss über den betroffenen Arealen darzustellen, dar (6). Für DAI, die mit petechialen Einblutungen einhergehen, ist die T2*-Wichtung (Gradient-Echo-Sequenz) sehr sensitiv. Hämosidderin-bedingte Veränderungen können auch noch Jahre nach der Verletzung nachgewiesen werden (5).

Schlussfolgerung

DWI-Sequenzen sind hoch sensibel für ischämische und zytotoxisch-ödematöse Läsionen, welche bei DAI auftreten. DWI erweitert die Sensitivität der konventionellen MRT bezüglich der Darstellung traumatischer Zerebralläsionen und hilft Kinder mit erhöhtem Risiko für posttraumatische Defektzustände zu erkennen und entsprechende Therapie- und Rehabilitationsentscheidungen zu modifizieren.

An das Vorliegen von DAI sollte klinisch auch immer dann gedacht werden, wenn die Schwere der klinischen Symptomatik nicht zu den CT-Befunden passt.

Literatur

1. Adams JH, Doyle D, Ford I, Gennarelli TA, Graham DI, McLellan DR (1989) Diffuse axonal injury in head injury: definition, diagnosis and grading. Histopathology 15:49–59
2. Beaulieu C, D'Arceuil H, Hedehus M, de Crespigny A, Kastrup A, Moseley ME. (1999) Diffusion-weighted magnetic resonance imaging: theory and potential applications to child neurology. Semin Pediatr Neurol 6:87–100
3. Blumbergs PC, Scott G, Manavis J, Wainwright H, Simpson DA, McLean AJ (1994) Staining of amyloid precursor protein to study axonal damage in mild head injury. Lancet 344:1055–1056

4. Case ME, Graham MA, Handy TC, Jentzen JM, Monteleone JA (2001) National Association of Medical Examiners Ad Hoc Committee on Shaken Baby Syndrome. Position paper on fatal abusive injuries in infants and young children. Am J Forensic Med Pathol 22:112–122
5. Hermier M, Nighoghossian N, Derex L, Berthezene Y, Blanc-Laserre K, Trouillas P, Froment JC (2001) MRI of acute post-ischemic cerebral hemorrhage in stroke patients: diagnosis with T2*-weighted gradient-echo sequences. Neuroradiology 43:809–815
6. Ito H, Isshi K, Onuma T et al (1997) Cerebral perfusion changes in traumatic diffuse brain injury; IMP SPECT studies. Ann Nucl Med 11:167–172
7. Liu AY, Maldjian JA, Bagley LJ, Sinson GP, Grossman RI (1999) Traumatic brain injury: diffusion-weighted MR imaging findings. Am J Neuroradiol 20:1636–1641
8. Paterakis K, Karantanas AH, Komnos A, Volikas Z (2000) Outcome of patients with diffuse axonal injury: the significance and prognostic value of MRI in the acute phase. J Trauma 49:1071–1075
9. Schaefer PW (2001) Diffusion-weighted imaging as a problem-solving tool in the evaluation of patients with acute strokelike syndromes. Top Magn Reson Imaging 11:300–309
10. Suh DY, Davis PC, Hopkins KL, Fajman NN, Mapstone TB (2001) Nonaccidental pediatric head injury: diffusion-weighted imaging findings. Neurosurgery 49:309–318
11. Takayama H, Kobayashi M, Sugishita M, Mihara B (2000) Diffusion-weighted imaging demonstrates transient cytotoxic edema involving the corpus callosum in a patient with diffuse brain injury. Clin Neurol Neurosurg 102:135–139
12. Wilson JT, Hadley DM, Wiedmann KD, Teasdale GM (1995) Neuropsychological consequences of two patterns of brain damage shown by MRI in survivors of severe head injury. J Neurol Neurosurg Psychiatry 59:328–331

6. Pathophysiologie und Behandlung der Infantilen Zerebralparese

Impaired motor programming in children with Cerebral Palsy

H. Forssberg

Introduction

Cerebral palsy (CP) is an umbrella diagnosis for diseases with various types of motor symptoms emerging during early life. The symptoms are caused by lesions in the immature, developing brain, which result in damage of various cortical and subcortical parts of the sensorimotor system. The motor symptoms of CP depends on the site and extent of the lesion, as well as on the developmental stage at which the lesion occurs. Clinically the cerebral palsies are mainly divided according to the most predominating symptoms, i.e., in spastic and dyskinetic syndromes. The spastic syndromes are classified depending on which parts of the body are involved, e.g. hemiplegia, quadriplegia, and diplegia, or bilateral spastic hemiplegia.

In contrast, from a motor control perspective CP can be characterized as a group of movement disorders with various types of motor dysfunction. The major motor dysfunctions in CP are presented in Table 1. A subject with CP may have his/her unique individual blend of these motor dysfunctions. There are several reasons for applying a motor control perspective. One reason is that a CP-syndrome seldom presents itself in a pure form. Usually a child with CP exhibits a mixture of spastic, dyskinetic and other symptoms. Secondly, and more importantly, this functional approach attempts to understand the neural deficits underlying the movement disorder, thereby offering a good base for the planning of individually tailored therapy.

Table 1:

Cerebral palsy Movement Disorder Syndromes	
+	–
– Spasticity	– Paresis
– Musculoskeletal Malformations	– Central Dyscoordination
– Dyskinesis	
– Hyperreflexia	
– Retained Developmental Reactions	
– Co-contractions	
– Mirror movements	

Basically, the motor dysfunctions of CP can be divided into two categories. One category consists of pathological features, which are added to the motor behaviour. These »extra« motor properties are marked with a (+) in the table. These are the dysfunctions included in most textbook chapters on CP. However, recent research has shown that the motor behaviour of children with CP also is characterized by an improper coordination, indicating deficiencies of sensorimotor control. Such an abnormal programming of motor behaviour may be as deleterious to motor activity as the »extra« (+) pathological motor properties. The central dyscoordination stands for a deficient neural control and reflects a failure to develop proper sensorimotor mechanisms. Therefore it is marked with a (–). Likewise, paresis is marked with a (–) since it is also due to a lack of proper neural control. In this context it represents a deficient capacity to produce a powerful muscle contraction during voluntary movements. In this chapter I will briefly discuss the motor dysfunctions in CP following the disposition of the table. In particular, I will focus on the central dyscoordination in two crucial movement behaviours, i.e., locomotion and fine motor skills.

Spasticity

Some clinicians use spasticity in a general manner letting the term cover several of the symptoms presented in table 1. However, from a motor control perspective the definition by Lance is more accurate (Lance 1980). According to Lance spasticity denotes »a motor disorder characterized by a velocity dependent increase in the tonic stretch reflexes (»muscle tone«) with exaggerated tendon jerks, resulting from hyperexcitability of the stretch reflex«. In CP the other motor dysfunctions usually are existing in combination with spasticity but they are not caused by the spasticity and they are due to different neural deficits than the spasticity.

Musculoskeletal malformations

Spasticity mainly involves the antigravity muscles, i.e. the extensor and adductor muscles in the leg and the flexor muscles in the upper extremities. The increased tone in one of the antagonistic muscles around a joint leads to an imbalance and a shortening of the hypertonic muscle. In addition to changed contractile properties of the muscle as a direct effect of the spasticity, the shortening in itself leads to impaired growth of sarcomeres and eventually to fibrosis and manifest contractures when the muscle cannot any longer be stretched to its natural length. The contractures reduce the range of movement (ROM) in the affected joints and hampers the performance of movements.

The imbalance between the antagonistic muscles exerts a continuous tension on the bone and on the joints. Especially in young children where the bone and soft tissues are growing the constant tension affects the anatomy of the bone and leads to severe malformations, which further restrict the movement around the joints and the possibility to use the limbs in functional movements.

Dyskinesia

Dyskinesia denotes the presence of involuntary motor activity. In a minority of children with cerebral palsies (about 10%) dyskinesia constitutes the major motor problem. The causes of this dyskinetic form of CP include genetic mutation with or without inborn errors of metabolism, asphyxia around term age and – in former days – hyperbilirubinaemia, resulting in the clinical picture of »kern icterus«. In general, dyskinesia is not an isolated phenomenon, but is present together with the other dysfunctions of CP, in particular spasticity. The major forms of dyskinesia are athetosis, chorea, dystonia and ataxia.

Persisting infantile reactions

During the first postnatal months healthy infants show specific reaction patterns, such as neonatal stepping, rooting, the Moro reaction, the palmar and the plantar grasp reactions, Asymmetrical Tonic Neck Reflex (ATNR) posturing and the crossed extensor reflex. These response patterns are transient, with the majority of responses disappearing during the first postnatal year. The response patterns are known by various names, such as neonatal reflexes, primary reflexes, primitive reflexes or as infantile reactions (Touwen 1984).

In severe forms of CP, the infantile reactions are not suppressed, but may rather be aggravated. Especially Moro- or startle like reactions may brake through the voluntary motor control and completely disrupt the ongoing movement. Similarly, the ATNR may be easily elicited and thereby influencing the goal directed movements of the upper arms.

Paresis

Paresis means a deficient capacity to generate sufficient muscle force, particularly during voluntary movements. The paresis can be tested by measuring the maximal voluntary muscle force. The poor force generation in children with CP is primarily due to deficient recruitment of the motoneurons. Partly this is due to improper motor programming and could thus be included in the central dyscoordination. In addition, the lack of proper muscle activation induces an atrophy of the muscle's contractile components. When the voluntary force generation in various muscles is tested, the subject induces activity through corticospinal pathways. Experiments with transcranial magnetic stimulation (TMS) in congenital hemiplegia showed absent or low responses in the paretic arm when the damaged motor cortex, contralateral to the arm, was stimulated (Carr et al. 1993).

The voluntary force production is also due to the synchronisation of synergistic motor units, i.e. muscles that work in concert to produce a high force. The synchronisation is due to a common drive presumably through branching of the corticospinal tract. In recent studies Gibbs et al (Gibbs et al. 1999) found a reduced motor unit synchronisation in the short and long thumb muscles in children with CP. To what degree this lost synchronization of synergistic muscles contributes to the poor muscle activation in CP is, however, not clear.

A low force production may also be due to coactivation of antagonistic muscles, which will counteract the force produced in the agonistic muscles. There is a high degree of antagonistic coactivation in several motor patterns in CP. Another study, which used a similar cross-correlogram technique as used by Gibbs and colleagues, revealed that children with spastic diplegia exhibited clear evidence of a synchronization between soleus and tibialis anterior motor units in the lower extremities (Brouwer and Smits 1996). The same children also demonstrated strong activation of both soleus and tibialis anterior in response to TMS. These data suggest that abnormal corticospinal projections or a pathological modulation of the spinal inteneurons may contribute to the co-activation of antagonistic muscles. However, a more recent study could not confirm the existence of abnormal synchronisation between antagonistic leg muscles (Gibbs et al. 1999).

In H-reflex experiments, the excitability in the antagonistic calf muscle of standing children with CP was recorded while they lifted their toes (standing on their heels) by activating the pretibial muscles (Fig. 1). Instead of a reduction, the children with CP displayed an enhanced excitability level in the calf muscle motoneurons (Leonard et al. 1990). This experiment indicates an impaired reciprocal inhibition in children with CP. Normally, corticospinal pathways inhibit – via the inhibitory Ia and Renshaw inteneurons – the calf muscle motoneurons about 50 ms prior to inducing the activity in the pretibial muscle. If this is a general principle in other types of voluntary movements, deficient reciprocal inhibition will contribute to the reduction of the force generation and to the paresis in children with CP. In which way an impaired transcallosal inhibition contributes to the paresis is unclear (Heinen et al. 1999).

Central dyscoordination

Control of innate and learned movements

In order to perform fluent and smooth movements the muscle contractions have to be coordinated in very precise spatial and temporal patterns. Studies in motor control laboratories during the last decades have shown that children with cerebral palsies exhibit impaired coordination patterns (Forssberg 1999). Schematically the human movement repertoire can be divided in innate behaviours that develop spontaneously, and learned movements that has to be learned and trained.

The innate movements are basically essential for the survival of the species and can be traced from the beginning of the evolution. They take care of the basic needs such as respiration, feeding, and protective reactions including blinking, coughing and withdrawal reactions. Locomotion immediately after birth is also a prerequisite for survival in many species. It includes the generation of the basic locomotor rhythm and postural control mechanisms maintaining balance while moving. Typically, these innate movement patterns emerge already during the fetal life, around the 10th week of human gestation, being prepared to be regu-

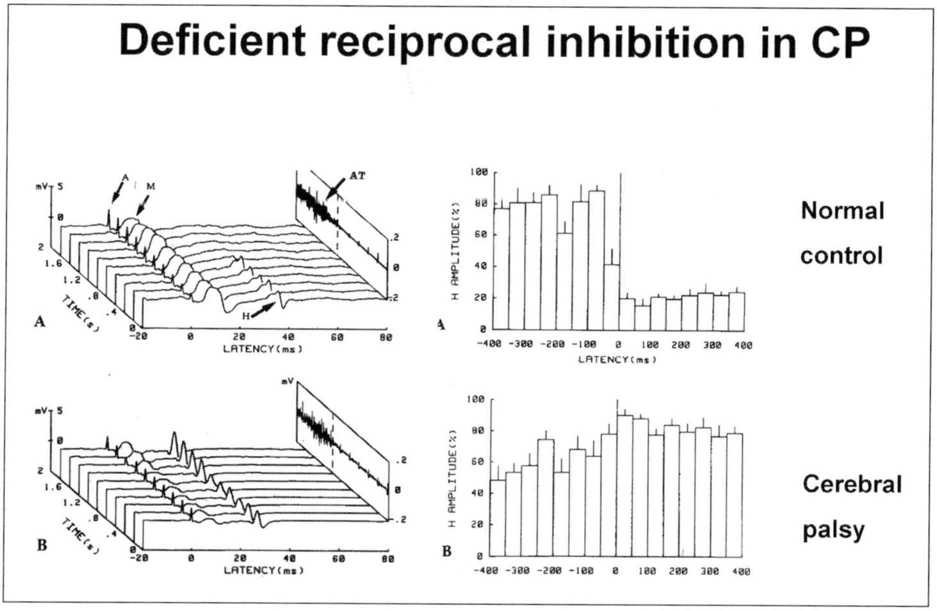

Fig. 1: Reciprocal inhibition evaluated by H-reflex testing.
Left hand panels: Representation of single two-second trials during H-reflex testing of gastrocnemius-soleus (GS) muscle during dorsiflexion of the foot of standing subjects. The test stimulus was applied to the posterior tibial nerve every 200 ms. Ten stimulations are displayed behind each other in successive order, with the time-scale for onset of stimulation on the left. At time zero the subject initiated the dorsiflexion movement, which results in an activation of the anterior tibialis muscle (AT, displayed on the right of the graph). At the top: Recording in a 16-year non-disabled subject. The H-wave in GS decreased from 3.90 to 0.96 mV 48 ms before the onset of AT EMG-activity. At the bottom: Recording in a 14-year old boy with spastic diplegia. Here the H-wave amplitudes increased after the onset of AT-activation. A = stimulus artifact; M = M-wave; H = H-wave.
Right hand panels: Pooled data of GS H-reflex amplitude changes before, during and after dorsiflexion of the foot in 6 non-disabled children (C) and 6 children with CP (D). Time zero indicates the onset of AT-activity. The graph represents the pooled normalized data of the six children of each group for each 50 ms interval. Note the decrease in H-reflex 50 ms before the onset of AT-activity in the non-disabled children (C) and the increase in H-reflex after AT-onset in the children with CP (D). (Modified from Leonard et al. 1990.)

larly used directly after birth. The innate movements are controlled by networks of neurons that are organised in a way that they produce a specific pattern of nerve signals to the muscles. These neural networks can be called central pattern generators or CPGs. The CPGs are located in the phylogenetically old parts of the CNS, i.e. the spinal cord and brain stem, and seem to be conserved both regarding their location and the properties of the neurons and the synaptic transmission.

While the neural networks generating innate movement patterns are organized in lower parts of the CNS, learned movements are controlled by neural circuits in the cortical motor areas, basal ganglia and cerebellum. Although a particular voluntary motor task can be performed in various ways by different means of muscle activation patterns, well learned movements become automatised and invariant. The Russian scientist Bernstein discussed this phenomenon of motor equivalence and argued that the motor system has too many degrees of freedom to be controlled by a single controller. He proposed that the CNS solves this problem by the organization of muscle synergies rather than by separate commands for individual muscles. The grouping into synergies would reduce the complexity of the control system. In contrast to the CPG's, which consists of more hard wired circuits of neurons with fixed coupling to the motoneurons that are activated, the synergies seem to be more adaptable and can be used to control different muscles in various limbs.

Locomotion

Locomotor movements are generated by central pattern generators located in the spinal cord. The application of modern molecular and electrophysiologial techniques has allowed a detailed exploration of the neural networks in several lower vertebrates, e.g., the lamprey.

There is less detailed knowledge about the spinal CPG-networks in mammals compared with lower vertebrates. Yet, the existence is evident since locomotor movements can be induced in cats after transecting the spinal cord, in particular in young kittens and when the hindlimbs are trained to walk on a treadmill (Forssberg et al. 1980). Several groups have recently been able to induce locomotion in humans after incomplete spinal lesions (Barbeau et al. 1992). The locomotor capacity improves by training on a treadmill with the body suspended in a harness supporting part of the body weight. While it seems that the spinal cord controls many aspects of locomotion also in humans, several functions required for a purposeful locomotion are controlled by supraspinal circuits.

Development of human locomotion

During evolution humans have developed a bipedal plantigrade gait, which is unique. Although other primates can walk on two legs they have not adopted the specific plantigrade gait pattern. The plantigrade gait pattern is characterised by certain plantigrade determinants, which are not present in non-human primate gait and in newborn stepping (Table 2). These, contribute to increase the stability of the bipedal gait and to save the energy expenditure. The development of a prominent heel strike is of special significance.

Children go through several phases during their locomotor development (Table 3). The first locomotor-like movements occur in the fetus at 10–12 weeks of gestation. The postnatal continuation of the fetal locomotor-like movements is the infant stepping, which can be elicited a few minutes after birth when the child is held erect over a horizontal surface and slowly pulled forwards. The stepping

Table 2: Plantigrade determinants

1. Foot movement: heel strike – push off
2. Knee movement: flexion of supporting leg
3. Intralimb coordination: joint movements out of phase
4. Pelvic movement: rotation, tilt, translation
5. Muscle acitivity: specific temporal pattern

Table 3: Stages of human locomotor development

1. Fetal locomotor-like movements
2. Infant stepping
3. Supported locomotion
4. Free walking
5. Transformation to plantigrade gait

movements can be elicited during the neonatal period, and diminish in most infants after a couple of months.

The infant stepping lacks all the plantigrade determinants (Forssberg 1985). One characteristic is the lack of segment-specific movements, i.e., the leg tends to flex-extend as one unit. Other attributes are the lack of heel strike and the uniform EMG pattern with pronounced antagonistic coactivation. Flexor- and extensor muscles tend to be active simultaneously, with large bursts at foot contact and lift-off. The activity of the calf muscles prior to foot contact plantar flexes the foot and contributes to a digitigrade gait, i.e. there is no heel strike and instead the toes or the fore foot contact ground first. After foot contact a large EMG peak often occurs, more pronounced in extensor than in flexor muscles.

Supported locomotion emerges at 7–9 months of age. The movement now appears to be voluntarily induced and goal directed. Between 9–18 months the infant starts to walk independently, i.e., without any external support. This event is often mentioned as a »milestone«, and is used clinically to monitor the progress of locomotor development. But this motor milestone is rather depending on postural development.

Throughout all these stages the infant has an immature locomotor pattern, i.e., lacking all the plantigrade determinants. After some months of independent walking the quality of walking changes and the step length and the duration of single support increases. Several of the plantigrade determinants emerge before the child is 2 years old. First after 2 years of age children develop a prominent heel strike, including an active dorsiflexion of the foot. The uniform muscle activity is gradually changed to the specific plantigrade locomotor pattern, in which each muscle is activated during a certain period of the step cycle. The reflex EMG potentials following foot contact disappear at the same time as the wide distribution of the myotatic reflex is reduced to mainly the stretched muscle. The joint movements become desynchronized with the ankle joint getting out of phase with the knee and hip joints. The maturation of the gait pattern is mainly completed by 4 years, but measurements have shown that children up to the age of 12 years expend more energy than adults, which may indicate that the final development may take even more time.

Locomotion development in children with CP

Children with CP, who establish bipedal gait, do not develop the plantigrade determinants. The muscle activation pattern and the locomotor movements of the children with CP during supported locomotion do not differ in comparison with those during normal development. They use the same immature pattern which

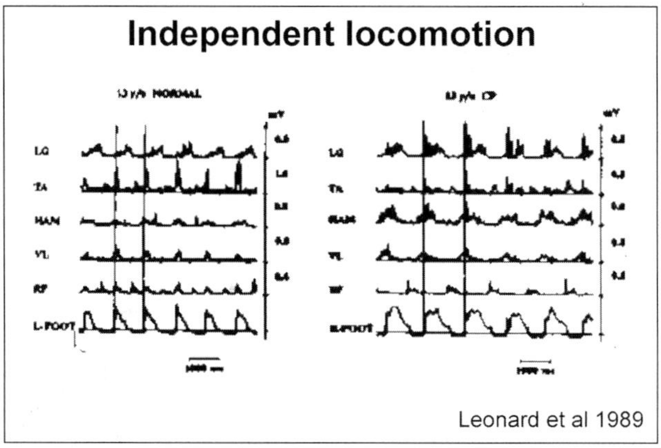

Fig. 2: EMG-recordings from two 13-year old boys: A a control and B a child with spastic diplegia. In A the typical plantigrade pattern has evolved, while the pattern in B displays short reflex activity particularly in the gastrocnemius muscle after contact, premature activation of the gastrocnemius muscle prior to contact, lacking bi-modal activity in the tibialis anterior muscle.

resembles that of infant stepping. However, while normal children start to develop the plantigrade determinants after they have established independent gait, children with CP do not (Berger et al. 1984, Leonard et al. 1991). This means maintenance of antagonistic coactivation and persistence of short latency reflex responses at foot contact (Fig. 2). The calf muscle activity is not shifted towards the middle of the stance phase, but continue to be activated already during the swing phase, which results in a premature plantar flexion of the foot before it is placed on the ground. This contributes to the toe gait pattern, characteristic for children with CP. Many of these children can stand with their whole foot sole contacting ground, which indicates that the toe walking is not due to shortened muscle-tendons. As soon as they start to walk, they rise on their toes. Clinically it is important to consider that the toe-walking pattern often is due to an immature motor program for locomotion, and not to spasticity and contractures. This also explains the rather unsuccessful results after tendon lengthening surgery.

The spasticity also contributes to the impaired gait. The stretching of spastic muscles induce reflex activity, which normally is suppressed (Crenna et al. 1992). This additional, non-programmed muscle activity disturbs the balance around the joints and interferes with the movement. Shortened muscle tendons and malformations of the joints may of course also severely disturb the gait.

Manual skills

Children with CP often have impaired fine motor skills. The manipulation of objects in one hand or between hands is controlled by complex interaction of sensory information and motor commands (Johansson 1996).

Sequential coordination of movement phases: In well coordinated prehension a series of movement phases are linked to each other in a smooth and well coordinated manner. Each phase is characterized by a particular goal (e.g. to establish contact, to lift the object off the support, to transport the object), and a mechanical event that marks that the goal has been completed. The first goal is to reach out and transport the hand to a position with the tips of the digits onto the contact surface of the object and to establish a stable grasp. The contact elicits a brisk activation of several types of mechano-receptors in the fingers, informing the CNS that the first reaching phase has been completed. The next goal is to generate the necessary forces to lift the object. When the load force overcomes the weight of the object it starts to move into the desired position. At lift off there is again a brisk discharge in some of the fast adapting mechano-receptors, signalling that the target load force for lifting the object has been reached. Hence, the grasping behaviour is produced by a series of prestructured motor commands (one for each phase), in which subsequent motor commands are released by the sensory information from the mechanical events signalling goal completion.

Grip-lift synergy: Grasp stability during the initial phase of the lift is obtained by a small grip force increase followed by a parallel increase in the grip and load

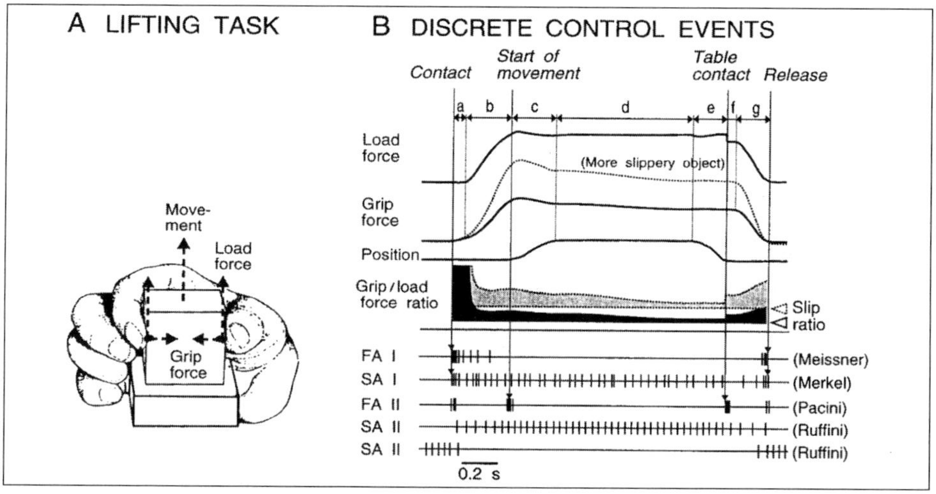

Fig. 3: Schematic representation of the instrumented object used to study the isometric fingertip forces during lifts with the precision grip (A). The load force (tangential to the grip surface) and the grip force (normal force) are recorded together with the vertical movement. In B, the load and grip forces and the vertical movement are displayed together with the afferent responses in the four types of tactile afferent units in the human glabrous skin. The ratio between the grip force and load force is calculated, and the minimum grip:load force ratio to prevent slips is indicated by the slip ratio for sandpaper (lower) and silk (upper). The safety margin to prevent slips is indicated by hatching. The recordings show typical lifts when a subject grasps the object, lifts it from the table, holds it in the air, and then replaces it. After contact with the object, demarcated by initial tactile responses, the grip force increases during a short period (a), before the lifting drive is released when the grip and load force increase in parallel during isometric conditions (b). This increase continues until lift-off (demarcated by burst response in FAII), when the load force overcomes the force gravity. The object is lifted to the intended position (c) and a static hold phase (d) is reached. After the replacement of the object on the table (e), there is a short delay (f) before the two forces decline in parallel and the object is released (tactile responses). The force trajectories show lifts during two conditions; i.e. when the grip surfaces are covered by sandpaper or silk. Note that the slip ratio is higher for silk, and that the grip force is increased accordingly to produce an adequate safety margin. (Adapted by permission from Johansson 1991).

forces during the loading phase. The coupling of the two forces ensures adequate grip force also when the weight of the object is changed, and prevents the object from slipping. This type of invariant, task-related behaviour represents the output from functional synergies (or coordinative constraints) that simplifies the demands on the CNS by reducing the number of degrees of freedom that have to be controlled. In addition, the coupling of the grip and load forces forms the basis for adaptation to the physical properties of the lifted object.

Adaptation of the forces to the physical properties of the object: The grip force has to be properly adjusted to the object to prevent slips or damage of fragile objects. Adults automatically adjust the grip force (i.e. the Grip Force to Lift Force ratio, GF:LF ratio) to the *frictional condition* of the object, i.e. they use less grip force when lifting an object with high friction (sand paper) compared with an object covered by silk (low friction). By this adaptation people keep a rather constant safety margin (the margin above the slip ratio) independent of the friction between the object and the skin. The tactile receptors in the fingertips are crucial for this adaptation. In experiments with local finger anaesthesia the adjustment to the friction is abolished. Instead the subjects use excessive grip forces rendering in a high safety margin and less skilled manipulation of the object.

The adaptation of the grip force is based on memory representations of the object, which are intermittently updated. In addition to the compensations of the ongoing lift the updated memory representation of the friction can be used for anticipatory control of the GF:LF ratio, i.e. the grip force increase is programmed prior to the lift based on the sensory information derived from the previous lift.

People also adapt their force output to the *weight* of an object, i.e. the grip and load force output is larger for heavy than for light objects. Adults program the whole force increase in one pulse, which results in a uni-modal or a bell-shaped force rate trajectory, (i.e. the first time derivatives of the grip force and load force). During a well programmed lift both the load and the grip force rate are targeted to the weight of the object. Since explicit information of an objects weight can not be acquired until at lift off, the adaptation of the grip and load force output has to rely on memory representations of the objects weight achieved during previous lifts.

Ontogeny of the sensorimotor control of grasping and manipulation

Sequential coordination of movement phases: In children, the various movement phases of the precision lift are much longer especially in children below 2 years of age (Forssberg et al. 1991). This is partly due to prolonged delays from the mechanical events signalling the termination of one phase and the onset of the next phase. The delay from the first contact with the object indicating the end of the reaching phase, and the onset of the load force increase indicating the initiation of the loading phase, is twice as long in children below three years than they are in adults. This probably reflects an inability to quickly use the tactile information obtained during finger contact to release the motor command for the lifting drive. Similarly, the shift from the loading phase to the transition phase after

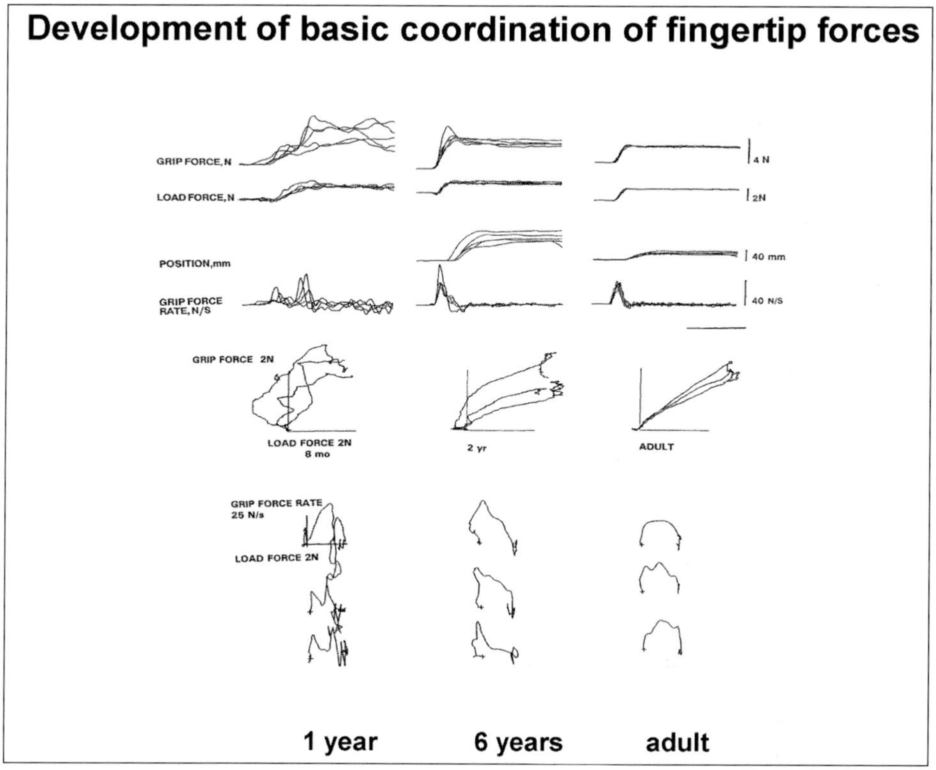

Fig. 4: Development of the Grip-Lift synergy while lifting an instrumented object. At the top, the grip force, load force, vertical position of the object, and grip force rate are plotted as a function of time in 1 and 6 years old children and an adult. The trials are synchronized from the onset of positive load force. In the middle, the grip force is plotted versus the load force and at the bottom the grip force rate is plotted versus the load force for the same subjects. The grasps show a decrease in the variation of the force within a trial and between subsequent trials; a change from a sequential to a more synchronous initiation of the grip force and load force; an increased parallel increase of grip force and load force best seen in the middle figures, and development of single peaked grip force rate trajectories targeted to the weight of the object (best seen in lower graphs). (Modified from Forssberg et al 1991.)

lift-off in the youngest children is not smooth, as shown by a longer delay between lift-off and the termination of the grip force increase.

Grip-lift synergy: The global strategy to couple the grip force and load force is not present when children start to use their hands for grasping (Forssberg et al. 1991). By the onset of positive load force there is already a large grip force, indicating a sequential rather than simultaneous onset. This strategy will provide a high grip stability with a large safety margin, avoiding that the grasped object slips out of the hand. On the other hand, it will not allow a delicate sensorimotor control of the grip force.

During the latter part of the second year, the grip and load force start to be initiated more simultaneously and to be increased in parallel, and the coupling between them increases until adolescence. At the same time the large variation of the force output between trials diminishes, and children start to develop an invariant pattern. The large variability in the young children may serve as an adaptive strategy to develop efficient movement patterns. It may allow the CNS to explore and evaluate the outcome of the various movement patterns, and to select efficient patterns and discard less efficient, according to the »Neuronal group selection theory« (Sporns and Edelman 1993).

Adaptation to the physical condition of the object: Young children quickly start to adapt the GF:LF ratio according to the frictional condition of the finger-object interface (Forssberg et al. 1995). However, they use an excessive grip force rendering in a high safety margin. The rationale for the excessive grip force is uncertain but it may be a compensatory mechanism to avoid slips due to large oscillations of the grip force. The unstable grip force would require higher safety margin to not loose the object during the lowest point of the grip force. The high safety margin could also be a strategy to compensate for the slower and smaller grip responses to sudden loading and slips (see previous section).

The force increase for young children during the loading phase occurs in small increments, with multi peaked force rate profiles. This indicates that children do not program the entire force pulse to target the weight of the object, but rather use a feed back based »probing strategy«. During the later part of the second year, the force rate profiles become increasingly bell-shaped with small irregularities. Subsequent development is gradual and approximate adult like coordination by the time children reach 6–8 years of age, with subtle improvements until adolescence.

Yet, there is clear evidence that children already before 2 years of age start to adapt the grip force to the friction at the finger object interface not only during the lift, but also during the subsequent lift. A similar scaling of both the grip force and load force according to the weight of the object is also seen at this age (Eliasson et al. 1992a, Forssberg et al. 1995). This suggests that the anticipatory control emerges sometimes during the second year of life, but at individual points in time.

Development of the control of grasping and manipulation in children with CP

Sequential coordination of movement phases: In children with cerebral palsy the movement phases of the precision lift continue to be long also after 2 years of age when the duration of the phases normally shortens. This is partly due to maintained long delays from the mechanical events which signal the termination of one phase and the onset of the next, i.e. from finger contact to the onset of the lift force drive. There is also a long delay from the lift off to the termination of the grip force increase. These results indicate that children with CP have a deficient sensory motor integration (Eliasson et al. 1991). The complex interaction between prestructured motor commands and mechanical events signalling the completion of one phase and the triggering of the next command is not functioning as rapid and smooth as in other children of the same age. Probably this is an impairment

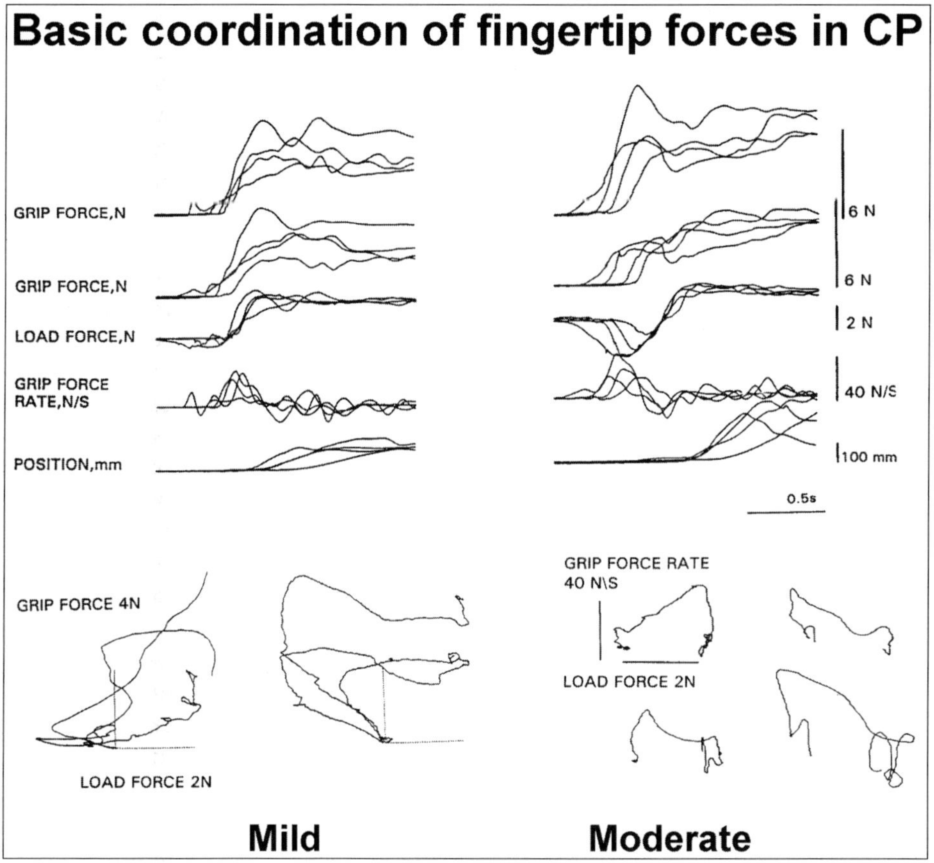

Fig. 5: The Grip-Lift synergy in children with spastic hemiplegic cerebral palsy. See figure 4 for details. The trajectories show large variation of the force within a lift and between subsequent lifts; sequential initiation of grip force and load force; negative load force in which the object is pressed against the support; no parallel increase of grip force and lift force, and the grip force rate is not targeted towards the weight of the object in a single peak trajectory. (From Eliasson et al 1991.)

occurring in children with CP in all complex movement behaviours composed of sequences of submovements interacting with external objects.

Grip-lift synergy: The global strategy to couple the grip force and load force does not develop properly in many children with CP (Eliasson et al. 1991) (Fig. 5). Several children do not only maintain the sequential onset of grip force followed by load force but also develop a strong negative load force at the beginning of the lift, i.e. they press the object against the surface while they initiate and increase the grip force. This is a clearly abnormal force coordination pattern, but may indeed be functional since it provides a high grip stability. Yet, these studies show that children with CP are unable to develop the basic motor components, which form the basis for manual skills. The developmental stage of the grip lift synergy also significantly correlates with the motor performance in various clinical tests of the hand function (Forssberg et al. 1999).

The stage of development of the grip-lift synergy was further correlated with the distribution of brain lesions recorded with MRI scans (Forssberg et al. 1999). The (aberrant) stage of the grip-lift synergy was especially correlated with the overall extension of the brain lesion. In addition, lesions in the deep white matter and lesions of the basal ganglia/thalamus had a strong effect on the grip-lift synergy. These results indicate that the manipulation of objects involves a large neural circuitry including most of the known sensory and motor areas. This may be advantageous when restricted lesions occur early during development, as such a situation might offer a large capacity for plastic compensatory mechanisms which could take over the function of the lost neural tissue.

Adaptation to the physical condition of the object: While most children with CP are capable of adjusting their grip forces to the object's weight and texture, their forces are often excessive and variable, with less adaptation than in age matched control children (Eliasson et al. 1992b, Eliasson et al. 1995). Yet children with hemiplegia can use anticipatory control based on both the weight and texture of the object, but they require a greater number of trials than other children of the same age. The initial lack of anticipatory control and the need for repeated lifts indicate a disturbed capacity to form a memory representation of the object's physical properties. This is supported by the finding that sensory information from the non-involved hand can be used for anticipatory scaling of the isometric force increase during subsequent lifts with the contralateral involved hand (Gordon et al. 1999, Gordon and Duff 1999).

Therapeutical considerations – implications of the motor control perspective

When the motor disorders of CP are viewed from a motor control perspective, a complicated mixture of impaired motor functions emerges. In addition to the well-known pathological symptoms added to the motor behaviours, i.e. spasticity, secondary musculoskeletal malformations, retained infantile reactions and dyskinesis, there is also a lack of neural control mechanisms resulting in paresis and dys-coordination. Currently there are few evidence-based methods for treating the movement disorders in CP. The largest arsenal of therapies is addressed to reduce the muscle hypertonus in spastic muscles, e.g. Botulinum toxin A, selective dorsal rhizotomy, intrathecal Baclofen infusion. For both Botulinum toxin and selective dorsal rhizotomy there is a growing number of randomized studies, showing that the treatment indeed may reduce the spasticity. However, when the motor behaviour is studied in these children, there is little if any functional improvement of the anti-spasticity therapy (McLaughlin et al. 1998, Corry et al. 1997). Two major conclusions can be drawn from these results. The first is that the spasticity is not the only, and not even the most influential, dysfunction that hamper the motor performance in the group of children treated in these studies, i.e. in children with mild to moderate types of cerebral palsy.

Consequently, this means that for these children there are other factors which are more important contributors to the impaired motor performance. The second conclusion is that the treatment has to be directed towards the underlying causes of the motor dysfunctions, which means that there is no rationale for general cookbook receipts.

To be able to make an effective therapeutic plan it is thus necessary to first carefully investigate the blend of impaired motor functions which is unique for each child. In general, there are some »clusters« of combinations, but yet, the inter individual variation of dysfunctions is large also in these groups. For example, in children with spastic diplegia, spasticity might be the dominating symptom in some children, while in others a deficient programming of the muscle activation pattern or paresis of the muscles may be the main cause. In the future there is a need for much better diagnostic tools aimed to reveal the underlying pathophysiological factors. Yet, this will only be a first step. A second and more critical step will be to develop new strategies to improve the impaired motor function. Presently there are only a few therapeutical methods which have been proven to be effective according to usual scientific criteria. In addition to the treatment against spasticity and musculoskeletal malformations, training of muscle force seems to be beneficial. Few studies have been published in which specific motor functions have been trained in children with CP. Recent studies on adult monkeys have shown a great plastic capacity in both sensory and motor cortex depending on the activity of the monkeys, e.g. tactile discrimination tasks or finger sequencing tasks. There is thus reason to believe that a focussed training of specific functions, which are impaired due to losses of neural substrates, may influence the neural reorganisation and improve the behaviour.

References

1. Barbeau H, Dannakas M, Arsenault B. (1992) The effects of locomotor training in spinal cord injured subjects: a preliminary study. *Restorative Neurol and Neurosci* **12**: 93–6.
2. Berger W, Altenmueller E, Dietz V. (1984) Normal and impaired development of children's gait. *Human Neurobiology (Berlin)* **3**: 163–70.
3. Brouwer B, Smits E. (1996) Corticospinal input onto motor neurons projecting to ankle muscles in individuals with cerebral palsy. *Developmental Medicine & Child Neurology* **38**: 787–96.
4. Carr LJ, Harrison LM, Evans AL, Stephens JA. (1993) Patterns of central motor reorganisation in hemiplegic cerebral palsy. *Brain (London)* **116**: 1223–47.
5. Corry IS, Cosgrove AP, Walsh EG, McClean D, Graham HK. (1997) Botulinum toxin A in the hemiplegic upper limb: a double-blind trial. *Developmental Medicine and Child Neurology* **39**: 185–93.
6. Crenna P, Inverno M, Frigo C, Palmieri R, Fedrizzi E. (1992) Pathophysiological Profile of Gait in Children with Cerebral Palsy. In: Forssberg H , Hirschfeld H (editors.) *Movement Disorders in Children.* Basel: Karger.p 186–98.
7. Damiano DL, Abel MF. (1998) Functional outcomes of strength training in spastic cerebral palsy. *Archives of Physical Medicine & Rehabilitation* **79**: 119–25.
8. Eliasson AC, Forssberg H, Kinoshita H, Johansson RS, Westling G, Gordon AM. (1992a) Development of human precision grip II: Anticipatory control of isometric forces targeted for object's weight. *Experimental Brain Research (Berlin)* **90**: 393–8.

9. Eliasson AC, Gordon AM, Forssberg H. (1991) Basic coordination of manipulative forces in children with cerebral palsy. *Developmental Medicine and Child Neurology* **33**: 661–70.
10. Eliasson AC, Gordon AM, Forssberg H. (1992b) Impaired anticipatory control of isometric forces during grasping by children with cerebral palsy. *Developmental Medicine and Child Neurology* **34**: 216–55.
11. Eliasson AC, Gordon AM, Forssberg H. (1995) Tactile control of isometric fingertip forces during grasping in children with cerebral pares. *Developmental Medicine and Child Neurology* **37**: 72–84.
12. Forssberg H. (1985) Ontogeny of human locomotor control. I. Infant stepping, supported locomotion and transition to independent locomotion. *Experimental Brain Research* **57**: 480–93.
13. Forssberg H. (1999) Neural control of human motor development. *Current Opinion in Neurobiology* **9**: 676–82.
14. Forssberg H, Eliasson AC, Kinoshita H, Johansson RS, Westling G. (1991) Development of human precision grip I: Basic coordination of force. *Experimental Brain Research (Berlin)* **85**: 451–7.
15. Forssberg H, Eliasson AC, Kinoshita H, Westling G, Johansson RS. (1995) Development of human precision grip IV: Tactile adaptation of isometric finger forces to the frictional condition. *Experimental Brain Research (Berlin)* **104**: 323–30.
16. Forssberg H, Eliasson AC, Redon-Zouiiteni C, Mercuri E, Dubowitz LM. (1999) Impaired grip-lift synergy in children with unilateral brain lesions. *Brain (London)* **122**: 1157–68.
17. Forssberg H, Grillner S, Halbertsma J. (1980) The locomotion of the spinal cat. I. Coordination within a hindlimb. *Acta Physiologica Scandinavica (Stockholm)* 269–81.
18. Gibbs J, Harrison LM, Stephens JA, Evans AL. (1999) Does abnormal branching of inputs to motoneurones explain abnormal muscle contraction in cerebral palsy? *Developmental Medicine & Child Neurology* **41**: 472.
19. Gordon AM, Charles J, Duff SV. (1999) Fingertip forces during object manipulation in children with hemiplegic cerebral palsy. II: bilateral coordination. *Developmental Medicine & Child Neurology* **41**: 176–85.
20. Gordon AM, Duff SV. (1999) Fingertip forces during object manipulation in children with hemiplegic cerebral palsy. I: anticipatory scaling. *Developmental Medicine & Child Neurology* **41**: 166–75.
21. Heinen F, Kirschner J, Fietzek U, Glocker FX, Mall V, Korinthenberg R. (1999) Absence of transcallosal inhibition in adolescents with diplegic cerebral palsy. *Muscle & Nerve* **22**:255–7.
22. Johansson RS. (1996) Sensory control of dexterous manipulation in humans. In: Wing AM, Haggard P, Flanagan JR (editors.) *Hand and Brain: The neurophysiology and psychology of hand movements.* San Diego: Academic Press.p 381–414.
23. Lance JW. (1980) Spasticity: Disordered motor control. In: Feldman RG, Young RR, Koella WP (editors.) *Symposium synopsis.* Chicago: Year Book Publ.p 485–500.
24. Leonard CT, Hirschfeld H, Forssberg H. (1991) The development of independent walking in children with cerebral palsy. *Developmental Medicine and Child Neurology* 567–77.
25. Leonard CT, Moritani T, Hirschfeld H, Forssberg H. (1990) Deficits in reciprocal inhibition in children with cerebral palsy as revealed by H reflex testing. *Developmental Medicine and Child Neurology* **32**: 974–84.
26. McLaughlin JF, Bjornson KF, Astley SJ, Graubert C, Hays, RM, Roberts TS, Price R, Temkin N. (1998) Selective dorsal rhizotomy: efficacy and safety in an investigator-masked randomized clinical trial (see comments). (Review) (62 refs). *Developmental Medicine & Child Neurology* **40**: 220–32.
27. Sporns O, Edelman GM. (1993) Solving Bernstein's problem: a proposal for the development of coordinated movement by selection. *Child Development* **64**: 960–81.
28. Touwen BC. (1984) Primitive reflexes – conceptional or semantic problem? In: Prechtl HFR (editor.) *Conitinuity of neural functions: from prenatal to postnatal life.* Philadelphia: Blackwell Scientific Publications Ltd.p 115–25.

H-Reflex-Modulation während des Gehens bei Kindern mit Cerebralparese

M. Faist, M. Hodapp, C. Klisch, W. Berger

Zusammenfassung

Bereits 6-10jährige Kinder zeigen eine rhythmische Modulation spinaler Reflexe während des Gehens. Mit zunehmendem Alter werden die Reflexe durch supraspinale Einflüsse immer stärker unterdrückt. Cerebralparetische Kinder mit einer sehr früh in der Entwicklung stattfindenden, bilateralen supraspinalen Schädigung, die *vor* dem Erwerb des Gehens auftritt, zeigen ebenfalls eine rhythmische Modulation, eine Weiterentwicklung mit Unterdrückung der Reflexe bleibt jedoch aus. Die Reifung der supraspinalen inhibitorischen Mechanismen ist gestört.

Einleitung

Die Eigenreflexe der Beinextensoren werden bei gesunden Erwachsenen während des Gehens rhythmisch moduliert. Während der Standphase steigt die Reflexamplitude an und erreicht ihr Maximum in der späten Standphase. Während der Schwungphase wird der Reflex unterdrückt. Dies ist funktionell sinnvoll, da die Reflexe in der Standphase zur Stabilisierung der Haltung und zur Kraftentwicklung beitragen können, während sie in der Schwungphase die Gelenkbeugung eher stören würden (CAPADAY & STEIN 1986, 1987). Die Eigenreflexe werden durch verschiedene spinale Mechanismen wie präsynaptische Hemmung (FAIST et. al. 1996) oder reziproke Hemmung (SINKJAER et al. 1996) beeinflusst, die wiederum unter supraspinaler Kontrolle stehen. Bei Erwachsenen mit einer Schädigung des ersten Motorneurons ist die Kontrolle der spinalen Reflexmodulation gestört. Bisher ist nicht bekannt, ob bei Kindern die Reflexmodulation während des Gehens bereits vorhanden ist und ob diese einer Entwicklung unterliegt. Bei Kindern mit Cerebralparese kommt es zu einer bilateralen supraspinalen Schädigung bevor das Nervensystem ausgereift ist. BERGER et al. (1984) zeigten, dass das ältere cerebralparetische Kind ein ähnliches Gangmuster wie ein gesundes Kleinkind aufweist. Es kommt zu einer Koaktivierung der Extensoren und Flexoren während der Standphase, einer geringen Extensorenaktivität und großen biphasischen Reflexen des M. triceps surae zu Beginn der Standphase. Daraus wurde gefolgert, dass bei cerebralparetischen Kindern die Reifung des normalen Gehens ausbleibt. Bislang ist nicht bekannt, ob sich dies auch in einer gestörten Entwicklung der Reflexmodulation widerspiegelt. In dieser Studie wurden folgende Fragen untersucht:

1. Unterliegt die Reflexmodulation gesunder Kinder einer altersbedingten Entwicklung?
2. Wie unterscheidet sich die Reflexmodulation cerebralparetischer Kinder von der altersentsprechender gesunder Kinder?

Patienten und Methoden

Während des Gehens auf einem speziellen Laufband wurden H-Reflexe des M. soleus, Elektromyogramme (EMG) verschiedener Beinmuskeln und Gelenkwinkel aufgezeichnet. Untersucht wurden 36 gesunde Kinder im Alter von 7–16 Jahren und 9 Kinder mit Cerebralparese im Alter von 6–16 Jahren, sowie 10 gesunde Erwachsene im Alter von 22–33 Jahren. Die gesunden Probanden gingen mit einer Geschwindigkeit von 1,2 und 3,0 km/h, die cerebralparetischen mit einer Geschwindigkeit von 0,6–1,0 km/h, entsprechend ihren Möglichkeiten. Gereizt wurde unipolar mit der Kathode in der Kniekehle über dem N. tibialis und einer 7 x 5 cm großen Anode über der Patella. Nach der Bestimmung der Schwellen für H-Reflex und M-Antwort sowie der maximalen M-Antwort (Mmax) wurde die Reizstärke für die Untersuchung so festgelegt, dass eine kleine M-Antwort ausgelöst wurde. Über die Größe dieser M-Antwort, die in der gesamten Untersuchung konstant gehalten wurde, kann die tatsächliche Reizstärke am Nerven kontrolliert werden. Durch Anpassung der Stromstärke wurde somit in allen Schrittphasen eine gleichbleibende tatsächliche Reizstärke am Nerven gewährleistet. Jeder Schritt wurde in acht gleich lange Phasen unterteilt. In jeder dieser Phasen wurden in randomisierter Reihenfolge jeweils mindestens zwölf Reflexe aufgezeichnet (Einzelheiten zur Methode siehe FAIST et al. 1996).

Die Größe eines H-Reflexes hängt wesentlich von der jeweiligen EMG-Aktivität eines Muskels ab. Da der M. soleus in den einzelnen Schrittphasen sehr unterschiedlich aktiviert wird, wurden als Kontrolle Reflexe im Sitzen (und teilweise auch im Stehen) mit unterschiedlicher willkürlicher Muskelaktivität des M. soleus ausgelöst, bis für jede Gangphase eine Kontrollbedingung mit ähnlicher EMG-Aktivität im M. soleus vorlag. Dadurch konnte überprüft werden, ob die Veränderungen des H-Reflexes während des Gehens nicht allein durch Veränderungen der Aktivität des M. soleus bedingt sind. Für jede der acht Schrittphasen wurde die mittlere Reflexamplitude aus denjenigen Reflexen bestimmt, bei denen die M-Antwort und somit die tatsächliche Reizstärke konstant war. Die Abschätzung der Soleus EMG-Aktivität in den einzelnen Schrittphasen und während der Kontrolluntersuchungen erfolgte durch Aufsummieren des gleichgerichteten EMG. Das Integral des EMG diente als Maß der EMG-Aktivität. Somit konnte den einzelnen Schrittphasen jeweils eine Kontrollbedingung mit ähnlichem Soleus EMG zugeordnet werden. Berechnungen wurden mit laboreigener Sofware und Microsoft EXCEL durchgeführt. Die Absolutwerte der Reflexamplituden wurden als Prozentsatz von Mmax ausgedrückt. Das Hintergrund-EMG für jede Schrittphase wurde als Prozentsatz der mittleren Aktivität während des gesamten Schrittzyklus dargestellt. Diese Normierung erlaubt einen Vergleich zwischen den einzelnen Probanden. Die Mittelwerte aller

Probanden wurden für den gesamten Schrittzyklus graphisch dargestellt. Zur Darstellung der altersabhängigen Entwicklung wurde die Gruppe der gesunden Kinder zunächst in 3 Altersgruppen eingeteilt. Um noch sinnvolle Gruppengrößen zu erhalten wurden, die 9 cerebralparetischen Kinder in zwei Altersgruppen aufgeteilt und die gesunden Kinder für den direkten Vergleich ebenso. Die Zustimmung der lokalen Ethikkommission lag vor.

Ergebnisse

Die Ergebnisse von gesunden Erwachsenen zeigt Abbildung 1. Es sind die Gruppenmittelwerte der H-Reflexamplitude und des Hintergrund-EMG für die einzelnen Schrittphasen dargestellt. Zusätzlich sind die Reflexamplituden einer korrespondierenden Kontrolluntersuchung im Stehen aufgetragen. Anders als bei den Kindern wurden 16 Schrittphasen abgeleitet, um eine höhere Auflösung der Modulation zu erzielen. Es zeigt sich eine rhythmische Modulation der Reflexamplitude mit einem Maximum gegen Ende der Standphase und einem starken Abfall bis zu einer weitgehenden Unterdrückung während der Schwungphase. Auf den ersten Blick folgen die Veränderungen der Reflexamplitude während des Gehens den Änderungen des Hintergrund-EMG. Anhand der Kontrollreflexe mit ähnlicher EMG-Aktivität wird jedoch deutlich, dass nur ein Teil der Modulation hierdurch erklärt werden kann. Darüber hinaus liegt während des Gehens insgesamt eine Unterdrückung der Reflexamplitude vor, und insbesondere in der Schwungphase ist der Reflex nahezu nicht auslösbar.

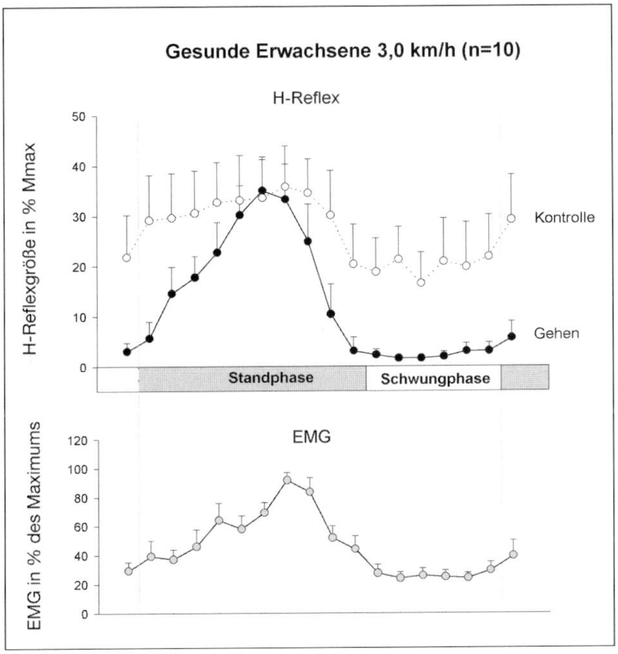

Abb. 1: H-Reflexmodulation von gesunden Erwachsenen während des Gehens. Die H-Reflexe sind in % der maximalen M-Antwort (Mmax) und das Hintergrund-EMG in % der maximalen Hintergrund-Aktivität dargestellt. Als Kontrolle dienen Reflexe, die im Stehen bei einer der jeweiligen Schrittphase ähnlichen, willkürlich hervorgerufenen Muskelaktivität im M. soleus ausgelöst wurden.

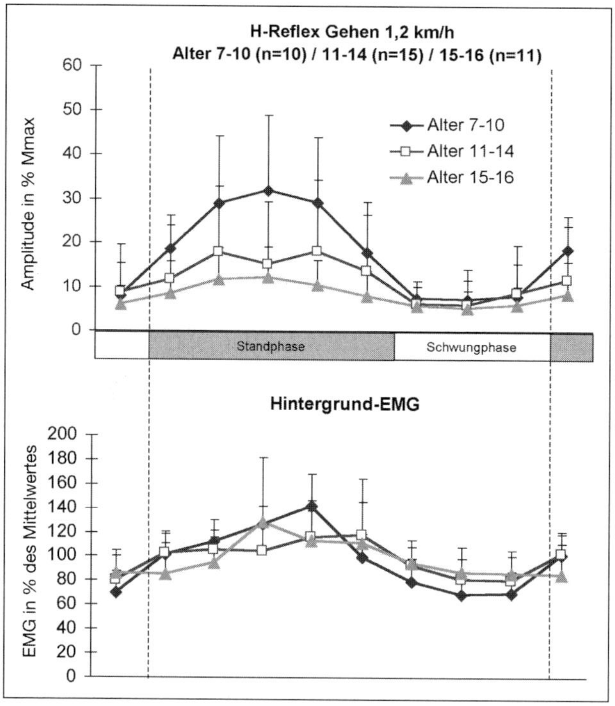

Abb. 2: Dargestellt sind die Mittelwerte der H-Reflexe gesunder Kinder für die einzelnen Altersgruppen in % der maximalen M-Antwort und das Hintergrund-EMG normiert als % der mittleren Hintergrund-Aktivität beim Gehen mit 1,2 km/h jeweils mit Standardabweichung. In der Standphase sind die Reflexe der jüngeren Kinder deutlich größer, während sich der Verlauf des Hintergrund-EMG kaum unterscheidet.

Analog hierzu zeigt Abbildung 2 die Entwicklung der Reflexmodulation bei gesunden Kindern, aufgeteilt in 3 Altersgruppen von 7–10, 11–14, 15–16 Jahren. Die Kurven sind übereinandergelegt. Bereits mit 7 Jahren ist wie bei Erwachsenen die rhythmische Modulation vorhanden, allerdings nimmt mit zunehmendem Alter die Reflexamplitude in der Standphase deutlich ab. Es kommt also zu einer zunehmenden Unterdrückung des Reflexes, was bereits bei den 11–14jährigen Kindern deutlich zu sehen ist.

Abbildung 3 zeigt die Ergebnisse der Kinder mit Cerebralparese, aufgeteilt in 2 Altersgruppen von 6–10 und 11–16 Jahren. Anders als bei den gesunden Kindern zeigt sich hier keine wesentliche Unterdrückung nach dem 11. Lebensjahr. In Abbildung 4 werden die Kinder mit Cerebralparese und die altersentsprechenden Kontrollgruppen einander gegenübergestellt. Im linken Teil der Abbildung 4 sind die 6–10jährigen Kinder aufgetragen. Es zeigt sich bei diesen jüngeren Kindern kein wesentlicher Unterschied. Die Differenz am Übergang der Standphase zur Schwungphase ist durch die relativ längere Standphase der Kinder mit Cerebralparese erklärt. Im rechten Teil der Abbildung 4 sind die 11–16jährigen gesunden Kinder in einer Gruppe zusammengefasst. Es zeigt sich eine deutliche Unterdrückung des Reflexes im Vergleich zu den Kindern mit Cerebralparese. Das Hintergrund-EMG ist jedoch ähnlich.

In Abbildung 5 ist das Ausmaß der Reflexunterdrückung im Vergleich zu einer Kontrollbedingung im Sitzen mit ähnlicher Willkürkontraktion wie in der jeweiligen Schrittphase dargestellt. Hierzu wurde der Quotient von Gangreflex

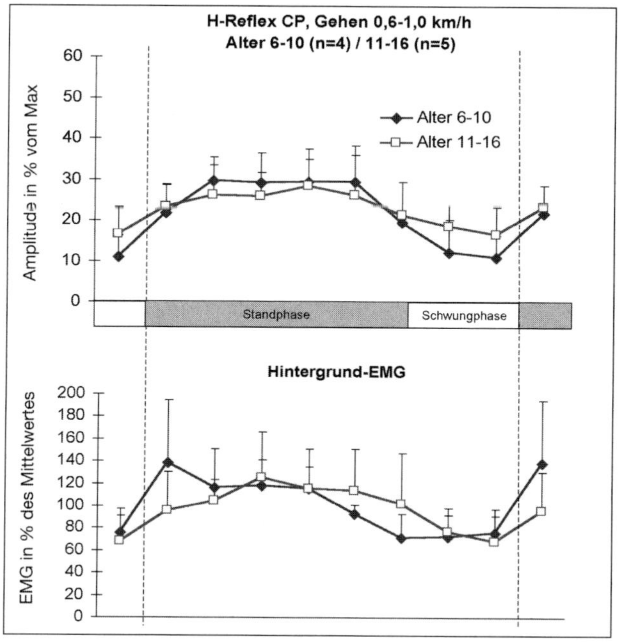

Abb. 3: Vergleich zweier Altersgruppen von Kindern mit Cerebralparese (CP). H-Reflex beim Gehen in % der maximalen M-Antwort und Hintergrund-EMG in % der mittleren Hintergrund-Aktivität. Die Reflexe sind in beiden Altersgruppen ähnlich groß.

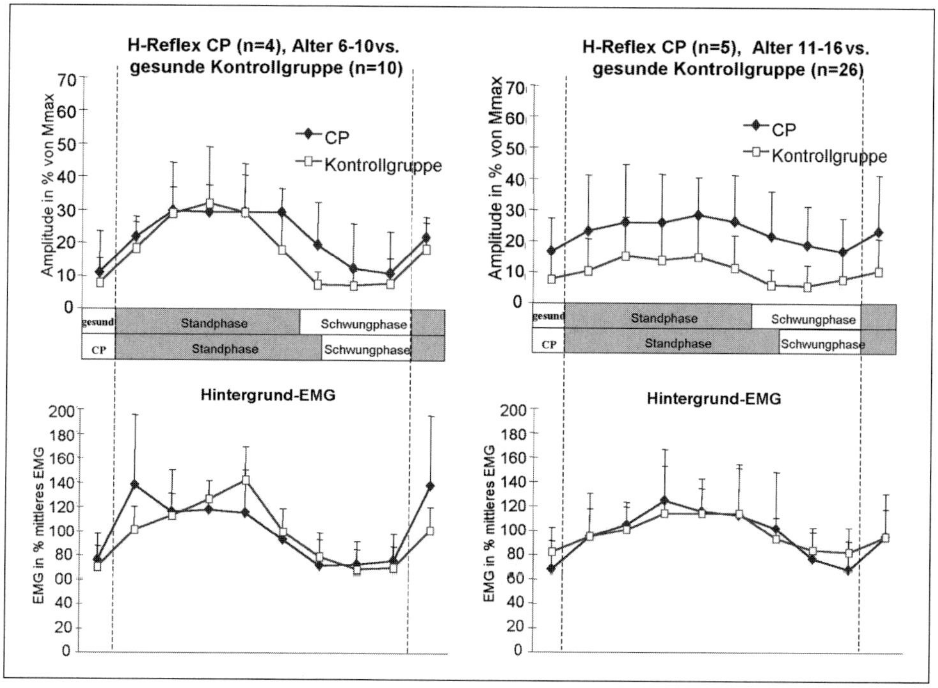

Abb. 4: Vergleich zwischen cerebralparetischen Kindern und gesunder Kontrollgruppe: Die CP-Kinder haben im Vergleich zur gesunden Kontrollgruppe eine längere Standphase und die Modulation ist weniger stark ausgeprägt. Bei den 6–10jährigen sind die Reflexe in der Standphase in etwa gleich groß, bei den 11–16jährigen liegen die Reflexe der CP-Kinder deutlich über denen der gesunden Kontrollgruppe.

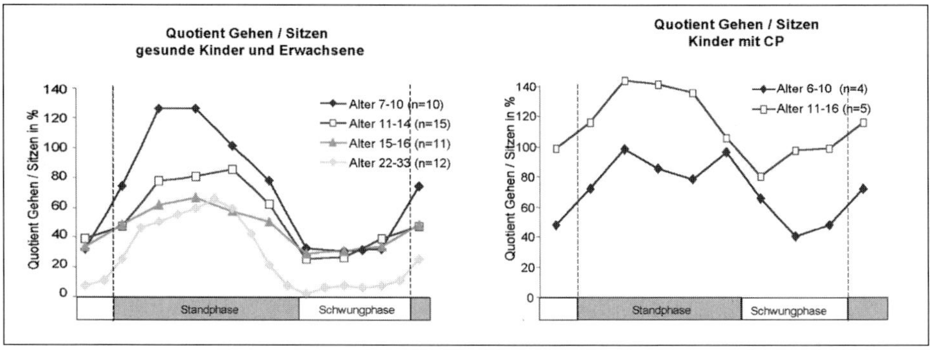

Abb. 5: Dargestellt sind links die Quotienten Gehen/Sitzen für die drei untersuchten Altersgruppen gesunder Kinder und der Quotient einer erwachsenen gesunden Kontrollgruppe. Die Gangreflexe werden mit zunehmendem Alter im Vergleich zur Sitzkontrolle immer stärker unterdrückt. Rechts sind die Quotienten Gehen/Sitzen bei CP-Kindern dargestellt. Anders als bei gesunden Kindern werden die Reflexe mit zunehmendem Alter nicht stärker unterdrückt.

und Sitzkontrolle gebildet. Werte deutlich kleiner als 100% spiegeln eine deutliche, vom EMG unabhängige Hemmung wider. Bei den gesunden Kindern und Erwachsenen zeigt sich eine deutliche altersabhängige Entwicklung. Der Quotient Gehen/Sitzen nimmt von den 6–10jährigen bis zum Erwachsenenalter ab (Abb. 5 links), d.h. die Reflexe im Gehen werden im Vergleich zum Sitzen immer stärker gehemmt, während das rhythmische Muster mit Maximum in der Standphase und Minimum in der Schwungphase bereits bei den jüngsten untersuchten Kindern vorhanden ist. Auf der rechten Seite von Abbildung 5 sind die Quotienten der Kinder mit Cerebralparese dargestellt. Hier zeigt sich bei beiden Altersgruppen zwar eine rhythmische Modulation, jedoch liegt der Quotient Gehen/Sitzen bei den älteren Kindern sogar höher als bei den jüngeren. Der Grund für die Zunahme des Quotienten erklärt sich folgendermaßen: Die absolute Größe der Gangreflexe bleibt im Altersverlauf etwa gleich, während die Reflexe im Sitzen deutlich kleiner werden. Somit gibt es zwar auch bei cerebralparetischen Kindern eine Hemmung der Reflexe mit zunehmendem Alter. Diese findet allerdings nur bei tonischer Kontraktion statt, unter der dynamischen Bedingung des Gehens bleibt sie hingegen aus.

Diskussion

Zusammenfassend lässt sich sagen, dass die rhythmische Reflexmodulation während des Gehens bei gesunden Kindern bereits bei den 6–10jährigen dem Muster gesunder Erwachsener gleicht, jedoch unterliegt die Reflexgröße einer altersabhängigen Entwicklung. Mit zunehmendem Lebensalter kommt es im Vergleich zur Kontrolluntersuchung im Sitzen zu einer stärkeren Unterdrückung der Reflexe in der Standphase. Mit der Reifung des ZNS werden ab dem Alter von 10–14 Jahren diese spinalen Reflexe vermutlich durch supraspinale

Reifungsmechanismen unterdrückt. Auch die cerebralparetischen Kinder zeigen eine Modulation der Reflexe während des Gehens, die Unterdrückung der Reflexe in der Standphase im Altersverlauf bleibt jedoch aus. Schon frühere Studien an cerebralparetischen Kindern, in denen EMG-Aktivität (Berger et al. 1982, 1984, Leonard et al. 1991), Schrittparameter (Norlin & Odenrick 1986), posturale Antwort (Brogren et al. 1996, 1998, Hadders-Algra et al. 1999) und cerebrospinale Bahnen durch transkranielle Magnetstimulation (Brouwer & Ashby 1991, Brouwer & Smits 1996) untersucht wurden, zeigten eine fehlende Weiterentwicklung frühkindlicher Gangmuster.

Bei erwachsenen Patienten mit Paraparese nach spinalem Trauma mit bilateraler Schädigung ist keine Modulation von Eigenreflexen zu erkennen (Yang et al. 1991, Faist et al. 1999). Die Reflexamplituden bleiben während des gesamten Schrittzyklus auf ähnlichem Niveau, die Unterdrückung der Reflexe und auch das rhythmische Modulationsmuster fehlen. Andererseits sind bei einer unilateralen cerebralen Schädigung nach einem cerebralen Insult ein großer Teil der rhythmischen Modulation und auch die Unterdrückung der Eigenreflexe während des Gehens noch erhalten (Faist et al. 1999). Aufgrund der Ergebnisse nach spinalem Trauma kann gefolgert werden, dass Teile der Modulation von supraspinal reguliert werden, während die Ergebnisse von hemiparetischen Patienten nahelegen, dass eine intakte unilaterale cerebrospinale Projektion ausreicht, um sowohl das rhythmische Muster, als auch die Reflexunterdrückung zu gewährleisten.

Nach den Ergebnissen der vorliegenden Studie mit Kindern besteht die rhythmische Modulation sehr früh und ist auch bei einer frühen cerebralen Schädigung, vor dem Erwerb des Gehens, vorhanden. Andererseits entwickelt sich die Hemmung erst mit zunehmendem Alter, und diese Entwicklung einer Unterdrückung von Eigenreflexen während einer funktionellen Bewegung ist bei Kindern mit einer frühen bilateralen cerebralen Schädigung gestört. Dies spricht für eine ausbleibende Reifung der hierfür verantwortlichen cerebrospinalen Bahnen bei diesen Kindern. Ferner kann aus der Zusammenschau der vorliegenden Ergebnisse gefolgert werden, dass die rhythmische Modulation und die Unterdrückung der Reflexe in unterschiedlichen anatomischen Regionen oder unterschiedlichen Entwicklungsstadien reguliert werden. Die fehlende Unterdrückung der Reflexe während des Gehens spricht dafür, dass die rhythmische Modulation in Arealen generiert wird, die von der frühkindlichen Schädigung nicht betroffen sind. Zwar wird vermutet, dass es spinale Rhythmusgeneratoren auch beim Menschen gibt (Dietz et al. 1994), dennoch spricht die deutliche Störung der gesamten Modulation auch bei inkompletten spinalen Läsionen für einen starken supraspinalen Einfluss auf diese spinalen Zentren, die an der rhythmischen Komponente der Modulation beteiligt sein könnten.

Literatur

1. Berger W., Quintern J. & Dietz V. (1982). Pathophysiology of gait in children with cerebral palsy. *Electroencephalography and Clinical Neurophysiology* **53**: 538–548
2. Berger W., Altenmüller E. & Dietz V. (1984). Normal and impaired development of children's gait. *Human Neurobiology* **3**: 163–170
3. Brogren E., Hadders-Algra M. & Forssberg H. (1996). Postural control in children with spastic diplegia: muscle activity during pertubations in sitting. *Developmental Medicine and Child Neurology* **38**: 379–388
4. Brouwer B. & Ashby P. (1991). Altered corticospinal projections to lower limb motoneurones in subjects with cerebral palsy. *Brain* **114**: 1395–1407
5. Brouwer B. & Smits E. (1996). Coticospinal input onto motor neurons projecting to ankle muscles in individuals with cerebral palsy. *Developmental Medicine and Child Neurology* **38**: 787–796
6. Capaday C. & Stein R.B. (1986). Amplitude of the soleus H-reflex in the human during walking and standing. *Journal of Neuroscience* **6**: 1308–1313
7. Capaday C. & Stein R.B. (1987). Difference in the amplitude of the human soleus H reflex during walking and running. *Journal of Physiology (London)* **392**: 513–522
8. Dietz V., Colombo G. & Jensen L. (1994). Locomotor activity in spinal man. *Lancet* **344**: 1260–3.
9. Faist M., Dietz V. & Pierrot-Deseilligny E. (1996). Modulation, probably presynaptic in origin, of monosynaptic Ia excitation during human gait. *Exprimental Brain Research* **109**: 441–449
10. Faist M., Ertel M., Berger W. & Dietz V. (1999). Impaired modulation of the quadriceps tendon jerk reflex during spastic gait: differences betweeen spinal and cerebral lesion. *Brain* **122**: 567–579.
11. Hadders-Algra M., Brogren E. & Forssberg H. (1996). Ontogenity of postural adjustments during sitting in infancy: variation, selection and modulation. *Journal of Physiology (London)* **493**: 273–288
12. Leonard C.T., Hirschfeld H. & Forssberg H. (1991a). The development of independent walking in children with cerebral palsy. *Developmental Medicine & Child Neurology* **33**: 567–577
13. Norlin R. & Odenrick P. (1986). Development of gait in spastic children with cerebral palsy. *Journal of Pediatric Orthopedics* **6**: 674–680
14. Sinkjaer T., Andersen J.B. & Larsen B. (1996). Soleus stretch reflex modulation during gait in humans. *Journal of Neurophysiology* **76**: 1112–1120
15. Yang J.F., Stein R.B. & James K.B. (1991). Contribution of peripheral afferents to the activation of the soleus muscle during walking in humans. *Experimental Brain Research,* **87**: 679–687

Kortikale Reorganisation bei Patienten mit Cerebralparese

M. Staudt, J. Stitz, W. Grodd, C. Gerloff, I. Krägeloh-Mann

Einleitung

Das unreife, kindliche Nervensystems besitzt eine höhere Kompensationsfähigkeit nach fokalen Schädigungen als das reife Gehirn eines Erwachsenen. Diese Beobachtung wird als das »Kennard-Prinzip« bezeichnet, nach einer Studie zur motorischen Erholung nach experimentellen Läsionen beim Affen (Kennard, 1936). Beim Menschen wurde nach frühen unilateralen Läsionen eine kompensatorische Rekrutierung neuraler Strukturen in der intakten Hemisphäre als ein wichtiges Prinzip der Reorganisation des sensomotorischen Systems identifiziert, wie etwa durch den Nachweis von abnormen ipsilateralen motorischen Projektionen aus der intakten Hemisphäre zur paretischen Hand bei kongenitaler Hemiparese (Benecke et al., 1991; Farmer et al., 1991; Carr et al., 1993; Maegaki et al., 1997; Nezu et al., 1999). Allerdings fand man solche Projektionen keineswegs bei allen betroffenen Patienten; auch zeigten Studien, die sich mit dem kortikalen Ursprung dieser Projektionen oder mit deren Leitungsgeschwindigkeiten beschäftigten, divergierende Ergebnisse für unterschiedliche Gruppen von Patienten (Benecke et al., 1991; Farmer et al., 1991; Carr et al., 1993; Maegaki et al., 1995, 1997; Nirrko et al., 1997; Watson and Colebatch, 1997; Macdonell et al., 1999; Nezu et al., 1999; Thickbroom et al., 2001). Funktionell-bildgebende Untersuchungen beschrieben zudem eine erhebliche Variabilität in der Topographie kortikaler Aktivierung während aktiver Bewegungen der paretischen Hand, mit Rekrutierung von primär-motorischen, prämotorischen, und auch parietalen Arealen in beiden Hemisphären (Cao et al., 1994; Nirrko et al., 1997; Müller et al., 1997, 1998a, 1998b; Macdonnell et al., 1999; Bernasconi et al., 2000; Staudt et al., 2001; Thickbroom et al., 2001).

Diese Heterogenität der Reorganisation nach frühen Läsionen erklärt sich möglicherweise durch den Einfluss von verschiedenen Faktoren, die diesen Prozess beeinflussen können. Am häufigsten werden die Faktoren Art, Lokalisation und Größe der Läsion, sowie der Reifegrad des ZNS zum Zeitpunkt der Schädigung genannt (Woods and Teuber, 1978; Carr et al., 1993; Maegaki et al., 1997; Müller et al., 1997; Nezu et al., 1999; Thickbroom et al., 2001). Wie diese Faktoren aber im Einzelnen Reorganisation beeinflussen, ist noch weitgehend unbekannt, vor allem deshalb, weil bisherige Studien in der Regel verschiedene Arten von Pathologie umfassten, oder sogar Patienten einschlossen, von denen keine zerebrale Bildgebung verfügbar war.

Für die hier vorgestellte Studie (Staudt et al., 2002) wurde ein homogeneres Kollektiv an Patienten rekrutiert, nämlich junge Erwachsene mit kongenitaler Hemiparese aufgrund von unilateralen Läsionen des periventrikulären Marklagers. Dadurch konnten die Faktoren »Art« und »Lokalisation« der Läsion relativ konstant gehalten werden; außerdem kann die Entstehung von Läsionen diesen Typs dem frühen dritten Trimenon der Schwangerschaft (24.–36. Schwangerschaftswoche) zugeordnet werden, einer Zeit, in der solche Schädigungen entweder als Komplikationen bei Frühgeburtlichkeit, oder als – oft unbemerkt verlaufende – intrauterine Affektionen bei Reifgeborenen entstehen (Krägeloh-Mann et al., 1995; Volpe, 1995). Dadurch kann das von uns untersuchte Patientenkollektiv als homogen in Bezug auf Art, Lokalisation und Entstehungszeit der Läsionen betrachtet werden, so dass es möglich wird, die Auswirkungen unterschiedlicher Läsions*größen* auf sensomotorische Reorganisation zu untersuchen.

Patienten und Methoden

Die Studie umfasste 12 Patienten mit kongenitaler Hemiparese (Tab. 1), bei denen strukturelle MRT-Untersuchungen unilaterale Läsionen des periventrikulären Marklagers gezeigt hatten. Alle 12 Patienten wurden mittels fMRT untersucht, während TMS nur bei 9 durchgeführt werden konnte, nachdem zwei Patienten diesem Teil der Studie nicht zustimmten, und eine Frau vor der geplanten TMS-Untersuchung schwanger geworden war. Die Kontrollgruppe umfasste 10 gesunde Rechtshänder (6 Frauen; Alter: 19–33 Jahre; fMRT bei 6, TMS bei 7).

Tab. 1: Demographische Daten und Perinatalanamnese der 12 Patienten

Patient	Geschlecht	Alter bei Untersuchung (Jahre)	Seite der Hemiparese	Frühgeburtlichkeit/ SSW	Geburtsgewicht (g)	Prä-/perinatale Komplikationen
# 1	w	16	l	–	3640	–
# 2	m	23	r	–	3800	Cerclage in 33. SSW
# 3	w	20	r	–	3040	–
# 4	m	17	r	–	3650	–
# 5	m	20	l	–	3130	–
# 6	m	22	r	33	2380	–
# 7	w	21	r	–	3400	–
# 8	w	20	r	–	3340	–
# 9	w	21	r	–	3070	–
#10	m	18	r	–	2300	pathol. CTG, Sectio
#11	m	19	r	32	1300	pathol. CTG, Sectio
#12	w	25	r	36	2500	–

SSW = Schwangerschaftwoche; CTG = Cardiotokogramm

Klinische Untersuchung

Die motorische Beeinträchtigung der oberen Extremität wurde anhand einer 4-Punkt-Skala vorgenommen (Tab. 2), adaptiert nach Krägeloh-Mann et al, 1993, und Staudt et al, 2000.

Viele der Patienten zeigten während unimanueller Bewegungen unwillkürliche Mitbewegungen der jeweils anderen Hand. Der Ausdruck »Spiegelbewegungen« blieb dabei reserviert für Patienten, bei denen diese Mitbewegungen reproduzierbar und phasisch waren sowie eine Amplitude von mindestens 10 mm an den Fingerspitzen aufwiesen. Bei Patienten ohne sichtbare Mitbewegungen wurde die Abwesenheit von subklinischer Muskelaktivität mittels Oberflächen-EMG dokumentiert.

Tab. 2: Stufeneinteilung der motorischen Beeinträchtigung der paretischen Hand

Motorische Beeinträchtigung der oberen Extremität	
Grad 0	keine neurologischen Zeichen der spastischen CP
Grad 1	Sequentielle Fingeropposition nicht wesentlich eingeschränkt
Grad 2	Sequentielle Fingeropposition verlangsamt / unvollständig
Grad 3	keine Einzelfingerbewegungen, jedoch erhaltene Greiffunktion
Grad 4	kein aktives Greifen

Transkranielle Magnetstimulation (TMS)

TMS wurde mit einer fokalen »Schmetterlingsspule« durchgeführt (2 x 70 mm, Magstim 200); motorisch evozierte Potentiale (MEP) wurden mittels Oberflächen-Klebeelektroden von beiden Unterarmen über entspannten Fingerextensoren registriert. Beide Hemisphären wurden nach Stimulationspositionen für kontra- und ipsilaterale Antworten abgesucht, und für jede Antwort wurden die »optimal points«, die motorischen Schwellen sowie die Latenzen bestimmt.

Das Fehlen von ipsi- und/oder kontralateralen Antworten wurde durch Stimulation mit 200% der motorischen Schwelle bzw. mit maximalem Stimulator-Output in 2 cm Umkreis um den »optimal point« dokumentiert; waren aus der geschädigten Hemisphäre keinerlei Antworten evozierbar, so wurde dieses Stimulationsareal etwa symmetrisch zum »optimal point« der intakten Hemisphäre gewählt.

Strukturelle MRT

Die genaue Methodik der Rekonstruktion von Semikoronarschnitten entlang anatomischer Landmarken der somatotopen Gliederung des Pyramidenbahnsystems wurde im Detail in unserer früheren Studie (Staudt et al., 2000)

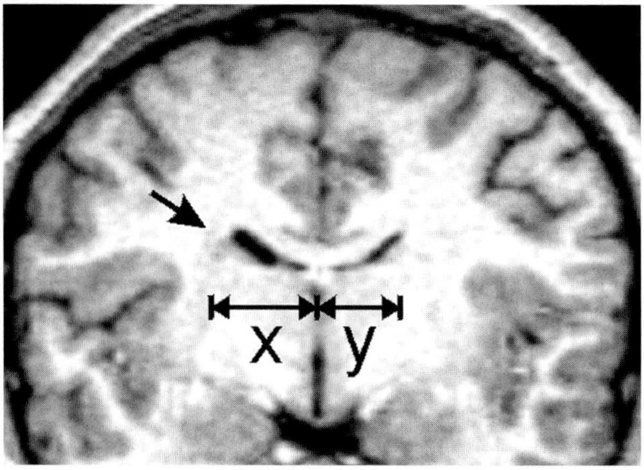

Abb. 1: Semikoronarschnitt entlang handmotorischer Projektionen der Pyramidenbahn.
Die Relevanz der periventrikulären Läsion (Pfeil) wird quantifiziert durch das laterale Ausmaß der Läsion (x), geteilt durch die Ventrikelweite der gesunden Seite (y), so dass ein Läsions- (Asymmetrie-)Index L = x/y entsteht.

beschrieben und soll hier nur kurz angerissen werden (Abb. 1, aus Staudt et al, 2000):

Für jede Extremität wurde ein solcher Schnitt rekonstruiert. Dabei dienten als Landmarken für Handprojektionen der »hand knob« des Gyrus praecentralis sowie das vordere Drittel des Hinterschenkels der Capsula interna, für Projektionen zur unteren Extremität der mantelkantennahe Abschnitt des Sulcus centralis sowie das mittlere Drittel des Hinterschenkels der Capsula interna. Die Rekonstruktion der Semikoronarebene erfolgte nun derart, dass die zwei Landmarken für die jeweilige Extremität in dieser Ebene enthalten waren, so dass diese Schnitte den Verlauf entsprechender Projektionen des kortiko-spinalen Systems vom Gyrus praecentralis (= Sitz der Perikarya der 1. Motoneurone) zur Capsula interna in etwa abbilden. Dadurch kann auf diesen Schnitten die Relevanz einer periventrikulären Läsion für motorische Projektionen zu dieser Extremität abgeschätzt werden. Diese Schwere der Läsion wurde über einen Läsions-(Asymmetrie-)Index L erfasst, der umso höher ist, je weiter die Läsion in dieser Ebene nach lateral in die weiße Substanz hineinreicht (Abb. 1).

Funktionelle MRT

Die funktionellen MRT-Messungen erfolgten an einem konventionellen 1.5 Tesla Siemens Vision Gerät mit EchoPlanarImaging (EPI) Sequenzen (TR 8 s, TA 4.87 s, TE 84 ms, 1 mm gap, 27 axiale Schichten, 2 x 2 x 5 mm Voxelgröße; vgl. Klose et al., 1999). Die Experimente waren im »Block Design« aufgebaut, mit 4 Epochen von repetitivem Öffnen/Schließen der paretischen Hand im Wechsel mit 4 Epochen von Ruhe; jede dieser Epochen umfasste 6 Scans = 48 s. Zur Bildnachverarbeitung und Auswertung wurde SPM99 Software benutzt (Statistical Parametric Mapping, Wellcome Department of Cognitive Neurology, University College London), und umfasste die Schritte Realignment, nicht-lineare Normalisierung, Smoothing, und statistische Analyse.

Aus den fMRT Daten wurden zunächst individuelle Aktivierungsmaps für jeden einzelnen Patienten berechnet, mit einer Schwelle von p < 0,05 (korrigiert für multiple Vergleiche) und einer zusätzlichen »extent threshold« von 5 Voxeln.

Im nächsten Schritt wurden voxel-basierte Vergleiche zwischen Gruppen von Patienten und Kontrollen angestellt (»random-effect« Analyse; Friston et al., 1999). Für diese aufgrund der geringen Fallzahl weniger sensitiven Berechnungen wurde eine liberalere Aktivierungsschwelle von p < 0,005 benutzt, und die Korrektur für multiple Vergleiche erfolgte erst auf Cluster-Ebene (p < 0,05).

Ergebnisse

Tab. 3: Ergebnisse von struktureller MRT, klinischer Untersuchung, TMS und fMRI

Pt	MRI Läsions-index	Motor. Beeintr. der paret. Hand	Spiegel-bewe-gungen	TMS (Latenz; MS)			fMRI (aktivierte Voxel)			
				Hemi (geschädigt)	Hemi (intakt)		Bewegung der paretischen Hand			
				MEP in der paretischen Hand	MEP in der paretischen Hand	MEP in der nicht-paret. Hand	Hemi (ge-schädigt)	Hemi (intakt)	MFC	CBM
# 1	0.82	1	–	17.0 ms; 43%	–	17.8 ms; 49%	547	–	–	–
# 2	0.90	1	–	20.3 ms; 43%	–	19.2 ms; 43%	1214	532	453	129
# 3	1.20	1	–	16.9 ms; 41%	–	15.4 ms; 33%	1880	104	493	–
# 4	1.32	1	–	17.3 ms; 39%	–	17.7 ms; 41%	1300	128	222	201
# 5	1.37	2	–	19.0 ms; 48%	16.4 ms; 36%	16.4 ms; 35%	208	–	–	–
# 6	1.51	2	(+)	16.9 ms; 43%	18.8 ms; 57%	18.5 ms; 37%	84	–	68	–
# 7	1.61	2	+	n.d.	n.d.	n.d.	577	42	9	–
# 8	1.63	2	+	–	16.9 ms; 59%	16.4 ms; 57%	695	25	–	–
# 9	1.69	2	+	–	17.2 ms; 45%	17.6 ms; 45%	1511	143	186	–
#10	1.82	3	+	–	17.1 ms; 32%	16.5 ms; 29%	*	*	*	*
#11	2.14	3	+	n.d.	n.d.	n.d.	1215	45	194	–
#12	2.63	2	+	n.d.	n.d.	n.d.	1394	179	124	–
Alle Patienten (MW ± SA)				17.9 ms ± 1.4; 42.8% ± 3.0%	17.3 ms ± 0.9; 45.8% ± 12.1%	17.3 ms ± 1.2; 41.0% ± 8.7%	1054.1 ± 490.9	108.9 ± 153.8	157.5 ± 177.5	30.0 ± 72.1
Kontrollen (MW ± SA)				17.5 ms ± 1.2; 43.8% ± 6.7#			480.0 ± 357.1	0	7.1 ± 10.2	34.4 ± 42.2
Statistische Signifikanz				n.s.	n.s. #	n.s.	< 0.05	< 0.01	< 0.1	< 0.1

(+) Patient #6 zeigte keine sichtbaren Spiegelbewegungen, jedoch phasische EMG-Aktivität in der Unterarmmuskulatur der nicht-paretischen Hand während repetitivem Faustschluss der paretischen Hand. (*) fMRT während Bewegung der paretischen Hand zeigte keine überschwellige Aktivierung bei Patient #10, wahrscheinlich aufgrund von Kopfbewegungen. (#) Keine Kontrollperson zeigte ipsilaterale MEP, so dass die Latenzen und motorischen Schwellen der ipsilateralen MEP bei den Patienten nur mit denen der kontralateralen MEP der Kontrollen verglichen werden konnten.
MS = motorische Schwelle, Hemi = Hemisphäre, MEP = motorisch evoziertes Potential, MFC = mesialer frontaler Cortex, CBM = Cerebellum.

Die Ergebnisse für die klinische Untersuchung, strukturelle MRT, TMS und funktionelle MRT sind in Tabelle 3 dargestellt. Wie schon in unserer früheren Studie gezeigt wurde (Staudt et al., 2000), bestand eine enge Korrelation zwischen der Schwere der Schädigung pyramidaler Projektionen (bestimmt auf rekonstruierten Semikoronarschnitten) und der resultierenden handmotorischen Beeinträchtigung ($r = 0.855$, $p < 0.001$, Spearman rank, einseitig).

Zwei verschiedene Gruppen von Patienten konnten unterschieden werden (Abb. 2, nach Staudt et al., 2002):

Gruppe SL (»small lesions«)

Patienten mit nahezu unbeeinträchtigter Handfunktion (Grad 1; n = 4) wiesen die geringste Schädigung handmotorischer Pyramidenbahnprojektionen auf (Läsionsindex < 1.32). MEP der paretischen Hand waren nur durch Stimulation der geschädigten Hemisphäre auslösbar.

Gruppe LL (»large lesions«)

Patienten mit deutlicherer handmotorischer Beeinträchtigung (Grad 2–3) und mit Spiegelbewegungen hatten die ausgedehntesten Läsionen handmotorischer Fasern des Pyramidenbahnsystems (Läsionsindex > 1.61). TMS der geschädigten Hemisphäre evozierte keinerlei MEP; TMS der intakten Hemisphäre evozierte hingegen bilaterale MEP mit ähnlichen »optimal points«, Latenzen und motorischen Schwellen.

Die Patienten #5 und #6 mit Läsionsgrößen zwischen den beiden anderen Gruppen wiesen eine Kombination der klinischen und neurophysiologischen Charakteristika der beiden anderen Gruppen auf: Wie Gruppe SL zeigten sie keine Spiegelbewegungen, obwohl die handmotorische Beinträchtigung (Grad 2) im Bereich von Gruppe LL lag. Außerdem konnten MEP in der paretischen Hand sowohl bei Stimulation der geschädigten Hemisphäre (wie in Gruppe SL) als auch bei Stimulation der intakten Hemisphäre (wie in Gruppe LL) ausgelöst werden.

Funktionelle MRT zeigte bei allen Kontrollpersonen eine kräftige Aktivierung der kontralateralen Zentralregion, sowie, in variablem Ausmaß, zusätzliche Aktivierung von prämotorischen, supplementär-motorischen und zerebellären Regionen. In keinem Fall war jedoch überschwellige Aktivierung in der Hemisphäre ipsilateral zur bewegten Hand zu sehen. Eine solche ipsilaterale Aktivierung wurde bei 8/11 Patienten nachgewiesen (bei Patient #10 war das fMRT-Experiment fehlgeschlagen), wobei die kontralaterale Hemisphäre in jedem Fall

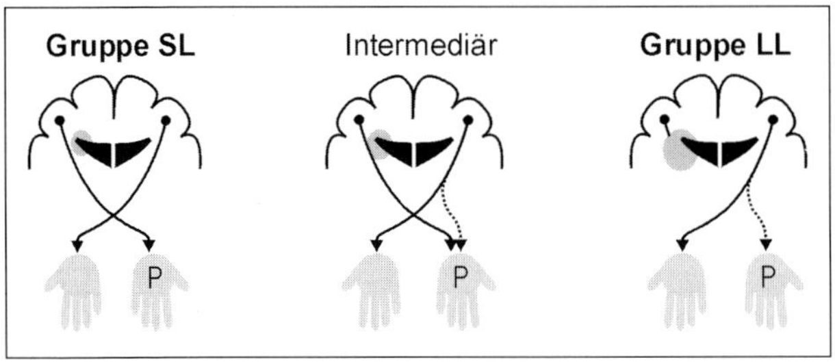

Abb. 2: Schematische Darstellung von TMS-Konstellationen im untersuchten Kollektiv.
Grauer Kreis = periventrikuläre Läsion, P = paretische Hand.

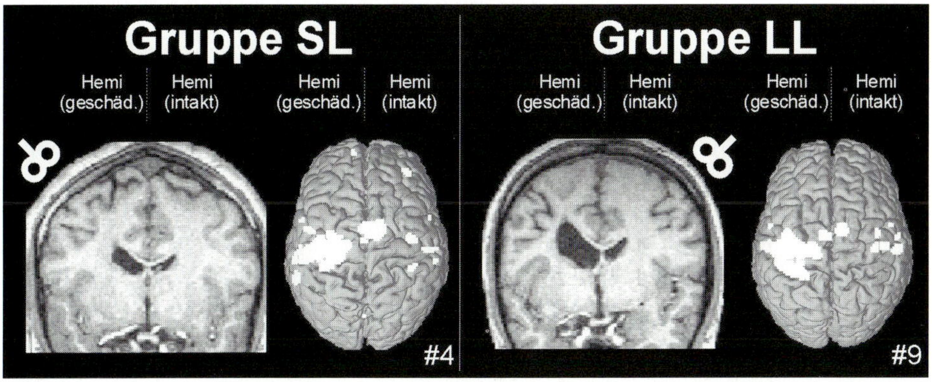

Abb. 3: Zusammenstellung von strukturellen MRT, TMS, und fMRT-Befunden von je einem Patienten aus Gruppe SL und LL. Auf den rekonstruierten Semikoronarschnitten (links) markiert die weiße »TMS-Spule« diejenige Hemisphäre, von der aus motorisch evozierte Potentiale (MEP) in der paretischen Hand auslösbar waren. Rechts werden fMRT-Aktivierungen (SPM99, $p < 0{,}05$ korrigiert, in weiß) während Bewegungen der paretischen Hand gezeigt, projiziert auf individuelle, normalisierte Oberflächenrekonstruktionen.

eine noch stärkere und auch ausgedehntere Aktivierung zeigte. Abgesehen davon waren die individuellen Aktivierungsmuster sehr variabel; auch konnten anhand der individuellen Aktivierungsmuster keine systematischen Unterschiede zwischen den beiden Gruppen festgestellt werden (Abb. 3).

Erst in den voxel-basierten Gruppenvergleichen (Random-Effekt-Analysen; Abb. 4) fanden sich solche Unterschiede: Gruppe LL zeigte im Vergleich mit Kontrollen wie mit Gruppe SL eine signifikante Mehraktivierung der Zentralregion der intakten Hemisphäre (primär sensomotorischer Kortex); Gruppe SL zeigte Mehraktivierung im Vergleich mit Kontrollen dagegen in inferioren prämotorischen Arealen (Brodmann Area 6).

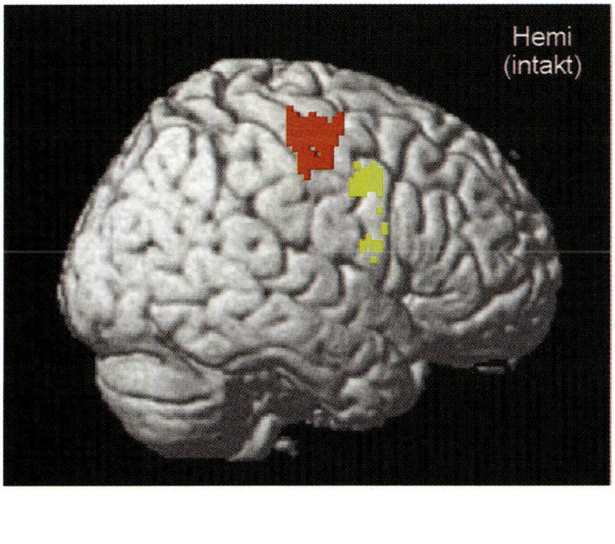

Abb. 4: Mehraktivierung von Patienten aus Gruppe SL (gelb) und Gruppe LL (rot) im Vergleich zur Kontrollgruppe (SPM99 random-effect Gruppenanalyse). Signifikante Mehraktivierung findet sich in der intakten Hemisphäre im primär-sensomotorischen Kortex in Gruppe LL, in Gruppe SL hingegen im inferioren Sulcus praecentralis (prämotorischer Kortex).

Diskussion

Patienten mit unilateralen Hirnläsionen können kompensatorisch Areale der intakten Hemisphäre für die motorische Kontrolle der paretischen Hand rekrutieren, vor allem wenn die Läsionen früh entstehen. In der hier vorgestellten Studie werden zwei völlig unterschiedliche Arten von ipsilateraler Rekrutierung nachgewiesen, die mittels klinischer Kriterien sowie den Befunden aus TMS, struktureller und funktioneller MRT klar unterschieden werden konnten:

Patienten mit erhaltener kortikaler Repräsentation des primär-motorischen Areals in der geschädigten Hemisphäre wiesen nur eine geringe handmotorischer Beeinträchtigung auf, in Übereinstimmung mit entsprechenden Berichten anderer TMS-Studien (Gruppe D in Carr et al., 1993; Maegaki et al., 1997; Gruppe C in Nezu et al., 1999). Bei diesen Patienten konnten wir mit Hilfe der fMRT erhöhte Aktivierung eines motorischen Netzwerks in der intakten Hemisphäre, also ipsilateral zur paretischen Hand, nachweisen. Dabei waren bei TMS dieser intakten Hemisphäre keine kortiko-spinalen Projektionen zur paretischen Hand nachweisbar. Diese ipsilateralen Aktivierungen sind damit offensichtlich nicht-primär motorischer Natur, und der gemeinsame Nenner dieser ipsilateralen Rekrutierung war tatsächlich im inferioren Sulcus praecentralis, also im prämotorischen Kortex (Brodmann Area 6) zu finden. Daher wurde diese Art von Rekrutierung der intakten Hemisphäre als Reorganisation vom *»prämotorischer Typ«* bezeichnet.

Bei Patienten mit schwererer motorischer Beeinträchtigung und deutlichen Spiegelbewegungen waren motorisch evozierte Potentiale dagegen nur durch TMS der intakten, nicht aber der geschädigten Hemisphäre nachweisbar – wiederum in Übereinstimmung mit früheren Studien, die Patienten mit ähnlichen Charakteristika beschrieben hatten (Farmer et al., 1991; Gruppe A in Carr et al., 1993; Maegaki et al., 1997; Gruppe A in Nezu et al., 1999). Nachdem dieser TMS-Befund impliziert, dass bei solchen Patienten die primär-motorische Repräsentation der paretischen Hand abnorm in der Zentralregion der intakten Hemisphäre, also ipsilateral organisiert ist, wurde diese Konstellation als Reorganisation vom *»primär-motorischen Typ«* bezeichnet. Überraschend war hier der Nachweis von fMRT-Aktivierung in der geschädigten Hemisphäre, die bei allen Patienten sogar stärker ausgeprägt war als die Aktivierung ihres ipsilateral reorganisierten primär-motorischen Kortex. Die Entstehungsmechanismen und funktionelle Relevanz dieser Aktivierung der geschädigten Hemisphäre sind bislang unklar und werden Gegenstand zukünftiger Untersuchungen sein.

Die unterschiedlichen TMS-Befunde der beiden Patientengruppen korrelierten eng mit der Schwere der strukturellen Schädigung handmotorischer Projektionen der Pyramidenbahn, die auf MRT-Rekonstruktionen abgeschätzt wurde: Intakte kreuzende Projektionen waren nur bis zu einem Asymmetrie-Index von 1.51 nachweisbar, und abnorme ipsilaterale Projektionen aus der intakten Hemisphäre bei allen Patienten mit Indices von 1.37 oder höher. Die Relevanz verschieden schwerer Schädigungen des pyramidalen Systems wird zusätzlich untermauert durch die beiden Patienten im »Überlappungsbereich«

der beiden TMS-Phänomene, mit Asymmetrie-Indices von 1.37 und 1.51, die in der Tat klinische und neurophysiologische Charakteristika beider Gruppen aufwiesen.

Literatur

1. Benecke R, Meyer BU, Freund HJ. Reorganisation of descending motor pathways in patients after hemispherectomy and severe hemispheric lesions demonstrated by magnetic brain stimulation. Exp Brain Res 1991; 83: 419–26.
2. Bernasconi A, Bernasconi N, Lassonde M, Toussaint PJ, Meyer E, Reutens DC, et al. Sensorimotor organization in patients who have undergone hemispherectomy: a study with (15)O-water PET and somatosensory evoked potentials. Neuroreport 2000; 11: 3085–90.
3. Cao Y, Vikingstad EM, Huttenlocher PR, Towle VL, Levin DN. Functional magnetic resonance studies of the reorganization of the human hand sensorimotor area after unilateral brain injury in the perinatal period. Proc Natl Acad Sci USA 1994; 91: 9612–6.
4. Carr LJ, Harrison LM, Evans AL, Stephens JA. Patterns of central motor reorganization in hemiplegic cerebral palsy. Brain 1993; 116: 1223–47.
5. Farmer SF, Harrison LM, Ingram DA, Stephens JA. Plasticity of central motor pathways in children with hemiplegic cerebral palsy. Neurology 1991; 41: 1505–10.
6. Friston KJ, Holmes AP, Price CJ, Büchel C, Worsley KJ. Multisubject fMRI studies and conjunction analyses. NeuroImage 1999; 10: 385–96.
7. Kennard MA. Age and other factors in motor recovery from precentral lesions in monkeys. Am J Physiol 1936; 115: 137–46.
8. Klose U, Erb M, Wildgruber D, Müller E, Grodd W. Improvement of the acquisition of a large amount of MR images on a conventional whole body system. Magn Reson Imaging 1999; 17: 471–74.
9. Krägeloh-Mann I, Petersen D, Hagberg G, Vollmer B, Hagberg B, Michaelis R. Bilateral spastic cerebral palsy – MRI pathology and origin. Analysis from a representative series of 56 cases. Dev Med Child Neurol 1995; 37: 379–97.
10. Krägeloh-Mann I, Hagberg G, Meisner C, Schelp B, Haas G, Eeg-Olofsson KE, Selbmann HK, Hagberg B, Michaelis R: Bilateral spastic cerebral palsy – a comparative study between south-west Germany and western Sweden. I: Clinical patterns and disabilities. Dev Med Child Neurol 1993; 35: 1037–47.
11. Macdonell RA, Jackson GD, Curatolo JM, Abbott DF, Berkovic SF, Carey LM, et al. Motor cortex localization using functional MRI and transcranial magnetic stimulation. Neurology 1999; 53: 1462–7.
12. Maegaki Y, Maeoka Y, Ishii S, Shiota M, Takeuchi A, Yoshino K, et al. Mechanisms of central motor reorganization in pediatric hemiplegic patients. Neuropediatrics 1997; 28: 168–74
13. Müller RA, Rothermel RD, Behen ME, Muzik O, Chakraborty PK, Chugani HT. Plasticity of motor organization in children and adults. Neuroreport 1997b; 8: 3103–8.
14. Müller RA, Chugani HT, Muzik O, Mangner TJ. Brain organization of motor and language functions following hemispherectomy: a [(15)O]-water positron emission tomography study. J Child Neurol 1998a; 13: 16–22.
15. Müller RA, Watson CE, Muzik O, Chakraborty PK, Chugani HT. Motor organization after early middle cerebral artery stroke: a PET study. Pediatr Neurol 1998b; 19: 294–8.
16. Nezu A, Kimura S, Takeshita S, Tanaka M. Functional recovery in hemiplegic cerebral palsy: ipsilateral electromyographic responses to focal transcranial magnetic stimulation. Brain Dev 1999; 21: 162–5.
17. Nirkko AC, Rösler KM, Ozdoba C, Heid O, Schroth G, Hess CW. Human cortical plasticity: functional recovery with mirror movements. Neurology 1997; 48: 1090–3.
18. Staudt M, Grodd W, Gerloff C, Erb M, Stitz J, Krägeloh-Mann I: Two types of ipsilateral reorganization in congenital hemiparesis: a TMS and fMRI study. Brain 2002, in Druck.

19. Staudt M, Niemann G, Grodd W, Krägeloh-Mann I. The pyramidal tract in hemiparesis – relationship of morphology and function in congenital periventricular lesions. Neuropediatrics 2000; 31: 257–64.
20. Staudt M, Pieper T, Grodd W, Winkler P, Holthausen H, Krägeloh-Mann I: Functional MRI in a 6-year-old boy with unilateral cortical malformation: concordant representation of both hands in the unaffected hemisphere. Neuropediatrics 2001; 32: 159–61.
21. Thickbroom GW, Byrnes ML, Archer SA, Nagarajan L, Mastaglia FL. Differences in sensory and motor cortical organization following brain injury early in life. Ann Neurol 2001; 49: 320–7.
22. Volpe JJ. Neurology of the Newborn. Philadelphia: Saunders, 1995: 211–372.
23. Watson SRD, Colebatch JG. Pathophysiology of congenital mirror movements. J Clin Neurosci 1997; 4: 69–74.
24. Woods BT, Teuber HL. Mirror movements after childhood hemiparesis. Neurology 1978; 28: 1152–7.

Läsionen der Pyramidenbahn bei bilateraler PVL korrelieren mit Schwere der motorischen Behinderung

M. Staudt, M. Pavlova, S. Böhm, W. Grodd, I. Krägeloh-Mann

Einleitung

Die bilaterale periventrikuläre Leukomalazie (PVL) ist ein typisches Schädigungsmuster nach zerebralen Komplikationen bei Frühgeborenen, die sich klinisch häufig in einer beinbetonten bilateralen spastischen Zerebralparese äußert. Dabei besteht ein Zusammenhang zwischen der ultrasonographisch oder MR-tomographisch bestimmten Ausdehnung solcher Läsionen mit der resultierenden motorischen Behinderung (1, 2, 4, 5, 7).

In einer früheren Studie konnten wir anhand von *unilateralen* periventrikulären Läsionen zeigen, dass eine solche Morphologie-Funktions-Beziehung besser gelingt, wenn anstelle einer unspezifischen, globalen Abschätzung der Läsionsgröße die Schwere der Schädigung kortiko-spinaler Projektionen auf 3D-MRT-Rekonstruktionen bestimmt wird (6). Ziel der hier vorgestellten Untersuchung war die Überprüfung dieses Konzepts bei Patienten mit *bilateraler* PVL.

Patienten und Methoden

13 ehemalige Frühgeborene (27.–33. Schwangerschaftswoche) im Alter von 14–16 Jahren nahmen an der Untersuchung teil. Als Kontrolle dienten 11 ehemalige Frühgeborene und 9 Reifgeborene gleichen Alters mit unauffälligen klinisch-neurologischen und MR-tomographischen Befunden.

Klinische Untersuchung

Alle Patienten wurden einer standardisierten klinisch-neurologischen Untersuchung unterzogen. Die Einteilung der motorischen Behinderung erfolgte anhand einer 4-Punkt-Skala (Tab. 1), adaptiert nach Krägeloh-Mann et al. (3) und Staudt et al. (6).

Magnetresonanztomographie und 3D-Rekonstruktion

Von allen Teilnehmern wurden axiale T2-gewichtete Aufnahmen (35 Schichten, TR 4800 sec, TE 85 ms, 4 mm Schichtdicke) sowie T1-gewichtete 3D-Datensätze akquiriert (TR 9.7ms, TE 4ms, Schichtdicke sagittal 1.5 mm). Die

Tab. 1: Stufeneinteilung der funktionellen Beeinträchtigung von oberer und unterer Extremität. Die Beurteilung erfolgt für jede Extremität getrennt, mit Ausnahme von Grad 4 der unteren Extremität, die für eine schwere Beeinträchtigung beider Beine vergeben wird

	Obere Extremität	**Untere Extremität**
Grad 0	keine neurologischen Zeichen der spastischen CP	keine neurologischen Zeichen der spastischen CP
Grad 1	Sequentielle Fingeropposition nicht wesentlich eingeschränkt	Fersengang möglich
Grad 2	Sequentielle Fingeropposition verlangsamt / unvollständig	Fersengang nur mit intermittierendem Vorfuß-Boden-Kontakt
Grad 3	keine Einzelfingerbewegungen, jedoch erhaltene Greiffunktion	Vorfuß kann nicht vom Boden abgehoben werden
Grad 4	kein aktives Greifen	kein freies Gehen

Datenanalyse und 3D-Rekonstruktion erfolgte mittels SPM99 (Statistical Parametric Mapping, Wellcome Department of Cognitive Neurology, University College London).

In einem ersten Schritt wurde eine lineare Normalisierung durchgeführt. Diese Methode schafft einheitliche Dimensionen (Länge, Breite, Höhe) für alle Gehirne, ohne andere physiologische oder pathologische Eigenarten der individuellen Anatomie zu verändern. Dadurch können alle morphometrischen Daten in Absolutwerten verglichen werden. Dies ist deshalb notwendig, weil bei bilateralen Läsionen – anders als bei den unilateralen Läsionen der Vor-Studie – eine intakte Hemisphäre als »interne Referenz« zur Errechnung von Asymmetrie-Quotienten nicht zur Verfügung steht.

In diesen normalisierten Daten wurden zwei Arten von Quantifizierung der Läsion durchgeführt: Zum einen als manuelle Volumetrie der Seitenventrikel auf T2-gewichteten Aufnahmen, einschließlich aller Areale erhöhten T2-Signals (= periventrikuläre Gliosen), zum anderen auf rekonstruierten Semikoronarschnitten (aus T1-gewichteten 3D-Datensätzen) zur Abschätzung der strukturellen Schädigung hand- bzw. beinmotorischer Pyramidenbahnprojektionen. Diese Methode wird im Beitrag »Kortikale Reorganisation bei Patienten mit Zerebralparese« kurz erläutert, für Details verweisen wir auf (Staudt et al., 2000).

Im Unterschied zu der Studie bei unilateralen Läsionen konnte allerdings bei bilateraler PVL oft die laterale Ausdehnung der Läsion nicht genau bestimmt werden, nachdem der Übergang zu Gewebe mit normaler Signalgebung häufig fließend war. Außerdem waren in einigen Fällen, und anders als bei den unilateralen periventrikulären Läsionen, Areale pathologischer Signalgebung durch »Brücken« scheinbar intakter weißer Substanz vom Seitenventrikel abgetrennt (Abb. 1). Daher wurde hier stattdessen die laterale Ausdehnung des Seitenventrikels auf T1-gewichteten Rekonstruktionen als Maß für die Schwere der Läsion verwendet, so dass gliotische Bezirke unberücksichtigt blieben.

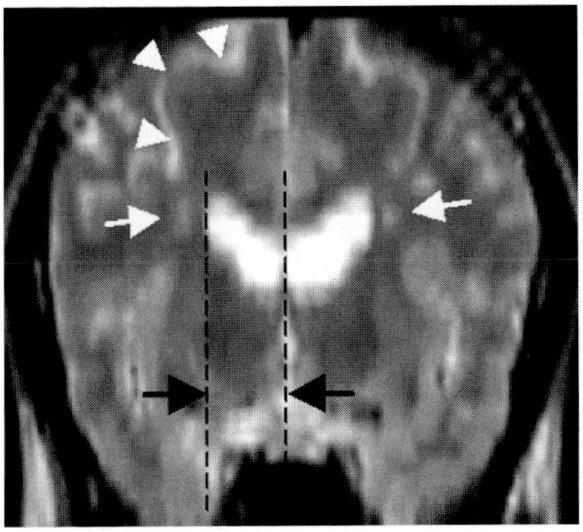

Abb. 1: Beispiel einer semikoronaren T2-Rekonstruktion für Handprojektionen der linken Hemisphäre bei einer Patientin mit bilateraler PVL.
Beachte die »Brücken« intakt erscheinenden Gewebes zwischen Ventrikelwand und Gliose!

Pfeilspitzen = Sulcus centralis am »Hand knob«; weiße Pfeile = periventrikuläre Gliosen; schwarze Pfeile = laterale Ventrikelweite als Maß für die Schwere der periventrikulären Schädigung pyramidaler Projektionen zur kontralateralen Hand.

Ergebnisse und Diskussion

Spearman Rank Analysen zeigten enge Korrelationen zwischen der motorischen Beeinträchtigung jeder der vier Extremitäten und der Pyramidenbahnläsion auf der entsprechenden Semikoronarebene. Weniger stark korrelierten die volumetrisch bestimmten Läsionsgrößen als unspezifisches Maß für die Läsionsschwere mit der motorischen Behinderung (Tab. 2; siehe Beispiele in Abb. 2).

Damit konnte die prinzipielle Anwendbarkeit der Methodik auch bei bilateraler PVL gezeigt werden. Allerdings waren die errechneten Korrelationen weniger stark als bei unilateralen Läsionen (Staudt et al., 2000), was zumindest teilweise auf die notwendigen Modifikationen der Methodik (Absolutmaße aus normalisierten Daten statt interne Referenz; keine Berücksichtigung von Gliosen) zurückzuführen sein dürfte.

Auch gelang keine differentielle Korrelation von Hand- und Beinfunktion mit entsprechenden Rekonstruktionen: Hand- und beinmotorische Behinderung korrelierten annähernd gleich stark mit der Schwere der Schädigung hand- wie beinmotorischer Projektionen. Dies ist offensichtlich eine Folge der relativ homogeneren Läsionsverteilung bei bilateraler PVL, mit in aller Regel parieto-okzipitalen Schwerpunkt und unterschiedlich starker Ausdehnung einerseits

Tab. 2:

Motorische Beeinträchtigung	**anteriore Ebene**	**posteriore Ebene**	**kontralaterales PVL Volumen**
L obere Extremität	0.647**	0.716**	0.472
R obere Extremität	0.767**	0.791**	0.613*
L untere Extremität	0.800**	0.798**	0.514*
R untere Extremität	0.828**	0.922**	0.626*

* $p<0.05$; ** $p<0.01$

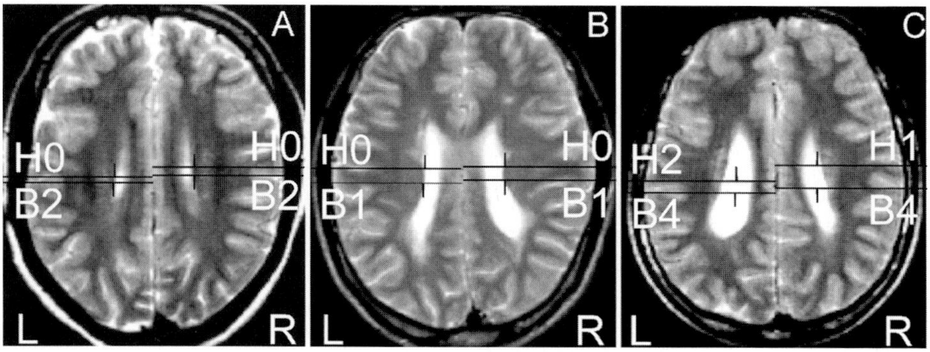

Abb. 2: Beispiele für Patienten mit unterschiedlich ausgedehnter bilateraler PVL (axiale T2). Ziffern = Grad der motorischen Beeinträchtigung für Hände (H) und Beine (B); Waagrechte schwarze Linien = Position der semikoronaren Rekonstruktionen (anterior = Hand, posterior = Bein); senkrechte schwarze Striche = obere Grenze der Norm der Ventrikelbreite (Mittelwert + 2 SD der Kontrollgruppe).
Beachte die relativ erhaltenen zentralen (»pyramidalen«) Abschnitte des periventrikulären Marklagers bei Patient B, was die Diskrepanz zwischen geringer motorischer Beeinträchtigung trotz ausgedehnter Läsion erklärt.

nach lateral, andererseits nach frontal. Erkennbar wird dies unter anderem an der Korrelation zwischen den Läsionsausmaßen auf den beiden rekonstruierten Ebenen (anterior und posterior) einer Hemisphäre (links: $r = 0{,}949$, $p < 0{,}001$; rechts: $r = 0{,}902$, $p < 0{,}001$; Pearson).

Schlussfolgerung

Auch bei bilateraler PVL besteht eine enge Morphologie-Funktions-Beziehung zwischen der periventrikulären Schädigung kortiko-spinaler Projektionen und der motorischen Beeinträchtigung von oberer und unterer Extremität.

Literatur

1. Costello, A. M., Hamilton, P. A., Baudin, J., Townsend, J., Bradford, B. C., Stewart, A. L., et al. Prediction of neurodevelopmental impairment at four years from brain ultrasound appearance of very preterm infants. Dev. Med. Child Neurol. 30, 711–722 (1988)
2. De Vries, L. S., Eken P., Groenendaal F., van Haastert, I. C. Meiners, L. C. Correlation between the degree of periventricular leukomalacia diagnosed using cranial ultrasound and MRI later in infancy in children with cerebral palsy. Neuropediatrics 24, 263–268 (1993)
3. Krägeloh-Mann I, Hagberg G, Meisner C, Schelp B, Haas G, Eeg-Olofsson KE, Selbmann HK, Hagberg B, Michaelis R: Bilateral spastic cerebral palsy – a comparative study between south-west Germany and western Sweden. I: Clinical patterns and disabilities. Dev Med Child Neurol 1993; 35: 1037–47.
4. Krägeloh-Mann, I., Toft, P., Lunding, J., Andresen, J., Pryds, O., Lou, H. C.: Brain lesions in preterms: origin, consequences and compensation. Acta Paediatr. 88, 897–908 (1999)
5. Melhem ER, Hoon AH Jr, Ferrucci JT Jr, Quinn CB, Reinhardt EM, Demetrides SW, Freeman BM, Johnston MV: Periventricular leukomalacia: relationship between lateral ventricular volume on brain MR images and severity of cognitive and motor impairment. Radiology 2000; 214: 199–204.
6. Staudt M, Niemann G, Grodd W, Krägeloh-Mann I. The pyramidal tract in hemiparesis – relationship of morphology and function in congenital periventricular lesions. Neuropediatrics 2000; 31: 257–64.
7. Yokochi, K., Aiba, K., Horie, M., Inukai, K., Fujimoto, S., Kodama, M., et al. Magnetic resonance imaging in children with spastic diplegia: correlation with the severity of their motor and mental abnormality. Dev. Med. Child Neurol. 33, 18–25 (1991)

Chronisch neurologische Erkrankungen im Kindesalter – Klassifikation, Gesundheitsökonomie und Forschung

F. Heinen, V. Mall

Einleitung

Die Klassifikation neurologischer Erkrankungen wird in der Regel als ein Unterfangen wahrgenommen, das die eigentliche ärztliche Tätigkeit der Patientenversorgung hemmt oder gar verdrängt. Ohne Zweifel ist eine exakte Klassifikation mit zeitlichem Aufwand verbunden. Ohne Zweifel ist dieser zeitliche Aufwand ein »add-on« zu einem zeitlich strapazierten Alltag und ohne Zweifel gibt es in der Medizin spannendere Dinge als die Durchführung oder Kontrolle einer Klassifikation. Im Wissen um diese Mühen ist es nun die Aufgabe dieser Darstellung, die hohe Bedeutung der Klassifikation darzulegen, sowohl für den Bereich der Versorgung, als auch für den Bereich der Forschung.

In Deutschland sind im Laufe der Jahre die Gesundheitsausgaben von 5% auf 10% des Bruttoinlandproduktes gestiegen. Der Dienstleistungsbereich Gesundheitsversorgung hat sich zu einem der wichtigsten Wirtschaftbereiche entwickelt. Im Jahre 1998 wurde in Deutschland mehr als das Doppelte des inländischen Gesamtumsatzes der Automobilindustrie für ambulante und stationäre medizinische Versorgung ausgegeben. Während sich in der Medizin selbst Technologie und Leistungsanforderungen stetig weiterentwickeln, nehmen die öffentlichen Finanzierungsmöglichkeiten ab. Die Gegenläufigkeit dieser Entwicklung führt zu gravierenden Spannungen, die sich besonders für die Versorgung von Kindern mit neurologischen Erkrankungen auswirken.

Der in Deutschland für diese Krankheitsbilder traditionell verbreitete Verzicht auf Klassifikation, d.h. Verzicht auf diagnostisch eindeutige Zuordnung, Verzicht auf zielorientierte Therapiedefinition und Verzicht auf eine Aufwand-Erfolg-Relation kontrollierende Strukturbewertung, hat dazu geführt, dass Daten fehlen, mit denen der therapeutische Aufwand, der therapeutische Nutzen und die strukturellen Notwendigkeiten spezifisch belegt werden könnten. Die Aufgabe der Neuropädiatrie, die klassifikatorische Pionierarbeit z.B. bei den Cerebralparesen (zusammenfassende Übersicht siehe bei 1) geleistet hat, ist es, diesen Ansatz nun auch auf Verlauf, Schwere und Interventionskontrolle neurologischer Erkrankungen im Kindesalter zu übertragen.

Es bedarf hierzu einer aktiven Positionierung der Therapieforschung, die Intervention, Longitudinalverlauf und Gesamtversorgung ebenso berücksichtigt wie Gesundheitsökonomie und Grundlagen.

Werden chronische neurologische Erkrankungen zum Fokus wissenschaftlicher Forschung, so ist hier eine eindeutige Klassifikation »conditio-sine-qua-non«. Je präziser die wissenschaftliche Fragestellung ist, umso trennschärfer kann der klassifikatorische Ansatz gewählt werden.

Fokus Cerebralparesen

Für die klassifikatorische Eingrenzung der CP stehen eine Reihe von Zugangswegen zur Verfügung, von denen hier nur zwei näher betrachtet werden:

(1) der Level der Behinderung, sowie
(2) der Level der Evidenz

Nicht eingegangen wird auf die phänomenologische Klassifikation der CP (1), die den Typ der CP festlegt, nicht eingegangen wird auf das Gross Motor Classification System (2), welches altersbezogen die Schwere der CP festlegt. Ebenso nicht eingegangen wird auf die Möglichkeiten sogenannter qualitativer Forschung als evidenzorientierter Vorgehensweise, die den individualisierten Krankheitsausprägungen wie sie für die CP typisch sind, gerecht zu werden versucht.

Die Organisationen, die im Grunde gleichlautend, wenn auch nicht in jedem Detail wortidentisch, die Level der Behinderung definieren sind

(1) die WHO (World Health Organisation), die mit der ICF (International Classification of Functioning, Disability and Health) die ICIDH-2 (International Classification of Functioning, Disability and Health) ablöst. Die ICF wird auf der Internet-Seite (www.who.int/classification/icf) eingehend dargestellt. Weiterhin die
(2) AACPDM (American Academy on Cerebral Palsy and Developmental Medicine), die mit dem AACPDM-Framework, die WHO-Klassifikation für die Cerebralparesen spezifiziert und dieses auf der AACPDM Homepage darstellt (www.aacpdm.org).

Kernpunkt der Klassifikationen ist die Definition des Levels der Behinderung. Hierfür stehen folgende Ebenen zur Verfügung:

- Pathophysiologie // Zelle
- Impairment // Organ
- Functional limitation // Activity // Individuum
- Disability // Participation // Befinden und Verhalten des Individuums
- Societal limitations // Context factors // Gesellschaftliche Rahmenbedingungen

Jede Aussage, ob über Therapie oder Forschung, muss sich auf eine dieser Ebenen beziehen, kann dort ihre Fragen stellen und ihre Ergebnisse verifizieren oder falsifizieren. Sie kann aber nicht den Fehlschluss perpetuieren, dass z.B. relevante Ergebnisse auf der Ebene der Zelle auch relevant auf der Ebene des Individuums sein müssten. Für die Cerebralparesen gilt hierbei, dass bis zur Ebene des Individuums (Level 3 / Activity) methodisch gute Arbeiten vorliegen, dass für die nächste Ebene (Level 4 / Participation) nur noch sehr eingeschränkt methodisch akzeptable Daten zur Verfügung stehen und das für die wiederum nächste Ebene (Level 5 / Societal limitations) (noch) nicht auf methodisch akzeptable Daten zurückgegriffen werden kann.

So notwenig bei chronisch neurologischen Erkrankungen also der Bezug zum Level der Behinderung ist, so notwendig ist auch die Klassifikation der Daten auf den verschiedenen Evidenzebenen (3–5). Diese gliedern sich wie folgt:

I Randomized controlled trial
II Non-randomized controlled trial
Prospective cohort study, concurrent control group
III Case-control study
Cohort study, historical control group
IV Case-series and registries without controls
V Descriptive case series or case reports
Anecdote
Expert opinion
Theory based on physiology, bench or animal research
Common sense

Für die in Deutschland meinungsbildenden Äußerungen zur CP finden sich ganz überwiegend Level V Daten, bei denen entweder die Individualität der Anekdote, oder die Aussagekraft der grundlagenorientierten Tierversuche überbewertet werden. Dies führt oft zu verallgemeinernden und simplifizierenden Fehlschlüssen. Auch in diesem Spannungsfeld hat die Neuropädiatrie die evidenzorientierte Positionierung als herausfordernde Aufgabe.

Selbst dort, wo ein Studiendesign eben nicht in der Lage ist, die sachbestimmte Komplexität einer Fragestellung aufzunehmen, fehlt häufig die eine qualitativ hochwertige Forschung auszeichnende Transparenz, die aktiv die Qualifikation des Untersuchers, seine Motivation, den Kontext seiner Erfahrung und die Interessen möglicher Sponsoren darstellt.

Beispiele

(1) Wenn in Deutschland über Physiotherapie gesprochen wird, so wird regelhaft eine methodisch-adäquate Evaluierung mit dem Argument abgelehnt, so könne man an diese erfahrungsabhängige Therapieform nicht herangehen und also erübrige sich die Messung der Effekte. Folge ist das Verharren in mehr oder weniger ideologisch geführten Diskussionen, deren Sinnhaftigkeit etwa der mittelalterlichen Diskussion entspricht, die Streit darüber führte, wie viele Engel denn nun auf eine Nadelspitze passen.
Kontrastierend zu dieser methodischen Historienmalerei zeigt die im AACPDM Treatment Outcome Committee Review Panel zusammengefasste Gruppe mit ihrer Wertung des Neurodevelopmental Treatment (NDT) – dem

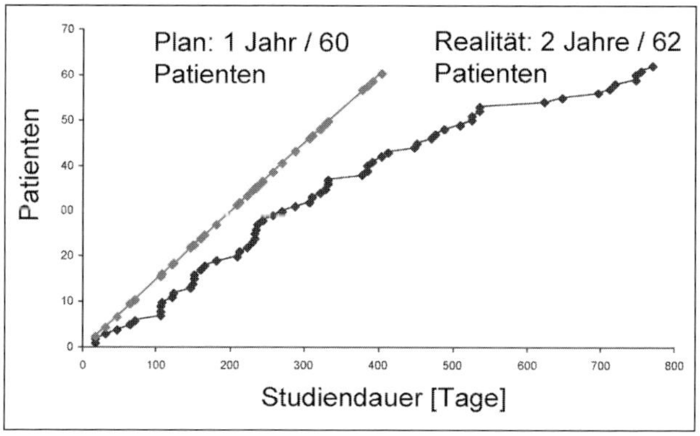

Abb. 1: Verlauf der Rekrutierung der Patienten bei der multizentrischen, plazebokontrollierten ABo1-Studie.

Bobath Konzept entsprechend –, dass in einer sehr sorgfältigen Metaanalyse eben keine überlegenen Spezifika dieser Therapieform erkennbar sind (6). Fazit ist: es geht also doch, methodisch adäquat, aufwendig und im Ergebnis jeder Form der Ideologie widersprechend.

(2) Die in Deutschland durchgeführte multizentrische, doppelblinde, plazebokontrolierte Studie zur Therapie des Adduktorenspasmus bei Cerebralparese (ABo1) zeigt als methodisch aufwendige Studie, dass sie auch mit dem ehrgeizigen Ziel von 60 behandelten Patienten durchführbar ist (7). Sie zeigt aber auch, dass die Rekrutierung dabei nicht ein, sondern zwei Jahre in Anspruch nahm (Abb. 1), dass zwischen erstem Entwurf des Studienprotokolls und Abschlussbericht fünf Jahre (!) liegen und dass ergo der Aufwand für den erfolgreichen Abschluss enorm war und in diesem Fall ohne Kooperation zur pharmazeutischen Industrie nicht möglich gewesen wäre.

Zusammenfassung

Die chronisch neurologischen Erkrankungen sind ein Hauptthema der Neuropädiatrie. Sowohl die therapeutischen als auch die forschenden Anliegen können nur mit einer adäquaten Klassifikation geleistet werden. Nur in diesem Dialog gelingt der Neuropädiatrie die Ressourcensicherung und gesundheitsökonomische Behauptung im Spannungsfeld von medizinischer Entwicklung und öffentlicher Mittelbegrenzung.

Einem Krankheitsbild wie dem der Cerebralparesen, per definitionem in seinen Anforderungen fächerübergreifend und chronisch, kann nur im Dialog von Neuropädiatrie, Sozialpädiatrie, Medizinischem Dienst der Krankenkassen, den Krankenkassen selbst und der Politik modern und zukunftsorientiert begegnet werden.

Literatur

1. Michaelis R, Niemann G. Entwicklungsneurologie und Neuropädiatrie. Stuttgart: Thieme, 2001.
2. Palisano R, Rosenbaum PL, Walter S, et al. Development and reliability of a system to classify gross motor function in children with cerebral palsy. Dev Med Child Neurol 1997; 39:214–223.
3. Greenhalgh T. Einführung in die Evidence-based Medicine. Kritische Beurteilung klinischer Studien als Basis einer rationalen Medizin. Bern, Hans Huber Verlag, 2000.
4. Heinen F, Bartens W., Hrsg. Das Kind und die Spastik. Bern: Hans Huber Verlag, 2001; 13–17.
5. Bassler D, Forster J, Antes G. Evidenz - basierte Pädiatrie. Praxisnahes EBM-Handbuch für pädiatrische Diagnose und Therapie. Grundwerk. Stuttgart, New York: Georg Thieme Verlag, 2001.
6. Butler C, Darrah J. Effects of neurodevelopmental treatment (NDT) for cerebral palsy: an AACPDM evidence report. Dev Med Child Neurol 2001; 43:778–790.
7. V Mall, Heinen F, W. Schulte-Matler, C. Bertram, J. Wissel, B. Dietz, W. Voss, B. Klowat, G. Göhlich-Ratmann, L. Döderlein, N. Breitbach, R. Korinthenberg. Multizentrische Studie zur Behandlung des Adduktoren-spasmus mit Botulinum Toxin A. In: *Aktuelle Neuropädiatrie* 1999, Hrsg. Millner, Nürnberg:Novartis Verlag, 2000, 277–282.

Handbücher und Web-Sites zur Klassifikation und Evaluation

1. Die WHO (World Health Organisation), www.who.int/classification/icf
2. AACPDM (American Academy of Cerebral Palsy and Developmental Medicine), www.aacpdm.org
3. Child & Brain Bonn Berlin GmbH, www.childbrain.de
4. Gross Motor Function Measure - GMFM-Handbuch in deutscher Sprache. McMaster University Ontario Canada Can Child Center for Childhood Disability Research. Autorisierte deutsche Übersetzung: Arbeitsgruppe Bewegungsstörungen, Zentrum für Kinderheilkunde und Jugendmedizin, Klinik für Neuropädiatrie und Muskelerkrankungen, Universität Freiburg i. Br., 2001
5. Gross Motor Function Classification System in deutscher Sprache. R. Palisano, P. Rosenbaum, S. Walter, D. Russel, E. Wood, and B. Galuppi., Br. Autorisierte deutsche Übersetzung: Arbeitsgruppe Bewegungsstörungen: Zentrum für Kinderheilkunde und Jugendmedizin, Klinik für Neuropädiatrie und Muskelerkrankungen, Universität Freiburg i. Br., 2001

Was ist erwiesen in der Frühtherapie der ICP?

H.G. Schlack

Zusammenfassung

Verbreiteten Vorstellungen zu Folge soll motorische Übungsbehandlung in Form verschiedener Methoden der Physiotherapie einen korrigierenden, wenn nicht sogar heilenden Einfluss auf das ZNS von Kindern mit Zerebralparese haben können. Diese Annahme wird von Evaluationsstudien nicht gestützt. Demgegenüber gibt es valide empirische Befunde, die dafür sprechen, dass die motorische Eigenaktivität des Kindes der entscheidende Faktor für die Entwicklung auch im Falle einer Zerebralparese ist. Die Anregung der motorischen Eigenaktivität muss daher in der Zielsetzung aller therapeutischen Interventionen (Physiotherapie, Hilfsmittelversorgung) eine herausragende Rolle spielen. Darüber hinaus ist ein systemischer Ansatz erforderlich, der die Auswirkung aller Interventionen auf die Interaktion zwischen dem Kind und seinen Bezugspersonen berücksichtigt.

Fragestellung

Das Thema des Beitrags enthält gleich drei definitorische Probleme:
- Welche Maßnahmen soll man unter den Begriff »Frühtherapie« subsumieren?
- Von welchem Alter an ist die Diagnose einer infantilen Cerebralparese (ICP) so eindeutig, dass man von einer spezifischen Behandlungsindikation sprechen kann?
- An welchen Outcome-Kriterien soll die Effektivität der eingesetzten Maßnahmen gemessen werden?

In den vorliegenden Publikationen wurde diesen Fragen überwiegend in folgender Weise begegnet:
1. Unter »Therapie« wird in der Mehrzahl der Evaluationsstudien Physiotherapie verstanden, offenbar unter der verbreiteten Vorstellung, dass bei einer motorischen Störung die Durchführung einer motorischen Übungsbehandlung eine angemessene und spezifische Maßnahme sei. Einige Publikationen sind auf spezielle Behandlungsmethoden fokussiert, insbesondere auf die Vojta- oder die Bobath-Methode.
2. Viele Publikationen beziehen sich auf einen Behandlungsbeginn ab Mitte des 1. Lebensjahres, einem Zeitpunkt also, zu welchem in vielen Fällen die Diagnose einer ICP noch nicht mit definitiver Sicherheit zu stellen ist. Eine Metaanalyse hat daher von vornherein zu berücksichtigen, dass die Gesamt-

stichprobe heterogen ist und dass Teile der Stichprobe auf etwas unsicherem diagnostischem Fundament stehen.

3. Als Kriterien des Behandlungserfolgs dienten in erster Linie die Ergebnisse standardisierter Entwicklungstests, teilweise solcher mit spezieller Ausrichtung auf motorische Fähigkeiten, oder aber qualitative Änderungen motorischer oder neurologischer Befunde.

Metaanalysen zur Wirksamkeit von Physiotherapie bei ICP

Aus den zurückliegenden 12 Jahren möchte ich 3 Metaanalysen zitieren, in welchen Publikationen zur Evaluation von Physiotherapie bei ICP vorzugsweise in den ersten Lebensjahren ausgewertet wurden (Tab. 1.). In diesen Metaanalysen wird versucht, nicht nur der Heterogenität von Stichproben und Outcome-Kriterien, sondern auch dem durchaus unterschiedlichen »Level of evidence« Rechnung zu tragen.

Tab. 1: Metaanalysen zur Effektivität von Physiotherapie in der Frühbehandlung

Tirosh & Rabino, AJDC 1989	9 Studien, davon 6 über Frühbehandlung
Turnbull, AJDC 1993	15 Studien, davon 12 über Frühbehandlung
Butler & Darrah, DMCN 2001	21 Studien, davon 10 ausschließlich und weitere 6 teilweise über Frühbehandlung

Aktuell ist eine weitere Metaanalyse über 50 Studien hinzugekommen (Siebes, Wijnroks u. Vermeer 2001), sie liegt noch nicht vollständig im Druck vor, sondern nur als Abstract und unveröffentlichtes Manuskript.
Summarisch stimmen die Aussagen dieser Metaanalysen in folgenden Punkten überein:

- Die Behandlungseffekte sind inkosistent: Tendenziell positive, aber überwiegend nicht signifikante positive Resultate stehen negativen gegenüber.
- Je strenger die methodischen Anforderungen an eine Studie waren, desto eher kamen die Untersucher zu einem negativen Ergebnis; eine besondere Bedeutung hatte dabei eine »blinde« Auswertung.
- Positive Ergebnisse hatten, soweit vorhanden, eine so geringe Effektstärke, dass sie nicht als spezifischer, gewissermaßen kurativer Erfolg einer bestimmten Methode gewertet werden können, zumal sich die verschiedenen Methoden in den nachweisbaren Effekten pauschal nicht unterschieden.

Nun kann man aus diesen Ergebnissen noch nicht schließen, dass Physiotherapie in der Frühbehandlung der ICP keinen bedeutsamen Effekt hätte. In der Literatur werden folgende Erklärungen für möglicherweise falsch-negative Evaluationsergebnisse diskutiert (Tab. 2):

Tab. 2: Erklärungen für möglicherweise falsch-negative Evaluationsergebnisse

– Inadäquates Untersuchungsdesign (eher Einzelfallstudien als Gruppenvergleiche sinnvoll wegen unvermeidlicher Heterogenität der Gruppen)
– Unzureichende Studienplanung (zu kleine Stichproben, zu kurze Laufzeit, mangelhafte Standardisierung des Programms)
– Interferenz mit anderen (insbesondere psychosozialen) Faktoren (»Auch in den besten Studien bestimmt das Behandlungsprogramm allenfalls 10% der Varianz des Outcome«, Halpern 1984).

Bedeutung anderer Interventionsformen

Auch wenn man diese Einwände berücksichtigen muss, scheint durch die Ergebnisse der Metaanalysen doch die Bedeutung der Physiotherapie relativiert zu werden, und es ist geboten, andere Interventionsformen in die Betrachtung einzubeziehen (Tab. 3)

Tab. 3. Interventionsformen bei Entwicklungsstörungen

Kindzentriert:
– Medizinisch orientierte Maßnahmen: Physiotherapie, Ergotherapie, Logopädie
– Pädagogisch-psychologische Maßnahmen: Lernprogramme, Verhaltensmodifikation
Elternzentriert:
– Information und Beratung
– Programmiertes Elterntraining
– Psychotherapie, soziale Stützung

Es liegt auf der Hand, dass zu diesem breiten Spektrum von Interventionsformen auch andere Outcome-Kriterien gehören als lediglich Entwicklungsquotienten oder motorische Indices. Adäquate Kriterien sind z.B. – je nach Fragestellung – Merkmale des Verhaltens und der Interaktion, der subjektiven Belastung der Eltern, der inner- und außerfamiliären Beziehungen und andere Faktoren der Lebensqualität. Ich wage die Behauptung, dass diesen Ziel- und Erfolgskriterien in der Medizin allgemein und auch in der Neuropädiatrie im Besonderen (noch) nicht die Wertigkeit zugebilligt wird, die ihnen aus der Sicht der betroffenen Kinder und Eltern zukommt.

Die unterschiedlichen Dimensionen der Maßnahmen zur Entwicklungsförderung und ihre Effektivität wurden in der m.W. umfangreichsten Metaanalyse auf diesem Gebiet von Dunst, Snyder und Mankinen (1989) untersucht, in welcher 105 Studien über Frühbehandlung und Frühförderung ausgewertet wurden. Diese Analyse bestätigt das Postulat eines positiven Effekts von Frühbehandlung und Frühförderung für Kinder mit Entwicklungsrisiken global, aber doch mit deutlichen Differenzierungen (Tab. 4).

Tab. 4: Metaanalyse von 105 Studien zur Effektivität früher entwicklungsfördernder Interventionen; Dunst, Snyder und Mankinen 1989

Deutliche positive Effekte
– bei jungen, psychosozial deprivierten Kindern
– durch Lernprogramme (psychologisch, pädagogisch)
– auf die Situation von Eltern bzw. Familie, auf die Interaktion
Geringe oder unsichere Effekte
– bei organisch bedingter, insbesondere schwerer Behinderung
– durch medizinisch orientierte Therapieformen

Auch wenn die Zielkriterien nicht durchweg vergleichbar sind, fällt doch auf, dass die auf Übungsbehandlung ausgerichteten Therapieformen aus dem medizinischen Bereich, wie Physiotherapie und Ergotherapie, auch in dieser Analyse im Vergleich zu pädagogisch oder psychologisch orientierten Interventionsformen schlechter abschneiden.

Auswirkung psychosozialer Faktoren

An dieser Stelle möchte ich die Interventionsstudien verlassen und den Blick auf Entwicklungsstudien lenken, in denen irgendwelche therapeutischen Interventionen *keine* Rolle spielten, sondern vielmehr der Entwicklungsfortschritt der Kinder in Abhängigkeit von bestimmten Qualitäten der Mutter-Kind-Interaktion untersucht wurde. Ich berichte über eine Analyse von 20 Studien, von denen sich je 6 auf Low-Risk-Kinder und auf Frühgeborene sowie 8 auf Kinder mit verschiedenen Behinderungen (Down-Syndrom, andere Formen mentaler Retardierung, Hörbehinderung, zerebrale Bewegungsstörung) beziehen, allesamt im Vorschulalter.

Aus dieser Auswertung sind zwei Aspekte besonders hervorzuheben: Zum einen sind die Outcome-Kritierien sehr einheitlich, nämlich der Verlauf der *funktionellen* Entwicklung, beurteilt nach standardisierten Entwicklungstests, in Abhängigkeit von *psychosozialen* Faktoren. Zum andern sind die Ergebnisse so einheitlich und tendenziell bei Kindern mit oder ohne Entwicklungsstörung so übereinstimmend, dass man von Evidenz sprechen kann. Bestimmte Verhaltensmerkmale der Bezugsperson zeigten signifikante Auswirkungen auf die Entwicklung der Kinder (Tab. 5).

An diesen Ergebnissen ist zweierlei bemerkenswert:
– Gemessen an relativ »harten« Kriterien (nämlich an den Resultaten standar-

Tab. 5: Einfluss der Mutter-Kind-Interaktion auf die funktionelle Entwicklung Schlack 1989 (Auswertung von 20 Entwicklungsstudien ohne Intervention)

Günstige Wirkung	Ungünstige Wirkung
– Responsivität	– Direktivität
– Verbale/emotionale Verstärkung	– Einengende Kontrolle
– Angebot adäquaten Spielzeugs	– Überstimulation

disierter Entwicklungstests) wird die funktionelle Entwicklung durch Faktoren der sozialen Umwelt stärker beeinflusst als durch vermeintlich spezifische therapeutische Maßnahmen,
- die fördernden und hemmenden Interaktionsformen lassen sich jeweils auf einen gemeinsamen Nenner bringen: Sie fördern bzw. hemmen die Eigenaktivität des Kindes.

Von der Empirie zur Arbeitshypothese

Aus diesen empirischen Daten lässt sich eine wegweisende Arbeitshypothese für die Frühbehandlung ableiten:

Die Anregung der motorischen Eigenaktivität des Kindes ist vermutlich das wichtigste Element früher Interventionen bei Zerebralparese.

In diesem Kontext ist auch das – häufig als paradox bezeichnete – Ergebnis der Palmer-Studie durchaus plausibel. Palmer et al. (1988) verglichen 2 Gruppen von Kindern mit spastischer Diplegie im 2. Lebensjahr. Die eine Gruppe erhielt über 12 Monate Physiotherapie nach der Bobath-Methode, die 2. Gruppe während der ersten 6 Monate eine heilpädagogische Förderung und in den folgenden 6 Monaten ebenfalls Physiotherapie. Die Gruppe mit der heilpädagogischen Förderung hatte nach 6 und nach 12 Monaten nicht nur einen höheren durchschnittlichen Entwicklungsquotienten, sondern wies *auch in der Motorik* die besseren Fortschritte auf, obwohl sie in der ersten Hälfte des Programms keine Physiotherapie erhalten hatte. Die Interpretation liegt nahe, dass die Kinder mit heilpädagogischer Förderung in ihrem gesamten Aktivitätsniveau angeregt wurden, so dass davon auch die motorischen Fähigkeiten profitierten.

Die Arbeitshypothese, dass es nicht nur in der normalen Entwicklung, sondern auch im Falle einer Schädigung des ZNS entscheidend auf die Anregung der Eigenaktivität und damit auf die Selbstübung der verbliebenen Fähigkeiten ankommt, ist konsistent mit den Vorstellungen über die Bedeutung der Motorik sowohl in den Konzepten der Entwicklungsneurologie als auch der Entwicklungspsychologie.

Zugleich zeigen die empirischen Befunde, dass bei allen Formen organischer Beeinträchtigung eines Kindes die Dominanz der erwachsenen Bezugsperson tendenziell zunimmt und dadurch die Eigenaktivität des Kindes gehemmt wird

(Sarimski 1986). Durch verordnete »Therapieprogramme« kann dieses Ungleichgewicht in der Eltern-Kind-Interaktion unversehens vergrößert werden. Das mag einen Teil möglicher Therapieeffekte neutralisieren.

Praktische Möglichkeiten der Anregung motorischer Eigenaktivität bei jungen Kindern mit ICP

Behandlungsansätze ergeben sich vor allem auf drei verschiedenen Ebenen:
- durch responsive Interaktion
- durch Stimulation im Rahmen der Physiotherapie
- durch frühe Hilfsmittelversorgung

Dazu sollen stichwortartig einige Erläuterungen gegeben werden:

Interventionsbereich »Interaktion«
- Anregungen müssen zurückhaltend und unter Berücksichtigung spontaner Initiativen des Kindes (»responsiv«) erfolgen. Selbstbestimmte Aktivitäten haben die größte Aussicht, zu subjektiven Erfolgserlebnissen zu führen und Kinder zu weiterer Anstrengung zu motivieren (Largo 1997).
- Bei allen Interventionen sind die meist verlangsamten Aufnahme- und Reaktionsmöglichkeiten des zerebralparetischen Kindes zu berücksichtigen. Andernfalls resultiert eine Überstimulation, bei welcher Aktion und Reaktion nicht mehr im Sinne wechselseitiger Verstärkung auf einander abgestimmt sind mit der Folge verringerter Eigenaktivität (Field 1980).
- Psychische und emotionale Belastungen der Familie beeinträchtigen die emotionale Zuwendung und die Responsivität. Die Berücksichtigung und Beeinflussung solcher Stressbedingungen sind deshalb ein essentieller Teil des Interventionskonzepts (Schlack 2000).

Interventionsbereich »Stimulation durch Physiotherapie«

Die Vorstellung, dass eine früh praktizierte Physiotherapie auf »neurophysiologischer Grundlage« eine gewissermaßen kurative Wirkung auf das ZNS habe, wird – wie dargestellt – von den Evaluationsergebnissen nicht gestützt. Das schließt aber einen wichtigen Beitrag der Physiotherapie zur Anregung der Eigenaktivität nicht aus (Schlack 1998), und zwar durch
- Kompensation des Defizits somatosensorischer Afferenzen als Folge der Bewegungsarmut, z.B. durch taktile und kinaesthetische Stimulation,
- damit verbunden Anhebung der Vigilanz mit Verbesserung des motorischen Antriebs
- und Verhinderung unerwünschter Habituation.

Interventionsbereich »Hilfsmittel«

Eine frühe, d.h. schon im ersten Lebensjahr einsetzende Versorgung mit orthopädischen Hilfsmitteln kann wesentliche Beiträge zur Anregung der Eigenaktivität leisten, z.B.

- über die Verbesserung der Aufnahme visueller und auditiver Reize und der Kommunikation durch aufrechte Körperhaltung (Sitzhilfen),
- durch Erleichterung (teil-)selbständiger Fortbewegung,
- durch Prophylaxe von Sekundärschäden auf neuroorthopädischem Gebiet (insbesondere Kontrakturen).

Erwähnt werden soll auch das Botulinumtoxin A als therapeutische Möglichkeit, die Spontanmotorik eines Kindes mit spastischer ICP zu erleichtern (Heinen et al. 2001). Sein Einsatz spielt aber in den ersten Lebensjahren – zumindest vorläufig – eine quantitativ untergeordnete Rolle.

Fazit

Die Annahme und Hoffnung, dass mit bestimmten motorischen Übungen eine gewissermaßen kurative Wirkung bei Kindern mit Zerebralparese ausgeübt werden könne, wird von den vorliegenden Publikationen nicht gestützt. Deshalb ist der Therapie-Begriff in diesem Kontext problematisch, weil er die Vorstellung von »Heilung« suggeriert (Bax 2001). Ich habe daher in diesem Beitrag den Begriff »Intervention« bevorzugt.

Es gibt auch keinen Anhalt dafür, dass einzelne Behandlungsmethoden sich in diesem Punkt grundsätzlich von einander unterscheiden, so dass Auseinandersetzungen zwischen Vertretern verschiedener Methoden über den richtigen Weg eher als Ausdruck subjektiver Überzeugungen denn als evidenzbasierte Aussagen gelten müssen. Keinesfalls ist es danach statthaft, solche Konflikte auf dem Rücken von Patienten und Eltern auszutragen.

Demgegenüber wird durch empirische Befunde die Annahme gestützt, dass die Eigenaktivität des Kindes mit ICP der entscheidende Faktor für eine – mehr oder weniger weit gehende – Kompensation der Störung und damit für die weitere Entwicklung ist. Bei der Förderung der Eigenaktivität können therapeutische Interventionen eine wichtige Rolle spielen, jedoch nicht in einer simplen, linear-kausalen Ursache-Wirkungs-Beziehung, sondern in komplexen Wechselwirkungen. Hierbei können unterschiedliche methodische Konzepte – und ebenso unterschiedliche Persönlichkeitsmerkmale der therapeutisch engagierten Fachleute – zu durchaus differenten Ergebnissen führen. Die Frage des richtigen Vorgehens ist also in dieser komplexeren, systemischen Sichtweise weiterhin relevant.

Systemische Sichtweisen sind in der Medizin theoretisch anerkannt, werden aber in der täglichen Praxis häufig vernachlässigt, weil man mit den einfacheren linear-kausalen Konzepten auszukommen scheint. Bei der Behandlung von Kindern mit ICP kommt man damit jedenfalls nicht aus. Die für die Umsetzung systemischer Konzepte notwendigen Fähigkeiten können (und müssen) ebenso erlernt werden wie z.B. die entwicklungsneurologische Diagnostik oder die Auswertung von EEG-Kurven. Angesichts der bedeutsamen Rolle, welche den Ärzten in der Diagnostik, Elternberatung und Behandlungsleitung zukommt, dürfen diese wichtigen Dimensionen notwendiger Interventionen nicht einfach dilettantisch gehandhabt oder an nichtärztliche Berufsgruppen delegiert werden.

Literatur

1. Bax M (2001) Does »therapy« have a future? (Editorial). Dev Med Child Neurol. 43:3
2. Butler C, Darrah J (2001) Effects of neurodevelopmental treatment (NDT) for cerebral palsy: an AACPDM evidence report. Dev Med Child Neurol 43:778–790
3. Dunst CJ, Snyder SW, Mankinen M (1989) Efficacy of early intervention. In Wang MC, Reynolds MC, Walberg HJ (eds) Handbook of special education, Vol 3. Pergamon, Oxford
4. Field T (1980) Interaction of high-risk infants: Quantitative and qualitative differences. In Sawin D (ed) Psychosocial risks in infant-environment transactions. Brunner & Mazel, New York
5. Halpern R (1984) Lack of effects for home-based intervention? Some possible explanations. Am J. Orthopsychiat 54:33–42
6. Heinen F et al (2001) Botulinum-Toxin A: Lokale Pharmakotherapie bei spastischen Bewegungsstörungen im Kindesalter. Kinderärztl Prax 72:18–32
7. Largo RH (1997) Wie entwickeln sich behinderte Kinder? Kinderärztl Prax 68:140–147
8. Palmer FB et al (1988) The effects of physical therapy on cerebral palsy. A controlled trial in infants with spastic diplegia. N Engl J Med 318:803–808
9. Sarimski, K (1986) Interaktion mit behinderten Kleinkindern. Reinhardt, München
10. Schlack HG (1989) I. Psychosoziale Einflüsse auf die Entwicklung. II. Wie spezifisch wirken »Therapie« und »Milieu« auf die Entwicklung behinderter Kinder? In Karch D, Michaelis R, Rennen-Allhoff B, Schlack HG (Hrsg) Normale und gestörte Entwicklung. Springer, Berlin-Heidelberg-New York.
11. Schlack HG (1998) Stimulation der Körperwahrnehmung – ein wichtiges Konzept in der Behandlung zerebralparetischer Kinder. In Schlack HG (Hrsg) Welche Behandlung nützt behinderten Kindern? Kirchheim, Mainz
12. Schlack HG (2000) Entwicklungsstörungen und Behinderungen. In Schlack HG (Hrsg) Sozialpädiatrie, 2. Aufl. Urban & Fischer, München
13. Siebes RC, Wijnroks L, Vermeer A (2001): Qualitative analysis of therapeutic intervention programmes for children with cerebral palsy. EACD abstracts. Dev Med Child Neurol 43, Suppl. 88, p. 34.
14. Tirosh E, Rabino S (1989) Physiotherapy for children with cerebral palsy. Am J Dis Child 143:552–555
15. Turnbull JD (1993) Early intervention for children with or at risk of cerebral palsy. Am J Dis Child 147:54–59.

Spättherapie der infantilen Zerebralparese (ICP) – Resultate wissenschaftlicher Studien

H. Bode

Zusammenfassung

Spättherapie bei infantiler Zerebralparese (ICP) wird als Therapie nach dem 5. Lebensjahr definiert, wenn die ICP eine definitive Diagnose ist. Therapiemodalitäten jenseits dieses Alters sind hauptsächlich Physiotherapie, Ergotherapie, Pharmakotherapie, Orthesen, orthopädische und neurochirurgische Operationen. In einem Überblick werden die Effekte dieser Therapiemodalitäten in Bezug auf evidenzbasierte Studien und Resultate neuerer wissenschaftlicher Publikationen beleuchtet.

Physiotherapie nach Bobath zeigt keine Vorteile gegenüber anderen physiotherapeutischen-, pädagogischen- und Stimulationsprogrammen. Möglicherweise ist die Art der Präsentation wichtiger als der Inhalt des Therapieprogramms. Wenige Studien zur Ergotherapie deuten auf positive Effekte bei konkreten Zielen hin. Unter den oralen Pharmaka mindert Baclofen die Spastizität. Botulinum Toxin A verbessert verschiedene Outcome-Dimensionen. Intrathekales Baclofen und die selektive dorsale Rhizotomie zeigen gewisse positive Effekte, die noch weiter belegt werden müssen. Orthesen und orthopädische Operationen werden häufig und individualisiert verwendet. Allgemeine anerkannte Therapiestandards müssen noch erarbeitet werden.

Therapien bei ICP müssen individualisiert und im familiären Kontext stattfinden. Ihre Effektivität steigt bei Orientierung auf spezifische Ziele, vermehrter unspezifischer motorischer Aktivierung und Feedback zwischen Eltern, Patient und Therapeuten.

Einleitung

Als Spättherapie der infantilen Zerebralparese (ICP) werden in dieser Übersicht Therapien nach dem 5. Lebensjahr definiert. Zu diesem Zeitpunkt ist nach internationalem Konsens die Diagnose einer ICP definitiv zu stellen.

Wissenschaftliche Studien zu diesem Thema stoßen auf verschiedene Schwierigkeiten: Die Häufigkeit der ICP ist mit etwa 2‰ relativ gering. Die in einzelnen Zentren betreuten Patienten sind nach Ursache, Art und Ausprägung der klinischen Symptome sehr heterogen und zeigen unterschiedliche, aber relevante Komorbiditäten. Die entwicklungsbedingten Veränderungen der Symptome und Therapieziele sind zu berücksichtigen. Therapien finden nicht isoliert unter Laborbedingungen statt, sondern als Bündel komplexer Maßnahmen im Alltagskontext. Die einzelnen Wirkfaktoren sind daher schwierig zu isolieren.

Außerdem erfolgen Therapien bei ICP selten standardisiert, sondern nach differentieller Therapie-Indikation und verschiedenen Therapie-Konzepten. Die fachliche Qualifikation der Therapeuten ist nicht hinreichend definiert und standardisiert. Selbst bei medikamentösen, orthopädisch nicht-operativen und operativen Verfahren existieren keine anerkannten Behandlungsstandards. Verschiedene Studien sind mithin schlecht vergleichbar. Auch werden Therapiedosis und Compliance selten erfasst.

In den letzten Jahren hat es allerdings Fortschritte bei der Standardisierung und Validisierung von Messverfahren gegeben. Man stimmt heute auch überein, dass in Folge der Komplexität von Therapiezielen eine Messung des Therapieerfolges auf verschiedenen Ebenen erfolgen muss.

Methoden

Für diese Übersicht werden verschiedene systematische Analysen, consensus statements, zahlreiche, überwiegend über MEDLINE abrufbare kontrollierte Gruppen- und Einzelfallstudien und schließlich Expertenmeinungen, die z.T. mit unkontrollierten klinischen Fallserien begründet werden, herangezogen. Es kann nur eine Auswahl von Resultaten zu wichtigen bzw. aktuell diskutierten Therapien dargestellt werden.

Die Bewertung der Studien benutzt die von der AACPDM definierten Evidenzlevels (13, 14). Dabei werden neben kontrollierten Gruppenvergleichsstudien auch Fallserien und Einzelfallstudien den bekannten Evidenzlevels I–V zugeordnet.

Ergebnisse

Physiotherapie

In einer aktuellen, sehr umfassenden Metaanalyse von 21 Studien, die spezifische Effekte der Bobath-Therapie bei ICP untersucht, zeigt sich mit Ausnahme einer kurzfristigen Verbesserung der Gelenkbeweglichkeit kein Vorteil der Bobath-Therapie gegenüber anderen Verfahren oder keiner Therapie (14). Es werden dabei in dieser Analyse Effekte der Bobath-Therapie überwiegend bei jüngeren Kindern untersucht, nur 4 Studien beziehen sich ausschließlich, 3 weitere zum Teil, auf die Spättherapie. Die Therapiedauer lag zwischen 2 Wochen und 12 Monaten, im Median bei etwa 3 Monaten. Die referierten Studien sind durch geringe Fallzahl (insgesamt 416 Kinder) und völlig fehlende Power-Berechnungen eingeschränkt. Der Therapieeffekt wird getrennt für die Dimensionen Pathophysiologie, Impairment/Organfunktion, funktionelle Einschränkungen/Aktivitäten, Behinderung/Partizipation und soziale Limitation/Kontextfaktoren untersucht. Die Autoren betonen, dass es in der vorgelegten Evidenz substantielle Lücken gibt (14).

Ähnlich enttäuschend sind die Ergebnisse einer prospektiven multizentrischen Studie über 18 Monate, die bei 56 Kindern mit spastischer Diplegie im

Alter von 3–12 Jahren keinen Effekt einer intensivierten Physiotherapie oder einer spezifischen Zielorientierung nachweisen konnten (Evidenzlevel I, 5).

Manuelle Therapie

Hierzu vorliegende Studien sind methodisch schwach. Es besteht Konsens, dass kurzfristige Effekte dieser Behandlung nachweisbar sind, indem durch die Mobilisierung der Weichteile und bestimmte Manipulationstechniken Muskeltonus und Körperhaltung positiv beeinflusst werden. Damit können Schmerz- und andere sekundäre Funktionsstörungen bei ICP gelindert werden. Die Langzeiteffekte dieser Therapien sind unklar (Evidenzlevel V, 27).

Neue Physiotherapiekonzepte

Hier zeigen sich erste hoffnungsvolle Ergebnisse. Ein *Krafttraining* der Beine bzw. Arme scheint Gehfähigkeit, Bewegungsgeschwindigkeit und die Rollstuhlbenutzung zu verbessern (Evidenzlevel IV, 8, 30, 33).

Überwiegend bei Kleinkindern wurde nachgewiesen, dass eine Orientierung der Physiotherapie auf kurzfristige Ziele sowie häusliche Bewegungsaktivierung die motorischen Fähigkeiten bei Kindern mit Bewegungsstörungen signifikant verbessern können (Evidenzlevel I, 4).

Ergotherapie

Diese hat wie die Physiotherapie in der Alltagspraxis für die Spättherapie der ICP eine anerkannte Indikation (12). Eine kontrollierte prospektive Studie konnte nachweisen, dass sensorisch-perzeptuell-motorisches Training über 3 Monate die körperlichen Fähigkeiten signifikant verbessert (Evidenzlevel II, 10). Konsequentes Selbständigkeitstraining junger Erwachsener mit ICP über 20 Tage verbessert ihre Fertigkeiten im Alltag und ihre Beschäftigungssituation (Evidenzlevel III, 25). Zu dem interessanten neuen Therapieprinzip »forced use« liegen für die ICP noch keine systematischen Studien vor.

Logopädie und Esstherapie

Diese sind in der Praxis der 3. Baustein der Therapie im Heilmittelkatalog (12). ICP-Kinder mit Ess-Störungen profitieren signifikant von einer systematischen 10wöchigen Esstherapie in definierten und validen Aspekten der Essfunktion (Evidenzlevel III, 21).

Pharmaka

Unter den *oralen Pharmaka* existieren randomisierte Studien zur Behandlung der ICP für Diazepam, Dantrolen und orales Baclofen.

Diazepam zeigte zwar bei 36% der behandelten Kinder eine Verbesserung des Muskeltonus und des Verhaltens, seine Anwendung war jedoch durch die bekannten Nebenwirkungen limitiert (Evidenzlevel I, 17).

Dantrolen hatte zwar in verschiedenen Studien bei etwa 50% der Patienten Effekte, allerdings ohne klare klinische Relevanz. Die Anwendung wird ebenfalls durch Nebenwirkungen und insbesondere durch eine Verminderung der Muskelkraft limitiert, so dass sie letztlich nur in ausgewählten Fällen erfolgreich ist (33).

Orales Baclofen verhinderte signifikant Muskeltonus und Spastik, dies war jedoch in keinem Fall funktionell bedeutsam (33).

Butolinumtoxin A (BTX-A), intramuskulär appliziert, hat in der klinischen Praxis in den letzten Jahren eine erhebliche Bedeutung in der Behandlung spezifischer Probleme von Kindern mit ICP erhalten. Eine Übersicht der Cochrane-Database im Jahre 2000 für 3 damals vorliegende randomisierte kontrollierte Studien (15, 20, 29) fand keine starke Evidenz, um BTX-A für die Therapie einer Spastizität der Beine bei ICP zu unterstützen oder abzulehnen (Evidenzlevel I, 1).

Eine systematische Übersicht über randomisierte kontrollierte Studien zu BTX-A bei ICP im Folgejahr hat einen positiveren Tenor (28). Auf der Ebene der Pathophysiologie konnte eine partielle Denervation des Muskels gezeigt werden (29), auf der Organebene (Impairment) fand sich beim spastischen Spitzfuß eine Zunahme der Dorsalflexion sowohl aktiv wie beim Gang. Passive Beweglichkeit und Kraftbedarf waren nicht verändert. Bei funktionellen Aktivitäten zeigten sich Gangfunktion und Gangbild verbessert (Evidenzlevel I, 29, 39, 41).

Bei präoperativer Gabe fand sich eine Reduktion postoperativer Schmerzen nach Adduktorentenotomie, der Krankenhausaufenthalt verkürzte sich (Evidenzlevel I, 3).

Studien mit BTX-A an den oberen Extremitäten mit kleinen Fallzahlen zeigten eine Verminderung des Muskeltonus in Hand- und Ellenbogengelenk, eine Verbesserung der Extension im Ellenbogen- und Daumengrundgelenk, der Handöffnung und Greiffunktion. Die funktionellen Möglichkeiten waren dadurch nur partiell verbessert, subjektiv wurde ein kosmetischer Gewinn gesehen (Evidenzlevel I bzw. II, 15, 19).

Die aktuellen Expertenempfehlungen zur Behandlung der ICP mit BTX-A beinhalten zwingend ein multimodales Behandlungskonzept (Evidenzlevel V, 23).

Die *intrathekale Baclofentherapie (ITB)* zur Therapie der Spastik bei ICP wurde kürzlich in einer Metaanalyse von 14 Studien untersucht. Bei 202 Patienten veränderte ITB die Spastik der unteren Extremitäten und verbesserte Alltagsfunktionen und Pflege. Die Effekte von ITB auf Kontrakturen, die aktive motorische Kontrolle und die Schmerzreduktion konnte bei geringer Fallzahl nicht gesichert werden. Die Effekte auf die soziale Funktion war uneinheitlich. Positive Effekte wurden nicht bei allen Patienten gesehen, es ergaben sich häufig medizinische Komplikationen, die Behandlung ist sehr teuer. Die vorliegenden Studien zeigen insgesamt eine positive, aber erst begrenzte Evidenz (Evidenzlevel I, 13).

Orthesen

In der Spätbehandlung der ICP haben Orthesen unterschiedliche Indikationen und Ziele, müssen individuell angepasst werden und sind sehr teuer. Sie sollten die Funktionen übernehmen, die der Patient selbst nicht erfüllen kann (6).

Aus aktuellem Anlass werden die *Unterschenkelorthesen* (= ankle-foot orthese = AFO) genauer besprochen. Sie bezwecken, dass beim spastischen Spitzfuß Tonus und Spastik kontrolliert und der Fuß in anatomischer Funktion gehalten wird. Es soll ein Fersen-Ballen-Gang erreicht werden, damit die motorische Funktion verbessert und der Energieverbrauch beim Laufen reduziert werden kann (7, 42). Die Terminologie wird uneinheitlich gehandhabt. Man unterscheidet steife (SAFO), klappbare (HAFO), bewegliche (Brunnerorthesen) sowie spiralige und dynamische (Hylton-) Unterschenkelorthesen.

In verschiedenen Kurzzeit-Studien mit kleinen Fallzahlen konnte man zeigen, dass Gangbild, Schrittlänge, Kadenz, Plantarflexion (HAFO und SAFO), sowie Energieeffizienz und funktionelle Mobilität (HAFO, Brunnerorthesen) durch Unterschenkelorthesen verbessert werden (Evidenzlevel III, IV, V, 7, 9, 11, 24, 31, 36). Eine Spitzfußprävention ist nur durch kniehohe Orthesen möglich (31).

Dynamische Sprunggelenk-Orthesen (Hyltonorthesen) werden kontrovers diskutiert. Sie verbesserten im Vergleich zum Zustand ohne Orthesen in einer kurzfristigen Studie bei 44 Kindern die grobmotorische Funktion im Zielbereich um etwa 10 Prozentpunkte, bei starker interindividueller Variabilität der Verbesserung (Evidenzlevel IV, 34).

Bei 8 vom 13 Kindern mit spastischer Diplegie zeigte sich mit Hyltonorthesen im Vergleich zum Barfußgang in der instrumentellen dreidimensionalen Ganganalyse eine Verbesserung der Raum-Zeit-Parameter, bei 11 von 26 Füßen auch in der Kinematik. Veränderungen an den Knien bzw. Hüften waren weniger deutlich bzw. selten. In einigen Fällen wurde eine Verschlechterung beobachtet (Evidenzlevel IV, 18).

Im Vergleich mit der Brunnerorthese schnitten die Hyltonorthesen bzgl. der Ziele Fersen-Ballengang und Dorsalflexion deutlich schlechter ab (Evidenzlevel III, 7).

Die den Hyltonorthesen zugeschriebenen tonusregulierenden Effekte müssen noch belegt werden. Im Vergleich mit konventionellen HAFO an 8 Kindern waren diese Effekte ohne funktionelle Bedeutung (16).

Bei Kindern mit geringeren Einschränkungen wurden Aktivitäten auf unebener Oberfläche (Klettern, Balancieren etc.) durch dynamische Sprunggelenkorthesen günstiger beeinflusst (31). Kontrollierte Untersuchungen zu den langfristigen Effekten verschiedener Unterschenkelorthesen fehlen (31).

Weitere Therapieverfahren

Lycra-Kompressionskleidung wird von Patienten oft nicht akzeptiert (35). Früher häufiger eingesetzte Seriengipse scheinen eine Operation nicht zu verhindern und werden daher insgesamt seltener empfohlen (42). Eine randomisierte kontrollierte Studie zeigte keine Wirkung einer therapeutischen Elektrostimulation. (Evidenzlevel I, 38). Eine Elektrostimulation in Kombination mit dynamischen Schienen zeigte dagegen in einer kleinen Studie positive Ergebnisse (37).

Die Kombination verschiedener Therapieverfahren ist häufige Praxis, sie erfolgt meist unstandardisiert. Es liegen keine aussagekräftigen Studien zur Wirksamkeit kombinierter Verfahren vor.

Orthopädische Operationen

Sie haben in der Spättherapie der ICP einen hohen Stellenwert. An Füßen, Knien, Hüften und Wirbelsäule können Sehnenverlängerungen, Sehnentransfers, andere Weichteileingriffe, Osteotomien und Arthrodesen durchgeführt werden. Kontrollierte prospektiv randomisierte Studien existieren nicht (maximale Evidenzlevel IV).

Zum operativen Vorgehen bei verschiedenen Problemen besteht kein allgemeiner Konsens. Häufig werden heute folgende Verfahren angewandt (40):

- Beim dynamischen pes equinovarus ein hälftiger Tibialis Posterior Transfer.
- Beim spastischen Knick-Senk-Fuß die extraartikuläre Versteifung des unteren Sprunggelenks nach Grice sowie die Kalkaneus-Verlängerungs-Osteotomie in Verbindung mit Weichteileingriffen.
- Bei Kniekontrakturen kombinierte Weichteileingriffe mit Transfer des Rectus Femoris.
- Bei Hüftluxation, die bei bis zu 50% der Kinder Schmerzen verursacht, anstatt der früher häufigeren Adduktorentenotomie vermehrt rezentrierende Operationsverfahren.
- Bei Skoliose eine Arthrodese mit Implantaten.

In der Vergangenheit etablierte Verfahren haben nicht selten zu Enttäuschungen und Komplikationen geführt. Die Auswirkung der neuen, funktionell orientierten Operationsverfahren muss im Langzeitverlauf noch untersucht werden. Dabei ist zu bedenken, dass erwachsene ICP-Patienten ihre Bedürfnisse in der Rangfolge: Kommunikation, Selbständigkeit im Alltag und Mobilität, allerdings nicht unbedingt beim Gehen, benennen (22).

Fazit

Evidenzbasierte Medizin (EBM) ist kein Ergebnis, sondern ein Prozess. Was heute gilt, ist morgen überholt. Bei allem Respekt gegenüber der Methodik der EBM sind einige Kritikpunkte und die Grenzen der EBM zu bedenken, die sich bei Fragen zur Spättherapie der ECP deutlich zeigen: Verschiedene Gremien verwenden unterschiedliche Evidenzkriterien. Metaanalysen selektieren (Publikationsbias). Patientenstichproben sind oft hoch selektiv und nicht repräsentativ. Eine nachgewiesene therapeutische Wirkung (efficacy) mag für den Alltag des Patienten unbedeutend oder nicht generalisierbar sein (effectiveness). Auch wirtschaftliche Faktoren haben Einfluss darauf, welche therapeutischen Fragen untersucht und welche Ergebnisse publiziert werden. EBM wird – gerade für die Spättherapie der ICP – nur in begrenztem Umfang das therapeutische Vorgehen beeinflussen (26).

Festzuhalten ist, dass unterschiedliche physiotherapeutische Konzepte bei der ICP keine spezifischen Vorteile zeigen. Historische Kontrollen und Beispiele nicht behandelter Kinder der dritten Welt belegen andererseits die Wirksamkeit von Physiotherapie. Spezifische therapeutische Maßnahmen, an konkreten und realistischen Therapiezielen orientiert, zeigen auch in wissenschaftlichen Studien nachweisbare Effekte (4), Neue Therapieprinzipien müssen wissenschaftlich untersucht werden (Kraft-, Ausdauer-, Laufbandtraining; forced use; gezielte Übung von Alltagsfertigkeiten).

Die Therapie mit BTX-A, die Versorgung mit Hilfsmitteln und orthopädische Operation müssen kombiniert und individuell adaptiert werden. Eine ICP kann nicht geheilt werden. Therapieziele müssen dann mehrdimensional formuliert werden und insbesondere eine Verbesserung von Funktion, Partizipation und Autonomie des Patienten beinhalten und dabei die Bedürfnisse der Patienten und ihrer Eltern berücksichtigen.

Bei vielen Fragen in der Spättherapie der ICP wird der Arzt und Therapeut auch künftig nicht auf Antworten der EBM rechnen können, sondern auf seine Beobachtungen und Erfahrungen angewiesen sein.

Literatur

1. Ade-Hall RA, Moore AP (2000) Botulinum toxin type A in the treatment of lower limb spasticity in cerebral palsy. Cochrane Database Syst Rev 2:1469–1493
2. Bakheit M et al (1999) Recommendations for minimum standards of healthcare in children with cerebral palsy. Hemi Help, London
3. Barwood S, Baillieu C, Boyd R et al (2000) Analgesic effects of botulinum toxin A: a randomized, placebo-controlled clinical trial. Dev Med Child Neurol 42:116–121
4. Bode H (2002) Indikation zur Behandlung von cerebralen Bewegungsstörungen und Evaluationsergebnisse. In: Aksu (Hrsg) Aktuelle Neuropädiatrie. Novartis Verlag Wehr
5. Bower E, Michell D, Burnett M, Campbell MJ, McLellan DL (2001) Randomized controlled trial of physiotherapy in 56 children with cerebral palsy followed for 18 month. Dev Med Child Neurol 43:4–15
6. Brunner R (2000) Welches Hilfsmittel für welche Bewegungsstörung? Physiotherapie – OST-Sonderheft Propriozeption, 50–51
7. Brunner R (2000) Dynamische Sprunggelenk-Fußorthesen oder konventionelle Unterschenkelorthesen? Physiotherapie – OST-Sonderheft Propriozeption, 47–49
8. Bütefisch CH, Hummelsheim H (1995) Repetive training of isolated movements improves outcome of motor rehabilitation of the centrally paretic hand. J Neurol Sci 130: 59–68
9. Buckon C, Thomas S, Jacobsen-Huston S, Moor M, Sussman M, Aiona M (2001) Comparison of three ankle-foot orthosis configurations for children with spastic hemiplegia. Dev Med Child Neurol 43:371–378
10. Bumin G, Kayihan H (2001) Effectiveness of two different sensory-integration programmes for children with spastic diplegic cerebral palsy. Disabil Rehabil 23:394–399
11. Burtner P, Woollacott MH, Qualls C (1999) Stance balance control with orthoses in a group of children with spastic cerebral palsy. Dev Med Child Neurol 41:748–757
12. Bundesausschuss der Ärzte und Krankenkassen (2001) Heilmittelkatalog Heilmittelrichtlinien. www.heilmittelkatalog.de.
13. Butler C et al (2000) Evidence of the effects of intrathecal baclofen for spastic and dystonic cerebral palsy. Dev Med Child Neurol 42:634–645
14. Butler C et al (2001) Effects of neurodevelopmental treatment (NDT) for cerebral palsy: an AACPDM evidence report. Dev Med Child Neurol 43:778–790
15. Corry IS, Cosgrove AP, Walsh EG, McClean D, Graham HK (1997) Botulinum toxin A in the hemiplegic upper limb: a double-blind trial. Dev Med Child Neurol 39:185–193
16. Crenshaw S, Herzog R, Castagno P, Richards J, Miller F, Michaloski G, Moran E (2000) The efficacy of tone-reducing features in orthotics on the gait of children with spastic diplegic cerebral palsy. J Pediatr Orthop 20(2):210–216
17. Denhoff E, Feldman S, Smith MG (1975) Treatment of spastic cerebral-palsied children with sodium dantrolene. Dev Med Child Neurol 17:736
18. Döderlein L, Metaxiotis D, Siebel A (2000) Zur Wirksamkeit sogenannter neuroreflektorischer Einlagen und Fußorthesen. Physiotherapie Ost-Sonderheft Propriozeption:42–46
19. Fehlings D, Rang M, Glazier J, Steele C (2000) An evaluation of botulinum-A toxin injections

to improve upper extremity function in children with hemiplegic cerebral palsy. J Pediatr 137:331–337
20. Flett PJ, Stern LM, Waddy H, Connell TM, Seeger JD, Gibson SK (1999) Botulinum toxin A versus fixed cast stretching for dynamic calf tightness in cerebral palsy. J Paediatr Child Health 35:71–77.
21. Gisel EG, Applegate-Ferrante T, Benson J, Bosma JF (1996) Oral-motor skills following sensorimotor therapy in two groups of moderately dysphagic children with cerebral palsy: aspiration vs nonaspiration. Dysphagia 11:59–71
22. Goldberg MJ (1991) Measuring outcomes in cerebral palsy. J Pediat Orthop 11:682–685
23. Graham HK, Aoki KR, Autti-Ramo I, Boyd RN, Delgado MR, Gaebler-Spira DJ, Gormley ME, Guyer BM, Heinen F, Holton AF, Matthews D, Molenaers G, Motta F, Garcia-Ruiz PJ, Wissel J (2000) Recommendations for the use of botulinum toxin type A in the management of cerebral palsy. Gait Posture 11:67–69
24. Hainsworth F, Harrison MJ, Sheldon TA, Roussounis SH (1997) A preliminary evaluation of ankle orthoses in the management of children with cerebral palsy. Dev Med Child Neurol 39:243–247
25. Healy H, Rigby P (1999) Promoting independence for teens and young adults with physical disabilities. Can J Occup Ther 66:240–249
26. Helmchen H (2002) Evidenz der evidenzbasierten Medizin? Der Nervenarzt 73:1–2
27. Karch D, Gross-Selbeck G, Hanefeld F, Ritz A, Schlack HG (1998) Behandlung motorischer Störungen mit manueller Therapie. Förster C (Hrsg) Aktuelle Neuropädiatrie 1997 Novartis Verlag, Wehr
28. Kirschner J, Berweck S, Mall V, Korinthenberg R, Heinen F (2001) Botulinumtoxin – Neue Therapieoption für Kinder mit Zerebralparese. Deutsches Ärzteblatt 1998 50:B2840–B2844
29. Koman LA, Mooney JF, Smith BP, Walker F, Leon JM (2000) Botulinum toxin type A neuromuscular blockade in the treatment of lower extremity spasticity in cerebral palsy: a randomized, double-blind, placebo-controlled trial. BOTOX Study Group. J Pediatr Orthop 20:108–115
30. MacPhail HE, Kramer JF (1995) Effect of isokinetic strength-training on functional ability and walking efficiency in adolescents with cerebral palsy. Dev Med Child Neurol 37:763–775
31. Morris C (2002) A review of the efficacy of lower-limb orthoses used for cerebral palsy. Dev Med Child Neurol 44:205–211
32. O'Connell DG, Barnhart R (1995) Improvement in wheelchair propulsion in pediatric wheelchair users through resistance training: a pilot study. Arch Phys Med Rehabil 76:368–372
33. O'Donnell ME, Armstrong R, Scheinberg A, Williams K (2000) Cerebral palsy. In: Mayer et al (Echo): Endence Based Pediatrics an Child Health. BMJ
34. Reime U, Lohse-Busch H (2001) Hylton-Orthese – eine Effektivitätsanalyse. http://www.ot-forum.de/Verlag-OT/Reime/adm.htm
35. Rennie D, Morton R, Nicholson J, Attfield C (2000) Lycra dynamic splints for children with motor disorders. Dev Med Child Neurol 42:Suppl 83, p29
36. Rethlefsen S, Tolo VT, Reynolds RA, Kay R (1999) Outcome of hamstring lengthening and distal rectus femoris transfer surgery. J Pediatr Orthop B 8:75–79
37. Scheker LR, Chesher SP, Ramirez S (1999) Neuromuscular electrical stimulation and dynamic bracing as a treatment for upper-extremity spasticity in children with cerebral palsy. J Hand Surg Br 24:226–232
38. Sommerfeld K, Markestad T, Berg K, Saetesdal I (2001) Therapeutic electric stimulation in cerebral palsy: A randomized, controlled, crossover trial. Dev Med Child Neurol 43:609–13
39. Sutherland DH, Kaufman KR, Wyatt MP, Chambers HG, Mubarak SJ (1999) Double-blind study of botulinum A toxin injections into the gastrocnemius muscle in patients with cerebral palsy. Gait Posture 10:1–9
40. Stücker R (2001) Neue Entwicklungen bei operativen Therapieverfahren. In: Heinen F, Bartens W (Hrsg) Das Kind und die Spastik. Verlag Hans Huber, Bern
41. Ubhi T, Bhakta BB, Ives HL, Allgar V, Roussounis SH (2000) Randomized double blind placebo controlled trial of the effect of botulinum toxin on walking in cerebral palsy. Arch Dis Child 83:481–487
42. Woo R (2001) Spasticity: Orthopedic Perspective. J Child Neurol 16:47–53

Jenseits wissenschaftlicher Studien – die Notwendigkeit der Behandlung von zerebralen Bewegungsstörungen

D. Karch

Zusammenfassung

Aus ethischen Gründen dürfen bei der Behandlung nur Verfahren eingesetzt werden, deren Wirksamkeit erwiesen (evident) und deren unerwünschten Wirkungen bekannt sind.

Die Ansprüche an die Methodik von Evaluationsstudien haben sich in den letzten Jahren ständig erhöht. Daher können zahlreiche erprobte Vorgehensweisen nicht mehr als »evidenzbasiert« angesehen werden – nicht nur bei der Behandlung von zerebralen Bewegungsstörungen –, und es wird immer schwieriger neue Behandlungsverfahren einzuführen. Die wissenschaftlich anerkannten Vorgehensweisen wie z.B. placebokontrollierte Studien oder Meta-Analysen sind aber nicht unumstritten. Selbst Studien, die den methodischen Ansprüchen am besten entsprechen, weisen nicht unerhebliche Schwächen bei der Durchführung und der Interpretation der Ergebnisse auf. Berücksichtigt man diese Kritik, kann man die Notwendigkeit der Behandlung trotz der unbefriedigenden Situation leichter begründen. Die Behandlung hat sich zu orientieren an den medizinisch, psychologisch, sozial und ethisch zu begründenden Wunsch der Patienten, ein möglichst selbstständiges Leben in unserer Gesellschaft führen zu können. Aber auch ökonomische Aspekte können nicht unberücksichtigt bleiben; die Solidargemeinschaft aller Versicherten darf durch überzogene Anforderungen von Interessengruppen nicht in Frage gestellt werden.

Einleitung

Eine kaum übersehbare Vielfalt von Konzepten und Verfahren wird bei der Behandlung von zerebralen Bewegungsstörungen angeboten. Die Auswahl der Verfahren, die in der konkreten Behandlungssituation eingesetzt werden, können die Ärzte zum Teil beeinflussen durch eine Verordnung entsprechend dem Heilmittelkatalog, wo im Bereich der Physiotherapie differenzierte Angaben gefordert werden. Im Bereich der Ergotherapie werden allerdings im Heilmittelkatalog nur die Festlegung der Ziele aber nicht die der Behandlungsmethoden verlangt. Die Therapeuten setzen je nach ihrer Ausbildung oder Weiterbildung und nach ihren persönlichen Erfahrungen bestimmte Methoden ein. Nur wenige Verfahren sind ausreichend evaluiert bzw. nur auf dem untersten Level der Evidenzhierarchie abgesichert (Siehe Beiträge Bode und Schlack in diesem Band). Oft werden von den Angehörigen aber auch von den Therapeuten nicht

Tab. 1: Behandlungsverfahren bei zerebralen Bewegungsstörungen (Auswahl)

Etablierte Verfahren
– Krankengymnastik »auf neurophysiologischer Grundlage« nach Bobath oder Vojta
– Botulinumtoxin Injektionen
– Konduktive Förderung nach Petö
– Selective dorsale Rhizotomie
– Manuelle Therapie (Chirotherapie)
Alternative Verfahren
– Laufbandtraining
– Hippotherapie
– Feldenkrais u.a.
Unübliche Verfahren
– Kraniosakrale Therapie
– Akupunktur
– Rolfing
– Reflexzonen und Bindegewebsmassagen u.a.
Abzulehnende Verfahren
– Doman und Delacato
– »Delphintherapie«
– Sauerstoff-Behandlungen
– Magnetfeldtherapie u.a.

nur die Anwendung sog. etablierter Methoden gewünscht, sondern zusätzlich Hippotherapie, Kraniosakrale Therapie, Feldenkrais wenn nicht sogar unkonventionelle Verfahren (Tab. 1).

Vor allem bei Kindern, die unter etablierten Behandlungsverfahren nur geringe Fortschritte zeigen, fällt es schwer, sich den Wünschen der Eltern ohne weiteres zu entziehen; schließlich werden im Einzelfall immer wieder überraschende Effekte beobachtet bzw. spektakulär in den Medien dargestellt. Es stellt sich daher nicht selten die Frage, inwieweit jenseits einer evidenzbasierten Medizin die Behandlung zu gestalten ist und inwieweit im Einzelfall sogar ein Recht auch auf eine ungewöhnliche Behandlung besteht, insbesondere dann wenn alles dafür spricht, dass positive Effekte erreicht worden sind. Vor Beantwortung dieser Fragen wird zunächst kritisch auf einige Probleme bei wissenschaftlichen Studien zur Evaluation einer Behandlung eingegangen werden.

Evidenzbasierte Medizin

Aus ethischen Gründen wurde die Forderung erhoben, dass zur Behandlung von Patienten nur Verfahren eingesetzt werden sollten, deren Wirksamkeit wissenschaftlich abgesichert worden ist (Sackett et al. 1997). Inzwischen sind größere Arbeitsgruppen und Institutionen entstanden, die dieser Forderung sehr systematisch nachgehen. Dabei zeigte sich, dass bei der Behandlung von vielen Krankheiten die bisherigen Konzepte verworfen oder zumindest modifiziert werden mussten. Es wird nun die Orientierung an Leitlinien gefordert, wo früher die persönliche Erfahrung und kasuistische Mitteilungen unser therapeutisches Handeln bestimmten. Leider ist durch die gesundheitspolitisch-ökonomischen Zwänge ein weiterer, viel schwerwiegender Grund hinzu gekommen weitgehend nach festgelegten Kriterien vorzugehen. Auch bei der Erstellung von Leitlinien wird immer rigider gefordert, wissenschaftlich abgesicherte Studien zu berücksichtigen, weniger aus ethischen, denn aus finanziellen Gründen (Ärztl. Zentralstelle Qualitätssicherung 1999).

Die wissenschaftlichen Kriterien dieser Studien wurden von Biostatistikern entwickelt, die sich vor allem mit der Evaluation einer pharmakologischen Therapie beschäftigt haben. Sackett (1981) war einer der ersten Autoren, welche die wichtigsten Voraussetzungen für Therapieevaluationsstudien beschrieb (Tab. 2). Den höchsten Rang in der Evidenzhierarchie nehmen randomisierte und kontrollierte Studien ein. Eine Forderung, die bei personenbezogenen Interventionen extrem aufwendig ist. Selbst bei Behandlungsverfahren, die abhängig sind von der direkten Interaktion von Therapeut und Patient, wird z.T. gefordert, dass nur doppel-blind oder placebo-kontrollierte Studien der Goldstandard seien. Bei der Behandlung von Kindern mit zerebralen Bewegungsstörungen ist dies aber nur bei technischen Eingriffen denkbar (z.B. Botulinumtoxin oder Extrakorporale Stoßwellen).

Placebo-Effekte

Die Erfassung der Effekte der Behandlung mit Scheinmedikamenten im Vergleich zu Verum-Medikamenten gelten bei der Erprobung von Pharmaka als eines der wichtigsten Kriterien zur Beurteilung der tatsächlichen Wirksamkeit. Diese allgemein akzeptierte Auffassung beruht auf der Annahme, dass etwa

Tab. 2: Statistische Voraussetzungen für Interventionsstudien (nach Sackett 1981)

– Randomisierung der Patienten in den Vergleichsgruppen (gematchte Patientengruppen)
– Repräsentative Auswahl der Patienten
– Detaillierte Beschreibung des Interventionsprogramms
– Keine zusätzlichen Behandlungsangebote
– Gesicherte Mitarbeit von Patient und Bezugspersonen
– Evaluation von evtl. zusätzlichen Effekten
– Sorgfältige Interpretation der Ergebnisse
– Prüfung der prognostischen Signifikanz

20–30% der Wirksamkeit einer medikamentösen Behandlung als sog. Placebo-Effekt gedeutet werden muss.

Nach Hrobjartsson und Götzsche (2001) muss diese Ansicht allerdings revidiert werden. Sie fanden bei der Auswertung von 114 Studien, in denen nicht nur eine Placebo-Gruppe sondern auch eine Gruppe ohne Medikamente verglichen worden sind, dass nur bei wenigen Therapieverfahren ein Placebo-Effekt nachzuweisen war! Daraus wird von den Autoren gefolgert, in Zukunft die Placebo-Kontrolle zu verlassen und stattdessen nur die tatsächlichen Effekte im Vergleich zu nichtbehandelten Patienten zu prüfen.

Diese Veröffentlichung stößt in das Zentrum der Diskussion vor, wie man die Evidenz eines Behandlungserfolges bei einem Behandlungsverfahren beweisen soll und kann. Wenn sich diese Fragen bei der pharmakologischen Behandlung nicht eindeutig beantworten lassen, so ist die Unsicherheit noch größer bei der Physiotherapie, Ergotherapie, Logopädie oder Psychotherapie.

Bei den meisten analysierten Evaluationsstudien wurden andere, sog. kontextuelle Effekte, nicht erfasst. Sie beziehen sich darauf, dass mit der Verordnung eines Medikamentes auch Untersuchungen, Beratungsgespräche und Zuwendung zum Patienten verbunden sind (Koch 2001). In der Schmerzforschung ist dieses Phänomen gut bekannt. Alleine durch die Beteiligung an einer Studie treten eindeutige Effekte auf, die z.T. stärker sind als die der verabreichten Medikamente. Blasi et al. (2001) analysierten Studien in denen diese Effekte überprüft wurden. Es zeigte sich, dass bei Ärzten, die ein emotionales Einfühlungsvermögen besaßen und sich ausreichend Zeit zur Patienteninformation nahmen, die Erfolge signifikant größer waren, als bei Ärzten, die eher verschlossen und sachlich agierten.

Meta-Analysen

Meta-Analysen gelten als ein wichtiges Forschungsinstrument zur Bewertung von unterschiedlichen Studien. Dabei besteht auch die Chance aus der Zusammenschau der vorliegenden Daten eigenständige oder neue Erkenntnisse zu gewinnen. Die entscheidenden Kriterien für die Qualität der Meta-Analysen selbst ist die Beurteilung der Vorgehensweise bei der Auswahl der zur Bewertung herangezogenen Studien und der selbstkritische Umgang mit den Ergebnissen. Arbeitsgruppen und Einrichtungen, die sich dieser Aufgabe stellen sind z.B. die COCHRANE Arbeitsgruppen (Cochrane Collaboration) und die QUORUM Gruppe (Quality of Reporting of Meta-analyses) (Cochrane 1972).

Auch Meta-Analysen finden aber nicht die »Wahrheit« sondern geben einen Überblick über den aktuellen Stand des Wissens (Siehe Beiträge von Bode und Schlack in diesem Band). Sie dienen als Hilfe für die Entscheidung über den Einsatz von Medikamenten oder Behandlungsverfahren. Dadurch soll die Chance für den Patienten vergrößert werden die bestmögliche Behandlung zu erhalten (Antes et al. 1999, The Lancet 1997). Die wissenschaftliche Beschäftigung mit der Qualität von Evaluationsstudien hat dazu geführt, dass renommierte Zeitschriften nur noch Arbeiten veröffentlichen, die bestimmten Ansprüchen genügen, wie sie z.B. in einer standardisierten Checkliste (Consort Statement) aufgeführt werden.

Interessant ist in diesem Zusammenhang das Ergebnis einer Meta-Analyse über den Einfluss der sog. grauen Literatur auf Meta-Analysen, d.h. von Studien, die nicht in international zugänglichen Journale publiziert worden sind. Mc Auley et al. (2000) wertete 135 zufällig ausgewählte Meta-Analysen aus, von den 33 auch Studienergebnisse aus der grauen Literatur erfasst hatten. Dabei zeigte sich, dass durch das Weglassen der grauen Literatur eine Überschätzung eines Interventionserfolges um durchschnittlich 12% verursacht worden wäre.

Anmerkungen zu einzelnen Evaluationsstudien

Selbst bei sehr gut geplanten Evaluationsstudien (»Level I–II Studien«) ergeben sich methodische Probleme, die Anlass geben, die Ergebnisse sehr vorsichtig zu interpretieren. Am Beispiel von zwei vorbildlichen Studien zur Behandlung von Kindern mit zerebralen Bewegungsstörungen lässt sich dies gut demonstrieren. Frau Bower (2001) führte eine randomisierte und kontrollierte Studie bei 56 Kindern mit ICP durch, die sehr überlegt angelegt worden war, da sie auf einer immensen Vorerfahrung beruhte. Es zeigte sich, dass die Effekte einer Intensivierung der Physiotherapie über einen Zeitraum von 6 Monaten keine Vorteile gegenüber der routinemäßigen Behandlung erbrachten.

Dennoch ist damit nicht ausgesagt, dass eine intensivere Behandlung generell nicht effektiv oder effizient sein kann. Die folgenden Einwände sind zu diskutieren:

- Die Studie wurde von 56 Therapeuten durchgeführt, die sicher nicht immer einheitlich die jeweils adäquaten Behandlungsschritte gewählt haben dürften; letztlich lässt sich dies bei der großen Zahl nicht ausschließen.
- Die Routine-Therapie kann bei den ausgewählten Patienten bereits zum bestmöglichen Ergebnis, gemessen an Alter und Entwicklungsstand der Kinder, geführt haben.
- Eine bloße Intensivierung der Behandlung durch dieselben Therapeuten, ohne wesentliche Änderung der Methode lässt nicht erwarten, dass entscheidende Fortschritte erzielt werden können, insbesondere, wenn es sich um sehr motivierte Therapeuten handelt, die sich aus eigenem Interesse zur Teilnahme an der Studie bereit erklärt haben.
- Ein Intensivierungsprogramm von 6 Monaten Dauer führt möglicherweise am Anfang zu dem oben genannten Effekt; die meisten Therapeuten und Kinder waren am Ende der Intensivperiode aber nicht mehr bereit in gleicher Intensität weiter zu verfahren.

Die Studie von Palmer et al. (1988) über die Behandlung von Kindern mit spastischen Diparesen genügt sehr hohen Ansprüchen der evidenzbasierten Medizin. 48 Kinder im Alter von 12–18 Monaten mit spastischer Diparese wurden erfasst und 12 Monate behandelt. Dabei erhielt eine Gruppe (A) durchgehende

Physiotherapie und eine Gruppe (B) zunächst 6 Monate ein multimodales Förderprogramm und wurde danach physiotherapeutisch behandelt. Es zeigte sich, dass die motorische Entwicklung in der rein physiotherapeutisch behandelten Gruppe signifikant langsamer verlief. Es bestand ein nicht zu unterschätzender Unterschied zwischen den Gruppen, nämlich die Kinder, die zunächst nach »ergotherapeutischen« Gesichtspunkten behandelt worden waren, hatten im Durchschnitt einen höheren mentalen EQ (66,1 vs. 62,0). Auch die Vorgaben für die physiotherapeutische Behandlung beeinflussten mit hoher Wahrscheinlichkeit das Ergebnis. Die Kinder wurden nur solange mehrfach pro Woche physiotherapeutisch behandelt bis sie die Fähigkeit erreicht hatten, sich aufzusetzen. In Sorge um negative Folgen einer zu frühen Vertikalisierung wurden sie entsprechend dem damaligen Bobath-Konzept nicht angehalten sich aufzustellen oder mit Unterstützung zu laufen. Die Unterschiede zwischen den beiden Gruppen waren aber gerade im Bereich der motorischen Entwicklung signifikant (freies Gehen, Gehen an einer Hand gehalten und rückwärts Gehen).

Da aus ethischen Gründen keine unbehandelte Gruppe mituntersucht wurde, kann über die Wirkung der Physiotherapie (nach dem Bobath Konzept) keine generelle Aussage getroffen werden. Es wurde nur der Unterschied zwischen zwei Vorgehensweisen geprüft, nicht inwieweit der »natürliche Verlauf« durch die Behandlungsprogramme verbessert wurde!

Es ist daher nicht richtig, die Ergebnisse der »Palmer-Studie« als Beweis für die Nichtwirksamkeit der Physiotherapie (nach dem Bobath-Konzept) zu zitieren. Man darf aber annehmen, dass beide Vorgehensweisen wirksam waren und dass sich das damalige Bobath-Konzept im Hinblick auf die Fortschritte bei der motorischen Entwicklung eher hinderlich auswirkte; die Qualität des Bewegungsablaufes wurde aber nicht geprüft.

Kritische Anmerkungen zu den Evaluationskriterien

Bei Kindern mit zerebralen Bewegungsstörungen sind die motorischen Fähigkeiten und die motorische Entwicklung das entscheidende Beurteilungskriterium für die Wirksamkeit der Behandlung. Hierfür stehen auch verlässliche Messverfahren zur Verfügung, insbesondere die Gross Motor Function Measure (GMFM). Nur bei wenigen Studien wurden die Effekte einer regelmäßigen Behandlung auf den Ebenen der »disability« (Behinderung) und der Teilhabe an der Gesellschaft ausreichend erfasst oder gar als wesentliches Therapieziel angesehen. Butler und Darrah (2001) fanden bei einer Meta-Analyse der Evaluationsstudien zur Behandlung nach dem Bobath-Konzept außerdem, dass in diesen Studien nur geringe positive Effekte in den Bereichen »disability« oder »participation« nachgewiesen worden sind. Auch bei der umfassenden Studie von Palmer et al. (1988, 1990) ließen sich keine signifikanten Unterschiede im Temperament des Kindes, der Mutter-Kind-Interaktion oder der häuslichen Versorgungssituation (Emotion, Responsivität, Erziehung, Spielangebote u.a.) finden, trotz der Unterschiede in der psychomotorischen Entwicklung zwischen der Gruppe A und B. Allerdings lässt sich dies aus den angegebenen Kriterien nur bedingt schließen, wie von den Autoren der Studie selbst eingeräumt wird.

Behandlung unter dem Aspekt des ICIDH

Wenn man unter dem Begriff »Behandlung« alle Aktivitäten von Angehörigen, Therapeuten und Ärzten gegenüber den Teilbereichen »Therapie« oder »Förderung« zusammenfasst, werden die kritischen Einwände gegenüber den bisherigen Evaluations-Studien verständlicher. Noch offensichtlicher wird die Problematik, wenn man das Leben der Kinder mit zerebralen Bewegungsstörungen unter dem Blickwinkel der Teilhabe an der Gesellschaft betrachtet. Hierfür werden unterschiedliche Begriffe verwendet: soziale Einschränkungen, Partizipation, sozialer Kontext usw. Die amerikanische Akademie für zerebrale Bewegungsstörung und Entwicklungsmedizin (AACPM) hat sich hierzu mehrfach geäußert. Butler et al. (1999) haben diesen Bereichen Behandlungsziele zugeordnet, die in exzellenter Weise beschreiben, worum es bei der Behandlung der chronisch kranken und behinderten Kinder geht:

1) Auf der Ebene pathophysiologischer und pathologisch-anatomischer Veränderungen sind selbst bei frühestmöglichem Behandlungsbeginn nur sehr begrenzte Effekte denkbar. Sie betreffen vor allem die grundsätzliche Fähigkeit des ZNS sich zu reorganisieren um die bestehenden Schädigungen zu kompensieren (»pathophysiology«).
2) Einschränkung der Gleichgewichts- und Haltungskontrolle und damit bei der Aufrichtung, der Kontrolle von zielgerichteten Bewegungsabläufen einschließlich überschießender Anspannung des Muskeltonus oder fehlendem Tonusaufbau, verminderte Belastbarkeit und Ausdauer sowie Störungen der Wahrnehmung, allerdings häufig nicht nur im Bereich der Perzeptuomotorik (»impairment«).
3) Funktionseinschränkungen im Bereich der Motorik, die sich an den unkoordinierten Bewegungsabläufen, der eingeschränkten Selbstständigkeit im Alltag und den verminderten kognitiven Leistungsfähigkeit zeigen (»functional limitation«).
4) Dies führt zu Lernstörungen, beschränkten sportlichen Betätigungen, Behinderung der gesamten familiären Aktionen, Abhängigkeit von fremder Hilfe oder Pflege, eingeschränkter Möglichkeit von Partnerschaften und sexueller Beziehungen usw. (»disability«)
5) Eingeschränkte Möglichkeiten am öffentlichen Leben teilzuhaben, nicht nur infolge der bestehenden Behinderung (wie z.B. durch die Rollstuhlabhängigkeit) sondern auch infolge ungeeigneter Wohngelegenheiten oder Ausschluss von Versicherung bestimmter Risiken bis hin zur Würdigung der eigenständigen Persönlichkeit und eigenen Anstrengungen und Leistungen zur Kompensation der Krankheitsfolgen (»societal limitation«).

Grundlagen der Behandlung von Kindern mit zerebralen Bewegungsstörungen

Die Behandlung von Kindern und Jugendlichen mit zerebralen Bewegungsstörungen kann sich daher nicht nur auf die eigentlich physiotherapeutisch relevanten Ziele beschränken. Grundlage einer erfolgversprechenden Behandlung sind daher (Karch 2002):

- eigenständige Tätigkeiten in alltagsrelevanten Aufgabenbereichen fördern,
- aktive motorische Lernprozesse planen und unterstützen,
- spezielle Fertigkeiten systematisch trainieren,
- Möglichkeiten der »Neuroplastizität« nutzen, sekundäre Veränderungen von Struktur und Funktionen des Muskel-Skelett-Systems vermeiden,
- psychosoziale Eingliederung fördern,
- sekundäre Verhaltensstörungen vermeiden.

Eigene Studie

Aus den genannten Überlegungen entschlossen wir uns, eine Studie zur Evaluation einer interdisziplinären Behandlung von Kleinkindern mit zerebralen Bewegungsstörungen auf der Eltern-Kind Station der Klinik für Kinderneurologie und Sozialpädiatrie in Maulbronn durchzuführen (Storck et al. 2000). Die Behandlungserfolge bei 22 Kindern mit zerebralen Bewegungsstörungen infolge frühkindlicher Hirnschädigung im Alter zwischen 2 bis 6 Jahren (im Mittel 3;4 Jahre) wurden evaluiert. Bei den meisten Kindern bestanden zusätzliche Verhaltensstörungen wie z.B. Schlafstörungen, Essstörungen, die nicht alleine durch die Bewegungsstörung verursacht waren. Sie wurden stationär mit einem Elternteil aufgenommen und drei Wochen lang intensiv behandelt. Die Angehörigen wurden in die Behandlung einbezogen, über Entwicklungsstand und Diagnose aufgeklärt und verhaltens- und familientherapeutisch psychologisch betreut. Zusammen mit ihnen wurden auch die Therapieziele erarbeitet. Zur Evaluation wurden die Kinder jeweils vor und nach der Baseline phase von 3 Monaten, der stationären Behandlungsphase von 3 Wochen und der Nachphase von 3 Monaten entwicklungsneurologisch untersucht und die motorischen Funktionen nach der GMFM erfasst. Über Fragebögen wurden zusätzlich erhoben: der elterliche Stress (Abidin), die Lebensqualität des Kindes (Goldbeck und Storck) und die soziale Orientierung der Eltern (Soebek).

Dabei fanden sich signifikante Effekte nicht nur Im Bezug auf die Lebensqualität sondern auf die motorischen Fähigkeiten, gemessen mit dem GMFM bei einem Vergleich der Entwicklung in der Baselinephase gegenüber der Nachphase, aber nicht gegenüber der dreiwöchigen Intensivtherapie. Die signifikanten Verbesserungen der motorischen Funktionen fanden sich in den Bereichen der GMFM, die vorher als Zielbereiche definiert worden waren.

Aufgaben einer neuropädiatrisch-sozialpädiatrischen Behandlung

Die Studie unterstützt den Anspruch der Kinder mit zerebralen Bewegungsstörungen auf eine umfassende Behandlung unter Einschluss aller Ebenen des ICIHD. Von einer englischen Arbeitsgruppe (»HemiHelp«) wurden die folgenden Empfehlungen für das Mindestmass an Versorgung von CP Patienten formuliert (Recommendations 1999):

- Detaillierte und einfühlsame Aufklärung der Angehörigen über die Diagnose (auch Verdachtsdiagnose) und Prognose der Erkrankung und ggfls. auch des Kindes, in Abhängigkeit vom Alter und der geistigen Entwicklung. Hilfe bei der Bewältigung der dabei auftretenden psychischen Belastungen in der Familie;
- Sozialpädiatrische Betreuung von Kind und Familie im Bezug auf seine soziale Eingliederung ebenso wie Beratung bei finanziellen Angelegenheiten einschließlich Hilfen im Umgang mit den entsprechenden Ämtern und Regularien;
- Umfassende medizinische Behandlung einschließlich Ernährung, Gedeihen, Wachstum, psychosomatischer Symptomatik, sekundärer Verhaltensstörungen. Individuell abgestimmte Förderung und Behandlung der somatischen, sensorischen, sprachlichen und kognitiven Entwicklung. Adäquate Behandlung der speziellen Probleme bei zerebralen Bewegungsstörungen bis hin zu operativen Maßnahmen;
- Therapeutische Versorgung durch speziell erfahrene Physiotherapeuten (lebenslang), Ergotherapeuten und Sprachtherapeuten (einschließlich nonverbaler Kommunikation) in Kooperation mit der Familie und den pädagogischen Förderprogrammen sowie unter Berücksichtigung der medizinischen Notwendigkeiten.

Um den berechtigten Ansprüchen der Patienten und ihrer Familie einerseits und den ökonomischen Bedingungen andererseits gerecht zu werden, erfordert die Behandlung von zerebralen Bewegungsstörungen eine hohe medizinisch-ärztliche Kompetenz bei der Diagnosestellung, der Abklärung der Ursache, der Überprüfung des psychomotorischen Entwicklungsstandes, der Erfassung der Interaktion mit den nächsten Angehörigen und der psychosozialen Bedingungen, in der das Kind aufwächst, der Indikationsstellung und Beendigung von Behandlungsmaßnahmen. Darüberhinaus ist eine enge Zusammenarbeit mit unterschiedlichen Behörden und öffentlichen Einrichtungen, dem Kindergarten, der Schule oder den Berufsausbildungsstätten erforderlich.

Die Stellungnahmen der Neuropädiatrischen Gesellschaft zu verschiedenen Behandlungsverfahren, die in der Regel mit viel zu hohen Erfolgsversprechungen eingeführt und propagiert werden, sind u.a. verfasst worden, um zumindest grundlegende Kenntnisse über den theoretischen Hintergrund, die praktische Durchführung und die wissenschaftliche Absicherung zu beschreiben und Studien über die Wirksamkeit der unterschiedlichen Behandlungsverfahren wissenschaftlich zu bewerten. Bei der Empfehlung oder Verordnung von Förder- und Therapiemaßnahmen sind aber auch ökonomische Aspekte zu berücksichtigen, nicht nur im Hinblick auf die finanziellen Ressourcen, sondern auch auf die zeitliche Belastung von Kind und Familie. In welchem Verhältnis Aufwand und Erfolg stehen, muss im Einzelfall ebenso geprüft werden, wie die Möglichkeit einer zu hohen psychische Belastung durch die Interventionen.

Nur durch großes fachliches Wissen und ein großes Einfühlungsvermögen kann der individuell günstigste Weg gefunden werden. Eine vertrauensvolle Zusammenarbeit wird nicht dadurch gefördert, dass ohne Nachzudenken allen Wünschen entsprochen wird, sondern durch ein deutlich erkennbares Engagement für Kind und Familie.

Anerkennung neuer Therapieverfahren

Vielfach wird argumentiert, dass neue oder nicht anerkannte Therapieverfahren ohne weiteres eingesetzt werden könnten und ihre Kosten von der Versichertengemeinschaft getragen werden müssten, da viele auch etablierte Verfahren nicht ausreichend wissenschaftlich evaluiert worden seien. Diesen Forderungen ist vor allem unter ethischen Aspekten entgegenzuhalten, dass Effekte neuer Konzepte zunächst mit denen der alten verglichen werden müssen, da der jahrzehntelange Umgang mit etablierten Therapie- und Förderverfahren zu einem hohen Erfahrungswert nicht nur hinsichtlich der Indikation und der Erfolgsaussichten sondern auch im Hinblick auf unerwünschte Wirkungen führt. Diese Überlegungen berücksichtigen auch die Richtlinien des Bundesausschusses Ärztekrankenkassen (1998, Tab. 3) für die Neuzulassung von therapeutischen Maßnahmen. Sie fordern nicht nur den Nachweis der Wirksamkeit, sondern auch eine Begründung für die Notwendigkeit, neue Verfahren einzuführen. Hierzu gehört u.a. der Nachweis, dass tatsächlich bessere Erfolge erzielt werden können, als mit den etablierten Verfahren. Auch das Gebot der Wirtschaftlichkeit ist mit Recht zu beachten. Selbst, wenn bessere Erfolge nachgewiesen worden sind, müssen sie im Verhältnis zum Aufwand gewertet werden.

Tab. 3: Richtlinien für die Neueinführung von Behandlungsverfahren (Bundesausschuss Ärzte und Krankenkassen 1998)

Nutzen:
Studien zum Wirkungsnachweis,
Abwägung von Nutzen und Risiken,
Bewertung erwünschter und unerwünschter Folgen,
Vergleiche zu erprobten Behandlungsverfahren
Notwendigkeit:
Häufigkeit und Relevanz der zu behandelnden Erkrankung
Spontanverlauf der Erkrankung
Wirtschaftlichkeit (Kosten-Nutzen-Analyse):
für einzelne Patienten,
für die Gesamtheit der Versicherten und
im Vergleich zu den bisherigen Therapien.

Literatur

1. Antes G, Bassler D, Glandi D (1999) Systematische Übersichtsarbeiten. Ihre Rolle in der Evidenz-basierten Gesundheitsversorgung. Dt Ärztebl 96:A-616–622 (Heft 10)
2. Ärztliche Zentralstelle Qualitätssicherung (1999). Das Leitlinien-Clearingverfahren. Dt Ärztebl 96: B–1706–1707 (Heft 33)
3. Blasi Z D, Harkness E, Ernst E, Georgiou A, Kleijnen (2001) Influence of context effects on health outcomes: a systematic review. Lancet 357:757– 762
4. Bower E, Mc Lellan Dl, Arney J, Campbell MJ (1996) A randomised controlled trial of different intensities of physiotherapy and different goal-setting procedures in 44 Children with cerebral palsy. Dev Med Child Neurol 38:226–237
5. Bower E, Michell D, Burnett M, Campbell MJ, Mc Lellan DL (2001) Randomized controlled trial of physiotherapy in 56 children with cerebral palsy followed for 18 months. Dev Med Child Neurol 43:4–15
6. Bundesausschuss Ärzte und Krankenkassen (1998) Richtlinien des Bundesausschusses der Ärzte und Krankenkassen über die Einführung neuer Untersuchungs- und Behandlungsmethoden und die Überprüfung erbrachter vertragsärztlicher Leistungen. Dt Ärztebl C-46-C-48 (Heft ½)
7. Butler C, Chambers H, Goldstein M, Harris S, Leach J, Campbell S, Adams R, Darrah J (1999) Evaluating research in developmental disabilities: a conceptual framework for reviewing treatment outcomes. Dev Med Child Neurol 41:55–59
8. Butler C, Darrah J (2001) Effects of neurodevelopmental treatment (NDT) for cerebral palsy: AACPM evidence report. Dev Med Child Neurol 43:778–790
9. Cochrane AL (1972) Effectiveness and Effiency. Random Reflections on Health Services. Nuffield Provincial Hospitals Trust. London
10. Hrobartsson A, Götzsche P (2001) Is the placebo powerless? An analysis of clinical trials comparing placebo with no treatment. New Engl J Med 344:1594– 1602
11. Jung K, Gawlik C, Gibis B, Pötsch R, Rheinberger P, Schmacke N, Schneider G (2000) Bundesausschuss der Ärzte und Krankenkassen. Ansprüche der Versicherten präzisieren. Dt Ärztebl 97:A-365–370 (Heft 7)
12. Karch D (2002) Aktuelle Konzepte zur motorischen Entwicklung und motorischen Kontrolle. In: Aksu F (Hrsg) Aktuelle Neuropädiatrie 2001. S. 713–721. Novartis Pharma Verlag Nürnberg
13. Koch K(2001) Ein Mythos wird entzaubert. Dt Ärztebl 98: B-1866–1867 (Heft34–35)
14. McAuley L, B Pham, P Tugwell, D Moher (2000) Does the inclusion of grey literature influence estimates of intervention effectivness reported in meta-analysis? Lancet 356: 1228–1231.
15. Palmer FB, Shapiro B, Wachtel RC, Allen MC, Hiller JE,Harryman SE, Mosher BS, Meinert CL, Capute AJ (1988) The effects of physical therapy on cereral palsy. A controlled trial in infants with spastic diplegia. N Engl J Med 318:803–808
16. Palmer FB, Shapiro BK, Allen MC, Mosher BS, Bilker SA, Harryman SE, Meinert CL, Capute AJ (1990) Infant stimulation curriculum for infants with cerebral palsy: effects on infant temperament, parent-infant interaction, and home environment. Pediatrics 58:411–415
17. Recommendations for minimum standards of healthcare in children with cerebral palsy. HemiHelp, London 1999
18. Sackett DL, Richardson WS, Rosenberg W, Haynes RB (1997) Evidence-Based Medicine. How to practice and teach EBM. Churchill Livingstone, NewYork, Edinourgh, London.
19. Sackett DL (1981) How to read clinical journals. V: to distinguish useful from useless or even harmful therapy. Can Med Assoc J 124:1156–1162
20. Storck M, Haug U, Karch D (2000) Effect of a three week interdisciplinary inpatient therapy on young children with cerebral palsy. Vortrag: Jahrestagung European Academy of Disabled Children, Tübingen
21. The Lancet Editorial (1997) Meta-analysis under scrutinity. Lancet 350:675

Anwendung von Botulinum Toxin A in der Pädiatrie: eine neue Behandlungsoption für den Masseterspasmus bei Kindern mit spastischen Bewegungsstörungen. Ein Fallbeispiel.

M. Linder, V. Mall, A. Schelle, J. Kirschner, F. Heinen, R. Korinthenberg

Zusammenfassung

Als Standardindikationen für die lokale Anwendung von Botulinum Toxin A (BTX/A) bei Kindern mit Cerebralparese gelten der dynamische Pes equinus und der Adduktorenspasmus. Eine vergleichsweise seltene Indikation stellen schmerzhafte Spastiken der Kaumuskulatur dar, die im Kindesalter zum Beispiel im Rahmen schwerer Tetraparesen auftreten können. Wir berichten von einem sieben Jahre alten männlichen Patienten mit einer spastischen Tetraparese, der an einem intermittierenden Masseterspasmus litt. Die reduzierte Kontrolle der Mundmotorik verursachte erhebliche funktionelle Beeinträchtigungen im Alltag (u.a. rezidivierende Verletzungen der Mundschleimhaut, Ernährungsschwierigkeiten). Die intramuskuläre Injektion von BTX/A in die Massetermuskulatur führte zu einer deutlichen Reduktion der Spastik und damit zu einer verbesserten Funktion der Mundmotorik im Alltag. Nebenwirkungen der Injektion wurden nicht beobachtet. Die lokale Behandlung des Masseterspasmus mit BTX/A stellt im Kindesalter ein neues Therapiekonzept dar. Bei Erwachsenen sind lokale Effektivität, funktionelle Gewinne und Sicherheit von BTX/A für die Behandlung der Spastik der Kaumuskulatur durch mehrere Einzelfallberichte und offene Studien aus der Neurologie und der Mund-, Kiefer- und Gesichtschirurgie belegt.

Einleitung

Bei der lokalen intramuskulären Injektion von Botulinum Toxin A (BTX/A) handelt es sich um ein effektives und nebenwirkungsarmes Therapieverfahren zur selektiven temporären Schwächung spastisch hyperaktiver Muskulatur. Zu den klassischen Indikationen in der Pädiatrie zählen mittlerweile der dynamische Pes equinus und der Adduktorenspasmus (Corry et al., 1998; Heinen et al., 1999; Koman et al., 2000; Sutherland et al., 1999; Ubhi et al., 2000).

Im Rahmen schwerer spastischer Bewegungsstörungen im Kindesalter kann gelegentlich das Auftreten einer schmerzhaften, intermittierenden Verkrampfung der Kaumuskulatur beobachtet werden. Die reduzierte Kontrolle der Mundmotorik führt dabei zu erheblichen funktionellen Beeinträchtigungen im Alltag.

Bei Erwachsenen ist die Wirksamkeit von BTX/A bei der Behandlung von oromandibulären Dyskinesien, myogenen mandibulären Dysfunktionsschmerzsyndromen und habituellen Kiefergelenksluxationen durch mehrere Einzelfallberichte und offene, prospektive Studien gut belegt (Blitzer et al., 1989 und 2001; Daelen et al., 1997; Freund et al., 2000; Moore et al., 1997; Roser et al., 1998; Tan et al., 1999). Im Kindesalter stellt der Masseterspasmus eine neue Indikation für die lokale Anwendung von BTX/A dar.

Fallbeispiel und Methode

Wir berichten von einem sieben Jahre alten, schwer mehrfach behinderten, männlichen Patienten mit Zustand nach neonataler Enzephalitis ungeklärter Ätiologie. Neben einer mentalen Retardierung, einer ausgeprägten spastischen Tetraparese (Gross Motor Function Classification Scale, GMFCS: IV) und einer therapieschwierigen Epilepsie (V.a. Lennox-Gastaut-Syndrom), trat seit dem 4. Lebensjahr intermittierend eine schmerzhafte Spastik der Kaumuskulatur auf. Provokationsfaktoren waren unspezifische orale Reize sowie positive oder negative emotionale Erregung. Die einschießende Spastik der Kaumuskulatur führte im Verlauf zu rezidivierenden Bissverletzungen an Lippen, Zunge und Mundschleimhaut. Das Füttern der Mahlzeiten mit einem Löffel war nicht mehr möglich, was anamnestisch als Belastung der Mutter-Kind-Interaktion empfunden wurde. Durch den schwierigen bis unmöglichen Gebrauch einer Zahnbürste konnte eine adäquate Mundhygiene nicht mehr durchgeführt werden. Zusätzlich war die logopädische Therapie durch die fehlende Toleranz einer Zahnspange zur Stimulation der Mundmotorik beeinträchtigt.

In der klinischen Untersuchung konnte die einschießende Spastik der Kaumuskulatur durch orale Stimulation mit einem Holzspatel zuverlässig provoziert werden, es zeigte sich eine deutliche spastische Hyperaktivität der Massetermuskulatur beidseits ohne Beteiligung der Mm. temporales.

Die intramuskuläre Injektion von BTX/A erfolgte nach Palpation des Muskelbauchs transcutan unter sonographischer und elektromyographischer Kontrolle in die Mm. masseteres beidseits. Eine lokale Anästhesie mit Eisspray war bei diesem Patienten ausreichend. Die verwendete Dosierung lag bei 75 Units Dysport® pro M. masseter.

Ergebnis

Nach der intramuskulären Injektion von BTX/A kam es innerhalb von drei Tagen zu einer deutlichen Reduktion der spastischen Hyperaktivität der Massetermuskulatur. Bei einem Kontrolltermin nach vier Wochen konnte durch die orale Stimulation mit einem Holzspatel keine Spastik der Kaumuskulatur provoziert werden. Im Verlauf heilten die Bissverletzungen an der Mundschleimhaut vollständig ab. Das Essen mit einem Löffel und die tägliche Zahnpflege waren wieder problemlos möglich. Dieses wurde von der Mutter als besonders positiv hinsichtlich der Lebensqualität ihres Sohnes bewertet. Es zeigte sich eine deutlich verbesserte Toleranz der Zahnspange.

Nebenwirkungen wie z.B. Dysphagie oder Dysarthrie traten nicht auf. Die klinische Wirkung hielt sechs Monate an. Danach wurde eine graduelle Zunahme der muskulären Hyperaktivität beobachtet, so dass eine komplikationslose Reinjektion von BTX/A in die Massetermuskulatur beidseitig durchgeführt wurde.

Schlussfolgerung

Die lokale BTX/A-Behandlung des Masseterspasmus stellt im Kindesalter ein neues Therapiekonzept dar. Bislang liegen zu dieser Indikation nur Fallberichte und offene Studien aus der Erwachsenenmedizin vor. Unsere Kasuistik demonstriert lokale Wirksamkeit, funktionelle Gewinne und Sicherheit dieser Therapie auch im Kindesalter. Zusätzlich zeigt sich durch die verbesserte Kontrolle der Mundmotorik ein positiver Effekt auf die Lebensqualität des betroffenen Patienten.

Literatur

1. Blitzer A, Sulica L (2001). Botulinum toxin: basic science and clinical uses in otolaryngology. Laryngoscope 111(2):218–226
2. Blitzer A, Brin MF, Greene PE, Fahn S (1989). Botulinum toxin injection for the treatment of oromandibular dystonia. Ann Otol Rhinol Laryngol 98:93–97
3. Corry IS, Cosgrove AP, Duffy CM, McNeill S, Taylor TC and Graham HK (1998). Botulinum Toxin A compared with stretching casts in the treatment of spastic equinus: a randomized prospective trial. J Pediatr Orthop 18: 304–311
4. Daelen B, Thorwirth V, Koch A (1997). Treatment of recurrent disolocation of the temporomandibular joint with type A botulinum toxin. Int J Oral Maxillofac Surg 26(6): 458–60
5. Freund B, Schwartz M, Symington JM (2000). Botulinum toxin: new treatment for temporomandibular disorders. Br J Oral Maxillofac Surg 38(5): 466–71
6. Heinen F, Linder M, Mall V, Kirschner J, Korinthenberg R (1999). Adductor spasticity in children with cerebral palsy and treatment with botulinum toxin type A: the parents' view of functional outcome. Eur J Neurol 6 (suppl):47–50
7. Koman LA, Mooney JF3rd, Smith BP, Walker F, Leon JM (2000). Botulinum toxin type A neuromuscular blockade in the treatment of lower extremity spasticity in cerebral palsy: a randomized, double-blind, placebo-controlled trial. BOTOX Study Group, J Pediatr Orthop 20(1): 108–15
8. Moore AP, Wood GD (1997). Medical treatment of recurrent temporomandibular joint dislocation using botulinum toxin A. Br Dent J 183(11–12):415–417
9. Roser M, Cornelius CP, Topka H (1998). Neuerungen in der MKG-Chirurgie: Lokale Injektionsbehandlung mit Botulinumtoxin A. Mund Kiefer GesichtsChir 2 (suppl 2):121–124
10. Sutherland DH, Kaufman KR, Wyatt MP, Chambers HG, Mubarak SJ (1999). Double-blind study of botulinum A toxin injections into the gastrocnemius muscle in patients with cerebral palsy. Gait Posture 10(1):1–9
11. Tan EK, Jankovic J (1999). Botulinum toxin A in patients with oromandibular dystonia: long-term follow-up. Neurology 53:2102–2107
12. Ubhi T, Bhakta BB, Ives HL, Allgar V, Roussounis SH (2000). Randomised double blind placebo controlled trial of the effect of botulinum toxin on walking in cerebral palsy. Arch Dis Child 83(6):481–7

Botulinumtoxin B (BTB) Therapie bei Kindern mit spastischen Bewegungsstörungen (CP) – Haben wir eine neue Therapieoption?

A. Schwerin, A. Francke, S. Berweck, A. Feldkamp, F. Heinen

Einleitung

Der Gebrauch von Botulinumtoxin A (BTA) ist etabliert bei der Therapie der infantilen Cerebralparese. In Übereinstimmung mit den Kriterien der evidence based medicine hat BTA einen lokalen und funktionellen Effekt bei spastischen Bewegungsstörungen im Kindesalter (1, 2). Die meisten therapeutischen Erfahrungen liegen mit zwei BTA Präparaten vor (Botox® und Dysport®). Für die Anwendung bei Kindern ist nur das Präparat Botox® mit der Beschränkung auf den Spitzfuß bei Kindern älter als zwei Jahre und für eine Dosis von 4 U/kg Körpergewicht zugelassen. So geschieht die weite Anwendung bei Multilevel-Behandlungen, M.-Psoas-Injektionen, Behandlungen der oberen Extremität etc. bei Kindern off-label. Das ist eine typische Situation im Bereich der Pädiatrie, wo bis zu 80% der medikamentösen Therapien off-label Anwendungen sind (3).

Kinder mit spastischen Bewegungsstörungen scheinen häufiger sekundäre non-response und Antikörper gegen BTA zu entwickeln (~20–30%, 4) verglichen mit erwachsenen Patienten, die an cervikaler Dystonie leiden (5%, 5). Dies kann durch die höheren Dosierungen pro kg Körpergewicht bei Kindern bedingt sein. Für Patienten mit Antikörpern gegen BTA ist der Therapieeffekt begrenzt und die Behandlung mit Botulinumtoxin B (BTB) stellt eine zweite Therapieoption dar. Kinder mit einer spastischen Tetraparese haben darüber hinaus häufig Schluckstörungen und vermehrten Speichelfluss, was eine zusätzliche soziale Stigmatisierung bedeutet.

BTB wird bereits bei Erwachsenen mit dystonen Bewegungsstörungen angewendet. Die Wirksamkeit wurde in placebo-kontrollierten, Doppel-Blind-Studien für de-novo Patienten wie für Patienten mit Antikörpern gegen BTA nachgewiesen (6). Verglichen mit BTA scheinen systemische anticholinergen Wirkungen besonders die Reduktion des Speichelflusses häufiger bei BTB aufzutreten (7).

Es stellen sich somit folgende erste Fragen, die Behandlung von Kindern mit BTB betreffend:

1. Was ist der lokale und funktionelle Effekt für de-novo Patienten?
2. Wie ist die anticholinerge Wirkung von BTB bei Kindern mit spastischer Cerebralparese und Hypersalivation?
3. Ist die Behandlung mit BTB wirksam bei Patienten mit sekundärer non-response aufgrund von Antikörpern gegen BTA?
4. Ist die Wirkungsdauer von BTB vergleichbar mit der von BTA?

Methode

18 Patienten (5 weibliche, 13 männliche, Durchschnittsalter: 7,4 Jahre) mit spastischer Bewegungsstörungen wurden mit BTB als individueller Heilversuch behandelt.

Die Patienten hatten folgende Bewegungsstörungen: 15 Patienten litten an einer spastischen Tetraparese, 2 an einer spastischen Hemiparese, 1 Patient an einer spastischen Diparese. Das Ausmaß der Behinderung erstreckte sich zwischen Level I und V in Anlehnung an die Gross Motor Function Classification System (8). 7 Patienten litten an einem ausgeprägten Speichelfluss.

10 Patienten waren de-novo Patienten. 8 Patienten hatten vorher eine Behandlung mit BTA. Zwei dieser Patienten hatten einen signifikanten Antikörper-Titer gegen BTA (in vitro nerve-muscle assay) (9). 5 Patienten zeigten ein abnehmendes oder ein unzureichendes Ansprechen auf die BTA Therapie. Bei einem Patienten wurde von BTA auf die Therapie mit BTB wegen schwerer Hypersalivation gewechselt.

BTB (Neurobloc®) wurde intramuskulär unter Analgosedierung (rektale Applikation von Midazolam und Pethidin) ultraschallgesteuert appliziert. Es wurde die Standardpräparation von Neurobloc® verwendet (1 ml = 5000 U). Da es keine offiziellen Empfehlungen für die Dosierungen bei Kindern gibt, adaptierten wir die veröffentlichten Dosisangaben für Erwachsene. Von den 18 Patienten erhielten 8 Patienten eine, 9 Patienten zwei und ein Patient drei Behandlungen mit BTB. Die Gesamtzahl der durchgeführten Behandlungen betrug 29.

Die Daten wurden durch telefonische Befragung der Eltern 4–6 Wochen nach der Injektion und durch eine klinische Re-evaluation nach vier Monaten erhoben. Die Evaluation schloss eine Abschätzung der funktionellen Wirkung nach der Goal Attainment Skala (GAS) und eine Befragung über die Nebenwirkungen ein (insbesondere: Mundtrockenheit, Dysphagie, Blasen-Darm-Störungen, systemische Nebenwirkungen). Die Goal Attainment Scale umfasst mehrere Stufen: 0 entspricht dem definierten und erreichten Therapieziel, -1 entspricht einem teilweise erreichten Therapieziel und -2 entspricht einem nicht erreichten Therapieziel bzw. dem Ausgangsbefund.

Ergebnisse

1. Lokale und funktionelle Wirkung (GAS)

Die Hälfte der Injektionen (18/29) waren zielbezogen erfolgreich (GAS 0). Weitere 7 Injektionen waren teilweise erfolgreich (GAS -1). 3 Patienten hatten keine Wirkung der Injektion (GAS -2).

2. Erwünschte anticholinerge Wirkungen

Speichelflussreduktion trat bei 6/7 Patienten ein. Ein Kind zeigte keine Reduktion des Speichelflusses nach der Injektion (217 U /kg Körpergewicht Neurobloc®).

3. Wirksamkeit der BTB Therapie bei BTA non-respondern

Die zwei Patienten mit nachgewiesenen Antikörpern gegen BTA sprachen auf eine Behandlung mit BTB an. Sie erreichten das therapeutische Ziel jedoch nicht vollständig (GAS -1). Fünf non-responder auf BTA zeigten eine Wirkung unter BTB (drei erreichten das Therapieziel, zwei zeigten eine teilweise Wirkung).

4. Unerwünschte Nebenwirkungen

Bei 6 von 29 Injektionen (20%) wurden unerwünschte Nebenwirkungen wie Mundtrockenheit (10%), Dysphagie (7%), Obstipation (10%), Diarrhoe (7%) und Übelkeit (1%) berichtet. Drei Patienten (10%) litten an generalisierter Muskeltonusreduktion. Alle Patienten mit unerwünschten Nebenwirkungen erhielten Gesamtdosen zwischen 12 000 und 20 000 U BTB. 3–4 Wochen nach der Injektion waren alle unerwünschten Nebenwirkungen wieder verschwunden. Alle Patienten setzten die Behandlung fort.

5. BTB (Neurobloc®) Dosierung

Kleinste Dosis pro Muskel war 250 U (M. brachioradialis), höchste Dosis pro Muskel war 8000 U (M. gastrocnemius). Die minimale Dosis pro kg Körpergewicht betrug 133 U/kg, die maximale 970 U/kg (mittlere Dosis 324 U/kg).

Diskussion

Diese individuellen Heilversuche geben Informationen über die therapeutische Wirksamkeit, die Dosisbreite und die Nebenwirkungen von BTB, jedoch limitiert die angewandte Methodik die Evidenz unserer Schlussfolgerungen. Da es nur wenige Erfahrungen über den Gebrauch von BTB bei Kindern mit spastischen Bewegungsstörungen gibt, erscheint es uns aber wichtig, die ersten, wenn auch vorläufigen, Ergebnisse zu diskutieren.

Die Wirkung von BTB für Kinder mit spastischen Bewegungsstörungen war suffizient bei de-novo Patienten und non-respondern auf BTA.

Im Vergleich mit Studien über Therapie mit BTB bei Erwachsenen ist bei den von uns behandelten Kindern die Rate an unerwünschten anticholinergen Nebenwirkungen geringer (14% Mundtrockenheit, 10% Obstipation, 7% Dyphagie). Dressler et al. fanden z.B. 86% Mundtrockenheit (42% extreme Mundtrockenheit) (7). Brashear et al. berichteten über eine dosisabhängige Häufigkeit der Mundtrockenheit, 14% bei 5000 U und 24% bei 10 000 U BTB (6). Entsprechend der Literatur und unseren Erfahrungen sind die anticholinergen Nebenwirkungen dosisabhängig.

Da gewisse anticholinerge Wirkungen von BTB bei einigen Patienten ausdrücklich erwünscht sind, wie z.B. Reduktion des Speichelflusses bei schwerer Tetraspastik und Hypersalivation, besteht das Ziel darin, die verwendete Dosis vorsichtig zwischen erwünschten und unerwünschten Wirkungen auszubalanzieren.

Um unerwünschte systemische Wirkungen zu vermeiden, geben wir unter Vorbehalt folgende sehr vorläufige Empfehlungen: maximal 500 U/kg Körpergewicht Neurobloc® und eine maximale Gesamtdosis von 10 000 U Neurobloc® pro Behandlung.

Effektivität von BTB bei de-novo Patienten, Dosisbreite, Wirkungsdauer, Nebenwirkungen und anticholinerges Potential sind wichtige Fragen, die in zukünftigen Studien beantwortet werden sollten. Kontrollierte Studien, die BTB und BTA vergleichen (wenn möglich, doppel-blind, randomisiert u.U. auch placebo-kontrolliert) sind notwendig, um evidenz-basierte Ergebnisse für BTB zu erhalten.

Abkürzungen

BTA	Botulinum toxin type A
BTB	Botulinum toxin type B
GAS	Goal Attaiment Scale
U	Units

Literatur

1. Kirschner J, Berweck S, Mall V, Korinthenberg R, Heinen F. Botulinum toxin treatment in cerebral palsy: evidence for a new treatment option. J Neurol 2001;248:28–30.
2. Kirschner J, Berweck S, Mall V, Korinthenberg R, Heinen F. Botulinumtoxin – Neue Therapieoptionen für Kinder mit Zerebralparese. Dt Ärztebl 2001; 98:A3375–3379.
3. Zylka-Menhorn V. Den Schwarzen Peter hat der Arzt. Dt Ärztebl 2001;98:B2877–B2880.
4. Hermann J, Mall V, Bigalke H, Geth K, Korinthenberg R, Heinen F. Secondary non-response due to development of of neutralizing antibodies to Botulinum Toxin A during treatment of children with cerebral palsy. Neuropediatrics 2000;31:333–4.
5. Kessler KR, Skutta M, Benecke R. Long-term treatment of cervical dystonia with botulinum toxin A: efficacy, safety, and antibody frequency. German Dystonia Study Group. J Neurol 1999;246:265–74.
6. Brashear A, Lew M, Dykstra D, Comella C. Safety and efficacy of NeuroBloc (Botulinum toxin type B) in type A-responsive cervical dystonia. Neurol 1999;53:1439–46.
7. Dressler D, Benecke R. Erste Erfahrungen mit der klinischen Anwendung von Botulinum-Toxin Typ B. Nervenarzt 2002;73:194–8.
8. Palisano R, Rosenbaum P, Walter S, Russell D, Wood E, Galuppi B. Development and reliability of a system to classify gross motor function in children with cerebral palsy. Dev Med Child Neurol 1997;39:214–23.
9. Göschel H, Wohlfarth K, Frevert J, Dengler R, Bigalke H. Botulinum A toxin therapy: neutralizing and nonneutralizing antibodies – therapeutic consequences. Exp Neurol 1997;147:96–102.

7. Neuropharmakologie

Wirkmechanismen antiepileptischer Substanzen

B. Schmitt

Einleitung

Wesentliche Elemente eines Anfalls sind eine abnorme zelluläre Erregbarkeit und Fehler im neuronalen Netzwerk. Beide Störungen können das Resultat komplexer Prozesse sein. Antiepileptische Substanzen lassen sich nach 3 Grundprinzipien unterteilen: a) Verminderung der Erregung, b) Beeinflussung der Erregungsausbreitung und c) Verstärkung der GABAergen Hemmung (15).

Verminderung der Erregung

Glutamat ist der wichtigste erregende Neurotransmitter im Gehirn. Nach Eintreffen des Aktionspotentials an der Präsynapse werden spannungsabhängige high-threshold Ca^{++}-Kanäle geöffnet, Ca^{++} strömt in die Präsynapse und führt zur Freisetzung von Glutamat in den synaptischen Spalt. Phenytoin, Barbiturate, Oxcarbazepin, Lamotrigin, Topiramat, Felbamat und möglicherweise auch Levetiracetam können diese Ca^{++}-Kanäle blockieren und die Neurotransmitter-Freisetzung vermindern (35, 15, 23).

Postsynaptisch werden 3 Glutamatrezeptoren unterschieden: metabotrope, die über second-messenger funktionieren und zwei ionotrope (AMPA/Kainat und NMDA), die an Ionen-Kanäle gekoppelt sind. Die Rolle der Glutamat-Rezeptoren bei der Epilepsie ist noch ungenügend geklärt. Insbesondere Anfälle nach akut neurologischen Ereignissen oder bei Stoffwechselkrankheiten könnten über eine vermehrte Freisetzung von Glutamat bzw. eine Übererregung von Glutamatrezeptoren verursacht sein (29, 28). Topiramat und Phenobarbital haben eine antagonistische Wirkung am AMPA/Kainat Rezeptor (12, 15). Tierexperimente zeigen eine antiepileptische Wirkung von Topiramat bei Hypoxie-induzierten Anfällen (12). Am NMDA-Rezeptor wirken Valproat (18) und Felbamat, wobei Felbamat die Glyzinanbindungsstelle des NMDA-Rezepors blockiert (15). Ebenfalls wirksam am NMDA-Rezeptor sind Memantin, Amantadin, Ketamin und Dextromethorphan, die aber keine klassischen Antiepileptika sind, in speziellen Fällen aber eine gute antiepileptische Wirkung haben können (28, 13).

Absencen entstehen durch abnorme oszillatorische Rhythmen in thalamo-cortico-thalamischen Verbindungen (Abb. 1a). Letztere bestehen aus sensorischen thalamischen Schaltneuronen und cortikalen Pyramidenzellen, die sich gegenseitig stimulieren. Sowohl die thalamocortico als auch die corticothalamischen Verbindungen sind exzitatorisch (glutaminerg) und geben kollaterale Axone an den Nucleus reticularis thalami (NRT) ab. Zwischen NRT und Schalt-

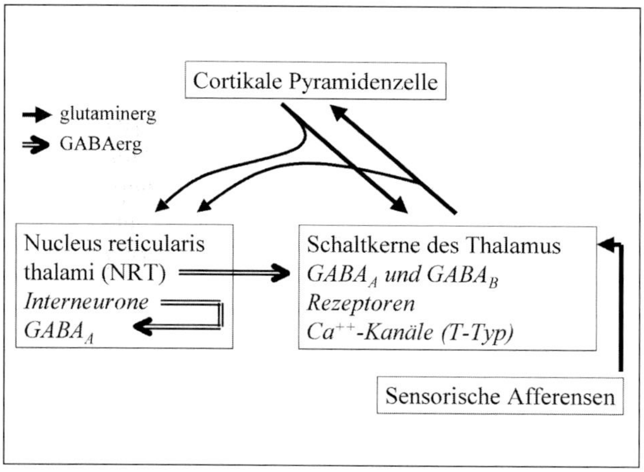

Abb. 1a: Thalamocorticaler Schaltkreis: Bei Absencen können T-Ca^{++}-Kanäle oder GABA$_B$-Rezeptoren gestört sein. Ethosuximid, Mesuximid und Zonisamid blockieren den T-Ca^{++}-Kanal. Clonazepam verstärkt über GABA$_A$-Rezeptoren die innere Selbstblockade im NRT und reduziert so die GABAerge Wirkung des NRT auf die GABA$_B$-Rezeptoren. Die glutaminerge Reizübermittlung kann durch Lamotrigin und durch NMDA-Rezeptorantagonisten reduziert werden.

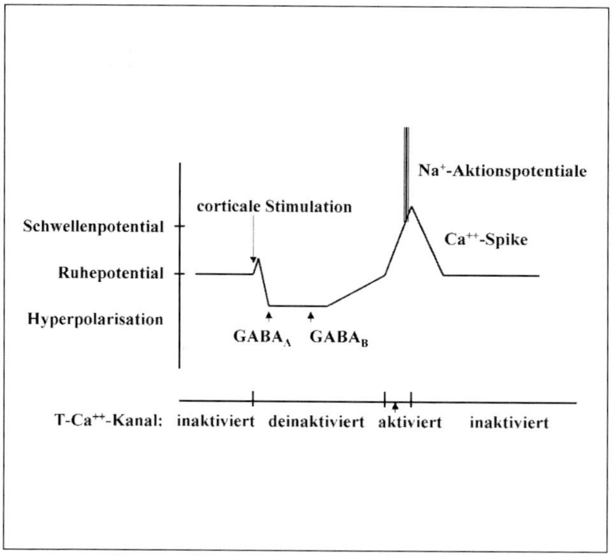

Abb. 1b: Schematisierter Funktionsablauf von low-voltage T-Ca^{++}-Kanälen: Bei Ruhepotential sind T-Ca^{++}-Kanäle inaktiviert. Ihre Deinaktivierung erfolgt durch eine prolongierte Hyperpolarisation (Aktivierung von GABA$_A$- und vor allem GABA$_B$-Rezeptoren). Im deinaktivierten Zustand genügt eine geringe Depolarisation, um den T-Ca^{++}-Kanal zu aktivieren und einen starken Ca^{++}-Einstrom zu bewirken. Der Einstrom verstärkt die Depolarisation (Ca^{++}-Spike) und löst nach Erreichen des Schwellenpotentials Na^+-abhängige Aktionspotentiale aus. T-Ca^{++}-Kanäle werden rasch inaktiviert.

kernen sind es GABAerge Neurone, die GABA$_A$ und GABA$_B$ Rezeptoren bedienen. Zusätzlich gibt es im NRT GABA-Interneurone, die im NRT selbst über GABA$_A$-Rezeptoren benachbarte GABA-Neurone blockieren. Thalamische Zellen zeigen im Schlaf eine oszillatorische und im Wachen eine tonische Aktivität. Für die oszillierende Aktivität spielen low-threshold Ca^{++}-Kanäle vom T-Typ eine Rolle. T-Ca^{++}-Kanäle sind im Wachen und bei Ruhepotential inaktiviert (Abb. 1b). Um sie zu deinaktivieren (was nicht gleichbedeutend ist mit aktivieren), braucht es eine prolongierte Hyperpolarisation durch GABA$_B$-Rezeptoren. Im deinaktivierten Zustand genügt eine geringe Depolarisation, um den T-Ca^{++}-Kanal zu öffnen (= aktivieren) und einen starken Ca^{++}-Einstrom zu bewirken. Der Einstrom verstärkt die Depolarisation (Ca^{++}-Spike) und löst durch Erreichen des Schwellenpotentials Na^+-abhängige Aktionspotentiale aus. Ca^{++}-Kanäle werden

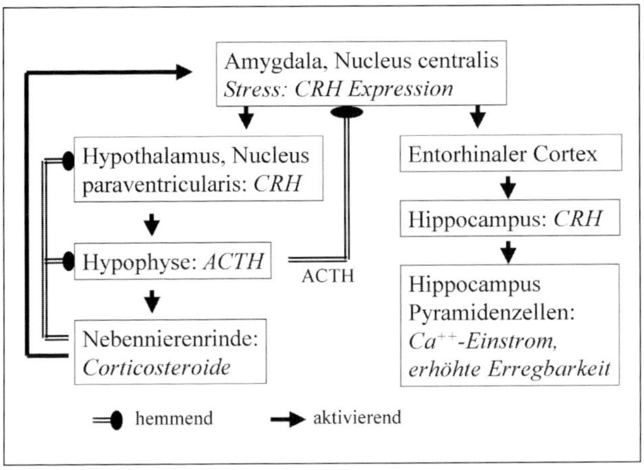

Abb. 2: Wirkprinzip von ACTH: Stress führt zur Expression von CRH im Nucleus centralis der Amygdala. CRH aktiviert eine neuroendokrine (links) und eine limbische (rechts) Achse. ACTH, aber nicht Glucocorticoide, binden an Melanocortin-Rezeptoren des Nucleus centralis der Amygdala und verhindern dort die Expression von CRH und damit die Aktivierung der neuroendokrinen und der limbischen Achse.

rasch inaktiviert (33, 7). Wie schon erwähnt, werden $GABA_A$- und $GABA_B$-Rezeptoren im Schaltkern durch GABAerge Neurone aus dem NRT aktiviert. Durch GABAerge Interneurone im NRT bremst der NRT seine eigene GABAerge Wirkung auf den Schaltkern (Selbstblockade).

Bei der Absencen-Epilepsie können T-Ca^{++}-Kanäle oder $GABA_B$-Rezeptoren gestört sein. Ethosuximid, Mesuximid und Zonisamid blockieren den T-Ca^{++}-Kanal und wirken so antiepileptisch (33, 7, 16). GABAerge Substanzen haben unterschiedliche Auswirkungen auf Absencen. Clonazepam verstärkt über $GABA_A$-Rezeptoren die innere Selbsthemmung des NRT, reduziert so die GABAerge Wirkung auf die $GABA_B$-Rezeptoren der Schaltkerne und wirkt damit antiepileptisch (33). Vigabatrin erhöht GABA, verstärkt damit auch den $GABA_B$-Rezeptor und kann so zur Verschlechterung der Absencen führen (33). Die glutaminerge Reizübermittlung lässt sich durch Lamotrigin (siehe unten) und durch NMDA-Rezeptorantagonisten reduzieren (33).

Einem anderen, altersabhängigen Wirkprinzip unterliegt ACTH. Obwohl umstritten, scheint ACTH bei der Behandlung der BNS-Epilepsie oralem Cortison überlegen zu sein (3), was eine spezifische antiepileptische Wirkung von ACTH beinhalten würde. Wichtige Aspekte dieses Konzepts waren die Entdeckung der exzitatorisch/epileptogenen Wirkung des Corticotropin-Releasing-Hormones (CRH) (2) und der Melanocortin-Rezeptoren (1). Im Nucleus centralis der Amygdala wird bei Stress CRH freigesetzt. Dieses CRH aktiviert eine neuroendokrine und eine limbische Achse (Abb. 2). Die neuroendokrine Achse führt über CRH-expremierende Neurone im Hypothalamus zur ACTH-Synthese in der Hypophyse und darüber zur Freisetzung von Glucocorticoiden in der Nebennierenrinde. Glucocorticoide haben einerseits eine negative feedback Wirkung auf die CRH Expression in Hypothalamus und Hippocampus, anderseits aber verstärken sie die Stress-induzierte CRH-Expression in der Amygdala.

In der limbischen Achse werden nach der CRH-Freisetzung in der Amygdala im Hippocampus CRH-expremierende Neurone aktiviert. In den Pyramidenzellen führt CRH über einen raschen Ca^{++}-Einstrom zu einer erhöhten Erregbarkeit. Die Wirkung von CRH ist im unreifen limbischen System viel ausgeprägter, als im reifen. Trifft auf die leichter erregbaren Neurone eine zusätzliche glutaminerge Erregung, kann dies zu einer epileptischen Entladung führen (2).

Warum wirkt ACTH in diesem Modell besser als Glucocorticoide? Natürliches ACTH reduziert über einen feedback Mechanismus durch Anbindung an Melanocortin-Rezeptoren im Nucleus centralis der Amygdala die Expression von CRH (6). Dies wirkt hemmend auf die neuroendokrine und die limbische Achse. Die Wirkung ist dosisabhängig und wird auch durch extern zugeführtes ACTH erreicht (6). Es genügt dafür ein ACTH-Fragment (4–10), welches nicht zur Freisetzung von Nebennierenrinden-Steroiden führt (3, 6). Für die Therapie der BNS-Epilepsie würde das bedeuten, dass a) ACTH eine bessere antiepileptische Wirkung besitzt als Steroide, b) für die antiepileptische Wirkung ACTH-Fragmente ausreichen, welche keine systemischen steroidalen Nebenwirkungen haben, und c) hohe Dosen wirksamer sind als niedrige.

Obwohl das Konzept Potential für Fortschritte in der Behandlung der BNS-Epilepsie besitzt, ist die Aussage, dass ACTH oralen Steroiden überlegen ist, bislang nicht zweifelsfrei belegt (10). Weitere Thesen zum Wirkprinzip von ACTH und Corticosteroiden sind a) Beschleunigung der Hirnreifung, b) Modulierung verschiedener Neurotransmittersysteme (GABA, Dopamin, Serotonin) und c) eine Wirkung über Immunsuppression (9).

Verminderung der Erregungsausbreitung

Postsynaptische erregende Potentiale verbunden mit membranendogenen Veränderungen (z.B. Öffnung von spannungsabhängigen Ca^{++}- oder Na^{+}-Kanälen) führen zu paroxysmalen Depolarisationen (paroxysmal depolarisation shift, PDS), die eine Serie hochfrequenter Aktionspotentiale auslösen (»burst«, epileptogene Entladungsmuster) (34, 8). Die spannungsabhängigen Ca^{++}-Kanäle sind prinzipiell die gleichen, wie diejenigen, die für die Neurotransmitterfreisetzung verantwortlich sind. Entsprechend ist auch hier ein antiepileptisches Wirkprinzip von Phenytoin, Phenobarbital, Oxcarbazepin, Lamotrigin, Topiramat, Felbamat und Levetiracetam denkbar (35, 15, 23).

Die Entstehung und Ausbreitung der Aktionspotentiale ist abhängig von spannungsabhängigen Na^{+}-Kanälen. Die Aktivierung spannungsabhängiger Na^{+}-Kanäle führt zum Na^{+}-Einstrom und zu einer starken Depolarisation (Aktionspotential). Gleichzeitig mit der Depolarisation wird a) der Na^{+}-Kanal inaktiviert und der weitere Na^{+}-Einstrom verhindert und b) verschiedene K^{+}-Kanäle aktiviert, die zur Re- bzw. Hyperpolarisation führen. Einer dieser K^{+}-Kanäle wird schon sehr früh bei der gleichen Spannung wie die Na^{+}-Kanäle aktiviert. Der so ausgelöste K^{+}-(Auswärts-)Strom (M-current) steuert der Depolarisation (Na^{+}-Einwärts-Strom) entgegen und limitiert das Entladen von Aktionspotentialen (27). Bei benignen familiären Neugeborenenkrämpfen ist dieser low-voltage K^{+}-Kanal gestört. Die Substanz Retigabine öffnet diesen K^{+}-Kanal und zeigt im Tierexperiment ein breites antiepileptisches Spektrum (27).

Die zur Verfügung stehenden Antiepileptika setzen hauptsächlich am spannungsabhängigen Na^+-Kanal an. Hierbei gilt es, physiologische Aktionspotentiale nicht zu beeinträchtigen und anfallsauslösende anhaltende Entladungen zu unterdrücken. Carbamazepin, Oxcarbazepin, Phenytoin, Topiramat, Felbamat, Lamotrigin, Zonisamid und Propofol tun dies über eine Stabilisierung, bzw. Verlängerung der Inaktivierungsphase des Na^+-Kanals. Das einzelne Aktionspotential wird dadurch nicht getroffen, wohl aber hochfrequente Aktionspotentiale (Entladungen) (19, 16, 32, 15). Sultiam reduziert den Na^+-Einstrom (20). Lamotrigin und Propofol wirken wahrscheinlich vorwiegend auf Na^+-Kanäle von glutamatsynthetisierenden Neuronen (26, 15, 17).

Bislang wurde nur für wenige Medikamente eine Wirkung an K^+-Kanälen gezeigt, die für die Repolarisation des Aktionspotentials verantwortlich sind. Eine Verstärkung der K^+-(Auswärts)-Ströme würde die Hyperpolarisation verstärken und damit hochfrequente Entladungen erschweren. Für Valproat (18), Carbamazepin und Oxcarbazepin (21) wird ein solcher Wirkmechanismus diskutiert.

Verstärkung der GABAergen Hemmung

GABA ist der wichtigste hemmende Neurotransmitter im Gehirn. Bei Pyridoxin-abhängigen Anfällen findet sich im Liquor ein reduzierter GABA- (14) und ein erhöhter Glutamat-Gehalt (4). Pyridoxin ist bei der Umwandlung von Glutamat zu GABA ein Coenzym der Glutamat-Decarboxylase und es wird angenommen, dass bei pyridoxinabhängigen Anfällen höhere Pyridoxinkonzentrationen notwendig sind, um die gestörte Cofaktor-Bindung an die Glutamat-Decarboxylase zu überwinden (31). Auch bei ketogener Diät wird eine vermehrte GABA-Bildung aus Glutamat diskutiert (36). Vigabatrin blockiert irreversibel die GABA-Transaminase in der Präsynapse, hemmt damit den GABA-Abbau und führt zu einem markanten Anstieg des GABA-Pools in den Synaptosomen (19). Topiramat und Gabapentin führen ebenfalls zu einem höheren GABA-Gehalt im Gehirn (24, 25). Der Mechanismus bei Topiramat ist unklar, bei Gabapentin wird eine vermehrte Synthese sowie ein verminderter Metabolismus von GABA diskutiert (15). Valproat bewirkt ebenfalls einen GABA-Anstieg in der Präsynapse und im extrazellulären Raum. Der Effekt ist regional unterschiedlich. Drei mögliche Wirkmechanismen werden diskutiert: a) Hemmung des GABA-Abbaus durch Inhibition der synaptosomalen GABA-Transaminase (ähnlich wie Vigabatrin), b) eine verstärkte GABA-Synthese und c) eine indirekte feedback Inhibition des GABA-Turnovers (18).

Im synaptischen Spalt hemmen Vigabatrin und Tiagabin die Aufnahme von GABA in die Gliazellen und Tiagabin darüber hinaus auch die Aufnahme von GABA in Neuronen (15). Die Blockade von Tiagabin ist auf einen GABA-Transporter (GAT-1) beschränkt und zeigt regional grosse Unterschiede mit Maximum in Cortex und Hippocampus (15).

Auf der postsynaptischen Seite werden 3 GABA-Rezeptoren unterschieden. Am besten untersucht ist die antiepileptische Wirkung am $GABA_A$-Rezeptor, ein ionotroper Rezeptor assoziiert mit einem Cl^--Kanal. Die Aktivierung von $GABA_A$-Rezeptoren führt über einen Einstrom von Cl^- zu einer Hyperpolarisation der Membran. Benzodiazepine, Phenobarbital, Topiramat und Felbamat potenzieren Cl^--Ströme durch den $GABA_A$-Rezeptor (15). Während Phenobarbital die Öffnungszeiten der Cl^--Kanäle verlängert, führen Benzodiazepine zu einer Erhöhung der Öffnungsfrequenz des Kanals. In beiden Fällen ist ein vermehrter Cl^--Fluss durch den GABA-Rezeptor die Folge (19, 32). Im Unterschied zu Benzodiazepinen können Barbiturate den GABA-Rezeptor auch ohne die Anwesenheit von GABA aktivieren (15). Auch Bromid wirkt möglicherweise über eine Potenzierung des GABA-Rezeptors (22). Bromid ist außerdem kleiner als Chlorid und kann schneller durch die Cl^--Kanäle in die Zelle fliessen. Bromid führt wie Chlorid zur Hyperpolarisation und damit zur Hemmung (5).

Sonstige Wirkprinzipien

Bislang nicht geklärt ist der antiepileptische Wirkmechanismus der ketogenen Diät (KD). Bei speziellen Erkrankungen, wie Pyruvatdehydrogenasemangel oder einem Glukosetransporter-(GLUT1)-Defekt ist der alternative Energiestoffwechsel das wesentliche Wirkprinzip (11). Ob auch bei anderen chronischen Epilepsien der alternative Energiemetabolismus der entscheidende Wirkmechanismus ist, ist unklar. Eine andere Theorie vermutet eine Stärkung der GABAergen Hemmung durch KD. Der Ketonkörper beta-Hydroxybutyrat hat strukturelle Ähnlichkeit mit GABA und lässt eine imitierende Wirkung am GABA-Rezeptor vermuten (30). Andere Untersuchungen sprechen für eine Erhöhung des GABA-Gehalts in der Präsynapse oder eine verminderte Aktivität des NMDA-Rezeptors durch die KD-induzierte Azidose. Allerdings scheint KD keine langfristige Veränderungen des pH im Gewebe zu bewirken (30). Andere vermuten in der Ketose das ausschlaggebende Wirkprinzip. Ketose bewirkt verschiedene Veränderungen des Hormonsystems, z.B. senkt es den Insulinspiegel. Insulin führt im ZNS über spezifische Insulinrezeptoren zu einer vermehrten neuronalen Erregbarkeit, reguliert den Neurotransmitter-Transporter-Mechanismus, beeinflusst die Steroidproduktion und moduliert die Wirkung von Glucocorticoiden. Die Senkung des Insulins hätte so evtl. eine antiepileptische Wirkung (30). Weiterhin diskutiert werden eine Wirkung über a) das erhöhte Cholesterol (Synthese neuroaktiver Moleküle), b) eine KD-assoziierte Dehydration, c) Einflüsse auf die Blut-Hirn-Schranke und d) Einflüsse auf die Genexpression (30). Es ist durchaus denkbar, dass bei verschiedenen Epilepsieformen unterschiedliche Wirkmechanismen zum Tragen kommen.

Obwohl verschiedene Medikamente dasselbe Wirkprinzip haben, können sie in der klinischen Anwendung unterschiedliche Wirkungen zeigen. Dies kann auf Unterschiede in Resorption und Metabolismus zurückzuführen sein, es gibt aber auch Gründe, die im ZNS selbst liegen. Ionenkanäle liegen in verschiedenen Varianten vor. Diese Varianten sind auf eine unterschiedliche Zusammensetzung der Untereinheiten zurückzuführen, was letztendlich die Eigenschaft des Kanals bestimmt. Die Varianten sind im Gehirn unterschiedlich verteilt. Ihre Verbreitung

Tab. 1: Wirkmechanismen antiepileptischer Substanzen

Substanz	**Na^+-Kanal**	**K^+-Kanal**	**Ca^{++}-Kanal T-Typ**	**Ca^{++}-Kanal andere**	**GABA-erg**	**AMPA**	**NMDA**	**Carboan-hydrase-hemmer**
Benzodiazepine					x			
Bromid					x			
Carbamazepin	x	(x)						
Ethosuximid			x					
Felbamat	(x)			(x)	(x)		x	
Gabapentin					x			
Lamotrigin	x			(x)				
Levetiracetam				(x)				
Oxcarbazepin	x	(x)		(x)				
Phenobarbital	x			(x)	x	x		
Phenytoin	x			(x)	(x)			
Propofol	x							
Sultiam	x							x
Tiagabin					x			
Topiramat	x			(x)	x	x		x
Vigabatrin					x			
Valproat	x	(x)			x		x	
Zonisamid	x		x					

oder Ausprägung ändert sich mit der Reifung des Gehirns und zeigt genetische und individuelle Unterschiede. Ein weiterer Faktor für die antiepileptische Wirkung einer Substanz ist die Kombination mehrerer Wirkprinzipien. Fast alle Antiepileptika haben mehrere antiepileptische Wirkmechanismen, und man kann davon ausgehen, dass für die meisten weitere Wirkmechanismen in Zukunft entdeckt werden.

Literatur

1. Adan RA, Gispen WH (2000) Melanocortins and the brain: from effects via receptors to drug targets. Eur J Pharmacol 405:13–24.
2. Baram TZ, Hatalski CG (1998) Neuropeptide-mediated excitability: a key triggering mechanism for seizure generation in the developing brain. Trends Neurosci 21:471–6.
3. Baram TZ, Mitchell WG, Tournay A, Snead OC, Hanson RA, Horton EJ (1996) High-dose corticotropin (ACTH) versus prednisone for infantile spasms: a prospective, randomized, blinded study. Pediatrics 97:375–9.
4. Baumeister FA, Gsell W, Shin YS, Egger J (1994) Glutamate in pyridoxine-dependent epilepsy: neurotoxic glutamate concentration in the cerebrospinal fluid and its normalization by pyridoxine. Pediatrics 94:318–21.

5. Browne T, R., Ascanape J, S. (1997) Diones, paraldehyde, phenacemide, bromides, and sulthiame. In: J Engel, J., TA Pedley (Herausg.) Epilepsy: A comprehensive textbook Lippincott-Raven, Philadelphia, New York, 1627–44.
6. Brunson KL, Khan N, Eghbal-Ahmadi M, Baram TZ (2001) Corticotropin (ACTH) acts directly on amygdala neurons to down-regulate corticotropin-releasing hormone gene expression. Ann Neurol 49:304–12.
7. Coulter DA (1997) Thalamocortical anatomy and physiology. In: J Engel, J., TA Pedley (Herausg.) Epilepsy: A comprehensive textbook Lippincott-Raven, Philadelphia, New York, 341–51.
8. Heinemann U, Eder C (1997) Control of neuronal excitability. In: J Engel, J., TA Pedley (Herausg.) Epilepsy: A comprehensive textbook Lippincott-Raven, Philadelphia, New York, 237–50.
9. Hrachovy R, A., Ascanape J, S. (1997) ACTH and steroids. In: J Engel, J., TA Pedley (Herausg.) Epilepsy: A comprehensive textbook Lippincott-Raven, Philadelphia, New York, 1463–73.
10. Hrachovy RA, Frost JD, Jr., Kellaway P, Zion TE (1983) Double-blind study of ACTH vs prednisone therapy in infantile spasms. J Pediatr 103:641–5.
11. Klepper J, Ecker D, Burkart P, Leiendecker P, Voit T, Baumeister F (2001) Indikation und Anwendung der ketogenen Diät im Kindesalter. Monatsschr Kinderheilkd 149:1383–90.
12. Koh S, Jensen FE (2001) Topiramate blocks perinatal hypoxia-induced seizures in rat pups. Ann Neurol 50:366–72.
13. Kurlemann G, Debus O, Schuierer G (1996) Dextromethorphan in molybdenum cofactor deficiency. Eur J Pediatr 155:422–3.
14. Kurlemann G, Loscher W, Dominick HC, Palm GD (1987) Disappearance of neonatal seizures and low CSF GABA levels after treatment with vitamin B6. Epilepsy Res 1:152–4.
15. Kwan P, Sills GJ, Brodie MJ (2001) The mechanisms of action of commonly used antiepileptic drugs. Pharmacol Ther 90:21–34.
16. Leppik IE (1999) Zonisamide. Epilepsia 40 Suppl 5:S23–9.
17. Lingamaneni R, Birch ML, Hemmings HC, Jr. (2001) Widespread inhibition of sodium channel-dependent glutamate release from isolated nerve terminals by isoflurane and propofol. Anesthesiology 95:1460–6.
18. Löscher W (1999) Valproate: a reappraisal of its pharmacodynamic properties and mechanisms of action. Prog Neurobiol 58:31–59.
19. Macdonald RL (1997) Cellular effects of antiepileptic drugs. In: J Engel, J., TA Pedley (Herausg.) Epilepsy: A comprehensive textbook Lippincott-Raven, Philadelphia, New York, 1383–91.
20. Madeja M, Wolf C, Speckmann EJ (2001) Reduction of voltage-operated sodium currents by the anticonvulsant drug sulthiame. Brain Res 900:88–94.
21. McLean MJ, Schmutz M, Wamil AW, Olpe HR, Portet C, Feldmann KF (1994) Oxcarbazepine: mechanisms of action. Epilepsia 35 Suppl 3:S5–9.
22. Meierkord H, Grunig F, Gutschmidt U, et al. (2000) Sodium bromide: effects on different patterns of epileptiform activity, extracellular pH changes and GABAergic inhibition. Naunyn Schmiedebergs Arch Pharmacol 361:25–32.
23. Niespodziany I, Klitgaard H, Margineanu DG (2001) Levetiracetam inhibits the high-voltage-activated Ca(2+) current in pyramidal neurones of rat hippocampal slices. Neurosci Lett 306:5–8.
24. Petroff OA, Hyder F, Rothman DL, Mattson RH (2000) Effects of gabapentin on brain GABA, homocarnosine, and pyrrolidinone in epilepsy patients. Epilepsia 41:675–80.
25. Petroff OA, Hyder F, Rothman DL, Mattson RH (2001) Topiramate rapidly raises brain GABA in epilepsy patients. Epilepsia 42:543–8.
26. Rehberg B, Duch DS (1999) Suppression of central nervous system sodium channels by propofol. Anesthesiology 91:512–20.
27. Rogawski MA (2000) KCNQ2/KCNQ3 K+ channels and the molecular pathogenesis of epilepsy: implications for therapy. Trends Neurosci 23:393–8.

28. Schmitt B, Netzer R, Fanconi S, Baumann P, Boltshauser E (1994) Drug refractory epilepsy in brain damage: effect of dextromethorphan on EEG in four patients. J Neurol Neurosurg Psychiatry 57:333–9.
29. Schmitt B, Steinmann B, Gitzelmann R, Thun-Hohenstein L, Mascher H, Dumermuth G (1993) Nonketotic hyperglycinemia: clinical and electrophysiologic effects of dextromethorphan, an antagonist of the NMDA receptor. Neurology 43:421–4.
30. Schwartzkroin PA (1999) Mechanisms underlying the anti-epileptic efficacy of the ketogenic diet. Epilepsy Res 37:171–80.
31. Scriver CR (2001) Disorders of beta- and gamma-amino acids in free and peptide-linked forms. In: CR Scriver, AL Beaudet, WS Sly, D Valle (Herausg.) The metabolic & molecular bases of inherited disease McGraw-Hill, New York, 2090.
32. Shank RP, Gardocki JF, Streeter AJ, Maryanoff BE (2000) An overview of the preclinical aspects of topiramate: pharmacology, pharmacokinetics, and mechanism of action. Epilepsia 41 Suppl 1:S3–9.
33. Snead OC, 3rd (1995) Basic mechanisms of generalized absence seizures. Ann Neurol 37:146–57.
34. Speckmann EJ, Straub H (1994) Pathogenese der Anfälle und Epilepsien. Neurophysiologische Grundlagen. In: W Fröscher, F Vassella (Herausg.) Die Epilepsien Walter de Gruyter, Berlin, New York, 89–104.
35. Stefani A, Spadoni F, Bernardi G (1997) Voltage-activated calcium channels: targets of antiepileptic drug therapy? Epilepsia 38:959–65.
36. Yudkoff M, Daikhin Y, Nissim I, Lazarow A (2001) Ketogenic diet, amino acid metabolism, and seizure control. J Neurosci Res 66:931–40.

Neuroprotektion

T.J. Feuerstein, B. Zucker

Zusammenfassung

Die Verhinderung des Untergangs von Neuronen ist therapeutisches Ziel bei akuter und chronischer Neurodegeneration. Beide Degenerationsformen hängen von ähnlichen ursächlichen Faktoren ab: Exzitotoxizität und intrazelluläre Calcium (Ca^{++}_i)-Erhöhung bedingen sich gegenseitig und spielen Hauptrollen bei der Schädigung von Neuronen. Sie tragen entscheidend zu Nekrose und/oder Apoptose von Nervenzellen bei. An Beispielen für Neuroprotektion in einem Modell der akuten Ischämie und im Modell einer chronischen, genetisch bedingten Schädigung, des M. Huntington, wird ein möglicherweise zukunftsträchtiges Neuroprotektivum vorgestellt, das synergistisch auf mehrere zelluläre Angriffspunkte zielt.

Was ist Neuroprotektion?

Die folgende Definition ist angelehnt an ein jüngst erschienenes Buch, Grundlagen der klinischen Neuroprotektion, von Ludolph und Schwarz (2001): Demnach versteht man unter Neuroprotektion »alle Maßnahmen, die langanhaltende günstige Effekte auf den Beginn oder Verlauf einer Erkrankung des Nervensystems haben, indem sie Ätiologie oder Pathogenese beeinflussen«. Ziel der Neuroprotektion ist also, den Untergang oder die Funktionsstörung von Neuronen zu verhindern, zu vermindern oder zu verzögern.

Offensichtlich wirken nicht nur pharmakologische Maßnahmen neuroprotektiv. Im folgenden beschränke ich mich als Pharmakologe jedoch auf pharmakologische Möglichkeiten.

Voraussetzung der Neuroprotektion ist eine bevorstehende oder bereits eingetretene Neurodegeneration. Hier haben wir zwischen akuten und chronischen Vorgängen bzw. Krankheiten zu unterscheiden. Die wichtigste akute Neurodegeneration betrifft den Schlaganfall; als Beispiel für eine chronische neurodegenerative Krankheit nenne ich den M. Huntington, nicht zuletzt deswegen, weil ich über eine neue, noch präklinische pharmakotherapeutische Entwicklung berichten möchte.

Exzitotoxizität spielt bei beiden Formen, der akuten und der chronischen Neurodegeneration, eine entscheidende Rolle. Exzitotoxizität hat mit einer zellulären Ca^{++}-Überladung zu tun, die entweder zum nekrotischen Zelltod führt oder Apoptose auslöst, und zwar unter Einbeziehung der Mitochondrien.

Die folgende Abbildung 1 zeigt den Circulus vitiosus des sich selbst erhöhenden extrazellulären Glutamatspiegels (Glu) und der daraus folgenden intrazellulären Ca^{++}-Überladung. Neben Glu wirkt auch Aspartat als Exzitotoxin.

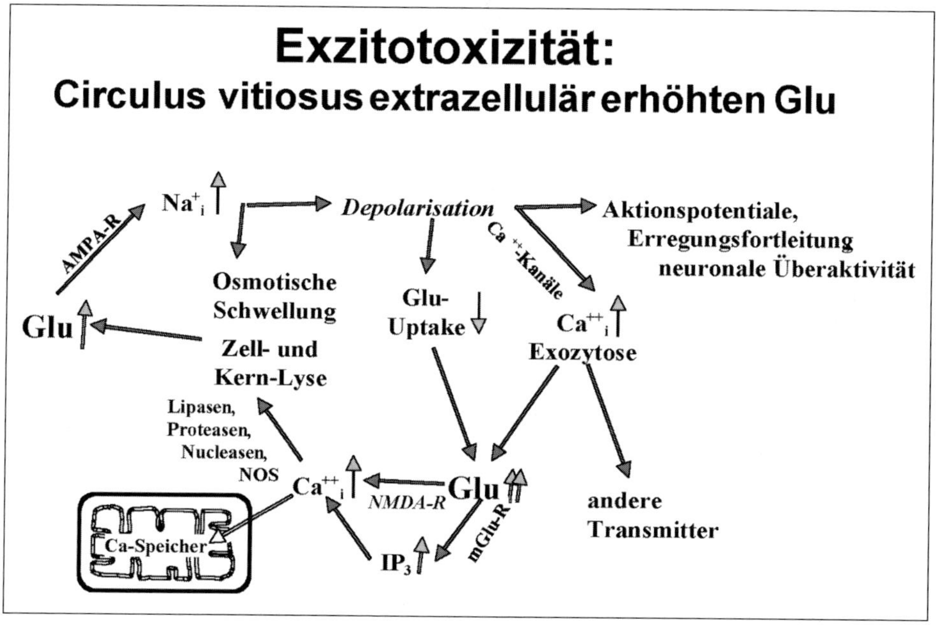

Abb. 1

Extrazelluläres Glu verstärkt sich selbst, es erhöht seine extrazelluläre zytotoxisch bedeutsame Konzentration folgendermaßen: Gehen wir von einer mäßig erhöhten Glu-Konzentration aus (links: Glu ↑). Die Aktivierung von AMPA-Rezeptoren auf Neuronen führt zu Na^{+}- und Wasser-Einstrom und damit zur Zellschwellung; im Extremfall kann dies bis zum Platzen der Zelle gehen, was typischerweise eine Zellnekrose bedeutet. Na^{+}-Einstrom führt auch zur Depolarisation, damit zu Aktionspotentialen, zu Erregungsfortleitung, zu neuronaler Überaktivität. Als weitere Folge der Depolarisation öffnen sich spannungsabhängige Ca^{++}-Kanäle, was Ca^{++}-Einstrom und Exocytose bedeutet. Exozytose des ohnehin schon erhöhten Glu, aber auch Ausschüttung anderer Transmitter. Depolarisation, also Verringerung des Na^{+}-Gradienten über Zellmembranen, heißt auch Verminderung der neuronalen und – noch bedeutungsvoller – der glialen Glu-Wiederaufnahme, was die extrazelluläre Glu-Konzentration weiter ansteigen lässt. Glu kann nun in dieser Situation der Depolarisation auch NMDA-Rezeptorkanäle öffnen, weiteres Ca^{++} strömt massiv in das Neuron ein. Die bereits erhöhte intrazelluläre Ca^{++}-Konzentration (Ca^{++}_{i}) steigt weiter an, wenn Glu zusätzlich metabotrope Glu-Rezeptoren der Gruppe I (Subtypen 1a, 5a) aktiviert, sodass sich über eine Aktivierung der Phospholipase C Inosittriphosphat bildet, das den intrazellulären Ca^{++}-Speicher des endoplasmatischen Reticulums öffnet. Weiterer Ca^{++}_{i}-Anstieg folgt, der Lipasen, Proteasen, Nucleasen und die Stickoxid-Synthase (NOS) aktiviert. Es kann zur akuten Zellnekrose kommen, sodass aus dem Intrazellulärraum weiteres Glu freigesetzt wird. Oder aber Ca^{++}_i wird in einem speziellen Ca^{++}-Speicher gepuffert, dem Mitochondrium, was evtl. zu einer anderen Schädigungform, der Apoptose (s.u.), führt.

Massive Zell- und Kernschwellung nach Aktivierung von Kern- und Zellmembran-zerstörenden Enzymen durch Ca^{++}_i bedeutet Nekrose oder akuter Zelltod. Freie Radikale aus zerfallenden, Energie-defizienten Mitochondrien tragen hierzu ebenfalls bei (Oxidation von Proteinen und DNA, Peroxidation von Membranlipiden). Die Entzündung räumt über Stunden bis Tage nekrotische Reste ab. Typischerweise wird ein Infarktkern nekrotisch.

Bleibt die Zell- und Mitochondrienschädigung subnekrotisch, wird das mitochondriale Todesprogramm eingeleitet, wenn die »Energievorräte« für das Überleben zu gering sind und zu hohe Ca^{++}_i-Spiegel die Pufferkapazität der Mitochondrien überfordern: Es resultiert der protrahierte, apoptotische Zelltod, der beim Hirninfarkt typischerweise in der Penumbra stattfindet, auch ausgelöst durch vermehrt gebildete reaktive Sauerstoffspezies (ROS) nach Reperfusion (»Reperfusionsschaden«).

Abbildung 2 zeigt den zeitlichen Ablauf der verschiedenen Schädigungen.

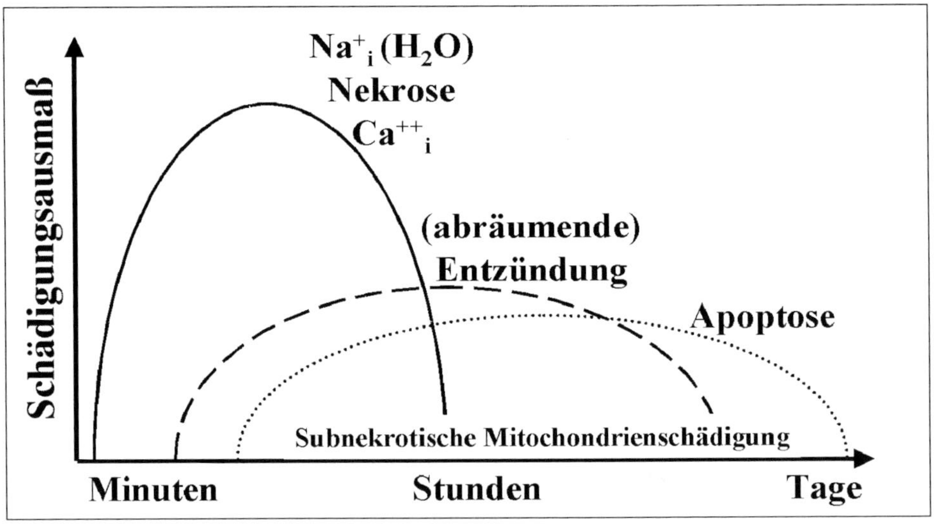

Abb. 2: Schädigungsverlauf bei Exzitotoxizität

Stoffwechselvorgänge mit hohem Energiebedarf disponieren bei mitochondrialer Vorschädigung oder Überlastung, z.B. durch zuviel sequestriertes Ca^{++}_i, zur Apoptose. Solche »anspruchsvollen« Stoffwechselvorgänge betreffen z.B. Ionenpumpen, die Ubiquitinierung von Proteinfragmenten zur Vorbereitung ihrer Beseitigung, und die DNA-Reparatur. An der Zellmembran führt ATP-Mangel aufgrund unzureichender Leistung der Ionenpumpen zu Depolarisation und, wie schon u.a. erwähnt (Abb. 1), zu verminderter Glu-Wiederaufnahme. Erhöhtes extrazelluläres Glu kann indirekt (rezeptorunabhängig) die ROS-Entgiftung in den Mitochondrien vermindern, indem Glu mit einer $EC_{50} < 100$ µM den Einwärtstransport der Aminosäure Cystein über den Cys/Glu-Antiporter in die

Zellen hemmt (Schubert und Piasecki 2001). Cystein steht damit für die Glutathion (GSH)-Synthese nicht mehr zur Verfügung, sodass Glutathion die Wasserstoffperoxid-Reduktion zu Wasser nicht mehr bewerkstelligen kann. Der Cys/Glu-Antiporter ist in Abbildung 3 eingezeichnet, welche auch die Vorgänge innerhalb einer Zelle und eines Mitochondrium bei der Apoptose zusammenfasst: Hier kann man zwischen einem physiologischen und einem pathophysiologischen Apoptoseweg unterscheiden. Der physiologische Weg, der u.a. während der Ontogenese eine wesentliche Rolle spielt, geht von »Todesliganden« an einem plasmamembranären »Todesrezeptor« aus. Dort wird eine Zelle also angewiesen, apoptotisch , das heißt u.a. ohne entzündliche Begleitreaktion, abzusterben, wenn sie nicht mehr gebraucht wird. Über eine Kaskade von Caspasen wird der Zelltod in die Wege geleitet, wobei Enzyme gespalten werden, die für die Integrität des Zytoskeletts, für den DNA-Stoffwechsel und sonstige lebensnotwendige Prozesse wichtig sind.

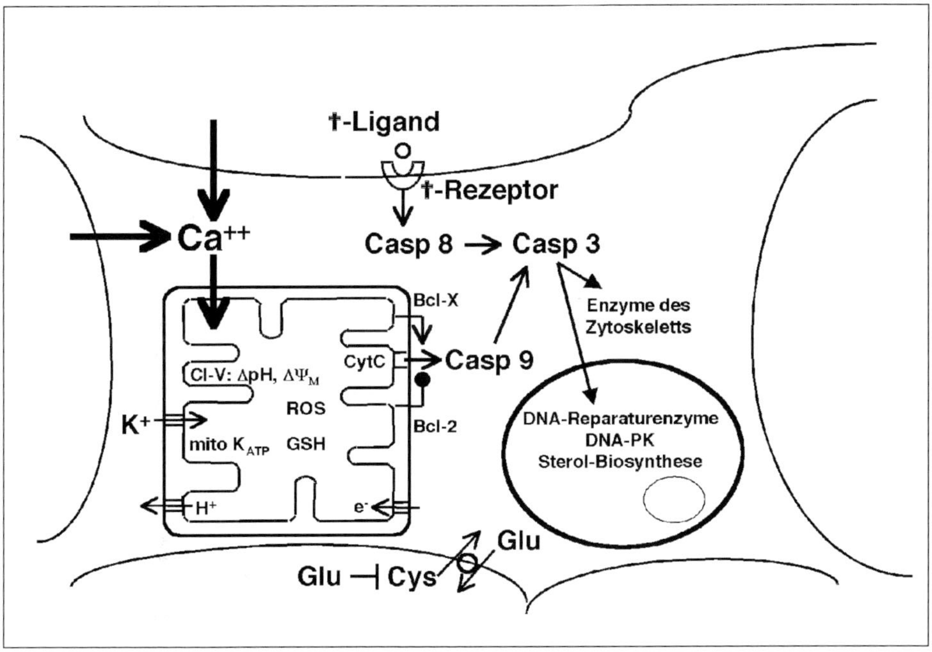

Abb. 3: Apoptose: physiologisch (ontogenetisch); pathophysiologisch

Der pathophysiologische Apoptoseweg beginnt in den Mitochondrien. Diese können – beispielsweise aufgrund einer Ca^{++}-Überladung – ihren Ladungs- ($\Delta\Psi_M$) und pH-Gradienten (ΔpH) und damit ihre Energieproduktion entlang der Komplexe I–V (CI–V)) nicht aufrechterhalten. Ihre Entgiftungskapazität für ROS reicht dann nicht mehr aus. ROS tragen nunmehr zur Öffnung einer Membranpore bei, die u.a. Cytochrom C (Cyt C) ausströmen lässt (Szewczyk und Wojtczak 2002). Dieser Ausstrom wird gefördert durch das Oncoprotein Bcl-X und gehemmt durch Bcl-2. Cyt C aktiviert über Zwischenschritte Caspase 9, was auf die bereits geschilderte Endstrecke des Apoptosewegs führt.

Wie die in Abbildung 3 ebenfalls aufgeführten mitochondrialen ATP-abhängigen K^+-Kanäle (mitoK_{ATP}-Kanäle) den pathophysiologischen Apoptoseweg »versperren«, wird später erläutert.

»Antiexzitotoxische Therapieprinzipien« betreffen sowohl akute als auch chronische neurodegenerative Prozesse, indem beide Prozesse durch erhöhte extrazelluläre Spiegel exzitatorischer Aminosäuren ausgelöst werden können.

Vor der Präsentation einer eigenen »neuroprotektiven« Substanzentwicklung zunächst ein Wort zu präklinischen Modellen und therapeutischen Erwartungen bei einigen repräsentativen Bildern der akuten und chronischen Neurodegeneration:

In präklinischen Modellen für den ischämischen Hirninfarkt, die anfallsbedingte (epileptische) Hirnschädigung und für traumatische ZNS-Läsionen wirken Antagonisten an AMPA-und NMDA-Rezeptoren durchaus günstig. Die klinische Realität, d.h. klinische Studien mit diesen Antagonisten, hat jedoch bislang entsprechende therapeutische Erwartungen enttäuscht. Die experimentellen Effekte waren nur mangelhaft auf Patienten übertragbar, was u.a. mit der zu großen »Heterogenität« klinischer Studienpopulationen im Vergleich zu homogenen, von sonstigen Erkrankungen freien Gruppen von Versuchstieren erklärt wurde.

In präklinischen Modellen chronischer neurodegenerativer Erkrankungen wurden zum Teil ebenfalls therapeutische Erwartungen geweckt, um sie klinisch wieder zu entmutigen. Einige Beispiele sollen die unterschiedliche Relation zwischen präklinischen Modellen und zugehörigen Krankheitsbildern verdeutlichen:

Der Neurolathyrismus, der durch die neurotoxische, in der Kichererbse vorkommende Aminosäure β-Oxalyl-aminoalanin (L-BOAA) verursacht wird, ist sowohl in Krankheitsmodellen, als auch – höchstwahrscheinlich – klinisch durch Weglassen des schädigenden Exzitotoxins zu verhindern oder zu bessern. Bei dieser pathogenetisch sehr aufschlussreichen Erkrankung verursacht L-BOAA als AMPA-Agonist eine Degeneration von Motoneuronen im Neocortex und im vorderen Lumbalmark mit typischer spastischer Paraparese, v.a. bei Männern. L-BOAA führt selektiv in diesen Neuronen zur Komplex I-Hemmung in Mitochondrien mit konsekutiver ROS-Bildung und Oxidation von SH-Gruppen in Proteinen. Dies lässt sich in einem Mausmodell durch das Antioxidans α-Liponsäure verhindern. Auch AMPA-Antagonisten verhindern in einem solchen Modell die Komplex-I-Hemmung: Die Glu-Toxizität ist wohl auch durch eine verminderte GSH-Synthese infolge einer Cystein-Aufnahmehemmung, also durch eine reduzierte ROS-Entgiftung bedingt, was zur mitochondrialen Dysfunktion führt.

Bei M. Friedreich, bei dem nach präklinischen Erkenntnissen vieles für eine mitverursachende Energiestoffwechselstörung spricht, wurde klinisch über eine Besserung der Kardiomyopathie unter Idebenon, einem Fänger freier Radikale, berichtet (Rustin et al. 1999). Aufgrund der geschilderten Zusammenhänge zwischen exzitotoxischen Aminosäuren und einer Überlastung mit ROS sollte bei dieser erblichen Neurodegeneration auch eine Therapie mit antiglutamatergen Substanzen in Betracht kommen (siehe z.B. Filla et al. 1993). Ein signifikanter und vor allem klinisch relevanter Effekt kann jedoch nur mit höheren Fallzahlen als den 12 Patienten in der erwähnten Studie von Filla et al. erwartet werden.

Die Amyotrophe Lateralsklerose (ALS) wird manchmal als Paradebeispiel der Bestätigung von präklinisch entstandenen Therapiehoffnungen durch eine klinisch wirksame Substanz dargestellt. Riluzol führt tatsächlich zu einer Steigerung der Lebenserwartung von ALS-Patienten (Lacomblez et al. 1996), deren Relevanz jedoch umstritten ist.

Bei M. Huntington wird ein zu hoher, die Mitochondrien überlastender Energieverbrauch durch Ubiquitinierung von abgelagerten Fragmenten des mutanten Genprodukts Huntingtin diskutiert. Dieser übersteigerte Energieverbrauch soll betroffene glutamaterg innervierte Neurone, beispielsweise des Striatums, anfällig gegenüber exzitotoxischen Aminosäuren machen. Unter anderem werden derzeit antiglutamaterge Therapieprinzipien (z.B. Riluzol) klinisch geprüft. Der nicht-kompetitive NMDA-Rezeptorantagonist Remacemide erwies sich jedoch nach einer jüngst in Neurology (The Huntington Study Group 2001) veröffentlichten klinischen Studie an »frühen« Huntington-Patienten als unwirksam.

Nach dem bisher Gesagten dürfte es sinnvoll sein, verschiedene Angriffsziele bei der therapeutischen Verhinderung bzw. Prophylaxe von Neurodegeneration miteinander zu kombinieren, evtl. in geeigneter zeitlicher Reihenfolge, da offensichtlich verschiedene Schädigungsmechanismen aufeinander folgen. Zum Beispiel bieten sich an: Verminderung extrazellulären Glu *plus* Verminderung der neuronalen Erregbarkeit *plus* Verhinderung der Apoptose.

Die folgende Darstellung einer eigenen, präklinisch erfolgreichen neuroprotektiven Substanz mit wahrscheinlich mehreren Angriffspunkten will nicht außer acht lassen, dass bisherige z.T. hochgestochene Erwartungen aus Therapieerfolgen an Tiermodellen in klinischen Studien allzuhäufig enttäuscht wurden.

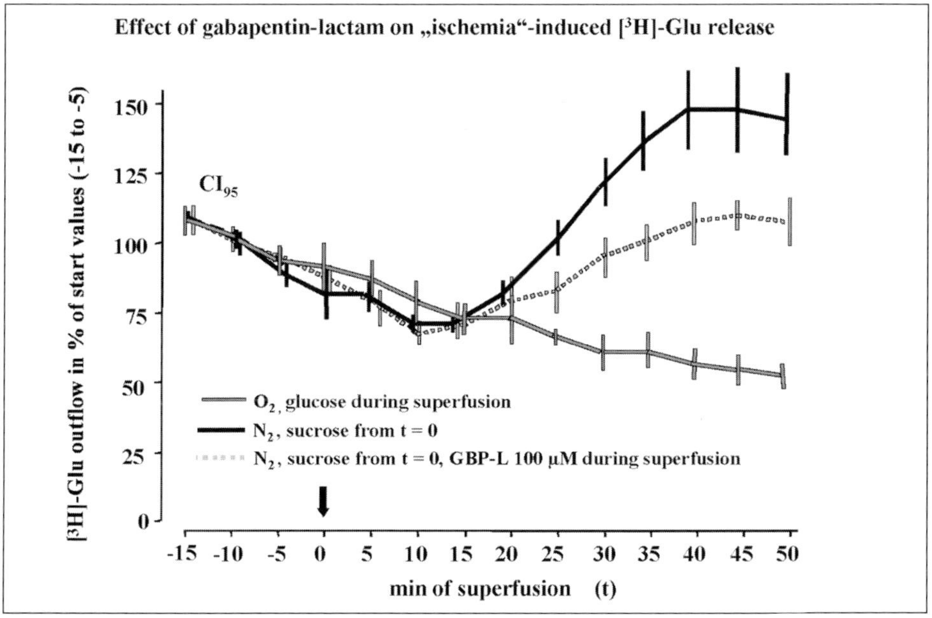

Abb. 4: Verminderung extrazellulären Glu

Abbildung 4, die der Veröffentlichung Jehle et al. (2000) entnommen wurde, zeigt die durch *»in vitro«*-Ischämie induzierte Glu-Ausschüttung in Hippocampusschnitten der Ratte. Diese *»in vitro«*-Ischämie wurde durch Ersatz von Glucose und Sauerstoff durch Sucrose und Stickstoff in der extrazellulären Flüssigkeit erzeugt. Die Entwicklungssubstanz Gabapentin-Lactam (GBP-L), ein Abkömmling des Antikonvulsivums Gabapentin (GBP), verminderte den Anstieg der extrazellulären Glu-Konzentration deutlich.

Gewissermaßen als erstes pathophysiologisches Ziel konnte GBP-L somit die »Ischämie«-bedingte extrazelluläre Glu-Konzentration senken.

Abbildung 5 stammt ebenfalls aus der Veröffentlichung Jehle et al. (2000). Sie vergleicht den Effekt von GBP-L mit demjenigen der Muttersubstanz GBP, das die »Ischämie«-evozierte Glu-Freisetzung ebenfalls reduzierte. Im weiteren zeigt diese Abbildung die Antagonisierbarkeit des Effektes von GBP-L durch den K_{ATP}-Kanalantagonisten Glibenclamid. GBP-L wirkt also als K_{ATP}-Kanal-Agonist. Ähnliches kann auch für GBP gezeigt werden (Freiman et al. 2001, in Abbildung 4 nicht dargestellt).

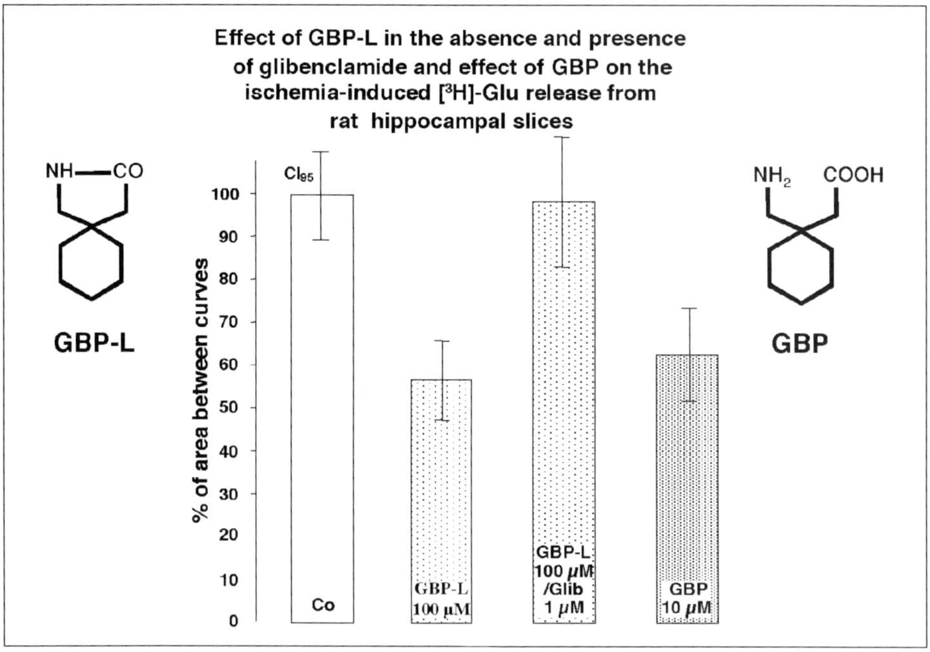

Abb. 5: Verminderung extrazellulären Glu

Wo liegt der Unterschied zwischen GBP und GBP-L?

Abbildung 6 erläutert diesen Unterschied anhand eines z.T. bereits bekannten zellulären Schemas (vgl. Abbildung 3). In dieser Zelle ist zusätzlich zu dem bereits erwähnten mitochondrialen K_{ATP}-Kanal ein weiterer K_{ATP}-Kanal in der Plasmamembran eingezeichnet. Öffnung dieses plasmamembranären Kanals lässt K^+ ausströmen, re- oder hyperpolarisiert damit die Zelle und führt zur Ver-

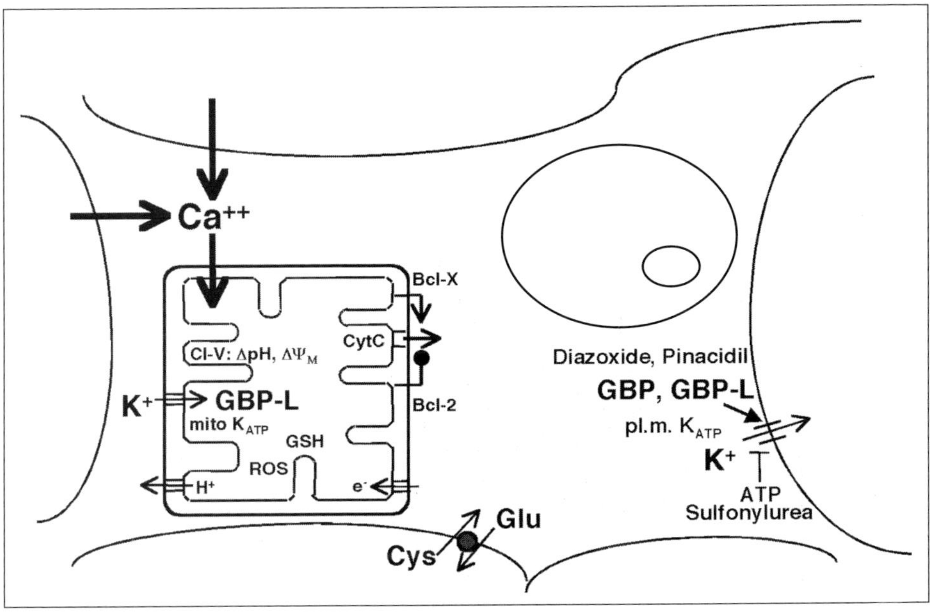

Abb. 6: Unterschiede zwischen GBP und GBP-L

minderung ihrer Erregbarkeit. Die verminderte Depolarisationsbereitschaft glutamaterger Neurone durch eine plasmamembranäre K_{ATP}-Kanalöffnung dürfte auch der Grund für die geringere »Ischämie-bedingte« Glu-Freisetzung aus den Hippocampusschnitten der Abbildungen 4 und 5 sein. Intrazelluläres ATP hingegen hemmt die Kanalöffnung und erlaubt die Depolarisation. Dies scheint energetisch sinnvoll, indem hohe intrazelluläre Energievorräte die depolarisationsbedingte Erregbarkeit oder Leistungsbereitschaft der Zelle auch verkraften können. Mangel an Energie bzw. an ATP öffnet jedoch die K_{ATP}-Kanäle; die so verminderte Erregbarkeit spart Energie. Die plasmamembranäre K_{ATP}-Kanalöffnung wirkt auch der Ischämie-bedingten Depolarisation entgegen und vermindert somit die Glu-Freisetzung.

Die aus der Diabetestherapie bekannten Sulfonyharnstoffe, z.B. der Antagonist Glibenclamid, hemmen ebenfalls die K_{ATP}-Kanalöffnung, die an der Plasmamembran durch klassische K_{ATP}-Kanalagonisten (Diazoxide, Pinacidil) und ebenfalls durch GBP und GBP-L gefördert wird.

Der mitochondriale K_{ATP}-Kanal wird jedoch nicht durch GBP, sondern nur durch GBP-L geöffnet; hierin liegt der Unterschied zwischen der Mutter- und der Tochtersubstanz (eigene, noch unveröffentlichte Egebnisse).

Was bedeutet dies für die angestrebte Neuroprotektion?

Dass die Verminderung einer exzitotoxisch bedingten Erregung durch Hyperpolarisation neuroprotektiv wirken kann, ist leicht nachvollziehbar. Warum aber sollte die Öffnung von mitochondrialen K_{ATP}-Kanälen eine antiapoptotische Wirkung entfalten, wie schon oben im Text zu Abbildung 3 behauptet wurde?

Tatsächlich imitieren Agonisten an mitochondrialen K_{ATP}-Kanälen den protektiven Effekt einer »ischämischen oder chemischen Präkonditionierung«. Mitochondriale K_{ATP}-Kanalantagonisten verhindern diese protektive Wirkung. Präkonditionierung ist eine leichte, dem eigentlichen Schädigungsereignis kurz vorausgehende funktionelle Beeinträchtigung, die z.B. durch kurzfristige Ischämie oder kurzfristige Applikation von Hemmern der mitochondrialen Atmungskette verursacht werden kann. Die Mechanismen der Präkonditionierung werden gegenwärtig nur unzureichend verstanden und wie mitochondriale K_{ATP}-Kanalagonisten eine solche neuroprotektive Funktionsbeeinträchtigung nachvollziehen können, ist ebenfalls unklar. Fest steht, dass sowohl die leichte Hemmung der Atmungskette als auch ein mitochondrialer K^+-Einstrom die intramitochondriale Elektronegativität und damit den elektrischen Gradienten ($\Delta\Psi_M$) vermindern. Dabei bleibt der pH-Gradient (ΔpH) für die ATP- und H_2O-Bildung am Komplex V erhalten oder wird sogar begünstigt (Szewczyk und Marban 1999). $\Delta\Psi_M$ ist wahrscheinlich die entscheidende treibende Kraft für den Einstrom von cytosolischem Ca^{++} in die Mitochondrien, die als Ca^{++}-Puffer eine cytosolische Ca^{++}-Überladung senken, um die unmittelbar »tödliche« Aktivierung von Lipasen, Proteasen, Nucleasen und der Stickoxid-Synthase zu verhindern. Zu hohes intramitochondriales Ca^{++} initiiert jedoch den pathophysiologischen Apoptoseweg und dies kann evtl. durch Abschwächung des Ca^{++}-Einstroms in die Mitochondrien oder durch veringerte Freisetzung von Ca^{++} aus seinen mitochondrialen Speichern infolge einer geringeren treibenden Kraft $\Delta\Psi_M$ unterbunden werden.

Wenn nun GBP-L an zwei neuroprotektiven Wirkorten, dem plasmamembranären *und* dem mitochondrialen K_{ATP}-Kanal angreift, GBP jedoch nur am plasmamembranären Kanal, dann sollte GBP-L dem GBP als Neuroprotektivum überlegen sein. Diese Überlegung wurde an zwei Krankheitsmodellen *in vivo* überprüft.

Abbildung 7 zeigt das erste Modell, die Druck-Ischämie der Retina an der Ratte: Hier wurde unter Narkose der intraokuläre Druck für eine Stunde über den systolischen Blutdruck erhöht, sodass die Retina nicht mehr durchblutet wurde, was man an dem weißen Fundus links im Vergleich zum unbeeinflussten

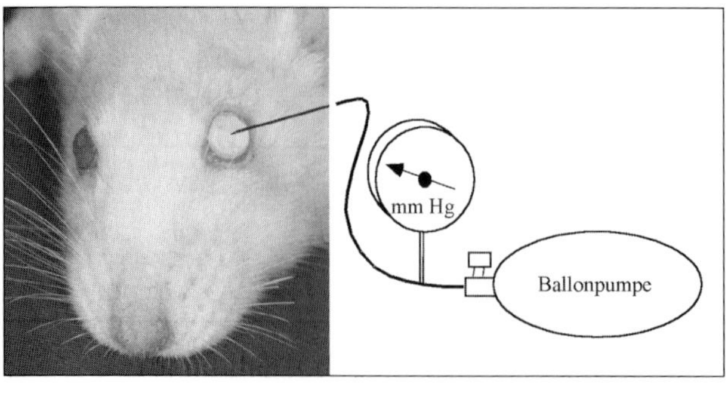

Abb. 7: Wirken GBP und GbP-L auch *in vivo?*
GBP und GBP-L (jeweils 50 mg/kg i.p.) unmittelbar vor und 5 h nach der 60 min-Druckischämie der Retina.

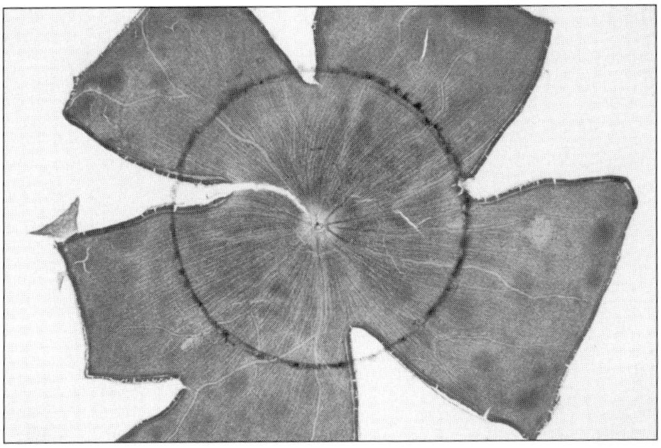

Abb. 8

Auge rechts erkennen kann. GBP und GBP-L wurden in den aufgeführten Dosierungen vor und nach der Druckischämie systemisch verabreicht. Die Ratten wurden 14 Tage später getötet, um histologisch die Dichte der retinalen Ganglienzellen im intraindividuellen Rechts-Links-Vergleich zu untersuchen. Die Frage dabei war, ob GBP oder GBP-L den Ischämie-bedingten Ganglienzellverlust reduzierte.

Zur Auswertung wurden pro Netzhaut acht rechtwinklige Felder aus der Region des in Abbildung 8 eingezeichneten Kreises ausgezählt.

Die nächste Abbildung 9 demonstriert an einem Beispiel, daß GBP-L den Ganglienzellverlust deutlich reduzierte, nicht jedoch GBP: das mittlere Bild steht für die nicht unterscheidbare Ganglienzelldichte nach Vehikel- oder GBP-Injektion. Das Bild rechts lässt den zytoprotektiven Effekt von GBP-L deutlich erkennen, wenn auch die dortige Ganglienzelldichte immer noch beträchtlich unter derjenigen eines Kontroll-Netzhautabschnitts im linken Bildteil liegt. Als Ganglienzellen sind nur die runden großen Neurone anzusehen, nicht die kleineren, häufig spindeligen Gliazellen.

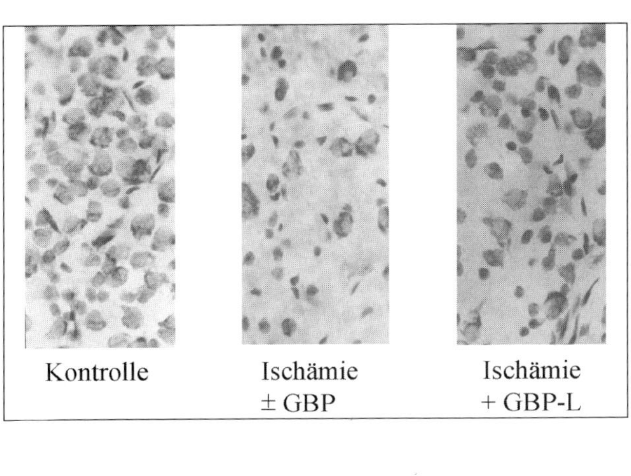

Abb. 9: Vergleich GBP vs. GBP-L.

Abbildung 10 quantifiziert die Effekte von GBP und GBP-L.

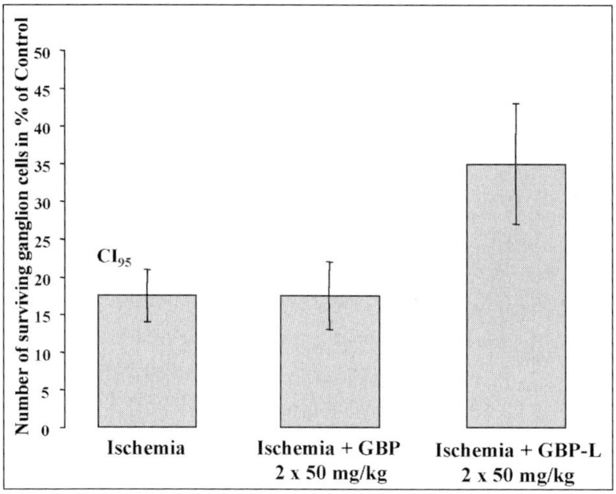

Abb. 10: Vergleich GBP vs. GBP-L.

Trotz eines deutlichen protektiven Effekts mit Verdoppelung des Anteils überlebender Ganglienzellen durch GBP-L ist aus den bisherigen Daten eine klinische Verwendbarkeit von GBP-L z.B. bei Schlaganfall noch nicht abzuleiten, da die Substanz bislang vor (und nach) dem Insult gegeben wurde. Dies entspricht der klinischen Realität nicht, bzw. weist allenfalls auf eine prophylaktisch verwertbare Wirkung hin.

Dementsprechend wurde eine Zeitwirkungskurve erstellt (Abb. 11; Lagrèze et al. 2001). Aus dieser Kurve ergibt sich ein überraschend breites Zeitfenster der postischämischen Wirksamkeit von GBP-L: Ein signifikanter und relevanter Effekt ist noch bei erstmaliger Gabe von GBP-L vier Stunden nach Ende der Ischämiephase deutlich.

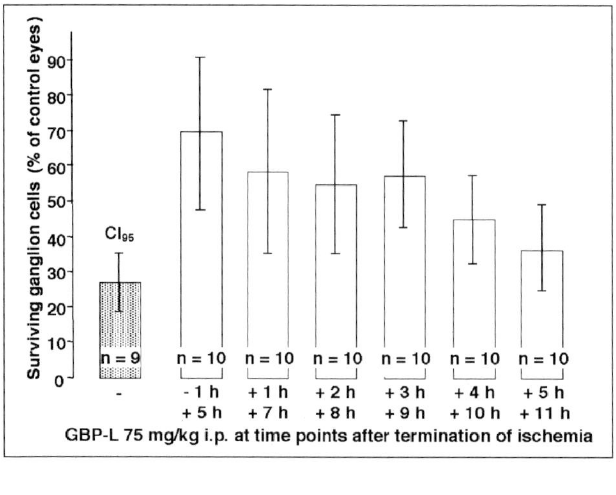

Abb. 11: Zeit-Wirkungskurve von GBP-L.

Eine Dosis-Wirkungskurve von GBP-L im selben Ischämiemodell zeigt Abbildung 12.

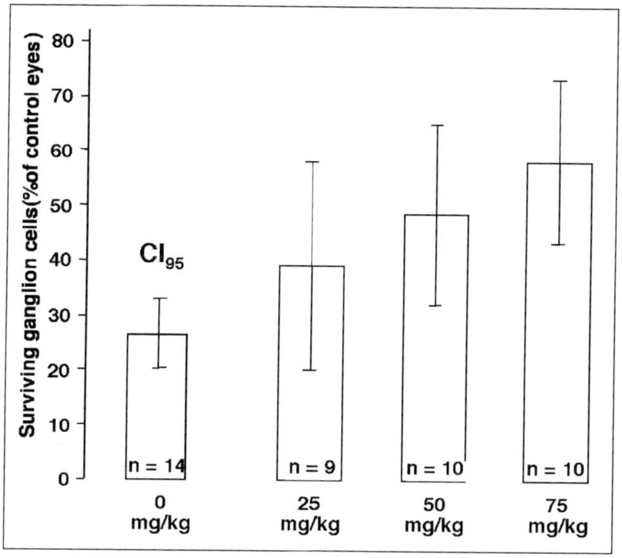

Abb. 12: Dosis-Wirkungskurve von GBP-L.

Im Gegensatz zu GBP scheint GBP-L aus folgenden Gründen als Neuroprotektivum bei akuter Neurodegeneration in Frage zu kommen:

GBP-L und GBP hemmten beide die »Ischämie«-evozierte [^{3}H]-Glu-Freisetzung in Hippocampusschnitten der Ratte als (plasmamembranäre) K_{ATP}-Kanalagonisten. GBP-L reduzierte jedoch zusätzlich den Ganglienzelluntergang nach retinaler Ischämie als mitochondrialer K_{ATP}-Kanalagonist, im Gegensatz zu GBP. Das Zeitfenster für die postischämische Applikation von GBP-L scheint hinreichend weit.

GBP-L wurde im Vergleich zu GBP auch bei chronischer Neurodegeneration, und zwar in einem Modell für die Huntington'sche Erkrankung, getestet.

Zum M. Huntington:

Der Erbgang dieser Erkrankung ist autosomal dominant. Klinisch unterscheidet man zwei Formen: (I) Die adulte Form, die im mittleren Alter beginnt und durch progressive Störungen der Motorik (v.a. Hyperkinesen), durch Psychosen, Reizbarkeit, aggressive Durchbrüche und eine dementielle Entwicklung gekennzeichnet ist. (II) Die juvenile Form, die bereits vor dem 20. Lebensjahr auftritt, und bei der Hypokinesen, ähnlich einem Parkinson-Syndrom, und epileptische Anfälle im Vordergrund stehen. Epidemiologisch zählt man 5–10 Krankheitsfälle der adulten Form pro 100.000 Einwohner und 0.5–1 Fall der juvenilen Form pro 100.000 Einwohner. Pathologisch findet sich ein generalisierter progressiver Neuronenverlust, v.a. im Striatum. Die Histologie zeigt neuronale, v.a. intranukleäre Einschlüsse. Die Ursache der Huntington'schen Erkrankung wurde erst in den letzten Jahren als Expansion der Basensequenz CAG (> 35 CAG-Wiederholungen) im Gen für das Protein Huntingtin auf Chromosom 4 entdeckt. Das zytoplasmatische Protein Huntingtin trägt dadurch überlange Polyglutaminketten, was zu Ablagerungen von Huntingtin-Fragmenten u.a. im Kern und zum Absterben der betroffenen Neurone führt. Die Ubiquitinierung der Huntingtin-Fragmente ist dabei als frustraner Selbstheilungsversuch der betroffenen Neurone anzusehen, um die fatalen Ablagerungen abbaubar zu machen. Eine Therapie ist nicht bekannt.

Bei dem verwendeten transgenen Tiermodell der Huntington'schen Erkrankung, dem R6/2-Mausmodell (Mangiarini et al. 1996), wurde ein Fragment des menschlichen Huntington-Gens in das Genom der Maus eingebaut. Die Lebenszeit solcher Mäuse ist auf 13–17 Wochen verkürzt. Verhaltensmäßig zeigen diese Mäuse ab der 7. Woche Störungen der Koordination und des Gleichgewichts, ab der 9. Woche epileptische Anfälle und Tremor und ab der 12. Woche einen kleinschrittigen Gang und dystoniforme Bewegungen. Die Pathologie ähnelt derjenigen beim Menschen mit Atrophie im Striatum und auch degenerierenden Neuronen in Neocortex und Cerebellum.

Wir verwendeten insgesamt 44 transgene Tiere (HD-Tiere). Ab der 6. Lebenswoche bis zum Tod erhielten sie GBP oder GBP-L oder Vehikel über Alzet-Pumpen verabreicht. Diese Pumpen der Größe 3 * 0.7 cm und einem Gewicht von 1.1 g wurden subcutan auf dem Rücken der Tiere implantatiert. Die untersuchten Gruppen umfassten neben der Vehikel-, der GBP- und der GBP-L-Gruppe zusätzlich eine unbehandelte Gruppe von HD-Mäusen (keine Alzet-Pumpen) und eine Gruppe von Wildtyp-Tieren (keine Alzet-Pumpen).

Abbildung 13 zeigt ein Tier mit Alzet-Pumpe und eines ohne.

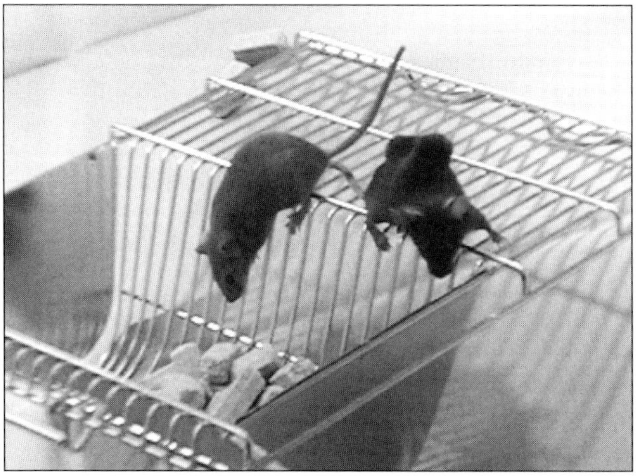

Abb. 13

Die motorische Leistung der Mäuse wurde zweimal wöchentlich durch Balkenlaufen geprüft. Der »schwierige« Balken hatte eine Breite von nur 5 mm, der leichte Balken war 14 mm breit. Die Balken waren 1 m lang. (Abb. 14). Nur der schmale, schwierige Balken erwies sich bei der Testung als »trennscharf«, d.h. als geeignet, zwischen verschiedenen Behandlungsgruppen zu unterscheiden.

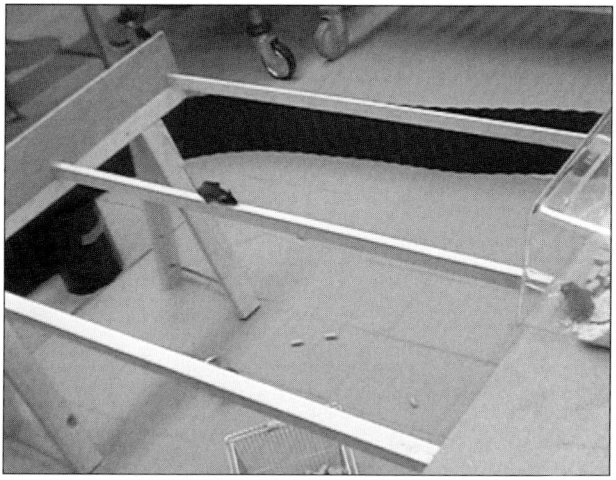

Abb. 14

In einer ersten Versuchsserie wurden Vehikel-HD-Tiere mit GBP-L-HD-Tieren verglichen (Abb. 15).

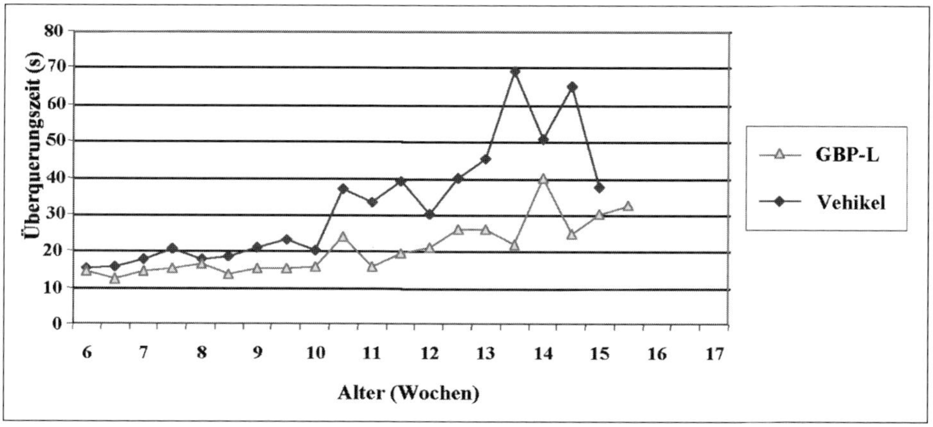

Abb. 15

Die mit zunehmendem Alter ansteigende mittlere Überquerungszeit zeigt funktionell die Krankheitsprogression an. Die Überquerungszeit wurde für jede Maus einzeln nach der Funktion $ln\ y = ax + b$ ausgewertet. Die Vehikelgruppe (n = 8) war deutlich schlechter als die GBP-L-Gruppe (n = 8; p = 0.004).

Eine zweite Versuchsserie verglich u.a. GBP-L-HD-Tiere mit GBP-HD-Tieren direkt (Abb. 16).

In diesem Fall schnitt die GBP-L-Gruppe (n = 8) deutlich besser als die GBP-Gruppe ab (n = 8, p = 0.008). GBP-L konnte bei HD-Tieren die progredienten motorischen Einschränkungen jedoch nicht beseitigen, was der Unterschied zur nicht kranken Wildtyp-Gruppe zeigt (n = 4, p = 0.001).

Die nächste im Sinne der Pathogenese der transgenen Mäuse zu stellende Frage war, ob GBP-L einen Einfluß auf die neuronalen intranukleären Ein-

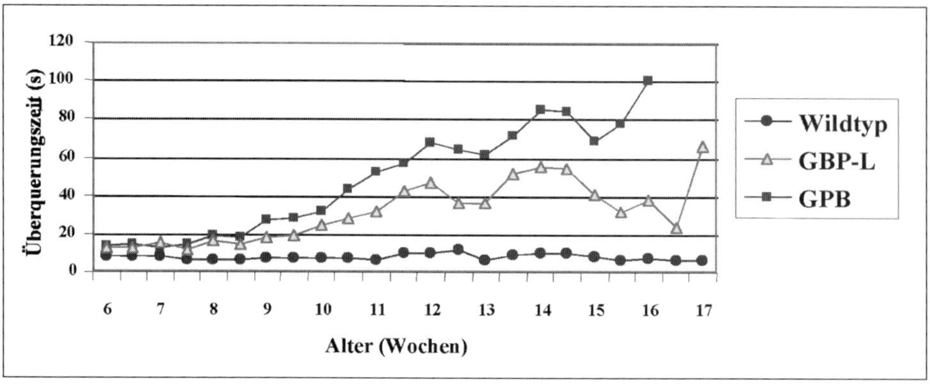

Abb. 16

schlüsse hatte. Histologisch weisen die Gehirne transgener Mäuse neuronale intranukleäre Einschlüsse auf. Diese enthalten Huntingtin und Ubiquitin und entstehen bereits vor dem Auftreten des Phänotyps. Sie gelten als Merkmale der Neurotoxizität.

Abbildung 17 zeigt solche immunhistochemisch mit einem Anti-Ubiquitin-AK (monoklonaler Maus-AK) gefärbte intranukleäre Einschlüsse. Die mittlere Fläche der ubiquitinierten Einschlüsse lag hier bei 7.6 μm^2.

Abbildung 18 demonstriert ebenfalls intranukleäre Einschlüsse in Hippocampusschnitten einer mit GBP behandelten HD-Maus. Die mittlere Fläche der ubiquitinierten Einschlüsse betrug 8.1 μm^2, war also gegenüber der unbehandelten Bedingung fast unverändert.

GBP-L reduzierte jedoch die intranukleären Einschlüsse sehr deutlich, wie Abbildung 19 zeigt. Die mittlere Fläche der Einschlüsse betrug nur noch 3.8 μm^2, was insgesamt einen hochsignifikanten und vor allem relevanten Effekt von GBP-L bedeutet. (Es wurden insgesamt 3600 Zellen mit intranukleären Einschlüssen ausgewertet, d.h. jeweils 100 Zellen pro Hirnregion und Maus).

Aufgrund der Ergebnisse in dem vorgestellten Modell für die Huntington'-sche Erkrankung scheint GBP-L als Neuroprotektivum auch bei chronischer Neurodegeneration infrage zu kommen, indem es die motorische Leistungsfähigkeit beim Balkenlaufen im Vergleich zu Vehikel-behandelten oder mit GBP behandelten HD-Tieren eindeutig verbesserte und die pathophysiologisch bedeutsamen intranukleären Einschlüsse erheblich reduzierte.

GBP-L verlängerte die Überlebenszeit bei Gabe ab der sechsten Woche nicht signifikant. Künftige Untersuchungen mit Verabreichung ab der ersten Lebenswoche sollten somit die Frage eines Einflusses auf die Überlebenszeit prüfen.

Ob GBP-L auch bei anderen neurodegenerativen »Polyglutamin-Erkrankungen« günstig wirkt bzw. ein generelles antiapoptotisches Prinzip darstellt sind offene und ebenfalls prüfungsbedürftige Fragen. Die Muttersubstanz GBP, ein Antikonvulsivum, das u.a. klinisch als Analgetikum bei chronischen Schmerzen häufig eingesetzt wird (Jensen 2002), enthält als Verunreinigung GBP-L in bis zu 1.4% (Knörle et al., Manuskript in Vorbereitung). Entgegen vielversprechender Ergebnisse in Tiermodellen (Gurney et al. 1996), blieb die klinische Anwendung

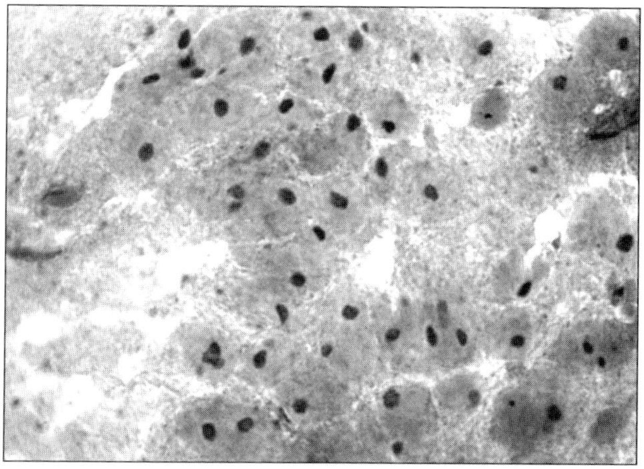

Abb. 17

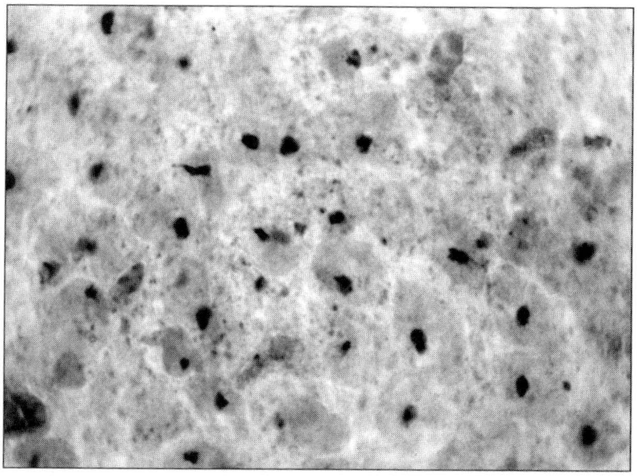

Abb. 18

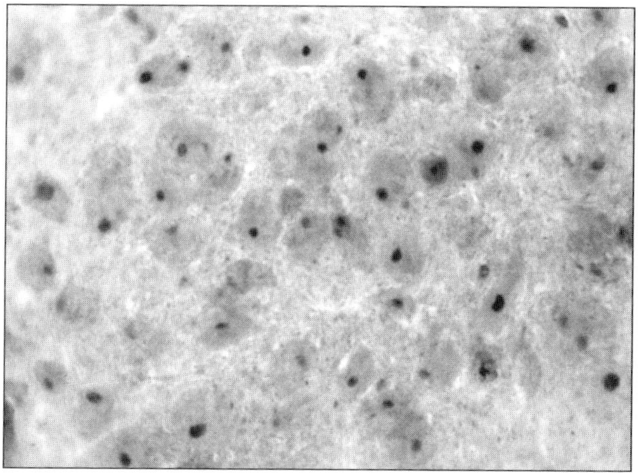

Abb. 19

von GBP bei neurodegenerativen Erkrankungen bisher enttäuschend (Miller et al. 2001). Möglicherweise reichte das Ausmaß der Verunreinigung der GBP-Kapseln mit GBP-L nicht aus, um einen neuroprotektiven Effekt der Tochtersubstanz deutlich werden zu lassen.

Danksagung

Wir bedanken uns bei Prof. Dr. R. Jackisch, Institut für Experimentelle und Klinische Pharmakologie und Toxikologie der Universität Freiburg, für seine kritische Durchsicht dieser Veröffentlichung.

Literatur

1. Feuerstein TJ, Zucker B (2002) Neuroprotection. Neuropediatrics 33:A8
2. Freiman TM, Kukolja J, Heinemeyer J, Eckhardt K, Aranda H, Rominger A, Dooley DJ, Zentner J, Feuerstein TJ (2001) Modulation of K^+-evoked [^{3}H]-noradrenaline release from rat and human brain slices by gabapentin: Involvement of K_{ATP} channels. Naunyn-Schmiedeberg's Arch Pharmacol 363:537–542
3. Filla A, De Michele G, Orefice G, Santorelli F, Trombetta L, Banfi S, Squitieri F, Napolitano G, Puma D, Campanella G (1993) A double-blind cross-over trial of amantadine hydrochloride in Friedreich's ataxia. Can J Neurol Sci 20:52–55
4. Gurney ME, Cutting FB, Zhai P, Doble A, Taylor CP, Andrus PK, Hall ED (1996) Benefit of vitamin E, riluzole and gabapentin in a transgenic model of familial amyotrophic lateral sclerosis. Ann Neurol 39:147–157
5. Jehle T, Lagrèze WA, Blauth E, Knörle R, Schnierle P, Lücking CH, Feuerstein TJ (2000) Gabapentin-lactam (8-aza-spiro[5,4]decan-9-on, GBP-L) inhibits glucose oxygen deprivation-induced [3H]-glutamate release and is a neuroprotective agent in a model of acute retinal ischemia. Naunyn-Schmiedeberg's Arch Pharmacol 362:74–81
6. Jensen TS Anticonvulsants in neuropathic pain: rationale and clinical evidence. Eur J Pain 6 (Suppl A):61–68
7. Knörle R, Feuerstein TJ, Schulze-Bonhage A (2002) Determination of gabapentin-lactam in serum of patients under gabapentin therapy, *submitted for publication*
8. Lacomblez L, Bensimon G, Leigh PN, Guillet P, Meininger V (1996) Dose-ranging study of riluzole in amyotrophic lateral sclerosis. Amyotrophic Lateral Sclerosis/Riluzole Study Group II. Lancet 347:1425–1431
9. Lagrèze W, Müller-Velten R, Feuerstein TJ (2001) The neuroprotective properties of gabapentin-lactam. Graefe's Arch Clin Exp Ophthalmol 239:845–849
10. Ludolph AC, Schwarz J (2001) Grundlagen der klinischen Neuroprotektion. 1. Auflage, UNI-MED, Bremen
11. Mangiarini L, Sathasivam K, Seller M, Cozens B, Harper A, Hetherington C, Lawton M, Trottier Y, Lehrach H, Davies SW, Bates GP (1996) Exon 1 of the HD gene with an expanded CAG repeat is sufficient to cause a progressive neurological phenotype in transgenic mice. Cell 87:493–506
12. Miller RG, Moore DH 2nd, Gelinas DF, Dronsky V, Mendoza M, Barohn RJ, Bryan W, Ravits J, Yuen E, Neville H, Ringel S, Bromberg M, Petajan J, Amato AA, Jackson C, Johnson W, Mandler R, Bosch P, Smith B, Graves M, Ross M, Sorenson EJ, Kelkar P, Parry G, Olney R (2001) Phase III randomized trial of gabapentin in patients with amyotrophic lateral sclerosis. Neurology 56: 843–848

13. Rustin P, von Kleist-Retzow JC, Chantrel-Groussard K, Sidi D, Munnich A, Rotig A (1999) Effect of idebenone on cardiomyopathy in Friedreich's ataxia: a preliminary study. Lancet 354:477–479
14. Schubert D, Piasecki D (2001) Oxidative glutamate toxicity can be a component of the excitotoxicity cascade. J Neurosci 21:7455–7462
15. Szewczyk A, Marban E (1999) Mitochondria: a new target for K channel openers? Trends Pharmacol Sci 4:157–161
16. Szewczyk A, Wojtczak L (2002) Mitochondria as a pharmacological target. Pharmacol Rev 54:101–127
17. The Huntington Study Group (2001) A randomized, placebo-controlled trial of coenzyme Q10 and remacemide in Huntington's disease. Neurology 57: 397–404

Neuropharmakologie: extrapyramidale Bewegungsstörungen

G.B. Landwehrmeyer

Einleitung

Extrapyramidale Bewegungsstörungen begegnen in der neuropädiatrischen Praxis nicht selten; da es sich oft um symptomatische Bewegungsstörungen handelt, ist eine korrekte ätiologische Einordnung von besonderer Bedeutung. In diesem Beitrag soll zunächst das gegenwärtige Verständnis der Funktion der Basalganglien und der Pathophysiologie der wichtigsten Syndrome mit prominenter Beteiligung der Basalganglien (Bradykinesie, Choreoathetose, Dystonie und Tremor) dargestellt werden; im Folgenden wird anhand der Leitsymptome Parkinsonsyndrom, Choreoathetose, Dystonie und Tremor die Differentialdiagnose und Differentialtherapie von Basalganglienerkrankungen diskutiert.

Basalganglien – Anatomie, Funktion und Pathophysiologie

Die Funktion der Basalganglien, zu denen üblicherweise das Striatum (mit den beiden Kerngebieten Nucleus caudatus und Putamen), das Globus pallidus mit der Substantia nigra pars reticulata, die dopaminerge Substantia nigra pars compacta sowie der Nucleus subthalamicus gerechnet werden, galt – um K. Wilson zu zitieren – lange als dunkel, passend zu ihrer Lage im »Keller« des Vorderhirns. Funktionell spielen die Basalganglien eine modulatorische Rolle, klinisch am besten fassbar in der Modulation der Motorik. Nach gegenwärtigem Verständnis dienen die Basalganglien der Verstärkung selektierter motorischer Programme bei gleichzeitiger Hemmung konkurrierender Programme (1). Eine unzureichende Verstärkung motorischer Programme führt zur Hypokinesie, eine fehlende Hemmung konkurrierender motorischer Programme zu Chorea/Choreoathetose (bei unzureichender Hemmung phasischer Innervationsmuster) oder zu dystonen Störungen (bei inadäquater Balance verschiedener tonischer Innervationsmuster). In sehr vereinfachter modellhafter Form wird ein motorisches Programm von einer Generatorstruktur (z.B. den supplementär-motorischen Arealen oder dem präfrontalen Cortex) parallel auf zwei verschiedenen Ebenen in die Basalganglien eingespeist, zum einen auf Ebene des Striatums, zum anderen auf Ebene des N. subthalamicus (Abb. 1). In der wesentlichen afferenten Struktur, dem Striatum, wird durch glutamaterge cortico-striatale Afferenzen eine umschriebene Gruppe inhibitorischer GABA-erger Projektionsneurone erregt, die ihrerseits einen hemmenden Einfluss auf spontanaktive inhibitorische GABA-erge Neurone des Globus pallidus internus/Substantia nigra pars reticu-

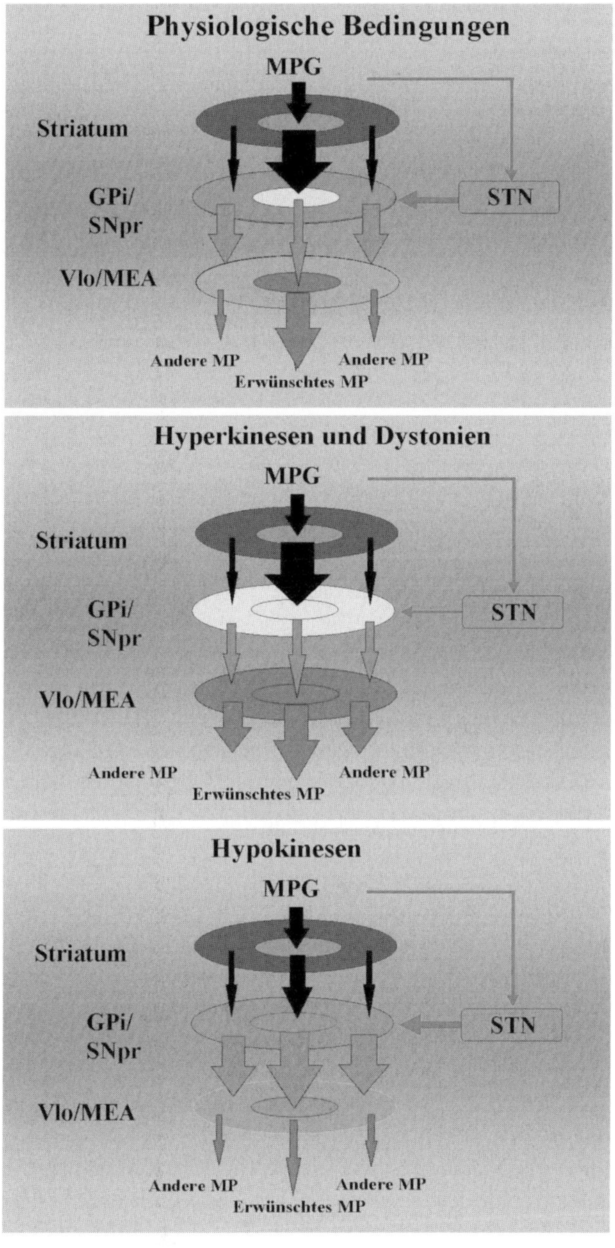

Abb. 1: Funktion der Basalganglien

lata als der wesentlichen efferenten Struktur der Basalganglien ausüben und dadurch eine Disinhibition thalamokortikaler Neurone bewirken; so werden erwünschte motorische Programme verstärkt. In der Nachbarschaft der Gruppe erregter Neurone (d.h. der Repräsentation gewünschter motorischer Programme) bildet sich im Striatum ein hemmendes Umfeld aus, das letztlich zu einer

Suppression unerwünschter, konkurrierender Motorprogramme auf Ebene des Thalamus führt. Vergleichbar einer Irisblende wird die Trennschärfe zwischen erwünschten und unerwünschten motorischen Programmen auf Ebene des Globus pallidus internus/Substantia nigra pars reticulata wesentlich durch erregende Neurone des Nucleus subthalamicus moduliert. Sind die Neurone des Nucleus subthalamicus nicht aktiv oder ganz ausgefallen, öffnet sich die Blende der Basalganglien weit: unerwünschte Bewegungsprogramme können nicht mehr suppremiert werden, es entstehen Hyperkinesen (z.B. bei einem Insult des Nucleus subthalamicus in Form eines Hemiballismus) oder dystone Störungen. Hypokinesen auf der anderen Seite sind vergesellschaftet mit einer erhöhten Aktivität von Neuronen des Nucleus subthalamicus; eindrucksvoll beweist die funktionelle Ausschaltung des Nucleus subthalamicus durch hochfrequente Stimulation mit Tiefenelektroden bei Patienten mit M. Parkinson, dass Hypokinesen vermittelt werden durch eine inadäquat gesteigerte, pathologische Aktivität der efferenten Strukturen der Basalganglien, dem Globus pallidus internus bzw. der Substantia nigra pars reticulata (2–4).

Hypokinetisch-rigide Syndrome = Parkinsonsyndrome

Hypokinetisch-rigide Syndrome sind bei Kindern selten; die Häufigkeit juveniler Parkinsonsyndrome (Symptombeginn vor dem 21. Lebensjahr) in der Fallserie von Schrag et al. betrug z.B. nur 10 von 149 Patienten mit Erkrankungsbeginn vor dem 40. Lebensjahr und lag somit bei etwa 5 pro 1.000.000 Einwohner (5). Die niedrige Prävalenz von Parkinsonsyndromen bei Kindern reflektiert vermutlich die Tatsache, dass der häufigste Grund für ein Parkinsonsyndrom bei Erwachsenen, die ideopathische Parkinsonerkrankung mit Lewy-Körperchen, eine altersabhängige Inzidenz zeigt. Patienten mit Symptombeginn zwischen dem 20. und 40. Lebensjahr zeigen autoptisch fast immer eine typische Lewy-Körperchen-Pathologie (6). In der Literatur sind dagegen nur 2 Patienten mit juvenilem Symptombeginn berichtet, die Lewy-Körperchen bei im übrigen eher atypischer Pathologie zeigten (7, 8), sodass eine ideopathische Parkinsonerkrankung bei Kindern ausserordentlich selten ist und möglicherweise gar nicht vorkommt. Zudem äussern sich beim reifenden Gehirn Läsionen der Basalganglien, die im Kontext des ausgereiften Gehirns zu einem Parkinsonsyndrom führen, oft als dystone Störung und nicht als hypokinetisch-rigides Syndrom. Ein Beispiel dafür sind die Dopaminsynthesestörungen, die sich bei Manifestation im Kindesalter in der Regel klinisch als Dystonie präsentieren (siehe dort), bei Manifestation im Erwachsenenalter hingegen als Parkinsonsyndrom (9). Pathophysiologisch liegt der abnorm gesteigerten Aktivität der inhibitorischen Basalganglienefferenzen – wie bei Erwachsenen – oft eine Störung der dopaminergen Neurotransmission zugrunde. Naturgemäß spielen Entwicklungsstörungen, die zu Fehlbildungen des Mittelhirns führen (siehe Tab. 1), bei Kindern eine besondere Rolle; der Nachweis struktureller Veränderungen im MRT ist hierbei diagnoseweisend. Eine ätiologische Differentialdiagnose von hypokinetisch-rigiden Syndromen bei Kindern ist in Tabelle 1 zusammengefasst.

Tab. 1: Ätiologie von juvenilen Parkinsonsyndromen

1. Strukturelle Läsionen: Fehlbildungen, Raumforderungen, vaskuläre Läsionen
Mittelhirn
  Fehlbildungen
    Pontocerebelläre Hypoplasie
    Rhombenzephalosynapsis
    Joubert-Syndrom
    Dandy-Walker-Malformation
  Intoxikationen
    Rotenon (Pflanzenschutzmittel)
Basalganglien
  CO-Intoxikation
  Mangan-Intoxikation
Andere Hirnregionen
  Vaskuläre Läsionen der SMA

2. Funktionelle Blockade der dopaminergen Neurotransmission als unerwünschte Arzneimittelwirkung (UAW)
Dopamine D_2-Rezeptor-Blockade
  Metoclopramid (z.B. in Paspertin)
  Calciumkanalantagonisten wie Flunarizin (z.B. Sibelium) und Cinnarizin (z.B. in Cinazet),
  Atypische Neuroleptika wie Risperdal, Olanzapin und Quetiapin
Isoniazid
Tetrabenzine, Reserpin
Methyldopa

3. Metabolische Störungen
Dopaminerge Neurotransmission
  GTP-Cyclohydroxylase-1-Mangel
  Tyrosinhydroxylase-Mangel
  Aromatische L-Aminosäuren-Decarboxylase-Mangel
Andere
  Kupferstoffwechsel: M. Wilson

4. Degenerative Erkrankungen
Hereditäre Parkinsonsyndrome (autosomal-rezessiv)
  Park2: Parkin-Mutationen
Triplet-Repeat-Erkrankungen (autosomal-dominant)
  Huntington-Erkrankung, Westphal-Variante
  SCA3
  Neuronal intranuclear inclusion disease (NIID)
Panthotenkinase-assoziierte Neurodegeneration (PKAN) = Hallervorden-Spatz
Niemann-Pick Typ C

Wie auch bei Erwachsenen ist ein häufiger Grund eines hypokinetisch-rigiden Syndroms eine unerwünschte Wirkung von Medikamenten, vor allem von Substanzen mit dopamin-D_2-rezeptor-antagonistischen Eigenschaften. Hierbei ist besonders zu erwähnen Metoclopramid (z.B. in Paspertin®), ein potenter Dopamin-D_2-Rezeptorantagonist, der im Regelfall die Bluthirnschranke nicht passiert, bei Kindern allerdings durchaus häufig zu einem hypokinetisch-rigiden Syndrom oder Frühdyskinesien führen kann sowie bestimmte Calciumkanalblocker wie Flunarizin (z.B. Sibelium®) und Cinnarizin (z.B. in Cinazet®).

Auch die als atypische Neuroleptika gehandelten partiellen oder schwachen Dopamin-D_2-Rezeptorantagonisten wie Risperidon (Risperdal®), Olanzapin (Zyprexa®) und Quetiapin (Seroquel®) können dosisabhängig zu einem Parkinson-Syndrom führen.

Neurodegenerative Erkrankungen mit Parkinsonsyndrom sind – wenn sie sich bereits im Kindesalter manifestieren – in der Regel genetisch bedingt. Eine positive Familienanamnese ist allerdings oft nicht zu erheben, da es sich meist um autosomal-rezessive Erkrankungen handelt. Ein wesentlicher Grund eines juvenilen Parkinsonsyndroms ist nach dem gegenwärtigen Stand der Dinge eine autosomal-rezessiven Form der Parkinsonerkrankung, Park2, die Folge von Mutationen im Parkin-Gen auf Chromosom 6 ist: bei 10 von 13 Patienten (77%) mit einem vor dem 20. Lebensjahr beginnenden sporadischen Parkinsonsyndrom waren Mutationen im Parkin-Gen nachweisbar; bei etwa der Hälfte der Familien mit familiärem Parkinsonsyndrom mit Beginn vor dem 45. Lebensjahr war das Parkinsonsyndrom auf eine Park2-Erkrankung zurückzuführen (10). Klinisch ist ein Parkinson-Syndrom infolge einer Parkinmutation durch eine eher symmetrische Ausprägung der Symptome, einer früh einsetzenden Dystonie (oft der unteren Extremitäten) sowie eine Hyperreflexie gekennzeichnet. Klinisch fällt es schwer, PARK2 von Dopa-sensitiven Dystonien (DSD; siehe dort) zu unterscheiden, da das Ansprechen auf L-DOPA bei beiden Erkrankungen sehr gut ist; allerdings zeigen sich – anders als bei den meisten Patienten mit DSD – oft früh L-DOPA-assoziierte Dyskinesien (9). Eine Behandlung mit Dopaminagonisten ist deshalb anzuraten, wobei zu dieser Frage allerdings keine kontrollierten Beobachtungen vorliegen. Eine definitive Diagnose eines PARK2 erfordert den (aufwändigen) Mutationsnachweis. Andere autosomal-rezessive Formen eines Parkinsonsyndroms, die mit dem Park6- und Park7- Lokus auf Chromosom 1 assoziiert sind, führen nach gegenwärtiger Kenntnis erst nach dem 25. Lebensjahr zu Symptomen (11, 12). Differentialdiagnostisch zu diskutierten sind – vor allem beim Nachweis deutlicher Okulomotorikstörungen wie einer supranukläre Ophthalmoplegie, die z.B. Cardoso (13) bei 5 seiner 6 Patienten mit juvenilem Parkinsonsyndrom fand – das Niemann-Pick-Syndrom Typ C (diagnoseweisend sind der Nachweis see-blauer Histiozyten in der Knochenmarksbiopsie [14, 15]), das Hallervorden-Spatz-Syndrom (HSS oder Panthotenkinase-assoziierte Neurodegeneration = PKAN; diagnoseweisend das MRI mit dem Nachweis eines »eye-of-the-tiger-Zeichens« [16, 17]), Triplet-Repeat-Erkrankungen wie die Westphal-Variante der Huntington-Erkrankung (18) sowie bestimmte autosomal-dominante spinocerebellären Ataxien (SCA), vor allem die Machado-Joseph-Erkrankung oder SCA3 (19, 20) (diagnoseweisend: positive Familienanamnese und Mutationsnachweis in Leukozyten-DNA), die sogenannte »neuronal intranuclear inclusion disease (NIID)« (21) sowie ein M. Wilson (diagnoseweisend erhöhtes freies Kupfer im Serum und erhöhte Kupferausscheidung im Urin [22]). Eine spezifische und kausale Behandlungsmöglichkeit ist bislang für keine dieser Erkrankungen mit Ausnahme der Wilson-Erkrankung etabliert (23).

Zur symptomatischen medikamentösen Behandlung von hypokinetisch-rigiden Syndromen steht ein ganzes Arsenal von Medikamenten zur Verfügung:

Dopamimetika, insbesondere L-DOPA kombiniert mit einem peripheren Decarboxylasehemmer (Carbidopa oder Benserazid) sowie Dopaminagonisten, MAO-B-Hemmer, COMT-Hemmer, Anticholinergika und NMDA-Rezeptorantagonisten. Um den Früheinsatz von L-DOPA besonders auch bei Kindern und Jugendlichen außerhalb von Störungen des Dopaminstoffwechsels, die in den Folgeabschnitten diskutiert werden, besteht eine lebhafte Kontroverse, da in vitro-Untersuchungen , vor allem in Zellkultur nahelegen, dass bei der Verstoffwechslung von L-DOPA zu Dopamin reaktive Sauerstoffradikale entstehen, die zu einer oxidativen Schädigung der bereits durch den primären Krankheitsprozess beeinträchtigten katecholaminergen Neurone führen könnten (24). Während zweifelsfrei etabliert ist, dass die frühzeitige Einnahme von L-DOPA mit einer erhöhten Inzidenz von DOPA-induzierten Hyperkinesen und Wirkfluktuationen vergesellschaftet ist, konnte bislang kein Beleg dafür erarbeitet werden, dass L-DOPA den natürlichen Verlauf von hypokinetisch-rigiden Syndromen ungünstig beeinflusst (25).

In den letzten Jahren besonders in den Vordergrund gerückt sind Dopaminagonisten, die sich nach ihrer chemischen Struktur in Mutterkornalkaloidderivate (Ergolinderviate) wie Alpha-Dihydroergocryptin (z.B. Almirid®), Bromocriptin (z.B. Pravidel®), Cabergolin (Cabseril®), Lisurid (Dopergin®) und Pergolid (Parkotil®) sowie Nicht-Ergolinderviate wie Pramipexol (Sifrol®) und Ropinerol (Requip®) unterscheiden lassen. Gemeinsam ist allen Dopaminagonisten eine Stimulation der Dopmin-D_2-Rezeptorfamilie, wobei die intrinsische Aktivität am Dopaminrezeptor mit der möglichen Ausnahme des nur parenteral verfügbaren Apomorphins als geringer eingeschätzt wird als die von L-DOPA. Durch eine parallele Stimulation der präsynaptisch lokalisierten Dopaminautorezeptoren kommt es neben einer Stimulation der postsynaptisch lokalisierten Dopaminrezeptoren zu einer Reduktion des Metabolismus der dopaminergen Neurone, womit ein möglicher neuroprotektiver Effekt von Dopaminagonisten begründet werden kann (26). Untersuchungen mit dem Surrogatmarker F-DOPA-PET stehen kurz vor der Veröffentlichung. Die verschiedenen zur Verfügung stehenden Dopaminagonisten unterscheiden sich vor allen Dingen durch ihre Halbwertzeit, die von 3–4 Stunden (Lisurid) bis zu mehr als 24 Stunden (Cabergolin) reicht. Daneben zeigen sich Unterschiede in der Rezeptoraffinität, deren klinische Relevanz zur Zeit ungeklärt ist. In der Erwachsenen-Neurologie hat sich gezeigt, dass der Einsatz von Dopaminagonisten das Dyskinesierisiko deutlich reduzieren (27); bei juvenilen Parkinson-Patienten vor allem mit der autosomal-rezessiven Parkinmutation, die unter Behandlung mit L-DOPA ein hohes Dyskinesierisiko zeigen, bietet sich deshalb eine Behandlung mit Dopaminagonisten an. Kontrollierte klinische Studien bei Kindern oder Jugendlichen mit Dopaminagonisten liegen allerdings nicht vor.

In Kombination mit L-DOPA werden COMT-Hemmer eingesetzt; COMT-Hemmer mit peripherem Wirkansatz (z.B. Entacapon = Comtess®) hemmen außerhalb der Bluthirnschranke den Abbau von L-DOPA und erhöhten somit die zur Verfügung stehende L-DOPA-Konzentration im Serum, die mit der Gewebskonzentration im Gehirn im Equilibrium steht. COMT-Hemmer werden vor allem bei Patienten mit fortgeschrittenem hypokinetisch-rigiden Syndrom eingesetzt. Weniger klar ist die Relevanz von MAO-B-Hemmern wie Selegilin (Movergan®, Deprenyl®); ein zunächst diskutierter neuroprotektiver Effekt der MAO-B-Hemmer konnte in kontrollierten klinischen Studien von einem symptomatischen Effekt durch Hemmung des Dopamin-Abbaus nicht getrennt werden (28, 29). Die Indikation von MAO-B-Hemmern ist vor allem bei juvenilem Parkinson-Syndrom unklar; kontrollierte Studien liegen nicht vor. Bei wenig ausgeprägtem Parkinsonsyndrom und bei L-DOPA-induzierten Dyskinesien werden NMDA-Antagonisten (Kanalblocker niedriger Affinität) wie Amantadin (z.B. PK-Merz®) eingesetzt (30); bei juvenilen Parkinson-Patienten spielt diese Substanzgruppe eine untergeordnete Rolle, auch wegen Bedenken einer möglichen Interferenz mit plastischen Vorgängen im sich entwickelnden Gehirn.

Bei der symptomatischen Therapie von Parkinson-Syndromen stellt sich die Frage, *wann mit welchem Medikament* und in *welcher Dosis* behandelt werden soll. Als allgemeines Prinzip lässt sich formulieren, dass bei im Alltag behindernden Beschwerden mit einer dopamimetischen Behandlung begonnen werden sollte, die nach klinischem Effekt dosiert werden muss, so dass mit der niedrigsten wirksamen Dosis ein möglichst unbehindertes Leben geführt werden kann.

Chorea

Unter Chorea werden unwillkürliche, unregelmäßige, abrupt auftretende, kurzzeitige, nicht repetitive und zufällig verteilte Bewegungen mit distaler Betonung verstanden. Als Choreoathetose werden mehr proximal lokalisierte Hyperkinesen bezeichnet, bei proximal betonter Ausprägung mit großem Bewegungsumfang spricht man von einem Hemiballismus. Pathophysiologisch stehen die Hyperkinesen den Dystonien insofern nahe, als beide Erkrankungen mit einer pathologisch erniedrigten Aktivität der efferenten Strukturen der Basalganglienefferenzen vergesellschaftet sind.

Anders als bei Erwachsenen, wo der häufigste Grund einer persistierenden oder progredienten Chorea die Huntington-Erkrankung ist, spricht eine choreatiforme Bewegungsstörung vor dem 10. Lebensjahr gegen die Annahme einer Huntington-Erkrankung (siehe »Parkinsonsyndrome«). Nach dem klinischen Bild können unterschieden werden zwischen persistierenden Hyperkinesen, transienten Hyperkinesen und paroxysmale Dyskinesien. Eine ätiologische Differentialdiagnose findet sich in Tabelle 2.

Die meisten Patienten mit *persistierender Chorea* mit Beginn im Kindesalter leiden an hereditären Erkrankungen. Die Diagnose einer benignen hereditären Chorea, die als autosomal-dominante Erkrankung vererbt wird, wurde in der Vergangenheit durchaus kontrovers diskutiert (31), bis es mit Koppelungsanalysen gelang, einen Defekt auf Chromosom 14 nachzuweisen (32). Typischerweise manifestiert sich die Erkrankung mit plötzlichen, choreatiformen Bewegungen kleiner Amplitude, die in der Regel im Alter von 1–5 Jahren beginnen und nicht zu einer Beeinträchtigung der kognitiven Leistungsfähigkeit führen sowie keine Progression zeigen (in einzelnen Fällen wurde sogar nach der Pubertät eine

Tab. 2: Ätiologie der juvenilen choreatischen Syndrome

Strukurell	
	Cerebralparalyse
	Kernikterus
Unerwünschte Arzneimittelwirkung (UAW)	
	Antikonvulsiva (Phenytoin, Carbamazepin)
	Orale Antikontrazeptiva
	Amphetamin-Derivate
Degenerativ/Hereditär	
	Benigne hereditäre Chorea (Chrom 14 und)
	Ataxia-teleangiectasia
	Panthotenkinase-assoziierte Neurodegeneration (PKAN) = Hallervorden-Spatz
	HARP-Syndrom
	M. Fahr
	(Huntingtonerkrankung)
Hereditär/paroxysmal	
	Paroxysmale kinesiogene Choreoathetose (PKC)
	Paroxysmale nicht-kinesiogene/dystone Choreoathetose (PDC)
	Paroxysmale exercise-induced Choreoathetose (PEC)
	Choreoathetose mit Spastizität, episodisch (CSE)
	Familiäre Dsykinesie mit facialer Myokymie (FDFM)
Metabolisch/hereditär	
	Mitochondriopathie (Leigh's)
	Wilson
	Lesch-Nyhan
	GM1-Gangliosidose
	Glutarazidurie Typ 1
	Acyl-CoA-Dehydrogenase Mangel
	Methylmalonazidurie
	Propionazidurie
	Hypoparathyreose
	Hyperthyreose
Metabolisch	
	Hyperglykämie
	Hypocalzämie
	Hypomagnesiämie
	Hyper- und Hyponatriämie
	Vitamin B1-Mangel
	Vitamin B12-Mangel
Autoimmun	
	Sydenham-Chorea
	Systemischer Lupus erythematodes (SLE)
	Antiphospholipd/Anticardiolipin-Antikörper-Syndrom
	Purpura Schönlein-Henoch

Verbesserung der Hyperkinesen beobachtet) und die die Lebenserwartung nicht einschränken (33). Ursache dieses Syndroms sind Mutationen im TITF-1-Gen, dem Thyroid-Transkription-Faktor-I-Gen, der eine wichtige Rolle für die Organogenese der Basalganglien spielt (34). Differentialdiagnostisch zu diskutieren sind andere hereditär-degenerativen Erkrankungen wie eine Ataxia teleangiectatica, die Pantothenat-Kinase-assoziierte Neurodegeneration (PKAN; früher Hallervorden-Spatz-Syndrom) und das dazu allelische HARP-Syndrom (**H**ypopraelipoproteinämie, **A**kanthozytose, **R**etinitis pigmentosa, **P**allidumdegeneration; [35]) sowie Stoffwechselstörungen, vor allem das Leigh-Syndrom und andere Mitochondriopathien (Leber'sche Optikusatrophie), die Glutarazidurie Typ I (Glutaryl-CoA-Dehydrogenase-Mangel; [36] und andere Organazidämien/-urien (Propionsäure bei Propionyl-CoA-Carboxylase-Mangel, Methylmalonsäure bei Methylmalonyl-CoA-Mutase-Mangel oder Synthesedefekten des essentiellen Kofaktors 5'-Deoxyadenosylcobalamin) sowie die Wilson'sche Erkrankung (siehe Tab. 2).

Als spezifische Therapie der PKAN wird eine Substitution phosphorylierter Panthothensäure zur Wiederherstellung der Biosynthese von Coenzyme A diskutiert (16). Die Zufuhr hoher Dosen von Pantothensäure scheint nur bei Patienten mit Restaktivität der Pantothen-Kinase hilfreich zu sein. Als spezifische Therapie bei Organazidurien wird eine Supplementierung der Nahrung mit 100 mg Carnitin /kg Körpergewicht/d empfohlen, da die meisten Patienten mit organischen Azidurien erniedrigte Plasmasiegel von Carnitin zeigen (vermutlich durch einen vermehrten renalen Verlust von Carnitin-Konjugaten mit organischen Aminosäuren). Es wird eine Proteinrestriktion auf 0.5–1.5 g/kg Körpergewicht/d angeraten. Der Wert einer diätetischen Beschränkung der Zufuhr der Aminosäuren, deren Stoffwechsel gestört ist, ist unklar; bereits bestehende neurologische Defizite scheinen nicht ausgleichen werden zu können. Zusätzlich wird empfohlen, die jeweiligen Kofaktoren zu substituieren, also bei Methylmalonyl-CoA-Mutase-Mangel Vitamin B_{12} (1000–2000 µg/d) und bei Propionyl-CoA-Carboxylase-Mangel Biotin (5–10 mg/d p.o.).

Bei *transienter Chorea* im Kindesalter mit raschem Beginn ist an immunvermittelte choreatische Syndrome zu denken, in erster Linie an die Sydenham-Chorea als Poststreptokokken-Erkrankung, die häufig mit obsessiv-kompulsiven Symptomen und Tics assoziiert ist (37). Der Verlauf der Syndenham-Chorea ist günstig; zur Akuttherapie wird eine Behandlung mit 3 x 1 Mio IE Penicillin oral für 10 Tage empfohlen, danach eine Prophylaxe mit 1–1,2 Mio IE/Monat für 5 Jahre. Als symptomatische Behandlung der Chorea, die in vielen Fällen nicht nötig ist, wird empfohlen eine Behandlung mit dem atypischen Neuroleptikum Tiaprid (z.B. Tiapridex®) in einer Dosierung von 150–300 mg/d oder eine Gabe von Valproat (z.B. Orfiril®) in einer Dosierung von 20 mg/kg Körpergewicht/Tag. Bei einer Persistenz der choreatischen Bewegungsstörung über ein Jahr oder bei klinisch beeinträchtigend assoziierter Zwangsstörung wird empfohlen, eine i.v. Immunglobulintherapie (oder eine Plasmapherese) zu durchzuführen (38). In den letzten Jahren ist das Konzept einer Poststreptokokken-Erkrankung im Sinne einer akut disseminierten Enzephalomyelitis mit präferentieller Beteiligung der Basalganglien und autoreaktiven Basalganglien-Antikörpern erheblich erweitert worden (39). Klinisch präsentieren etwa 50% der Betroffenen mit einer dystonen Bewegungsstörung, 70% zeigen Zeichen einer Verhaltensauffälligkeit im Sinne einer Zwangsstörung (39). Die Diagnose lässt sich sichern durch eine MR-Untersuchung des Gehirns, die bei etwa 80% der Patienten mit Post-Streptokokken-

Enzephalomyelitis in T2-Gewichtung hyperintense Signale in den Basalganglien zeigt, durch eine Streptokokken-Serologie sowie den Nachweis von Antikörpern gegen striatale Antigene [40].

Hereditär (autosomal dominant) oder sporadisch sind *paroxysmale dyskinetische Bewegungsstörungen* (41, 42). Bei Patienten mit paroxysmalen kinesiogenen Choreoathetosen (PKC; [43]) treten – ausgelöst durch Willlkürbewegungen (z.B. Aufstehen vom Sitzen) – kurz dauernde (Sekunden bis Minuten) dyskinetische Attacken auf, die häufig sind (bis zu 100 Attacken/d) und gut auf eine Behandlung mit Carbamazepin (z.B. Tegretal®) ansprechen; die PKC ist häufiger bei Knaben (ca. 4 : 1), kann mit epileptischen Anfällen vergesellschaftet sein (44) und ist vermutlich eine Ionenkanal-Erkrankung. Als paroxysmale nichtkinesiogene Choreoathetosen oder paroxysmale dystone Choreoathetosen (45) werden mehr dystone, länger andauernde (bis zu 6 Stunden) dyskinetische Attacken bezeichnet, die durch Kaffee, Tee, Alkohol, Erschöpfung oder mentale Belastung, nicht aber durch Willlkürbewegungen ausgelöst werden; Carbamazepin (z.B. Tegretal®) ist in der Regel nicht hilfreich, eher Clonazepam (z.B. Rivotril®) und Acetazolamid (z.B. Diamox®). Als »paroxysmal exercise induced choreoathetosis« (PEC) schließlich werden durch körperliche Beanspruchung induzierte, für ca. 1–2 Stunden anhaltende Attacken bezeichnet; für diese Form ist keine Behandlung etabliert. Weitere Sonderformen finden sich in der Tabelle 2.

Zur Klärung der Ätiologie von Choreasyndromen sind Zusatzuntersuchungen erforderlich, die in der Regel eine MR-Untersuchung des Kopfes einschließen sollten, um strukturelle Auffälligkeiten darzustellen sowie Laboruntersuchungen zum Nachweis einer Streptokokken-Infektion, einer eventuellen Vaskulitis sowie von Auto-Antikörpern und letztlich molekularbiologischer Untersuchungen zum direkten Nachweis hereditärer Störungen.

Bei der symptomatischen Behandlung einer Chorea ist zunächst zu bedenken, dass Chorea in vielen Fällen weniger die betroffenen Patienten als vielmehr deren Umgebung beeinträchtigt. Die Indikation zur medikamentösen Suppression sollte deswegen streng gestellt werden. Als pharmakologischer Ansatz kommen bei allen choreatischen Syndromen in Frage eine partielle Blockade von Dopamin-D_2-Rezeptoren, z.B. durch klassische Neuroleptika oder Substanzen wie Sulpirid (z.B. Dogmatil®) und Tiaprid (Tiapridex®) (46, 47). Alle Substanzen dieser Art führen dosisabhängig zu einer medikamentös induzierten Bradykinese, die (zumindest im Fall der Huntington-Erkrankung) krankheitstypisch vorbestehende Hypokinesen weiter verschlechtert. Da die Brady- und Hypokinese die eigentlich behindernde Komponente der Bewegungsstörung ist, sollte mit möglichst niedriger Dosis und wegen der Gefahr von Frühdyskinesien möglichst unter Verzicht auf typische Neuroleptika behandelt werden. Alternativ steht mit Tetrabenazin (z.B. Nitomane®) eine Reserpin-ähnliche Substanz zur Verfügung, die die Einspeicherung von Dopamin in synaptische Vesikel verhindert und damit choreatische Symptome von der präsynaptischen Seite durch eine Hemmung der Freisetzung von Dopamin mildert (48). Neben diesen Substanzen, die in erster Linie die dopaminerge Neurotransmission beeinflussen, haben sich Antikonvulsiva wie Valproat (z.B. Orfiril, 15–20 mg/kg/d) bei Patienten mit immunologisch verminderter Chorea als hilfreich und relativ gut verträglich gezeigt (49).

Dystonien

Unter Dystonien wird ein Syndrom anhaltender Muskelkontraktionen verstanden, die häufig zu verzerrenden und repetitiven Bewegungen oder abnormen Haltungen führen und damit zu einer Fehlfunktion bei der Bewegungs- und Haltungskontrolle führen. Elektrophysiologisches Kennzeichen von Dystonien ist eine Kokontraktion funktionell antagonistischer Muskeln. Die meisten primären Dystonien sind genetisch bedingt (50); bei Kindern ist die häufigste Form einer generalisierten Dystonie die autosomal dominante DYT-1, die auf eine GAG-Deletion auf Chromosom 9 zurückzuführen ist (51). Die DYT-1 beginnt früh, üblicherweise an den unteren Extremitäten und dehnt sich allmählich auf andere Glieder aus, wobei die kraniale Muskulatur selten, der Nacken gelegentlich betroffen sein kann. Nicht alle Mutationsträger erkranken; es besteht eine reduzierte Penetranz von 30–40% (52).

Von besonderer Bedeutung sind bei Kindern Dopamin-Stoffwechselstörungen als Ursache dystoner Symptome. Metabolische Beeinträchtigungen im Dopaminstoffwechsel zeichnen sich durch eine sehr deutliche und langanhaltende Wirksamkeit eher kleiner Dosen von L-DOPA ohne Wirkfluktuationen oder L-DOPA-induzierte Hyperkinesen aus (53). Die DOPA-responsiven Dystonien können verursacht werden durch Mutationen in mehreren Genen. Als häufigster Grund einer DOPA-responsiven Dystonie ist eine Mutation in einem Gen, das für die GTP-Cyclohydrolase I (GTPCH I), die das Schrittmacherenzym für die Synthese für Tetrahydrobiopterin (TH4) kodiert anzusehen (54). Tetrahydrobiopterin ist ein essentieller Co-Faktor für das Enzym Tyrosin-Hydroxylase (Schrittmacherenzym für die Bildung von L-DOPA), Phenylalanin-Hydroxylase (Bildung von Noradrenalin) sowie der Tryptophan-Hydroxylase (Bildung von Serotonin). Typischerweise finden sich bei Kindern mit DOPA-responsiver Dystonie belastungsabhängige Fußdystonien, wobei sich das dystone Bild ausdehnen kann oder auch abortiv verlaufen kann, so dass sich nur sehr diskrete klinische Auffälligkeiten finden lassen (9, 55). Im typischen Fall zeigen sich deutliche Fluktuationen im Tagesverlauf mit deutlicher Besserung nach Schlaf oder Ruhephasen (53). Nicht selten (ca. 20%) ist das klinische Bild bestimmt durch eine als spastische Paraplegie imponierende Bewegungsstörung (56). Kennzeichnend und diagnosesichernd für eine DOPA-responsive Dystonie ist das gute Ansprechen auf eine Behandlung mit L-DOPA. In den meisten Fällen sind bei Kindern kleine Dosen von 25–100 mg L-DOPA, kombiniert mit einem peripheren Decarboxylasehemmer erforderlich. Vielfach ist eine Besserung rasch zu beobachten; allerdings sollte zum Ausschluss einer L-DOPA-sensitiven Dystonie eine Behandlung über mindestens 3 Wochen mit einer Dosis von mindestens 300 mg erfolgen. Neben den häufigen Mutationen im GTPCH-I-Gen, die in einer größeren Studie bei 30 von 58 Patienten mit DOPA-responsiver Dystonie nachweisbar waren, auch Mutationen in anderen Genen spielen eine, vor allem im Gen für Tyrosin-Hydroxylase (56). Eine Lumbalpunktion mit Bestimmung der Dopaminkonzentrationen und der Dopaminmetaboliten sowie ein Phenylalanin-Belastungstest ist sinnvoll, um eine Beeinträchtigung der Dopaminbiosynthese nachzuweisen. Weitere Gene, z.B. DYT 14 auf dem langen Arm von Chromosom 14 führen ebenfalls zu einer DOPA-responsiven Dystonie, wobei das verantwortliche Gen noch nicht identifiziert ist (57). Gemeinsam ist allen DOPA-responsiven Dystonien, die vor allem bei Symptombeginn in höherem Lebensalter als hypokinetisch-rigides Syndrom imponieren, ein guter Erhalt der Anzahl dopaminerger Neurone in der Substantia nigra sowie im Locus coeruleus eine ebenfalls gut erhaltene Dichte dopaminerger Terminale im Striatum. Neben DOPA-responsiven Dystonien sind auch Dopamin-Agonisten responsive Dystonien beschreiben worden, die auf einen Defekt eines Enzyms (aromatische L-Aminosäure-Decarboxylase = AADC) zurückgehen, das L-DOPA in Dopamin umwandelt (58–60); es wird eine Behandlung mit einem Dopamin-Agonisten (z.B. Bromocriptin), Pyridoxin (Kofaktor der AADC) und MAO-Hemmer empfohlen.

Nach dem Ausschluss einer DOPA-sensitiven Dystonie (auch bei Kindern mit »spastischer« Paraplegie!) stehen als Behandlungsoption Anticholinergica, Baclofen, Benzodiazepine und Dopamin-Entspeicherer wie Tetrabenazin zur Verfügung. Als Anticholinergicum wird vor allem Trihexyphenidyl (z.B. Artane®) eingesetzt. Die Behandlung beginnt mit niedrigen Dosen (z.B. 0,25 mg/d); für einen antidystonen Effekt sind allerdings oft sehr hohe Dosen (50–100 mg/d) erforderlich, die bei einschleichender Dosissteigerung häufig erstaunlich gut toleriert werden. 40–50% der Patienten sprechen wenigsten moderat auf die Behandlung an (61, 62). Ist die Behandlung mit Anticholinergika nicht erfolgreich oder wird sie nicht vertragen, sollte Baclofen eingesetzt werden. Bei Kindern kann damit z. Teil eine deutliche Besserung erzielt werden (62, 63). Da der Erfolg einer bestimmten Medikation im Einzelfall nur empirisch geklärt werden kann, ist es allgemeine Praxis, Therapieversuche mit Tetrabenazine (Nitomane®; [48]), Benzodiazepinen, Valproat und Carbamazepin bei unbefriedigendem Effekt anzuschließen. Als experimentell ist der der Einsatz von Lokalanästhetika (speziell des oral verfügbaren Mexitelin = Mexitil®) zu betrachten, der bei cervikalen Dystonien zum Teil zu einer sehr deutlichen Verbesserung der Klinik führt (64). Die systemische Therapie kann bei Patienten mit fokal betonter (z.B. lokal schmerzhafter oder besonders behindernden) Dystonie durch Injektionen von Botulinum-Toxin A ergänzt werden. Bei sehr schweren generalisierten Dystonien ist ein Trippeltherapie mit dem Dopaminentspeicherer Tetrabenzine (Nitomane®), einem Dopamin-D_2-Rezeptor-Antagonisten (z.B. Pimozide – Orap®) und einem Anticholinergikum Trihexyphenidyl (Artane®) vorgeschlagen worden (65). Insgesamt kann die medikamentöse Therapie schwerer generalisierter Dystonien oft nicht befriedigen. Die hochfrequente bilaterale Tiefenstimulation im Globus pallidus führt (vor allem bei Patienten mit einer DYT1-Mutation) in einem hohen Prozentsatz zu einer deutlichen klinischen Verbesserung, die allerdings erst nach einer Latenz von mehreren Wochen deutlich zu Tage tritt (66–68). Die Standardtherapie fokaler Dystonien ist die lokale Chemodenervierung durch Injektion von Botulinum-Toxin A (Botox® oder Dysport®), neuerdings auch mit Botulinum-Toxin B (Neurobloc®); für eine detaillierte Darstellung der therapeu-

Tab. 3: Ätiologie der juvenilen Dystonien

Primäre (isolierte) Dystonien
- DYT1: AD Dystonie mit frühem (distalen) Beginn (Chromosom 9q)
- DYT4: AD Torsionsdystonie mit Dysphonie und kranialer Beteiligung
- DYT6: AD Torsionsdystonie mit Beginn bei Jugendlichen in Gliedern und cerviko-kranial (Chromosom 8p)

Dystonie-Plus-Syndrome
- DOPA-sensitive Dystonien
  - DYT 5: AD GTP-cyclohydrolase 1 (GTPCH-1; Chromosom 14q)
  - Tyrosinhydroxylase (TH; Chromosom 11p)
  - DYT 14: Chromosom 14
- Dopamin-Agonist responsive Dystonie (Aromatische L-Aminosäuren-Decarboxylase-Mangel; Chromosom 7p)
- DYT11: mit Myoklonus: Myoclonus-Dystonie (Chromosom 7q)
- DYT12: mit Parkinsonsyndrom rapid onset Dystonia-Parkinsonism (RDP; Chromosom 19q)

Paroxysmale Dystonien
- DYT8: paroxysmale nicht-kinesogene Dystonie (PNKD Chromosom 2q; [78])
- DYT10: paroxysmale kinesogene Choreoathetose (PKC; Chromosom 16q (auch: infantile convulsions and childhood athetosis ICCA) und 2q)
- PED paroxysmal exercise induced dystonia
- DYT9: Choreoathetose mit Spastizität, episodisch (CSE; Chromosom 1p)
- Familiäre Dsykinesie mit facialer Myokymie (FDFM; [79])

Heredodegenerative Dystonie
- Aicardi-Goutieres Syndrom
- Panthotenkinase-assoziierte Neurodegeneration (PKAN) = Hallervorden-Spatz-
- PARK2

Tripletrepeat-Erkrankungen:
- Huntington
- SCA3
- DRPLA
- Neuronal intranuclear inclusion disease (NIID)

Metabolisch/hereditär
- Mitochondriopathien
  - Leber's hereditäre Optikusneuropathie
  - Mohr-Tranebjaerg-Syndrom
  - Leigh's
- Wilson
- Biotin-responsive Basalganglienerkrankung
- Lesch-Nyhan
- GM1-Gangliosidose
- Glutarazidurie Typ 1
- Methylmalonazidurie
- Propionazidurie
- Acyl-CoA-Dehydrogenase Mangel
- Hypoparathyreose
- Hyperthyreose

Sekundäre Dystonien

tischen Erfahrungen mit Botulinum-Toxin bei Kindern sei auf Heinen et al. 1997 verwiesen (69).

Tremor

Unter einem Tremor werden unwillkürliche rhythmische, oszillierende (sinusoide) Bewegungen verstanden, deren elektrophysiologisches Korrelat reziprokalternierende Muskelaktivitäten in antagonistischen Muskelpaare darstellen (70). Nach Aktivierungsbedingungen (Ruhe, Halteinnervation, Zielbewegung) werden verschiedene Tremor-Syndrome unterschieden. Die häufigste im Jugendalter auftretende Tremorform ist der essentielle Tremor, der eine zweigipflige Altersverteilung mit einer ersten Häufung von Krankheitsfällen um das 10. Lebensjahr hat (71, 72). Klinisch zeigt sich beim essentiellen Tremor bilateral ein Tremor der oberen Extremitäten, kombiniert mit einem isolierten Kopftremor sowie in der Regel einer positiven Familienanamnese und – bei Erwachsenen – eine Alkoholsensitivität. Zur Differentialdiagnose der Tremores im Kindesalter sei auf die Tabelle 4 verwiesen.

Zur Therapie des essentiellen Tremors mit dem Zielsymptom Händetremor ist ein mehrstufiges Vorgehen anzuraten; Mittel der Wahl ist Propranolol, (z.B.

Tab. 4: Ätiologie der juvenilen Syndrome mit Tremor

Unerwünschte Arzneimittelwirkung (UAW) Lithium Valproat Trizyklische Antidepressiva Bronchodilatatoren Neuroleptika Cyclosporine Schilddrüsenhormon
Metabolisch Hyperthyreose Hepatische Enzephalopathie (Asterixe) Hypoglykämie Hypocalcämie Hypomagnesiämie
Entzündlich Enzephalomyelitis disseminata
Degenerativ M. Wilson M. Huntington Park2 Neuronal intranuclear inclusion disease (NIID) Tay-Sachs
Ideopathisch Essentieller Tremor Verstärkter physiologischer Tremor

Dociton®), in der 2. Wahl Primidon (z.B. Liskantin®) oder die Kombination von Propranolol und Primidon. Zur Eindosierung von Propranolol bei essentiellem Tremor ist zu beachten, dass der wirksamste Dosierbereich bei höheren Dosen (4–5 mg/kg Körpergewicht) liegt; eine Steigerung auf mehr als 5 mg/kg Körpergewicht allerdings scheint mit keinem zusätzlichen therapeutischen Vorteil verbunden zu sein (73). In 50–70% kann unter hochdosierter Propranolol-Gabe eine objektive Tremoramplitudenreduktion beobachtet werden, selten allerdings eine vollständige Suppression. Nach einem Jahr muss mit einem Wirkungsverlust bei etwa 12,5% der Patienten gerechnet werden. Alternativ kann Primidon eingesetzt werden; hier ist ein Beginn im Niedrigdosisbereich und eine schleichende Eindosierung essentiell. Bewährt hat sich die Gabe von 1 ml Liskantin®-Saft zur Nacht (20 mg) mit einer wöchentlichen Steigerung um höchsten 62,5 mg. Ähnlich wie bei Propranolol findet sich bei Monotherapie mit Primidon bei etwa 70% der Patienten eine objektive Tremorreduktion. Auch bei Behandlung mit Primidon tritt nach einem Jahr ein Wirkverlust bei ca. 30% der Patienten ein.

Bei unbefriedigendem Therapieeffekt sollte die Gabe von Gabapentin (Neurontin®) bis zu einer Tagesdosis von 2400 mg, die Gabe von Clonazepam (z.B. Rivotril®) in einer Dosierung von 1–6 mg sowie als Mittel der Reserve die Gabe von Clozapin (z.B. Leponex®) in niedriger Dosierung (12,5 bis 75 mg) erprobt werden. Bei einem unbefriedigendem Effekt dieser medikamentösen Therapieoptionen ist eine Thalamotomie (einseitig) bzw. eine Tiefenstimulation des Thalamus (beidseitig) zu überlegen (74, 75).

Ist das Zielsymptom bei der Therapie des essentiellen Tremors ein Kopf- und Stimmtremor, ist zunächst Propranolol und Primidon wiederum Mittel der ersten Wahl; in der 2. Stufe jedoch bei unbefriedigendem Ansprechen auf diese medikamentöse Therapie ist zu einer Botulinum-Toxin-Injektion im Bereich der Halsmuskulatur bzw. im Bereich der Stimmlippen zu raten (76). Botulinum-Toxin ist Mittel der Wahl bei einem dystonen Tremor und bei tätigkeitsspezifischen Tremores. Bei sehr ausgeprägten Tremor-Symptomen allerdings bieten neurochirurgische therapeutische Optionen (bilaterale Thalamus-Stimulationen) die besten langfristige Erfolgsaussicht (77).

Literatur

1. Mink, J.W., The basal ganglia: focused selection and inhibition of competing motor programs. Prog Neurobiol, 1996. 50(4): p. 381–425.
2. Bergman, H., T. Wichmann, and M.R. DeLong, Reversal of experimental parkinsonism by lesions of the subthalamic nucleus. Science, 1990. 249(4975): p. 1436–8.
3. Limousin, P., et al., Electrical stimulation of the subthalamic nucleus in advanced Parkinson's disease. N Engl J Med, 1998. 339(16): p. 1105–11.
4. Vingerhoets, F.J., et al., Subthalamic DBS replaces levodopa in Parkinson's disease: two-year follow-up. Neurology, 2002. 58(3): p. 396–401.
5. Schrag, A., et al., Young-onset Parkinson's disease revisited--clinical features, natural history, and mortality. Mov Disord, 1998. 13(6): p. 885–94.
6. Gibb, W.R. and A.J. Lees, A comparison of clinical and pathological features of young- and old- onset Parkinson's disease. Neurology, 1988. 38(9): p. 1402–6.

7. Olsson, J.E., et al., Dopa-responsive dystonia with depigmentation of the substantia nigra and formation of Lewy bodies. J Neurol Sci, 1992. 112(1–2): p. 90–5.
8. Yokochi, M., et al., Juvenile parkinsonism--some clinical, pharmacological, and neuropathological aspects. Adv Neurol, 1984. 40: p. 407–13.
9. Tassin, J., et al., Levodopa-responsive dystonia. GTP cyclohydrolase I or parkin mutations? Brain, 2000. 123(Pt 6): p. 1112–21.
10. Lücking, C.B., et al., Association between early-onset Parkinson's disease and mutations in the parkin gene. French Parkinson's Disease Genetics Study Group. N Engl J Med, 2000. 342(21): p. 1560–7.
11. Valente, E.M., et al., PARK6-linked parkinsonism occurs in several European families. Ann Neurol, 2002. 51(1): p. 14–8.
12. van Duijn, C.M., et al., Park7, a novel locus for autosomal recessive early-onset parkinsonism, on chromosome 1p36. Am J Hum Genet, 2001. 69(3): p. 629–34.
13. Cardoso, F. and S. Camargos, Juvenile parkinsonism: a heterogeneous entity. Eur J Neurol, 2000. 7(5): p. 467–71.
14. Carstea, E.D., et al., Niemann-Pick C1 disease gene: homology to mediators of cholesterol homeostasis. Science, 1997. 277(5323): p. 228–31.
15. Uc, E.Y., D.A. Wenger, and J. Jankovic, Niemann-Pick disease type C: two cases and an update. Mov Disord, 2000. 15(6): p. 1199–203.
16. Zhou, B., et al., A novel pantothenate kinase gene (PANK2) is defective in Hallervorden-Spatz syndrome. Nat Genet, 2001. 28(4): p. 345–9.
17. Swaiman, K.F., Hallervorden-Spatz syndrome. Pediatr Neurol, 2001. 25(2): p. 102–8.
18. Siesling, S., M. Vegter-van der Vlis, and R.A. Roos, Juvenile Huntington disease in the Netherlands. Pediatr Neurol, 1997. 17(1): p. 37–43.
19. Zhou, Y.X., et al., Machado-Joseph disease in four Chinese pedigrees: molecular analysis of 15 patients including two juvenile cases and clinical correlations. Neurology, 1997. 48(2): p. 482–5.
20. Tuite, P.J., et al., Dopa-responsive parkinsonism phenotype of Machado-Joseph disease: confirmation of 14q CAG expansion. Ann Neurol, 1995. 38(4): p. 684–7.
21. O'Sullivan, J.D., et al., Neuronal intranuclear inclusion disease and juvenile parkinsonism. Mov Disord, 2000. 15(5): p. 990–5.
22. Brewer, G.J., Recognition, diagnosis, and management of Wilson's disease. Proc Soc Exp Biol Med, 2000. 223(1): p. 39–46.
23. Brewer, G.J., et al., Treatment of Wilson's disease with zinc XVI: treatment during the pediatric years. J Lab Clin Med, 2001. 137(3): p. 191–8.
24. Agid, Y., Levodopa: is toxicity a myth? Neurology, 1998. 50(4): p. 858–63.
25. Simuni, T. and M.B. Stern, Does levodopa accelerate Parkinson's disease? Drugs Aging, 1999. 14(6): p. 399–408.
26. Le, W.D. and J. Jankovic, Are dopamine receptor agonists neuroprotective in Parkinson's disease? Drugs Aging, 2001. 18(6): p. 389–96.
27. Hubble, J.P., Long-term studies of dopamine agonists. Neurology, 2002. 58(4 Suppl 1): p. S42–50.
28. Impact of deprenyl and tocopherol treatment on Parkinson's disease in DATATOP subjects not requiring levodopa. Parkinson Study Group. Ann Neurol, 1996. 39(1): p. 29–36.
29. Impact of deprenyl and tocopherol treatment on Parkinson's disease in DATATOP patients requiring levodopa. Parkinson Study Group. Ann Neurol, 1996. 39(1): p. 37–45.
30. Metman, L.V., et al., Amantadine for levodopa-induced dyskinesias: a 1-year follow-up study. Arch Neurol, 1999. 56(11): p. 1383–6.
31. Schrag, A., et al., Benign hereditary chorea--entity or syndrome? Mov Disord, 2000. 15(2): p. 280–8.
32. de Vries, B.B., et al., Benign hereditary chorea of early onset maps to chromosome 14q. Am J Hum Genet, 2000. 66(1): p. 136–42.
33. Fernandez, M., et al., Hereditary benign chorea: clinical and genetic features of a distinct disease. Neurology, 2001. 57(1): p. 106–10.
34. Breedveld, G.J., et al., Mutations in TITF-1 are associated with benign hereditary chorea. Hum Mol Genet, 2002. 11(8): p. 971–9.

35. Ching, K.H., et al., HARP syndrome is allelic with pantothenate kinase-associated neurodegeneration. Neurology, 2002. 58(11): p. 1673–4.
36. Hoffmann, G.F. and J. Zschocke, Glutaric aciduria type I: from clinical, biochemical and molecular diversity to successful therapy. J Inherit Metab Dis, 1999. 22(4): p. 381–91.
37. Cardoso, F., et al., Chorea in fifty consecutive patients with rheumatic fever. Mov Disord, 1997. 12(5): p. 701–3.
38. Cardoso, F., et al., Persistent Sydenham's chorea. Mov Disord, 1999. 14(5): p. 805–7.
39. Dale, R.C., et al., Poststreptococcal acute disseminated encephalomyelitis with basal ganglia involvement and auto-reactive antibasal ganglia antibodies. Ann Neurol, 2001. 50(5): p. 588–95.
40. Church, A.J., et al., Anti-basal ganglia antibodies in acute and persistent Sydenham's chorea. Neurology, 2002. 59(2): p. 227–31.
41. Demirkiran, M. and J. Jankovic, Paroxysmal dyskinesias: clinical features and classification. Ann Neurol, 1995. 38(4): p. 571–9.
42. Bhatia, K.P., The paroxysmal dyskinesias. J Neurol, 1999. 246(3): p. 149–55.
43. Kertesz, A., Paroxysmal kinesigenic choreoathetosis. An entity within the paroxysmal choreoathetosis syndrome. Description of 10 cases, including 1 autopsied. Neurology, 1967. 17(7): p. 680–90.
44. Thiriaux, A., et al., Co-occurrence of infantile epileptic seizures and childhood paroxysmal choreoathetosis in one family: clinical, EEG, and SPECT characterization of episodic events. Mov Disord, 2002. 17(1): p. 98–104.
45. Lance, J.W., Familial paroxysmal dystonic choreoathetosis and its differentiation from related syndromes. Ann Neurol, 1977. 2(4): p. 285–93.
46. Deroover, J., et al., Tiapride versus placebo: a double-blind comparative study in the management of Huntington's chorea. Curr Med Res Opin, 1984. 9(5): p. 329–38.
47. Roos, R.A., et al., Tiapride in the treatment of Huntington's chorea. Acta Neurol Scand, 1982. 65(1): p. 45–50.
48. Jankovic, J. and J. Beach, Long-term effects of tetrabenazine in hyperkinetic movement disorders. Neurology, 1997. 48(2): p. 358–62.
49. Daoud, A.S., et al., Effectiveness of sodium valproate in the treatment of Sydenham's chorea. Neurology, 1990. 40(7): p. 1140–1.
50. Nemeth, A.H., The genetics of primary dystonias and related disorders. Brain, 2002. 125(Pt 4): p. 695–721.
51. Ozelius, L.J., et al., The early-onset torsion dystonia gene (DYT1) encodes an ATP-binding protein. Nat Genet, 1997. 17(1): p. 40–8.
52. Bressman, S.B., et al., The DYT1 phenotype and guidelines for diagnostic testing. Neurology, 2000. 54(9): p. 1746–52.
53. Segawa, M., et al., Hereditary progressive dystonia with marked diurnal fluctuation. Adv Neurol, 1976. 14: p. 215–33.
54. Ichinose, H., et al., Hereditary progressive dystonia with marked diurnal fluctuation caused by mutations in the GTP cyclohydrolase I gene. Nat Genet, 1994. 8(3): p. 236–42.
55. Steinberger, D., et al., Dopa-responsive dystonia: mutation analysis of GCH1 and analysis of therapeutic doses of L-dopa. German Dystonia Study Group. Neurology, 2000. 55(11): p. 1735–7.
56. Furukawa, Y., et al., Dopa-responsive dystonia simulating spastic paraplegia due to tyrosine hydroxylase (TH) gene mutations. Neurology, 2001. 56(2): p. 260–3.
57. Grötzsch, H., et al., Neuropathology of a case of dopa-responsive dystonia associated with a new genetic locus, DYT14. Neurology, 2002. 58(12): p. 1839–42.
58. Hyland, K. and P.T. Clayton, Aromatic amino acid decarboxylase deficiency in twins. J Inherit Metab Dis, 1990. 13(3): p. 301–4.
59. Maller, A., et al., Aromatic L-amino acid decarboxylase deficiency: clinical features, diagnosis, and treatment of a second family. J Child Neurol, 1997. 12(6): p. 349–54.
60. Korenke, G.C., et al., Aromatic L-amino acid decarboxylase deficiency: an extrapyramidal movement disorder with oculogyric crises. Europ J Paediatr Neurol, 1997. 1(2–3): p. 67–71.
61. Burke, R.E., S. Fahn, and C.D. Marsden, Torsion dystonia: a double-blind, prospective trial of high-dosage trihexyphenidyl. Neurology, 1986. 36(2): p. 160–4.

62. Greene, P., H. Shale, and S. Fahn, Analysis of open-label trials in torsion dystonia using high dosages of anticholinergics and other drugs. Mov Disord, 1988. 3(1): p. 46–60.
63. Greene, P.E. and S. Fahn, Baclofen in the treatment of idiopathic dystonia in children. Mov Disord, 1992. 7(1): p. 48–52.
64. Ohara, S., et al., Mexiletine in the treatment of spasmodic torticollis. Mov Disord, 1998. 13(6): p. 934–40.
65. Marsden, C.D., M.H. Marion, and N. Quinn, The treatment of severe dystonia in children and adults. J Neurol Neurosurg Psychiatry, 1984. 47(11): p. 1166–73.
66. Coubes, P., et al., Treatment of DYT1-generalised dystonia by stimulation of the internal globus pallidus. Lancet, 2000. 355(9222): p. 2220–1.
67. Krack, P. and L. Vercueil, Review of the functional surgical treatment of dystonia. Eur J Neurol, 2001. 8(5): p. 389–99.
68. Vercueil, L., et al., Deep brain stimulation in the treatment of severe dystonia. J Neurol, 2001. 248(8): p. 695–700.
69. Heinen, F., et al., Interventional neuropediatrics: treatment of dystonic and spastic muscular hyperactivity with botulinum toxin A. Neuropediatrics, 1997. 28(6): p. 307–13.
70. Deuschl, G., et al., The pathophysiology of tremor. Muscle Nerve, 2001. 24(6): p. 716–35.
71. Louis, E.D., L.S.t. Dure, and S. Pullman, Essential tremor in childhood: a series of nineteen cases. Mov Disord, 2001. 16(5): p. 921–3.
72. Louis, E.D., Clinical practice. Essential tremor. N Engl J Med, 2001. 345(12): p. 887–91.
73. Wasielewski, P.G., J.M. Burns, and W.C. Koller, Pharmacologic treatment of tremor. Mov Disord, 1998. 13(Suppl 3): p. 90–100.
74. Benabid, A.L., et al., Chronic electrical stimulation of the ventralis intermedius nucleus of the thalamus as a treatment of movement disorders. J Neurosurg, 1996. 84(2): p. 203–14.
75. Koller, W., et al., High-frequency unilateral thalamic stimulation in the treatment of essential and parkinsonian tremor. Ann Neurol, 1997. 42(3): p. 292–9.
76. Brin, M.F., et al., A randomized, double masked, controlled trial of botulinum toxin type A in essential hand tremor. Neurology, 2001. 56(11): p. 1523–8.
77. Schuurman, P.R., et al., A comparison of continuous thalamic stimulation and thalamotomy for suppression of severe tremor. N Engl J Med, 2000. 342(7): p. 461–8.
78. Fink, J.K., et al., Paroxysmal dystonic choreoathetosis linked to chromosome 2q: clinical analysis and proposed pathophysiology. Neurology, 1997. 49(1): p. 177–83.
79. Fernandez, M., et al., Familial dyskinesia and facial myokymia (FDFM): a novel movement disorder. Ann Neurol, 2001. 49(4): p. 486–92.

Neuroleptisch-antiandrogene Kombinationstherapie eines autistischen Patienten mit therapierefraktären Aggressionsdurchbrüchen bei vermutlich neuroleptikainduzierter Leberfunktionsstörung

H. Niederhofer, B. Hackenberg

Zusammenfassung

Es wird über einen 13jährigen Patienten berichtet, der zum insgesamt dritten Mal wegen rezidivierender, auf neuroleptisch-tranquilisierende Therapie nur unzureichend ansprechender Aggressionsdurchbrüche bei bekanntem frühkindlichem Autismus sowie bestehendem Leberschaden an unserer Klinik stationär aufgenommen wurde. Eine antiandrogen-neuroleptische Kombinationstherapie führte nach ca. 3monatiger Behandlungs- und Beobachtungsdauer zu einer deutlichen Besserung der Symptomatik, sodass der Patient wieder in häusliche Pflege und ambulante Therapie entlassen werden konnte.

Summary

We refer about a 13 years old patient who was admitted in our hospital for three times because of autism of the early childhood, liver damage and multiple aggressions. Tranquilizing medication did not show any sufficiant effect.

Combined neuroleptical – antiandrogenic medication caused a significant remmission of symptomatology. The patient could finally be dimitted and therapy could be continued in an ambulant setting.

Einleitung

Nach dem derzeitigen Kenntnisstand der Wissenschaft werden, neben vorrangig verhaltenstherapeutischen Maßnahmen – Patienten mit aggressiver Störung psychopharmakologisch mit Carbamazepin und Neuroleptika erfolgreich behandelt (Schulte et al, 1973; Riederer et al., 1992; Stahl, 1996; Hinterhuber et al., 1997; Faust, 1995). Generell wird jedoch von einer häufigen Therapieresistenz dieser Störungen, vor allem wenn sie mit einer Entwicklungsstörung einhergehen, berichtet (Scahill, 1999). Bei beiden Substanzklassen ist jedoch eine Lebertoxizität (Riederer, 1992; Kutcher, 1997) bekannt. Bei männlichen Patienten wird überdies eine Behandlung mit Antiandrogenen, welcher einer temporären hormonellen Kastration gleichkommt, angewandt (Schulte, 1973; Faust, 1996). Es kann angenommen werden, dass hohe Testosteronspiegel signifikant mit erhöhter Aggressionsbereitschaft korrelieren (Higley et al., 1996) und deren Erniedrigung somit zur Senkung des Aggressionspotentials beiträgt. Antiandrogene Medikation birgt zwar kein Risiko einer Lebertoxizität (Schulte, 1973; Kaiser et al., 1991) in sich, muss jedoch bezüglich Indikation strengstens abgewogen werden. Auch wurde eine Kombination dieser beiden Substanzklassen bisher noch nicht beschrieben, besonders nicht vor dem Hintergrund einer massiven Entwicklungsretardation. Der deutliche Erfolg dieser Kombination könnte für eine zumindest temporär durchzuführende aggressionsmindernde Therapiemöglichkeit sprechen.

Kasuistik

Zur Aufnahme kam ein 13jähriger türkischer Patient, welcher bislang als »Frühkindlicher Autismus« (ICD-10) (Dilling et al, 1993) diagnostiziert wurde. Hinsichtlich der Biographie ist zu berichten, dass der Patient drei ältere Geschwister hat, die Schwangerschaft und Geburt insofern kompliziert waren, als dass eine einmalige Nabelschnurumschlingung diagnostiziert wurde (APGAR allerdings 9/9/10). Die erste stationäre Aufnahme erfolgte im Alter von 3 Monaten wegen einer Tonsillopharyngitis in Kombination mit einer Otitis media beidseits und einer parenteralen Dyspepsie, welche unter konservativ-antibiotischer Therapie ohne Residuen nach drei Wochen abklangen. Die nächste stationäre Aufnahme erfolgte, als der Patient drei Jahre alt war. Neben Hinweisen auf eine mangelnde Förderung im sprachlichen Bereich fiel damals bereits eine deutliche Sprachentwicklungsverzögerung auf. Zu diesem Zeitpunkt beschrieben die Eltern des Patienten ein Sistieren der psychomotorischen Entwicklung im Alter von 9 Monaten. Die organische Abklärung (Audiogramm) erbrachte keinen auffälligen Befund. Auch der nächstfolgende stationäre Aufenthalt – der Patient war damals bereits sieben Jahre alt – wies den Patienten sowohl motorisch als auch kognitiv und sprachlich wie sozial als in der Altersstufe von zweijährigen befindlich aus. Auch fiel bereits ein deutlich erhöhtes Aggressionspotential auf. Die neurologisch-klinische Untersuchung erbrachte keine Hinweise auf eine organische Ursache der motorischen Entwicklungsretardation. Die Schilddrüsenfunktion war unauffällig, ebenso die genetische Untersuchung (Karyotyp 46, XY, kein Hinweis auf ein fragiles X-Chromosom).

Ab diesem Zeitpunkt besuchte der Patient eine Schule für sprachgestörte Kinder. Die abermalige stationäre Aufnahme an unserer Klinik erfolgte wegen rezidivierender Aggressionsdurchbrüche, die eine weitere ambulante Betreuung unmöglich machten. Zu diesem Zeitpunkt lagen, wie auch bei den Vorbefunden, im Rahmen derer mögliche Stoffwechselstörungen und gastroenterologische Erkrankungen wie z.B. ein Morbus Wilson umfassend abgeklärt wurden, die Leberwerte im Normbereich. Der Patient hatte bis zu dieser Aufnahme auch noch keine längerfristige und bekannterweise die Leber belastende, insbesondere aber keinerlei neuroleptische Medikation erhalten. Neben intensiver Einzelbetreuung erhielt der Patient initial 70 mg Chlorprothixen als orale Suspension per diem, wegen schlechter Wirksamkeit und einem Anstieg der GOT auf max. 30 U/l und der GPT auf 51 U/l wurde von einer weiteren Dosissteigerung abgesehen und stattdessen additiv Thioridazin in der Dosierung von 100 mg TD, peroral sowie Flupenthixol, ebenfalls peroral in der Dosis von 1 mg TD verabreicht. Unter dieser Medikation kam es unter zusätzlicher unspezifischer Tranquilisierung mit Lorazepam vorübergehend zu einer zufriedenstellenden Beruhigung des Patienten bei konstant erhöhter GOT und GPT, sodass er nach Vermittlung einer intensiven ambulanten Weiterbetreuung entlassen werden konnte.

Die neuerliche stationäre Aufnahme an unserer Klinik erfolgte abermals wegen rezidivierender, nicht beherrschbarer Aggressionsdurchbrüche bei unveränderter Entwicklungsretardation. Der Patient vermochte zwar Farben richtig zuzuordnen sowie Einzelheiten zum Ganzen richtig anzugeben, konnte jedoch weder Formen richtig einsetzen, Mengen richtig zuordnen oder Längen sortieren. Unter Anleitung gelang es ihm, einfache Alltagstätigkeiten

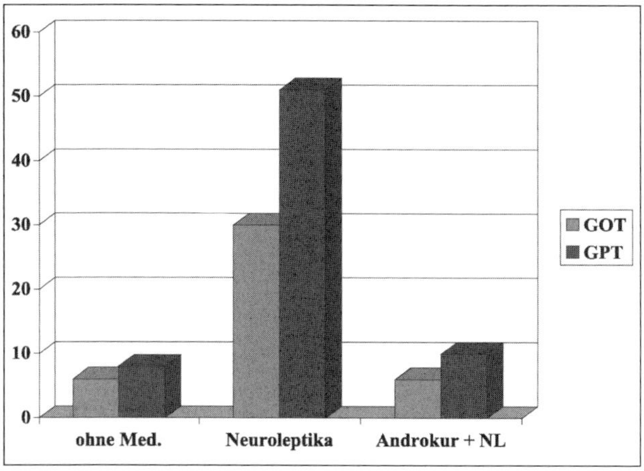

Abb. 1: Veränderung der Leberenzyme bei NL bzw. NL und Antiandrogentherapie.

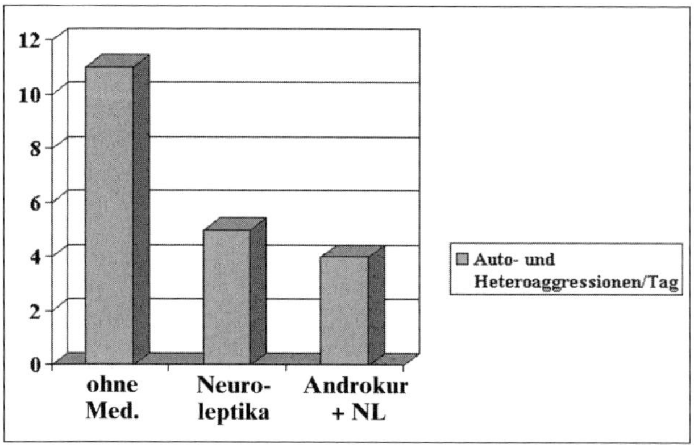

Abb. 2: Veränderung der Anzahl der Aggressionsdurchbrüche durch NL und NL+Antiandrogene.

und die Körperpflege zu verrichten. Zählen oder konzentriert Zuhören konnte er nicht; auch beherrschte er nicht alle Laute, was er jedoch mit einer Zeichensprache teilweise kompensieren konnte. Außerdem wies der Patient eine massiv defizitäre soziale Interaktionsfähigkeit auf. Er wiederholte oft minutenlang Tätigkeiten wie z.B. das Werfen von Messern gegen Wand oder Decke, schlug mit dem Kopf wiederholt gegen eine Betonwand, attackierte unmotiviert Betreuungspersonen und Mitpatienten, wobei auch deren Angst- und Fluchtreaktionen seine Aggressionen nicht zu stoppen vermochten. Eine verbale Kommunikation mit dem Patienten war praktisch unmöglich; seine größtenteils unverständlichen Äußerungen waren monoton, kaum moduliert und entbehrten jeglicher Begleitgestik. Besonders guten »Kontakt« hatte er zu Spielkarten, mit welchen er sich oft stundenlang beschäftigen konnte, indem er sie betastete oder daran roch. Äußerlich wies er Zeichen vorangegangener Selbstverletzungen auf. Sein Verhalten ließ jegliche Spontaneität vermissen. Auch war eine deutliche Hypersexualität zu beobachten. Unter Chlorprothixen-, Thioridazin-, Flupenthixol-, sowie schließlich stattdessen Zyclopenthixol und Laevopromazintherapie kam es zu keiner zufriedenstellenden Besserung der Symptomatik. Der Patient kam somit einerseits zur einstweiligen Entlastung des Betreuungssystems, andererseits zur neuerlichen aggressionsvermindernden Medikation zu uns. Nach kurzzeitiger Weiterführung der vorbestehenden Zyclopenthixol-Laevomepromazin-Kombinationsmedikation unter additiver unspezifisch tranquilisierender Therapie mit Lorazepam unter engmaschigem Leberfunktionsmonitoring (GOT und GPT blieben konstant stabil erhöht) verabreichten wir in der Folge Methylphenidat unter Beibehaltung der neuroleptischen Medikation. Es kam zu keiner zufriedenstellenden Abnahme des Aggressionspotentials des

Patienten. Wegen der bekannten Hepatotoxizität verzichteten wir auf die Verabreichung von Carbamazepin, Valproat, sowie atypischen Neuroleptika wie z.B. Olanzapin. Eine Lithiummedikation wurde von den Eltern abgelehnt. Wir stellten schließlich nach Messung des Serumtestosteronspiegels (mit 2,36 ng/ml im unteren Normalbereich gelegen) auf eine antiandrogene Therapie mit 100 mg Cyproteronazetat per diem (unter Beibehaltung der niedrigdosierten neuroleptischen Therapie mit Zyclopenthixol und Laevomepromazin) um. Nachdem beim Patienten extrapyramidalmotorische Nebenwirkungen (Muskeltonuserhöhung, oculogyre Krisen) festzustellen waren, stellten wir schließlich doch – wegen der zusätzlich sedierenden Komponente – unter engmaschigem Monitoring der Leberwerte auf Zotepin (200 mg TD) unter Beibehaltung der antiandrogenen Therapie nach Absetzen der Zyclopenthixol-Laevomepromazin-Kombination um. Eine neuerliche Messung des Serumtestosteronspiegels ergab mit 2,10 ng/ml einen etwas niedrigeren Wert als bei der ersten Untersuchung. Unter dieser Medikation konnte der Patient seine Impulse zunehmend besser kontrollieren, die Aggressionsdurchbrüche nahmen sowohl an Häufigkeit sowie auch an Intensität ab. Wegen der nach wie vor konstanten Erhöhung der Leberfunktionsparameter setzten wir die antiandrogene Medikation nicht ab, da wir eine neuerliche Zunahme der aggressiven Impulse befürchteten und diese infolge der Leberschädigung nicht durch eine kurzzeitig erhöhte Zotepintherapie beherrscht hätten werden können. Wir konnten den Patienten unter Beibehaltung der vorbestehenden intensiven heilpädagogischen Betreuung schließlich wieder in ambulante Therapie entlassen.

Die erhobenen Befunde wiesen auszugsweise folgende Auffälligkeiten aus: Serumphosphorspiegel 1,96 mmol/l, Creatininkinase 1428 U/l, Pyruvatserumspiegel im Normbereich, Serumamoniak- und Serumlaktatspiegel im Normbereich, ebenso Blutbild und antinukleäre Antikörper, Harn und Kälteagglutinine und Zytomegalievirusscreening. Das Thoraxröntgen und die cerebrale Magnetresonanztomographie waren unauffällig. Aufgrund der erhöhten Creatininkinase wurden eine Elektromyographie und eine Elektroneurographie durchgeführt, welche Hinweise auf ein mäßiggradig ausgeprägtes myopathisches Innervationsbild erbrachten. Die ebenfalls aus diesem Grunde durchgeführte abdominelle Sonographie war unauffällig.

Diskussion

Berichtenswert erschien uns dieser Kasus wegen der guten Wirksamkeit der Kombination von Zotepin und einem Testosteronantagonisten bei einem autistischen, therapierefraktär aggressiven Patienten mit einer additiven, vermutlich neuroleptikainduzierten Leberfunktionsstörung, welche eine höherdosierte neuroleptische Therapie als kontraindiziert schienen ließ. Ebendiese Leberfunktionsstörung machte auch eine additive Carbamazepinmedikation problematisch. Wir suchten daher nach leberschonenden Alternativen für eine aggressionsmindernde Therapie. Bezüglich der Interaktionen sogenannter »atypischer« Neuroleptika wie z.B. Zotepin in niedriger Dosierung mit Testosteronantagonisten liegen unsereres Wissens nach keine eindeutigen Ergebnisse vor. Diese Kombination unter engmaschigem Leberfunktionsmonitoring erwies sich als nur wenig lebertoxisch bei guter klinischer Wirksamkeit. Einerseits, so glauben wir, aus unserem Ergebnis ableiten zu können, kann durch die additive Kombination mit Antiandrogenen die Neuroleptikadosis deutlich erniedrigt werden, welcher Umstand die Hepatotoxizität verringert und außerdem die Wahrscheinlichkeit neuroleptikainduzierter Dyskinesien herabsetzt, was besonders bei Patienten mit einem tiefgreifenden psychomotorischen Entwicklungsrückstand von Bedeutung ist, andererseits trägt die additive Gabe eines »atypischen« Neuroleptikums zur

Verringerung der Antiandrogendosis bei, was besonders bei noch nicht vollständig abgeschlossener sexueller Entwicklung von Bedeutung ist. Es erscheint uns wichtig, auf diese zusätzliche Behandlungsmöglichkeit therapierefraktärer rezidivierender Aggressionsdurchbrüche hinzuweisen, wobei die als gering einzustufende Gefahr von Leberschäden und neuroleptikabedingten extrapyramidalmotorischen Symptomen diese Kombination nicht nur als ultima ratio anzuwendende Methode sinnvoll erscheinen lässt.

Literatur

1. Dilling, H., Mombour, W., Schmidt, M.H.: Internationale Klassifikation psychischer Störungen. Huber, Bern 1993.
2. Faust, W. (Hrsg.): Psychiatrie. G. Fischer, Stuttgart-Jena-New York 1995.
3. Higley, JD., Mehlman, PT., Poland, RE., Taub, DM., Vickers, J., Suomi, SJ., Linnoila, M.: CSF testosterone and 5-HIAA correlate with different types of aggressive behaviours. Biological Psychiatry 40 (11), 1067–82, 1996.
4. Hinterhuber, H., Fleischhacker, W.W.: Lehrbuch der Psychiatrie. Thieme, Stuttgart 1997.
5. Kaiser, E., Gruner, S.: Long-term studies with an anti-androgen/estrogen combination preparation of ist effectiveness, liver tolerance and lipid metabolism in females. Geburtshilfe Frauenheilkunde 51(4), 298–303, 1991.
6. Kutcher, S.P.: Child and Adolescent Psychopharmcology. W.B. Saunders Company, Philadelphia 1997.
7. Riederer, P., Laux, G., Pöldinger, W. (Hrsg.): Neuropsychopharmaka. Springer, Wien-New York 1992
8. Scahill, l., Koenig, K.: Pharmacotherapy in children and adolescents with pervasive developmental disorders. Journal of Child and Adolescence Psychiatric Nursery 12(1), 41–43, 1999
9. Schulte, W., Tölle, R.: Psychiatrie. Springer, Heidelberg 1973
10. Stahl, S. M.: Essential Psychopharmacology. Cambridge University Press, Cambridge 1996

8. Neuromuskuläre Erkrankungen

Drug Treatment In Duchenne Muscular Dystrophy: Practical and Experimental

A.Y. Manzur

The major advances in understanding of molecular genetics and pathogenesis of the Duchenne muscular dystrophy (DMD) have raised expectation of a curative treatment. This however is not yet available and symptomatic and palliative treatment is essential to enhance the patient's quality of life. Physical therapy for prevention of contractures and promotion of ambulation is the mainstay of treatment. Judicious surgical intervention may improve or stabilize motor function in carefully selected patients. Early detection and treatment of respiratory and cardiac complications reduces morbidity, improves quality of life and prolongs survival. This contribution focuses on the current role of drug therapies aimed at improving function and quality of life in muscular dystrophy.

Course of Duchenne muscular dystrophy

The presentation of Duchenne muscular dystrophy is with abnormal gait, inability to run and difficulty in rising from the floor, in the first 5 years of life (Emery 1993, Dubowitz 1995). The relentless progression of muscle weakness together with tendo Achilles and iliotibial band contractures, leads to loss of walking at a mean age of 9.5 years. Once wheelchair bound, there is development of scoliosis in 90% cases. The late teen years are marked by progression of respiratory muscle weakness, leading to nocturnal hypoventilation, respiratory failure and death in late teens or 20's. The associated cardiomyopathy may become symptomatic in approximately 20%. No curative treatment for Duchenne muscular dystrophy is available. The potential benefit of pharmacotherapy, especially glucocorticoids in Duchenne muscular dystrophy, has been recognized and will be discussed. The main expectations from a successful treatment are to prolong walking, preserve respiratory function and prolong survival, with enhancement of quality of life, but with minimal side effects.

Pathogenesis of DMD

Familiarity with the molecular genetics and the underlying pathogenesis of Duchenne dystrophy is essential in understanding the possible mechanisms of efficacy of the various drug treatments.

The cause of DMD is a mutation in the gene at Xp21, which results in a severe reduction or complete absence of dystrophin (Koenig et al 1987, Hoffman et al 1987) in the skeletal and cardiac muscle. In healthy subjects, dystrophin localises at the cytoplasmic side of the sarcolemma, and binds to a glycoprotein complex (Ahn & Kunkel 1993). The dystrophin-glycoprotein complex provides a link between the cytoskeleton in the muscle fibre and the extracellular matrix (Matsumura et al 1993). Lack of dystrophin compromises this link, and the ongoing contraction and relaxation of muscle is postulated to lead to damage of the sarcoplasma, increased influx of calcium, activation of proteases, degeneration of muscle fibres and their replacement by fibrous tissue (Burton and Davies 2001). Though DMD is not primarily an immune mediated disease, there is evidence raising the possibility of humoral and cellular immune responses contributing to the pathological processes. These include invasion of necrotic muscle fibres by macrophages and cytotoxic T-cells (Arahata and Engel 1984), complement activation with deposition of membrane attack complexes on necrotic fibres (Engel and Bissecker 1982), expression of HLA class I antigens on the dystrophic muscle fibres (McDouall et al 1990) making them susceptible to T-cell mediated damage.

Pharmacotherapy

Drug treatment trials in Duchenne muscular dystrophy have been reviewed (Dubowitz 1980, Heckmatt 1989, Emery 1993). Of all the medications studied, glucocorticoids, hold the maximal promise (Dubrovsky et al 1998, Manzur 2001, 2002). The terms steroids, corticosteroids and glucocorticoids have been used interchangeably in this context in neuromuscular literature, though strictly speaking glucocorticoids is the most appropriate descriptive term as it avoids confusion by excluding anabolic and androgenic steroids.

The availability of animal models (Nonaka 1998), has opened the possibility of therapeutic screening of potentially useful drugs. In a programme of preclinical screening in the mdx mouse, Granchelli et al (2000) reported improvement in whole body strength with prednisolone, glutamine, creatine, and anabolic hormone insulin like growth factor. The study confirms the feasibility of screening studies in animal model of muscular dystrophy prior to launching expensive and ethically difficult human therapeutic trials in the future.

The following drug therapies for DMD will be discussed:

- *Practical*
  Glucocorticoids
- *Experimental*
  Oxandrolone
  Cyclosporin
  Azathioprine
  Creatine
  Gentamicin

Glucocorticoids

The studies evaluating glucocorticoids in Duchenne muscular dystrophy over the last three decades are summarized in table 1. The preparation used in the in North American studies is prednisone, while the preparation often used in Europe is its hydroxylated form, prednisolone. Prednisone is broken down in the body to prednisolone and both preparations are equi-potent in glucocorticoid effect (Azarnoff 1975, Frey 1990). Deflazacort, an oxazoline derivative of prednisolone, has been used in a number of studies in the last decade. For purposes of comparison, 1 mg prednisone is equivalent in anti-inflammatory (glucocorticoid) effect to 1.2 mg deflazacort (British National Formulary).

The early open studies to document some benefit of glucocorticoid therapy in Duchenne dystrophy (Drachman 1974, Siegel 1974, Brooke 1987, DeSilva 1987) used prednisone in high doses ranging from 1.5 mg/kg/day to 5 mg/kg on alternate days. The open study by DeSilva et al (1987) used loss of walking ability as the primary end-point, and reported a prolongation of walking by approximately 2 years. The side effects of steroid treatment in this study were significant and included excessive weight gain in majority of the patients and also hyperactivity, cataracts and stress fracture. These studies lead to further randomized controlled trials to assess the efficacy and find the optimal dose regimes to minimize the side effects.

Three sequential randomized controlled studies of prednisone in Duchenne muscular dystrophy (Mendell 1989, Fenichel 1991, Fenichel 1991b) from four collaborating centres in the USA utilized a single cohort of 103 boys. These studies established Prednisone 0.75 mg/kg/day as a suitable starting dose and resulted in improvement in strength at 3 months followed by stabilization of muscle strength for up to a total of 3 years. The functional improvement to the subjects in these studies is difficult to ascertain, because of the wide age range (5–15 years) and because some of them were non-ambulant at entry to the study. The side effects were noted in over half of the patients and further reduction of the drug dose was required. Prednisone 0.65 mg/kg/day was considered to be the minimum effective dose and this could be tolerated by only half the subjects by the end of the study.

The dose response to prednisone and the time course of improvement was further evaluated by Griggs et al (1991). Prednisone 0.75 mg/kg/day was found to be more effective than 0.35 mg/kg/day and the improvement in strength was demonstrable as early 10 days after initiation of treatment. Though the duration of this study was only 6 months, 30% of the boys taking prednisone 0.75 mg/kg/day showed a weight gain of over 20 kg.

Daily dose glucocorticoid regimes have significant side effects in the longer term, with poor tolerability, and the need to reduce the steroid dosage. The long term result of a US prospective open follow-up study of patients reported in 1989, originally treated with daily prednisolone at a dose of 0.75 mg/kg/day, were reported at the World Muscle Society congress in Salt Lake City (Pandya 2001). Thirty patients were followed up for an average period of 10 years. Because of the systemic side effects, prednisone dose had to be reduced and over the long term, the mean prednisone dose tolerated was 0.35 mg/kg/day.

Table 1: Glucocorticoid trials in Duchenne muscular dystrohpy

Authors	Design	N =	Age (Years)	Glucocorticoid Regimen	Treatment Period	Outcome	Comments
Drachman 1974	Open	14	4 – 10.5	Prednisone 2 mg/kg/day for 3 months Then 2/3rds dose on alternate days	3 weeks – 28 months	Improvement	Side effects in 4
Siegel 1974	Double Blind	14	6 – 9	Prednisone 5 mg/kg alternate days	24 months	No benefit	
Brooke 1987	Open	33	5 – 15	Prednisone 1.5 mg/kg/day	6 months	Improvement	6 drop outs
DeSilva 1987	Open	16	3 – 10	Prednisone 2 mg/kg/day for 3 months Then 2/3rds dose on alternate days	1 – 11 years	Walking prolonged by 2 years	Excessive weight gain in 12 Cataracts in 2
Mendell 1989	Randomised double blind	103	5 – 15	Prednisone 0.75 mg/kg/day Prednisone 1.5 mg/kg/day	6 months	Improved at 3 months then stabilisation	30% boys had more than 20% weight gain
Fenichel 1991	Double blind	103	5 – 15	Prednisone 1.25 mg/kg/alternate day Prednisone 2.5 mg/kg/alternate day	6 months	Improved at 3 months	Similar side effects on daily and alternate day regimes
Fenichel 1991b	Open	92	5 – 15	Prednisone 0.75 mg/kg/day	2 years	Stabilisation for 2 years. Pred 0.65mg/kg/day least effect dose	Cataracts in 10 Glycosuria in 10 Significant weight gain
Griggs 1991	Randomised	99	5 – 15	Prednisone 0.3 mg/kg/day Prednisone 0.75 mg/kg/day	6 months	Strength improved at 10 days	30% boys had more than 20% weight gain
Mesa 1991	Double blind	28	5 – 11	Deflazacort 1 mg/kg/day	9 months	Improved till 6 months, then stable	35% cushingoid No significant weight gain
Griggs 1993	Randomised	107	5 – 15	Prednisone 0.75 mg/kg/day Azathioprine 2.5 mg/kg/day	18 months 12 months	Strength and function improved	No additional benefit of Azathioprine
Sansome 1993	Open	32	6 – 14	Prednisolone 0.75 mg/kg/day, for 10 days/months (10 days on 20 days off)	18 months	Strength improved at 6 months, slow decline at 18 months	Less side effects, but, 26% boys had more than 20% weight gain
Angelini 1994	Randomised	28	6.5 – 9	Deflazacort 2 mg/kg/alternate days	24 months	Stabilisation of strength	70% had >20% weight gain 1 pathological fracture
Backman 1995	Double blind crossover	37	4 – 19	Prednisone 0.3 mg/kg/day	12 months	Stabilisation for 1 year	Weight gain in 29%
Bonifati 2000	Randomised	18	5 – 14	Prednisolone 0.75 mg/kg/day Deflazacort 0.9 mg/kg/day	1 year	Prednisolone and deflazacort equally effective	Weight gain more significant in Prednisolone group
Biggar 2001	Open	30	7 – 15	Deflazacort 0.9 mg/kg/day	3.8 years (±SD 1.5)	Ambulation prolonged FVC preserved	Cataracts in 30%
Reitter 1995 (Data reported in Dubowitz 2000b)	Double Blind	100	5 – till ambulant	Prednisolone 0.75 mg/kg/day Deflazacort 0.9 mg/kg/day	2 years	Muscle function stabilised	Excessive weight gain in prednisolone group. Cataracts in 27% of deflazacort group
Dubowitz 2002	Open	2	4	Prednisolone 0.75 mg/kg/day, given 10 days on and 10 days off	5 years	Stabilization of motor function	Irritability in 1 patient

In order to lessen the adverse effects of long-term glucocorticoid treatment, Dubowitz (1991) recommended an intermittent regime of Prednisolone 0.75mg per kg per day for the first 10 days of every calendar month (cycles of 10 days on prednisolone treatment, 20 days off treatment). An open study of 32 patients at the Hammersmith Hospital demonstrated that this intermittent regime had a positive influence on strength at 6 months followed by a slow decline at 12 and 18 months (Sansome 1994); the weight gain and other side effects were much less than with continuous therapy. Subsequently, in order to increase the efficacy, the regime was modified to give prednisolone 0.75 mg/kg/day on a 10 days on treatment and 10 days off treatment. The long-term tolerability of the intermittent (10 days on treatment, 10 days off) regime of prednisolone has been further highlighted in a recent study by Dubowitz et al (2002). The 2 boys reported in this study were started on prednisolone at 4 years of age and followed up over a period of 5 years. These boys showed remarkable improvement, which was well sustained without the evidence of abnormal weight gain or demineralisation of bone or other signs of chronic prednisolone toxicity. This study, together with our observations in clinical practice, suggests that the beneficial effects of glucocoticoids appear to be greater when treated is initiated in the early ambulant phase.

Three recent studies have evaluated deflazacort (Angelini 1994, Bonifati 2000, Biggar 2001) and confirmed the beneficial effect of glucocorticoid therapy, in line with the findings of the previous prednisone studies. High dose deflazacort treatment over 24 months was reported to postpone loss of ambulation by 1.3 years, with only "modest" weight gain and slight behavioral changes in 54% (Angelini 1994). A small randomized comparative study of deflazacort versus prednisolone over the course of 1 year showed the two drugs to be equally effective, but the weight gain was more significant in the prednisolone group Bonifati et al (2000). The most impressive long-term functional outcome of deflazacort was reported in a retrospective study by Biggar et al (2001). They used deflazacort 0.9 mg/kg/day in 30 boys with Duchenne dystrophy (age 7–15 years) over 3.8 years (SD1.5) and reported prolongation of ambulation and remarkable preservation of pulmonary function (forced vital capacity) in the treated boys. Ten of the 30 boys in deflazacort treatment group developed asymptomatic cataracts.

A multicentre randomized trial comparing prednisolone (0.75 mg/kg/day) with deflazacort (0.9 mg/kg/day) in 100 boys with Duchenne muscular dystrophy has been completed and is awaiting publication (Reitter 1995, Dubowitz 1996, Dubowitz 2000). The preliminary data presented at the 75th European Neuromuscular Centre International workshop (Dubowitz 2000) showed that equipotent anti-inflammatory doses of prednisolone and deflazacort showed equal "effectiveness in almost completely preserving muscle performance" on testing manual muscle strength and timed motor functions. Weight gain was significantly higher in the prednisolone treated group, but 16 out of 44 boys treated with deflazacort developed cataracts (1/36 in the prednisolone group). On longer-term follow-up, cataracts became symptomatic in 2 boys in the deflazacort group, and required eye surgery with lens replacement (Dubowitz 2000).

The need for caution with the long-term use of glucocortcoids is necessary not only because of the high incidence of cataracts with deflazacort, but also the possibility of other adverse effects, including osteoporosis. Bothwell et al (2001) reported a cohort of 25 Duchenne boys treated with daily dose steroids for a median duration of 4.5 years. Overall, 10 of the 25 boys (40%) developed vertebral fractures. By 100 months of therapy, 75% had sustained a vertebral fracture.

The precise mechanism by which glucocorticoids increase strength in Duchenne dystrophy is not known but their beneficial effects include inhibition of muscle proteolysis (Rifai et al 1995, Elia et al 1981), stimulatory effect on myoblast proliferation (Bal 1980), anti-inflammatory / immunosuppressive effect (Kissel et al 1991) and upregulation of utrophin (Pasquini et al 1995).

It is difficult to formulate evidence-base guidelines for glucocorticoid use in DMD muscular dystrophy in spite of the number of studies available. There are uncertainties about the long-term use of glucocorticoid treatment in DMD, primarily relating to the quantum of functional benefit and the attendant adverse effects. An example of how controversial the issue is can be found in the recent review article by Dr. Susan Iannaccone (2001), who concludes – "oral steroids are not recommended for treatment of DMD on a routine basis." The long-term benefit, especially with regards prolongation of walking ability, and preservation of respiratory function, the optimal glucocorticoid regime with maximal efficacy and minimal side effects, still need to be established in clinical trials.

Current recommendations for clinical practice

The decision to start glucocorticoid treatment should be made by a physician experienced in management of DMD, after a full discussion with the affected child and the parents. The arrangements for long term follow up should be made at a clinic/centre with medical and physiotherapy facilities for monitoring of disease activity and glucocorticoid therapy are available. The intermittent prednisolone regime recommended by Dubowitz (1991, Sansome 1994, Dubowitz 2000, 2002) offers the possibility of long-term use with a lesser risk of pituitary adrenal axis suppression and other side effects, and is used in our clinical practice at the Hammersmith Hospital (repetitive cycles of prednisolone 0.75 mg/kg/day, 10 days on, 10 days off). Pre-existing diabetes mellitus, obesity, osteoporosis and a history of gastrointestinal haemorrhage are relative contraindications for glucocorticoid therapy in DMD. The decision to use glucocorticoids needs to be individualised depending on the child's age, motor status and parental wishes.

"Presymptomatic" phase (age range 0–4 years)

This group comprises of boys who are diagnosed early on the basis of family history or following incidental discovery of high CK or ALT/AST in the course of investigation of other medical problems. Though there may be a theoretical advantage in starting glucocorticoid treatment early, prior to major muscle cell necrosis and replacement by fibrosis, the clinical symptoms at this stage are absent or minimal. With the present state of research in this area, we are reluctant to expose boys to the long term side effects of steroid treatment at a relatively asymptomatic stage and therefore do not recommend use of prednisolone in this group.

Early ambulant phase (4–7 years)

There is an urgent need to clarify the functional benefit of such therapy in well designed clinical trials, to justify it's routine clinical use. We are setting up a United Kingdom multicentre randomised trial of this intermittent prednisolone schedule to specifically answer the questions of long-term benefits of prolongation of independent ambulation, and tolerability with acceptable side effects (International Standardized Randomised Control Trial Number 91883476).

There may be parents who wish for prednisolone treatment to be given to their affected sons in this age group, outside of any clinical trials. In this situation, the pros and cons of treatment and the equipoise in research over the use of steroids should be explained in full detail. If the facilities for long term monitoring of glucocorticoid therapy are available, it will be reasonable to offer this treatment.

Late ambulant phase (8 years till loss of walking)

These are boys who often have lost the ability to rise from the floor and their walking is deteriorating gradually or rapidly, with impending loss of ambulation. Glucocorticoids, in this "otherwise inevitable" situation are a reasonable option, provided the adverse effect profile is acceptable to the family and the physician. This again entails a full discussion with the family and the need for monitoring facilities.

Wheel chair dependent phase

There is little data, in this group, to support the initiation of glucocorticoid therapy, and at this stage, the adverse effects out-weigh any potential benefits.

Experimental drug treatments

Oxandrolone

Fenichel et al (1997) reported pilot study of oxandrolone 0.1 mg/kg/day for 3 months in 10 boys with Duchenne dystrophy. There was an improvement in the average muscle score as compared to natural history controls, and the magnitude of improvement was similar to that after prednisolone administration. No randomised controlled studies are available, and the use of this anabolic steroid is still experimental.

Azathioprine

Improvement in strength in Duchenne dystrophy with prednisolone raised the possibility of immunosuppression as the mode of its action. This hypothesis was tested by a randomised, controlled trial of prednisolone and azathioprine (Griggs et al 1993) to determine whether azathioprine alone, or in combination with prednisone, improves muscle strength. Azathioprine did not have a beneficial effect in this study and this also suggests that prednisone's beneficial effect is not due to immunosuppression.

Cyclosporin

Sharma et al (1993) investigated the effect of cyclosporin in force generation in Duchenne muscular dystrophy. Fifteen boys (age 5–10 years, 5 non-ambulant) were given oral cyclosporin in a dose of 5 mg/kg/day. An increase in tetanic force and maximum voluntary contraction strength in the tibialis anterior muscles was reported after 2 months of cyclosporin therapy, and this was largely lost following the 2 month wash-out phase. Functional benefit was not assessed. No further human studies have been reported.

Creatine

Creatine is a dietary component in meat-eaters and is also synthesised endogenously and stored in skeletal muscle. Creatine in the muscle is converted to phosphocreatine to build, and provide energy in the form of adenosine triphosphate (Jacobs 1999, Benzi 2000). Creatine may enhance the performance of high-intensity, short-duration exercise (Kamber et al 1999) but is not useful in endurance sports (Graham 1999). Despite this, creatine supplementation is widely taken by athletes to enhance muscular performance (Graham 1999). Creatine pre-treatment of mdx mice muscle cell cultures increases phosphocreatine levels, myotube formation and survival (Pulido et al 1998). Oral creatine supplementation was reported to improve muscle performance and intracellular creatine levels on gastrocnemius muscle 31P magnetic resonance spectroscopy in a 9 year old boy with Duchenne dystrophy (Felber et al 2000). Walter et al (2000) assessed the safety and efficacy of creatine monohydrate in various types of muscular dystrophies in a double-blind, crossover trial. The study included 8 patients with Duchenne dystrophy who were randomized to receive Creatine or placebo for 8 weeks. Mild improvement was reported in muscle strength and daily-life activities by Medical Research Council scales and the Neuromuscular Symptom Score. The beneficial effect of creatine has been so modest that it is not recommended as routine treatment in DMD.

Gentamicin

The mechanism of action of this aminoglycoside antibiotic is to cause misreading of the RNA code, allowing insertion of alternative amino acids at the site of the mutated codon, leading to transcription and protein formation (Mankin 1999). Barton-Davis et al (1999) reported restoration of dystrophin function to skeletal muscles of mdx mice with the use of gentamicin. The application in the human model is limited as this mechanism of action is possible only in patients with point mutation of a stop codon in the dystrophin gene (which comprises only a few percent of Duchenne patients).

Wagner et al treated 4 patients with Duchenne and Becker muscular dystrophy, with various stop codon sequences, with once daily intravenous gentamicin at 7.5 mg/kg/day for 2 weeks. No ototoxicity or nephrotoxicity was detected. Full-length dystrophin was not detected in pre- and post-treatment muscle biopsies. Currently, gentamicin treatment in DMD remains strictly experimental.

Summary

The pharmacological therapies, in particular glucocorticoids, hold some promise in Duchenne muscular dystrophy. While waiting for a curative treatment to become available, there is need for research studies to evaluate drug therapies and evidence based approach to integrate the use of effective and safe treatments in clinical practice.

References

1. Ahn AH. Kunkel LM. The structural and functional diversity of dystrophin. Nat Genet 1993;3:283–91
2. Angenlini C, Pegoraro E, Turella E. et al. Deflazacort in Duchenne dystrophy: Study of long-term effect. Muscle Nerve 1994;17:386–391
3. Arahata K, Engel AG. (1984) Monoclonal antibody analysis of mononuclear cells in myopathies. I: Quantitation of subsets according to diagnosis and sites of accumulation and demonstration and counts of muscle fibers invaded by T cells. Ann Neurol. 16:193–208.
4. Azarnoff DL. 1975. Steroid therapy. WB Saunders Co, Philadelphia PA
5. Backman E, Henriksson KG. Low-dose prednisolone treatment in Duchenne and Becker muscular dystrophy. Neuromuscul Disord. 1995 May;5(3):233–41.
6. Bal E, Sanwall W. A synergistic effect of glucocorticosteroids and insulin on the differention of myoblasts. J Cell Physiol 1980;102:27–36
7. Barton-Davis ER, Cordier L, Shoturma DI. et al. Aminoglycoside antibiotics restore dystrophin function to skeletal muscles of mdx mice. J Clin Invest 1999;104:375–381
8. Benzi G. Is there a rationale for the use of creatine either as nutritional supplementation or drug administration in humans participating in sport? Pharmacol Res 2000; 41:255–264
9. Biggar WD, Gingras M, Fehlings DL, Harris VA, Steele CA. Deflazacort treatment of Duchenne muscular dystrophy. J Pediatr 2001 Jan;138(1):45–50
10. Bonifati MD, Ruzza G, Bonometto P, Berardinelli A, Gorni K, Orcesi S, Lanzi G, Angelini C. A multicenter, double-blind, randomized trial of deflazacort versus prednisone in Duchenne muscular dystrophy. Muscle Nerve. 2000 Sep;23(9):1344–7.
11. British National Formularly.2000,British Medical Association and Royal Pharmaceutical Society of Great Britain. No 40
12. Brooke MH, Fenichel GM, Griggs RC, Mendell JR, Moxley RT 3d, Miller JP, Kaiser KK, Florence JM, Pandya S, Signore L, et al. Clinical investigation of Duchenne muscular dystrophy. Interesting results in a trial of prednisone. Arch Neurol. 1987 Aug;44(8):812–7.
13. Burton EA, Davies KE. The pathogenesis of Duchenne muscular dystrophy. From: Pathogenesis of neurodegenerative disorders Edited by MP Mattson, Humana Press Inc., Totowa., NJ
14. Carter GT, McDonald CM. Preserving function in Duchenne dystrophy with long-term pulse prednisone therapy. Am J Phys Med Rehabil. 2000 Sep-Oct;79(5):455–8.
15. Committee on Safety of Medicines, Medicines Control Agency,. Calcort (Deflazacort): advertising has been withdrawn. Curr Prob Pharmacovigilance. 1998;24:10
16. Demos J, Tuil D, Berthelon M, Katz P, Broyer M, Riberi P, Testard R, Rognon LM, Pillet J, Collin P. Progressive muscular dystrophy. Functional improvement after a renal allograft. J Neurol Sci. 1976 Nov;30(1):41–53.
17. DeSilva S, Drachman DB, Mellits D, Kuncl RW. Prednisone treatment in Duchenne muscular dystrophy. Long-term benefit. Arch Neurol. 1987 Aug;44(8):818–22.
18. Drachman DB, Toyka KV, Myer E. Prednisone in Duchenne muscular dystrophy. Lancet. 1974 Dec 14;2(7894):1409–12.
19. Dubowitz V, Heckmatt J. Management of muscular dystrophy. British Medical Bulletin 1980;36:139–144

20. Dubowitz V, Kinali M, Mercuri E, Muntoni F. Remission of clinical signs in early Duchenne muscular dystrophy on intermittent low dose prednisolone therapy. European Journal of Paediatric Neurology. 2002: 6;1
21. Dubowitz V. 47th ENMC International workshop: treatment of muscular dystrophy. 13–15 Dec,1996, Naarden, The Netherlands. Neuromusc Disord. 1997:7:261–267
22. Dubowitz V. 75th ENMC International workshop: Treatment of muscular dystrophy, Baarn 10–12 Dec, 1999. Neuromusc Disord 2000;10:313–320
23. Dubowitz V. Muscle Disorders In Childhood Second Edition, W B Saunders 1995.
24. Dubowitz V. Prednisolone in Duchenne dystrophy. Neuromusc Disord 1991;3:161–163
25. Dubrovsky AL, Corrado Angelini, Bonifati DM. Steroids in muscular dystrophy: Where do we stand? Neuromusc Disord 1998;8: 380–384
26. Elia M, Carter A, Bacon S. et al. Clinical usefulness of urinary 3-methylhistidine excretion in indicating muscle protein breakdown. Br Med J (Clin Res Ed) 1981;282(6261):351–4
27. Emery AEH. Duchenne muscular dystrophy. 2nd edition. Oxford Monographs on Medical Genetics, Vol 24. Oxford University Press 1993
28. Emery AEH. Neuromuscular Disorders: Clinical and Molecular Genetics. J Wiley & Sons, Chichester 1998
29. Engel AG, Biesecker G. Ann Neurol (1982) Complement activation in muscle fiber necrosis: demonstration of the membrane attack complex of complement in necrotic fibers. Sep;12(3):289–96
30. Felber S, Skladal D, Wyss M, Kremser C, Koller A, Sperl W. Oral creatine supplementation in Duchenne muscular dystrophy: a clinical and 31P magneticresonance spectroscopy study. Neurol Res. 2000 Mar;22(2):145–50.
31. Fenichel G, Pestornk A, Florence J. et al. A beneficial effect of oxandrolone in the treatment of Duchenne muscular dystrophy: A pilot study. Neurology 1997;48:1225–6
32. Fenichel GM, Florence JM, Pestornk A. et al. Long-term benefit from prednisolone in Duchenne muscular dystrophy. Neurology 1991;41:1874–1877,
33. Fenichel GM, Mendell JR, Moxley RT 3d, Griggs RC, Brooke MH, Miller JP, Pestronk A, Robison J, King W, Signore L, et al. A comparison of daily and alternate-day prednisone therapy in the treatment of Duchenne muscular dystrophy. Arch Neurol. 1991 Jun;48(6):575–9.
34. Frey BM, Frey FJ 1990. Clinical pharmacokinetics of prednisone and prednisolone. Clinical Pharmacokinetics 19:126–46
35. Graham AS, Hatton RC. Creatine: a review of efficacy and safety. J Am Pharm Assoc (Wash) 1999;39:803–10;
36. Granchelli JA, Pollina C, Hudecki MS. Pre-clinical screening of drugs using the mdx mouse. Neuromuscul Disord. 2000 Jun;10(4–5):235–9.
37. Griggs RC, Moxley RT, Mendell JR. et al. Duchenne dystrophy: randomized, controlled trial of prednisone (18 months) and azathioprine (12 months). Neurology. 1993;43:520–7
38. Griggs RC, Moxley RT, Mendell JR. et al. Prednisolone in Duchenne dystrophy: a randomised trial defining the time course and dose response. Arch Neurol 1991;48:383–388
39. Heckmatt JZ, Rodillo E, Dubowitz E. Management of children: Pharmacological and physical. Br Med Bulletin 1989;45:788–801
40. Hoffman EP, Brown RH Jr, Kunkel LM. Dystrophin: the protein product of the Duchenne muscular dystrophy locus. Cell:1987;51:919–928
41. Iannaccone ST, Nanjiani Z. (2001) Duchenne Muscular Dystrophy. Curr Treat Options Neurol 3:105–117.
42. Jacobs I. Dietary creatine monohydrate supplementation. Can J Appl Physiol 1999 Dec;24:503–14
43. Kamber M, Koster M, Kreis R. et al. Creatine supplementation – part I: performance, clinical chemistry, and muscle volume. Med Sci Sports Exerc 1999;12:1763–9
44. Kissel JT, Burrow K, Rammohan KW. et al. Mononuclear cell analysis of muscle biopsies in prednisolone and azathioprine treated Duchenne muscular dystrophy. Neurol 1991;41:667–672

45. Koenig M, Hoffman EP, Bertelson CH. et al. Complete cloning of Duchenne muscular dystrophy (DMD) cDNA and preliminary genomic organisation of the DMD gene in normal and affected individuals. Cell. 1987;50:509–517
46. Mankin AS, Liebman SW. Baby, don't stop! Nature Genet 1999;23:8–10
47. Manzur AY, Muntoni F. (2002) The management of Duchenne muscular dystrophy. Current Paediatrics (in press)
48. Manzur AY. (2001)"Treatment of muscular dystrophy" in Muscular dystrophy. Ed AEH Emery. Oxford Medical Publications.
49. Matsumura K, Ohlendieck K, Ionasescu VV. et al. The role of the dystrophin-glycoprotein complex in the molecular pathogenesis of muscular dystrophies. Neuromuscul Disord. 1993;3:533–5
50. McDouall RM, Dunn MJ, Dubowitz V. (1990) Nature of the mononuclear infiltrate and the mechanism of muscle damage in juvenile dermatomyositis and Duchenne muscular dystrophy. J Neurol Sci. 99:199–217.
51. Mendell JR, Moxley RT, Griggs RC. et al. Randomized controlled trial of prednisolone in Duchenne's muscular dystrophy. NEJM 1989;320:1592–1597,
52. Mesa LE, Dubrovsky AL, Corderi J, Marco P, Flores D. Steroids in Duchenne muscular dystrophy – deflazacort trial. Neuromuscul Disord. 1991;1(4):261–6.
53. Nonaka I. 1998. Animal models of muscular dystrophies. Lab Anim Sci 48: 8–17
54. Pandya S, Myers G and RT Moxley. Effect of daily prednisone on independent ambulation in patients with Duchenne muscular dystrophy treated up to 15 years. World Muscle Society Congress, Salt Lake City, Utah, 5–8th September 2001. Neuromuscular Disorders, 2001; 11, Abstract
55. Pasquini F, Guerin C, Blake D. et al. The effect of glucocorticoids on the accumulation of utrophin by cultured normal and dystrophic human skeletal muscle satellite cells. Neuromusc Disord 1995;5:105–114
56. Persky AM, Brazeau GA. (2001) Clinical pharmacology of the dietary supplement creatine monohydrate. Pharmacol Rev. Jun;53(2):161–76. Review.
57. Pulido-SM; Passaquin-AC; Leijendekker-W. et al. Creatine supplementation improves intracellular Ca2+ handling and survival in mdx skeletal muscle cells. FEBS-Lett. 1998; 439: 357–62
58. Reitter B. Deflazacort vs. prednisone in Duchenne muscular dystrophy: trends of an ongoing study. Brain Dev. 1995;17 Suppl:39–43.
59. Rifai Z, Welle E, Moxley RT. et al. Effect of prednisolone on protein metabolism in Duchenne muscular dystrophy. Am J Physiol 1995;268:E67–E74
60. Sansome A, Royston P, Dubowitz V. Steroids in Duchenne muscular dystropy; Pilot study of a new low-dosage schedule. Neuromusc Disord 1993;3:567–569
61. Sharma KR, Mynhier MA, Miller RG. Cyclosporine increases muscular force generation in Duchenne musculardystrophy. Neurology 1993;43:527–32
62. Siegel IM, Miller JE, Ray RD. Failure of corticosteroid in the treatment of Duchenne (pseudo-hypertrophic) muscular dystrophy. Report of a clinically matched three year double-blind study. IMJ Ill Med J. 1974 Jan;145(1):32–3
63. Tawil R, McDermot M, Pandya S. et al. A pilot trial of prednisolone in facioscapulohumeral dystrophy (FSHD). Neurology 1997;48:46–49
64. Wagner KR, Hamed S, Hadley DW, Gropman AL, Burstein AH, Escolar DM, Hoffman EP, Fischbeck KH.. Gentamicin treatment of Duchenne and Becker muscular dystrophy due to nonsense mutations. Ann Neurol 2001 Jun;49(6):706–11
65. Walter MC, Lochmuller H, Reilich P, Klopstock T, Huber R, Hartard M, Hennig M, Pongratz D, Muller-Felber W. (2000) Creatine monohydrate in muscular dystrophies: A double-blind, placebo-controlled clinical study. Neurology. 54:1848–50.
66. Winter K, Schara U, Mortimer J, Liersch R, Mortier W. Duchenne muscular dystrophy with long term steroid therapy. Absence of cardiac side effects. Acta Myologica 1999;III:159–162

Physiotherapie und orthopädische Behandlung bei neuromuskulären Erkrankungen

J. Forst

Zusammenfassung

Die orthopädische Behandlung von Muskelkranken hat sich im Laufe des letzten Jahrzehntes von einer Behandlung von bereits aufgetretenen Kontrakturen und Skoliosen durch Orthesen und Physiotherapie zu einer prophylaxeorientierten Behandlung entwickelt. Die Erkenntnisse über die maligne Hyperthermie und maligne Hyperthermie-Reaktion hat zu Narkoseverfahren geführt, bei denen heute das Narkoserisiko für die Patienten mit Muskelerkrankungen nicht wesentlich höher liegt als bei muskelgesunden Patienten. Zusätzliche Entwicklungen, wie z.B. die Anwendung des Sakralblockes bei Kindern haben zu einer geringeren Narkosebelastung bei Extremitäteneingriffen geführt. Zudem konnte die postoperative Schmerztherapie hierdurch wesentlich verbessert werden. Durch die in aller Regel Gips- und Orthesenfreie Nachbehandlung (Ausnahme knöcherne Eingriffe) konnte die postoperative Immobilisation der Patienten fast vollkommen reduziert werden. Die Patienten werden am ersten postoperativen Tag gemäß ihren motorischen Funktionen remobilisiert. Untersuchungen an großen Patientenkollektiven (100 Patienten), die die Wirksamkeit der durchgeführten operativen Maßnahmen untersucht haben, liegen lediglich für die Duchenne-Muskeldystrophie vor. Entsprechend strukturierte Untersuchungen sind für die spinale Muskelatrophie, Gliedergürtel-Muskeldystrophie oder FSH-Muskeldystrophie wegen der Heterogenität dieser Erkrankung bisher nicht durchgeführt worden. Die Empfehlung operativer Maßnahmen bei diesen Krankheitsbildern beziehen sich im allgemeinen auf die Beobachtung von wenigen Patienten und können daher nur im Einzelfall bei entsprechender Klinik indiziert werden. Einigkeit herrscht heute jedoch dahingehend, dass die frühzeitige operative Versorgung empfohlen wird, da hierbei in der Regel weniger invasive Eingriffe zur Anwendung gelangen und das funktionelle Ergebnis besser ist. Orthesen und Physiotherapie allein können bei Muskelerkrankungen weder das Auftreten von Deformitäten verhindern noch ihre Progredienz wesentlich beeinflussen.

Einleitung

Das orthopädische Behandlungskonzept von Patienten mit neuromuskulären Erkrankungen hat sich von der viele Jahrzehnte praktizierten »Sekundär-Prophylaxe« zu einer »Primär-Prophylaxe« gewandelt. Unter Sekundär-Prophylaxe versteht man die konservativen oder operativen Maßnahmen, mit denen versucht wurde, bereits bestehende Deformitäten der Bewegungsorgane zu behandeln. Bei der Primär-Prophylaxe strebt man dagegen an, all diejenigen Veränderungen die in Kenntnis des natürlichen Verlaufes der jeweiligen Erkrankung auftreten, vorzeitig durch orthopädische Maßnahmen zu behandeln und damit möglichst zu vermeiden.

Lange Zeit wurden insbesondere bei rasch progredienten Erkrankungen, wie z.B. der Duchenne-Muskeldystrophie, kaum operative Maßnahmen durchgeführt. In der Progression, dem hohen Narkoserisiko und den vermeintlich notwendigen langen Immobilisationszeiten sah man Faktoren, die gegen ein operatives Vorgehen sprachen. Heute wissen wir dagegen, dass durch moderne Anästhesie- und intensivmedizinische Verfahren sowie durch geeignete Operationstechniken sowohl das Narkose- als auch das Operationsrisiko für Patienten mit neuromuskulären Erkrankungen nicht unvertretbar erhöht ist.

Physiotherapie und Orthesen

So selbstverständlich die physiotherapeutische Behandlung als »wesentliches Therapieelement« in der symptomatischen Behandlung von Muskelerkankungen »schon immer« etabliert ist, so häufig wurde deren Effizienz im Laufe der Jahre durch zahlreiche Studien sowohl belegt als auch angezweifelt. Kritiker warnten vor allem vor der Gefahr einer Beschleunigung der progredienten Muskelschwäche durch Überlastung der Muskulatur. Bezüglich der »richtigen« physiotherapeutischen Behandlung bei der DMD wurden zahlreiche, z.T. sehr konträre Positionen bezogen und vehement vertreten. Während in Deutschland unter der Federführung von Beckmann und Teirich-Leube (1970) ausschließlich passive Übungsverfahren erlaubt waren und generell zur Schonung der Patienten geraten wurde, ähnlich wie Demos (1971) in Frankreich, werden heute, individuell am Patienten orientiert, statische und dynamische Übungen nebeneinander eingesetzt (Mortier 1994).

Abhängig vom klinischen Befund und dem angestrebten Behandlungsziel können im Verlaufe der Muskelerkrankung orthetische Maßnahmen gezielt eingesetzt werden. Finden sich bei muskelkranken Patienten beginnende Kontrakturen der Gelenke der unteren Extremitäten, könnten z.B. bei Kontraindikation gegen eine operative Behandlung dieser Kontrakturen und entsprechender Compliance des Patienten Redressionsorthesen eingesetzt werden. Archibald und Vignos (1959) hoben hervor, dass die Nachtschienen-Behandlung keine Alternative zur Physiotherapie sei, sondern beide Verfahren stets gemeinsam eingesetzt werden müssen. Scott et al. (1981) berichteten anhand einer Untersuchung von 59 DMD-Patienten (4–12 Jahre), dass eine Nachtschienen-Versorgung in Kombination mit konsequenter Dehnungstherapie möglicherweise bei sehr frühzeitigem Einsatz helfen könne, Spitzfußkontrakturen sinnvoll zu beeinflussen. Sie mussten aber auch die Erfahrung machen, dass über 60% dieser Versorgungen fehlschlugen, da die Patienten das nächtliche Tragen von Orthesen ablehnten. Redressionsorthetische Maßnahmen bei Kniegelenksbeugekontrakturen ab 15° und Spitzfüßigkeit ab 5° sind aber z.B. bei der DMD ohne jeden therapeutischen Effekt. Der Aufwand für den Patienten und der therapeutische Nutzen dieser Maßnahme stehen in keinem vertretbaren Verhältnis. Diller (1989) konnte keinen positiven Effekt bezüglich einer effizienten Spitzfußprophylaxe durch Nachtschienen nachweisen.

Oberschenkel-Orthesen dienen zur Stabilisierung der »Beinsäulen« beim Gehen und/oder Stehen. Meist ist vor einer solchen Versorgung gegen Ende der Gehfähigkeit der Patienten eine komplexe operative Kontrakturlösung an beiden unteren Extremitäten erforderlich, wenngleich auch über das Fortsetzen der Gehfähigkeit mit Bein-Orthesen ohne operative Vorbehandlung berichtet wurde. Orthesenversorgte, aber gehunfähige Patienten haben den Vorteil, dass sie aus dem Rollstuhl heraus an nahezu jedem beliebigen Ort – auch im Stehständer – zum Stand mobilisiert werden können. Ferner bieten orthesenversorgte Patienten für die sie betreuenden Personen den Vorteil, dass die Transferbewegungen, die im täglichen pflegerischen Umgang mit den Patienten anfallen, wesentlich einfacher und für die Wirbelsäule der Helfer schonender möglich sind.

Zur Therapie einer Skoliose ist eine Indikation zur Korsettbehandlung bei gehunfähigen Patienten mit rasch progredienten Muskelerkrankungen nur dann gegeben, wenn sie eine rechtzeitige operative Stabilisierung der Wirbelsäule zu Beginn der Rollstuhlphase ablehnen oder aber im Sinne einer Kompromisslösung in inoperablen Spätstadien. Diese Korsettversorgungen dienen einer Verbesserung der Sitzposition, haben jedoch keinen Einfluss auf die Progredienz der Skoliose.

Operative Behandlungsmaßnahmen

Patienten mit rasch progredienten Muskelerkrankungen entwickeln fast immer obligat auftretende Deformitäten insbesondere der unteren Extremitäten (sekundärer Klumpfuß bzw. Pes cavo-varo-adductus, Hüft- und Kniebeugekontrakturen, mitunter Hüftluxationen). Diese Deformitäten lassen sich durch frühzeitig durchgeführte Operationen, bei gerade beginnenden Überstreckverlusten der Gelenke der unteren Extremitäten bzw. noch schwach ausgebildeten Beugekontrakturen, zumeist vermeiden bzw. gegenüber nicht operierten Patienten deutlich mildern. Je früher diese Eingriffe durchgeführt werden können, um so weniger invasiv sind die notwendigen operativen Maßnahmen und um so geringer sind die physische und psychische Belastung der Patienten und ihrer Familien.

Von 231 Patienten mit Duchenne-Muskeldystrophie haben wir 88 Patienten in einem frühen Krankheitsstadium »prophylaktisch« und 143 Patienten gegen Ende der Gehfähigkeit operativ an beiden unteren Extremitäten behandelt. Die Operationskriterien für die Durchführung prophylaktischer Operationen sind beginnende Einschränkungen der Überstreckfähigkeit von Hüft-, Knie- und Sprunggelenken sowie als Folge einer Verkürzung des Tractus iliotibialis eine Adduktionsseinschränkung der Hüftgelenke. Die Gesamt-Muskelkraft muss 70%, die Quadricepskraft MRC 3 betragen. Die Gowers'-Zeit aus Rückenlage muss unter 5 sec. sein.

Im Vergleich zu einer Gruppe von 222 nicht operativ behandelten Patienten konnten wir zeigen, dass durch die operative Behandlung in beiden operierten Gruppen eine deutliche und anhaltende Verbesserung der Gelenkbeweglichkeit erzielt werden konnte. Insbesondere die bei nicht operierten Patienten obligat auftretenden Hüft- und Kniebeugekontrakturen von bis zu 90° sind bisher bei den operativ behandelten Patienten nicht aufgetreten. Auch die starken Abduktionskontrakturen der Hüftgelenke, die das Sitzen im Rollstuhl erschweren, waren bei den operativ behandelten Patienten im Langzeitverlauf bisher nicht zu verzeichnen. Im Vergleich der früh operierten Patienten mit den zum oder kurz nach Ende der Gehfähigkeit operierten Patienten konnten wir zeigen, dass die selbständige Gehfähigkeit und die Fähigkeit alleine vom Boden aufzustehen um ca. 2 Jahre verlängert werden konnte. Einigkeit herrscht heute über die Notwendigkeit einer operativen Stabilisierung der Wirbelsäule zu Beginn der Rollstuhlphase als Methode der Wahl zur fast immer auftretenden Skoliose bei Patienten mit Duchenne-Muskeldystrophie. Nach heutiger Auffassung sollten nachgewiesene progrediente Skoliosen ab einem Krümmungswinkel von 20° nach Cobb und erhaltener forcierter Vitalkapazität > 25% der Altersnorm vom 2. oder 3. Brustwirbel bis zum Sacrum operativ stabilisiert werden. Es werden ausschließlich Instrumentarien verwandt, die eine korsettfreie Nachbehandlung erlauben.

In der Langzeitbeobachtung von Patienten mit HMSN stellte sich heraus, dass keine konservative Behandlungsmethode dauerhaft die Entstehung und das Fortschreiten der Ballenhohlfußdeformität verhindern kann, so dass aus orthopädischer Sicht eine frühzeitige, symptomorientierte und damit ganz individuelle operative Korrektur des jeweils vorliegenden Muskelungleichgewichtes bzw. der Fußdeformität erfolgen sollte. Ziel der Therapie ist hierbei die muskuläre Ausbalancierung des Fußes bei noch flexiblen Veränderungen bzw. die knöcherne Korrektur fortgeschrittener Fußdeformitäten zur Wiederherstellung einer möglichst normalen Fußstatik und -biomechanik sowie Vermeidung von Folgeschäden wie einer frühzeitigen Arthrose durch einseitige Gelenkbelastungen. Durch eine genaue klinische Untersuchung wird zunächst festgestellt, wie sich das Muskelungleichgewicht jedes Fußes zusammensetzt und ob eine flexible oder fixierte Fußdeformität vorliegt (Lateral-block Test). Während des Wachstums werden in der Regel Weichteileingriffe und erst nach Erreichen der Skelettreife bei fixierten Deformitäten knöcherne Eingriffe, ggf. in Kombination mit Weichteileingriffen, vorgenommen. Liegt ein isolierter Spitzfuß vor, so kann eine Achillessehnenverlängerung durchgeführt werden. Eine Verkürzung der Plantarfaszie kann durch eine Plantarfaszienspaltung im Ansatzbereich am Fersenbein behandelt werden. Zur Kräftigung der Fußaußenrandhebung wird bei erhaltener Kraft des Peroneus longus ein Transfer auf den Peroneus brevis vorgenommen. Zur Stabilisierung des Sprunggelenkes und Stärkung der Fußhebung wird ein Tibialis posterior-Transfer empfohlen, bei der die Sehne von der Fußinnenseite auf den Fußrücken verlagert wird. Häufig ist eine Kombination dieser OP-Verfahren erforderlich, in den meisten Fällen werden beide Füße gleichzeitig operiert. Nach der Operation ist keine Gipsruhigstellung erforderlich, und die Patienten können vom ersten postoperativen Tag an mit dem Steh- und Gehtraining beginnen. Bei einigen Patienten ist trotz operativer Versorgung durch ein Fortschreiten der Muskelschwäche ein Wiederauftreten oder eine Verschlechterung einer Fußdeformität zu beobachten. Für diese Patienten und für solche, die sich erst mit einer fixierten Fußdeformität in orthopädische Betreuung begeben, kommen nur knöcherne Korrekturen in Frage. Neben Versteifungsoperationen bei Krallenzehen und Fersenbeinkorrekturen werden in der Literatur unterschiedliche Formen der Mittelfußosteotomie bis hin zur Tripleosteotomie beschrieben. Letztere sollte sehr schweren und rigiden Ballenhohlfüßen vorbehalten bleiben. Im klinischen Alltag hat sich aus unserer Sicht die sogenannte Imhäuser-Osteotomie bewährt. Dabei wird eine dreidimensionale Fußkorrektur durch die Entnahme eines nach außen und oben offenen Knochenkeiles aus dem Mittel- bzw. Rückfuß erreicht. Postoperativ muss zur Stabilisierung der Korrektur eine 12-wöchige Entlastung des Beines im Unterschenkelgips erfolgen. Als Vorteile dieser OP-Methode sind die Stabilisierung des Sprunggelenkes, die Wiederherstellung der normalen Fußausrichtung, die postoperativ häufig spontane Zehenstreckung und die nicht seltene Möglichkeit zum Tragen normaler Konfektionsschuhe aufzuführen.

Literatur

1. Archibald KC, Vignos PJ (1959) A study of contractures in muscular dystrophy. Arch Phys Med Rehabil 39: 150–157
2. Blietz, R (1982) Erfahrungen in der Sekundärprophylaxe von hereditären Muskeldystrophien. Z Phys Med Baln Med Klim 11: 191–195
3. Diller KG (1989) Zur Wirkung von Nachtlagerungsschienen bei Kontrakturen infolge von Muskeldystrophie Duchenne. Inaugural-Dissertation Univiversität Mainz
4. Emery AEH (Hrsg.) (2001) The Muscular Dystrophies. Oxford University Press, New York (ISBN 0-19-263291-4)
5. Forst J (1999) Bedeutung orthopädisch-operativerer Behandlungsmaßnahmen an den unteren Extremitäten für den Verlauf der Duchenne-Muskeldystrophie. Wissenschaftsverlag Mainz, Aachen (ISBN 3-86073-719-8)
6. Forst R (2000) Die orthopädische Behandlung der Duchenne-Muskeldystrophie. Enke im Thieme Verlag, Stuttgart, New York (ISBN 3-13-117941-4)
7. Imhäuser G (1984) Die Behandlung des schweren Hohlklumpfußes bei der neuralen Muskelatrophie. Z Orthop 122: 827–834
8. Mortier W (1994) Muskel- und Nervenerkrankungen im Kindesalter. Georg Thieme Verlag, Stuttgart, New York (ISBN 3-13-128801-9)
9. Scott OM, Hyde SA, Goddard C, Dubowitz V (1981) Prevention of deformity in Duchenne muscular dystrophy. A prospective study of passive stretching and splintage. Physiotherapy 67: 177–180

Konzept und Ergebnisse der nichtinvasiven Heimbeatmung bei Muskelkranken

K.H. Wollinsky, A. Erhard, H.-H. Mehrkens

Einleitung

Muskelerkrankungen führen über einen ungewissen Zeitraum zu einer Abnahme bis zum Verlust motorischer Funktionen. Der Verlust der Gehfähigkeit zwingt zur sofortigen Anpassung von Hilfsmitteln. Einschränkungen des respiratorischen Systems bleiben oft lange Zeit verborgen, weil sie sich schleichend entwickeln und unter Ruhebedingungen lange kompensiert werden können. Ein banaler Infekt der oberen Luftwege kann über Komplikationen wie Sekretverhalt, Atelektasen und Pneumonie, lebensbedrohend für Muskelkranke werden und die schwere respiratorische Insuffizienz demaskieren. Zusammenhänge zwischen Abnahme der Muskelkraft und der Vitalkapazität (Lyager et al. 1995), Skoliose und Rollstuhlpflicht mit weiterer funktioneller Verschlechterung, sind bekannt (Yamashita et al. 2001). Die Idee, neben orthopädischen operativen Techniken und konservativer Hilfsmittelversorgung auch die Atmung zu unterstützen, ist nicht neu. So sind bei den großen Polioepidemien Negativdruckverfahren eingesetzt worden, die Eisernen Lungen. Viele Poliopatienten haben ihr Überleben diesen Geräten zu verdanken. Diese Geräte sind aber eher ein Käfig als ein modernes Hilfsmittel, das dem Muskelkranken seine Mobilität erhalten kann. Ab einem stärkeren Skoliosegrad ist die Nutzung der eisernen Lunge gar nicht mehr möglich. Bereits in den frühen 80er Jahren ist sie auch bei Duchenne Dystrophie empfohlen worden (Curran 1981). Französische (Rideau et al. 1983) und amerikanische Rehabilitationsmediziner (Bach et al. 1983) haben eine adäquate moderne respiratorische Hilfsmittelversorgung eingeführt. Diese sind sehr wichtige Bausteine in der Rehabilitation von Muskelkranken. Zunächst wurde neben der Eisernen Lunge die invasive Beatmung über Tracheostoma favorisiert (Frates et al. 1985, Gilgoff et al. 1989, Heckmatt et al. 1989). Dank mobiler Beatmungsgeräte, die unabhängig von Druckluft betrieben werden, wurden Muskelkranke zunehmend nichtinvasiv über nasale Masken beatmet. Diese Techniken sind anfangs sehr in Zweifel gezogen worden, sei es wegen der eingesetzten nichtinvasiven Technik, der Durchführung der Beatmung durch Laien oder wegen der nicht unerheblichen Kosten des Equipments. Im Laufe der Zeit ist die Überlegenheit dieser Beatmungstechnik im Vergleich zur Eisernen Lunge klar gezeigt worden. (Ellis et al.1987). Zunächst wurde die Anwendung der nichtinvasiven Beatmung bei Jugendlichen und Erwachsenen akzeptiert (Bach et al. 1995, Wang et al. 1994). Die anfängliche Skepsis gegenüber der Anwendung der nasalen Beatmung bei Kindern unter 10 Jahren (Heckmatt et al. 1990) wurde überwunden durch positive Rückmeldung bei der Anwendung im Kindesalter (Birnkrant et al. 1997, Buhr-Schinner et al. 1999, Paditz 1997, Simonds et al. 2000,

Wollinsky et al. 1995). Entscheidend aber war die Akzeptanz durch die Betroffenen selbst. So stand der Empfehlung durch die Muskelgesellschaften und Muskelzentren und neuropädiatrischen Zentren (v. Moers et al. 2000), diese Techniken anzuwenden, nichts mehr im Wege. In Deutschland sind Heimbeatmungszentren entstanden, die teils an die Muskelzentren, teils an pneumologische oder Rehabilitations-Kliniken angeschlossen sind. Diese Kliniken haben Erfahrung mit der Betreuung von chronisch respiratorisch insuffizienten Patienten und Patienten mit schlafbezogenen Störungen. Basierend auf Europäischen Empfehlungen (Robert et al. 1993) entstanden in Deutschland Richtlinien zur Heimbeatmung (Laier-Groeneveld et al. 1993).

Diagnostik

Zur Erfassung von respiratorischen Störungen untersuchen wir unsere Patienten in der Beatmungssprechstunde des Muskelzentrums zunächst ambulant. In einer eingehenden Anamnese fragen wir gezielt nach Symptomen, die auf eine chronisch ventilatorische Störung hinweisen können (Tab. 1). Das sind z.B. erschwerte Atmung, Tagesmüdigkeit, Atemnot, Schlafstörungen, Aufwachen nachts, Lagerung und Lagerungswechsel, Depressionen, Kopfschmerzen. Massive Atemnot kann am Tag noch fehlen und im Schlaf bereits manifest sein. Die Häufigkeit von pulmonalen Infekten, bereits erforderliche ambulante oder stationäre Behandlungen wegen Pneumonien, Antibiotikagaben, evtl. durchgeführte Antibiotika-Prophylaxen werden ebenfalls erfragt. Wichtig ist uns auch die Kenntnis von bereits vorhandenen und genutzten Hilfsmittel wie Verneblern, Absaugegeräten, Pulsoximetern und Sauerstoffkonzentratoren.

Bei der klinischen Untersuchung wird auf knöcherne Veränderungen wie Trichterbrust, Brustkorbdeformierung, Skoliose sowie Grad und Ausmaß der muskulären Atrophie, interkostale Einziehungen, Atemmechanik, Zwerchfellatmung (SMA) und Hilfsmuskeleinsatz geachtet (Abb. 1). Die Auskultation kann bereits Hinweise auf Komplikationen wie Atelektasen oder Pneumonien ergeben.

Die klinische Untersuchung wird ergänzt durch Röntgenaufnahmen des Thorax, EKG, Bestimmung der pulsoxymetrischen Sauerstoffsättigung, des endexspiratorischen oder transkutanen CO_2 und einer Blutgasanalyse. (Wir bevorzugen die arterielle Abnahme nach Vorbereitung durch Lokalanästhesiesalbe (EMLA®)). Ferner wird die Lungenfunktion und ggf. die inspiratorische Kraft bestimmt. Allerdings können bei Kleinkindern und Säuglingen diese Untersuchungen, entsprechend der Kooperation, nur bedingt eingesetzt werden. Ergeben sich geringste Hinweise auf eine respiratorische Störung, sollte unbedingt eine Kontrolle der Parameter im nächtlichen Schlaf durchgeführt werden. Eine komplette Schlaflaboruntersuchung bei diesen Patienten wird nur in ganz wenigen Kliniken angeboten. Sie ist, unserer Meinung nach, bei den neuromuskulären Erkankungen nicht so entscheidend wie bei Patienten mit Schlafstörungen (wie der Schlafapnoe), wo sie unerlässlich ist. Wir sehen in der SO_2 Messung bei Muskelkranken (Abb. 2) einen hochsensiblen Parameter, der selbst frühe Störungen sehr gut darstellt (Wollinsky et al. 1991).

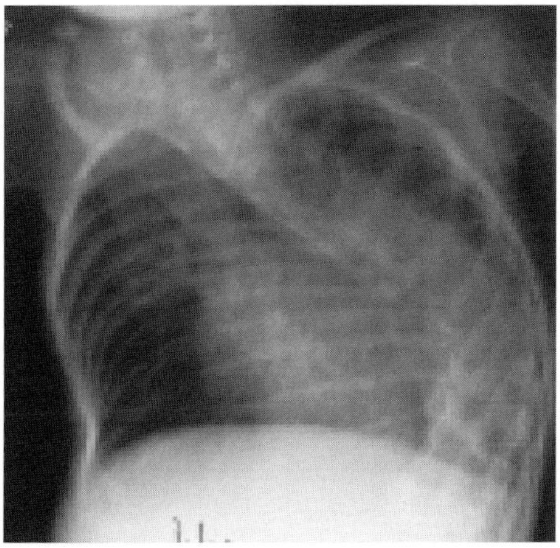

Abb. 1: SMA Kind mit schwerster thorakolumbaler Skoliose.

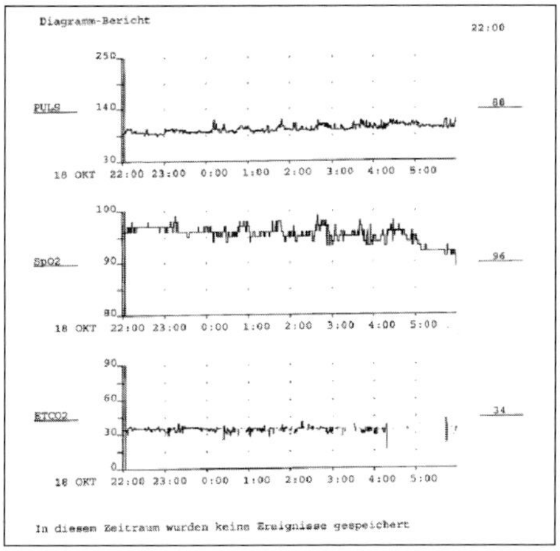

Abb. 2: Nächtliche Auswertung von Puls, Sauerstoffsättigung und endexspiratorischem CO_2 (Abnahme der SO_2 gegen morgen).

Tab. 1: Symptome einer chronischen Ateminsuffizienz ⇒ Alarmzeichen (Abb. 1 und 2)

Veränderte Atmung
Müdigkeit
Konzentrationsstörung
Schlafstörungen
häufiges Aufwachen
Alpträume
Depression
Schnarchen
Kopfschmerzen
muskuläre Schmerzen (Hilfsmuskulatur)
Schwitzen

In einer kürzlich durchgeführten Untersuchung bei ALS Patienten konnten wir folgendes zeigen: Von 24 Patienten mit schwerster chronischer Ateminsuffizienz hatte einer eine leichte, 23 Patienten eine starke Reduktion im nächtlichen SO_2. Dagegen hatten nur 10 von 24 ein pathologisch erhöhtes pCO_2 (Butz et al. 2000).

Werden die frühen Alarmzeichen für eine respiratorische Erschöpfung der Atempumpe übersehen, können manifeste Symptome einer Ateminsuffizienz mit Atemnot entstehen (Tab. 2).

Das führende Symptom, wenn auch manchmal am Tage nicht richtig fassbar, ist die Atemnot, die bei einigen Patienten erst im Liegen und in der Nacht auftritt. Eine Hypercapnie kann bei SMA I Kindern durchaus fehlen. Im schlechtesten Fall können die muskelkranken Patienten in einer akuten Infektsituation dekompensieren (Tab. 3).

In dieser Situation ist eine notfallmäßige Aufnahme auf der Intensivstation nicht zu umgehen.

Tab. 2: Symptome einer chronischen Ateminsuffizienz ⇒ Manifestation (Abb. 3)
massive Atemnot
Tachypnoe
Hypoxämie mäßig bis stark
Normo- bis Hypercapnie
Sprechpausen
gehäufte Infekte
Pneumonien
Abhustprobleme
Atelektase
Gewichtsabnahme
Gedeihstörung

Tab. 3: Symptome einer chronischen Ateminsuffizienz ⇒ Dekompensation (Abb. 4)
Entgleiste pulmonale Parameter
Cyanose
schwerste Hypoxämie
schwerste Hypercapnie
Cor pulmonale
Herzinsuffizienz
Ödeme
Tachycardie
Bradycardie
Herz-Rhythmusstörungen

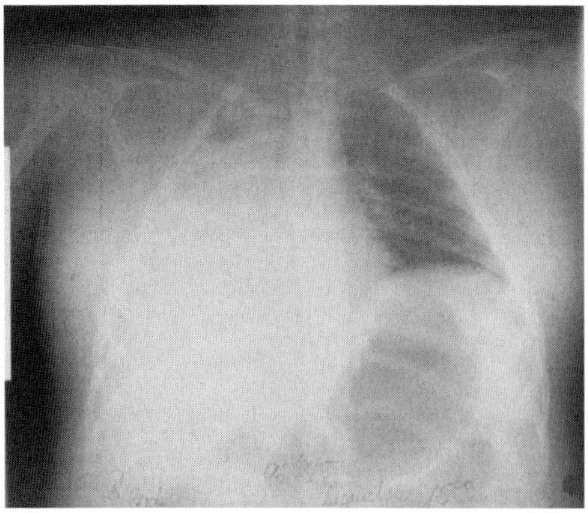

Abb. 3: Manifestation einer chron. Ateminsuffizienz mit Atelektase re. und Pneumonie re.

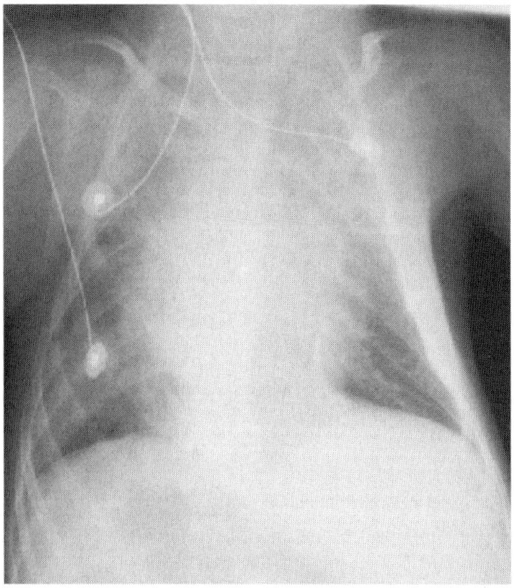

Abb. 4: Dekompensation einer chronischen Ateminsuffizienz – Cor pulmonale.

Indikation zur Beatmung

Eine Indikation für den Beginn einer respiratorischen Unterstützung sehen wir bei mindestens einem der in der Tabelle 4 aufgeführten Kriterien. Bei Zweifeln, aber klinischer Symptomatik, sollte eine Beatmung getestet werden, um zu sehen, ob die Krankheitssymptome sich bessern. Schwierig ist es, den optimalen Zeitpunkt für den Beginn der Beatmung zu treffen. Prophylaktische Beatmung scheint Nachteile zu haben.

Tab. 4: Indikation Beatmung

Klinische Symptome
Vitalkapazität < 20%
Sauerstoffsättigung im Schlaf < 90%
arterielles pO_2 < 55 mm Hg
arterielles pCO_2 > 45 mm Hg
Endexspiratorisches CO_2 > 45 mm Hg

Die Indikation zur Beatmung ergibt sich aus Erfüllung der bereits aufgeführten anamnestischen, klinischen und objektivierten Störungen der Atempumpe. Wichtig ist dabei die Behandlung der Pumpfunktionsstörung durch das extern eingesetzte Beatmungsgerät. Spontanatmung unterstützende Beatmungsmodi wie CPAP führen zu keiner Entlastung der Atempumpe. Teilentlastende Verfahren wie BIPAP oder druckunterstützte Modi können nur bei Patienten mit relativ gut erhaltener Kraft der Atempumpe eingesetzt werden. Eine volle Entlastung der Atempumpe wird jedoch nur durch volumenkontrollierte oder druckkontrollierte Beatmung erreicht. (Criée et al. 1997) In diesem Zusammenhang muss nochmals dringend gewarnt werden vor der immer noch weit verbreiteten Praxis, die Verordnung von Sauerstoff und dessen Anwendung unter Erhalt der Spontanatmung. Dies ist nicht die richtige Therapie der chronisch ventilatorischen Insuffizienz. Wie Gay et al. (1991) zeigen konnten, steigt bei Sauerstoffapplikation ein bereits erhöhtes art. pCO_2 noch an, eine Entlastung der Atempumpe wird nicht erreicht. Zudem verzögert die insuffiziente alleinige O_2 Gabe die definitive Respirator-Versorgung bei den Patienten um Monate und verschlechtert damit das Langzeitergebnis. Wir konnten dies bei mehreren Patienten beobachten.

Völlig problemlos kann eine Beatmung in einer noch stabilen Phase begonnen werden. Ohne zeitlichen Druck wird stundenweise der Umgang mit dem für viele Patienten zunächst ungewohnten Beatmungsgerät trainiert. Schwieriger ist der Start bei bereits erfolgter Dekompensation, denn die klinische Situation zwingt zu einer schnellen Steigerung der Beatmungszeiten, zusätzlich oft zu Sauerstoffgabe und PEEP Anwendung. In schweren Fällen muss, als Zwischenlösung, eine invasive Beatmung über Endotrachealtubus für einige Tage eingesetzt werden.

Verschiedene neuromuskuläre Erkrankungen führen zu vergleichbaren Symptomen. Die Behandlungsstrategien sind ähnlich. Am Beispiel der Duchenne Dystrophie lassen sich Ablauf und Durchführung der Heimbeatmung sehr gut darstellen. Gerade diese Patientengruppe ist eine der zahlenmäßig größten. Zur Effizienz der Heimbeatmung bei Duchenne Dystrophie liegen die meisten Daten vor. Besonderheiten sind für die SMA zu beachten, auf die im Einzelnen eingegangen wird.

Für die Aufnahme in ein Heimbeatmungsprogramm zwingend erforderlich ist eine Kooperation der behandelnden Neuropädiater, Pädiater, Hausärzte, Neurologen, Orthopäden, Internisten, Pneumologen, Anästhesisten, Physiotherapeuten, Ergotherapeuten, Medizintechniker, Eltern, Pflegedienste und der Selbsthilfegruppen (meist die Deutsche Gesellschaft Muskelkranker). Ein Beatmungszentrum und der Medizintechnikdienst muss bei Problemen rund um die Uhr bereit sein und bei infektbedingter Verschlechterung muss immer die Möglichkeit einer stationären Aufnahme bestehen. Ein Kontakt zu anderen Betroffenen, die bereits eine Beatmung durchführen, ist günstig. Denn positive Erfahrungen anderer Muskelkranker können Ängste nehmen und motivieren.

Durchführung

In Abhängigkeit vom zeitlichen Verlauf der Muskelerkrankung und dem Schweregrad der Restriktion hat sich ein Stufenschema bewährt.

Tab. 5: Basismaßnahmen

Physiotherapie
Atemtraining (Vojta)
Lagerungsmaßnahmen insbesondere Bauchlage
Sekretmobilisation
Abhusthilfe, Vibrax, Magic Hand®, Absaugen

Die Basismaßnahmen sollten durchgeführt werden bevor es zu respiratorischer Erschöpfung kommt.

Regelmäßige Physiotherapie, in allen Schweregraden, hat eine besondere Bedeutung. Kontrakturen werden dadurch vermieden, die Rückenmuskulatur wird beübt und die respiratorische Funktion so effektiv wie möglich unterstützt. Die Vojta Techniken haben sich dabei bei SMA Kindern besonders bewährt.

Tab. 6: Atemtherapie

Intermittierende Überdruckinhalation mit Atemtherapiegeräten z.B. AERO-LIFE,® täglich 4–6 x 5–10 Minuten

Überdruckatemtherapie sehen wir als geeignet an, um Kinder bei grenzwertiger, stagnierender oder langsam nachlassender Vitalkapazität aktiv zu beüben, ehe die Phase der Atempumpenstörung erreicht wird. Ältere Kinder können ein Mundstück verwenden, jüngere Kinder akzeptieren eher eine oronasale weiche aufblasbare Wulstmaske (VBM®). Die intermittierende Therapie stellt eine kurzfristige Erholung dar, und kann Komplikationen wie Atelektasen verhindern. Wir haben im Langzeitverlauf bei SMA Kindern gesehen, dass ein trapezförmiger knöcherner Thorax sich günstig erweitern kann. Auch nimmt die Gefahr regelmäßig wiederkehrender Infekte durch ein aktives Training ab. Wie Mellies et al. (dieser Band) zeigen konnte, kann mit Hilfe der Nutzung solcher Geräte die zum Husten notwendige Kraft wesentlich gesteigert werden. Bei Bedarf können zusätzlich Medikamente vernebelt werden. Im infektfreien Intervall genügt die Zumischung von Kochsalz bei niedriger Verneblerstärke, bei Infekten können Sympathikomimetika und Corticosteroide eingesetzt werden. Ein weiterer Effekt der Überdruckatemtherapie ist die langsame Akzeptanz von Geräten zur Verbesserung der Atmung und ein Zeitgewinn von einigen Monaten bis die weitere Progredienz der Muskelerkrankung zur nasalen Beatmung zwingt.

Tab. 7: Nasale nichtinvasive Beatmung (Abb. 5)

Beatmung mit mobilem Heimrespirator(volumen-oder druckgesteuert) mit Masken

Als effektive Entlastung einer geschwächten Atemmuskulatur gilt die Beatmung über nasale Maske (Abb. 6). Eine oro-nasale Beatmung führt bei den meisten Kindern eher zu Panik, da sie unter der Maske nicht mehr nach den Eltern oder Betreuern rufen können. Die nasale Beatmung kann letztlich an alle

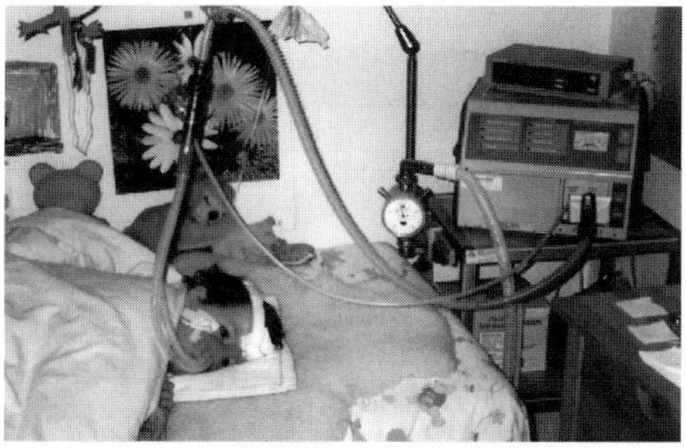

Abb. 5: Nasale Beatmung zu Hause bei SMAI Kind mit Massmaske (Dr. Mindé) und volumengesteuertem Gerät Typ Breas PV 501®, Kindervolumeter Dräger® und Pulsoxymeter Nellcore®.

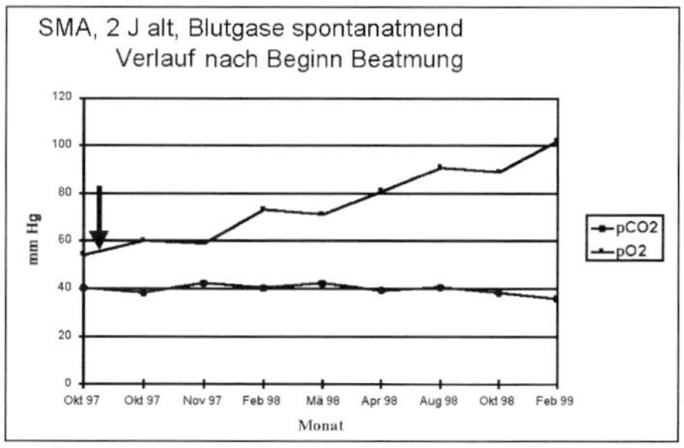

Abb. 6: Verbesserung der Blutgase unter Beatmung.

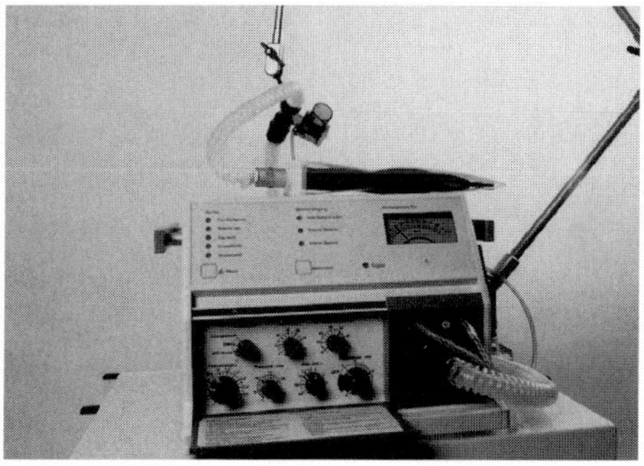

Abb. 7: Volumengesteuertes Beatmungsgerät Typ Dräger EV 801®.

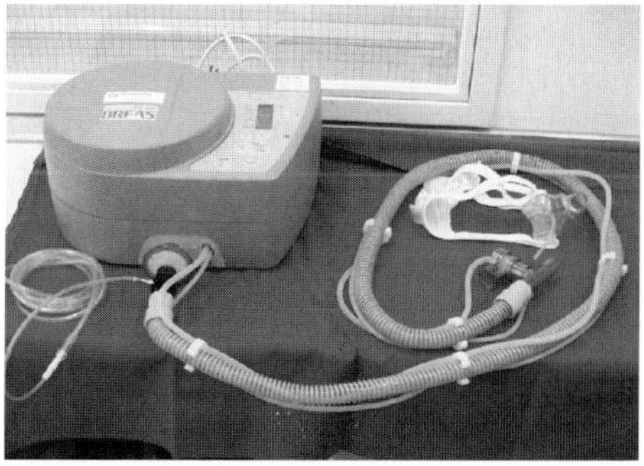

Abb. 8: Druckgesteuertes Beatmungsgerät Typ BREAS PV 401®.

mobilen Heimbeatmungsgeräte angeschlossen werden. Volumengesteuerte Geräte (BREAS PV 501®, Abb. 5, Dräger EV 800/801®, Abb. 7); Life Care PLV 100®) haben ein relativ begrenztes aber völlig ausreichendes Spektrum von Beatmungsmustern. Im Allgemeinen können das Tidalvolumen, die Atemfrequenz, das Atemzeitverhältnis oder die Inspirationszeit, der Trigger und die Alarmgrenzen eingestellt werden. Der am Patient erreichte Druck wird mit einem Manometer überwacht.

Neuerdings kommen vermehrt druckgesteuerte Beatmungsgeräte auf den Markt (BREAS PV 401, Abb. 8), Dräger Respicare und im neuesten Trend Geräte die sowohl druck-, als auch volumengesteuerte Modi ermöglichen (BREAS PV 403, Dräger VV®). Im Gegensatz zu den volumengesteuerten Geräten wird ein Beatmungsdruck vorgegeben, daneben Atemfrequenz, Inspirationszeit, Trigger, und ein Druckplateau eingestellt. Das Volumen wird hochgerechnet. Alarme reagieren auf Volumina und Atemfrequenzen.

Alle Geräte werden mit Strom angetrieben, einige haben einen eingebauten Akku als Notversorgung, dieser sichert für begrenzte Zeit die Beatmung bei Stromausfall. Andere können zusätzlich über einen externen Powerpack für mehrere Stunden Energie liefern. Manche Geräte können auch an externe Stromquellen wie der Rollstuhlbatterie oder einer Autobatterie (Zigarettenanzünder) angeschlossen werden. Somit erlauben die Heimbeatmungsgeräte eine sehr große individuelle Mobilität.

Tab. 8: Vergleich der Beatmungszugänge: Vor- und Nachteile

invasive Technik	**nichtinvasive Technik**
Tracheostoma	**nasale Maske**
geringe Akzeptanz	hohe Akzeptanz
Absaugen erforderlich	kein Absaugen erforderlich
Infektgefahr hoch	Infektgefahr niedrig
Trachealschäden	Luftinsufflation in den Magen
Sprechen erschwert	Sprechen normal
kein Leck	Lecks bis 50%
Beatmung 24 Std	Beatmung auch bis max. 24 Std
Eigenatmung nicht erforderlich	Rest Eigenatmung erforderlich

Beatmung mit Zubehör (Sauerstoff und PEEP)

In Phasen einer pulmonalen Dekompensation ist Beatmung mit Raumluft nicht mehr ausreichend. In alle Heimbeatmungsgeräte kann Sauerstoff eingespeist werden, meist über ein T-Stück. Auch ein positiv endexspir. Druck kann durch Aufstecken eines PEEP Ventils in das Exspirationsventil erreicht werden. Während eines Infektes kann vorübergehend eine invasive Beatmung erforderlich werden. Nach Erholung vom Infekt sollte erneut eine nasale Beatmung versucht werden. Eine Tracheostomiebeatmung ist primär nicht das Ziel einer Heimbeatmung.

Fehlt der eigene Atemantrieb über wesentliche Strecken des Tages (> 16 Std) kann ein invasiver Zugang erforderlich werden. Ist Beatmung unter Zumischung von Sauerstoff erforderlich, sollte, der Mobilität wegen, Flüssigsauerstoff verordnet werden. Sauerstoffkonzentratoren eignen sich nur bei stationärem Betrieb, zum Beispiel wenn ein mit Raumluft beatmetes Kind im Infektfall sauerstoffangereicherte Luft benötigt (max FIO2 von 0,4–0,5).

Überwachung

Pulsoxymeter sind bei allen Säuglingen und Kleinkindern eine wesentliche Erleichterung (Abb. 5). Pulsoxymeter dienen der Kontrolle der Ventilation und Früherkennung von Problemen wie Infekten oder nicht mehr adäquater Respiratoreinstellungen. Bei volumengesteuerten Beatmungsgeräten ist ein Volumeter günstig, vor allem wenn bei Kleinkindern Ventile zur Reduktion des Tidalvolumens benötigt werden. CO_2 Messgeräte dagegen halten wir im Routinefall nicht für erforderlich. Ebenso scheint die Mehrzahl der stabilen Duchenne Patienten kein Pulsoxymeter zu benötigen. Wird aber eine Beatmung über Tracheostoma durchgeführt, ist eine Überwachung mit Pulsoxymeter dringend erforderlich. Ein Gerätealarm (z.B. bei Diskonnektion oder zu hoher Beatmungsdrucke durch Sekret) kann bei Patienten mit geringer Eigenatmung als Fernalarm zu Angehörigen geschaltet werden und somit die Überwachung verbessern.

Bei geringer Eigenatmung, großer Abhängigkeit vom Respirator und Beatmungszeiten von mehr als 12 Stunden täglich oder an mehreren Orten (Schule/zu Hause oder Rollstuhl/Schlafzimmer), ist eine Versorgung mit Zweitgerät angezeigt.

Praxis

Die Einstellung der Beatmung erfolgt entweder auf einer Intensivstation oder bei stabileren älteren Kindern auf der Allgemeinstation. Die Anpassung auf der Allgemeinstation dauert im Allgemeinen deutlich länger (1–3 Wochen). Zunächst wird die Beatmung mit Konfektionsmasken und einem Leihgerät begonnen. Die Konfektionsmasken werden in verschiedenen Grössen und Weiten angeboten. Neue Masken mit Rändern aus Gel haben die primäre Einstellung von respiratorisch insuffizienten Patienten deutlich erleichtert. Gerade bei Muskelkranken hängt die Effizienz einer nichtinvasiven Beatmung ganz besonders vom Komfort und der Dichtigkeit der Maske ab. Auf Grund vielfacher Veränderung der Anatomie (muskulär knöchern, Zahn- und Bissfehlstellungen) sehen wir für die meisten Muskelkranken eine Maske nach Individualabdruck als unerlässlich an. Bei Ateminsuffizienz anderer Genese (z.B. COPD Patienten) ist inzwischen weitgehend die Gelmaskenversorgung üblich. Leider ist die Genehmigungspraxis der Kostenträger bei einer solchen Versorgung häufig sehr zeitraubend. So müssen muskelkranke Patienten teilweise bis zu neun Monate auf grünes Licht für eine Maske nach Maß warten. Bei Haltbarkeit der Masken von bis zu sieben Jahren amortisiert sich ihr ursprünglich höherer Aufwand im Ver-

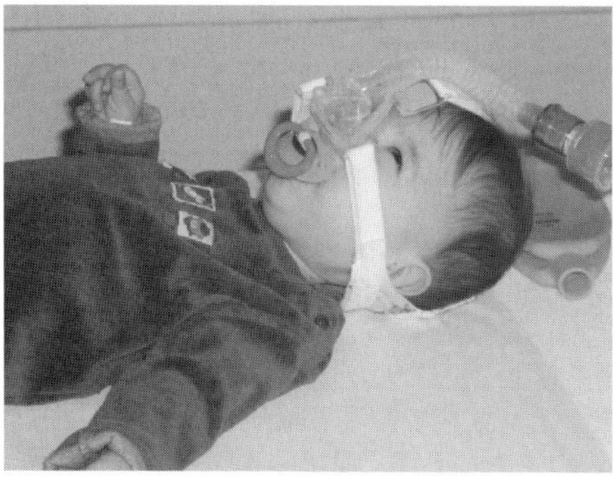

Abb. 9: Säugling mit Konfektionsmaske Respironics Infant® modifiziert.

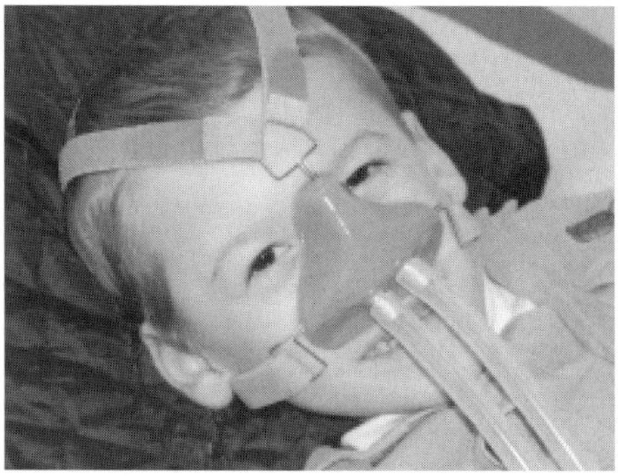

Abb. 10 a und b: Beatmung eines Kleinkindes mit Maßmaske (Dr. Mindé).

Tab. 9: Hilfsmittel und Kostenaufstellung

Konfektionsmaske aus Gel z.B. Respironics Gold seal® ca. 250 €
Maske nach Maß 1500–2500 €
Beatmungsgerät 10 000–15000 € z.B. BREAS PV 403/ 501®
Bedarfsorientiert pflegerische Betreuung (Behandlungspflege: 10000–20000 € Monat)

gleich zu konfektionierten Gelmasken, die teilweise mehrfach im Jahr gewechselt werden müssen rasch.

Ein Abdruck bei Säuglingen und Kleinkindern ist ohne Überwachung oder Schutzmaßnahmen bei Atemproblemen, gegen Verschlucken oder Aspiration von Abdruckmaterial nicht möglich. Ein Säugling lässt im Allgemeinen keine solche Maßnahme ohne Sedierung an sich durchführen. Wir halten die Abdrucknahme in Sedierung, ggf. Anästhesie unter Intensivüberwachung für erforderlich. Anbieter, die ohne ärztliche Kontrolle am Patienten arbeiten und Abdrucke zu Hause machen, stellen unserer Meinung nach eine Gefährdung der Patienten dar.

Nasale Beatmung ist inzwischen ein weitgehend anerkanntes effektives Verfahren zur Beatmung. Allerdings sollte man mögliche Probleme kennen. Leckagen durch Entweichen von Luft an den Rändern der Masken vor allem bei Beatmungsdrucken von mehr als 15 mm Hg sind häufig. Die am Nasenrücken entweichende Luft kann Konjunktivitiden hervorrufen. Ferner muss mit Druckstellen bei Konfektionsmasken gerechnet werden. Sie treten häufig auch bei Gelmasken auf und sind durch die erheblichen Fehlstellungen des knöchernen und weichteiligen Gesichtsschädels zu erklären. (Druckulcera können durch unterlegen von dünnster Varihesive® Folie behandelt werden). In einzelnen Fällen ist eine antibiotische Therapie erforderlich. Die oben genannten Probleme sind durch Maßmasken zu beheben.

Leckagen finden auch über den geöffneten Mund statt. Die druckgesteuerten Beatmungsgeräte können hier den Flow nachregulieren und somit einen Teil der Lecks kompensieren. Sollte keine suffiziente Beatmung möglich sein, können Kinnbänder und in Ausnahmefällen auch Gesichtsmasken, die über Mund und Nase reichen, eingesetzt werden. Unsere Erfahrung nach waren aber Gesichtsmasken ausschließlich bei Erwachsenen mit bulbärer Symptomatik erforderlich, nie bei Kindern.

Eine Mittelgesichtshypoplasie bei Beatmung ab Kindesalter ist beschrieben. (Li et al. 2000). Wir sehen eine leichter verlaufende Störung bei einem Mädchen mit mitochondrialer Myopathie, das seit dem 4. Lebensjahr nasal beatmet wird und bereits vor Beatmungsbeginn eine Progenie aufwies. Die Hypoplasie wird z.Zt. im Rahmen einer Kieferorthopädisch-kieferchirurgischen Therapie korrigiert. Ernste Komplikationen wie eine Aspiration konnten wir, entgegen unserer anfänglichen Bedenken, bisher nicht beobachten. Eine Luftansammlung im Magen kann gelegentlich Probleme bereiten und mit SAB simplex Tropfen® behandelt werden. Falls möglich sollten die Beatmungsdrucke reduziert werden.

Besonderheiten ergeben sich in der Beatmung von SMA Säuglingen und Kleinkindern. Hohe Atemfrequenzen, kleine Tidalvolumina und die Atemmechanik, die vom Zwerchfell geprägt ist, erschweren die Anpassung und Adaptation an ein Beatmungsgerät. Bei Verwendung der volumgesteuerten Geräte ist zur Reduktion der Tidalvolumina unter 200 ml ein zusätzliches Druckminderungsventil einzusetzen. Das Einstellen der optimalen Beatmungsvolumina kann nur indirekt über endexspiratorischen SO_2, Sauerstoffsättigung und Blutgase erfolgen. Die druckgesteuerten Geräte erlauben hier eine wesentlich einfachere Gewöhnung an das Gerät, so kann ggf. eine druckunterstützte Beatmung mit Freigabe der eigenen hohen Atemfrequenzen bis 50/Minute zum Beginn der Beatmung eingesetzt werden. Wird das Gerät toleriert, so gelingt der Übergang auf eine druckgesteuerte entlastendere Beatmung besser. Einige SMA Kleinkinder werden in Zeiten ohne Infekt druckunterstützt, in Infektzeiten druckkontrolliert beatmet.

Wesentlich erscheint uns bei Beatmung von SMA-I Kindern das Gesamtkonzept. In erster Linie soll eine PEG-Anlage die Ernährung und Flüssigkeitssubstitution des Kindes sicherstellen. Durch Vermeiden der gehäuften Aspirationsgefahr bei SMA I Säuglingen und Kleinkindern hat sich dieses Vorgehen bewährt. Adäquate Flüssigkeitszufuhr, Mukolytika bei Neigung zu Sekreteindickung, Antibiotika bei jedem Infekt der oberen Luftwege, regelmäßige Vojta-Technik und intensive Nutzung der Bauchlagerung sind wichtig. Viele dieser Kinder müssen regelmäßig aktiv im Nasen-Rachenraum abgesaugt werden. Dennoch stellt uns diese Patientengruppe bei jeder äußeren Störung wie Zahndurchbruch, Virusinfekte des Magen-Darm-Traktes vor Probleme und erfordert, zumindestens kurzfristig, eine erneute stationäre Aufnahme. Hier muss noch einmal auf das sehr wichtige Zusammenspiel der ambulant betreuenden Neuropädiater und Pädiater mit dem Beatmungszentrum hingewiesen werden.

Ergebnisse

Aus der Beatmungssprechstunde wurden in einer Langzeitstudie bis Ende 2000 über 58 muskelkranke Patienten überprüft. Detaillierter darstellen möchten wir die zahlenmäßig größten Gruppen, nämlich die Duchenne Dystrophie und die Spinale Muskelatrophie, die auch am ehesten mit Ergebnissen aus der Literatur verglichen werden können.

Duchenne Dystrophie

Von 38 Patienten, die an DMD erkrankt sind, waren 11 bisher noch völlig ohne Zeichen einer chronischen Ateminsuffizienz, 5 erhielten bei sonst tolerabler Situation eine IPPB Atemtherapie mit Überdruckgeräten. 22 wurden in die Heimbeatmung eingeschlossen. Die meisten Knaben waren im Alter zwischen 16 und 20 Jahren ateminsuffizient geworden (median 18 Jahre). 4 von 22 Patienten wurden in einer Dekompensation bei Infekt an die Beatmung genommen, 18 in einer stabilen Phase mit reiner Atempumpenstörung. Die Vitalkapazität bei Beatmungsbeginn war auf 0,88 Liter im Median eingeschränkt. Die Beatmung erfolgte zunächst ausschließlich während der Nacht zwischen 5–9 Stunden täglich (median 8 Stunden). Im 4. Jahr nach Beginn der Beatmung sank die Vitalkapazität weiter ab auf etwa 300 ml durch Progression der Dystrophie und Zunahme der Skoliose. Unterschiede zwischen Wirbelsäulenoperierten DMD Patienten und nichtoperierten konnten noch nicht herausgearbeitet werden, da nur 4 der 22 Patienten operiert sind. Es scheint aber die resp. Insuffizienz, wenn die Skoliose operiert wurde, später aufzutreten und die Vitalkapazität weniger stark abzufallen als bei den nichtoperierten Patienten.

21/22 Patienten wurden mit volumgesteuerten Geräten (Typ Dräger EV 800/801®) 19x, Breas PV 501® 1x, Lifecare PLV 100® 1x) beatmet. Mit Progression der Muskeldystrophie nimmt die Beatmungszeit pro Tag zu, das heisst neben der nächtlichen Beatmung müssen die Patienten auch am Tage stundenweise beatmet werden.

Respiratorische Parameter wie die Sauerstoffsättigung (Abb. 11), das endexspiratorische CO_2 (Abb. 12) sowie arterielles pO_2 und pCO_2 können von anfangs pathologischen Werten über Jahre relativ stabil in physiologischen Bereichen gehalten werden.

Eine zunehmende Cardiomyopathie, Herzinsuffizienz, Herzrhythmusstörungen, Kammerflimmern, aber auch Pneumonien stellen die Grenzen der Beatmung dar. Die Dauer der Beatmung bewegt sich zwischen einem Monat und über 10 Jahren (Abb. 13). 9 der 22 DMD Patienten sind zwischenzeitlich verstorben, meist an der Progression der Erkrankung, 4 unter dem Bild eines cardialen Versagens, 5 unter dem Bild pulmonaler Störungen. 2 der 5 Patienten, die an Pneumonien starben, verstarben bereits einen und fünf Monate nach Beginn der Beatmung, nicht zuletzt deshalb, weil das erforderliche Steigern der täglichen Beatmungszeit nicht schnell genug gelungen war.

Spinale Muskelatrophie

Von 20 Patienten mit einer spinalen Muskelatrophie waren 4 so stabil, dass keine Beatmung notwendig wurde, 4 erhielten bei noch tolerabler Lungenfunk-

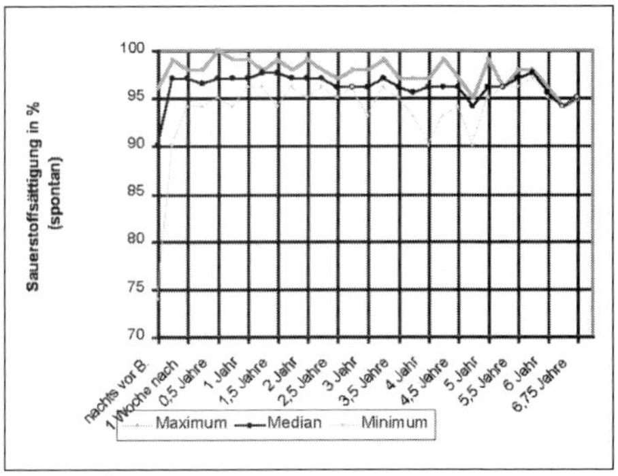

Abb. 11: DMD Sauerstoffsättigungsverläufe über Jahre.

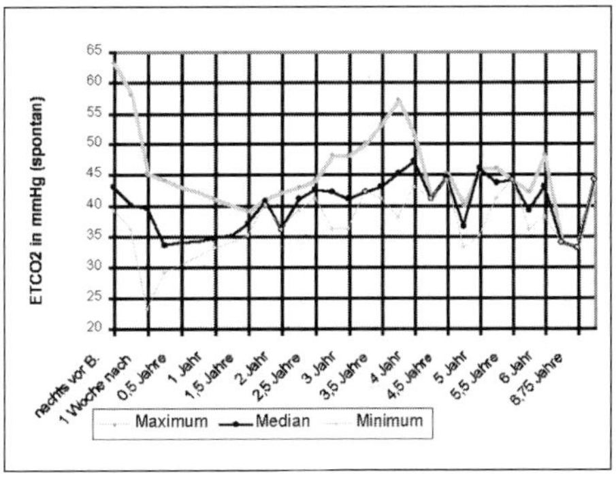

Abb. 12: DMD Endexspiratorische CO_2 Verläufe über Jahre.

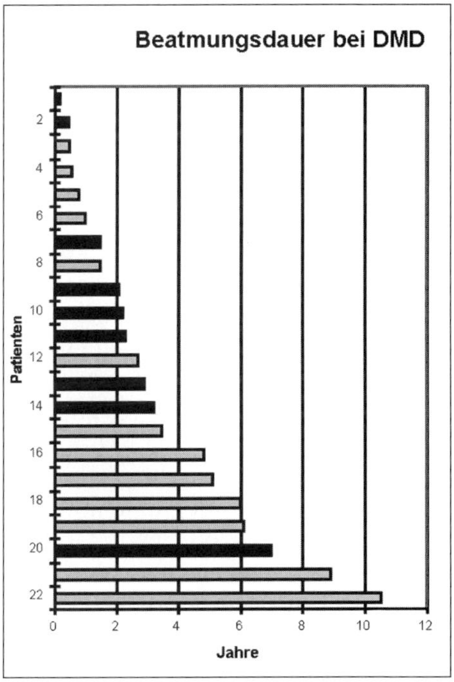

Abb. 13: Dauer der Beatmung bei DMD Patienten (n = 22) (schwarze Balken: Patient verstorben).

tion eine IPPB Atemtherapie und 12 wurden in die Heimbeatmung genommen, darunter 6 mit SMA I (Alter im Median 16 Monate), 2 mit SMA II (Alter im Median 4 Jahre) und 4 mit SMA III (Alter im Median 16 Jahre).

Für die Einstellung einer Heimbeatmung bei SMA Patienten gibt es einige Besonderheiten. Die Einstellphase ist schwieriger, da es sich um Säuglinge und Kleinkinder handelt. Hohe Atemfrequenzen und die gestörte Atemmechanik können nur mit Tricks umgangen werden. In der Anfangsphase beatmeten wir 8 von 12 SMA Kindern mit volumgesteuerten Geräten (6x Dräger EV 800/801®, 1x BREAS PV 501®, 1x Lifecare PLV 100®), teilweise unter Einsatz von Überdruckventilen zur Reduktion der Tidalvolumina, da Volumina unter 200 ml anders nicht eingestellt werden konnten. Weiter bereiteten die hohen Atemfrequenzen Kopfzerbrechen, denn Werte > 40/Min. sind bei den volumgesteuerten Geräten nicht zu erreichen. Die Geräteeinstellung muss im Regelfall indirekt erfolgen, das heißt die optimale Respiratoreinstellung kann nur über Pulsoxymetrie, endexspiratorischen CO_2 Messung und BGA erreicht werden. Zur Totraumverkleinerung müssen Kinderschlauchsysteme eingesetzt werden und kürzere Verbindungsstücke.

Eine wesentliche Erleichterung gerade bei den SMA Kindern brachten uns die druckgesteuerten Geräte. So können höhere Atemfrequenzen erreicht werden. Im Modus druckunterstützte Beatmung kann versucht werden, die hohe Atemfrequenz des Kindes > 50 zu erlauben, bis es sich an das Gerät gewöhnt hat. Danach und bei Ermüdung lässt es sich dann eher auf druckkontrollierten Modus umstellen. Die Beatmung erfolgt oft in einer Infektphase. Deshalb ist beim Start der Beatmung bei SMA I Kindern meist eine Zumischung von Sauerstoff erforderlich.

Größere Probleme macht die geringe Auswahl an geeigneten konfektionierten Masken für den Beginn der Beatmung, da selbst Päd Masken meist zu groß sind. Für die Benutzung bei Respiratoren mit Exspirationsventilen müssen die Überdrucköffnungen von Infant CPAP Masken (von Neugeborenen) mit Folien verschlossen werden. Die Anpassung einer Maske nach Maß ist bei diesen Kinderm elementar, da fast immer erhebliche Biss-Zahnfehlstellungen bestehen.

Respiratorische Parameter: Im Gegensatz zu DMD ist die Vitalkapazität bei den SMA I Kleinkindern nicht bei Beginn erhebbar gewesen. Die Sauerstoffsättigung ist bei den SMA I Gruppe (6 Kinder) teilweise dramatisch erniedrigt besonders im Schlaf (Median 88%). Bereits nach einer Nacht durchgehender Beatmung steigt die SO_2 (Abb. 14) auf physiologische Werte (Median 99%). Auch bei der SMA II Gruppe waren die nächtlichen SO_2 Werte vor Beatmung erniedrigt (Median 89%) und nach der ersten Nacht bereits gebessert (Median 94%). Die Erholung dauert aber insgesamt länger als bei den SMA I Kleinkindern.

Bei den SMA I Säuglingen und Kleinkindern war das nächtliche endexspiratorische CO_2 auf 53 mm Hg erhöht (Median). Nach nur einer Nacht Beatmung

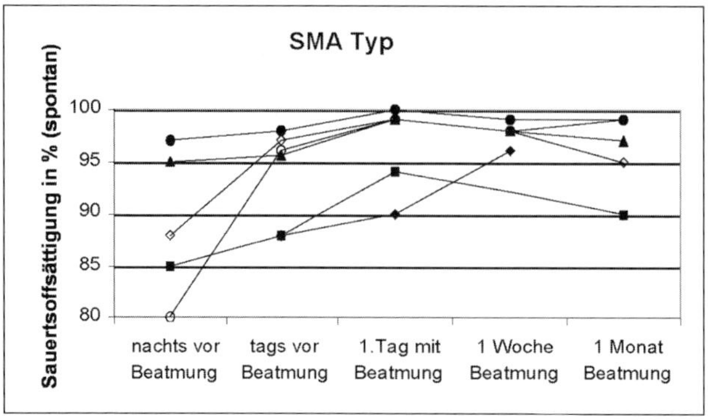

Abb. 14: Verlauf Sauerstoffsättigung bei SMA Typ I (n = 6).

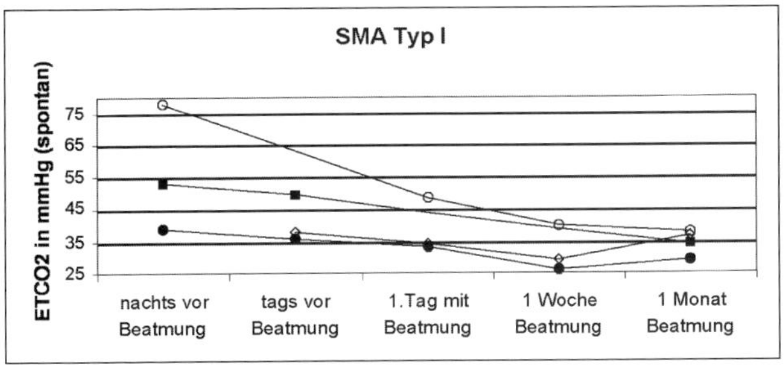

Abb. 15: Verlauf Exdexspiratorisches CO_2 bei SMA Typ I (n = 4).

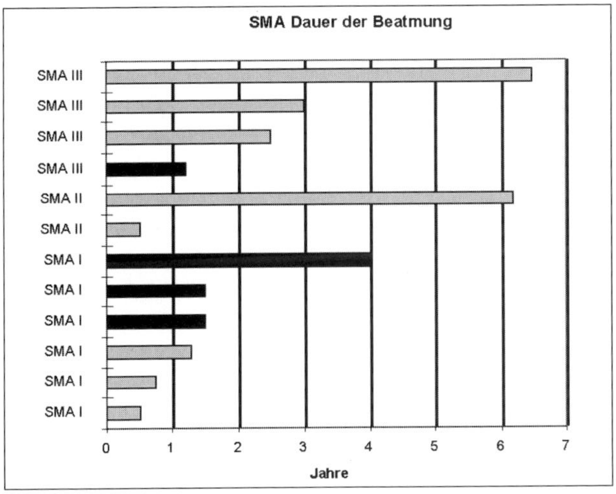

Abb. 16: Dauer der Beatmung bei SMA Patienten (SMA I: n = 6, SMA II: n = 2, SMA III: n = 4) (schwarze Balken: Patient verstorben).

konnte der Wert abgesenkt werden auf 34 mm Hg (Median) (Abb. 15). Die Blutgase zeigen einen Monat nach Beatmung Werte im Bereich 35 mm Hg für pCO_2 und >75 mm Hg für pO_2.

Bei den SMA II Kindern war das arterielle pO_2 63,5 mm Hg (Median) vor und 70,5 mm Hg direkt nach Beginn der Beatmung (Median).

Die teils eklatant erhöhten pCO_2 Werte bei SMA I vor Beatmung (Median 44 mm Hg) wurden nach Beatmung in physiologische Bereiche abgesenkt (Median 33 mm Hg). Bei SMA II Kindern war der pCO_2 vor Beatmung 40 (Median) und nach Beatmung 30 mm Hg (Median).

Die Beatmung wurde zwischen einigen Monaten und mehreren Jahren durchgeführt (Abb. 16). Ein Säugling mit SMA I schwerster Ausprägung wurde ab dem 11. Monat und über mehr als vier Jahre erfolgreich nichtinvasiv beatmet. Lediglich ein kurzer stationärer Aufenthalt war in dieser Zeit erforderlich.

Diskussion

Die Verbesserung der Lebensqualität durch die Heimbeatmung ist bereits von Rideau et al.(1983) als essentiell dargestellt worden. Sie ist inzwischen als wesentlicher Baustein im Gesamtkonzept der Versorgung von Muskelkranken eingeführt. Dass sich damit auch die Überlebenszeit verlängert, wird meistens berichtet (v. Moers). Lediglich Raphael et al. (1994) haben in einer Studie mit prophylaktischer Frühbeatmung bei DMD eine höhere Mortalität als in der noch nicht beatmeten Gruppe bei DMD gezeigt. Allerdings mögen in dieser Studie die sehr unterschiedliche Erfahrung der einzelnen Zentren (die teilweise sehr wenige Patienten mit Muskelkranken betreuten) und die häufige Anwendung von Sauerstoff das outcome in den Gruppen beeinflusst haben. DMD Patienten sterben bei respiratorischer Stabilisierung auch weiterhin an cardialer Dekompensation.

Unsere Erfahrung zeigt, in Bestätigung des allgemeinen Trends, eine nachhaltige Verbesserung der respiratorischen Situation unter Beatmung, wenn die Akzeptanz gut ist und die Nachsorge regelmäßig durchgeführt wird (Wollinsky 1994). Bei Nachlassen der muskulären Kraft muss die Beatmungszeit pro Tag angepasst werden. Nach wie vor sind schwere Pneumonien (bei niedrigster Vitalkapazität 300 ml und weniger) und vor allem cardiale Dekompensation lebensbegrenzend. In den ersten Jahren der Beatmung ist die Mobilität und Lebensqualität der Patienten deutlich verbessert, was an beruflichen Aktivitäten (Berufsausbildung, Studium) und am Aktionsradius bei Reisen abgelesen werden kann. Am besten scheinen die Ergebnisse im Gesamtkonzept mit einer orthopädisch operativen Korrektur zu sein.

Für Kleinkinder mit Ateminsuffizienz insbesondere SMA ist die Beurteilung der Beatmung in der Literatur widersprüchlich. Neben positiven Langzeiterfahrungen bei einzelnen, meist älteren Betroffenen (Bach et al. 1995, Gilgoff et al. 1989, Wang 1994) stehen Einwände wegen technischer Probleme in der Beatmung (Heckmatt et al. 1990) und kurzer Überlebenszeit (Birnkrant et al. 1998) sowie ethischer Bedenken (Ignatius et al. 1994, Thomas et al. 1994) im Vordergrund. Unsere eigenen Erfahrungen sind im wesentlichen mit den zuletzt vorgestellten Ergebnissen von Bach et al. (2000) bei 11 Kindern SMA I in Einklang zu bringen. Eine Umfrage bei japanischen Ärzten, die Kinder mit SMA beatmeten, zeigte, dass in den meisten Fällen Eltern und Ärzte die Entscheidung für die Beatmung gemeinsam trafen und nur in Ausnahmefällen eine Beatmung auf Wunsch der Eltern nicht begonnen wurde (Sakakihara et al. 2000). Auch Paditz (1997) resumiert grundsätzlich eine positive Einstellung zur Beatmung bei SMA. Allerdings muss klar sein, dass SMA I Kinder eine insgesamt kürzere Lebenserwartung haben und eine Reihe von Komplikationen im Verlauf der Behandlung dieser Kleinkinder auftreten kann.

Entscheidend bleibt unseres Erachtens, alle möglichen Verläufe und Prognosen (Ignatius et al. 1994, Thomas et al. 1994, Iannaccone et al. 1998, Russman et al. 1992, Zerres et al. 1995) sehr kritisch mit den Eltern bei Beginn der Beatmung zu erörtern. Hilfreich sind Kontakte mit Eltern, die ihr Kind über Jahre betreut haben.

Unsere Erfahrungen in der Heimbeatmung von Muskelkranken sind durchweg positiv. Das Ziel einer Verbesserung der Lebensqualität für die Betroffenen und ihre Familienangehörigen wurde vielfach erreicht (Abb. 17). Auch bei schwersten Verlaufsformen zeigt sich eine Akzeptanz der Beatmung durch die

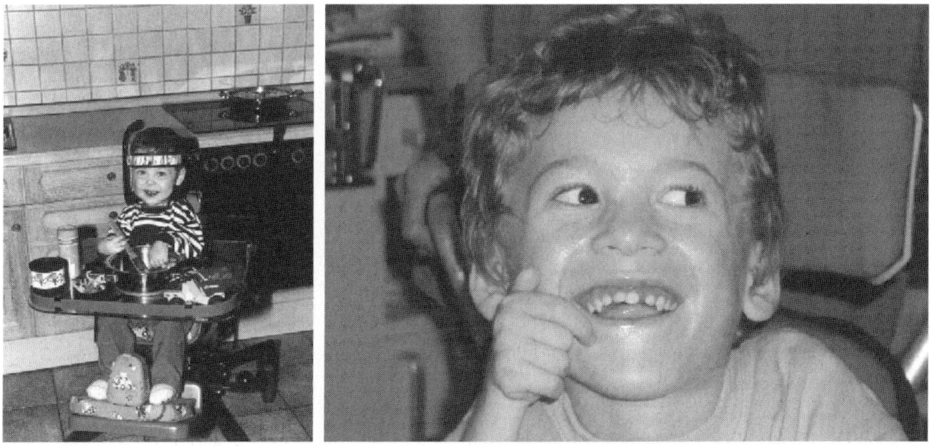

Abb. 17 a und b: Lebensqualität SMA I/II unter Beatmung.

betroffenen Kinder, die wir selbst in dieser Form nicht erwartet haben. Bestätigt wurde dies durch Paditz et al. (2000) in einer Untersuchung, wonach Kinder sich viel weniger durch die Beatmung gestört fühlten, als die Eltern dachten und viel zufriedener damit waren.

Literatur

1. Bach J, Alba A, Lee M, Rideau Y (1983) Long-term respiratory rehabilitation in the treatment of neuromuscular disease. Ann Réadapt Méd Phys 26:101–109
2. Bach JR, Wang T-G (1995) Noninvasive long-term ventilatory support for individuals with Spinal Muscular Atrophy and functional bulbar musculature. Arch Phys Med Rehabil 76: 213–217
3. Bach JR, Niranjan V, Weaver B (2000) Spinal muscular atrophy type I: A noninvasive respiratory management approach. Chest 117:1100–1105
4. Birnkrant DJ, Pope JF Eiben RM (1997) Pediatric noninvasive nasal ventilation. J Child Neurol 12: 231–236.
5. Birnkrant DJ, Pope JF, Martin JE, Repuicci AH, Eiben RM (1998) Treatment of type I spinal muscular atrophy with noninvasive ventilation and gastrostomy feeding. Pediatric Neurology 18: 407–410
6. Buhr-Schinner H, Laier-Groeneveld H, Criée CP (1999) Die nichtinvasive intermitterende Selbstbeatmung bei Kindern. Med Klin 94: Sondernummer 1, 73–76
7. Butz M, Wollinsky KH, Wiedemuth-Catrinescu U, Sperfeld A, Ludolph AC, Schreiber H (2000). Effect of intermittent non-invasive nasal ventilation (INNV) on symptoms of alveolar hypoventilation and pulmonary function in patients with amyotrophic lateral sclerosis. Akt Neurol 27: Suppl 91
8. Criée C-P, Laier-Groeneveld G (1997) Die nichtinvasive Beatmung-Überblick. In: Paditz E: Nasale Maskenbeatmung im Kindes- und Erwachsenenalter. Springer Verlag Berlin Heidelberg New York 15–25
9. Curran FJ (1981) Night ventilation by body respirators for patients in chronic respiratory failure due to late stage Duchenne muscular dystrophy. Arch Phys Med Rehab 62: 270–274
10. Ellis ER, Bye PTP, Bruderer JW, Sullivan CE. (1987) Treatment of respiratory failure during sleep in patients with neuromuscular diseases. Am Rev Resp Dis 135:148–152

11. Frates RC, Splaingard ML, Smith EO, Harrison GM (1985) Outcome of home mechanical ventilation in children. J Pediatr 106: 850–856
12. Gay PC, Patel AM, Viggiano RW, Hubmayr RD (1991) Nocturnal nasal ventilation for treatment of patients with hypercapnic respiratory failure. Mayo Clin Proc. 66: 695–703
13. Gibson B (2001) Long-term ventilation for patients with Duchenne dystrophy. Chest 119: 940–46
14. Gilgoff IS, Kahlstrom E, Mac Laughlin E, Keens Th (1989) Long-term ventilatory support in spinal muscular atrophy. J Pediatr 115:904–909
15. Heckmatt JZ, Loh L, Dubowitz V (1989) Nocturnal hypoventilation in children with nonprogressive neuromuscular disease. Pediatrics 83: 250–255
16. Heckmatt JZ, Loh L, Dubowitz V (1990) Night-time nasal ventilation in neuromuscular diseases. Lancet 335: 579–582
17. Iannaccone ST (1998) Spinal muscular atrophy. Sem Neurol18:19–26
18. Ignatius J (1994) The natural history of severe spinal muscular atrophy- further evidence for clinical subtypes. Neuromusc Disord 4: 527–528
19. Laier-Groeneveld für die Arbeitsgruppe Heim- und Langzeitbeatmung (1993) Richtlinien zur Indikation und Durchführung der intermittierenden Selbstbeatmung (ISB). Med Klin 88: 509–510
20. Li KK, Riley RW, Guilleminault C (2000) An unreported risk in the use of home nasal continuous positive airway pressure and home nasal ventilation in children. Chest 117: 916–918.
21. Lyager S, Steffensen B, Juhl B (1995) Indicators of need for mechanical ventilation in Duchenne muscular dystrophy and spinal muscular atrophy. Chest 108:779–85
22. Moers v A, Hartmann A, Grieben U (2000) Heimbeatmung bei Kindern mit Muskeldystrophien. Kinderärztliche Praxis 6: 366–375
23. Paditz E (1997) Nasale Beatmung im Kindes- und Jugendalter. In: Paditz E: Nasale Maskenbeatmung im Kindes- und Erwachsenenalter Springer Verlag Berlin Heidelberg New York 26–42
24. Paditz E, Zieger S, Bickhardt J, Bockelbrink A, Grieben U, Hammer J, Kemper A, Knape H, Laier-Groeneveld G, Mellies U, Regneri W, Scholle S, Schönhofer B, Weise M, Wiebel M, Windisch W, Wollinsky KH et al. (2000) Lebensqualität unter Heimbeatmung im Kindes, Jugend- und jungen Erwachsenenalter: unterschiedliche Sichtweisen von Eltern und Kindern. Somnologie 4: 13–19
25. Raphael J-C, Chevret S, Chastang C, Bouvet F(1994) Randomised trial of preventive nasal ventilation in Duchenne muscular dystrophy .Lancet 343:1666–1604
26. Rideau Y, Gatin G, Bach J, Gines G (1983) Prolongation of Life in Duchenne's dystrophy. Acta Neurol 5:1187–1124
27. Robert D, Willlig TN, Paulus J (1993) Long-term nasal ventilation in neuromuscular disorders: report of a Consensus Conference. Eur Resp J 6: 599–606
28. Russman BS, Iannacone ST, Buncher CR, Samaha FJ, White M, Perkins B, Zimmermann L, Smith C, Burhans K, Barker L (1992) Spinal muscular atrophy: new thoughts on the pathogneensis and classification scheme. J Child Neurol 7:347–353
29. Sakakihara Y., Kubota M, Kim S. Oka A (2000) Long-term ventilator support in patients with Werdnig-Hoffmann disease. Pediatrics Int 42: 359–363
30. Simonds AK, Ward S, Heather AS, Bush A, Muntoni F (2000) Outcome of paediatric domiciliary mask ventilation in neuromuscular and skeletal disease. Eur Resp J 16: 476–481
31. Thomas H, Dubowitz V(1994) The natural history of Type I (severe) Spinal muscular atrophy. Neuromusc Disord 4: 497–502
32. Wang T-G, Bach JR, Avilla C, Augusta AS, Yang G-F W (1994) Survival of individuals with Spinal muscular atrophy on ventilatroy support. Am J Phys Med Rehabil 73: 207–211
33. Wollinsky KH, Hülser P-J, Mehrkens H-H, Geiger P, Weindler M, Naumann Th (1991) Nächtliche Hypoxie und Hypercapnie bei Patienten mit Duchennescher Muskeldystrophie. In: Schläfke M: Schlaf und schlafbezogene autonome Störungen aus interdisziplinärer Sicht. Universitätsverlag Dr. N. Brockmeyer-Bochum 247–251

34. Wollinsky KH, Mindé A, Geiger P, Gelowicz-Maurer M, Hülser P-J, Naumann Th, Mehrkens H-H (1994) Nasale nächtliche Beatmung bei Muskelkranken: Kann sie Lebensqualität verbessern und Leben verlängern? Med Klin 89: Sondernr 1, 23–25
35. Wollinsky KH, Mindé A, Schreiber H, Kluger P, Mehrkens H-H (1995) Effektivität der Heimbeatmung bei Kleinkindern und Säuglingen. Med Klin 90: Sondernr 1, 57–59
36. Yamashita T, Kanaya K, Yokogushi K, Ishikawa Y Minami R (2001) Correlation between progression of spinal deformity and pulmonary function in Duchenne muscular dystrophy. J Pediatr Orthop 21:113–116
37. Zerres K, Rudnik-Schöneborn S, Dubowitz V, Emery AEH, Forst R, Granata C, Haverkamp F, Merlini L, Mielke U, Mokrusch Th, Mortier W, Nix WA, Rüdel R, Voit Th, Wollinsky KH, Zierz S, Röhrig D (1995) Guidelines für symptomatic therapy in Spinal muscular atrophy (SMA). Acta Cardiomyol 7: 61–66

Verbesserung des maximalen Hustenstoßes bei Kindern und Jugendlichen mit neuromuskulären Erkrankungen durch Hyperinsufflations-assistierte Hustenmanöver

C. Schwake, U. Mellies, R. Ragette, T. Voit, H. Teschler

Zusammenfassung

Patienten mit neuromuskulären Erkrankungen (NME) sind aufgrund ihrer respiratorischen Muskelschwäche durch Komplikationen wie Pneumonien und Atelektasen nicht selten vital bedroht. Ziel der Studie war es, den Einfluss von Hyperinsufflations-assistierten Hustenmanövern auf den maximalen Hustenstoß zu messen.

Vierzehn Kinder und Jugendliche mit NME und einem maximalen Hustenstoß < 160 l/min oder anamnestisch häufigen Atemwegsinfekten wurden in die Studie eingeschlossen. Mittels intermittierender Überdruck-Beatmung, einem volumen-gesteuerten Beatmungsgerät oder einem Ambu-Beutel wurden die Lungen passiv über die Inspiratorische Vitalkapazität (IVC) hinaus überbläht (Maximale Insufflations-Kapazität MIC). Dabei konnte das Lungenvolumen bei jedem einzelnen Patienten und im Durchschnitt von 570 ± 362 ml (IVC) auf 960 ± 485 ml (MIC) gesteigert werden ($p < 0{,}001$). Der maximale Hustenstoß PCF wurde mit einem Peak-Flow-Meter vor und unmittelbar nach Durchführung des Manövers gemessen und ebenfalls bei allen Patienten von 112 ± 57 l/min auf 199 ± 85 l/min ($p < 0{,}001$) verbessert.

Hyperinsufflations-assistierte Hustenmanöver führen zu einer deutlichen Steigerung des maximalen Hustenstoßes und können somit durch verbesserte Sekret-Clearance zu einer wirksamen Pneumonie- und Atelektasen-Prävention beitragen.

Einleitung

Neuromuskuläre Erkrankungen wie die Spinale Muskelatrophie (SMA), Duchenne Muskeldystrophie (DMD) oder Congenitale Muskeldystrophien (CMD) führen häufig schon im Kindes- und Jugendalter zu schwerwiegenden Komplikationen des respiratorischen Systems wie Pneumonien und Atelektasen (siehe Abb. 1a). Pneumonien treten deutlich häufiger als bei Gesunden auf. Im fortgeschrittenen Stadium kommt es z.B. bei DMD zu einer Inzidenz von ca. einer Lungenentzündung pro Jahr (1). Pathophysiologisch scheint ein insuffizienter Hustenstoß bei leichten Infekten der oberen Atemwege eine wesentliche Rolle zu spielen. Eine unzureichende Sekret-Clearance ist die Folge. Bei Gesunden ist

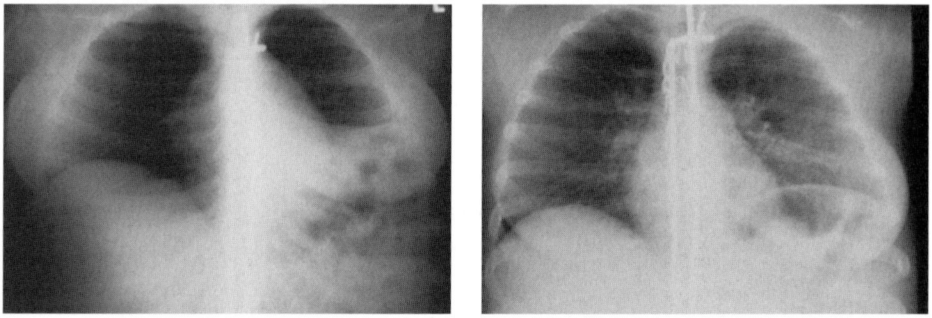

Abb. 1a und b: Atelektase des linken Unterlappens bei einer 13jährigen Patientin mit HSMN und vollständige Rückbildung nach intensivierten Hyperinsufflations-assistierten Hustenmanövern.

der Hustenstoß durch drei wesentliche Mechanismen determiniert: 1) Nach tiefer Einatmung kommt es 2) zum Glottis-Verschluss, und 3) wird durch Anspannung der exspiratorischen Atemmuskulatur der Hustenstoß generiert. Bei den meisten Patienten mit fortgeschrittenen NME ist weder eine tiefe Insufflation (messbar als IVC) noch eine effektive Aktivierung der Exspirationsmuskulatur (messbar als maximaler Exspirationsdruck PEmax) möglich. Hingegen funktioniert der Glottis-Verschluss außer bei Patienten mit Bulbärparese, z.B. bei Amyotropher Lateralsklerose zumeist noch hinreichend.

Eine Verbesserung des Hustenstoßes sollte also bei den Punkten 1) und 3) (s. o.) ansetzen. Durch Hyperinsufflation über das patienteneigene Vermögen hinaus (> IVC) werden die Lungen überbläht. Die gesteigerte passive Vordehnung führt über die pulmonalen elastischen Rückstellkräfte zu einem höheren Atemfluss, der in einem verbesserten Hustenstoß genutzt werden kann. Die exspiratorische Muskulatur wird zusätzlich durch manuelle abdominothorakale Kompression unterstützt.

Die vorliegende Studie beschreibt die Durchführung von Hyperinsufflations-assistierten Hustenmanövern und untersucht den Einfluss auf den maximalen Hustenstoß PCF bei Kindern und Jugendlichen mit neuromuskulären Erkrankungen.

Methoden

Insgesamt vierzehn Patienten mit neuromuskulären Erkrankungen (5 DMD, 5 SMA, 2 CMD, 1 Hereditäre sensomotorische Neuropathie, 1 Glykogenose II; Alter 15,2 ± 6,1 Jahre) wurden in die Studie eingeschlossen. Bei allen wurde eine Spirometrie (IVC, FEV1) und eine Atemmuskelfunktion (maximale In- und Exspirationsdrücke PImax, PEmax) durchgeführt, sowie der maximale Hustenstoß (PCF) gemessen. Zu diesem Zweck erhielten die Patienten ein Peak-Flow-Meter und wurden aufgefordert, mit maximalem Kraftaufwand hinein zu husten.

Bei allen wurden Hyperinsufflations-Manöver eingeübt. Zwölf erhielten ein IPPB-Gerät, ein Patient einen Ambu-Beutel und eine Patientin benutzte ihr volumen-gesteuertes Beatmungsgerät. Die Patienten wurden aufgefordert, die

Lungen mit den entsprechenden Hilfsmitteln passiv aufblähen zu lassen, »wie einen Luftballon«. In das Schlauchsystem wurde ein Pneumotachygraph zwischengeschaltet, an dem das Volumen, auch für den Patienten sichtbar, abgelesen werden konnte. Insofern hatte auch der Einzelne ein Feedback über den »Erfolg« der Hyperinsufflation. Das insufflierte maximale Volumen (Maximale Insufflationskapazität MIC) wurde notiert.

Im nächsten Schritt erlernten die Patienten den Glottis-Verschluss, d.h. die eingeatmete Luft in den Lungen zu halten. Durch ein erneutes maximales Hustenmanöver in das Peak-Flow-Meter hinein wurde PCF1 gemessen. Alle Patienten hatten mindestens zwei Tage Zeit, das assistierte Husten zu erlernen.

Die Daten werden als Durchschnittswerte ± Standardabweichung präsentiert. Die statistische Auswertung der Vorher-Nachher-Vergleiche erfolgte mittels Wilcoxon-Test für Paardifferenzen.

Ergebnisse

Alle Patienten zeigten eine schwere restriktive Ventilationsstörung (IVC 22,3 ± 13,0%) und erniedrigte maximale Inspirations- und Exspirationsdrücke (PImax 2,4 ± 1,1 kPa, PEmax 2,0 ± 0,9 kPa). Dreizehn der Kinder und Jugendlichen hatten eine Skoliose, elf waren bereits einmal stationär aufgrund einer Pneumonie.

Durch die Hyperinsufflation der Lungen konnte die maximale Insufflations-Kapazität MIC bei allen Patienten über die Vitalkapazität hinaus um knapp das Doppelte gesteigert werden (IVC 570 ± 372 ml gegenüber MIC 960 ± 485 ml; $p < 0,001$). Im Anschluss an die Überblähung der Lungen wurde der maximale Hustenstoß erneut gemessen. Im Durchschnitt kam es zu einer Verbesserung des PCF von 112 ± 57 auf 199 ± 85 l/min ($p < 0,001$).

Diskussion

In unserer Studie konnte gezeigt werden, dass mittels Hyperinsufflations-assistierten Hustenmanövern bei Patienten mit restriktiven Ventilationsstörungen und geschwächter exspiratorischer Muskulatur der maximale Hustenstoß auf etwa das Doppelte gesteigert wurde. Insofern scheint diese Therapie ein wirkungsvoller Mechanismus für eine verbesserte Sekret-Clearance zu sein.

In der Literatur sind unterschiedliche Methoden zur Steigerung des PCF fast ausschließlich bei Erwachsenen beschrieben. Alle beruhen auf einer passiven Hyperinsufflation der Lungen, entweder mittels Überdruck (IPPB, In-Exsufflator) oder gesteigertem Volumen (Ambu-Beutel, Beatmungsgerät oder »glossopharyngeal breathing«) (2, 3, 4, 5). Bis auf zwei Patienten erhielten alle an unserer Studie teilnehmenden ein IPPB-Gerät, ursprünglich entwickelt zur Inhalation bei Erwachsenen mit Chronisch Obstruktiver Bronchitis.

Was sind die Vorteile des »Intermittent positive pressure breathing (IPPB)«? 1) Im Infekt besteht die Möglichkeit des gleichzeitigen Inhalierens mit Kochsalz oder bei Obstruktion der Atemwege mit Bronchospasmolytika. 2) Die Übungen können auch bei gering erhaltener Muskelkraft der Extremitäten vom Patienten allein durchgeführt werden, bzw. die Hilfsperson kann sich darauf konzentrieren, zusätzlich durch abdominothorakale Kompression die Effektivität zu steigern. 3) Gerade im Kindesalter scheint es einfacher zu sein, die Atemmanöver mit Hilfe von Überdruck zu koordinieren, als z.B. durch einen Ambu-Beutel die Luft mehrfach hintereinander anzuhalten, um entsprechend wirkungsvolle Volumina zu insufflieren.

Bisher eine einzige Studie (4) untersuchte den Effekt der Steigerung des PCF mittels IPPB-assistierter Hustenmanöver. Eine signifikante Verbesserung konnte nur bei Patienten mit respiratorischer Muskelschwäche ohne Skoliose gezeigt werden. Dieses Ergebnis widerspricht dem unserer Untersuchungen, da hier fast alle (13/14) eine Skoliose hatten. Der Unterschied ist wahrscheinlich dadurch erklärbar, dass in der Studie von Sivasothy et al. (4) die Patienten mit Skoliose noch einen effektiven Hustenstoß von im Durchschnitt 350 l/min hatten und somit eine Verbesserung aus klinischen Gesichtspunkten nicht notwendig war.

Assistierte Hustenmanöver können nicht nur aus prophylaktischer Sicht zur Verhinderung von Pneumonien wichtig sein. Auch im akuten Fall führt die intensive Durchführung zu einer effektiven Sekret-Clearance und zusammen mit einer zielgerichteten Antibiose zur Ausheilung von Pneumonie und Atelektase (siehe Abb. 1b).

Schlussfolgerung

Zur Beurteilung der respiratorischen Funktion bei Patienten mit Neuromuskulären Erkrankungen sollte neben Lungen- und Atemmuskelfunktion auch die Messung des maximalen Hustenstoßes gehören. Bei einem Hustenstoß von < 160 l/min oder anamnestisch häufigen Infekten und Problemen, pulmonales Sekret abzuhusten, sollten Hyperinsufflations-assistierte Hustenmanöver erlernt werden. Im infektfreien Intervall ist das ein- bis zweimalige Durchführen für ca. 10 Minuten zu empfehlen, während eines Infektes ist, je nach Bedarf, auf bis zu 10mal täglich zu intensivieren.

Literatur

1. Bach JR, Rajaraman R, Ballanger F, Tzeng AC, Ishikawa Y, Kulesa R, Bansal T (1998): Neuromuscular ventilatory insufficiency: Effect of home mechanical ventilator use v oxygen therapy on pneumonia and hospitalization rates. Am J Phys Med Rehabil; 77: 8–19
2. Bach JR (1993): Mechanical Insufflation-Exsufflation. Comparison of Peak Expiratory flows with manually assisted and unassisted coughing techniques. Chest; 104: 1553–62
3. Kang SW, Bach JR (2000): Maximum insufflation capacity. Chest; 118: 61–65
4. Sivasothy P, Brown L, Smith IE, Shneerson JM (2001): Effect of manually assisted cough and mechanical insufflation on cough flow of normal subjects, patients with chronic obstructive pulmonary disease (COPD), and patients with respiratory muscle weakness. Thorax; 56(6): 438–44
5. Tzeng AC, Bach JR (2000): Prevention of pulmonary morbidity for patients with neuromuscular disease. Chest; 118: 1390–1396

Der Phänotyp der »Rippling«-Muskelerkrankung im Kindesalter

U. Schara, M. Vorgerd, K. Ricker, W. Mortier

Abstrakt

Die »Rippling«-Muskelerkrankung ist eine seltene, überwiegend autosomal-dominant vererbte, jedoch auch sporadisch auftretende Erkrankung. Die Erstbeschreibung erfolgte durch Torbergsen 1975; kürzlich konnte sie durch den Nachweis von Mutationen im *Caveolin-3* Gen als Caveolinopathie klassifiziert werden. Während Daten zur Klinik im Erwachsenenalter schon ausführlich beschrieben sind, können wir erstmals Symptome im Kindesalter zusammenfassen. Erste Auffälligkeiten waren Gangstörungen mit häufigem Hinfallen, erschwertem Hackengang sowie ein Zehengang mit Myalgien und »warm-up« Phänomen, darüberhinaus eine Wadenhypertrophie und eine Erhöhung der Kreatinkinase im Serum. Druck-/Perkussion-induzierte rasche Kontraktionen und ein schmerzhaftes Muskel-»Mounding« konnten schon im Kindesalter, das Muskel-»Rippling« in unserem Kollektiv erst nach dem 10. Lebensjahr beobachtet werden. Die Diagnosesicherung erfolgt durch die Mutationsanalyse im *Caveolin-3* Gen. Die Muskelbiopsie kann bei den Patienten ohne Muskelschwäche oder sichere Zeichen der mechanischen Übererregbarkeit hilfreich sein, um die »Rippling«-Muskelerkrankung von der autosomal-dominanten, progredienten Gliedergürtel-Muskeldystrophie 1C abzutrennen.

Einleitung

Die »Rippling«-Muskelerkrankung ist eine seltene, überwiegend autosomal-dominant vererbte Erkrankung, charakterisiert durch mechanisch induzierte unwillkürliche Bewegungen (5,19,20,23,27,28). Sporadische Fälle sind mitgeteilt (29). Die Erstbeschreibung erfolgte durch Torbergsen 1975 (26). 1989 wurde über 2 deutsche Familien berichtet und der Begriff »Rippling muscle disease« geprägt (19). Seitdem wurden weitere Familien beschrieben (5, 20, 23, 28). »Rippling« illustriert die Tatsache, dass bei plötzlicher Dehnung der Muskulatur nach vorheriger Kontraktion wellenartige Bewegungen in diesen Muskeln auftreten; z.B. kommt es bei abrupter Beugung im Kniegelenk nach vorheriger Streckung zu Wellenbewegungen über den M. quadriceps femoris, im Oberschenkel häufig von oben lateral nach unten medial. Die »Rippling«-Muskelerkrankung ist genetisch heterogen; in einer Familie aus Oregon wurde die Erkrankung an den Genort auf Chromosom 1q41 gekoppelt (23); der genetische Defekt ist bisher nicht identifiziert. Kürzlich konnten für die »Rippling«-Muskelerkrankung in den 5 europäischen Familien Mutationen im *Caveolin-3* Gen als molekulare Ursache des

Phänotyps identifiziert werden (3, 29). Aufgrund der nachgewiesenen Mutationen im *Caveolin-3* Gen und der daraus resultierenden Caveolin-3 Reduktion im Muskelgewebe konnte die »Rippling«-Muskelerkrankung in europäischen Familien als Caveolinopathie identifiziert werden (3, 29). Neben dieser gut definierten Erkrankung wurden andere Krankheitsentitäten mit einer mechanischen Übererregbarkeit der Muskulatur in Kombination mit einer Myasthenia gravis und Thymom (2) oder mit verzögertem Knochenalter und Kleinwuchs (10) beschrieben. Klinische Symptome im Erwachsenenalter sind ausführlich mitgeteilt (5, 19, 20, 23, 27, 28, 29) und diagnostische Kriterien zusammengestellt worden (28). Wir können erstmals klinische Daten von 7 Kindern mit autosomal-dominanter »Rippling«-Muskelerkrankung aufgrund einer Mutation im *Caveolin-3* Gen berichten.

Patienten und Methode

Klinische und laborchemische Daten von 7 Kindern aus 5 Familien mit autosomal-dominanter »Rippling«-Muskelerkrankung konnten zusammengestellt werden (Tab. 1). Bei allen Kindern wurde die Diagnose durch den Mutationsnachweis im *Caveolin-3* Gen gesichert. Alle Kinder wurden durch die Autoren untersucht.

Ergebnisse

Symptome der »Rippling«-Muskelerkrankung zeigten 7 Patienten, untersucht im Alter von 5 bis 16 Jahren. Die klinischen Daten dieser Patienten sind in Tabelle 1 zusammengefasst.

Erste Symptome, die von Patienten und/oder Eltern berichtet wurden, waren Gangauffälligkeiten mit häufigem Hinfallen, erschwertem Hackengang sowie ein Zehengang mit Myalgien und einem »warm-up« Phänomen (d.h. nach Ruhephasen kommt es zunächst zu einem schmerzhaften Zehengang für ca. 2–3 Minuten, der durch die wiederholten Bewegungen gemildert wird oder ganz abklingt). Häufig beklagen Betroffene auch belastungsabhängige Myalgien (6/7), eine Belastungsintoleranz, eine Muskelsteifheit nach Ruhe oder Belastung (6/7) und zeigen eine generalisierte Muskel- oder Wadenhypertrophie (5/7). Bei der Untersuchung konnten bei allen Kindern Druck-/Perkussion-induzierte rasche Kontraktionen (PIRC) ausgelöst werden; ein schmerzhaftes Muskel-»Mounding« (bei Druck auf oder Stossen an die Muskulatur kommt es an dieser Stelle zu einer schmerzhaften, »hügelartigen« Verhärtung für die Dauer von 5–10 Sekunden) zeigten 4 von 7 Patienten. Das Muskel-»Rippling« konnte bei 3 von 7 Kindern im Alter von 12 bis 16 Jahren beobachtet werden. Die Kreatinkinase (CK) war bei allen Kindern erhöht (max. 8000 E/l, Norm $\leq$ 100 E/l). Das Elektromyogramm (EMG) bei 5 Kindern zeigte, trotz erhöhter mechanischer Muskelerregung, keine myotonen Entladungen.

Einige Symptome wurden nur in Einzelfällen beobachtet. Bei einem Patienten wurde eine beidseitige, bei einem weiteren eine rechtseitige Hüftdysplasie

Tab. 1: Symptome der »Rippling«-Muskelerkrankung im Kindesalter

Patient Nr.	**1**	**2**	**3**	**4**	**5**	**6**	**7**
Geschlecht	männlich	weiblich[1]	männlich[1]	männlich[3]	weiblich[3]	weiblich[3]	männlich[2]
Alter bei Untersuchung (Jahre)	14	14	14	5	12	3	16
Alter zu Beginn (Jahre)	2	1	14	4	3	3	8
Erste Symptome	Zehengang nach Ruhephasen	Zehengang	Waden-hypertrophie PIRC, Mounding	Zehengang nach Ruhephasen	Myalgien in der Wadenmuskulatur	Häufiges Hinfallen	Verlangsamte Bewegungen nach Ruhe
Zehengang nach Ruhe mit Myalgien und »warm-up«	ja	ja	nein	ja	ja	ja	ja
Muskelsteifheit	ja	ja	nein	nein	nein	ja	ja
Myalgien	ja	ja	nein	ja	ja	ja	ja
PIRC[4]	ja	ja	ja	ja	ja	ja	ja
Mounding	ja	ja	ja	nein	nein	ja	ja
Rippling	ja	nein	nein	nein	ja	nein	ja
Wadenhypertrophie	ja	nein	ja	nein	ja	ja	ja
Erschwerter Hackengang	ja	nein	nein	ja	ja	ja	nein
Häufiges Hinfallen	ja	ja	nein	nein	ja	ja	nein
Percussion-/ Greif- induzierte Myotonie-artige Reaktion	ja	ja	nein	nein	ja	nein	ja
Erhöhte CK[5] (U/l)	8000	312	900	346	400	945	388

[1]Mitglied der Familie beschrieben von Vorgerd; [2]Mitglied der Familie beschrieben von Torbergsen; [3]Mitglied der Familie beschrieben von Ricker; die Nummern beziehen sich auf die Literaturzitate; [4]PIRC = Druck- / Perkussion-induzierte rasche Kontraktionen; [5]CK = Kreatinkinase

berichtet. Drei Kinder konnten nach kräftigem Händedruck die Hände nur verzögert öffnen, ähnlich wie bei einer Greifmyotonie. Ein anderer Patient zeigte bei Perkussion des Thenars eine Adduktion des Daumens, ähnlich wie bei der Perkussionsmyotonie bei Myotonia congenita. Schmerzhafte Myalgien der Bauchwand- und/oder der Thoraxwandmuskulatur wurden bei 3 Kindern berichtet; dies führte in einem Fall aufgrund einer vermuteten Appendizitis zu weiterer chirurgischer Intervention. Ein Mädchen beklagte Episoden mit plötzlich auftretender Einschränkung der Augenmotilität.

Diskussion

Wir konnten klinische Daten von 7 Kindern aus 5 Familien mit autosomal-dominanter »Rippling«-Muskelerkrankung, verursacht durch Mutationen im *Caveolin-3* Gen, zusammenfassen. Eine Kombination typischer Symptome, auch schon im Kindesalter (Tab. 1), lassen eine »Rippling«-Muskelerkrankung annehmen. Häufig, mit Beginn des freien Laufens, zeigen die Kinder einen Zehengang mit Myalgien besonders nach Ruhephasen; nach ca. 2–3 Minuten Laufen ist die Symptomatik gemildert oder ganz abgeklungen (»warm-up« Phänomen). Alle Kinder zeigten PIRC und eine erhöhte CK im Serum. Zusätzlich war ein schmerzhaftes »Mounding« bei 5 von 7 Patienten zu beobachten. Muskel-»Rippling« konnte bei nur 3 von 7 Patienten im Alter von 12 bis 16 Jahren ausgelöst werden, nicht bei jüngeren Patienten. Wenn junge Patienten alle Kriterien für die »Rippling«-Muskelerkrankung wie PIRC, »Mounding«, »Rippling« und die erhöhte CK erfüllen (28), dann muss in der Differentialdiagnostik noch die autosomal-rezessive Erkrankung mit »Rippling«, verzögertem Knochenalter und Kleinwuchs berücksichtigt werden (10). Molekulargenetische Analysen im *Caveolin-3* Gen können die Diagnose sichern. Unspezifische erste Symptome in früher Kindheit oder später inkomplett auftretende Symptome führen zu einer breiteren Differentialdiagnostik (Tab. 2). Eine erhöhte CK, eine Wadenhypertrophie mit verzögerter motorischer Entwicklung und/oder Gangstörungen mit häufigem Hinfallen, erschwertem Hackengang und Myalgien können auf eine Dystrophinopathie, besonders auf eine Becker-Muskeldystrophie, hinweisen. Gangstörungen mit einer relativ kurzen Anamnese von Wochen oder Monaten zusammen mit einer erhöhten CK und Myalgien können auf eine Myositis hinweisen. Um unnötige Untersuchungen zu vermeiden, sind CK-Bestimmungen zusätzlich zur ausführlichen Anamnese und klinischen Untersuchung der Patienten und deren Eltern notwendig. Die Familienanamnese kann einen autosomal-dominanten Erbgang oder das Auftreten eines sporadischen Falls belegen. Vier von 7 Kindern zeigten Perkussion-/oder Greif-induzierte Kontraktionen, die schwierig von einer Myotonie zu differenzieren waren. Um hereditäre Erkrankungen mit Myotonien von der »Rippling«-Muskelerkrankung zu trennen, kann das EMG hilfreich sein; dieses zeigt keine myotonen Entladungen während des Muskel-»Mounding« und/oder -»Rippling« (19, 26). Das Ausmaß der CK-Erhöhung bei der »Rippling«-Muskelerkrankung ist variabel (Tab. 1). Besonders bei nur leichter Erhöhung der CK müssen hereditäre Myotonien in der Differentialdiagnostik berücksichtigt werden.

Kürzlich konnte die »Rippling«-Muskelerkrankung als Caveolinopathie identifiziert werden. Mutationen im Caveolin-3 Gen wurden sowohl bei allen 7 Kindern und deren betroffenen Familienmitgliedern als auch bei einem sporadischen Fall nachgewiesen (3, 29). Die »Rippling«-Muskelerkrankung ist genetisch heterogen, wie es auch ein Fall mit »Rippling« und moderater CK-Erhöhung, gefolgt von einer Myasthenie zeigt (2); hier konnte keine Mutation im *Caveolin-3* Gen gefunden werden (29). In der von Stephan beschriebenen Familie aus Oregon (23) wurde eine Kopplung an Chromosom 1q41 berichtet; der Gendefekt ist bisher aber nicht identifiziert. In der von So beschriebenen Familie (20)

Tab. 2: Differentialdiagnose der »Rippling«–Muskelerkrankung im Kindesalter

	Myotonie: Klinisch*	Myotonie: EMG	PIRC	Rippling	»warm-up« Phänomen	Muskel-Steifheit	Myalgien	Muskel-schwäche	Erhöhte CK (U/l)
»Rippling« – Muskel-erkrankung	–	–	+	(+)	+	(+)	(+)	–	–
Myotonische Dystrophie Steinert	(+)	(+)	–	–	–	–	–	Dist.++ / Prox. +	+/–
Myotonia congenita									
Chloridkanal	+	+	–	–	+	+	–	+/prox.	+/–
Natriumkanal	+	+	–	–	–	+K.i.	–	(+)	+/–
Metabolische Myopathien									
Muskuläre Glykogenosen	–	–	–	–	–	+	+	+/prox.	+/–
Lipid-Myopathien	–	–	–	–	–	–	+	+/prox.	+/–
Myoadenylat-deaminase Defizienz	–	–	–	–	–	+	+	+/prox.	+/–
Becker Muskel-dystrophie	–	–	–	–	–	–	+	+/prox.	+/–

*Greif- und Perkussions-Myotonie, verzögertes Lidöffnen, eingeschränkte Augenbewegungen; Warm-up Phänomen = Zehengang für einige Minuten nach Ruhephasen; PIRC = Perkussion-induzierte rasche Kontraktionen; K.i. = Kälte induziert; CK = Kreatinkinase; + = Symptom bei allen Patienten vorhanden; (+) = Symptom möglich; ((+)) = Symptom selten; – = Symptom nicht vorhanden; +/– = Symptom vorhanden oder nicht vorhanden

wurde die Region auf Chromosom 1q41 ausgeschlossen. Mutationsanalysen im *Caveolin-3* Gen wurden bisher in diesen beiden Familien (20, 23), bei dem sporadischen Fall mit Myasthenie und Thymom (2) und bei Erkrankungen mit Muskel-»Rippling« in Kombination mit anderen Symptomen (10, 18), nicht mitgeteilt.

Die durch Mutationen im *Caveolin-3* Gen bedingte Caveolin-3 Defizienz zeigt eine klinische Heterogenität: die progrediente Gliedergürtel-Muskeldystrophie Typ 1C (8, 12, 14), die idiopathische CK-Erhöhung (6), eine besondere Form einer distalen Myopathie (26) und die »Rippling«-Muskelerkrankung (3, 29). Patienten mit einer »Rippling«-Muskelerkrankung zeigen im Gegensatz zur Gliedergürtel-Muskeldystrophie Typ 1C normalerweise keine Muskelschwäche (5, 19, 20, 23, 27, 28, 29); in der Literatur wird nur in wenigen Fällen eine Muskelschwäche berichtet (20). Bei unseren Patienten im Kindesalter wurde keine Muskelschwäche beobachtet. Zeichen der mechanischen Muskelübererregbarkeit wie PIRC, »Mounding« und »Rippling« sind schon im Kindesalter zu beobachten; letzteres Symptom ist aber häufiger im Jugend- und Erwachsenenalter auszulösen. Auf der anderen Seite kann der im Kindesalter oft zu beobachtende

Zehengang mit »warm-up« Phänomen im Erwachsenenalter wieder vollständig abgeklungen sein.

Bei den Patienten mit nachgewiesener Mutation im *Caveolin-3* Gen, aber fehlender Muskelschwäche bzw. inkonstanten und/oder nicht überzeugenden Symptomen der mechanischen Muskelübererregbarkeit, kann die Muskelbiopsie hilfreich sein, um zwischen der Gliedergürtel-Muskeldystrophie 1C und der »Rippling«-Muskelerkrankung zu unterscheiden. Sie zeigt eine reduzierte Caveolin-3 Expression (12) und degenerative Veränderungen bei einigen Patienten (8) bei der Gliedergürtel-Muskeldystrophie 1C, während letztere bei der »Rippling«-Muskelerkrankung fehlen. Im Mausmodel verursacht die Caveolin-3 Defizienz auch degenerative Veränderungen der Muskulatur (7). Die Gliedergürtel-Muskeldystrophie 1C ist eine progredient verlaufende Erkrankung (14); die »Rippling«-Muskelerkrankung zeigt normalerweise keine Progredienz und eine relativ gute Prognose (5, 19, 20, 23, 27, 28, 29). Verlaufsuntersuchungen von asymptomatischen Kindern mit CK-Erhöhung sind notwendig, um eventuell eine Zuordnung zum Phänotyp einer Gliedergürtel-Muskeldystrophie 1C, einer »Rippling«-Muskelerkrankung oder einer distalen Myopathie zu ermöglichen.

Die Pathophysiologie der Caveolinopathien, besonders deren verschiedene Phänotypen bei gleichem Genotyp, ist noch unklar. In der Skelettmuskelfaser interagiert Caveolin-3 direkt mit der neuronalen Nitritoxid-Synthase (nNOS); um die normale Muskelfunktion aufrecht zu erhalten wird die katalytische Aktivität von nNOS durch Caveolin-3 gehemmt (13, 29). Zahlreiche biologische Prozesse im Muskel werden durch Nitritoxid beeinflusst (9, 17, 22, 24). Die nNOS Expression war im Muskelgewebe eines unserer Patienten normal, was mit Untersuchungen an Muskelgewebe von anderen Patienten mit der »Rippling«-Muskelerkrankung im Einklang ist (3, 29). Die normale nNOS Expression und die erhöhte Induzierbarkeit von nNOS können Gründe für die muskuläre Übererregbarkeit sein (3, 29). Im transgenischen Mausmodel mit erhöht induzierter nNOS Aktivität wurden myopathische Symptome, verzögertes Wachstum, eine Kyphose und ein auffälliges Gangbild beobachtet (25). Im Gegensatz dazu konnte eine herabgesetzte nNOS Aktivität bei der Gliedergürtel-Muskeldystrophie 1C (14) und bei der Duchenne-Muskeldystrophie (4) nachgewiesen werden. nNOS-knock-out Mäuse hingegen zeigen keinen myopathischen Phänotyp (15). Eine Caveolin-3 Defizienz und eine erhöht induzierte nNOS Aktivität können den Phänotyp einer »Rippling«-Muskelerkrankung verursachen, während eine schwere Reduktion von Caveolin-3 und ein sekundärer Verlust von nNOS zu dem Phänotyp der Gliedergürtel-Muskeldystrophie mit dystrophem Gewebsbild führen können (29). Das Ausmaß der nNOS Expression scheint funktionell wichtig zu sein, aber offensichtlich in Abhängigkeit von anderen strukturellen und/oder funktionellen Faktoren.

Caveolin-3 und nNOS sind in der Skelettmuskelfaser mit dem Dystrophin-Glykoprotein-Komplex verbunden (17, 21, 28). In dem Muskelgewebe eines unserer Patienten war die Expression von α-Dystroglykan normal; in dem von Vorgerd beschriebenen sporadischen Fall (29) war α-Dystroglykan leicht reduziert. Ein kompletter Verlust von α-Dystroglykan wurde bei Gliedergürtel- (12) und anderen Muskeldystrophien (16, 21) beschrieben. So scheint auch das

Ausmaß der Reduktion von α-Dystroglykan funktionell wichtig zu sein, und möglicherweise kann dadurch der Phänotyp mit beeinflusst werden (29).

Mutationen im *Caveolin-3* Gen als Ursache für die Rippling-Muskelerkrankung implizieren eine wichtige Rolle des Caveolin-3 in der Physiologie der Muskelkontraktion. Der exakte Mechanismus bleibt noch offen und weitere Untersuchungen von Caveolin-3 und die Zusammenhänge mit anderen zellulären Funktionen sind notwendig.

Zusammenfassend zeigt unsere Untersuchung, dass Symptome der »Rippling«-Muskelerkrankung auch schon im Kindesalter auftreten können. Bei Kindern mit Zehengang und »warm-up« Phänomen mit/ohne Myalgien oder anderen Gangstörungen, einer Wadenhypertrophie und CK-Erhöhung ist diese Erkrankung zu berücksichtigen. Eine sorgfältige klinische Untersuchung von Patienten und deren Eltern, inklusive der CK-Bestimmung und eine Familienanamnese, führen zur Verdachtsdiagnose. Die molekulargenetische Analyse im *Caveolin-3* Gen kann die Diagnose sichern; dies erlaubt Informationen über eine relativ gute Prognose für die Patienten und deren Familien. Eine Muskelbiopsie kann bei den Patienten mit nachgewiesener Mutation im *Caveolin-3* Gen, aber ohne sichere Zeichen einer muskulären Übererregbarkeit oder einer Muskelschwäche, hilfreich sein, um eine Differenzierung zwischen der progredient verlaufenden Gliedergürtel-Muskeldystrophie 1C und der »Rippling«-Muskelerkrankung zu ermöglichen.

Literatur

1. Alberca R, Rafel E, Castilla JM et al.: Increased mechanical muscle irritability syndrome. Acta Neurol Scand 1980; 62:250–254
2. Ansevin CF, Agamanolis DP: Rippling muscles and myasthenia gravis with rippling muscles. Arch Neurol 1996; 53:197–199
3. Betz RC, Schoser BGH, Kasper D et al.: Mutations in the CAV3 cause mechanical hyperirritability of skeletal muscle in rippling muscle disease. Nature Genet 2001; 28:218–219
4. Brenman JE, Chao DS, Xia H et al.: Nitric oxide synthase complexed with dystrophin and absent from skeletal muscle sarcolemma in Duchenne muscular dystrophy. Cell 1995; 82:743–752
5. Burns RJ, Bretag AH, Blumbergs PC et al.: Benign family disease with muscle mounding and rippling. J Neurol Neurosurg Psychiatry 1994; 57:344–347
6. Carbone I, Bruno C, Sotgia F et al.: Mutation in the CAV3 gene causes partial caveolin-3 deficiency and hyperCKemia. Neurology 2000; 54:1373–1376
7. Hagiwara Y, Sasaoka T, Araishi K et al. : Caveolin-3 deficiency causes muscle degeneration in mice. Hum Mol Genet 2000; 9:3047–3054
8. Herrmann R, Straub V, Blank M et al.: Dissociation of the dystroglycan complex in caveolin-3-deficient limb girdle muscular dystrophy. Hum Mol Genet 2000; 9:2335–2340
9. Kaminski HJ, Andrade HA: Nitric oxide: biologic effects on muscle and role in muscle diseases. Neuromuscul Disord 2001; 11:517–524
10. Koul RL, Chand RP, Chacko A et al.: Severe autosomal recessive rippling muscle disease. Muscle Nerve 2001; 24:1542–1547
11. Lim LE, Campell KP: The sarcoglycan complex in limb-girdle muscular dystrophy. Curr Opin Neurol 1998; 11:443–452
12. McNally EM, de Sa Moreira E, Duggan DJ et al.: Caveolin-3 in muscular dystrophy. Hum Mol Genet 1998; 7: 871–877

13. Michel T, Feron O: Nitric oxide synthases: which, where, how and why? J Clin Invest 1997; 100:2146–2152
14. Minetti C, Sotgia F, Bruno C et al.: Mutations in the caveolin-3 gene cause autosomal dominant limb-girdle muscular dystrophy. Nature Genet 1998; 18:365–368
15. Nelson RJ, Demas GE, Huang PL et al.: Behavioural abnormalities in male mice lacking neuronal nitric oxide synthase. Nature 1995; 378:383–386
16. Ohlendieck K, Matsumura K, Ionasescu VV et al.: Duchenne muscular dystrophy: deficiency of dystrophin-associated proteins in the sarcolemma. Neurology 1993; 43:795–80
17. Rando TA: The dystrophin-glycoprotein complex, cellular signaling, and the regulation of cell survival in the muscular dystrophies. Muscle Nerve 2001; 24:1575–1594
18. Rao KR, Hafford JM, Grunnet M et al.: Electrically silent muscle contractions, myoedema and myopathy. Electroenceph Clin Neurophysiol 1987; 66:S85
19. Ricker K, Moxley RT, Rohkamm R: Rippling muscle disease. Arch Neurol 1989; 48:405–408
20. So YT, Zu L, Barraza C et al.: Rippling muscle disease: Evidence for phenotypic and genetic heterogeneity. Muscle Nerve 2001; 24:340–344
21. Sotgia F, Lee JK, Das K et al.: Caveolin-3 directly interacts with the C-terminal tail of beta-dystroglycan. Identification of a central WW-like domain within caveolin family members. J Biol Chem 2000; 275:38048–38058
22. Stamler JS, Meissner G: Physiology of nitric oxide in skeletal muscle. Physiol Rev 2001; 81:209–237
23. Stephan DA, Buist NRM, Chittenden AB et al.: A rippling muscle disease gene is localized to 1q41: Evidence for multiple genes. Neurology 1994; 44:1915–1920
24. Sunada Y, Ohsawa Y, Murakami T et al.: Caveolin-3 and muscular dystrophy. Acta Myologica 2001; XX:162–167
25. Sunada Y, Ohi H, Hase A et al.: Transgenic mice expressing mutant caveolin-3 show severe myopathy associated with increased nNOS activity. Hum Mol Genet 2001; 10:173–178
26. Tateyama M, Aoki M, Nishino I et al.: Mutation in the caveolin-3 gene causes a peculiar form of distal myopathy. Neurology 2002; 58:323–325
27. Torbergsen T: A family with dominant hereditary myotonia, muscular hypertrophy, and increased muscular irritability, distinct from myotonia congenita Thomsen. Acta Neurol Scand 1975; 51:225–232
28. Vorgerd M, Bolz H, Patzold MD et al.: Phenotypic variability in rippling muscle disease. Neurology 1999; 52:1453–1459
29. Vorgerd M, Ricker K, Ziemssen F et al.: A sporadic case of rippling muscle disease caused by a de novo caveolin-3 mutation. Neurology 2001; 57:2273–2277

Glykosylierungsdefekte bei Kongenitalen Muskeldystrophien

V. Straub, R. Herrmann, A. Steinbrecher, T. Voit

Zusammenfassung

Viele Muskeldystrophien entstehen durch funktionelle Veränderungen von Membranproteinen oder Proteinen der extrazellulären Matrix. Mehrere von ihnen sind mit dem sogenannten Dystrophin-Glykoprotein-Komplex assoziiert (DGC), welcher in quergestreiften Muskelfasern Laminin in der extrazellulären Matrix mit dem F-Aktin-Zytoskelett verbindet. Ein Schlüsselmolekül des Komplexes ist das aus einer extrazellulären α- und einer transmembranösen β-Untereinheit bestehende Dystroglycan. Dystroglycan spielt eine entscheidende Rolle beim Aufbau der Basalmembran und in der Pathogenese kongenitaler Muskeldystrophien (CMD). Kürzlich konnte gezeigt werden, dass verschiedene Formen von CMD durch Glykosylierungsdefekte verursacht werden. Die fehlerhafte Glykosylierung führt möglicherweise zu den bei diesen Erkrankungen beschriebenen Schädigungen der Basalmembran. Sekundäre Veränderungen im Expressionsmuster von Laminin α2 und α-Dystroglycan spiegeln diese Schädigungen wider.

Einleitung

Die kongenitalen Muskeldystrophien (CMD) umfassen eine Gruppe von Krankheiten (Tab. 1), die durch Muskelschwäche und Muskelhypotonie bei Geburt oder in den ersten Lebensmonaten auffallen und genetisch determiniert sind (Voit, 1998). In der Skelettmuskelbiopsie zeigen sich die charakteristischen Zeichen einer Muskeldystrophie mit Skelettmuskelfaserdegeneration und -regeneration, Schwankungen im Faserkaliber, einer Zunahme an zentralen Kernen und bereits im frühen Stadium eine endo- und perimysiale Fibrose. Das histologische Bild weist zwar auf das Vorliegen einer Muskeldystrophie hin, ist jedoch nicht spezifisch genug, um eine Erkrankung von der anderen abzugrenzen.

Neben der Skelettmuskelpathologie weisen mehrere der CMD auch Veränderungen im Bereich des peripheren und zentralen Nervensystems und der Augen auf (Muntoni and Guicheney, 2002). Alle Formen zeigen einen progredienten und viele von ihnen einen sehr schwerwiegenden Verlauf. Die geschätzte Prävalenz der CMD in der kaukasischen Bevölkerung unter 16 Jahren beträgt 2,5 x 10^{-5} (Darin and Tulinius, 2000). Bereits vor der Identifizierung und Charakterisierung der primären Defekte wurde in verschiedenen Formen von CMD der Verdacht auf das Vorliegen von Veränderungen in der extrazellulären Matrix geäußert. Dieser Verdacht gründete sich vor allem auf die feingeweblich zu beobachtende Fibrose in der Skelettmuskulatur und auf elektronenmikroskopische Veränderungen von Basalmembranen im ZNS und im Skelettmuskel (Hayashi et al., 1993; Ishii et al., 1997). Diese Beobachtungen führten zu der Vermutung, dass Mutationen in Genen, die Bestandteile der extrazellulären Matrix kodieren, primär für diese Gruppe von Erkrankungen verantwortlich sind. Im Rahmen von Expressionsstudien konnte erstmals bei der in Japan am häufigsten vorkommenden Form der CMD, der CMD vom Typ Fukuyama (FCMD), eine Expressionsverminderung von Laminin α2, einer Komponente der Basalmembran, in der Skelettmuskulatur gefunden werden (Hayashi et al., 1993). Dieser initiale Befund führte schließlich zur ersten molekulargenetischen Charakterisierung einer CMD, der Laminin α2-defizienten CMD 6q22 (Tome et al., 1994).

Die primäre Laminin α2-Defizienz (MDC 1A, MIM # 156225) ist die häufigste autosomal rezessive CMD weltweit und liegt etwa 50% aller CMD-Fälle in der kaukasischen Bevölkerung zugrunde (Jones et al., 2001). Patienten mit komplettem Proteinverlust zeigen einen relativ homogenen klinischen Phänotyp mit ausgeprägter Muskelschwäche, einer deutlich erhöhten Creatin-Kinase-Aktivität im Serum und charakteristischen Veränderungen der weißen Substanz in der Kernspintomographie. Aufgrund der Muskelschwäche erlangen die Patienten keine eigenständige Gehfähigkeit. Zunehmend werden auch Patienten mit primärem Partialmangel von Laminin α2 berichtet, die einen variablen klinischen Phänotyp zeigen und erst im Jugendlichen- und Erwachsenenalter symptomatisch werden (Jones et al., 2001). Neben der Skelettmuskelsymptomatik können Patienten mit Laminin α2-Defizienz auch eine mentale Retardierung, eine Epilepsie, neuronale Migrationsdefekte und cardiale Beeinträchtigungen zeigen (He et al., 2001; Jones et al., 2001).

Gemeinsam mit Laminin β1 und Laminin γ1 bildet Laminin α2 das in der Skelettmuskulatur überwiegend vorkommende heterotrimere Laminin-2, das früher Merosin genannt wurde (Burgeson et al., 1994). Laminin-2 wird aber auch in anderen Geweben, wie Plazenta, Haut, Schwann-Zellen und der Basalmem-

Tab. 1: Die Tabelle gibt eine Übersicht über die derzeit gültige Nomenklatur und die bekannten Genorte bei CMD. AR, autosomal rezessiv.

Erkrankung	Erbgang	Genlocus	Protein
MDC 1A	AR	6q2	Laminin α2
MDC 1B	AR	1q42	
MDC 1C	AR	19q13.3	Fukutin related protein
FCMD (Typ Fukuyama)	AR	9q31–q33	Fukutin
Muscle-Eye-Brain-disease (MEB)	AR	1p32–p34	POMGnT1
CMD with rigid spine (RSMD1)	AR	1p35–36	Selenoprotein N1
CMD with integrin deficiency	AR	12q13	Integrin α7
UCMD (Typ Ullrich)	AR	21q22.3, 2q3	Kollagen VI (COL6A1/A2/A3)

bran von Blutgefäßen im ZNS und in der Glia limitans des Gehirns expremiert (Ehrig et al., 1990; Ringelmann et al., 1999; Sewry et al., 1998; Vuolteenaho et al., 1994). Es ist daher nicht überraschend, dass Patienten mit Laminin α2-defizienter CMD neben der Einschränkung der Skelettmuskelfunktion auch weitere pathologische Befunde zeigen. Fokale kortikale Migrationsstörungen im ZNS von Patienten legen die Vermutung nahe, dass die Glia limitans eine Rolle in der Regulation der neuronalen Migration spielt (Pini et al., 1996).

Neben dem primären Expressionsverlust von Laminin α2 kommt es bei betroffenen Patienten in der Skelettmuskulatur auch zu einem sekundären Expressionsverlust der Laminin-Rezeptoren α-Dystroglycan und Integrin α7 (Cohn et al., 1999; Hodges et al., 1997).

Sekundäre Laminin α2-defiziente CMD

Eine neue Gruppe von CMD sind Erkrankungen mit sekundärem Laminin α2-Mangel. Entsprechende Patienten wurde unabhängig von der zugrunde liegenden klinischen Symptomatik aufgrund einer unregelmässigen und reduzierten Expression von Laminin α2 und seinem Rezeptor α-Dystroglycan in der Skelettmuskulatur diagnostiziert (Abb. 1). Für drei dieser Erkrankungen, die im folgenden näher charakterisiert werden sollen, wurden inzwischen die verantwortlichen Gene charakterisiert, die allesamt Glykosyltransferasen kodieren. Damit gehören diese Formen der CMD gleichfalls zu den angeborenen Störungen der Glykosylierung, besser bekannt als CDG-Syndrome (congenital disorders of glycosylation).

Fukuyama-CMD (FCMD, MIM # 253800)

Es wurde bereits seit Längerem vermutet, dass Veränderungen der Basalmembran wahrscheinlich eine entscheidende Rolle in der Pathogenese der nur bei Personen japanischer Herkunft vorkommenden FCMD spielen (Ishii et al.,

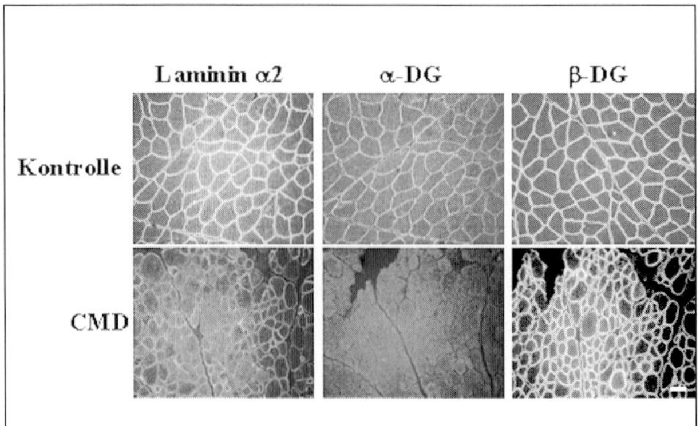

Abb. 1: Die Abbildung zeigt 6 µm dünne Kryostatschnitte von Skelettmuskulatur, die mit Antikörpern gegen Laminin α2, α-Dystroglycan (α-DG) und β-Dystroglycan (β-DG) gefärbt wurden. Der Patient (CMD), der per Kopplungsanalyse vom Genort für Laminin α2 (6q2) ausgeschlossen wurde, zeigt eine sekundäre Expressionsverminderung von Laminin α2 und α-Dystroglycan (Balken entspricht 50 µm).

1997). FCMD zeichnet sich durch die Kombination von Muskeldystrophie, ZNS-Veränderungen mit Micropolygyrie und Augenveränderungen aus (Fukuyama, 1999). In der Skelettmuskulatur von FCMD Patienten wurde eine deutliche Expressionsverminderung von Laminin α2 und α-Dystroglycan beschrieben (Hayashi et al., 1993; Hayashi et al., 2001). Eine verminderte Expression von Laminin α2 und β-Dystroglycan wurde zudem im Rückenmark eines FCMD-Feten beobachtet (Yamamoto et al., 1997). Kürzlich wurde das für die FCMD verantwortliche Gen auf Chromosom 9q31 kloniert und gezeigt, dass das Genprodukt Fukutin in die extrazelluläre Matrix sezerniert wird (Kobayashi et al., 1998). Die meisten Patienten sind für die gleiche Gründermutation, eine Insertion eines Retrotransposons im 3' nicht codierenden Bereich, homozygot. Die genaue Funktion von Fukutin ist weiterhin unklar, aber Sequenzanalysen lassen darauf schliessen, dass es sich beim Fukutin um eine Glycosyltransferase mit Homologie zur *fringe*-like Glycosyltransferase handelt . Die sekundären Expressionsveränderungen von Laminin α2 und Dystroglycan spiegeln möglicherweise eine Veränderung der Glykosylierung wider.

MDC 1C (MIM # 606612)

Obwohl es FCMD kaum außerhalb von Japan gibt, so finden sich doch CMD Patienten mit einer sekundären Expressionsverminderung von Laminin α2 und α-Dystroglycan (Talim et al., 2000; Villanova et al., 2000). Sequenzanalysen führten dazu, Gene mit Homologien zum Fukutin zu identifizieren und diese als Kandidatengene für CMD Syndrome mit sekundärem Laminin α2- und Dystroglycan-Mangel zu untersuchen. So wurde ein neues Mitglied der Fukutin-Proteinfamilie, Fukutin-related protein (FKRP), charakterisiert, welches durch ein Gen auf Chromosom 19q13.3 kodiert wird (Brockington et al., 2001a). Wie Fukutin, so weist auch FKRP Sequenzmotive auf, die es als Glykosyltransferase ausweisen. Mutationen im FKRP-Gen wurden kürzlich bei einer schweren Form von CMD mit sekundärem Laminin α2- und α-Dystroglycan-Mangel nachgewiesen (MDC 1C) (Brockington et al., 2001a). Anhaltende Mutationsanalysen haben das phänotypische Spektrum von FKRP-defizienten Patienten inzwischen deutlich erweitert. Neben Patienten mit einer kongenitalen Form der Erkrankung finden sich auch Patienten bei denen sich FKRP-Mutationen klinisch in Form einer Gliedergürtel Muskeldystrophie (LGMD 2I) mit Krankheitsbeginn im Jugend- und zum Teil im Erwachsenenalter manifestieren (Brockington et al., 2001b). Der klinische Phänotyp hängt möglicherweise von der verbleibenden Enzymaktivität ab. Interessanterweise zeigen Patienten mit einer Nullmutation und einer Missensemutation den schweren MDC 1C-Phänotyp, wohingegen Patienten mit zwei Missensemutationen einen milderen Gliedergürtel-Phänotyp ausbilden. Bisher wurden keine Patienten mit zwei Nullmutationen identifiziert, was darauf schliessen lässt, dass dies zu einem embryonal-letalen Phänotyp führen könnte. Möglicherweise spielt FKRP, ebenso wie Fukutin eine Rolle bei der Prozessierung von α-Dystroglycan und Laminin α2, und Mutationen in den entsprechenden Genen führen zu einer abnormen Glykosylierung dieser Proteine.

Muscle-Eye-Brain Disease (MEB, MIM # 253280)

In Finnland haben Santavuori und Mitarbeiter eine Form von CMD mit Pachygyrie, Polymicrogyrie, Hirnstammhypoplasie, cerebellärer Dysgenesie und Augenveränderungen beschrieben und diese Muscle-Eye-Brain Disease (MEB) genannt (Santavuori et al., 1989). Nachdem das MEB-Gen einem Genort auf Chromosom 1p32–34 zugeordnet werden konnte (Cormand et al., 1999), gibt es zunehmend Anhalt dafür, dass MEB häufig auch außerhalb von Finnland vorkommt. Die Kombination von neuronalen Migrationsstörungen, strukturellen Veränderungen der Augen und elektronenmikroskopischen Veränderungen in der Basalmembran von Skelettmuskelfasern legt die Vermutung nahe, dass es sich bei MEB wie bei FCMD um eine zugrunde liegende Erkrankung der Basalmembran handelt. Neuropathologische Untersuchungen haben deutliche Strukturveränderungen im Bereich des cerebralen und cerebellären Kortex mit Aufhebung der horizontalen Lamination gezeigt. Die Hirnoberfläche zeigt aufgrund der Migration von radiären Neuronen durch die Glia limitans ein charakteristisches Kopfsteinpflasteraussehen (cobblestone lissencephaly) (Haltia et al., 1997). Kürzlich wurde darüber berichtet, dass Mutationen im Gen für die Protein O-gebundene Mannose β1,2-N-Acetylglucosaminyltransferase (POMGnT1) MEB verursachen (Yoshida et al., 2001). POMGnT1 ist ein Enzym, das an der Synthese von O-mannosylierten Glykanen beteiligt ist. Auch bei MEB Patienten konnte eine sekundäre Expressionsverminderung von α-Dystroglycan gefunden werden (Kano et al., 2002), was möglicherweise auf eine fehlerhafte Glykosylierung des peripheren Membranproteins zurückzuführen ist. Diese Beobachtung ist ein weiterer Hinweis darauf, dass verschiedenen Muskeldystrophien durch Glykosylierungsdefekte von Basalmembranproteinen und ihren Rezeptoren verursacht werden, und dass α-Dystroglycan eine wichtige Rolle in der Pathogenese dieser Erkrankungen spielt.

Unklassifizierte CMD-Syndrome mit sekundärer Laminin α2-Defizienz

Neben den beschriebenen CMD-Syndromen mit definierten genetischen Defekten gibt es auch Familien mit CMD und sekundärer Laminin α2-Defizienz in der Skelettmuskulatur, die von den bisher beschriebenen Genorten per Kopplungsanalyse ausgeschlossen werden konnten. Einige dieser Familien zeigen eine Kopplung zu Chromosom 1q42 (Brockington et al., 2000), wohingegen andere auch von diesem Genort ausgeschlossen wurden. Unter den Familien, die von allen bisher bekannten CMD-Genorten ausgeschlossen wurden, finden sich sowohl Patienten mit der klassischen Form einer CMD, bei der klinisch primär die Muskeldystrophie imponiert, als auch Patienten mit zusätzlichen Augen- und Hirnveränderungen, wie sie bei MEB beobachtet werden. Zu den letzteren Erkrankungen gehört das Walker-Warburg-Syndrom, bei dem der klinische Phänotyp besonders schwer ist. Neben Gyrierungsstörungen tritt häufig ein shuntpflichtiger Hydrocephalus auf. Die Patienten lernen bestenfalls Sitzen, sind blind oder schwer sehbehindert und haben eine deutlich eingeschränkte Lebenserwartung (Cormand et al., 2001). Neben der Expressionsverminderung von Laminin α2 findet sich auch bei dieser Gruppe von CMD-Syndromen eine sekundäre Expressionsverminderung von α-Dystroglycan. Aufgrund der klinischen, histologischen und immunhistochemischen Untersuchungen liegt die Vermutung nahe, dass es sich auch bei diesen Erkrankungen um angeborenen Störungen der Glykosylierung handelt, und Mutationen in Glykosyltransferasen möglicherweise als ursächlich anzusehen sind.

Zusammenfassung

Veränderungen in Strukturproteinen galten bisher als eines der charakteristischen Merkmale in der Pathogenese vieler Muskeldystrophien. Da die Skelettmuskulatur zu den mechanisch am stärksten beanspruchten Geweben zählt, wurde insbesondere der Aufrechterhaltung und Integrität der Plasmamembranstruktur eine wichtige Funktion beigemessen. Der Dystrophin-Glykoprotein-Komplex (DGC) gilt dabei als eine entscheidende molekulare Struktur. In der Skelettmuskelfaser dient der DGC als Verbindungselement zwischen der extrazelluären Matrix und dem subsarkolemmalen Zytoskelett. Untersuchungen der letzten Jahre haben gezeigt, dass primäre Defekte in bisher 6 verschiedenen integralen Bestandteilen des oligomeren Komplexes für unterschiedliche Formen von Muskeldystrophien verantwortlich sind (Straub and Campbell, 1997). Als Schlüsselelement im DGC gilt Dystroglycan, das sich aus dem transmembranösen β-Dystroglycan und dem peripheren Membranprotein α-Dystroglycan zusammensetzt. Beide Proteine werden gemeinsam von einem Gen transkribiert, posttranslational modifiziert und ubiquitär expremiert. Das stark glykosylierte α-Dystroglycan dient als Rezeptor für verschiedene Basalmembranproteine, u.a. Laminin α1, Laminin α2, Agrin und Perlecan (Henry and Campbell, 1999). In Mäusen führen gezielte Mutationen im Dystroglycan-Gen zur frühen embryonalen Letalität (Williamson et al., 1997), was eine Begründung dafür sein kann, dass menschliche Dystroglycan-Mutationen bisher nicht beschrieben sind. Eine sekundäre Expressionsverminderung von α-Dystroglycan wurde in der Skelettmuskulatur verschiedener CMD-Syndrome beschrieben. Interessanterweise konnten Mutationen in Glykosyltransferasen, Enzymen, die für die Glykosylierung von Glykoproteinen und Glykolipiden verantwortlich sind, in verschiedenen Formen von CMD charakterisiert werden. Damit gehören diese CMD-Syndrome, FCMD, MEB und MDC 1C, definitionsgemäß zu den CDG-Syndromen, den angeborenen Störungen der Glykosylierung. Möglicherweise führt eine fehlerhafte Glykosylierung von α-Dystroglycan zur Expressionsverminderung des Proteins und trägt entscheidend zur Pathogenese der CMD-Syndrome mit Glykosylierungsdefekten bei.

Literatur

1. Brockington, M., Blake, D.J., Prandini, P., Brown, S.C., Torelli, S., Benson, M.A., Ponting, C.P., Estournet, B., Romero, N.B., Mercuri, E., Voit, T., Sewry, C.A., Guicheney, P., and Muntoni, F. (2001a). Mutations in the fukutin-related protein gene (FKRP) cause a form of congenital muscular dystrophy with secondary laminin alpha2 deficiency and abnormal glycosylation of alpha-dystroglycan. Am J Hum Genet. 69:1198–209.
2. Brockington, M., Sewry, C.A., Herrmann, R., Naom, I., Dearlove, A., Rhodes, M., Topaloglu, H., Dubowitz, V., Voit, T., and Muntoni, F. (2000). Assignment of a form of congenital muscular dystrophy with secondary merosin deficiency to chromosome 1q42. Am J Hum Genet. 66:428–35.
3. Brockington, M., Yuva, Y., Prandini, P., Brown, S.C., Torelli, S., Benson, M.A., Herrmann, R., Anderson, L.V., Bashir, R., Burgunder, J.M., Fallet, S., Romero, N., Fardeau, M., Straub, V., Storey, G., Pollitt, C., Richard, I., Sewry, C.A., Bushby, K., Voit, T., Blake, D.J., and Muntoni, F. (2001b). Mutations in the fukutin-related protein gene (FKRP) identify limb girdle muscular dystrophy 2I as a milder allelic variant of congenital muscular dystrophy MDC1C. Hum Mol Genet. 10:2851–2859.
4. Burgeson, R.E., Chiquet, M., Deutzmann, R., Ekblom, P., Engel, J., Kleinman, H., Martin, G.R., Meneguzzi, G., Paulsson, M., Sanes, J., and et al. (1994). A new nomenclature for the laminins. Matrix Biol. 14:209–11.
5. Cohn, R.D., Mayer, U., Saher, G., Herrmann, R., van der Flier, A., Sonnenberg, A., Sorokin, L., and Voit, T. (1999). Secondary reduction of alpha7B integrin in laminin alpha2 deficient congenital muscular dystrophy supports an additional transmembrane link in skeletal muscle. J Neurol Sci. 163:140–52.
6. Cormand, B., Avela, K., Pihko, H., Santavuori, P., Talim, B., Topaloglu, H., de la Chapelle, A., and Lehesjoki, A.E. (1999). Assignment of the muscle-eye-brain disease gene to 1p32-p34 by linkage analysis and homozygosity mapping. Am J Hum Genet. 64:126–35.
7. Cormand, B., Pihko, H., Bayes, M., Valanne, L., Santavuori, P., Talim, B., Gershoni-Baruch, R., Ahmad, A., van Bokhoven, H., Brunner, H.G., Voit, T., Topaloglu, H., Dobyns, W.B., and Lehesjoki, A.E. (2001). Clinical and genetic distinction between Walker-Warburg syndrome and muscle-eye-brain disease. Neurology. 56:1059–69.
8. Darin, N., and Tulinius, M. (2000). Neuromuscular disorders in childhood: a descriptive epidemiological study from western Sweden. Neuromuscul Disord. 10:1–9.
9. Ehrig, K., Leivo, I., and Engvall, E. (1990). Merosin and laminin. Molecular relationship and role in nerve-muscle development. Ann N Y Acad Sci. 580:276–80.
10. Fukuyama, Y. (1999). Congenital muscular dystrophies: an update. J Child Neurol. 14:28–30.
11. Haltia, M., Leivo, I., Somer, H., Pihko, H., Paetau, A., Kivela, T., Tarkkanen, A., Tome, F., Engvall, E., and Santavuori, P. (1997). Muscle-eye-brain disease: a neuropathological study. Ann Neurol. 41:173–80.
12. Hayashi, Y.K., Engvall, E., Arikawa-Hirasawa, E., Goto, K., Koga, R., Nonaka, I., Sugita, H., and Arahata, K. (1993). Abnormal localization of laminin subunits in muscular dystrophies. Journal of the Neurological Sciences. 119:53–64.
13. Hayashi, Y.K., Ogawa, M., Tagawa, K., Noguchi, S., Ishihara, T., Nonaka, I., and Arahata, K. (2001). Selective deficiency of alpha-dystroglycan in Fukuyama-type congenital muscular dystrophy. Neurology. 57:115–21.
14. He, Y., Jones, K.J., Vignier, N., Morgan, G., Chevallay, M., Barois, A., Estournet-Mathiaud, B., Hori, H., Mizuta, T., Tome, F.M., North, K.N., and Guicheney, P. (2001). Congenital muscular dystrophy with primary partial laminin alpha2 chain deficiency: molecular study. Neurology. 57:1319–22.
15. Henry, M.D., and Campbell, K.P. (1999). Dystroglycan inside and out. Curr Opin Cell Biol. 11:602–7.
16. Hodges, B.L., Hayashi, Y.K., Nonaka, I., Wang, W., Arahata, K., and Kaufman, S.J. (1997). Altered expression of the alpha7beta1 integrin in human and murine muscular dystrophies. J Cell Sci. 110:2873–81.

17. Ishii, H., Hayashi, Y.K., Nonaka, I., and Arahata, K. (1997). Electron microscopic examination of basal lamina in Fukuyama congenital muscular dystrophy. Neuromuscul Disord. 7:191–7.
18. Jones, K.J., Morgan, G., Johnston, H., Tobias, V., Ouvrier, R.A., Wilkinson, I., and North, K.N. (2001). The expanding phenotype of laminin alpha2 chain (merosin) abnormalities: case series and review. J Med Genet. 38:649–57.
19. Kano, H., Kobayashi, K., Herrmann, R., Tachikawa, M., Manya, H., Nishino, I., Nonaka, I., Straub, V., Talim, B., Voit, T., Topaloglu, H., Endo, T., Yoshikawa, H., and Toda, T. (2002). Deficiency of alpha-dystroglycan in muscle-eye-brain disease. Biochem Biophys Res Commun. 291:1283–6.
20. Kobayashi, K., Nakahori, Y., Miyake, M., Matsumura, K., Kondo-Iida, E., Nomura, Y., Segawa, M., Yoshioka, M., Saito, K., Osawa, M., Hamano, K., Sakakihara, Y., Nonaka, I., Nakagome, Y., Kanazawa, I., Nakamura, Y., Tokunaga, K., and Toda, T. (1998). An ancient retrotransposal insertion causes Fukuyama-type congenital muscular dystrophy. Nature. 394:388–92.
21. Muntoni, F., and Guicheney, P. (2002). 85th ENMC International Workshop on Congenital Muscular Dystrophy. 6th International CMD Workshop. 1st Workshop of the Myo-Cluster Project 'GENRE'. 27-28th October 2000, Naarden, The Netherlands. Neuromuscul Disord. 12:69–78.
22. Pini, A., Merlini, L., Tome, F.M., Chevallay, M., and Gobbi, G. (1996). Merosin-negative congenital muscular dystrophy, occipital epilepsy with periodic spasms and focal cortical dysplasia. Report of three Italian cases in two families. Brain & Development. 18:316–322.
23. Ringelmann, B., Roder, C., Hallmann, R., Maley, M., Davies, M., Grounds, M., and Sorokin, L. (1999). Expression of laminin alpha1, alpha2, alpha4, and alpha5 chains, fibronectin, and tenascin-C in skeletal muscle of dystrophic 129ReJ dy/dy mice. Exp Cell Res. 246:165–82.
24. Santavuori, P., Somer, H., Sainio, K., Rapola, J., Kruus, S., Nikitin, T., Ketonen, L., and Leisti, J. (1989). Muscle-eye-brain disease (MEB) [see comments]. Brain Dev. 11:147–53.
25. Sewry, C.A., Uziyel, Y., Torelli, S., Buchanan, S., Sorokin, L., Cohen, J., and Watt, D.J. (1998). Differential labelling of laminin alpha 2 in muscle and neural tissue of dy/dy mice: are there isoforms of the laminin alpha 2 chain? [published erratum appears in Neuropathol Appl Neurobiol 1998 Apr;24(2):166]. Neuropathol Appl Neurobiol. 24:66–72.
26. Straub, V., and Campbell, K.P. (1997). Muscular dystrophies and the dystrophin-glycoprotein complex. Curr Opin Neurol. 10:168–75.
27. Talim, B., Kale, G., Topaloglu, H., Akcoren, Z., Caglar, M., Gogus, S., and Elkay, M. (2000). Clinical and histopathological study of merosin-deficient and merosin-positive congenital muscular dystrophy. Pediatr Dev Pathol. 3:168–76.
28. Tome, F.M., Evangelista, T., Leclerc, A., Sunada, Y., Manole, E., Estournet, B., Barois, A., Campbell, K.P., and Fardeau, M. (1994). Congenital muscular dystrophy with merosin deficiency. Comptes Rendus de l Academie des Sciences – Serie Iii, Sciences de la Vie. 317:351–357.
29. Villanova, M., Mercuri, E., Bertini, E., Sabatelli, P., Morandi, L., Mora, M., Sewry, C., Brockington, M., Brown, S.C., Ferreiro, A., Maraldi, N.M., Toda, T., Guicheney, P., Merlini, L., and Muntoni, F. (2000). Congenital muscular dystrophy associated with calf hypertrophy, microcephaly and severe mental retardation in three Italian families: evidence for a novel CMD syndrome. Neuromuscul Disord. 10:541–7.
30. Voit, T. (1998). Congenital muscular dystrophies: 1997 update. Brain Dev. 20:65–74.
31. Vuolteenaho, R., Nissinen, M., Sainio, K., Byers, M., Eddy, R., Hirvonen, H., Shows, T.B., Sariola, H., Engvall, E., and Tryggvason, K. (1994). Human laminin M chain (merosin): complete primary structure, chromosomal assignment, and expression of the M and A chain in human fetal tissues. J Cell Biol. 124:381–94.
32. Williamson, R.A., Henry, M.D., Daniels, K.J., Hrstka, R.F., Lee, J.C., Sunada, Y., Ibraghimov-Beskrovnaya, O., and Campbell, K.P. (1997). Dystroglycan is essential for early embryonic development: disruption of Reichert's membrane in Dag1-null mice. Hum Mol Genet. 6:831–41.

33. Yamamoto, T., Shibata, N., Kanazawa, M., Kobayashi, M., Komori, T., Ikeya, K., Kondo, E., Saito, K., and Osawa, M. (1997). Localization of laminin subunits in the central nervous system in Fukuyama congenital muscular dystrophy: an immunohistochemical investigation. Acta Neuropathol (Berl). 94:173–9.
34. Yoshida, A., Kobayashi, K., Manya, H., Taniguchi, K., Kano, H., Mizuno, M., Inazu, T., Mitsuhashi, H., Takahashi, S., Takeuchi, M., Herrmann, R., Straub, V., Talim, B., Voit, T., Topaloglu, H., Toda, T., and Endo, T. (2001). Muscular dystrophy and neuronal migration disorder caused by mutations in a glycosyltransferase, POMGnT1. Dev Cell. 1:717–24.

IGHMBP2: das zweite Gen für eine Form der spinalen Muskelatrophie ist identifiziert

K. Grohmann, M. Schuelke, A. Diers, K. Hoffmann, C. Adams, E. Bertini, H. Leonhardt-Horti, F. Muntoni, R. Ouvrier, R. Rossi, L. Van Maldergem, J.M. Wilmshurst, S. Rudnik-Schöneborn, K. Zerres, C. Hübner

Die klassische spinale Muskelatrophie (SMA) ist eine autosomal rezessive Erkrankung, die durch Mutationen im *SMN1* (Survival of Motor Neuron)-Gen verursacht wird (1). Nicht durch Mutationen im *SMN1*-Gen auf dem humanen Chromosom 5q wird eine weitere Form der spinalen Muskelatrophie verursacht, die spinale Muskelatrophie mit respiratory distress Typ 1 (SMARD1, MIM*604320). Diese unterscheidet sich klinisch am deutlichsten von der klassischen SMA durch eine sehr frühe Beteiligung des Zwerchfells (2–5). Die Lähmung des Zwerchfells, die häufig schon nach 4–6 Lebenswochen symptomatisch wird, führt bei den betroffenen Kindern zu einer Ateminsuffizienz, die in der Regel eine dauerhafte Beatmung zur Folge hat. Meist zeitgleich oder im Verlauf entwickeln die Patienten eine generalisierte Muskelschwäche, die Kinder zeigen das Bild eines »floppy infant«. Im Gegensatz zur klassischen SMA ist die Muskelschwäche bei den SMARD1-Patienten oft distal betont. Vor allem fällt eine ausgeprägte Greifschwäche und an den unteren Extremitäten eine Fußmuskellähmung mit Fußdeformitäten auf.

Durch einen Whole Genome Linkage Scan, einer genetischen Untersuchung des gesamten autosomalen Genoms mit spezifischen Mikrosatellitenmarkern, konnten wir den Genort der SMARD1 auf dem humanen Chromosom 11q13-q21 lokalisieren (6). Es wurden drei Familien untersucht, von denen zwei Familien mit einer nicht-kongenitalen Form der SMARD in diese chromosomale Region kartierten, eine deutsche Familie und eine konsanguine Familie libanesischen Ursprungs. Eine dritte Familie aus Italien mit einer kongenitalen Form der SMARD zeigte keine Kopplung zu den untersuchten Markern auf Chromosom 11q. Damit stellt die SMARD eine heterogene Krankheitsgruppe dar und die SMARD, die auf 11q13-q21 kartiert, wurde im OMIM als SMARD Typ 1 (SMARD1) aufgenommen.

In der Folge konnten wir viele weitere potentielle SMARD1-Familien klinisch und genetisch untersuchen, den zuvor noch großen Genlokus auf Chromosom 11q13-q21 auf 9 cM verkleinern, und das für die SMARD1 verantwortliche Gen identifizieren. Es ist das *IGHMBP2* (Immunoglobulin μ-bindende Protein 2)-Gen, welches auf Chromosom 11q13 liegt. Wir wiesen Mutationen im *IGHMBP2*-Gen (MIM*600502) bei 6 SMARD1- Familien mit insgesamt 11 Patienten und 21 gesunden Geschwistern und Eltern nach (Tab. 1).

Die Familien stammen aus unterschiedlichen Herkunftsländern, und keine der Mutationen wurde zweimal gefunden. Wir identifizierten drei Missense-, zwei Nonsense-, eine Frameshift- und eine Splice Donor Site-Mutation in verschie-

Tab. 1: Mutationen im *IGHMBP2*-Gen

Familie	Herkunftsland	Mutationen	Lokalisation	Aminosäuren-Austausch	Art der Mutation
1	Süditalien	1540G→A	Exon 11	E514K	Missense
2	Libanon	638A→G	Exon 5	H213R	Missense
3	Türkei	1738G→A	Exon 12	V580I	Missense
4	Deutschland	121C→T 675delT	Exon 2 Exon 5	Q41X –	Nonsense Frameshift
5	Libanon	707T→G	Exon 5	L236X	Nonsense
6	Sizilien	IVS13+1G→T	Intron 13	–	Splice Donor Site

denen Exons des *IGHMBP2*-Gens (7). Mittlerweile können wir an der Charité/ Berlin eine SMARD1-Diagnostik für Patienten sowie eine Pränataldiagnostik für die betroffenen Familien anbieten.

Das *IGHMBP2*-Gen wird in jeder Körperzelle exprimiert und gehört damit zu den sog. Haushalts (Housekeeping)-Genen. Warum Mutationen dieses Haushaltsgens nun spezifisch zu einem Motoneuronenuntergang im Rückenmark führen, ist Inhalt und Herausforderung weiterer Untersuchungen. Interessant ist in diesem Zusammenhang die Analogie zum *SMN1*-Gen der klassischen spinalen Muskelatrophie: Auch hier verursachen Mutationen eines Haushaltsgens spezifisch einen Motoneuronenuntergang.

Das Genprodukt IGHMBP2 besteht aus 993 Aminosäuren und wird durch 15 Exons kodiert. Die genaue Funktion des Proteins ist bislang nicht aufgeklärt. Strukturelle Simulationen *(http://smart.embl-heidelberg.de)* weisen verschiedene funktionelle Domänen auf (Abb. 1).

Zum einen findet sich eine sog. DEAD-Box Domäne. Es handelt sich bei IGHMBP2 um eine putative RNA-Helikase, die Funktionen zum Beispiel beim Aufbau des spliceosomalen Apparates übernehmen könnte (8). Überlappend findet sich eine ATPase-Domäne, die z.B. für die Energiegewinnung zur Ausführung der Helikasefunktion wichtig ist. Weiter C-terminal findet sich eine sog. R3H-Domäne, welche eine Struktur für die Bindung von Einzelstrang- DNA beinhaltet. Auch ein benachbartes Zinkfinger-Motiv lässt Rückschlüsse auf eine mögliche Funktion als Transkriptionsfaktor ziehen (9–11). Wieder deckt der Vergleich zum SMN der klassischen spinalen Muskelatrophie Parallelen auf. SMN bindet an DNA und RNA (12), aktiviert die Transkription durch Assoziation mit dem viralen nukleären Transkriptionsfaktor E2 (13) und ist an der prä-mRNA-Prozessierung beteiligt (14–15). Obwohl SMN selber keine Helikasemotive enthält, ist es am Aufbau des spliceosomalen Apparates beteiligt, der die RNA-Helikase DP103/Gemin 3 enthält (16–18).

Angesichts des schweren, letalen Verlaufes der Erkrankung ist jede Forschung zu der Funktion des Proteins, des Pathomechanismus und dem Verlauf der Erkrankung für die betroffenen Familien wichtig, damit die erlangten Erkenntnisse in Zukunft sowohl für eine Prognosestellung als auch vielleicht für die Entwicklung einer spezifischen Therapie eingesetzt werden können.

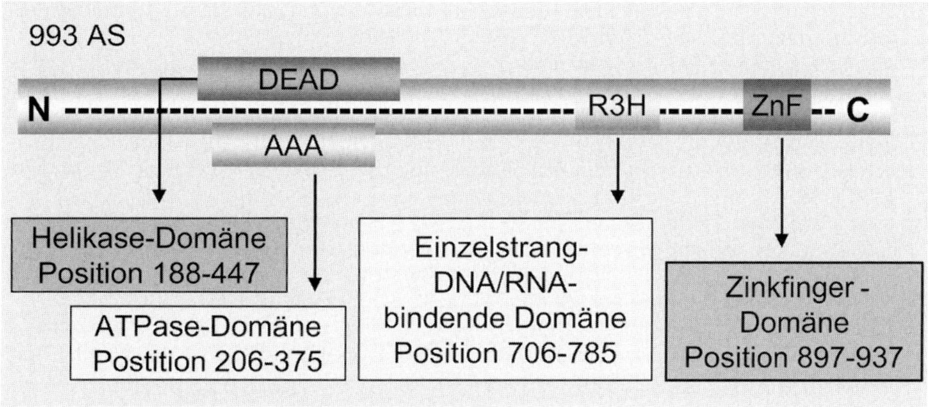

Abb. 1: Funktionelle Domänen des IGHMBP2.

Literatur

1. Lefebvre S, Burglen L, Reboullet S et al. (1995) Identification and characterization of a spinal muscular atrophy-determining gene. Cell 80:155–165
2. Mellins RB, Hays AP, Gold AP, Berdon WE and Bowdler JD (1974) Respiratory distress as the initial manifestation of Werdnig-Hoffmann disease. Pediatrics 53:33–40
3. Bertini E et al. (1989) Distal infantile spinal muscular atrophy associated with paralysis of the diaphragm: a variant of infantile spinal muscular atrophy. Am J Med Genet 33:328–335
4. Rudnik-Schöneborn S, Forkert R, Hahnen E, Wirth B, Zerres K (1996) Clinical spectrum and diagnostic criteria of infantile spinal muscular atrophy: further delineation on the basis of SMN gene deletion findings. Neuropediatrics 27:8–15
5. Zerres K and Davies KE (1999) 59th ENMC International Workshop: Spinal Muscular Atrophies: recent progress and revised diagnostic criteria 17–19 April 1998, Soestduinen, The Netherlands. Neuromuscular Disord 9:272–278
6. Grohmann K, Wienker TF, Saar K, Rudnik-Schöneborn S, Stoltenburg-Didinger G, Rossi R, Novelli G, Nürnberg G, Pfeufer A, Wirth B, Reis A, Zerres K, Hübner C (1999) Diaphragmatic spinal muscular atrophy with respiratory distress is heterogeneous, and one form is linked to chromosome 11q13-q21. Am J Hum Genet 65:1459–1462
7. Grohmann K, Schuelke M, Diers A, Hoffmann K, Lucke B, Adams C, Bertini E, Leonhardt-Horti H, Muntoni F, Ouvrier R, Pfeufer A, Rossi R, Van Maldergem L, Wilmshurst JM, Wienker TF, Sendtner M, Rudnik-Schöneborn S, Zerres K, Hübner C (2001) Mutations in the gene encoding immunoglobulin m-binding protein 2 cause spinal muscular atrophy with respiratory distress type 1. Nat Genet 29:75–77
8. Molnar GM et al. (1997) Association of the mammalian helicase MAH with the pre-mRNA splicing complex. P Natl Acad Sci USA 94:7831–7836
9. Chen NN, Kerr D, Chang CF, Honjo T and Khalili K (1997) Evidence for regulation of transcription and replication of the human neurotropic virus JCV genome by the human Sμbp-2 protein in glial cells. Gene 185:55–62
10. Zhang Q, Wang YCJ and Montalvo EA (1999) Sμbp-2 represses the Epstein-Barr virus lytic switch promoter. Virology 255:160–170
11. Miao M, Chan SL, Fletcher GL and Hew CL (2000) The rat ortholog of the presumptive flounder antifreeze enhancer-binding protein is a helicase domain-containing protein. Eur J Biochem 267:7237–7245
12. Lorson CL and Androphy EJ (1998) The domain encoded by exon 2 of the survival motor neuron protein mediates nucleic acid binding. Hum Mol Genet 7:1269–1275

13. Strasswimmer J et al. (1999) Identification of survival motor neuron as a transcriptional activator-binding protein. Hum Mol Genet 8:1219–1226
14. Meister G et al. (2000) Characterization of a nuclear 20S complex containing the survival of motor neurons (SMN) protein and a specific subset of spliceosomal Sm proteins. Hum Mol Genet 9:1977–1986
15. Pellizzoni L, Charroux B, Rappsilber J, Mann M and Dreyfuss G (2001) A functional interaction between the survival motor neuron complex and RNA polymerase II. J Cell Biol 152:75–85
16. Charroux B et al. (1999) Gemin3: a novel DEAD box protein that interacts with SMN, the spinal muscular atrophy gene product, and is a component of gems. J Cell Biol 147:1181–1193
17. Campbell L et al. (2000) Direct interaction of Smn with dp103, a putative RNA helicase: a role for Smn in transcription regulation? Hum Mol Genet 9:1093–1100
18. Grundhoff AT et al. (1999) Characterization of DP103, a novel DEAD box protein that binds to the Epstein-Barr virus nuclear proteins EBNA2 and EBNA3C. J Biol Chem 274:19136–19144

Arthrogryposis multiplex congenita und Relaxatio diaphragmatica bei initial subklinischer maternaler Myasthenia gravis

G. Willig, M. Heckmann, I. Reiss , B.A. Neubauer

Einleitung

Die Assoziation von maternalen Acteylcholin-Rezeptor Autoantikörpern und einer fetalen Arthrogryposis multiplex congenita (AMC) ist selten aber gut belegt. Bei insgesamt 32 Schwangerschaften von 13 in der Literatur berichteten Frauen mit Symptomen einer Myasthenia gravis (MG) wurde die Diagnose einer fetalen AMC gestellt (1, 2). Es liegt aber nur ein Fallbericht einer asymptomatischen Mutter vor, deren Schwangerschaften durch eine fetale AMC kompliziert wurden (3, 1).

Bei der von uns vorgestellten Patientin, deren Mutter ebenfalls zunächst keinerlei Symptome einer MG aufwies, lag neben der AMC zusätzlich eine hochgradige – bisher in dieser Ausprägung unbeschriebene – Relaxatio diaphragmatica rechts vor.

Kasuistik

Anamnese:

Unsere Patientin wurde in der 35+4. SSW spontan entbunden (Geburtsgewicht 2.200 g, Apgar 5/6/6, Nabelschnur-pH 7,3). In der Schwangerschaft bestand ein Polyhydramnion unklarer Ursache. Eine Amniocentese erbrachte einen normalen weiblichen Karyotyp, die pränatale Sonographie gab keinen Hinweis auf Fehlbildungen. Bei der Mutter, einer 23jährigen II G, I P, bestand kein Anhalt auf eine akute oder abgelaufene Infektion, die Familienanamnese war unauffällig.

Befunde:

Das Kind wurde direkt postnatal bei ausgeprägter Dyspnoe intubiert. Es lag eine Relaxatio diaphragmatica rechts mit einer kaum nachweisbaren Zwerchfellbeweglichkeit und begleitender Lungenhypoplasie vor. An den Fingern beider Hände bestanden Beugekontrakturen, der Muskeltonus war erheblich reduziert, die Muskeleigenreflexe nicht auslösbar. Im weiteren Verlauf zeigte sich eine ausgeprägte Schluckstörung.

Die zu diesem Zeitpunkt völlig beschwerdefreie Mutter wies eine unauffällige neurologische Untersuchung inklusive der bildgebenden und neurophysiologischen Diagnostik auf.

Es wurden deutlich erhöhte Acetylcholin-Rezeptor-Antikörper bei Mutter (270 nMol/l, Referenz < 0,2 nMol/l) und Kind (4 nMol/l) nachgewiesen.

Therapie und Verlauf:

Nach der Extubation am zweiten Lebenstag benötigte das Kind über Monate hinweg intermittierend immer wieder N-CPAP mit wechselndem Sauerstoffbedarf. Radiologisch fanden sich rezidivierende Dystelektasen. Neben der durch die konnatale Zwerchfellrelaxation bedingten Lungenhypoplasie wurde die kardiorespiratorische Situation des Kindes noch durch eine pulmonale Hypertension kompliziert, die systemische PA-Drücke erreichte.

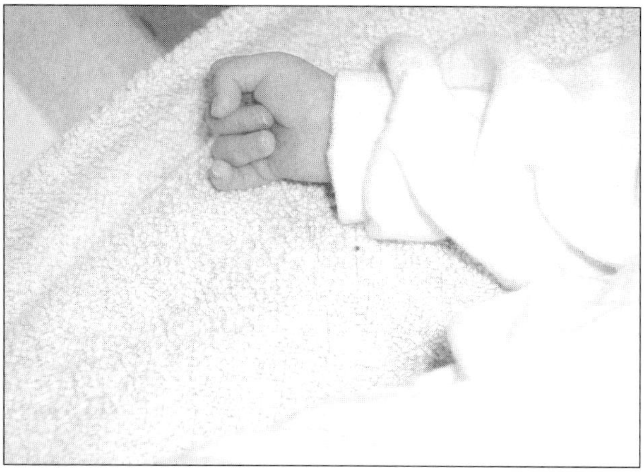

Abb. 1: Hand der Patientin mit Beugekontrakturen.

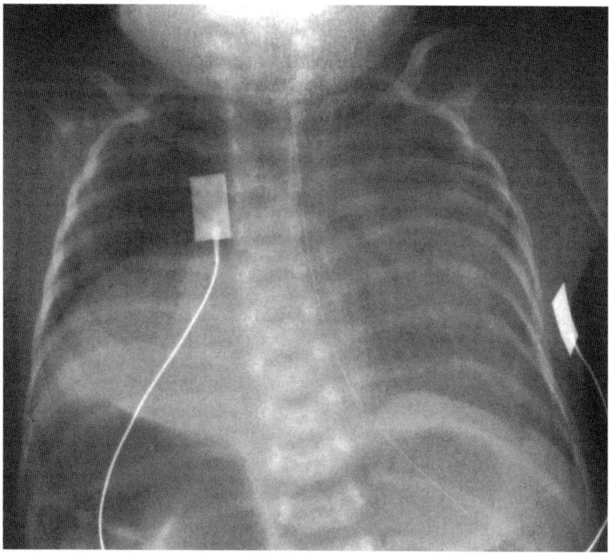

Abb. 2: Röntgenbild des Thorax mit Relaxatio diaphragmatica rechts.

Ein initialer Therapieversuch mit Pyridostigminbromid musste aufgrund erheblicher Nebenwirkungen eingestellt werden.

Schluck- und Atemstörung besserten sich nur langsam, während Muskeltonus und Motorik bereits ab dem dritten Lebensmonat und darüber hinaus deutliche Fortschritte machten.

Die Patientin konnte im Alter von 7 Monaten entlassen werden. Sie erhält weiterhin kontinuierlich Sauerstoff. Der orale Nahrungsaufbau macht erfreuliche Fortschritte, das Kind wird nur noch teilweise sondiert. Die psychomotorische Entwicklung des Mädchens ist noch um 2–3 Monate retardiert.

Zum Zeitpunkt der Entlassung deuteten die uns vorliegenden Untersuchungsbefunde der Mutter auf eine subklinische maternale Myasthenia gravis hin. Vor kurzem jedoch wurde die bisher beschwerdefreie Frau symptomatisch, und die erneut durchgeführte neurologische Untersuchung bestätigt eine Manifestation der Erkrankung.

Diskussion

Polyhydramnion, Arthrogryposis multiplex congenita, muskuläre Hypotonie und respiratorische Insuffizienz mit ausgepägter diaphragmaler Beteiligung sind mögliche Komplikationen einer maternalen Myasthenia gravis, wobei die Mutter völlig asymptomatisch sein kann.

Bisher liegen nur einzelne Berichte über ein positives kindliches Outcome im Zusammenhang mit einer Therapie der maternalen MG vor. In einem Fall verhinderte eine Thymektomie und die Verabreichung von Pyridostigmin das Auftreten einer AMC. Prednisolon, Azathioprin und die Thymektomie erreichten ein ähnliches Ergebnis in einem zweiten Fall. Plasmaaustausch und die Gabe von IgG führten bei einem weiteren Kind ebenfalls zum Erfolg (1).

Das Wiederholungsrisiko für das erneute Auftreten einer AMC bei weiteren Schwangerschaften kann bis zu 100% bei ausbleibender Therapie betragen. Ein vergleichbarer Phänotyp ist auch bei Mutationen im Gen der Acetylcholin-Rezeptor-delta Untereinheit zu beobachten (4).

Zusammenfassend sollte im Rahmen der Differentialdiagnose der Arthrogryposis multiplex congenita auch bei asymptomatischer Mutter die Bestimmung von Acetylcholin-Rezeptor Autoantikörpern erfolgen.

Literatur

1. Polizzi A, Huson SM, Vincent A. 2000. Teratogen update: Maternal myasthenia gravis as a cause of congenital arthrogryposis. Teratology 62:332–341
2. Barnes PR et al . 1995. Recurrent congenital arthrogryposis leading to a diagnosis of myasthenia gravis in an initially asymptomatic mother. Neuromusc Disord 5:59–65
3. Bruteon LA et al. 2000. Asymptomatic maternal myasthenia as a cause of the Pena-Shokeir phenotype. Am J Med Genet 92:1–6
4. Brownlow S et al. 2001. Acetylcholine receptor δ subunit mutations underlie a fast-channel myasthenic syndrome and arthrogryposis mutliplex congenita. J Clin Invest 108:125–130

9. Therapie mit Immunglobulinen bei neurologischen Erkrankungen im Kindesalter

Wirkmechanismen und Nebenwirkungen der Therapie mit intravenösen Immunglobulinen

R. Gold, A. Weishaupt, M. Mäurer

Zusammenfassung

Immunglobuline vermitteln sowohl Funktionen der erworbenen als auch der angeborenen humoralen Immunität. Sie dienen der Erkennung und schließlich der Elimination von pathogenen Erregern sowie ihrer Metaboliten. Zudem können Fraktionen der Immunglobuline und die in den Präparationen enthaltenen aktiven, löslichen Immunmoleküle eine regulatorische Funktion auf die zelluläre und humorale Immunität des menschlichen Organismus ausüben. Dadurch können sie zur Begrenzung von Entzündungsreaktionen beitragen. Aus diesem Grund haben Immunglobulinpräparate mittlerweile einen breiten Eingang in die Therapie verschiedener Autoimmunerkrankungen gefunden. Die zur Therapie von Autoimmunerkrankungen gegebenen intravenösen 7S-Immunglobuline (IgG) besitzen *in-vivo* eine Halbwertszeit von drei bis vier Wochen. Wir besprechen im folgenden die Vielzahl der Wirkmechanismen, die *in-vitro, ex-vivo* und *in-vivo* beschrieben wurden. Von einer vergleichenden Bewertung der therapeutischen Relevanz der Mechanismen in der Neuroimmunologie möchten wir absehen, weil unserer Ansicht nach bei der klinischen Anwendung von Immunglobulinpräparaten immer alle Wirkungen zum Zuge kommen können und die Relevanz einzelner Mechanismen letztlich vom Status des Empfängers abhängt. Das Zusammenwirken der vielfältigen Mechanismen macht es erst möglich, dass die wohl eher milden Einzeleffekte sich zu einer therapeutischen Bedeutung summieren können.

Einleitung

Die stetige, rasche und effiziente Abwehr von Krankheitserregern ist in einem großen, vielzelligen Organismus wie dem Menschen nur durch eine lebenslange Anpassungsfähigkeit des Immunsystems möglich. Dies leistet die erworbene Immunität. Sie beruht auf zellulären und humoralen Mechanismen. Eine wesentliche Säule der humoralen Immunität stellt die Bildung von Immunglobulinen durch reife B-Lymphozyten dar, die aufgrund spezieller Rekombinationsmechanismen auf DNS-Ebene mehr als 10^7 Antikörper mit unterschiedlicher Spezifität abgeben können. Immunglobuline können immunogene Strukturen *(Antigene)* auf eindringenden Mikroorganismen erkennen und durch Aktivierung des Komplementsystems und Stimulation phagozytierender Zellen zur Elimination des Erregers führen. In Abhängigkeit davon, wie viele B-Lymphozyten über ihre Tochterzellen die Immunreaktion vermitteln, kommt es zu einer *polyklonalen* (Beitrag vieler Ursprungszellen), *oligoklonalen* (Beitrag nur weniger Zellklone), oder *monoklonalen (Beitrag einzelner Zellklone) Immunantwort.* Oligoklonale und vor allem die seltenen monoklonalen Antworten machen sich meist durch eine klinische Abnormität bemerkbar.

Am Anfang fast aller Herstellungsverfahren zur Immunglobulingewinnung steht auch heute noch eine der vielen Abwandlungen der Cohn'schen Kälte-Ethanolfraktionierung des gepoolten Serums von 5.000 bis 60.000 Spendern (Cohn et al. 1946; Olivares-Villagómez et al. 2000; Geng et al. 2000), gefolgt von weiteren, herstellerspezifischen Reinigungsschritten und speziellen nachgeschalteten Methoden zur Verhinderung der spontanen Aktivierung von Komplement und Zellen durch Aggregatbildung. Die modernen Präparate besitzen durch verbesserte Herstellungsbedingungen und Selektion der Spender eine hohe Sicherheit gegen Übertragung infektiöser Erreger; so wird das Risiko der Hepatitis C Virus-Übertragung bei korrekter Anwendung der Good Manufacturing Practice (GMP) heute auf etwa 1:2.000.000 geschätzt.

In den so gewonnenen Präparaten besitzen die IgG-Moleküle mit einer Sedimentationskonstante von 7S, soweit sie bei den nachgeschalteten Methoden nicht chemisch modifiziert wurden, volle biologische Aktivität und entsprechen den Anforderungen der Weltgesundheitsorganisation (Clinical Immunology Committee 1982). Daneben enthalten die Immunglobulinpräparationen herstellungsbedingt weitere immunaktive Moleküle, die möglicherweise zu den in Zellkultur und experimentell beschriebenen Eigenschaften der Immunglobuline beitragen (s.u.). Unklar ist auch, inwieweit die durch unterschiedliche Herstellungsprozesse hervorgerufenen Unterschiede in den immunbiologischen Funktionen, die in *in vitro Experimenten* und in Tiermodellen nachweisbar sind (siehe z.B. (Romer et al. 1982)), eine Relevanz für die therapeutische Wirkung der Präparationen besitzen.

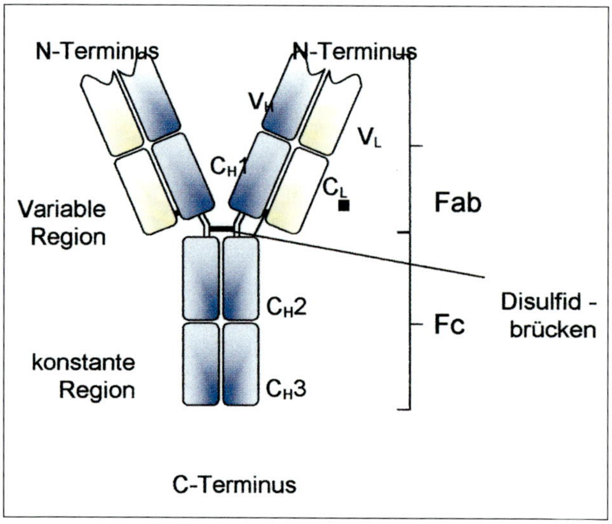

Abb. 1: Struktur des Immunglobulinmoleküls. V = variable Region, C = konstante Region, H = schwere Kette, L = Leichtkette, Fab = antigenbindendes Fragment, Fc = konstantes Fragment.

Allgemeine Struktur und Funktion des Immunglobulinmoleküls

Antikörper sind Proteine, die aus jeweils zwei identischen leichten (L) und schweren (H) Polypeptidketten zusammengesetzt sind (Toyka et al. 1987, Frazer und Capra 1999) (Abb. 1). Die Erkennung von Antigen ist an den N-terminalen, variablen Teil der Leicht- und Schwerketten gebunden *(Idiotypen)*. Dort liegen auch die hypervariablen Regionen (CDR = complementarity determining residues), die durch Mutationen und somatische Rekombination entstehen und die Spezifität des Immunglobulins bestimmen. Jedes Molekül besitzt an seiner schweren Kette in Richtung des freien C-terminalen Endes einen konstanten Teil (Isotyp), der die Zugehörigkeit zu einer bestimmten Hauptgruppe, auch Immunglobulin-Klasse genannt, determiniert. Daneben ist an den *Isotyp* hauptsächlich das Vermitteln von Effektorfunktionen durch Bindung an sogenannte Fc-Rezeptoren auf Immunzellen im Organismus gekoppelt (Späth 1999; Frazer und Capra 1999;Toyka et al. 1987). Über den konstanten Teil der Immunglobuline kann auch das Komplementsystem aktiviert werden (Späth 1999). Durch spezifische Proteasen wie Papain kann das IgG-Molekül in Untereinheiten, den Fc-Teil und in die spezifischen Fab-Teile, zerlegt werden.

Beim Menschen existieren fünf Immunglobulin-Klassen, nämlich IgG, IgA, IgM, IgD und IgE. Für die therapeutische Anwendung bei Autoimmunerkrankungen haben nur IgG-Präparate eine besondere Bedeutung erlangen können. Etwa 80% des körpereigenen Immunglobulins besteht aus IgG (Roitt 1989). IgG hat ein Molekulargewicht von ca. 150.000. Im Gegensatz zu anderen Immunglobulinen passieren alle IgG-Subklassen die Plazentarschranke und vermitteln so die Neugeborenenimmunität.

Zusammensetzung von intravenösen Immunglobulinpräparationen (IVIg) und Dosierung bei neurologischen Autoimmunerkrankungen

Präparate für den intravenösen Einsatz bestehen fast ausschließlich aus IgG und enthalten nur noch Spuren von anderen Immunglobulinen oder Aggregaten (Kaveri et al. 1991). Die IgG Subklassenverteilung entspricht meist der des normalem Serums, nämlich ca. 65% IgG_1, 20% IgG_2 und kleinere Anteile von IgG_3 und IgG_4 (Roitt 1989; Toyka et al. 1987). Man nimmt an, dass die IgG Subklassen, mit Ausnahme des rascher abgebauten IgG_3, in-vivo eine Halbwertszeit von bis zu 3 Wochen besitzen (Kaveri et al. 1991; Drews 1986). Durch die hohe Zahl von Spendern enthalten die gepoolten, polyvalenten Präparationen eine Vielfalt von Antikörpern, die das Repertoire eines einzelnen Menschen bei weitem übersteigt.

Neben Immunglobulinen kommen in den kommerziell verfügbaren Präparationen noch weitere, potentiell immunregulatorische Inhaltsstoffe wie lösliche HLA und CD4 Moleküle (Blasczyk et al. 1993; Grosse-Wilde et al. 1992) oder Zytokine (Kekow et al. 1998) vor. Da ihr Gehalt je nach Hersteller und Präparation stark schwanken kann und nicht gesondert angegeben wird, sind Aussagen über die Bedeutung dieser »Kontaminationen« für die therapeutische Wirksamkeit z.Z. nicht möglich. Am ehesten sehen wir eine Rolle solcher Moleküle im Zusammenhang mit den IVIg vermittelten Mechanismen und nicht als relevanten Einzeleffekt. Auch die in IVIg-Präparaten enthaltenen Stabilisatoren, wie Zucker (Glucose, Sucrose und Maltose) oder auch Aminosäuren (Glycin), können z.B. die Proliferationsantwort von Leukozyten auf mitogene Lektine wie das Phytohämagglutinin oder auf T-Zellrezeptoraktivierung deutlich vermindern (Alder et al. 1996).

Die gebräuchlichste Dosierung von IVIg, nämlich 0,4 g/kg Körpergewicht über 3–5 Tage, folgt jener für die idiopathische (immun) thrombozytopenische Purpura (ITP). Diese Dosierung wurde zunächst empirisch festgelegt (Imbach et al. 1981), jedoch später durch große kontrollierte Therapiestudien (van der Meche et al. 1992) bestätigt. Letztlich existiert aber keine Dosisfindungsstudie, die zeigt, dass die Therapie mit 0,4 g/kg über 3 bis 5 Tage wirklich optimal ist. Es gibt Hinweise darauf, dass eine immunmodulatorische Wirkung mit hohen Einzeldosen besser erzielbar ist als wenn die Gesamtdosis auf mehrere Gaben verteilt wird. Dies ist z.B. für die Behandlung des Kawasaki-Syndroms entscheidend (Newburger et al. 1991). Auch für die Therapie der akuten ITP wurde die Dosis von 5 x 0,4 g/kg KG (Körpergewicht) bereits durch die einmalige Gabe von 0,8 g/kg KG abgelöst. Man empfiehlt nach der Infusion eine abwartende Haltung für drei Tage, um dann zu entscheiden, ob eine zweite Infusion notwendig ist. Dieses Vorgehen stellt eine Individualisierung der IVIg-Therapie dar, die über kurz oder lang bei anderen Anwendungen auch angestrebt werden sollte.

Ein 70 kg schwerer Patient erhält nach o.g. Schema innerhalb von drei bis fünf Tagen ca. 90 g IVIg. Dies stellt etwa die doppelte Menge des im Plasma vorhandenen körpereigenen IgG (circa 40 g) dar und entspricht in etwa der Hälfte des Gesamtgehalts an IgG im Extrazellulärraum (170 g). Somit wird kurzzeitig der IgG Gehalt im Plasma verdoppelt (Fateh-Moghadam et al. 1984) und normalisiert sich innerhalb der nächsten drei bis vier Wochen durch Umverteilung mittels Diffusion ins Interstitium (Besinger et al. 1987). Die relativ lange Halbwertszeit ermöglicht es mit hohen Dosen unter klinisch annehmbaren Bedingungen zu arbeiten.

Immunmodulation durch Immunglobuline – mögliche Wirkmechanismen

Autoimmunerkrankungen werden als Ausdruck einer Dysregulation des Immunsystems angesehen, die zu einer fehlgesteuerten Immunreaktion gegen körpereigenes Gewebe führt. In diesem fehlgesteuerten Netzwerk aus Helfer- und Suppressor-T Lymphozyten und davon abhängigen B-Zellen, können exogen zugeführte polyvalente Immunglobuline auf mehreren Stufen modulierend eingreifen (Übersicht in Dalakas 1999). Für die Immunmodulation durch Immunglobulinpräparate werden folgende Effekte verantwortlich gemacht:

- *anti-idiotypische Antikörper* (Übersicht in (Kaveri et al. 1991)),
- *Neutralisierung von Komplement-vermittelten Effekten* (Basta et al. 1989) (Frank et al. 1992)

- *Hemmung der überschießenden Komplementaktivierung* (Lutz et al. 1996),
- *Hemmung der pathogenen Antikörperproduktion von B-Zellen* (Ballow et al. 1989)
- *erhöhte Katabolie von pathogenem IgG über protektive Fc Rezeptoren* (Yu und Lennon 1999),
- *Internalisation von Fc Rezeptoren* (Sinclair 1991),
- *Inhibition von CD5+ B-Zellen durch anti-CD5 Antikörper* (Vassilev et al. 1993), *lösliche HLA Klasse II, CD4 Moleküle und Zytokine* (Grosse-Wilde et al. 1992; Blasczyk et al. 1993),
- *Neutralisierung von Superantigenen und infektiösen Erregern* (Takei et al. 1993; Masson 1993),
- *anti-idiotypische (-klonotypische) Effekte auf T-Zellen* (Marchalonis et al. 1992)
- *Verminderung der Produktion von proinflammatorischen Zytokinen wie IL-1, IL-6, IFN-γ* (Andersson und Andersson 1990; Andersson et al. 1993; Svenson et al. 1993).

Die Vielzahl der möglichen, sich ergänzenden Wirkmechanismen ist verwirrend. Wahrscheinlich sind nur einige wenige für die therapeutische Wirkung relevant (Stangel et al. 1999b):

Durch kontrollierte Studien wurde die *Neutralisierung von aktivierten Komplementprodukten* bei der Dermatomyositis eindeutig belegt. Durch die Gabe von IVIg (Dalakas et al. 1993) wurde die lokale Komplementablagerung zumindest vorübergehend fast völlig verhindert (Basta und Dalakas 1994). Die Dermatomyositis stellt praktisch die einzige neurologische Autoimmunerkrankung dar, bei der der Effekt von IVIg-Gaben direkt mit einem Rückgang der Komplementaktivierung im Serum korreliert (Basta und Dalakas 1994). Die Verminderung der $C3b_n$-haltigen Immunkomplexe nach IVIg-Gabe konnte *in vivo* bei der Dermatomyositis gezeigt werden (Frigerio et al. 2000). Auch bei der experimentellen Neuritis spielt wahrscheinlich die Modulation der Komplementablagerung eine zentrale Rolle (Miyagi et al. 1997).

Eine weitere zentrale Rolle nehmen Fc Rezeptor-vermittelte Wirkungen ein. Viele der IVIg-Wirkungen sind am ausgeprägtesten bei der Verwendung von intaktem 7S IgG zu beobachten. Man geht davon aus, dass die konstante Region von 7S IgG an die Fc Rezeptoren von B und T Zellen binden kann und regulatorisch auf die Lymphozyten wirkt. Dabei scheint es sich nicht um eine einfache Blockade der der Fc-Rezeptoren durch Immunkomplexe zu handeln. Kürzlich konnte am Tiermodell der ITP nachgewiesen werden, dass über Fc Rezeptoren inhibitorische Signale vermittelt werden (Samuelsson et al. 2001). Auch bei der experimentellen Neuritis, dem Tiermodell für das humane Guillain-Barré-Syndrom (GBS), spielen Fc-vermittelte Effekte von IVIg möglicherweise eine zentrale Rolle (Miyagi et al. 1997). Neben den klassischen Fc Rezeptoren wird die Wirkung der sog. protektiven Fc Rezeptoren FcRp zunehmend diskutiert. Diese stellen Transportmoleküle für IgG in endozytotische Vesikel dar und können IgG Moleküle auf diese Weise vor Degradation schützen und rezirkulieren (Übersicht in Yu und Lennon 1999). Durch die exogene Gabe von IVIg kommt es wahrscheinlich zur Übersättigung dieses Rezirkulationssystems und damit relativ zu einer vermehrten Katabolie körpereigener, autoreaktiver Immunglobulinmoleküle. Diese Konzepte konnten bereits in knockout-Modellen bestätigt werden. Weiterhin wurde ein humanes Homolog zu dem zunächst nur in Nagetieren beschriebenen Rezeptor identifiziert (Yu und Lennon 1999).

Kürzlich gelang an einem *in-vitro* Modell für synaptische Übertragung der Nachweis von *anti-idiotypischen Antikörpern.* Dies sind Antikörper, die die Antigenerkennungsregion (»Idiotyp«) von pathogenetisch relevanten Patientenantikörpern erkennen. Anti-idiotypische Antikörper wurden erstmals 1984 von Sultan et al. *in vivo* und in IVIg Präparationen nachgewiesen (Sultan et al. 1984). Anti-Idiotypen neutralisieren autoaggressive Antikörper (Abdou et al. 1981) und begünstigen wahrscheinlich ihre nachfolgende Elimination über Fc Rezeptoren. Diese »Anti-Antikörper« (Übersicht in Kaveri et al. 1991) sollen eine inhärente Komponente der Immunregulation sein, kommen bei Gesunden und somit auch im Spenderpool für IVIg, vor und bieten einen natürlichen Schutz vor pathologischen Autoantikörpern. Ein indirekter Hinweis auf idiotypische Wechselwirkungen von IgG Molekülen leitet sich aus elektronenmikroskopischen Untersuchungen ab. In Abhängigkeit von der Poolgröße liegen bis gegen 20% der Immunglobuline eines Spenderpools in dimerer Form vor (Roux und Tankersley 1990; Hauser et al. 2000). Anti-Idiotypen sind allerdings bisher nur in der Rekonvaleszenz-Phase einiger weniger Immunkrankheiten sicher nachgewiesen worden. Einzelne Befunde bei der chronisch-entzündlichen Polyneuritis (CIDP) (van Doorn et al. 1990) , bei Patienten mit Guillain-Barré-Syndrom (GBS) (Lundkvist et al. 1993) und bei Patienten mit Lupus erythematodes (Ronda et al. 1994) sprechen aber durchaus für Effekte auf dieser Ebene. Bei zwei Patienten mit akuter sensomotorischer axonaler Neuropathie (AMSAN), einer axonalen Unterform des GBS, gelang es *in-vitro,* einen funktionell anti-idiotypischen Effekt von IVIg mit der sog. Makro-Patchclampmethode zu demonstrieren (Buchwald et al. 2002).

Bedeutung der Remyelinisierung durch Immunglobuline

Die Vorstellung, dass durch IVIg eine Remyelinisierung gefördert werden könnte, wurde aus der Wirkung polyklonaler Immunoglobuline gegen Rückenmarkshomogenat am Modell der Theilervirus-Enzephalitis abgeleitet (Rodriguez und Lennon 1990), einem virus-vermitteltem Modell für die multiple Sklerose. In Nachfolgestudien konnte der Hinweis erbracht werden, dass diese remyelinisierende Wirkung auf Antikörpern gegen basisches Myelinprotein beruhen dürfte (Rodriguez et al. 1996). Schließlich gelang es Rodriguez und Mitarbeitern ein Hybridom zu etablieren, das einen monoklonalen IgMκ Antkörper sezernierte, der Remyelinisierung vermitteln konnte (Miller et al. 1994), die Entzündungsreaktion unterdrückte und auch in einem Modell einer toxisch-bedingten Demyelinisierung wirksam war (Pavelko et al. 1998). Die weitere Charakterisierung dieses Antikörpers ergab, dass er polyreaktiv war und Antigene auf der Oberfläche und im Zytoplasma von Oligodendrozyten und anderen Gliazellen

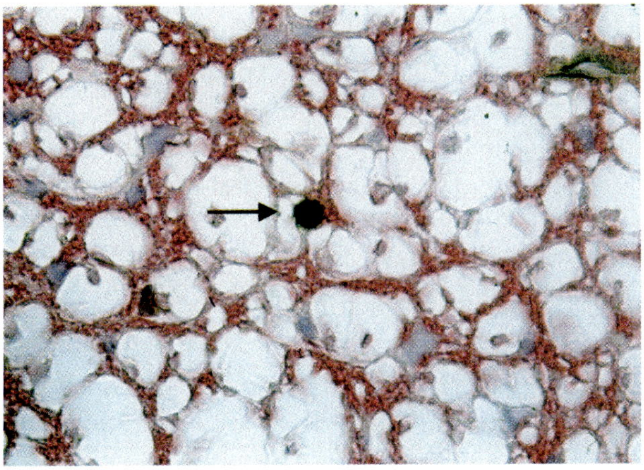

Abb. 2: Apoptotischer Zelltod von Oligodendrozyten im Tiermodell der MS. Durch IVIg konnte in diesem Modell keine Protektion erreicht werden.
Pfeil = apoptotischer Zellkern eines Oligodendrozyten, rot = Myelinprotein MOG.

erkannte (Asakura et al. 1996). Von den verschiedenen möglichen Wirkmechanismen zur Förderung der Remyelinisierung stellt die Modulation von Oligodendrozyten das schlüssigste Konzept dar. Gleichzeitig wird damit aber auch die traditionelle Ansicht in Frage gestellt, dass Antikörper gegen Myelinbestandteile grundsätzlich pathogen sind und Demyelinisierung vermitteln. Remyelinierungsfördernde Wirkungen von IVIg wurden auch am Modell der experimentellen Neuritis postuliert. Nachdem allerdings zwei sorgfältig geplante, plazebokontrollierte Studien zur Remyelinisierung bei MS negativ verliefen (Noseworthy et al. 2001; Noseworthy et al. 2000), scheint die Wirkung von IVIg bei der MS eher auf direkten immunologischen Angriffspunkten (s.o.) zu beruhen. Auch konnten Untersuchungen aus der Arbeitsgruppe von Compston keinen Effekt auf Proliferation und Differenzierung von Oligodendrozyten belegen (Abb. 2) (Stangel et al. 1999a). Es wurde allerdings ein Schutz vor Komplement-vermittelter Zytotoxizität nachgewiesen(s.o.) (Stangel et al. 2000).

Nebenwirkungen von Immunglobulinpräparaten

Mit dem zunehmenden Einsatz von IVIg bei neurologischen Autoimmunerkrankungen ist auch die Zahl der berichteten Nebenwirkungen angestiegen. In den meisten Fällen handelt es sich dabei nur um Kasuistiken, so dass aufgrund fehlender prospektiver Untersuchungen die tatsächliche Häufigkeit nur schwer abgeschätzt werden kann. Aufgrund unserer Erfahrung liegt die Frequenz der Nebenwirkungen jedoch deutlich unter den in retrospektiven Analysen angegebenen (Bertorini et al. 1996; Brannagan, III et al. 1996) Zahlen. Gerade die häufig vorkommenden Probleme nach Gabe von IVIg sind in den meisten Fällen leichter Natur, *schwere Zwischenfälle* treten selten oder nur bei Nichtbeachtung entsprechender Sicherheitsbestimmungen und Kontraindikationen ein. Dabei sind meist ältere und kardiovaskulär vorgeschädigte Patienten gefährdet.

Schwere Nebenwirkungen: Kardiovaskuläre Komplikationen, Thrombembolien, renale Funktionsstörungen, Infektion

IVIg-Präparate werden häufig als Alternative zur Plasmapherese eingesetzt, wenn es sich um ältere Patienten, oder Patienten mit septischen Komplikationen oder kardiovaskulären Vorerkrankungen handelt. Gerade bei Letzteren kann die Vergrößerung des Plasmavolumens durch IVIg zu einer Dekompensation einer vorbestehenden Herzinsuffizienz führen. Die Vergrößerung des Plasmavolumens sowie erhöhte Plasma- und Blutviskosität begünstigen auch ein akutes Nierenversagen (s.u.) und akute Blutdruckkrisen. Desweiteren können thrombembolische Ereignisse ausgelöst werden, die zu ischämischen Hirninfarkten und Lungenembolien führen (Dalakas 1994; Steg und Lefkowitz 1994). Obwohl die Häufigkeit solcher Nebenwirkungen nach Literaturangaben nur ca. 3% beträgt, sind sie doch ausreichend schwer und müssen dem Patienten im Aufklärungesgespräch mitgeteilt werden.

Als seltene, aber schwere Nebenwirkung von IVIg-Behandlung kann es zu einem akuten Nierenversagen kommen. Meist tritt dies bei Patienten mit vorbestehender kompensierter Niereninsuffizienz auf (Tan et al. 1993; Ahsan et al. 1994). In vielen Fällen ist eine vorübergehende Dialysebehandlung erforderlich. Bioptisch konnte eine Schwellung und Vakuolisierung des proximalen Tubulusepithels als Hinweis auf einen osmotischen Schaden nachgewiesen werden (Tan et al. 1993; Ahsan et al. 1994). Hinweise für ein immunologisch vermitteltes Geschehen fanden sich hingegen nicht. Eine mögliche Erklärung ist, dass osmotisch wirksame Stabilisatoren in IVIg-Präparaten wie Sucrose oder Mannose die Nephropathie auslösen. Präparate mit Glycin als Stabilisator sind diesbezüglich unproblematisch. In Einzelfällen sind auch transiente Proteinurien nach IVIg beschrieben worden. Aus der Literatur und nach unserer Erfahrung gibt es keine klaren Hinweise für eine kumulative Schädigung der Nierenfunktion durch Langzeitbehandlung mit IVIg. Als Sicherheitsmaßnahme empfiehlt es sich, das Serum-Kreatinin vor und während einer IVIg-Therapie zu kontrollieren.

Gerade zu Beginn der 90er Jahre wurde durch eine bestimmte Charge von Immunglobulin die infektiöse Hepatitis C übertragen (Bjoro et al. 1994; Flora et al. 1996). Diese Probleme traten nur bei einem Hersteller auf, bevor dieser sein Reinigungsprotokoll um einen Zwischenschritt zur Inaktivierung von Lipidumhüllten Viren erweitert hatte. Die Übertragung von HIV- und anderen viralen Infektionen oder Prionenerkrankungen trat bisher unter Immunglobulintherapie nicht auf.

Als Zeichen einer Hypersensitivitätsreaktion kann es innerhalb einer Stunde nach IVIg-Infusion zu Tachykardie und Blutdruckabfall kommen, wobei diese Nebenwirkungen meist durch Unterbrechen der Infusion gestoppt werden kann (Ratko et al. 1995).

Leichte Nebenwirkungen: Kopfschmerzen und aseptische Meningitiden, Leberenzymanstiege, Allgemeinreaktionen

Die häufigsten leichten Nebenwirkungen von IVIg stellen Kopfschmerzen dar. Ursprünglich dachte man, dass sie bei weniger als 5% der Patienten auftreten, jedoch wurde in einzelnen Studien eine Inzidenz von bis zu 48% berichtet

(Brannagan, III et al. 1996). Meist sind die Symptome nur leicht ausgeprägt und können durch eine Verlangsamung der Infusionsrate bewältigt werden. Gelegentlich werden auch Analgetika benötigt (Casteels-van Daele et al. 1990). Möglicherweise sind Patienten mit Migräne-Neigung zur Entwicklung von Kopfschmerzen besonders disponiert. Auch in Fällen mit schweren Kopfschmerzen gab es keine Langzeitfolgen, und in allen Fällen trat rasche Erholung der Patienten ein. Daher sehen wir Kopfschmerzen zwar als relevante, aber nicht als schwerwiegende Nebenwirkung von Immunglobulin an. Der pathogenetische Mechanismus ist ungeklärt, möglicherweise beruht die Nebenwirkung auf dem hohen Anteil proinflammatorischer Zytokine in IVIg Präparationen. In zwei Fällen wurde auch eine encephalopathische Reaktion beschrieben, wobei eine davon mit intrazerebralen Vasospasmen vergesellschaftet war (Voltz et al. 1996; Harkness et al. 1996). Bei beiden Patienten traten keine Spätfolgen auf.

Zu den Allgemeinreaktionen kann man Myalgien, Arthralgien, Rücken- und Thorax-Schmerzen, Fieber, Übelkeit und Erbrechen sowie Pruritus zählen. Bei Patienten, die besonders hohe Dosen an IVIg erhielten, traten häufiger Dermatitiden auf (Sorensen et al. 1998;Whittam et al. 1997). Leichte, klinisch nicht relevante Anstiege der Leberenzyme sind oft präparateabhängig.

Die anderen Nebenwirkungen manifestieren sich meist innerhalb der ersten Infusionsstunden und sind üblicherweise selbstlimitierend. Man kann sie deutlich reduzieren, indem man die Infusionsgeschwindigkeit verringert und vorübergehend die Infusion unterbricht. In schweren Fällen werden Analgetika, Antihistaminika oder Glukokortikosteroide eingesetzt. Es ist wichtig, zu unterscheiden, ob die potentiellen Nebenwirkungen nicht auch durch die Grunderkrankung bedingt sein können, wie dies z.B. für Rückenschmerzen beim Guillain-Barré-Syndrom zutrifft.

Literatur

1. Abdou MI, Wall H, Lindsley HB, Hasley JF, Susuki T. (1981) Network theory in autoimmunity: in vitro suppression of serum anti-DNA antibody binding to DNA by anti-idiotypic antibody in systemic lupus erythematosus. J Clin Invest 67: 1297–1304.
2. Ahsan N, Palmer BF, Wheeler D, Greenlee RG, Toto RD. (1994) Intravenous immunoglobulin-induced osmotic nephrosis. Arch Int Med 154: 1985–1987.
3. Alder LBA, Morgan LA, Spickett GP. (1996) Contribution of stabilizing agents present in intravenous immunoglobulin preparations to modulation of mononuclear cell proliferation in vitro. Scand J Immunol 44: 585–591.
4. Andersson JP, Andersson UG. (1990) Human intravenous immunoglobulin modulates monokine production in vitro. Immunology 71: 372–376.
5. Andersson UG, Björk L, Skansen-Saphir U, Andersson JP. (1993) Down-regulation of cytokine production and interleukin-2 receptor expression by pooled human IgG. Immunology 79: 211–216.
6. Asakura K, Miller DJ, Murray K, Bansal R, Pfeiffer SE, Rodriguez M. (1996) Monoclonal autoantibody SCH94.03, which promotes central nervous system remyelination, recognizes an antigen on the surface of oligodendrocytes. J Neurosi Res 43: 273–281.
7. Ballow M, White W, Desbonnet C. (1989) Modulation of in vitro synthesis of immunoglobulin and the induction of suppressor activity by therapy with intravenous immune globulin. J Allergy Clin Immunol 84: 595–602.

8. Basta M, Dalakas MC. (1994) High-dose intravenous immunoglobulin exerts its beneficial effect in patients with dermatomyositis by blocking endomysial deposition of activated complement fragments. J Clin Invest 94: 1729–1735.
9. Basta M, Kirshbom P, Frank MM, Fries LF. (1989) Mechanism of therapeutic effect of high-dose intravenous immunoglobulin. Attenuation of acute, complement-dependent immune damage in a guinea pig model. J Clin Invest 84: 1974–1981.
10. Bertorini TE, Nance AM, Homer LM, Greene W, Gelfand MS, Jaster SH. (1996) Complications of intravenous gammaglobulin in neuromuscular and other diseases. Muscle & Nerve 19: 388–391.
11. Besinger U, Fateh-Moghadam A, Knorr-Held S, Wick M, Kissel H, Albitz M. (1987) Immunomodulation in myasthenia gravis by high-dose intravenous 7S-immunoglobulins. Ann NY Acad Sci 505: 828–831.
12. Bjoro K, Froland SS, Yun Z, Samdal HH, Haaland T. (1994) Hepatitis C infection in patients with primary hypogammaglobulinemia after treatment with contaminated immune globulin. N Engl J Med 331: 1607–1611.
13. Blasczyk R, Westhoff U, Grosse Wilde H. (1993) Soluble CD4, CD8, and HLA molecules in commercial immunoglobulin preparations. Lancet 341: 789–790.
14. Brannagan TH, III, Nagle KJ, Lange DJ, Rowland LP. (1996) Complications of intravenous immune globulin treatment in neurologic disease. Neurology 47: 674–677.
15. Buchwald B, Ahangari R, Weishaupt A, Toyka KV (2002) Intravenous immunoglobulins neutralize blocking antibodies in Guillain-Barre syndrom. Ann Neurol 51: 673–680.
16. Casteels-van Daele M, Wijndaele L, Hunninck K, Gillis P. (1990) Intravenous immune globulin and acute aseptic meningitis. N Engl J Med 323: 614–615.
17. Clinical Immunology Committee IUoISaWHO. (1982) Appropriate uses of human immunoglobulin in clinical practice. Bull WHO 60: 43–47.
18. Cohn EJ, Strong LE, Hughes WL, et al. (1946) Preparation and properties of serum and plasma proteins. I. A system for the separation into fractions of the protein and lipoprotein components of biological issues and fluids. J Am Chem Soc 68: 459–475.
19. Dalakas MC. (1994) High-dose intravenous immunoglobulin and serum viscosity: risk of precipitating thromboembolic events. Neurology 44: 223–226.
20. Dalakas MC. (1999) Intravenous immunoglobulin in the treatment of autoimmune neuromuscular diseases: Present status and practical therapeutic guidelines. Muscle and Nerve 22: 1479–1497.
21. Dalakas MC, Illa I, Dambrosia JM et al. (1993) Efficacy of high-dose intravenous immunoglobulin in the treatment of dermatomyositis: a double-blind, placebo-controlled study. N Engl J Med 329: 1993–2000.
22. Drews J. Immunpharmakologie. Berlin-Heidelberg: Springer Verlag, 1986.
23. Fateh-Moghadam A, Wick M, Besinger U, Geursen RG. (1984) High-dose intravenous gammaglobulin for myasthenia gravis. Lancet 1: 848–849.
24. Flora K, Schiele M, Benner K et al. (1996) An outbreak of acute hepatitis C among recipients of intravenous immunoglobulin. Ann Allergy Asthma Immunol 76: 160–162.
25. Frank MM, Basta M, Fries LF. (1992) The effects of intravenous immune globulin on complement – dependent immune damage of cells and tissues. Clin Immunol Immunopathol 62: S82–S86.
26. Frazer JK, Capra JD. Immunoglobulins: Structure and function. In: Paul WE, editor. Fundamental Immunology. New York: Raven Press, 1999: 37–74.
27. Frigerio S, Silei V, Ciusani E, Massa G, Lauro GM, Salmaggi A. (2000) Modulation of Fas-Ligand (Fas-L) on human microglial cells: an in vitro study. J Neuroimmunol 105: 109–114.
28. Geng YM, Shane RB, Berencsi K et al. (2000) Chlamydia pneumoniae inhibits apoptosis in human peripheral blood mononuclear cells through induction of IL-10. J Immunol 164: 5522–5529.
29. Grosse-Wilde H, Blasczyk R, Westhoff U. (1992) Soluble HLA class I and class II concentrations in commercial immunoglobulin preparations. Tissue Antigens 39: 74–77.
30. Harkness K, Howell SJ, Davies-Jones GAB. (1996) Encephalopathy associated with intravenous immunoglobulin treatment for Guillain-Barre syndrome. J Neurol Neurosurg Psychiatry 60: 586.

31. Hauser SL, Oksenberg JR, Lincoln R et al. (2000) Interaction between HLA-DR2 and abnormal brain MRI in optic neuritis and early MS. Neurology 54: 1859–1861.
32. Imbach P, Barandun S, d'Apuzzo V et al. (1981) High dose intravenous gammaglobulin for idiopathic thrombocytopenic purpura. Lancet I: 1228–1231.
33. Kaveri SV, Dietrich G, Hurez V, Kazatchkine MD. (1991) Intravenous immunoglobulins (IVIg) in the treatment of autoimmune diseases [published erratum appears in Clin Exp Immunol 1992 May;88(2):373]. Clin Exp Immunol 86: 192–198.
34. Kekow J, Reinhold D, Pap T, Ansorge S. (1998) Intravenous immunoglobulins and transforming growth factor b. Lancet 351: 184–185.
35. Lundkvist I, van Doorn PA, Vermeulen M, Brand A. (1993) Spontaneous recovery from the Guillain-Barre syndrome is associated with anti-idiotypic antibodies recognizing a cross-reactive idiotype on anti-neuroblastoma cell line antibodies. Clin Immunol Immunopathol 67: 192–198.
36. Lutz HU, Stammler P, Jelezarova E, Nater M, Spath PJ. (1996) High doses of immunoglobulin G attenuate immune aggregate-mediated complement activation by enhancing physiologic cleavage of C3b in C3bn-IgG complexes. Blood 88: 184–193.
37. Marchalonis JJ, Kaymaz H, Dedeoglu F, Schluter SF, Yocum DE, Edmundson AB. (1992) Human autoantibodies reactive with synthetic autoantigens from T- cell receptor β chain. Proc Natl Acad Sci USA 89: 3325–3329.
38. Masson PL. (1993) Elimination of infectious antigens and increase of IgG catabolism as possible modes of action of IVIg. J Autoimmun 6: 683–689.
39. Miller DJ, Sanborn KS, Katzmann JA, Rodriguez M. (1994) Monoclonal autoantibodies promote central nervous system repair in an animal model of multiple sclerosis. J Neurosci 14: 6230–6238.
40. Miyagi F, Horiuchi H, Nagata I et al. (1997) Fc portion of intravenous immunoglobulin suppresses the induction of experimental allergic neuritis. J Neuroimmunol 78: 127–131.
41. Noseworthy JH, O'Brien PC, Petterson TM et al. (2001) A randomized trial of intravenous immunoglobulin in inflammatory demyelinating optic neuritis. Neurology 56: 1514–1522.
42. Noseworthy JH, O'Brien PC, Weinshenker BG et al. (2000) IV immunoglobulin does not reverse established weakness in MS. Neurology 55: 1135–1143.
43. Olivares-Villagómez D, Wensky AK, Wang YJ, Lafaille JJ. (2000) Repertoire requirements of $CD4^+$ T cells that prevent spontaneous autoimmune encephalomyelitis. J Immunol 164: 5499–5507.
44. Pavelko KD, van Engelen BGM, Rodriguez M. (1998) Acceleration in the rate of CNS remyelination in lysolecithin- induced demyelination. J Neurosci 18: 2498–2505.
45. Ratko TA, Burnett DA, Foulke GE, Matuszewski KA, Sacher RA. (1995) Recommendations for off-label use of intravenously administered immunoglobulin preparations. University Hospital Consortium Expert Panel for Off-Label Use of Polyvalent Intravenously Administered Immunoglobulin Preparations. JAMA 273: 1865–1870.
46. Rodriguez M, Lennon VA. (1990) Immunoglobulins promote remyelination in the central nervous system. Ann Neurol 27: 12–17.
47. Rodriguez M, Miller DJ, Lennon VA. (1996) Immunoglobulins reactive with myelin basic protein promote CNS remyelination. Neurology 46: 538–545.
48. Roitt IM. Leitfaden der Immunologie. Darmstadt: Steinkopff Verlag, 1989.
49. Romer J, Spath PJ, Skvaril F, Nydegger UE. (1982) Characterization of various immunoglobulin preparations for intravenous application. II. Complement activation and binding to staphylococcus protein A. Vox Sang 42: 74–80.
50. Ronda N, Haury M, Nobrega A, Coutinho A, Kazatchkine MD. (1994) Selectivity of recognition of variable (V) regions of autoantibodies by intravenous immunoglobulin (IVIg). Clin Immunol Immunopathol 70: 124–128.
51. Roux KH, Tankersley DL. (1990) A view of the human idiotypic repertoire. Electron microscopic and immunologic analyses of spontaneous idiotype-anti-idiotype dimers in pooled human IgG. J Immunol 144: 1387–1395.
52. Samuelsson A, Towers TL, Ravetch JV. (2001) Anti-inflammatory Activity of IVIG Mediated Through the Inhibitory Fc Receptor. Science 291: 484–486.

53. Sinclair NRS. (1991) Fc-receptor-mediated immunomodulation. Immunology Today 12: 46.
54. Sorensen PS, Wanscher B, Jensen CV et al. (1998) Intravenous immunoglobulin G reduces MRI activity in relapsing multiple sclerosis. Neurology 50: 1273–1281.
55. Späth PJ (1999) Structure and function of immunoglobulins. Sepsis ; 3: 197–218.
56. Stangel M, Compston A, Scolding NJ. (1999a) Polyclonal immunoglobulins for intravenous use do not influence the behaviour of cultured oligodendrocytes. J Neuroimmunol 96: 228–233.
57. Stangel M, Compston A, Scolding NJ. (2000) Oligodendroglia are protected from antibody-mediated complement injury by normal immunoglobulins (»IVIg«). Journal of Neuroimmunology 103: 195–201.
58. Stangel M, Toyka KV, Gold R. (1999b) Mechanisms of high-dose intravenous immunoglobulins in demyelinating diseases. Arch Neurol 56: 661–663.
59. Steg RE, Lefkowitz DM. (1994) Cerebral infarction following intravenous immunoglobulin therapy for myasthenia gravis. Neurology 1180–1181.
60. Sultan Y, Kazatchkine MD, Maisonneuve P, Nydegger UE. (1984) Anti-idiotypic suppression of autoantibodies to factor VIII (antihaemophilic factor) by high-dose intravenous gammaglobulin. Lancet 2: 765–768.
61. Svenson M, Hansen MB, Bendtzen K. (1993) Binding of cytokines to pharmaceutically prepared human immunoglobulin. J Clin Invest 92: 2533–2539.
62. Takei S, Arora YK, Walker SM. (1993) Intravenous immunoglobulin contains specific antibodies inhibitory to activation of T cells by staphylococcal toxin superantigens [see comment]. J Clin Invest 91: 602–607.
63. Tan E, Hajinazarian M, Bay W, Neff J, Mendell JR. (1993) Acute renal failure resulting from intravenous immunoglobulin therapy. Arch Neurol 50: 137–139.
64. Toyka KV, Hartung HP, Hohlfeld R. Klinische Neuroimmunologie. Diagnostik, Pathophysiologie, Therapie. Weinheim: VCH Verlagsgesellschaft, 1987.
65. van der Meche FGA, Schmitz PIM, and the Dutch Guillain-Barre study group. (1992) A randomized trial comparing intravenous immune globulin and plasma exchange in Guillain-Barre syndrome. N Engl J Med 326: 1123–1129.
66. van Doorn PA, Rossi F, Brand A, van Lint M, Vermeulen M, Kazatchkine MD. (1990) On the mechanism of high-dose intravenous immunoglobulin treatment of patients with chronic inflammatory demyelinating polyneuropathy. J Neuroimmunol 29: 57–64.
67. Vassilev T, Gelin C, Kaveri SV, Zilber MT, Boumsell L, Kazatchkine MD. (1993) Antibodies to the CD5 molecule in normal human immunoglobulins for therapeutic use (intravenous immunoglobulins, IVIg). Clin Exp Immunol 92: 369–372.
68. Voltz R, Rosen FV, Yousry T, Beck J, Hohlfeld R. (1996) Reversible encephalopathy with cerebral vasospasm in a Guillain-Barre syndrome patient treated with intravenous immunoglobulin. Neurology 46: 250–251.
69. Whittam LR, Hay RJ, Hughes RAC. (1997) Eczematous reactions to human immune globulin. Br J Dermatol. 137: 481–482.
70. Yu ZY, Lennon VA. (1999) Mechanism of intravenous immune globulin therapy in antibody-mediated autoimmune diseases. N Engl J Med. 340: 227–228.

Immunglobuline bei peripher neurologischen Erkrankungen – eine evidenzbasierte Übersicht

J. Kirschner, R. Korinthenberg

Zusammenfassung

Die intravenöse Gabe von Immunglobulinen (IVIG) gehört mittlerweile zur Therapie der Wahl beim schweren Guillain-Barré Syndrom. Ob eine frühe Therapie möglicherweise einen schweren Krankheitsverlauf verhindert, konnte bisher nicht gezeigt werden. Bei der chronischen imflammatorischen demyelinisierenden Polyneuropathie gehören die IVIG neben den Steroiden ebenfalls zu den zur Primärtherapie geeigneten Medikamenten. Bei der juvenilen Myasthenia gravis und der Dermatomyositis hingegen scheint eine Therapie mit IVIG erst bei Versagen anderer Therapieoptionen, bei nicht tolerierbaren Nebenwirkungen oder zur besonderen Krisenintervention gerechtfertigt. Bei keiner der genannten Erkrankungen konnte eine Überlegenheit der Plasmapherese gegenüber der IVIG nachgewiesen werden.

Einleitung

Der Einsatz von Immunglobulinen wird bei einer Reihe von peripher neurologischen Erkrankungen im Kindes- und Jugendalter diskutiert. Die verfügbare Evidenz beruht zumeist auf entsprechenden kontrollierten klinischen Studien aus dem Erwachsenenalter. Für das Kindesalter liegen bisher nur wenige, meist unkontrollierte Studien oder Fallserien zum Einsatz von Immunglobulinen bei peripher neurologischen Erkrankungen vor. Ziel dieser Arbeit ist es, die relevanten Publikationen aus dem Erwachsenenalter sowie entsprechende Erfahrungen für das Kindesalter zusammenstellen, um so eine Hilfestellung für Therapieentscheidungen im klinischen Alltag zu geben. Im Einzelnen soll auf folgende für die Neuropädiatrie besonders relevante Krankheitsbilder eingegangen werden:

- Guillain-Barré Syndrom (GBS)
- Chronisch inflammatorische demyelinisierende Polyneuropathie (CIDP)
- Juvenile Myasthenia gravis
- Dermatomyositis

Guillain-Barré Syndrom (GBS)

Bei dem Guillain-Barré Syndrom handelt es sich um eine akute demyelinisierende Polyneuropathie die klinisch mit einer aufsteigenden Lähmung teilweise

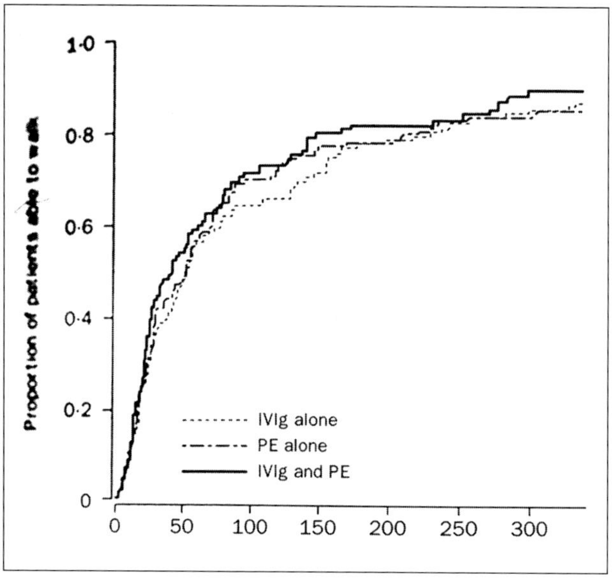

Abb. 1: Überlebenskurven für das Wiedererlangen der freien Gehfähigkeit bei Erwachsenen Patienten (n = 379). Vergleich von IVIG, Plasmapherese und einer Kombination von beiden (3).

bis zur Atemmuskulatur einhergeht. Auch wenn das verantwortliche Antigen noch unbekannt ist, konnte eine Beteiligung des humoralen und cellulären Immunsystems nachgewiesen werden. (1)

Nachdem die intravenöse Gabe von Immunglobulinen bei der CIDP Erfolge gezeigt hatte, wurde sie auch in mehreren kontrollierten Studien bei erwachsenen Patienten mit GBS geprüft (2, 3). Zusammenfassend führte die Gabe von 2 g IVIG/kg Körpergewicht über 5 Tage zu einer klinischen Wirksamkeit, die mit der der Plasmapherese vergleichbar ist. Exemplarisch sind in Abbildung 1 die Ergebnisse der GBS Trial Group für 379 nicht mehr frei gehfähige Patienten dargestellt.

Für die Behandlung des GBS im Kindesalter liegen bisher keine kontrollierten Studien vor. Auch hier lassen aber retrospektive Vergleiche eine ähnliche Effektivität von IVIG und Plasmapherese vermuten (4–7). Eine retrospektive Studie kam zu dem Schluss, dass die Gabe von 2 g IVIG/kg Körpergewicht über 2 Tage effektiver sein könnte als die Gabe über 5 Tage (8).

In einer eigenen kürzlich abgeschlossenen randomisierten Multizenterstudie zeigte sich jedoch in einer vorläufigen Auswertung bei der Behandlung nicht mehr gehfähiger Kinder kein Unterschied zwischen der Gabe über zwei oder fünf Tage (Abb. 2).

Bei den noch gehfähigen Patienten wurde in dieser Studie die Therapie mit IVIG mit einer Kontrollgruppe ohne Therapie verglichen. Bei einer relativ kleinen Patientenzahl (n = 16) zeigte sich hier kein signifikanter Unterschied, so dass der Nutzen einer frühen Therapie bei noch gehfähigen Patienten bisher noch nicht nachgewiesen werden konnte.

Zusammenfassend lässt sich sagen, dass der Einsatz von IVIG (2 mg/kg Körpergewicht über 2–5 Tage) bei nicht mehr gehfähigen Kindern und Jugend-

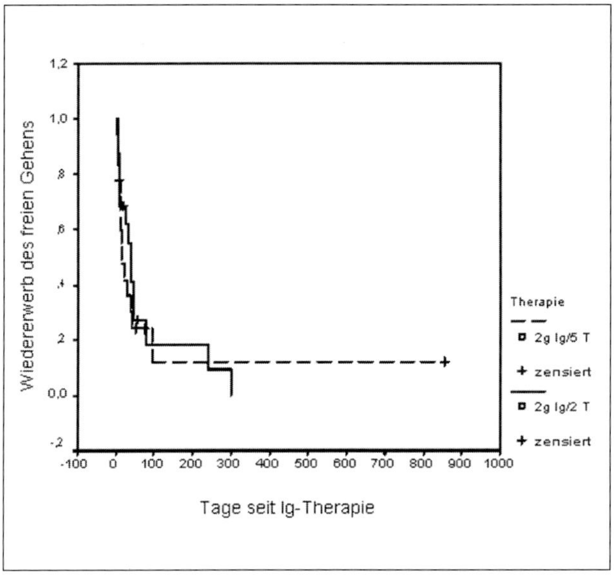

Abb. 2: Wiedererwerb der freien Gehfähigkeit bei Kindern und Jugendlichen (n = 34). Vergleich von 2 g/kg IVIG über 2 Tage und über 5 Tage (vorläufige, bisher nicht publizierte Ergebnisse der Freiburger Multizenterstudie).

lichen mit GBS weit verbreitet ist und aufgrund einer mindestens vergleichbaren Wirksamkeit und einer besseren Durchführbarkeit der Plasmapherese vorzuziehen ist. Ob auch niedrigere Dosierungen von IVIG ähnlich effektiv sind wäre in weiteren Studien zu prüfen.

Chronisch inflammatorische demyelinisierende Polyneuropathie (CIDP)

Bei der CIDP handelt es sich um eine erworbene demyelinisierende Neuropathie, die klinisch durch eine langsam über Wochen bis Monate progrediente Schwäche, Areflexie und Sensibilitätsstörungen gekennzeichnet ist. Immunpathogenetisch liegen vermutlich ähnliche Mechanismen wie beim GBS zugrunde. Während es bei Erwachsenen häufig zu einem chronisch progredienten oder remittierendem Verlauf kommt (9) scheint die Prognose im Kindesalter günstiger zu sein (10).

Im Gegensatz zum GBS zeigen die Steroide bei der CIDP eine gute Wirksamkeit. Ihr Einsatz ist jedoch bei chronischem Verlauf durch Nebenwirkungen und ein mögliches sekundäres Therapieversagen limitiert. Bezüglich der IVIG konnte bei Erwachsenen mit CIDP in doppelblinden Studien die Überlegenheit gegenüber Placebo (11, n = 30) und eine ähnliche Wirksamkeit wie bei Steroiden (12, n = 32) nachgewiesen werden.

Für das Kindesalter liegen bisher nur Fallserien zur Behandlung der CIDP vor (siehe Tab. 1). In diesen Publikationen sind insgesamt 38 Patienten enthalten, die mit IVIG behandelt wurden. Davon zeigten 30 Patienten (79%) eine klinische Verbesserung, wobei die IVIG nicht immer als Initialtherapie eingesetzt wurden.

Tab. 1: Fallserien zur Behandlung der CIDP im Kindes- und Jugendalter (k.A. = keine Angabe)

Publikation	Patienten n	Steroide behandelt/ verbessert	IVIG behandelt/ verbessert	PE behandelt/ verbessert
Colan 1980	5	5/5	k.A.	k.A.
Sladky et al. 1986	6	6/6	k.A.	k.A.
Beydoun et al. 1990	2	k.A.	k.A.	2/2
Uncini et al. 1991	5	4/4	k.A.	k.A.
Vedanarayanan et al. 1991	4	k.A.	4/4	k.A.
Baba et al. 1993	6	6/6	k.A.	k.A.
Nevo et al. 1996	13	13/13	3/6	3/3
Simmons 1997	12	5/7	7/8	4/4
Hattori 1998	10	7/9	1/2	1/2
Korinthenberg 1999	21	8/11	12/14	k.A.
Ryan et al. 2000	16	11/11	3/4	1/1
Summe	**100**	**65/72 (90%)**	**30/38 (79%)**	**11/12 (92%)**

Aufgrund der günstigeren Kosten-Nutzen Relation scheinen zur Initialtherapie der CIDP im Kindesalter die Steroide gut geeignet. IVIG kommen vor allem bei drohenden Nebenwirkungen oder bei Nichtansprechen auf Steroide in Kombination oder als Monotherapie zum Einsatz. Bei chronischem Verlauf ist gegebenenfalls die wiederholte Gabe im Abstand von drei bis vier Wochen erforderlich. Die Dosis kann dann dem individuellen Therapieerfolg angepasst werden.

Myasthenia gravis

Bei der Myasthenia gravis handelt es sich um einen Prototyp der Autoimmunerkrankungen mit einem bekannten Antigen (Acetylcholinrezeptor) und krankheitsverursachenden IgG-Antikörpern, die im Serum der betroffenen Patienten nachgewiesen werden können. Klinisch ist das Krankheitsbild durch okuläre Symptome (Doppelbilder, Ptose) und eine belastungsabhängige, meist proximal betonte Muskelschwäche charakterisiert.

Die Therapie erfolgt meist durch Thymektomie und Cholinesterasehemmer. Ergänzend kommen Corticosteroide, Azathioprin und Cyclosporin zum Einsatz. Der Wert der IVIG zur Behandlung der Myasthenia gravis ist umstritten. Zahlreiche offene Studien berichten von einem Ansprechen auf IVIG bei bis zu 78% der Patienten (13). In einer großen offenen randomisierten Studie von Gajdos et al. (14, n = 87) zeigten IVIG zur Behandlung einer akuten Exazerbation eine gleich gute Wirksamkeit wie die Plasmapherese.

Für das Kindes- und Jugendalter liegt eine Fallserie mit 10 Patienten mit Mysthenia gravis vor, die nicht ausreichend auf Cholinesterasehemmer ansprachen (15). Acht Patienten zeigten eine klinische Verbesserung, wobei der Akuteffekt deutlicher war als der Erhaltungseffekt. Interessant ist auch die Beobachtung, dass drei Patienten in dieser Studie kurz nach Therapiebeginn von der Beatmung entwöhnt werden konnten. Die Autoren ziehen daraus den Schluss, dass IVIG effektiv zur Kurzzeittherapie der Myasthenia gravis, bei myasthenen Krisen oder zur Vorbereitung von Patienten für Operationen eingesetzt werden können. Der Nutzen für die Langzeittherapie scheint jedoch eingeschränkt zu sein.

Dermatomyositis

Die Dermatomyositis ist eine erworbene Myopathie mit proximal betonter Muskelschwäche und einer Hautbeteiligung (z.B. Gesichtserythem, Teleangiektasien, Hyperkeratosen am Nagelfalz). Histologisch ist sie durch eine Entzündungsreaktion mit Kapillardestruktion und Schädigung der parafaszikulären Muskelfasern gekennzeichnet. Initial zeigen die Patienten oft ein gutes Ansprechen auf eine Steroidtherapie. Für sekundäre Therapieversager werden auch Azathioprin, Methotrexat oder Cyclosporin A eingesetzt.

Für das Erwachsenenalter liegt bisher eine placebo-kontrollierte Studie zum Wirksamkeitsnachweis der IVIG bei der therapierefraktären Dermatomyositis vor (16). Bei 15 Patienten konnte in einem cross-over design ein signifikanter Effekt im Hinblick auf die Verbesserung der Muskelkraft nachgewiesen werden. Der klinische Erfolg zeigte sich etwa zwei Wochen nach Therapiebeginn. Wiederholte Muskelbiopsien bestätigten den klinischen Effekt im Sinne einer Zunahme der Muskelfaserdurchmesser, einer Revaskularisierung und einer Abnahme der Entzündungsreaktion. Für das Kindes- und Jugendalter liegen nur unkontrollierte Berichte zum Einsatz von IVIG bei der Dermatomyositis vor. Die größte Serie von 18 Patienten mit steroid-refraktärer Dermatomyositis wurde von Al-Mayouf et al. publiziert (17). In der retrospektiven Analyse zeigten 12 Patienten (66%) eine klinische Verbesserung mit der Möglichkeit einer Steroidreduktion um mehr als 50% für mindestens drei Monate. Bei den übrigen 6 Patienten konnte dieses Therapieziel durch die IVIG nicht erreicht werden.

Da die Dermatomyositis in der Regel gut auf eine Steroidtherapie anspricht, ist eine IVIG-Therapie vor allem bei den Patienten in Erwägung zu ziehen, deren Krankheitsaktivität mit einer Kombination von Steroiden mit Methotrexat oder Azathioprin nicht ausreichend zu kontrollieren ist.

Literatur

1. Hartung HP, Pollard JD, Harvey GK, Toyka KV (1995) Immunopathogenesis and treatment of the Guillain-Barré syndrome – part II. Muscle Nerve 18:154–164.
2. van der Meche FGA, Schmitz PIM, and the Dutch Guillain-Barré Study Group (1992) A randomized trial comparing intravenous immune globulin and plasma exchange in Guillain-Barré syndrome. N Engl J Med 326:1123–1129.

3. Plasma Exchange/Sandoglobulin Guillain-Barré Syndrome Trial Group (1997) Randomized trial of plasma exchange, intravenous immunoglobulin, and plasma exchange followed by intravenous immunoglobulin in Guillain-Barré syndrome. Lancet 349:225–230.
4. Chun MR, Graf WD (1992) Comparison of plasmapheresis and intravenous immunoglobulin in the treatment of childhood Guillain-Barré syndrome. Ann Neurol 32:440.
5. Gürses N, Uysal S, Cetinkaya F, Islek I, Kalayci AG (1995) Intravenous immunoglobulin treatment in children with Guillain-Barré syndrome. Scand J Infect Dis 27:241–243.
6. Vajsar J, Sloane A, Wood E, Gordon Murphy E (1994) Plasmapheresis vs intravenous immunoglobulin treatment in childhood Guillain-Barré syndrome. Arch Paediatr Adolesc Med 148:1210–1212.
7. Wang CH, Trifiletti R, Gold AP, DeVivo DC (1992) Plasma exchange versus intravenous immunoglobulin as treatment for childhood-onset Guillain-Barré syndrome. Ann Neurol 32:440.
8. Kanra G, Uzon A, Vajsar J, Castagna L, Secmeer G, Topaloglu H (1997) Intravenous immunoglobulin treatment in children with Guillain-Barré syndrome. Eur J Pediatr Neurol 1:7–12.
9. Simmons Z, Albers JW, Bromberg MB, Feldman EL (1995) Long-term follow-up of patients with chronic imflammatory demyelinating polyradiculoneuropathy, without and with monoclonal gammopathy. Brain 118:359–368.
10. Korinthenberg R (1999) Chronic inflammatory demyelinating polyradiculoneuropathy in children and their response to treatment. Neuropediatrics 30:190–196.
11. Hahn AF, Bolton CF, Zochodne D et al (1996) Intravenous immunoglobulin treatment in chronic inflammatory demyelinating polyneuropathy – a double-blind, placebo-controlled, cross-over study. Brain 119:1067–1077.
12. Hughes R, Bensa S, Willison H, Van den Bergh P, Comi G, Illa I, Nobile-Orazio E, van Doorn P, Dalakas M, Bojar M, Swan A. (2001) Randomized controlled trial of intravenous immunoglobulin versus oral prednisolone in chronic inflammatory demyelinating polyradiculoneuropathy. Ann Neurol 50:195–201.
13. Dalakas MC (1997) Experience with IVIg in the treatment of patients with myasthenia gravis. Neurology 48 (suppl):64–69.
14. Gajdos PH, Chevret S, Clair B, Tranchant C, Chastang C (1997) Clinical trial of plasma exchange and high-dose intravenous immunoglobulin in myasthenia gravis. Ann Neurol 41:789–796.
15. Selcen D, Dabrowski ER, Michon AM, Nigro MA (2000) High-dose intravenous immunoglobulin therapy in juvenile myasthenia gravis. Pediatr Neurol 22:40–43.
16. Dalakas MC, Illa I, Dambrosia JM, Soueidan SA,STein DP, Otero C, Dinsmore ST, McCrosky S (1993) A controlled trial of high-dose intravenous immunoglobulin infusions as treatment for dermatomyositis. N Engl J Med 329:1993–2000.
17. Al-Mayouf SM, Laxer RM, Schneider R, Silverman ED, Feldman BM (2000) Intravenous immunoglobulin therapy for juvenile dermatomyositis: efficacy and safety. J Rheumatol 27:2498–503.

Immunglobuline bei Erkrankungen des zentralen Nervensystems

D. Pohl, F. Hanefeld

Zusammenfassung

Immunglobuline werden in der Therapie einer Vielzahl großteils entzündlicher oder autoimmunologischer neurologischer Erkrankungen des ZNS eingesetzt. Wenngleich für einige wenige Indikationen ein positiver Therapieeffekt in Doppelblindstudien gezeigt werden konnte, so für die Multiple Sklerose, das PANDAS- und das Stiff-Person-Syndrom, steht für die meisten ZNS-Erkrankungen ein wissenschaftlich fundierter Beleg für die Wirksamkeit einer Immunglobulin-Behandlung noch aus. Dies gilt unter anderem für die Epilepsie, die Rasmussen-Enzephalitis, die akute disseminierte Enzephalomyelitis, das Opsoklonus-Myoklonus-Syndrom und die Vaskulitiden mit ZNS-Beteiligung. Aufgrund widersprüchlicher bzw. großteils negativer Studienergebnisse äußerst zweifelhaft erscheint ein Einsatz von Immunglobulinen bei Autismus, Adrenoleukodystrophie und Chronic Fatigue Syndrom. Trotz der potentiell vielfältigen Einsatzmöglichkeiten ist somit eine Immunglobulin-Therapie bei Erkrankungen des zentralen Nervensystems in den meisten Fällen keine Evidenz-basierte Medizin und daher auch nicht zuletzt angesichts der hohen Kosten, die insbesondere bei einer immunmodulatorischen Dauertherapie entstehen können, zum jetzigen Zeitpunkt eher kritisch zu beurteilen.

Abkürzungen

ADEM	akute disseminierte Enzephalomyelitis
ALD	Adrenoleukodystrophie
Ig	Immunglobuline
IVIG	intravenöse Immunglobuline
MS	Multiple Sklerose
PANDAS	pediatric autoimmune neuropsychiatric disorders associated with streptococcal infections

Einleitung

Seit den 70er Jahren des vergangenen Jahrhunderts stehen Immunglobulinpräparate für den klinischen Einsatz zur Verfügung. Ursprünglich für die Therapie von Immundefizienzen vorgesehen, wiesen bald Zufallsbeobachtungen auf einen breiteren Indikationsbereich hin, der insbesondere autoimmunologische Erkrankungen einschließt. Darüber hinaus wurden Immunglobuline schon früh auch zur Behandlung von Erkrankungen des zentralen Nervensystems ohne gesicherte autoimmunologisch-entzündliche Pathomechanismen eingesetzt, hier insbesondere zur Behandlung therapierefraktärer Epilepsien. Trotz dieser teilweise bereits über zwei Jahrzehnte umfassenden Therapieerfahrungen fehlen valide, wissenschaftlich glaubwürdige Studien zur Anwendung von Immunglobulinen bei ZNS-Erkrankungen. In Abhängigkeit von der Evidenz vorliegender Publikationen ist die folgende Übersicht der Anwendungsmöglichkeiten von Immunglobulinen in mögliche, unsichere und zweifelhafte Indikationen gegliedert.

Mögliche Indikationen (Wirksamkeitsnachweis durch Doppelblindstudie)

Lediglich für drei ZNS-Erkrankungen liegen durch Doppelblindstudien gesicherte Ergebnisse zur Immunglobulintherapie vor, für die Multiple Sklerose (MS), das PANDAS-Syndrom (pediatric autoimmune neuropsychiatric disorders associated with streptococcal infections) und das Stiff-Person-Syndrom.

Multiple Sklerose

Bei der MS-charakteristischen Myelin-Destruktion sind neben T-Zell vermittelten Prozessen auch Antikörper-vermittelte autoimmunologische Vorgänge von Bedeutung (1). Ein positiver Effekt einer Therapie mit Immunglobulinen erscheint somit denkbar. Tatsächlich konnte in drei Doppelblindstudien unabhängig voneinander gezeigt werden, dass Immunglobuline in der Therapie der schubförmig-remittierenden MS ähnlich wirksam scheinen wie die zugelassenen immunmodulatorischen Therapien mit Beta-Interferonen oder Glatirameracetat: Immunglobuline führen bei der MS zu einer Reduktion der Schubrate um 27–47% (2–4). In allen 3 Studien zeigte sich auch ein signifikant höherer Prozentsatz schubfreier Patienten als in den Plazebogruppen. Bezüglich eines Effektes auf die Behinderungsprogression ließ sich eine signifikant positive Wirkung lediglich in Studie von Fazekas finden (2). Dies verwundert allerdings angesichts der zumeist langsamen Behinderungsprogression und der relativ kleinen Fallzahl bzw. der zusätzlich kurzen Studiendauer von maximal 2 Jahren nicht. Eine systematische Erfassung der cerebralen Kernspintomografie wurde nur in der Studie von Sörensen durchgeführt, hier fanden sich unter Immunglobulinbehandlung jeweils signifikant weniger Kontrastmittel-anreichernde Läsionen als in der Plazebo-Gruppe (4).

Bemerkenswert erscheint bei aller Ähnlichkeit der Ergebnisse der drei Studien, dass sich die verabreichten IVIG-Dosierungen um eine Zehnerpotenz unterschieden: In den Studien von Achiron und Fazekas wurden etwa 0,2 g/kg/Monat verwendet (2, 3), während in der Sörensen-Studie 2 g/kg/Monat gegeben wurden (4). Wenngleich sich die Sörensen-Studie insbesondere aufgrund des anderen Designs (Crossover) nicht direkt mit den Ergebnissen der anderen beiden Studien vergleichen lässt, sticht doch die deutlich höhere Rate unerwünschter Wirkungen, die in dieser Studie mit über 50% mindestens zehnmal höher ist als in den beiden Niedrigdosis-Studien, ins Auge. Für eine langjährige immunmodulatorische Therapie erscheint somit die für andere Indikationen durchaus etablierte IVIG-Dosis von 2 g/kg eher nicht geeignet, allenfalls vielleicht im Rahmen einer kurzen Induktionsbehandlung bei niedriger dosierter Erhaltungstherapie.

Trotz der sicherlich überzeugenden Studienergebnisse, die auf eine zumindest gleichwertige therapeutische Potenz der Immunglobuline im Vergleich zu den Beta-Interferonen und dem Glatirameracetat hindeuten, sind die Immunglobuline noch nicht für die Behandlung der MS zugelassen. In Einzelfällen von den Kassen genehmigte Indikationen sind die Behandlung von MS-kranken Frauen während der Schwangerschaft und Stillzeit, denn wenngleich es bisher zu keinen berichteten Schädigungen durch Beta-Interferon oder Glatirameracetat in der Schwangerschaft gekommen ist, dürfen diese Substanzen während der Schwangerschaft nicht eingesetzt werden. Eine zumindest denkbare Indikation für einen Therapieversuch mit Immunglobulinen bei der MS-Behandlung ist eine Therapieresistenz gegenüber Beta-Interferon und Glatirameracetat oder eine Unverträglichkeit dieser Substanzen bei einzelnen Patienten.

Für die Behandlung der MS im Kindes- und Jugendalter erscheint eine Therapie mit Beta-Interferonen oder Glatirameracetat, auch wenn diese Substanzen nur für Erwachsene zugelassen sind, angesichts der insgesamt guten Verträglichkeit durchaus möglich (5,6). Dennoch gibt es, wenn auch für andere Indikationen, insgesamt mehr Erfahrungen mit dem Einsatz von Immunglobulinen in dieser Altersgruppe, so dass insbesondere bei sehr jungen Kindern ein Einsatz von Immunglobulinen zur Behandlung der MS eine sinnvolle therapeutische Alternative darstellt.

PANDAS

Das eingängige Akronym PANDAS steht für »pediatric autoimmune neuropsychiatric disorders associated with streptococcal infections«. 1998 wurde erstmals eine Gruppe von Kindern mit Tic- und Zwangsstörungen, die eine auffällige Assoziation ihrer Symptome mit Streptokokken-Infektionen zeigten, unter der Diagnose PANDAS beschrieben (7). Für das PANDAS-Syndrom gelten folgende diagnostische Kriterien: Neben dem Vorliegen einer Tic- oder Zwangsstörung mit Manifestation vor der Pubertät muss ein schubförmiger Verlauf der Erkrankung bzw. ein abrupter Beginn der Symptomatik erkennbar sein. Beginn oder Exazerbationen der Symptomatik müssen im Abstand von weniger als 6 Wochen zu einer vorangegangenen Streptokokken-Infektion (durch Rachenabstrich oder Titeranstieg gesichert) auftreten. Des Weiteren müssen die Kinder neben den psychischen Auffälligkeiten auch assoziierte neurologische Symptome zeigen, typischerweise in Form einer Bewegungsstörung mit hyperaktiven und teilweise choreatiformen Bewegungsmustern.

Es wird angenommen, dass es sich bei PANDAS um eine postinfektiös-autoimmunologische Symptomatik handelt, die vielleicht eine forme fruste oder atypische Ausprägung einer Chorea Sydenham darstellen könnte. Aufbauend auf der Hypothese, dass es sich bei PANDAS um eine Autoimmunerkrankung handelt, wurde an einer Gruppe von 30 Kindern mit PANDAS-Symptomatik in einer Doppelblindstudie die Wirksamkeit von Immunglobulinen versus Plazebo untersucht (8). Es zeigten sich signifikant positive Behandlungseffekte der Immunglobuline im Hinblick auf die Zwangssymptomatik, das Ausmaß der globalen Beeinträchtigung, der psychosozialen Fähigkeiten, der Angst, der Depressivität und der emotionalen Labilität. Beeindruckenderweise war dieser positive Therapieeffekt auch noch nach einem Jahr erkennbar, wobei nur 2 der 9 Kinder einen zweiten IVIG-Behandlungspuls erhalten hatten.

Es bleibt zu bedenken, dass es sich vermutlich nur um eine sehr kleine Untergruppe aller Kinder mit Tic- und Zwangsstörungen handeln dürfte. So wurden die 30 Studien-Kinder innerhalb von 4 Jahren aus allen Teilen der USA rekrutiert. Auch bezüglich des langfristig erscheinenden Therapieeffektes gibt es noch Unklarheiten, da für die 1-Jahres-Daten keine Plazebo-Gruppe existiert (die Studienblindung war nach einem Monat aufgehoben worden und alle Patienten hatten eine Behandlung erhalten). Es bleibt somit zweifelhaft, ob es sich bei PANDAS nicht um eine ohnehin gutartige, auch spontan rückläufige Symptomatik handeln könnte. Zur Zeit werden zwei weitere Studien zur PANDAS-Therapie durchgeführt, deren Ergebnisse sicherlich abgewartet werden sollten.

Stiff-Person-Syndrom

Beim Stiff-Person-Syndrom handelt es sich um eine ZNS-Erkrankung unklarer Genese, bei der es zu einer progredienten Versteifung von Rumpf- und proximaler Extremitätenmuskulatur kommt. Des Weiteren werden schmerzhafte Muskelspasmen beobachtet, die insbesondere nach exogenen Reizen auftreten. Die Krankheit kann zu ausgeprägter Behinderung bis hin zu totaler Pflegebedürftigkeit führen. Der konventionelle Therapieansatz mit Diazepam zeigt häufig nur einen unzureichenden Effekt, wobei die benötigten Dosierungen (bis zu 60 mg/d) sehr oft zu intolerablen Nebenwirkungen führen. Stiff-Person-Patienten zeigen einige immunologische Auffälligkeiten, so finden sich häufig assoziiert andere Autoimmunerkrankungen oder subklinisch erhöhte Auto-Antikörper-Titer (9). Charakteristisch für die Erkrankung scheint der Nachweis des Glutamat-Decarboxylase-Antikörpers GAD65 zu sein (10). GAD65 wird intrathekal produziert und inhibiert die Aktivität und Synthese des inhibitorischen Neurotransmitters GABA. Bei Stiff-Person-Patienten werden erniedrigte GABA-Liquorspiegel gefunden, so dass die muskulären Dauerkontraktionen Folge eines immunmediierten Mangels an zentraler GABA-Inhibition sein könnten (11). Es handelt sich beim Stiff-Person-Syndrom also um eine wahrscheinlich Autoantikörper vermittelte Erkrankung, bei der eine Wirksamkeit von Immunglobulinen prinzipiell denkbar erscheint.

In einer randomisierten, doppelblinden Crossover-Studie wurde der Therapieeffekt einer jeweils dreimonatigen IVIG-Behandlung von Stiff-Person-Patienten untersucht (12). In der Verum-Gruppe fand sich eine signifikante Besserung des sogenannten »stiffness-scores«, die zwischen 6 Monaten und einem Jahr anhielt. Beim Stiff-Person-Syndrom erscheint somit, insbesondere vor dem Hintergrund der möglichen massiven Beeinträchtigung durch die Erkrankung und die beschränkten konventionellen therapeutischen Möglichkeiten, ein Therapieversuch mit Immunglobulinen gerechtfertigt.

Unsichere Indikationen (Wirksamkeitshinweis durch offene Studien/Fallberichte)

Schwierig und potentiell anfechtbar ist die Beurteilung der Therapieindikation für die Gruppe der therapierefraktären Epilepsien sowie für eine heterogene Krankheitsgruppe entzündlich-autoimmunologischer ZNS-Erkrankungen, für die noch keine validen Studien zur Immunglobulintherapie vorliegen und somit auf offene Studien oder schlimmstenfalls wenige Einzelfallberichte zurückgegriffen werden muss.

Therapierefraktäre Epilepsien

Die Immunglobulin-Behandlung therapierefraktärer Epilepsien geht auf eine Zufallsbeobachtung aus dem Jahr 1977 zurück: Pechadre hatte zur Behandlung einer saisonalen Allergie Immunglobuline (i.m.) eingesetzt und bei dem Kind eine deutliche Besserung seines Anfallsleidens bemerkt. Er führte daraufhin eine offene Studie mit 10 Kindern mit schwerer Epilepsie durch, und 8 dieser 10 Kinder zeigten eine Besserung ihrer Anfallssituation und ihres EEG (13).

Es folgten zahlreiche Einzelfallberichte und kleinere offene Studien. In einer 1996 erschienenen Übersichtsarbeit von Duse wurden 30 bis dahin erschienene Publikationen zur Immunglobulinbehandlung von Epilepsien analysiert (14). Bemerkenswerterweise fand sich bei 179 der insgesamt 383 mit Immunglobulinen behandelten Kinder, das heißt bei 47%, eine Verbesserung der Anfallssituation.

Wenngleich die publizierten Fallberichte eine Wirksamkeit der Immunglobulinbehandlung bei therapierefraktären Epilepsien nahe legen, ließ sich in der einzigen Doppelblindstudie zur Immunglobulinbehandlung von Epilepsien kein signifikant positiver Effekt für die Gesamtgruppe zeigen, lediglich für eine Untergruppe von Patienten mit Partialepilepsie (15). Einschränkend muss jedoch gesagt werden, dass in dieser Studie ein etwas ungewöhnliches Therapieschema mit 4 Infusionen in der ersten Woche und jeweils einer Infusion in der 2., 3., und 6. Woche angewendet wurde (drei Dosisgruppen: 100, 250 und 400 mg/kg).

Sicherlich ist bei der Immunglobulin-Behandlung von Epilepsien noch nicht von einem gesicherten Therapieeffekt auszugehen, solange es keine erfolgreichen Doppelblindstudien insbesondere auch zur Anwendung bei Landau-Kleffner-, Lennox-Gastaut- und West-Syndrom gibt. In Einzelfällen scheinen Therapieerfolge möglich zu sein, wobei der Wirkmechanismus noch völlig unklar ist.

Rasmussen-Enzephalitis

Die Rasmussen Enzephalitis ist eine seltene, zumeist im Kindesalter beginnende unilaterale chronisch progrediente Enzephalitis unklarer Genese, die charakteristischerweise zu therapieresistenten fokalen cerebralen Krampfanfällen und einer Hemiparese führt. Als Hinweis auf eine autoimmunologische Genese finden sich bei der Rasmussen-Enzephalitis Glutamat-Rezeptor-Antikörper im Serum (16). Therapeutisch ist die ultima ratio bei therapieresistentem Anfallsleiden und bereits manifester Hemiparese die Hemisphärektomie. Auf der Suche nach neuen, schonenderen Therapieansätzen, wurden aufbauend auf der Autoimmunhypothese der Pathogenese einige Patienten mit Immunglobulinen behandelt.

Es gibt bisher drei kleinere Fallsammlungen mit insgesamt 15 behandelten Patienten: In der ersten offenen Studie wurden Patienten mit Rasmussen-Enzephalitis und therapieresistentem Anfallsleiden mit i.v. Immunglobulinen oder Steroiden behandelt (17). Es zeigte sich ein positiver Therapieeffekt bei 8 von 9 mit IVIG behandelten Patienten und bei 10 von 17 mit Steroiden behandelten Patienten. In einer zweiten Veröffentlichung wird von zwei erwachsenen Patienten mit Rasmussen-Enzephalitis berichtet, die sich unter einer initialen Steroid-Therapie verschlechtert, unter Immunglobulinbehandlung jedoch anhaltend verbessert haben (18). In einer kleinen Fallsammlung von 4 Kindern mit Rasmussen-Enzephalitis wurde jedoch nur in einem Fall eine deutliche Verbesserung unter Immunglobulin-Behandlung beobachtet (19). Des Weiteren findet sich noch ein Einzelfallbericht über ein 14-jähriges Mädchen mit Rasmussen-Enzephalitis, die unter regelmäßigen IVIG-Pulsen eine Befundstabilisierung zeigte (20).

Zusammengefasst lässt sich aus diesen 16 Fällen sicherlich noch keine Evidenz-basierte Medizin ableiten, dennoch erscheint bei einem so therapieschwierigen Krankheitsbild wie der Rasmussen-Enzephalitis in Einzelfällen, insbesondere bei Nicht-Ansprechen auf Steroide und bei noch nicht bestehender Indikation zur Hemisphärektomie, ein Therapieversuch mit Immunglobulinen durchaus zu rechtfertigen.

Akute disseminierte Enzephalomyelitis (ADEM)

Die ADEM ist eine häufig postinfektiös auftretende akute, disseminierte Leukenzephalopathie mit oft enzephalitischem Krankheitsbild und ausgedehnten, häufig die Periventrikulärregion relativ aussparenden MRT-Veränderungen der weißen Substanz. Als Standard-Therapie kommen zumeist Steroide zum Einsatz, jedoch gibt es auch Berichte über die Anwendung von Immunglobulinen.

Insgesamt wurden bisher 19 Immunglobulin-behandelte Patienten mit ADEM publiziert, zumeist als Einzelfallberichte. Die größte Gruppe von 4 Patienten stammt von Pradhan, der bei allen Patienten eine Verschlechterung unter Methylprednisolon-Therapie und eine deutliche Verbesserung unter IVIG-Behandlung gesehen hat (21). Bei allen anderen publizierten Immunglobulinbehandelten Patienten ist es ebenfalls sehr früh, das heißt bereits am 2.–5. IVIG-Behandlungstag, zu einer Befundbesserung gekommen, auch wenn, wie bei 11 dieser 16 Patienten, eine vorangegangene Steroid-Therapie erfolglos gewesen war (22–33).

Eine denkbare Indikation für die Immunglobulin-Therapie bei ADEM ist somit eine Therapieresistenz gegenüber Steroiden. Eine Primärbehandlung mit Immunglobulinen kann aber auch dann sinnvoll erscheinen, wenn in der Frühphase der Erkrankung noch diagnostische Unsicherheiten bestehen und insbesondere eine erregerbedingte Enzephalitis differentialdiagnostisch zu erwägen ist.

Opsoklonus-Myoklonus

Das Opsoklonus-Myoklonus Syndrom tritt bei Kindern zumeist idiopathisch (postinfektiös?) auf. Des Weiteren kommt es auch beim Neuroblastom zum paraneoplastischen Auftreten von Opsoklonus-Myoklonus, hierbei kann diese Symptomatik der Neuroblastom-Manifestation um Monate vorausgehen. Beim Opsoklonus-Myoklonus treten unkontrollierte, schnelle, chaotische Augenbewegungen, auch umschrieben als »dancing eyes«, auf. Beim Vollbild der Erkrankung sind auch arrhythmische, aktionsverstärkte Polymyokloni und eine rumpfbetonte Ataxie sowie Dysarthrie zu beobachten. Immunologisch finden sich bei Opsoklonus-Myoklonus Patienten Purkinje-Zell-Antikörper im Serum (34), so dass für die Erkrankung eine Autoimmungenese angenommen wird.

Über die Anwendung von Immunglobulinen bei pädiatrischem Opsoklonus-Myoklonus gibt es eine Fallsammlungen von 5 Patienten, die nach Immunglobulin-Behandlung eine deutliche Besserung von Sprache, Grob- und Feinmotorik zeigten (35). Des Weiteren finden sich noch 7 Einzelfallberichte mit unterschiedlichen Ergebnissen – in drei Fällen kam es nach Immunglobulin-Behandlung zu einer Restitutio ad integrum (36–38), in einem dieser drei Fälle jedoch erst nach 12 Therapiezyklen (38). Bei zwei anderen Fällen war der Therapieerfolg weniger eindeutig, wobei nur die Kombination mit Dexamethason zu einer Restitutio (39) bzw. mit ACTH zu einer Besserung (40) führten. Zwei Publikationen berichten von einem Therapieversagen der Immunglobulinbehandlung bei jeweils einem 21 und einem 22 Monate alten Mädchen mit postinfektiösem Opsoklonus-Myoklonus (41, 42).

Zusammenfassend bleibt zu sagen, dass Immunglobuline beim Opsoklonus-Myoklonus-Syndrom in Einzelfällen eine sinnvolle Ergänzung zur besser etablierten und kostengünstigeren Steroid-Therapie darstellen können, insbesondere dann, wenn Steroide nicht zum gewünschten Therapieerfolg führen.

Vaskulitiden mit ZNS-Beteiligung

Zur Behandlung von ZNS-Vaskulitiden mit Immunglobulinen gibt es nur sehr wenige publizierte Erfahrungen. Es finden sich vier Veröffentlichungen mit insgesamt 5 Patienten: Zwei Mädchen mit einem systemischen Lupus erythematosus und akuter Parkinson-Symptomatik zeigten unter Methylprednisolon- und Cyclophosphamid-Therapie keine Besserung, unter Immunglobulin-Behandlung aber eine Restitutio ad integrum (43). Bei einer 28-jährigen Lupus-Patientin mit akuter Lupus-Enzephalitis wurden aufgrund der differentialdiagnostischen Möglichkeit einer ZNS-Infektion primär Immunglobuline eingesetzt, und auch hier zeigte sich unter IVIG-Therapie eine rasche Befundbesserung und eine neurologische Restitutio innerhalb von 5 Tagen (44). Eine Patientin mit einer Wegener-Granulomatose und einer akuten ZNS-Symptomatik mit starken Kopfschmerzen und rezidivierenden cerebralen Krampfanfällen zeigte kein Ansprechen auf eine Methylprednisolon- und Cyclophosphamid-Therapie. Erst unter einer Immunglobulin-Behandlung kam es zu neurologischer Beschwerdefreiheit (45). Schließlich wird noch von einer 59-jährigen Patientin mit Sjögren-Syndrom und ZNS-Vaskulitis berichtet, die nach IVIG-Behandlung mehrerer Schübe ihrer ZNS-Symptomatik jeweils rasche und komplette Remissionen zeigte (46).

Aufgrund der nur sehr beschränkten Erfahrungen mit Immunglobulinen bei ZNS-Vaskulitiden ist es sicherlich nicht möglich, eine allgemeine Therapieempfehlung auszusprechen. Bei Therapieresistenz gegenüber Steroiden und Cyclophosphamid sollte jedoch in Einzelfällen ein Therapieversuch mit Immunglobulinen in Betracht gezogen werden.

Zweifelhafte Indikationen (widersprüchliche, großteils negative Publikationen)

Wenngleich für diese Gruppe von Erkrankungen auch Berichte positiver Effekte einer Immunglobulin-Therapie vorliegen, überwiegen Studien mit negativen Ergebnissen, so dass eine Wirksamkeit der IVIG-Therapie bei den folgenden Diagnosen sehr fragwürdig erscheint.

Autismus

Aufbauend auf einigen immunologischen Auffälligkeiten autistischer Kinder (47) wurden offene Studien zur Immunglobulin-Behandlung von Kindern mit Autismus durchgeführt. Hierbei zeigte die erste Studie die eindrücklichsten Ergebnisse mit einer deutlichen Besserung bei 5 der 10 IVIG-behandelten Kinder (48). In einer zweiten Studie mit ebenfalls 10 Kindern zeigte nur noch ein Kind eine deutliche Besserung unter Immunglobulinen (49), in der dritten Studie ließ sich für die Gesamtgruppe kein signifikanter Therapieeffekt nachweisen (50). Zusammenfassend gibt es somit zum jetzigen Zeitpunkt sicherlich keine ausreichenden Hinweise auf eine Wirksamkeit von Immunglobulinen bei der Behandlung von Autismus.

Chronic Fatigue Syndrom

Bei 4 Doppelblindstudien zur Behandlung des Chronic Fatigue Syndroms mit Immunglobulinen (51–54) zeigte sich lediglich in der erste Studie ein Therapieerfolg (51), so dass eine IVIG-Behandlung dieser Erkrankung nicht gerechtfertigt erscheint.

Adrenoleukodystrophie (ALD)

Angeregt durch einen positiven Einzelfallbericht, in welchem es unter Immunglobulinbehandlung zu einer Befundstabilisierung bei einem ALD-kranken Jungen gekommen war (55), untersuchten Cappa et al. die Wirksamkeit von IVIG versus Plazebo bei insgesamt 12 ALD-Patienten (56). Nach einem Behandlungszeitraum von einem Jahr fand sich bezüglich der Krankheitsprogression kein signifikanter Unterschied zwischen der Verum- und der Plazebogruppe. Eine Indikation für eine IVIG-Therapie der ALD lässt sich somit nicht ableiten.

Zusammenfassung

Im Gegensatz zur Immunglobulin-Anwendung bei einigen Erkrankungen des peripheren Nervensystems gibt für Erkrankungen des zentralen Nervensystems noch keine gesicherten, zugelassenen Indikationen für Immunglobuline als Therapeutikum der ersten Wahl. Allerdings gibt es drei Diagnosen, für die die

Wirksamkeit einer Immunglobulin-Behandlung in Doppelblindstudien gezeigt werden konnte: Die Multiple Sklerose, das PANDAS-Syndrom und das Stiff-Person-Syndrom. Aufgrund positiver Erfahrungen in offenen Studien oder Fallberichten ist im Einzelfall auch ein Einsatz von Immunglobulinen bei folgenden Krankheitsbildern zu erwägen: Bei therapieschwierigen Epilepsien, bei der Rasmussen-Enzephalitis, bei der akuten disseminierten Enzephalomyelitis, dem Opsoklonus-Myoklonus Syndrom sowie bei ZNS-Vaskulitiden. Keine Indikation besteht nach jetzigem Wissensstand für die Behandlung des Autismus, des Chronic Fatigue Syndroms und der Adrenoleukodystrophie.

In zukünftigen Studien bleiben noch viele offene Fragen zu klären. Selbst bei den klassischen Autoimmunerkrankungen ist der Wirkmechanismus von Immunglobulinen noch nicht geklärt, erst recht nicht bei Krankheiten wie der Epilepsie. Für sehr wenige Indikationen gibt es gute Dosisfindungsstudien, so dass teilweise, wie bei der Immunglobulinbehandlung der MS, bis zu 10-fach unterschiedliche Dosierungen gegeben werden. Unabhängig von der Gesamtdosis ist auch noch unklar, ob es Unterschiede zwischen verschiedenen Applikationsschemata gibt, und fraglich ist auch, in welchem Abstand ein Immunglobulin-Puls bei einer chronischen Erkrankung wiederholt werden sollte. Ganz wesentlich ist natürlich auch die Frage nach der Dauer der Therapie, insbesondere angesichts der zumeist hohen Kosten. Bei manchen Erkrankungen scheint ein einzelner Behandlungspuls ausreichend, so z.B. beim PANDAS-Syndrom, bei anderen wie der MS handelt es sich nach jetzigem Wissensstand um eine Dauertherapie. Die wichtigste Frage bleibt jedoch diejenige nach der prinzipiellen Wirksamkeit von Immunglobulinen für die verschiedenen Indikationen, zu deren Klärung dringend weitere Studien erforderlich erscheinen.

Literatur

1. Archelos JJ, Storch MK, Hartung H-P (2000) The role of B cells and autoantibodies in multiple sclerosis. Ann Neurol 47:694–706
2. Fazekas F, Deisenhammer F, Strasser-Fuchs S, Nahler G, Mamoli B (1997) Randomised placebo-controlled trial of monthly intravenous immunoglobulin therapy in relapsing-remitting multiple sclerosis. Lancet 349:589–593
3. Achiron A, Gabbay U, Gilad R et al (1998) Intravenous immunoglobulin treatment in multiple sclerosis. Neurology 50:398–402
4. Sorensen PS, Wanscher B, Jensen CV et al (1998) Intravenous immunoglobulin G reduces MRI activity in relapsing multiple sclerosis. Neurology 50:1273–1281
5. Adams AB, Tyor WR, Holden KR (1999) Interferon beta-1b and childhood multiple sclerosis. Pediatr Neurol 21:481–483
6. Mikaeloff Y, Moreau T, Debouverie M et al (2001) Interferon-beta treatment in patients with childhood-onset multiple sclerosis. J Pediatr 193:443–446
7. Swedo SE, Leonard HL, Garvey M et al (1998) Pediatric autoimmune neuropsychiatric disorders associated with streptococcal infections: Clinical description of the first 50 cases. Am J Psychiatry 155:264–271
8. Perlmutter SJ, Leitman SF, Garvey MA et al (1999) Therapeutic plasma exchange and intravenous immunoglobulin for obsessive-compulsive disorder and tic disorders in childhood. Lancet 354:1153–1158

9. Dalakas MC, Fujii M, Li M, McElroy B (2000) The clinical spectrum of anti-GAD antibody-positive patients with stiff-person syndrome. Neurology 55:1531–1535
10. Ellis TM, Atkinson MA (1996) The clinical significance of an autoimmune response against glutamic acid decarboxylase. Nat Med 2:148–153
11. Dalakas MC, Li M, Fujii M, Jocobowitz DM (2001) Stiff person syndrome: quantification, specificity and intrathecal synthesis of GAD65 antibodies. Neurology 57:780–784
12. Dalakas MC, Fujii M, Li M et al (2001) High-dose intravenous immune globulin for stiff person syndrome. N Engl J Med 345:1870–1876
13. Pechadre JC, Sauvezie B, Osier C, Gibert J (1977) Traitement des encéphalopathies épileptiques de l'enfant par les gamma-globulines. Rev EEG Neurophysiol 7 :443–447
14. Duse M, Notarangelo LD, Tiberi S et al (1996) Intravenous immune globulin in the treatment of intractable childhood epilepsy. Clin Exp Immunol 104:71–76
15. Van Rijckevorsel-Harmant K, Delire M, Schmitz-Moorman W, Wieser HG (1994) Treatment of refractory epilepsy with intravenous immunoglobulins. Results of the first double-blind/dose finding clinical study. Int J Clin Lab Res 24:162–166
16. Rogers SW, Andrews PI, Gahring LC et al (1994) Autoantibodies to glutamate receptor GluR3 in Rasmussen's encephalitis. Science 265:648–651
17. Hart YM, Cortez M, Andermann F et al (1994) Medical treatment of Rasmussen's syndrome (chronic encephalitis and epilepsy): Effect of high-dose steroids or immunoglobulins in 19 patients. Neurology 44:1030–1036
18. Leach JP, Chadwick DW, Miles JB, Hart IK (1999) Improvement in adult-onset Rasmussen's encephalitis with long-term immunomodulatory therapy. Neurology 52:738–742
19. Topcu M, Turanli G, Aynaci FM et al (1999) Rasmussen encephalitis in childhood. Child's Nerv Syst 15:395–403
20. Wise MS, Rutledge SL, Kuzniecky RI (1996) Rasmussen syndrome and long-term response to gamma globulin. Pediatr Neurol 14:149–152
21. Pradhan S, Gupta RP, Shashank S, Pandey N (1999) Intravenous immunoglobulin therapy in acute disseminated encephalomyelitis. J Neurol Sci 165:56–61
22. Kleiman M, Brunquell P (1995) Acute disseminated encephalomyelits: response to intravenous immunoglobulin. J Child Neurol 10:481–483
23. Hahn JS, Siegler DJ, Enzmann D (1996) Intravenous gammaglobulin therapy in recurrent acute disseminated encephalomyelitis. Neurology 46 :1173–1174
24. Finsterer J, Grass R, Stöllberger C, Mamoli B (1998) Immunoglobulins in acute, parainfectious disseminated encephalomyelitis. Clin Neuropharmacol 21:258–261
25. Spieker S, Petersen D, Rolfs A et al (1998) Acute disseminated encephalomyelitis following Pontiac fever. Eur Neurol 40:169–172
26. Assa A, Watemberg N, Bujanover Y, Lerman-Sagie T (1999) Demyelinative brainstem encephalitis responsive to intravenous immunoglobulin therapy. Pediatrics 104:301–304
27. Nishikava M, Ichiyama T, Hayashi T, Ouchi K, Furukawa S (1999) Intravenous immunoglobulin therapy in acute disseminated encephalomyelitis. Pediatr Neurol 21:583–586
28. Revel-Vilk S, Hurvitz H, Klar A, Virozov Y, Korn-Lubetzki I (2000) Recurrent acute disseminated encephalomyelitis associated with acute Cytomegalovirus and Epstein-Barr virus infection. J Child Neurol 15:421–424
29. Sahlas DJ, Miller SP, Guerin M, Veilleux M Francis G (2000) Treatment of acute disseminated encephalomyelitis with intravenous immunoglobulin. Neurology 54:1370–1372
30. Andersen JB, Rasmussen LH, Herning M, Paerregaard A (2001) Dramatic improvement of severe acute disseminated encephalomyelitis after treatment with intravenous immunoglobulin in a three-year-old boy. Dev Med Child Neurol 43:136–140
31. Jaing T-H, Lin K-L, Chiu C-H, Lo W-C, Wu P-L (2001) Acute disseminated encephalomyelitis in autoimmune hemolytic anemia. Pediatr Neurol 24:303–305
32. Pittock SJ, Keir G, Alexander M, Brennan P, Hardiman O (2001) Rapid clinical and CSF response to intravenous gamma globulin in acute disseminated encephalomyelitis. Eur J Neurol 8:725–731
33. Riedel K, Kempf VAJ, Bechtold A, Klimmer M (2001) Acute disseminated encephalomyelitis (ADEM) due to Mycoplasma pneumoniae infection in an adolescent. Infection 29:240–242

34. Conolly AM, Pestronk A, Mehta S, Pranzatelli MR, Noetzel MJ (1997) Serum autoantibodies in childhood opsoclonus-myoclonus syndrome: An analysis of antigenic targets in neural tissues. J Pediatr 130:878–884
35. Mitchell WG, Davalos-Gonzalez BA, Brumm VL et al (2002) Opsoclonus-ataxia caused by childhood neuroblastoma: Developmental and neurological sequelae. Pediatrics 109:86–98
36. Sugie H, Sugie Y, Akimoto H, Endo K, Shirai M, Ito M (1992) High-dose iv human immunoglobulin in a case with infantile opsoclonus polymyoclonia syndrome. Acta Paediatr 81:371–372
37. Fisher PG, Wechsler DS, Singer HS (1994) Anti-Hu antibody in a neuroblastoma-associated paraneoplastic syndrome. Pediatr Neurol 10:309–312
38. Petruzzi MJ, De Alarcon PA (1995) Neuroblastoma-associated opsoclonus-myoclonus treated with intravenously administered immune globulin G. J Pediatr 127:328–329
39. Veneselli E, Conte M, Biancheri R, Acquaviva A, De Bernardi B (1998) Effect of steroid and high-dose immunoglobulin therapy on opsoclonus-myoclonus syndrome occuring in neuroblastoma. Med Pediatr Oncol 30:15–17
40. Borgna-Pignatti C, Balter R, Marradi P, Colamaria V (1996) Treatment with intravenously administered immunoglobulins of the neuroblastoma-associated opsoclonus-myoclonus. J Pediatr 129:179–180
41. Penzien JM, Speck S, Vassella F (1993) Opsoclonus polymyoclonia syndrome. Acta Paediatr 82:319–320
42. Yiu VWY, Kovithavongs T, McGonigle LF, Ferreira P (2001) Plasmapheresis as an effective treatment for opsoclonus-myoclonus syndrome. Pediatr Neurol 24:72–74
43. Kwong KL, Chu R, Wong SN (2000) Parkinsonism as unusual neurological complication in childhood systemic lupus erythematosus. Lupus 9:474–477
44. Sherer Y, Levy Y, Langevitz P, Lorber M, Fabrizzi F, Shoenfeld Y (1999) Successful treatment of systemic lupus erythematosus cerebritis with intravenous immunoglobulin. Clin Rheumatol 18:170–173
45. Taylor CT, Buring SM, Taylor KH (1999) Treatment of Wegener's granulomatosis with immune globulin: CNS involvement in an adolescent female. Ann Pharmacother 33:1055–1059
46. Canhao H, Fonseca JE, Rosa A (2000) Intravenous gammaglobulin in the treatment of central nervous system vasculitis associated with Sjögren's syndrome. J Rheumatol 27:1102–1103
47. Gupta S (2000) Immunological treatments for autism. J Autism Dev Disord 30:475–479
48. Gupta S, Aggarwal S, Heads C (1996) Brief report: Dysregulated immune system in children with autism: Beneficial effects of intravenous immune globulin on autistic characteristics. J Autism Dev Disord 26:439–452
49. Plioplys AV (1998) Intravenous immunoglobulin treatment of children with autism. J Child Neurol 13:79–82
50. DelGiudice-Asch G, Simon L, Schmeidler J, Cunningham-Rundles C, Hollander E (1999) Brief report: A pilot open clinical trial of intravenous immunoglobulin in childhood autism. J Autism Dev Disord 29:157–160
51. Lloyd A, Hickie I, Wakefield D, Boughton C, Dwyer J (1990) A double-blind, placebo-controlled trial of intravenous immunoglobulin therapy in patients with chronic fatigue syndrome. Am J Med 89:561–568
52. Peterson PK, Shepard J, Macres M et al (1990) A controlled trial of intravenous immunoglobulin G in chronic fatigue syndrome. Am J Med 89:554–560
53. Rowe KS (1997) Double-blind randomized controlled trial to asssess the efficacy of intravenous gammaglobulin for the management of chronic fatigue syndrome in adolescents. J Psychiatr Res 31:133–147
54. Vollmer-Conna U, Hickie I, Hadzi-Pavlovic D et al (1997) Intravenous immunoglobulin is ineffective in the treatment of patients with chronic fatigue syndrome. Am J Med 103:38–43
55. Miike T, Taku K, Tamura T et al (1989) Clinical improvement of adrenoleukodystrophy following intravenous gammaglobulin therapy. Brain Dev 11:134–137
56. Cappa M, Bertini E, Del Balzo P, Cambiaso P, Di Biase A, Salvati S (1994) High dose immunoglobulin IV treatment in adrenoleukodystrophy. J Neurol Neurosurg Psychiatr 57(S):69–70

10. Stoffwechselleiden und Genetik

Rett Syndrom bei Jungen: Göttinger Erfahrungen

P. Huppke, F. Hanefeld, F. Laccone

Einleitung

Lange Zeit galt das Rett Syndrom als eine Erkrankung, die ausschließlich bei Mädchen auftritt. Bis zur Beschreibung der ersten Gendefekte im *MECP2* Gen 1999, wurden nur wenige Jungen mit einem dem Rett Syndrom ähnlichen Krankheitsbild beschrieben (1). Es wurde vermutet, dass der Gendefekt bei Jungen letal ist, sie also schon im Mutterleib sterben. Eine Untersuchung von Trappe et al. zeigte jedoch, dass die defekten Allele fast ausschließlich vom Vater stammen (2). Da die Erkrankung X chromosomal ist, sind fast nur Mädchen betroffen. Inzwischen gibt es auch einige Beschreibungen von Jungen mit Rett Syndrom (Tab.1). Diese scheinen sich in 3 verschiedene Gruppen aufzuteilen:

1. Jungen mit schwerer epileptischer Enzephalopathie. Sie tragen Mutationen, die bei Frauen zum klassischen Rett Syndrom führen.
2. Jungen mit klassischem Rett Syndrom. Sie tragen ebenfalls Mutationen, die bei Frauen zum klassischen Rett Syndrom führen, haben jedoch zusätzlich ein Mosaik oder ein Klinefeltersyndrom.
3. Jungen mit mentaler Retardierung und unterschiedlichen neurologischen Störungen. Bei diesen finden sich Mutationen, die bisher bei Mädchen mit klassischem Rett Syndrom nicht gefunden wurden.

Fragestellung und Methoden

Ziel der Untersuchung war es, herauszufinden ob Mutationen im MECP2 Gen eine häufige Ursache von neurologischen Störungen bei Jungen sind.

30 Jungen wurden ausgewählt. Diese zeigten Symptome des Rett Syndroms oder Symptome, wie sie bei anderen Jungen mit Mutationen im *MECP2* Gen beschrieben wurden. Die gesamte kodierende Sequenz sowie die Exon-Intron-Übergänge wurden sequenziert.

Ergebnisse und Diskussion

Bei zwei Jungen konnten Veränderungen im *MECP2* Gen nachgewiesen werden. Der eine Junge wurde vorgestellt mit schwerer epileptischer Encephalopathie, sekundärer Mikrocephalie und periodischer Atmung. Die Symptome ähneln denen eines Jungen, der 1998 von Schanen und Francke beschrieben wurde (3). Der bei ihm nachgewiesene c.1282G->A Austausch führt zu einer

Tab. 1: Beschriebene Phänotypen bei Jungen mit MECP2 Mutationen

1. Jungen mit schwerer epileptischer Enzephalopathie

- Villard et al. (5) beschreiben 2 Brüder mit schwerer neonataler Enzephalopathie und Apnoen, die im ersten Lebensjahr verstarben. Die Schwester leidet am Rett Syndrom.
  Mutation: T158M
- Wan et al. (6) beschreiben einen Jungen mit schwerer neonataler Enzephalopathie, der früh verstarb. Seine Schwester leidet an einem Rett Syndrom.
  Mutation: 806delG

2. Jungen mit klassischem Rett Syndrom

- Hoffbuhr et al. (7) beschreiben einen Jungen mit Klinefeltersyndrom und klassischem Rett Syndrom.
  Mutation: T158M
- Clayton-Smith et al. (8) beschreiben einen Jungen mit Rett Syndrom.
  Mutation: Somatische Mutation (Mosaik) 241–242del
- Topcu et al. et al. (9) beschreiben einen Jungen mit Rett Syndrom.
  Mutation: Somatische Mutation (Mosaik) R270X
- Schwarzman et al. (10) beschreiben einen Jungen mit Klinefeltersyndrom und klassischem Rett Syndrom.
  Mutation: Y141K
- Monros et al. (11) beschreiben einen Jungen mit klassischem Rett Syndrom
  Mutation: R133H

3. Jungen mit mentaler Retardierung und unterschiedlichen neurologischen Symptomen

- Orrico et al. (12) beschreiben 4 Brüder mit schwerer mentaler Retardierung, Sprachstörungen und Ruhetremor
  Mutation: A140V
- Klauck et al. (13) beschreiben eine Familie mit 6 betroffenen männlichen Mitgliedern mit mentaler Retardierung, Psychose (manisch-depressiv), Pyramidenbahnläsionen und Makroorchie.
  Mutation: A140V
- Cohen et al. (14) beschreiben einen Jungen mit Sprachentwicklungsverzögerung und Schizophrenie.
  Mutation: A140V
- Imesseaoudene et al. (4) beschreiben einen Jungen mit mentaler Retardierung und Verhaltensauffälligkeiten.
  MutationG428S
- Meloni et al. (15) beschreiben eine Familie mit zwei männlichen Mitgliedern mit mentaler Retardierung, Paraplegie, bilateralen Katarakten und Epilepsie
  Mutation: E406V
- Yntema et al. (16) beschreiben eine Familie mit 3 männlichen Mitgliedern mit unspezifischer mentaler Retardierung.
  Mutation: 1161-1400del
- Couvert et al. (17) beschreiben eine Familie mit 9 betroffenen Mitgliedern mit mentaler Retardierung und Sprachstörungen.
  Mutation: E137G
- In einer weiteren Familie beschreiben sie 4 männliche Mitglieder mit mentaler Retardierung, Ruhetremor und Adipositas.
  Mutation: R167W
- Watson et al. (18) beschreiben einen Jungen mit mentaler Retardierung, Ataxie und Epilepsie
  Mutation: 241-242del

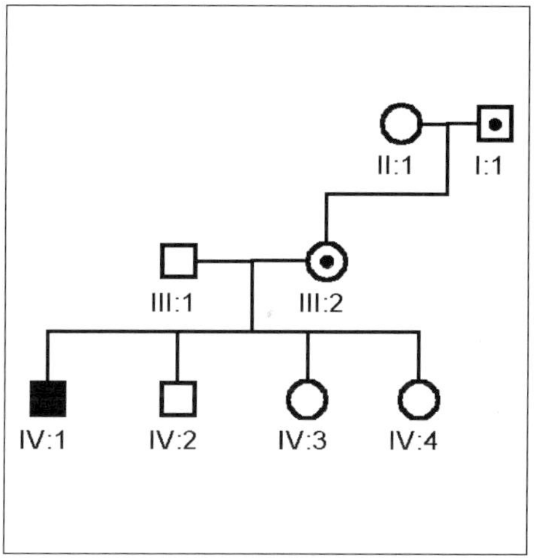

Abb. 1

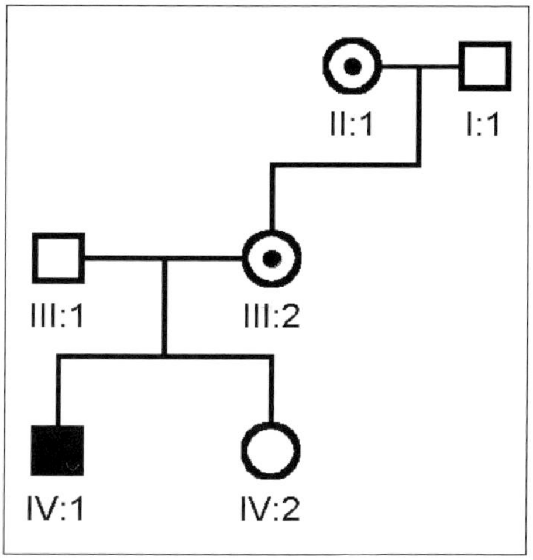

Abb. 2

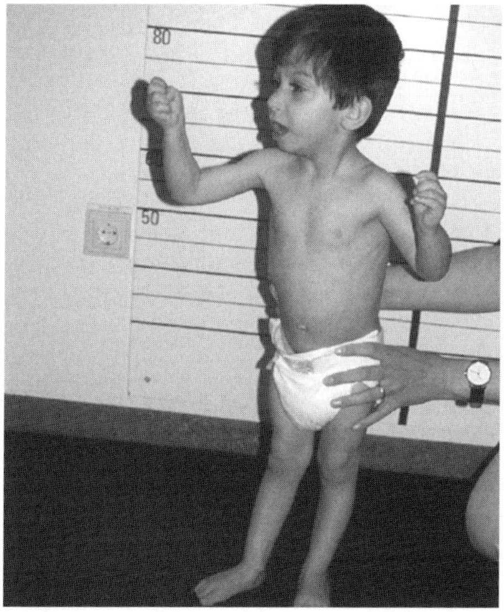

Abb. 3

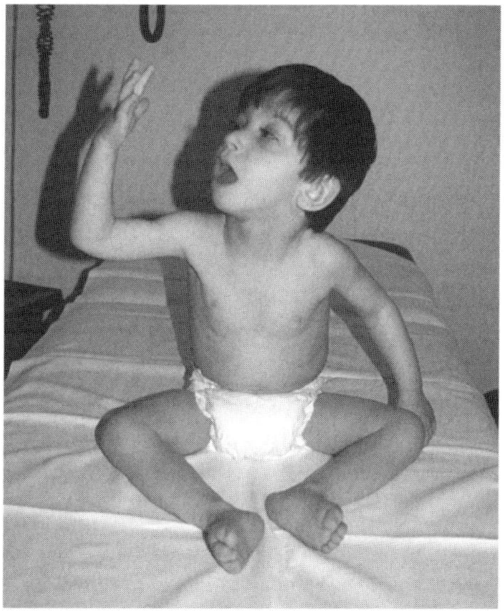

Abb. 4

Substitution des Glycin 428 durch Serin. Imessaoudene et al. beschreiben diese Mutation bei einem Jungen mit primärer globaler Entwicklungsverzögerung (4). Die Untersuchung der Familie unseres Patienten zeigte, dass auch die Mutter und der Großvater Träger dieser Genveränderung sind (Abb. 1). Da wir den Basenaustausch bei einem gesunden Mann, dem Großvater, nachweisen konnten, handelt es sich wahrscheinlich um einen Polymorphismus, der nicht für die Erkrankung ursächlich ist. Bei dem zweiten Jungen, bei dem wir eine Veränderung im *MECP2* Gen nachweisen konnten, bestand eine globale Entwicklungsverzögerung, eine Mikrozephalie und Handstereotypien (Abb. 3, 4). Die Genanalyse ergab einen c.1030C->T Austausch, der zu einer Substitution von

Arginin 344 durch Cystin führt. Die gleiche Veränderung war auch bei seiner Mutter und seiner Großmutter nachweisbar (Abb. 2). Da dieser Aminosäureaustausch bisher noch nicht beschrieben wurde, bleibt unklar, ob er für seine Erkrankung ursächlich ist. Fazit: Veränderungen im *MECP2* Gen sind auch bei Jungen nicht selten. Eine Vielzahl unterschiedlicher Phänotypen wurden dabei beschrieben. Bisher ist es jedoch häufig nicht möglich, zwischen Polymorphismen und Mutationen zu unterscheiden. Besonders wichtig ist daher die Untersuchung weiterer Familienmitglieder.

Literatur

1. Christen HJ, Hanefeld F. Male Rett variant. Neuropediatrics 1995;26(2):81–2.
2. Trappe R, Laccone F, Cobilanschi J, Meins M, Huppke P, Hanefeld F, et al. MECP2 mutations in sporadic cases of Rett syndrome are almost exclusively of paternal origin. Am J Hum Genet 2001;68(5):1093–101.
3. Schanen C, Francke U. A severely affected male born into a Rett syndrome kindred supports X-linked inheritance and allows extension of the exclusion map. Am J Hum Genet 1998;63(1):267–9.
4. Imessaoudene B, Bonnefont JP, Royer G, Cormier-Daire V, Lyonnet S, Lyon G, et al. MECP2 mutation in non-fatal, non-progressive encephalopathy in a male. J Med Genet 2001;38(3):171–4.
5. Villard L, Kpebe A, Cardoso C, Chelly PJ, Tardieu PM, Fontes M. Two affected boys in a Rett syndrome family: clinical and molecular findings. Neurology 2000;55(8):1188–93.
6. Wan M, Lee SS, Zhang X, Houwink-Manville I, Song HR, Amir RE, et al. Rett syndrome and beyond: recurrent spontaneous and familial MECP2 mutations at CpG hotspots. Am J Hum Genet 1999;65(6):1520–9.
7. Hoffbuhr K, Devaney JM, LaFleur B, Sirianni N, Scacheri C, Giron J, et al. MeCP2 mutations in children with and without the phenotype of Rett syndrome. Neurology 2001;56(11):1486–95.
8. Clayton-Smith J, Watson P, Ramsden S, Black GC. Somatic mutation in MECP2 as a non-fatal neurodevelopmental disorder in males. Lancet 2000;356(9232):830–2.
9. Topcu M, Akyerli C, Sayi A, Toruner GA, Kocoglu SR, Cimbis M, et al. Somatic mosaicism for a MECP2 mutation associated with classic Rett syndrome in a boy. Eur J Hum Genet 2002;10(1):77–81.
10. Schwartzman JS, Bernardino A, Nishimura A, Gomes RR, Zatz M. Rett syndrome in a boy with a 47,XXY karyotype confirmed by a rare mutation in the MECP2 gene. Neuropediatrics 2001;32(3):162–4.
11. Monros E, Armstrong J, Aibar E, Poo P, Canos I, Pineda M. Rett syndrome in Spain: mutation analysis and clinical correlations. Brain Dev 2001;23 Suppl 1:S251–3.
12. Orrico A, Lam C, Galli L, Dotti MT, Hayek G, Tong SF, et al. MECP2 mutation in male patients with non-specific X-linked mental retardation. FEBS Lett 2000;481(3):285–8.
13. Klauck SM, Lindsay S, Beyer KS, Splitt M, Burn J, Poustka A. A Mutation Hot Spot for Nonspecific X-Linked Mental Retardation in the MECP2 Gene Causes the PPM-X Syndrome. Am J Hum Genet 2002;70(4):1034–7.
14. Cohen D, Lazar G, Couvert P, Desportes V, Lippe D, Mazet P, et al. MECP2 mutation in a boy with language disorder and schizophrenia. Am J Psychiatry 2002;159(1):148–9.
15. Meloni I, Bruttini M, Longo I, Mari F, Rizzolio F, D'Adamo P, et al. A mutation in the rett syndrome gene, MECP2, causes X-linked mental retardation and progressive spasticity in males. Am J Hum Genet 2000;67(4):982–5.
16. Yntema HG, Oudakker AR, Kleefstra T, Hamel BC, van Bokhoven H, Chelly J, et al. In-frame deletion in MECP2 causes mild nonspecific mental retardation. Am J Med Genet 2002;107(1):81–3.
17. Couvert P, Bienvenu T, Aquaviva C, Poirier K, Moraine C, Gendrot C, et al. MECP2 is highly mutated in X-linked mental retardation. Hum Mol Genet 2001;10(9):941–6.

Neurotransmitterbefunde: Einige Tücken bei der Interpretation

B. Assmann, C. Bräutigam, G.F. Hoffmann

Zusammenfassung

Anhand von authentischen Fallbeispielen soll demonstriert werden, dass die Interpretation der Messergebnisse von Metaboliten des Neurotransmitterstoffwechsels – hier der biogenen Amine Serotonin und Dopamin – nicht einfach durch den Vergleich der gefundenen Werte mit den altersentsprechenden Referenzwerten erfolgen kann. Es sind Kenntnisse der Pathophysiologie der jeweiligen Transmittersysteme sowie gute Informationen über die Symptomatik des Patienten erforderlich. In manchen Fällen ist auch unter optimalen Bedingungen eine eindeutige Zuordnung nicht möglich. Hier sind Nachpunktionen einige Monate später oder nach Überwindung einer akuten Enzephalopathie oft hilfreich.

Einleitung

Aufschlüsse über Vorgänge und Störungen im Gehirn sind bei lebenden Patienten nur über indirekte Wege zu erhalten. Neben großen Fortschritten in der bildgebenden Diagnostik des Gehirns einschließlich funktioneller Aspekte sowie elektrophysiologischen Techniken, haben auch erhebliche Verbesserungen der biochemisch-analytischen Möglichkeiten im Liquor cerebrospinalis das »Fenster zum Gehirn« in den letzten 3 Jahrzehnten etwas geöffnet. Hieraus entstand neben der Möglichkeit auch eine Verpflichtung, behandelbare Erkrankungen frühzeitig zu diagnostizieren. Insbesondere Biosynthesestörungen des Dopamins lassen sich meist gut medikamentös behandeln oder zeigen zumindest einen positiven Effekt auf spezifische Therapie. Eine Übersicht über Pathophysiologie, Leitsymptome und diagnostische Strategien findet sich z.B. in Hoffmann et al. (3) sowie in der »Aktuellen Neuropädiatrie 2001« (4).

Die Probleme bei der Erstellung von altersentsprechenden Referenzwerten aus Liquor cerebrospinalis von Kindern sollen hier nicht im Einzelnen erörtert werden. Die sorgfältige Ermittlung an ausreichend großen Kollektiven und Beachtung der Altersabhängigkeit sind Voraussetzung für die Interpretation. In einem Ringversuch zwischen 11 Laboren zur Ermittlung der Vergleichbarkeit von Neurotransmitterbestimmungen zeigte sich, dass Richtigkeit und Präzision der Analysen überwiegend sehr gut waren (1). Die angegebenen Referenzbereiche waren jedoch unterschiedlich (1). In allen Labors werden unterschiedlich definierte Altergruppen zusammengestellt, deren Messwerte jeweils gesondert statistisch ausgewertet werden, um die Grenzen des Referenzbereiches zu definieren.

Zur Frage, inwieweit die Analyse von lumbal gewonnenem Liquor Rückschlüsse über Vorgänge im Gehirn und insbesondere in den Basalganglien erlaubt, wurden seit den frühen 1970iger Jahren Untersuchungen an Tieren und Menschen publiziert (6, 2). Eine ausführliche Diskussion mit entsprechenden Literaturzitaten findet sich in dem Buch »Cerebrospinal Fluid in Neurology and Psychiatry« (5), insbesondere Kapitel 2 und 3. Die Problematik des kraniocaudalen Gradienten der Metabolitkonzentrationen ist in den jeweiligen Originalpublikationen über Referenzwerte der verschiedenen Metabolite im Kindesalter sowie ebenfalls im Kapitel »Störungen der Neurotransmission« der »Aktuellen Neuropädiatrie 2001« (4) dargestellt. Aufgrund des kraniocaudalen Gradienten, der sich in unterschiedlicher Ausprägung für die verschiedenen Metabolite nachweisen lässt, sollten die Liquorproben zur Analyse der Neurotransmitter nach den Angaben des untersuchenden Labors in numerierten Röhrchen abgenommen werden. Zur Stabilisierung der Pterine ist das Auffangen des Liquors in speziell präparierten und lichtgeschützten Röhrchen erforderlich. Grundsätzlich soll der Liquor immer direkt am Patientenbett tiefgefroren werden (flüssiger Stickstoff oder Trockeneis). Unterschiedlich starkes Pressen beim Weinen sollte keine relevanten Verfälschungen verursachen, da mit dem Mandrin der Liquorfluss etwas gebremst werden kann.

Bei den folgenden Falldarstellungen sollen die beiden stabilen Endprodukte von Serotonin → 5- Hydroxyindolessigsäure, abgekürzt HIAA und von Dopamin → Homovanillinsäure, abgekürzt HVA, in den Mittelpunkt gestellt werden. Zur Biosynthese der beiden obengenannten biogenen Amine ist auch Tetrahydrobiopterin, abgekürzt BH_4, als Kofaktor erforderlich (3,4), dessen eigene Synthese und Recycling in unseren Routinemessungen mit einigen Metaboliten ebenfalls untersucht wird. Zur Orientierung seien hier die in verschiedenen Altersgruppen erhobenen Referenzwerte für HIAA und HVA tabellarisch dargestellt, die in unserem Zentrum ermittelt wurden (1) und zur Beurteilung der Patientenbefunde dienen (Tab. 1). Durch die getrennte statistische Auswertung der Altersgruppen entstehen im flacheren Bereich der Mittelwertkurve »Stufen« bei den Grenzwerten. Dies entspricht wahrscheinlich nicht genau den tatsächlichen biologischen Verhältnissen (die nur angenähert werden können), ist jedoch für die Interpretation der Befunde nicht ausschlaggebend, da neben klinischen Gesichtspunkten insbesondere auch der Quotient zwischen HVA und HIAA berücksichtigt wird. Beide Metabolite zeigen eine stabile Korrelation über den kraniokaudalen Gradienten hinweg und erlauben so eine Aussage über das Gleichgewicht zwischen dopaminergem und serotoninergem System. Nach der Konvention wird die HVA Konzentration in nmol/l im Zähler durch die HIAA Konzentration im Nenner geteilt, da hierbei im Normalfall Werte über 1 entstehen (siehe Tab. 1).

Falldarstellungen

Bei den im Folgenden skizzierten Fällen beschränken wir uns auf die Aspekte, die unmittelbar mit der Neurotransmitterdiagnostik und ihrer Interpretation

Tab. 1: Referenzwerte für HIAA, HVA und den Quotienten HVA/HIAA (1)

Alter [Jahre]	HIAA [nmol/l]	HVA [nmol/l]	HVA/HIAA
< 0.3	302 – 952	484 – 1446	1.0 – 2.6
0.3 – ≤ 0.7	159 – 528	427 – 989	1.2 – 2.9
0.7– ≤ 1	170 – 412	403 – 919	1.8 – 3.0
1– ≤ 2	155 – 359	364 – 870	1.6 – 3.9
2 – ≤ 5	130 – 362	313 – 824	1.5 – 4.1
5 – ≤ 8	87 – 247	240 – 713	1.8 – 4.1
8 – ≤ 12	101 – 237	285 – 560	1.7 – 3.7
12 – ≤ 15	82 – 203	217 – 507	1.5 – 3.9
> 15	51 – 204	115 – 455	1.1 – 3.7

bzw. der aus diesem Fall ableitbaren »Lehre« in Zusammenhang stehen. Familienanamnese, weitere Untersuchungsergebnisse, Therapien usw. werden demzufolge nur teilweise dargestellt.

Fall 1

Anamnese:

26 Monate altes Mädchen mit ausgeprägter hypoton-dystoner Bewegungsstörung. Die mentale Beeinträchtigung schien geringer zu sein.

Neurotransmitterbefunde:

HIAA *301* nmol/l (Referenzbereich *130–362* nmol/l, vgl. Tab. 1), HVA *319* nmol/l (Referenzbereich *313–824* nmol/l), Quotient *1.1* (Referenzbereich *1.5–4.1).*

Interpretation/ Diagnose:

Anhand des erniedrigten Quotienten ist eine Beeinträchtigung des dopaminergen Systemes zu erkennen. (Wenn das Kind 3 Monate früher diesbezüglich untersucht worden wäre, hätte es zur Altersgruppe darunter gehört und man hätte wahrscheinlich die HVA unterhalb des angegebenen Referenzwertes (vgl. Tab. 1) gefunden.) In der anschliessenden molekulargenetischen Untersuchung konnte ein *Tyrosinhydroxylasemangel* gefunden werden. Es ist bemerkenswert, dass die HVA Konzentration zumindest in der Nähe des Referenzbereiches lag, während bei diesem Defekt üblicherweise stark reduzierte HVA Konzentrationen gemessen werden.

Fall 2

Anamnese:

27 Monate alter Junge mit Enzephalitisartigem Krankheitsbild. Im Vordergrund standen schwer beherrschbare Krampfanfällen, Koma und Fieber. Computertomographie am 2. Krankheitstag unauffällig. Liquor zur Neurotransmitteranalytik vom 3. Krankheitstag.

Neurotransmitterbefunde:

HIAA *102* nmol/l (Referenzbereich *130–362),* HVA *69* nmol/L (Referenzbereich *310–820).* Quotient HVA/HIAA *0.7* (Referenzbereich *1.5–4.1).*

Interpretation/Diagnose:

Die HIAA Konzentration zeigte eine leicht (bis mässig) ausgeprägte Erniedrigung, während HVA mit 69 nmol/l (313–824) extrem erniedrigt war. Insbesondere der sehr erniedrigte Quotient zeigte einen ausgeprägten intrazerebralen Dopaminmangel an. Von den in unsererem analytischen Programm gemessenen Metaboliten (die Biosynthese und Abbau der biogenen Amine sowie Biosynthese und »Recycling« des Tetrahydrobiopterin erfassen) zeigte sich lediglich Neopterin sehr stark und Dihydrobiopterin deutlich erhöht. Dieses kann durch massive Aktivierung der zellulären Immunabwehr entstehen. Tetrahydrobiopterin lag im Normbereich, so dass ein »Verbrauch« des Kofaktors zur Synthese der biogenen Amine nicht als Erklärung für die erniedrigten Konzentrationen herangezogen werden kann. Insgesamt ist hier von sekundären Veränderungen im Rahmen eines Entzündungsprozesses auszugehen.

Fall 3

Anamnese:

Zwillings-Frühgeborenes der 33. SSW, CTG (Cardiotokogramm) pathologisch, postnatal ausgeprägte Multiorgansymptomatik bzw. Multiorganversagen, Hirnstammsymptome, Überstreckung mit schraubenden Bewegungen, MRT (Magnetresonanztomographie) des Gehirns normal.

Neurotransmitterbefunde:

HIAA *192* nmol/l (Referenzbereich ≥ *300–950),* HVA *29* nmol/l (Referenzbereich ≥ *480–1450),* Quotient HVA/HIAA *0.1* (Referenzbereich *1.0–2.6*).

Interpretation/Diagnose:

Zusätzlich war Neopterin deutlich erhöht, jedoch nicht so stark wie bei Fall 2, Dihydrobiopterin und Tetrahydrobiopterin waren normal. Hier ist möglicherweise eine Hypoxie Ursache der Neopterinerhöhung (Hypoxie verursacht u.a. akute Freisetzung von immunmodulatorischen Substanzen, nekrotisches Gewebe wird später von Makrophagen beseitigt). Das Spektrum der von uns gemessenen Metabolite zeigte in Abwesenheit einer Hyperphenylalaninämie keinen Hinweis auf eine monogene Störung im Soffwechsel der Pterine oder der biogenen Amine, so dass die exzessive Dopaminverarmung ebenfalls als sekundär interpretiert werden muss.

Im Gegensatz zu den Fällen 2 und 3, die insbesondere eine deutliche, sekundäre Dopaminreduktion zeigen, sollen die nächsten drei Fälle demonstrieren, dass auch sekundär erhöhte Konzentrationen der biogenen Amine gefunden werden können.

Fall 4

Anamnese:

6 Monate altes Mädchen mit progredienter Entwicklungsverzögerung, Hypotonie, Dysmyelinisierung im MRT sowie nahrungsabhängiger Laktatazidose.

Neurotransmitterbefunde:

HIAA *1130* nmol/l (Referenzbereich *159–528),* HVA *2327* nmol/l (Referenzbereich *427–989),* Quotient HVA/ HIAA *2.1* (Referenzbereich *1.3–3.1).*

Interpretation/Diagnose:

Die hier gefundenen, auf jeweils gut das Doppelte der oberen Norm erhöhten Metabolite der biogenen Amine (Vorstufen der biogenen Amine, Pterine und 5-Methyltetrahydrofolat waren normal) sind mit keinem der bekannten monogenen Defekte im Stoffwechsel der biogenen Amine oder der Folsäure zu vereinbaren. In diesem Fall passen die klinischen Befunde auch gut zu einer anderen neurodegenerativen Erkrankung, so dass mit großer Wahrscheinlichkeit von sekundären Veränderungen auszugehen ist.

Fall 5

Anamnese:

17 Monate altes Mädchen mit ursprünglich ausgeprägter muskulärer Hypotonie, dann einschiessendem Opisthotonus und schließlich überwiegend konstantem Opisthotonus, ohne jede psychomotorische Entwicklung. Es bestanden Hinweise darauf, dass der Opisthotonus Ausdruck eines epileptischen Geschehens war.

Neurotransmitterbefunde:

HIAA *603* nmol/l (Referenzbereich *155–359),* HVA *1020* nmol/l (Referenzbereich *364*–870), Quotient HVA/HIAA *1.7* (Referenzbereich *1.6–3.9)*

Interpretation/Diagnose:

Beide biogene Amine sowie alle Pterine (einschließlich Tetrahydrobiopterin) wurden oberhalb des Referenzbereiches gefunden, das gleiche galt in geringerem Ausmaß für die Vorstufen der biogenen Amine. Auch außerhalb der biogenen Amine wurden zahlreiche pathologische Laborbefunde erhoben. Auch in diesem Fall können die Befunde nicht mit einem monogenen Defekt im Stoffwechsel der biogenen Amine oder des Folates erklärt werden. Wahrscheinlich müssen sie entweder als sekundäre Steigerung der Biosynthese – oder mangelnde »Nutzung« der Neurotransmitter bei dysfunktionellen postsynaptischen Rezeptoren (?) im Rahmen einer sehr aktiven Epilepsie interpretiert werden.

Fall 6

Anamnese:

26 Monate altes Kind mit »kongenitalem Fehlbildungssyndrom«, Retardierung, Hypotonie, Myelinisierungsverzögerung.

Neurotransmitterbefunde:

HIAA *710* nmol/l (Referenzbereich *130–362),* HVA *2516* nmol/l (Referenzbereich *313–824),* Quotient HVA/HIAA *3.5* (Referenzbereich *1.5–4.1)*

Interpretation/Diagnose:

Der Serotoninmetabolit HIAA ist auf gut das Doppelte der oberen Norm, der Dopaminmetabolit HVA auf das Dreifache der oberen Norm erhöht, der Quotient liegt noch im Normalbereich. Auch hier muss eher an eine sekundäre Veränderung gedacht werden. Ein Defekt, der diese biochemische Konstellation erklären könnte, ist nicht bekannt.

Fall 7

Anamnese:

7.9 Jahre alter Junge mit dem klinischen Bild einer epileptischen Enzephalopathie, in dessen Verlauf sich eine ursprünglich spastisch-ataktische Bewegungsstörung in einen dominierenden Parkinsonismus verwandelte. Da die Epilepsie nicht auf konventionelle Medikationen ansprach, wurden über einen längeren Zeitraum nur alternative Therapien versucht, dann Topiramat, das ebenso wirkungslos blieb.

Neurotransmitterbefunde:

HIAA *56* nmol/l (Referenzbereich für Kinder *5–8 Jahre 87–247, 8–12 Jahre 101–237* nmol/l), HVA *144* nmol/l (Referenzbereich für Kinder *5–8 Jahre 240–713, 8–12 Jahre 285–560* nmol/l), Quotient HVA/HIAA *2.6* (Referenzbereich für Kinder 5–8 Jahre *1.8–4.1,* 8–12 Jahre *1.7–3.7)*

Interpretation/Diagnose:

Beide biogene Amine waren deutlich erniedrigt ohne Hinweise auf monogene Störungen im Stoffwechsel der biogenen Amine (oder der Folate). Ein Therapieversuch mit L-Dopa/-Carbidopa führte nicht zu einer Besserung, eher zu einer Zunahme der Dystonie im rechten Fuß im dritten Monat nach Therapiebeginn, woraufhin es langsam abgesetzt wurde (maximale Dosis knapp 10 mg/kg/Tag). Eine Therapie der Anfälle mit Phenobarbital wurde dann von den Eltern akzeptiert und führte – zumindest zeitgleich – zu einer deutlichen Besserung von Vigilanz und Bewegungsstörung. Es liegt auch hier die Vermutung nahe, dass die aktive Epilepsie die Biosynthese der biogenen Amine negativ beeinflusst hat. Im Gegensatz zu diesem Patienten ist der Einsatz von L-Dopa/Carbidopa bei manchen anderen Patienten mit ebenfalls höchstwahrscheinlich sekundären Dopaminmangelsituationen hilfreich. Dies sollte an dieser Stelle erwähnt werden.

Fall 8

Anamnese:

Ein Junge mit psychomotorischer Retardierung, BNS Anfällen, Hypotonie mit fraglich dystonen Handbewegungen sowie einer corticalen Dysplasie (MRT-Befund) wurde insgesamt drei Mal lumbal punktiert (LP). Nach der ersten LP im Alter von 10 Monaten wurde aufgrund einer deutlich erniedrigten HVA Konzentration L-Dopa/Carbidopa verordnet. Daraufhin wurde nur eine fragliche Besserung beobachtet. Deswegen erfolgte eine zweite Analyse der Neurotransmittermetabolite. In dieser, unter laufender L-Dopa/Carbidopa Medikation (45 mg/Tag bei uns unbekanntem Gewicht) im Alter von 19 Monaten, fand sich lediglich eine subnormale HVA Konzentration bei ansonsten unauffälligem Profil. Es wurde eine Steigerung der L-Dopa/Carbidopa Dosis empfohlen, die aber keine weitere Besserung der Bewegungsstörung und/oder der Entwicklungsverzögerung zur Folge hatte. Nachdem die molekulargenetische Analyse des Tyrosinhydroxylasegens einen Normalbefund erbracht hatte, wurde die Medikation letztlich im Alter von 33 Monaten abgesetzt und einen Monat später erneut eine Neurotransmitteranalyse durchgeführt. Die Ergebnisse der Lumbalpunktionen (LP) 1 und 3 sind in Tabelle 2 aufgelistet.

Neurotransmitterbefunde:

Tab. 2: Messwerte des Patienten *Fall 8* im Verlauf

LP Alter [Jahre]	**0.8**	**2.8**
HIAA [nmol/l] (Referenzbereich)	**148** (170 – 412)	**176** (130 – 362)
HVA [nmol/l] (Referenzbereich)	**150** (403 – 919)	**517** (313 – 824)
HVA/ HIAA Quotient (Referenzbereich)	**1.0** (1.8 – 3.0)	**2.9** (1.5 – 4.1)

Interpretation/Diagnose:

Die deutliche Beeinträchtigung des dopaminergen Systemes im Säuglingsalter kann hier ebenfalls nicht durch eine monogene Störung im Stoffwechsel der biogenen Amine erklärt werden, wie die Lumbalpunktion im Alter von 2.8 Jahren beweist. Es liegen uns keine genauen Angaben über die Aktivität der BNS Epilepsie zum Zeitpunkt der ersten LP vor, jedoch wurde die LP wahrscheinlich im Rahmen der ätiologischen Abklärung durchgeführt. Somit könnte auch hier die Anfallsaktivität zur Unterdrückung der Dopaminsynthese (in geringem Ausmaß auch der Serotoninsynthese) geführt haben. Auch bei diesem Patienten hat die L-Dopa/Carbidopa Substitution keinen überzeugenden Effekt gezeigt.

Fall 9

Anamnese:

10 Jahre altes Mädchen mit progredienter Demenz, Epilepsie, Dysarthrie, und seit kurzem zunehmenden Dyskinesien. In zwei verschiedenen Kliniken wurden Neurotransmitter im Abstand von ca. 2 Monaten untersucht. Die Ergebnisse sind in Tabelle 3 gelistet.

Neurotransmitterbefunde:

Tab. 3: Messwerte der Patientin *Fall 9* im Verlauf

LP Alter [Jahre]	**10.7**	**10.9**
HIAA [nmol/l] (Referenzbereich)	**99** (101 – 237)	**134** (101 – 237)
HVA [nmol/l] (Referenzbereich)	**187** (285 – 560)	**459** (285 – 560)
HVA/ HIAA Quotient (Referenzbereich)	**1.9** (1.7 – 3.7)	**3.4** (1.7 – 3.7)

Interpretation/Diagnose:

Hier zeigt sich zunächst eine leichte Erniedrigung des Dopaminmetaboliten HVA bei knapp normaler HIAA. Der Quotient liegt allerdings noch im unteren Normbereich. Bei der Nachpunktion konnten trotz klinischer Progredienz Normalwerte mit einem Quotienten eher im oberen Normalbereich gefunden werden. Dieses, sowie die anschließend im Knochenmark nachgewiesenen Speicherzellen zeigt, dass auch hier dem Krankheitsbild nicht eine primäre monogene Störung des Stoffwechsels der biogenen Amine zugrunde lag.

Fall 10

Anamnese:

Ein Säugling, der mit Hypotonie, cerebralen Krampfanfällen und rezidivierenden Pneumonien sowie einer Gedeihstörung auffiel. Im Alter von 11 Monaten war der Tonus an den oberen Extremitäten deutlich erhöht bei weiter fehlender Kopfkontrolle, wobei das Kind nun aufmerksam und interessiert wirkte. Im Weiteren Persistenz der beschriebenen Symptome. Es wurde wiederholt Liquor (von zwei verschiedenen Kliniken) zur Analyse an uns geschickt. Die Ergebnisse sind in Tabelle 4 zusammengefasst.

Neurotransmitterbefunde:

Tab. 4: Messwerte des Patienten *Fall 10* im Verlauf

LP Alter [Jahre]	**0.5**	**1.3**	**1.5**	**3.3**
HIAA [nmol/l] (Referenzbereich)	**331** (159 – 528)	**237** (155 – 359)	**309** (155 – 359)	**238** (130 – 362)
HVA [nmol/l] (Referenzbereich)	**482** (427 – 989)	**373** (364 – 870)	**450** (364 – 870)	**276** (313 – 824)
HVA/ HIAA Quotient (Referenzbereich)	**1.5** (1.2 – 2.9)	**1.6** (1.6 – 3.9)	**1.5** (1.6 – 3.9)	**1.2** (1.5 – .41)

Interpretation/Diagnose:

Nach der zweiten Lumbalpunktion wurde in Anbetracht der Dystonie bei biochemisch grenzwertigen Befunden eine probatorische Therapie mit L-Dopa/Carbidopa angeraten, die nicht umgesetzt wurde (wegen Umzuges der Eltern?). Nach der 4. Untersuchung mit nun biochemisch eindeutiger Dopaminmangelsituation wurde L-Dopa/Carbidopa vorsichtig eindosiert und das Kind zeigte deutliche Entwicklungsfortschritte. Die molekulargenetischen Untersuchungen sind noch nicht abgeschlossen.

Schlussfolgerungen

Die hier gezeigte Auswahl an Patienten verdeutlicht, dass die Interpretation von Neurotransmittermetaboliten in verschiedener Hinsicht komplex ist und auch unter optimalen Bedingungen letztlich nicht immer zu sicheren Diagnosen führt. Neben der *korrekten präanalytischen Behandlung* der Probe (vgl. (4)) ist für die Interpretation der Befunde und die Ableitung von Therapieempfehlungen ein guter Informationsaustausch zwischen den behandelnden und den befundenden Ärztinnen und Ärzten essentiell. Wenn dies nicht zu einer Diagnose führt, sind *Nachpunktionen* sehr hilfreich bzw. notwendig, wie die Fallbeispiele 8–10 zeigen. (In Bezug auf einen Diskussionsbeitrag im Anschluss an den Vortrag sei hier noch einmal klar gestellt, dass hierfür nur Patienten aufgenommen wurden, bei denen keinerlei Hinweise auf präanalytische oder analytische Probleme bestanden).

Auf die Problematik der *Referenzbereiche* wurde in der Einleitung schon hingewiesen. Im Gegensatz zu vielen anderen neurometabolischen Erkrankungen können die Veränderungen der Metabolitenkonzentrationen auch bei nachgewiesenen Defekten nur geringgradig ausgeprägt sein (Fall 1). Einige der Patienten demonstrieren, dass unterschiedliche biologische bzw. pathophysiologische Prozesse zu *sekundären* Veränderungen der messbaren Metabolite führen. Diese sind zu einem bestimmten Zeitpunkt im Einzelnen häufig nicht offensichtlich. Darüberhinaus kann man aus der Erniedrigung von HVA z.B. nicht zuverlässig schließen, dass eine Therapie mit L-Dopa/Carbidopa eine Besserung der Symptomatik zur Folge haben wird. Dies wird durch die Fallbeispiele 7 und 8 verdeutlicht, wobei der Fall 7 den Verdacht stützt, dass eine aktive Epilepsie die Neurotransmitterfunktion über unbekannte Mechanismen beeinflussen kann. Umgekehrt zeigen die Fälle 1 und 10, dass eine doparesponsive Erkrankung nicht immer schnell und einfach zu diagnostizieren sein muss. Bei Fall 10 ist noch nicht gesichert, ob es sich um eine primäre Störung im Stoffwechsel des Dopamins handelt. Manchmal zeigen Patienten eine Besserung unter L-Dopa/Carbidopa, auch wenn es sich mit an Sicherheit grenzender Wahrscheinlichkeit um einen sekundären Dopaminmangel handelt (z.B. pränataler Insult) oder biochemisch ein Dopaminmangel nicht nachweisbar ist (Fälle, die nicht Bestandteil dieser Auswahl sind).

Aus den im letzten Absatz skizzierten Unwägbarkeiten folgt auch, dass eine *Rückmeldung* über den *Verlauf* bei Patienten mit unklaren Diagnosen oder für die Diagnose untypischen Befunden sehr hilfreich für die Einschätzung weiterer Fälle ist. Es ist noch vieles ungeklärt in der cerebralen Informationsverarbeitung und Bewegungssteuerung, so dass die empirische Erfahrung mit Patienten einen extrem hohen Stellenwert sowohl für die effiziente Betreuung weiterer Patienten als auch im Hinblick auf die weitere Erforschung der cerebralen Netzwerke hat. An dieser Stelle sei unseren Einsendern für die erfolgten Informationen und Rückmeldungen herzlich gedankt.

Literatur

1. Bräutigam C (2001) Störungen der Neurotransmission: Standardisierung der Neurotransmitteranalytik zur Diagnostik und Behandlungskontrolle von angeborenen Defekten im Stoffwechselweg der biogenen Amine- biochemische und molekulare Charakterisierung. Dissertation, Fachbereich Pharmazie, Philipps-Universität Marburg
2. Garelis E, Young SN, Lal S, Sourkes TL (1974) Monoamine metabolites in lumbar CSF: the question of their origin in relation to clinical studies. Brain Res 79:1–8
3. Hoffmann GF, Surtees RA, Wevers RA (1998) Cerebrospinal fluid investigations for neurometabolic disorders. Neuropediatrics 29:59–71.
4. Hoffmann GF, Assmann B, Bräutigam C, Wevers RA (2001) Neurotransmitterstörungen: Klinik, Biochemie, Molekularbiologie und therapeutische Ansätze. In: Aksu F (Hrsg.) Aktuelle Neuropädiatrie 2001, Novartis Pharma Verlag 2002 , Nürnberg
5. McConnel H, Bianchine J, (1994) Cerebrospinal fluid dynamics (chapter 2) and CSF as a reflection of cerebral metabolism (chapter 3). In: McConnel H, Bianchine J (Hrsg.) Cerebrospinal fluid in Neurology and Psychiatry, 1st edition, Chapman and Hall Medical, London
6. Moir ATB, Ascroft GW, Crawford TBB, Eccleston D, Guldberg HC (1970) Cerebral metabolites in cerebrospianl fluid as a biochemical approach to the brain. Brain 93: 357–368

Pathogenese der X-chromosomalen Adrenoleukodystrophie: Funktionelle Charakterisierung von Mutationen im *ALD*-Gen

A. Klusmann, T. Dehmel, P. Roehrig, J. Gärtner

Einführung

Peroxisomen kommen in fast allen menschlichen Zellen vor und spielen eine essentielle Rolle in einer Vielzahl von Stoffwechselwegen, insbesondere des Fettstoffwechsels (1). Beispiele sind die β-Oxidation überlangkettiger Fettsäuren, der Abbau von Wasserstoffperoxid und die Cholesterinsynthese. Die X-chromosomale Adrenoleukodystrophie (X-ALD) ist die häufigste erbliche peroxisomale Stoffwechselerkrankung. Unter der männlichen Bevölkerung beträgt die Inzidenz 1:15.000 bis 1:100.000. Das für die Erkrankung verantwortliche *ALD*-Gen liegt auf Chromosom Xq28. Mutationen führen zu einer gestörten β-Oxidation und einer Anhäufung von überlangkettigen Fettsäuren in Körperflüssigkeiten und Geweben (2). Die Pathogenese der X-ALD ist bisher unklar.

Klinischer Phänotyp

Der Phänotyp ist variabel, abhängig von Erkrankungsalter, Organmanifestation und Progress der neurologischen Symptome. Man unterscheidet mindestens sechs verschiedene Phänotypen. Hierzu gehören die schwere zerebrale Adrenoleukodystrophie, die Adrenomyeloneuropathie, die einfache Addison-Variante, die asymptomatische Form des Erwachsenenalters und symptomatische Überträgerinnen. Die typischen klinischen Merkmale sind Wesensveränderungen, Konzentrationsstörungen, Demenz, Sprachstörungen, Seh- und Hörminderung, Parästhesien, Spastik, Blasen-/Mastdarmschwäche und häufig eine Nebenniereninsuffizienz. Ihr Auftreten variiert mit dem klinischen Phänotyp (3).

Biochemischer Phänotyp

Die Diagnose erfolgt über die biochemische Bestimmung der überlangkettigen gesättigten Fettsäuren (VLCFA: »very long chain fatty acids«). Die VLCFA werden normalerweise aus dem Zytosol durch die peroxisomale Membran in die peroxisomale Matrix transportiert und dort über die β-Oxidation metabolisiert (Abb. 1) (4). Aus Hefestudien geht hervor, dass das ALD-Protein eine Rolle im peroxisomalen Transport der VLCFA zu spielen scheint. Die Hydrolyse von ATP zu ADP liefert die Energie dafür. Da bei Patienten mit X-chromosomaler Adrenoleukodystrophie die Transportfunktion des ALD-Proteins und damit

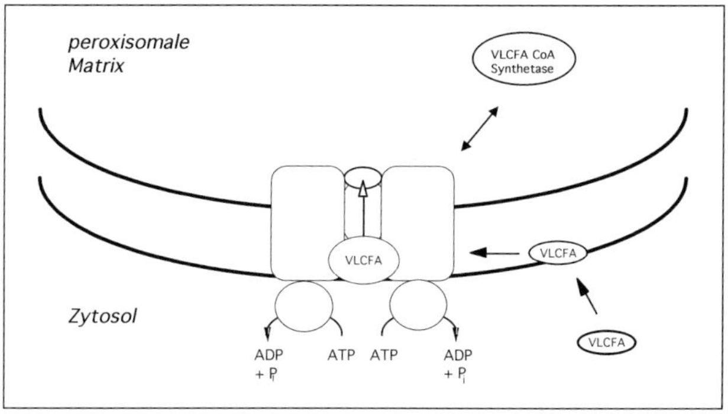

Abb. 1: Hypothetisches Modell zur Funktion des ALD-Proteins. Überlangkettige Fettsäuren werden mit Hilfe des Adrenoleukodystrophieproteins durch die peroxisomale Membran transportiert. Sie können dann durch die in der peroxisomalen Matrix stattfindende β-Oxidation abgebaut werden. VLCFA = very long chain fatty acids.

auch die peroxisomale β-Oxidation gestört ist, kommt es zu einer Anhäufung der überlangkettigen Fettsäuren vor allem in der weißen Substanz des Gehirns und Rückenmarks, in der Nebennierenrinde und den Hoden (5).

ALD-Gen und ALD-Protein

Das für die Erkrankung verantwortliche Gen wurde 1993 von Mosser und Mitarbeitern auf dem langen Arm des X-Chromosoms bei q28 identifiziert (6). Das *ALD*-Gen kodiert ein peroxisomales Membranprotein aus der Familie der ATP-Bindungs- und Transporter-Proteine (ABC-Transporter). Mutationen im *ALD*-Gen sind die primäre Erkrankungsursache der X-ALD. Es wird vermutet, dass diese die Stabilität des ALD-Proteins oder seine Eigenschaft, ATP zu binden und zu hydrolysieren, beeinflussen (6, 7).

In mehr als 250 betroffenen Familien konnte eine Vielzahl von Mutationen im *ALD*-Gen nachgewiesen werden. Die bisher beschriebenen Mutationen, zu denen Splice Site-Mutationen, Deletionen, Insertionen, Nonsense- und Missense-Mutationen zählen, sind über alle funktionellen Domänen des ALD-Proteins verteilt (Abb. 2). Diese heterogene Verteilung der Mutationen deutet daraufhin, dass ganz unterschiedliche Mechanismen zu einer Fehlfunktion des ALD-Proteins führen können.

Wir haben Wildtypkonstrukte sowie Mutationskonstrukte mit den bekannten Patienten-Mutationen G512S und S606L hergestellt. Die normale und die bei Patienten veränderte Nukleotidbindungsfalte des ALD-Proteins wurde in Fusion mit dem Maltose-Bindenden-Protein überexprimiert und gereinigt. Nach Markierung mit radioaktivem 8-azido-ATP zeigten alle Fusionsproteine eine starke spezifische ATP-Bindung. Dies zeigt die deutliche Affinität zu ATP und bestätigt die Rolle des Adrenoleukodystrophieproteins als ATP-Bindungsprotein.

Die ATPase-Aktivität der Fusionsproteine wurde anschließend mit einem spektrometrischen Assay gemessen. Beim Auftragen der gemessenen ATPase-Aktivität gegen die eingesetzte ATP-Konzentration zeigte sich eine typische Michaelis-Menten-Kurve. Die unterschiedlichen Kurvenverläufe der Wildtyp-

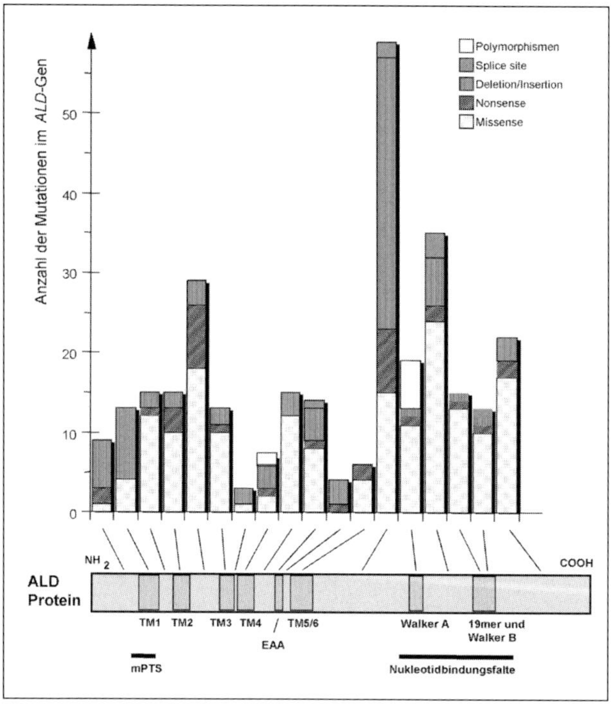

Abb. 2: Zuordnung von Mutationen im *ALD*-Gen zu den funktionellen Domänen des ALD-Proteins. Es zeigt sich eine heterogene Verteilung der Mutationen über alle ALD-Proteindomänen mit einer Clusterbildung im Bereich der Nukleotidbindungsfalte. Transmembrandomäne, mPTS = peroxisomale Signalsequenz, EAA = Fettsäurebindungsmotiv.

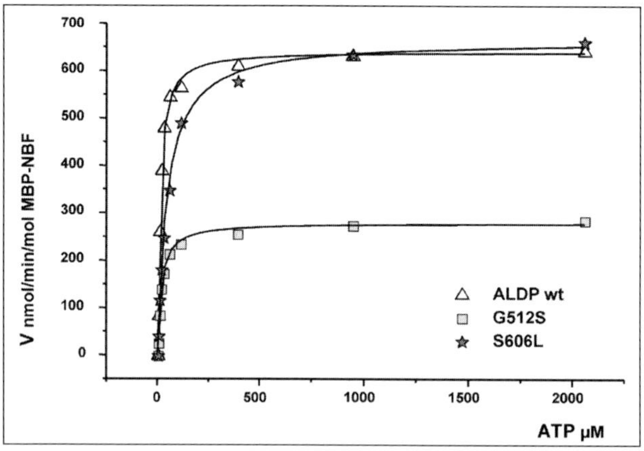

Abb. 3: ATPase-Aktivität der Nukleotidbindungsfalte des ALD-Proteins. Dargestellt sind die ermittelten Michaelis-Menten Kurven der Fusionsproteine des Wildtyps und der *ALD*-Genmutationen. Die Mutation G512S führt zu einer reduzierten maximalen Reaktionsgeschwindigkeit der ATPase und S606L zu einer verminderten ATP-Bindung (veränderte Steilheit des Kurvenanstiegs).

konstrukte und der Mutationskonstrukte weisen darauf hin, dass die untersuchten Patientenmutationen in der Nukleotidbindungsfalte zu einer veränderten ATP-Bindung und Verwertung führen. Die Mutation G512S reduziert die maximale Reaktionsgeschwindigkeit der ATPase-Aktivität. Dagegen führt die Mutation S606L zu einer verminderten ATP-Bindung (Abb. 3). Momentan untersuchen wir die funktionellen Konsequenzen in der Nukleotidbindungsfalte des Proteins, zu denen die vier im *ALD*-Gen bereits beschriebenen Patientenmutationen D629H, Q544R, R591Q und P560L zählen.

Zusammenfassung

Die Nukleotidbindungsfalte des ALD-Proteins ist eine ATP-spezifische Untereinheit, die eine ATPase-Aktivität aufweist und ATP hydrolysiert. Patientenmutationen im *ALD*-Gen, die zu einer veränderten Nukleotidbindungsfalte führen, verursachen entweder eine reduzierte ATP-Bindung oder eine veränderte ATPase-Aktivität. Durch das hier beschriebene rekombinante Modell kann die Funktion des ALD-Proteins und damit die Pathogenese der Erkrankung näher untersucht werden. Die Tatsache, dass ein und dieselbe *ALD*-Genmutation innerhalb eines Stammbaums zu unterschiedlichen Phänotypen führen kann, legt die Vermutung nahe, dass über den primären Gendefekt hinaus auch epigenetische Faktoren eine Rolle in der Pathogenese spielen (8). Daher sollen zu den rekombinanten ALD-Proteinmodellen auch mögliche epigenetische Faktoren addiert und ihr Einfluss auf die ALD-Proteinfunktion anschließend geprüft werden.

Literatur

1. Gould SJ, Raymond GV, Valle D (2001). The peroxisome biogenesis disorders. In: Scriver CR, Beaudet AL, Valle D, Sly WS (Hrsg) The metabolic and molecular bases of inherited disease. McGraw-Hill New York, S 3181–3217
2. Moser HW, Smith KD, Watkins PA, Powers J, Moser AB (2001) X-linked adrenoleukodystrophy. In: Scriver CR, Beaudet AL, Sly WS, Valle D (Hrsg) The metabolic and molecular bases of inherited disease. McGraw-Hill New York, pp 3257–3301
3. Gärtner J, Braun A, Holzinger A, Roehrig P, Lenard HG, Roscher AA (1998) Clinical and genetic aspects of X-linked adrenoleukodystrophy. Neuropediatrics 29:3–13
4. Shani N, Valle D (1998) Peroxisomal ABC transporters. Methods Enzymol 292: 753–776
5. Menkes J, Corbo L (1977) Adrenoleukodystrophy: Accumulation of cholesterol esters with very long chain fatty acids. Neurology 27: 928–932
6. Mosser J, Douar AM, Sarde CO, Kioschis P, Feil R, Moser H, Poustka AM, Mandell JL, Aubourg P (1993) Putative X-linked adrenoleukodystrophy gene shares unexpected homology with ABC transporters. Nature 361 (6414): 726–30
7. Higgins CF (1995) The ABC of channel regulation. Cell 82: 693–696
8. Gärtner J (2000) X-Chromosomale Adrenoleukodystrophie – Genetik und Epigenetik. In: Stephanie U (Hrsg) Aktuelle Neuropädiatrie. Novartis Pharma Verlag, Nürnberg, S 432–436

Unklare Leukoenzephalopathien: Genetische Heterogenität innerhalb von Krankheitsentitäten

N. Preuß, M. Henneke, V. Engelbrecht, J. Gärtner

Einleitung

Leukoenzephalopathien oder Leukodystrophien sind erworbene oder angeborene Erkrankungen, bei denen Fehler im Aufbau oder der Erhaltung des Myelins, d.h. der weißen Substanz des Gehirns und des Rückenmarks, vorliegen. Die angeborenen Leukodystrophien werden in der Regel in zwei Gruppen eingeteilt (van der Knaap und Valk 1995), die »klassischen Leukodystrophien« mit bekanntem und die »unklaren Leukodystrophien« mit unbekanntem Defekt (Abb. 1). Die Gruppe der »klassischen Leukodystrophien« bilden angeborene neurometabolische Erkrankungen, deren Einteilung nach den subzellulären Strukturen bzw. Organellen erfolgt, in denen die defekten Stoffwechselwege lokalisiert sind. Hierzu zählen lysosomale Erkrankungen wie die metachromatische Leukodystrophie und der Morbus Krabbe, mitochondriale Erkrankungen wie Defekte der Atmungskette und peroxisomale Erkrankungen wie die X-chromosomale Adrenoleukodystrophie und das Zellweger Syndrom (Gärtner 1998).

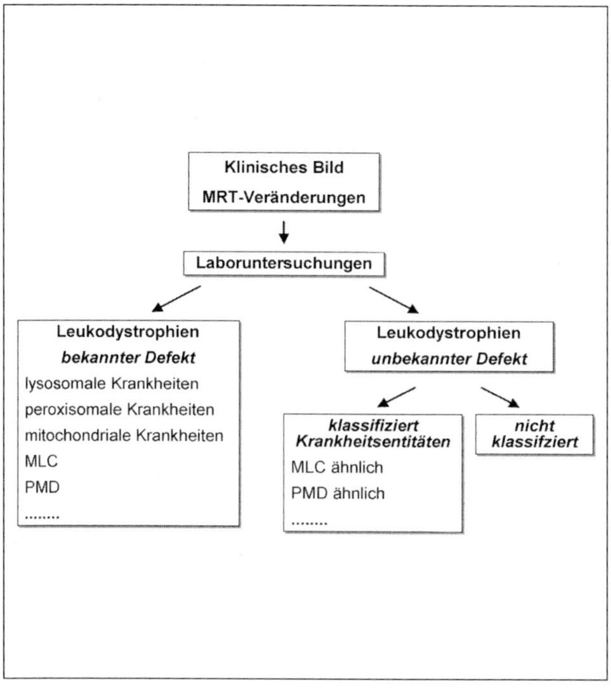

Abb. 1: Klassifikation von Leukodystrophien. Die anhand des klinischen Bildes und der Veränderungen in der Magnetresonanztomographie (MRT) und ggf. lokalisierten Protonenspektroskopie (MRS) des Schädels diagnostizierten Leukodystrophien können anhand von spezifischen Laboruntersuchungen weiter abgeklärt und die Diagnose einer »klassischen Leukodystrophie« gestellt werden. Führen diese Laboruntersuchungen nicht zu einer Diagnosestellung, liegt eine »unklare Leukodystrophie« vor. Leukodystrophien mit unbekanntem Defekt können wiederum anhand klinischer und neuroradiologischer Kriterien klassifiziert und so in Krankheitsentitäten eingeteilt werden, oder aber sie sind nicht klassifizierbar.

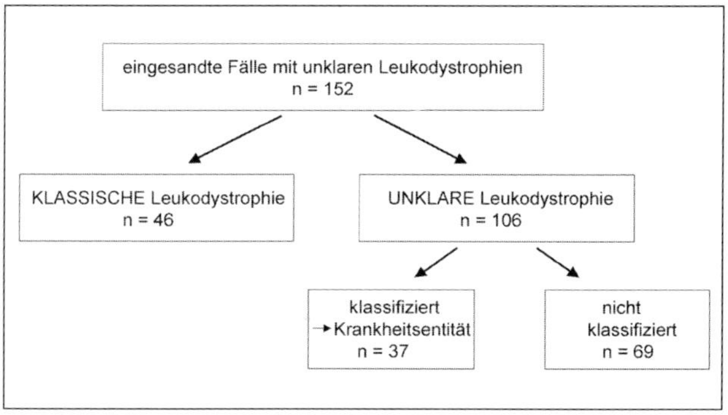

Abb. 2: Anzahl der Patienten mit unklaren Leukodystrophien, die dem Forschungsschwerpunkt bis April 2002 gemeldet wurden und deren Zuordnung in unterschiedlichen Leukodystrophiekategorien.

Die Gruppe der »unklaren Leukodystrophien« bilden diejenigen angeborenen Erkrankungen, deren klinische und radiologische Befunde einer klassischen Leukodystrophie ähnlich sind, deren primäre biochemische oder molekulargenetische Ursache derzeit jedoch unbekannt ist.

Mehrere internationale Arbeitsgruppen haben Datenbanken für unklare Leukoenzephalopathien erstellt und die Patienten nach klinischen, radiologischen und elektrophysiologischen Kriterien eingeteilt. Bisher konnten so mehr als acht verschiedene Krankheitsentitäten voneinander abgegrenzt werden. Die diesen Krankheitsentitäten zugrunde liegenden Genotypen scheinen auch innerhalb einer Krankheitsentität heterogen zu sein. Zwei dieser Entitäten mit heterogenem Genotyp, einem einerseits bekannten und andererseits noch unbekannten Gendefekt, sind die megalencephale Leukoenzephalopathie mit subcorticalen Zysten (MLC) und die Pelizaeus Merzbacher Erkrankung (PMD) bzw. das PMD-ähnliche Syndrom mit Hypomyelinisierung (van der Knaap et al. 1995, Seitelberger 1995, Wong et al. 2000, Ziereisen et al. 2000).

Ergebnisse

Stand des Forschungsschwerpunktes »Unklare Leukodystrophien«

Der Forschungsschwerpunkt »Unklare Leukodystrophien« (www.aps-med.de, Link: LEUKONET »UNKLAR«) befasst sich seit 1999 mit der Datensammlung klinischer, neuroradiologischer, laborchemischer und molekulargenetischer Befunde von vorwiegend an deutschen Kliniken betreuten Patienten mit ungeklärten Leukodystrophien. Die eingesandten Fälle werden interdisziplinär ausgewertet. Bis April 2002 wurden die Daten von 152 Patienten erfasst (Abb. 2). In 46 Fällen führte die Aufarbeitung der Fälle zur Diagnose einer klassischen Leukodystrophie. Von den 106 unklar gebliebenen Fällen konnten 37 Fälle anhand klinischer und kernspintomographischer Befunde klassifiziert und in Krankheitsentitäten eingeteilt werden. Ziele des Forschungsschwerpunktes sind es, die molekularen Grundlagen und die Pathogenese bislang unklarer, aber bereits klassifizierter Leukodystrophien zu untersuchen. Darüber hinaus sollen durch die Erhebung klinischer, radiologischer und biochemischer Daten weiterer

Tab. 1: Phänotyp und Genotyp von Patienten mit MLC

Phänotyp / Genotyp	Patient 1	Patient 2	Patient 3
jetziges Alter (Jahre, Monate)	4,7	15,7	15,6
Geschlecht (m: männlich, w: weiblich)	m	w	m
Herkunft	deutsch	italienisch	italienisch
Eltern konsanguin	–	–	–
Alter bei Diagnose (Monate)	6	<12	<12
Makrozephalie	+	+	+
Verschlechterung motorischer Fähigkeiten	–	+	+
Verschlechterung kognitiver Fähigkeiten	–	(+)	+
Ataxie	–	+	–
Epilepsie	–	+	+
ML C1-Genmutation	?	Splice / Del.	Miss. /–

+: vorhanden; –: nicht vorhanden; ?: nicht bekannt; (): geringgradig

Patienten neue Krankheitsentitäten gebildet und anschließend wissenschaftlich bearbeitet werden.

Genetische Heterogenität bei megalenzephaler Leukoenzephalopathie mit subcorticalen Zysten (MLC)

Der MLC konnten drei Patienten italienischer bzw. deutscher Herkunft zugeordnet werden (Tab. 1). Die Patienten waren bei Diagnosestellung jünger als zwölf Monate, ihr jetziges Alter variiert von vier Jahren und sieben Monaten bis hin zu 15 Jahren und sieben Monaten. Alle Patienten entwickelten in den ersten Lebensjahren eine Makrozephalie. Die zwei älteren Patienten zeigten eine langsame Verschlechterung ihrer motorischen Fähigkeiten und entwickelten auch eine Verschlechterung ihrer kognitiven Leistungen. Ein weiteres Symptom der älteren Patienten sind Krampfanfälle. Die kernspintomographischen Befunde aller drei Patienten sind identisch. Das Gehirn erscheint geschwollen mit diffus veränderter weißer Substanz und bilateralen subcorticalen Zysten. Ein Beispiel zeigt die Abbildung 3. Mutationen im *MLC1*-Gen wurden als primärer Defekt für diese Krankheitsentität beschrieben (Leegwater et al. 2001). Jedoch konnte nur bei einem der hier beschriebenen drei Patienten in beiden Allelen eine *MLC1*-Genmutation nachgewiesen werden.

Genetische Heterogenität bei Pelizaeus Merzbacher Erkrankung (PMD) und PMD-ähnlichem Syndrom mit Hypomyelinisierung

Dem PMD-ähnlichen Syndrom konnten drei weibliche und fünf männliche Patienten türkischer, kroatischer bzw. deutscher Herkunft zugeordnet werden (Tab. 2). Die Patienten waren bei Diagnosestellung zwischen einem Monat und 20 Monaten alt. Zwei der Patienten verstarben im Alter von sechs Monaten bzw. zwei Jahren und sechs Monaten. Das jetzige Alter der Patienten liegt zwischen fünf Jahren und sieben Monaten und 15 Jahren und 11 Monaten. Bei sechs der

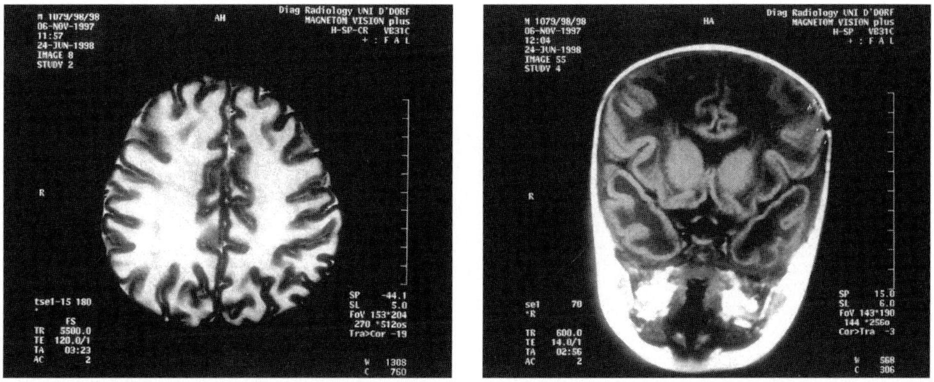

Abb. 3a/b: Magnetresonanztomographie bei einem sieben Monate alten Jungen mit MLC. (a) Axiales T2 -gewichtetes Bild mit diffus verändertem, geschwollenem Marklager. (b) Koronares T1 -gewichtetes Bild mit fronto-temporal gelegenen Zysten.

Tab. 2: Phänotyp und Genotyp von Patienten mit PMD-ähnlichem Syndrom

Phänotyp / Genotyp	**Patient** 1	**2**	**3**	**4**	**5**	**6**	**7**	**8**
jetziges Alter (†=verstorben; Jahre, Monate)	2,6†	8	13,11	8,6	14,11	5,5	0,6†	5,7
Geschlecht (m: männlich, w: weiblich)	m	m	m	m	w	w	m	w
Herkunft	türk.	dtsch.	dtsch.	türk.	türk.	türk.	kroat.	dtsch.
Eltern konsanguin	+	–	–	+	?	–	?	–
Alter bei Diagnose (Monate)	< 1	< 12	< 12	3	20	5	< 1	< 3
Nystagmus	–	+	+	+	+	–	+	+
Hypotonie	–	+	–	+	–	+	+	+
Entwicklungsverzögerung mental	+	+	+	+	–	+	+	+
Entwicklungsverzögerung motorisch	+	+	+	+	–	+	+	+
Epilepsie	+	–	+	–	–	–	–	–
Erkrankungsverlauf (stat: stationär, progr: progredient)	stat.	stat.	prog.	prog.	stat.	stat.	prog.	stat.
PLP-Genmutation /-Linkage	–/–	–/–	–/–	–/–			–/–	
X-Inaktivierungsmuster regelrecht					+	+		+

+: vorhanden; –: nicht vorhanden; ?: nicht bekannt

acht Patienten war das Auftreten eines Nystagmus eines der initialen Symptome, fünf von acht Patienten zeigten initial eine Hypotonie, sieben der acht Patienten entwickelten eine langsam progrediente psychomotorische Entwicklungsverzögerung. Die Krankheitsverläufe der einzelnen Patienten waren entweder stationär oder progredient (Tab. 2). Die MRT-Bilder der Patienten entsprechen denen von PMD-Patienten mit nachgewiesener *PLP*-Genmutation und zeigen eine diffuse Hypomyelinisation. Ein Beispiel zeigt die Abbildung 4. Im Gegensatz zur klassischen PMD, die X-chromosomal vererbt wird, folgt das PMD-ähnliche Syndrom wahrscheinlich einem autosomal rezessiven Erbgang (Ziereisen et al. 2000). Hierfür sprechen sowohl die Konsanguinität der Eltern der Patienten als auch ein nahezu ausgewogenes Verhältnis zwischen weiblichen und männlichen Betroffenen in der hier aufgeführten Patientengruppe. Die für alle männlichen Patienten durchgeführte Mutationsanalyse des *PLP*-Gens ergab keine Auffälligkeiten und darüber hinaus konnte ein Linkage zum *PLP*-Genlocus ausgeschlossen werden. Alle weiblichen Patienten zeigten ein normales X-Inaktivierungsmuster. Somit kann eine Mutation im X-chromosomalen *PLP*-Gen nicht ursächlich für den Phänotyp dieser Patienten sein.

Diskussion

Sowohl bei der megalenzephalen Leukoenzephalopathie mit subcorticalen Zysten (MLC) als auch bei der Pelizaeus Merzbacher Erkrankung (PMD) bzw. dem PMD-ähnlichen Syndrom mit Hypomyelinisierung liegt eine Krankheitsentität vor, innerhalb derer unterschiedliche Genotypen zu identischen klinischen Phänotypen führen. Bisher bekannte Genotypen für diese beiden Krankheitsentitäten sind Mutationen in dem *MLC1*-Gen bzw. dem *PLP*-Gen. Bei Patienten mit nicht nachweisbarer *MLC1*- bzw. *PLP*-Genmutation müssen daher andere, bisher noch unbekannte Gendefekte ursächlich sein, die zu einem identischen klinischen und radiologischen Phänotyp führen.

Dass unterschiedliche Genotypen zu identischen klinischen Phänotypen führen können, ist auch für zahlreiche andere neurometabolische Erkrankungen

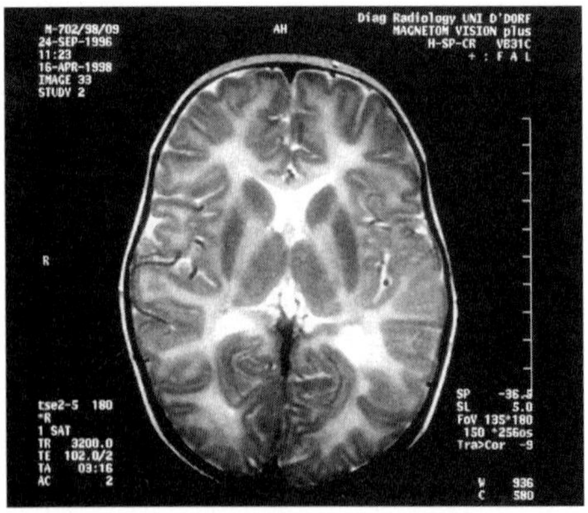

Abb. 4: Magnetresonanztomographie bei einem 18 Monate alten Mädchen mit PMD-ähnlichem Syndrom. Axiales T2 -gewichtetes Bild mit Amyelination.

bekannt. Ein Beispiel hierfür sind die in die Gruppe der klassischen Leukodystrophien einzuordnenden Peroxisomenbiogenesedefekte, wie das Zellweger Syndrom, die neonatale Adrenoleukodystrophie, die Rhizomelia chondrodysplasia punctata und der Morbus Refsum, bei denen mindestens zwölf unterschiedliche Genotypen zu einem klinisch, biochemisch und radiologisch identischen klinischen Phänotyp führen können (Gould et al. 2001). Diese Erkrankungen sind auf Mutationen in unterschiedlichen *PEX*-Genen zurückzuführen, die alle für die Bildung von Peroxisomen bedeutend sind. In vergleichbarer Weise lassen sich die Krankheitsentitäten megalencephale Leukoenzephalopathie mit subcorticalen Zysten (MLC) und Pelizaeus Merzbacher Erkrankung (PMD) bzw. PMD-ähnliches Syndrom mit Hypomyelinisierung auf Mutationen im *MLC1*- bzw. *PLP*-Gen und auch in anderen für die Bildung und Erhaltung des Myelins bedeutenden Genen zurückführen.

Die Einordnung von Patienten mit unklaren Leukoenzephalopathien in Krankheitsentitäten und deren wissenschaftliche Bearbeitung, beispielsweise anhand von Linkage-Studien, wird zur Identifizierung neuer Leukodystrophien verursachender Gendefekte führen und die Gruppe der bekannten »klassischen Leukodystrophien« erweitern. Darüber hinaus können die von Leukodystrophiegenen kodierten Proteine funktionell charakterisiert werden und so die Mechanismen der Bildung und Erhaltung des Myelins und die Pathogenese der Leukodystrophien näher beschrieben werden. Diese pathogenetischen Erkenntnisse sollen schließlich zur Entwicklung von Therapieansätzen genutzt werden.

Danksagung

Wir danken Herrn PD Dr. T. Bettecken (GSF Neuherberg) sowie Herrn Prof. Dr. A. Gal und Frau U. Orth (Institut für Humangenetik, Universitätskrankenhaus Hamburg-Eppendorf) für die molekulargenetischen Analysen. Wir danken Frau PD Dr. U. Burck-Lehmann (Praxis für Kinderheilkunde und Medizinische Genetik, Köln), Herrn Prof. Dr. T. Voit (Universitätskinderklinik, Essen), Frau Dr. G. Uziel (Instituto Neurologico C. Besta Milano, Italien) sowie Frau Dr. V. Printz und Frau Dr. S. Maron (Rummelsberger Kliniken, Garmisch-Partenkirchen) für die eingesandten Fälle.

Literatur

1. Gärtner J (1998): Unklare Leukodystrophien und Myelinationsstörungen – Klinisches Spektrum und Strategie. In: Bentele KHP und Kohlschütter A (Herausg.) Aktuelle Neuropädiatrie, Novartis Pharma Verlag, Nürnberg, Seiten 47–55
2. Gould SJ, Raymond GV, Valle D (2001). The Peroxisome Biogenesis Disorders. In: Scriver CR, Beaudet AL, Sly WS, Valle D (Herausg.) The Metabolic and Molecular Bases of Inherited Disease. McGraw-Hill Information Services Company, New York, Seiten 3181–3217
3. van der Knaap MS, Valk J (1995). Magnetic resonance of myelin, myelination, and myelin disorders. Springer-Verlag, Berlin, Heidelberg, New York, Seiten 1–5 und 18–21

4. Leegwater PAJ, Yuan BQ, van der Steen J, Mulders J, Konst AAM, Ilja Boor PK, Mejaski-Bosnjak V, van der Maarel SM, Frants RR, Oudejans CBM, Schutgens RBH, Pronk JC, van der Knaap MS (2001) Mutations of MLC1 (KIAA0027), encoding a putative membrane protein, cause megalencephalic leukoencephalopathy with subcortical cysts. Am J Hum Genet 68:831–838
5. Seitelberger F (1995): Neuropathology and genetics of Pelizaeus Merzbacher disease. Brain Pathol 5:267–273
6. Wong K, Armstrong RC, Gyure KA, Morrison AL, Rodriguez D, Matalon R, Johnson AB, Wollmann R, Gilbert E, Le TQ, Bradley CA, Crutchfield K, Schiffmann R (2000) Foamy cells with oligodendroglial phenotype in childhood ataxia with diffuse central nervous system hypomyelination syndrome. Acta Neuropathol 100:635–646
7. Ziereisen F, Dan B, Christiaens F, Deltenre P, Boutemy R, Christophe C (2000) Connatal Pelizaeus-Merzbacher disease in two girls. Pediatr Radiol 30:435–438

Neuroradiologische Befunde beim Marinesco-Sjögren Syndrom

A. Reinhold, I. Scheer, R. Lehmann, L. Neumann, T. Michael, R. Varon-Mateeva, A. von Moers

Zusammenfassung

Das Marinesco-Sjögren-Syndrom (MSS) ist eine seltene autosomal rezessiv vererbte, neurodegenerative Erkrankung. Die häufig beschrieben Kleinhirnatrophie bei MSS ist kein konstanter Befund, und ein nahezu normales kraniales MRT ist mit der Diagnose vereinbar. Offensichtlich lässt sich das MSS in eine primär myopathisch, zerebellär betonten Typ und eine neuropathischen Typ mit nur diskreten Veränderungen der hinteren Schädelgrube differenzieren. Häufiger beobachtete morphologische Auffälligkeiten der Hypophyse bei MSS-Patienten gehen meist nicht mit einer Funktionsstörung einher.

Einleitung

Das Mariensco-Sjögren-Syndrom (MSS) (MIM 248800) ist eine seltene autosomal rezessiv vererbte Erkrankung, die durch bilaterale Katarakte, eine zerebellare Ataxie, statomotorische Entwicklungsverzögerung und eine mentale Retardierung sehr unterschiedlichen Ausmaßes charakterisiert ist (1, 2). Weitere fakultative Symptome sind Minderwuchs, Skelettdeformitäten, Hypogonadismus und verschiedene neuromuskuläre Symptome wie eine Myopathie (3–5) oder eine motorische und sensorische Neuropathie (6, 7). Die Myopathie kann chronisch sein oder sich als akute parainfektiöse Rhabdomyolyse manifestieren (8). Die Erkrankung kommt in allen ethnischen Gruppen vor. MSS ist genetisch identisch mit dem congenital cataract facial dysmorphism neuropathy (CCFDN) syndrome (9). CCFDN (MIM 604168) ist eine autosomal rezessiv vererbte Erkrankung mit kongenitalen Katarakten, Neuropathie und charakteristischen Gesichtsdysmorphien, die primär bei bulgarischen Roma-Familien gefunden wurde (10). Das MSS/CCFDN-Gen ist auf dem Chromosom 18q23 lokalisiert (11, 9). Das Gen dieser Multisystem-Erkrankung ist noch unbekannt. Die Diagnose basiert auf der Familienanamnese, klinischen und neuroradiologischen Befunden, diagnostische Laborbefunde gibt es nicht. Eine niedrige Vitamin E-Konzentrationen im Serum aufgrund einer Chylomikronenretentions-Erkrankung wurde bei 2 italienischen MSS-Patienten beschrieben (12). Als wichtigster neuroradiologischer Befund wird in der Literatur eine ausgeprägte Kleinhirnatrophie mit kleiner hinterer Schädelgrube (Abb. 1) beschrieben (13, 14). Weitere supratentorielle Veränderungen in Form einer diffusen Hirnatrophie, Läsionen der weißen Substanz und Auffälligkeiten der Hypophyse können vorhanden sein

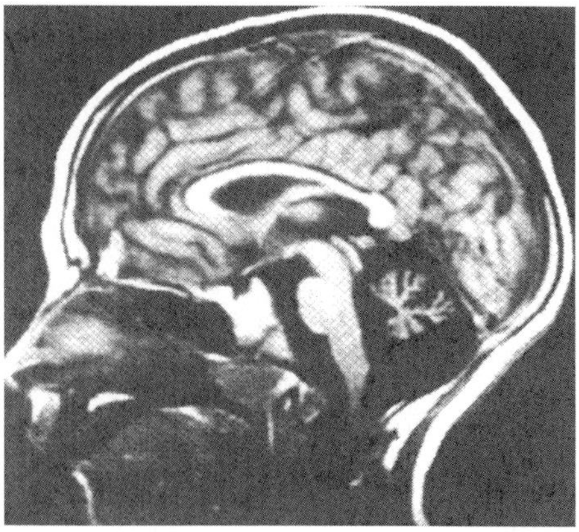

Abb. 1: Sagittales T1-gewichtetes cMRT eines MSS-Patientenmit Klienhirnatrophie und fehlendem Hypersignal der Neurohypophyse. Aus (14).

(14, 15). Die MRT-Befunde werden als wichtiger Bestandteil in der Diagnosefindung beim Marinesco-Sjögren-Syndrom angesehen (14). Insbesondere die Kleinhirnatrophie scheint ein relativ konstanter Befund mit nur wenigen beschriebenen Ausnahmen zu sein. Die beschriebenen Fallzahlen sind jedoch meist gering, so dass die Untersuchung einer größeren Patientengruppe erforderlich ist, um diese Schlussfolgerungen zu bestätigen.

Patienten

In den Jahren 1986 bis 2001 wurde in Kinderklinik der Charité bei 14 Patienten die Diagnose MSS gestellt. Alle Patienten sind Roma, die aus der selben Region in Serbien nördlich von Belgrad stammen. In diesen Familien besteht ein hohes Maß an Konsanguinität. Die Erkrankung zeigt einen autosomal rezessiven Vererbungsmodus, und wir konnten bei allen Patienten einen identischen, konservierten Haplotyp in der Region des MSS-Gens nachweisen.

Aktuell wurde bei 5 Patienten im Alter zwischen 5 und 19 Jahren umfangreiche Diagnostik zum Ausschluss einer Fettstoffwechselstörung oder endokrinologischen Störung sowie ein karniales MRT durchgeführt. Alle Patienten hatten bilaterale Katarakte, die in den ersten Lebensmonaten operativ entfernt wurden. Alle wiesen eine verzögerte statomotorische Entwicklung, eine leichte mentale Retardierung und deutliche Zeichen einer zentralen Bewegungsstörung mit unsicherem breitbasigen Gangbild, Dysarthie und extrapyramidalmotorischer Bewegungsstörung auf. Die Muskeleigenreflexe waren abgeschwächt oder erloschen. Die Nervenleitgeschwindigkeit war verlangsamt als Zeichen einer demyelinisierenden Neuropathie. Die CK im Serum war normal, keiner der Patienten hatte anamnestisch Episoden parainfektiöser Myalgien/Myoglobinurien. Bei keinem der Patienten ergab sich ein Anhalt für eine Hypophysenfunktionsstörung. Eine Fettstoffwechselstörung und ein Vitamin E-Mangel konnte bei allen Patienten ausgeschlossen werden. Die Vitamin E Serumkonzentrationen lagen zwischen 18,2 und 40,7 µmol/l (Referenzbereich 12–46 µmol/l).

Tab. 1: cMRT-Befunde bei 5 MSS-Patienten

Patienten MRT-Befund	**Patient 1 (5 J.)**	**Patient 2 (6 J.)**	**Patient 3 (9 J.)**	**Patient 4 (12 J.)**	**Patient 5 (19 J.)**
Kleinhirnatrophie	–	–	–	(+) Vermis	(+) Vermis
verbreiterte zerebellomedulläre Zisterne	+	+	–	–	–
Kortikale Atrophie	–	–	(+)	–	+
Leukenzephalopathie	–	–	–	unilateral 2 Herde juxta-kortikal	bilateral periventrikulär und juxta-kortikal
Hypoplastische Adenohypophyse	–	–	–	+	+
Hypersignal der Neurohypophyse	n.b.	–	n.b.	–	–

n.b. = nicht beurteilbar

Methode

Die kraniale MRT-Untersuchung wurde mit einem 1,5T *GE Medical Systems* MRT-Gerät durchgeführt. Es wurden native axiale T1-, T2- und PD-gewichtete Sequenzen, sagittale T1- oder T2-gewichtete Sequenzen und koronare Flair-Sequenzen aufgenommen. Die Größe des Kleinhirnwurmes und der Kleinhirnhemisphären wurde als normal oder kleiner als normal bewertet.

Ergebnisse

Die MRT-Befunde sind in Tabelle 1 zusammengestellt und ausgewählte Bilder erscheinen in Abbildung 2 bis 4.

Patient 4 und 5 weisen eine diskrete Kleinhirnatrophie mit betonter Furchung insbesondere im Bereich des Oberwurmes auf (Abb. 2). Die übrigen Patienten haben keine Kleinhirnatrophie, sowohl Kleinhirnwurm als auch die Hemisphären stellen sich normal groß und normal konfiguriert dar. Bei Patient 1 und 2 ist die zerebellomeduläre Zisterne verbreiteret (Abb. 3), ohne dass eine Kleinhirnatrophie vorliegt. Patient 4 und 5 haben eine Leukenzephalopathie mit periventrikulär und juxtakortikal herdförmigen Läsionen in der T2-/Flair-Wichtung (Abb. 4). Bei Patient 5 liegt zusätzlich eine kortikal-subkortikale Atrophie vor. Der Hypophysenvorderlappen ist hypoplastisch bei Patient 4 und 5. Das Hypersignal der Neurohypophyse in der T1-Wichtung fehlt bei den Patienten 2, 4 und 5 (Abb. 2). Bei den übrigen Patienten ist dies aufgrund fehlender sagittaler T1-Schichten nicht beurteilbar.

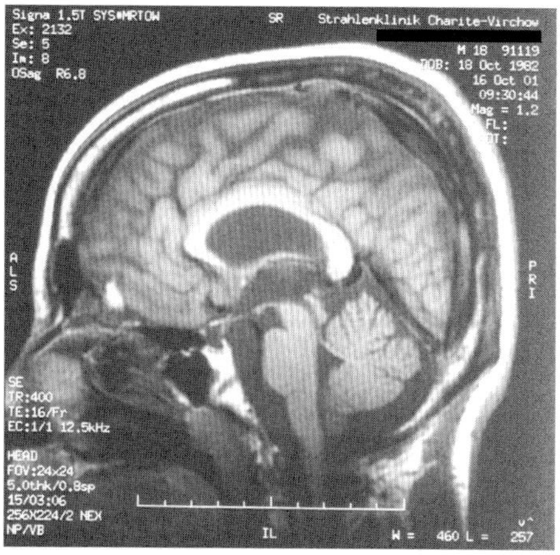

Abb. 2: Sagittales T1-gewichtetes cMRT: diskrete Kleinhirnatrophie im Bereich des Oberwurmes. Das Hypersignal der Neurohypophyse fehlt, die Adenohypophyse erscheint zu klein.

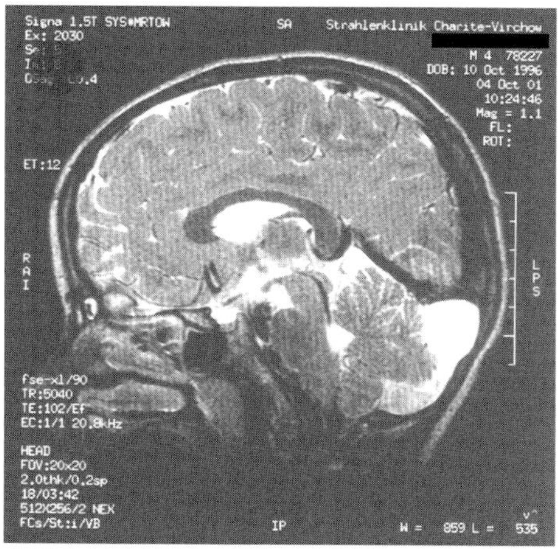

Abb. 3: Sagittales T2-gewichtetes cMRT. Die zerebellomedulläre Zisterne ist verbreitert und reicht bis unter das Tentorium. Es liegt keine Kleinhirnatrophie vor.

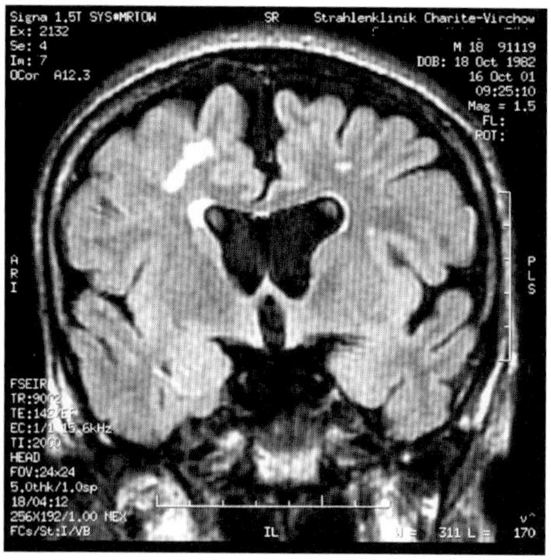

Abb. 4: Koronare Flair-Sequenz, cMRT: In der weißen Substanz stellen sich bilateral fleckförmige Signalintensitätsanhebungen dar.

Diskussion

Als klassischer neuroradiologischer Befund beim Marinesco-Sjögren-Syndrom gilt eine deutliche Kleinhirnatrophie insbesondere des Vermis. In der Literatur sind nur wenige Ausnahmen berichtet, allerdings sind die beschriebenen Fallzahlen zumeist klein (Tab. 2). Häufig handelt es sich nur um Einzelfallberichte, bei denen die Patienten alle eine ausgeprägte Kleinhirnatrophie aufwiesen (3, 12, 16, 17). McLaughlin et al. (14) und Georgy et al. (13) berichteten über die neuroradiologischen Befunde bei 3 bzw. 8 MSS-Patienten. Alle diese Patienten hatten einen kleinen Kleinhirnwurm und 9 dieser 11 Patienten hatten kleine Kleinhirnhemispheren. Georgy et al. zeigte zudem bei 4 Patienten, dass die

Tab. 2: Auswahl von MSS-Patienten in der Literatur: MRT-Befunde und Vorhandensein von Neuropathie und/oder Myopathie

Mrt und klinische Befunde Artikel	Zerebellare Atrophie	Kortikale Atrophie	Leukenze-phalopathie	Auffälligkeiten der Hypophyse	Neuro-pathie	Myopathie
Sasaki et al. (3) 1996 n = 1	1/1	–	–	?	–	1/1
Farah et al. (20) 1997 n= 2	2/2	2/2	–	?	2/2	2/2
Ishikawa et al. (17) 1993 n=1	1/1	–	–	?	–	1/1
Bromberg et al. (15) 1990 n=2	1/2	2/2	2/2	?	2/2 (mild)	2/2 (mild)
Superneau et al. (4) 1987 n = 17	17/17	–	–	?	–	17/17
McLaughlin et al. (14) 1996 n = 3	3/3	1/3	1/3	3/3	–	–
Georgy et al. (13) 1998 n = 8	8/8	–	–	?	–	8/8
Müller-Felber et al. (8), 1997 n = 4	2/4	–	–	?	4/4	,4/4 (akut)
Aguglia et al. (12) 2000 n = 2	2/2	–	–	?	2/2	–

Kleinhirnatrophie über eine Zeitspanne von 7 Jahren nicht progressiv war (13). Diese Autoren schlussfolgerten beide, dass die MRT-Untersuchung sehr hilfreich für eine frühe Diagnosestellung dieser Erkrankung ist. Durch die vorliegende Untersuchung und vereinzelte Befunde in der Literatur wird gezeigt, dass es sich um kein essentielles Kriterium bei MSS handelt. Die nur diskrete Ausbildung der Kleinhirnatrophie bei den von uns untersuchten und bei den von Müller-Felber et al. (8) beschriebenen Patienten könnte Ausdruck der Variabilität des Phänotyps bei MSS sein. Der CCFDN Phänotyp zeigt große Überlappung mit MSS (11). Die Neuropathie ist eines der Kardinalsymptome bei CCFDN und ein fakultatives Symptom bei MSS, andererseits ist die zerebellare Beteiligung nur gering und nicht obligat für die Diagnose CCFDN (10). Als neuroradiologische Befunde bei CCFDN sind eine zerebrale und spinale Atrophie sowie gelegentlich fokale Läsionen beschrieben (11). Diese Unterschiede begründeten ursprünglich die

Klassifikation in 2 verschiedene Krankheitsentitäten. Kürzlich wurde die genetische Identität dieser beiden Syndrome gezeigt (9). Die Analyse bisher publizierter MSS-Fälle mit Berücksichtigung von CCFDN-Fällen legt nahe, dass es beim Mariensco-Sjögren–Syndrom einen primär myopathischen, zerebellär betonten Typ und einen neuropathischen Typ mit nur diskreten Veränderungen der hinteren Schädelgrube gibt.

Die Neurohypophyse ist im T1-gewichteten MRT-Bild als ein umschriebenes hyperintses Signal dargestellt (18). Bei 3 der 5 MSS-Patienten fehlte das Hypersignal der Neurohypophyse, aufgrund fehlender sagittale T1-Schichten war dies bei den übrigen Patienten nicht beurteilbar. Keiner dieser 3 Patienten hatte Zeichen eines Diabetes insipidus centralis. In solchen Fällen liegt die Neurohypophyse meist dystop an der Basis des Hypothalamus (19). Bei den 2 Patienten mit hypoplastisch erscheinender Adenohypophyse konnte eine relevante Funktionsstörung ausgeschlossen werden. Diese Befunde wurden bereits bei 3 MSS-Patienten beschrieben (14).

Eine kortikale Atrophie, die wir bei 2 der 5 Patienten fanden, und periventrikuläre Läsionen der weißen Substanz, auch bei 2 der 5 Patienten, wurden ebenfalls bei MSS und CCFDN beschrieben (10, 14). In Übereinstimmung mit der Literatur (14) sind diese Befunde bei dem ältesten von uns untersuchten Patienten am stärksten ausgeprägt. Aufgrund fehlender Verlaufsuntersuchungen bleibt jedoch offen, ob es sich tatsächlich um progrediente Veränderungen handelt. Die Pathogenese der Leukenzephalopathie ist bisher unbekannt.

Literatur

1. Marinesco G, Draganesco S, Vasiliu D (1931): Nouvelle maladie familiale caracterisée par une cataracte congénitale et un arret du développement somato-neuro-psychique. Encephale; 26: 97–109.
2. Sjögren T (1950): Hereditary congenital spinocerebellar ataxia accompanied by congenital cataract and oligophrenia. Confinia Neurol; 10: 293–308.
3. Sasaki K, Suga K, Tsugawa S, et al (1996).: Muscle pathology in Marinesco-Sjögren syndrome: a unique ultrastructural feature. Brain Dev; 18: 64–67.
4. Superneau DW, Wertelecki W, Zellweger H, Bastian F (1987): Myopathy in Marinesco-Sjogren Syndrome. Eur Neurol; 26: 8–16.
5. Torbergsen T, Stalberg E, Aasly J, Lindal S (1991): Myopathy in Marinesco-Sjogren syndrome: an electrophysiological study. Acta Neurol Scand; 84(2): 132–138.
6. Hakamada S, Sobue G, Watanabe K, Kumagai T, Hara K, Miyazaki S (1981): Peripheral neuropathy in Marinesco-Sjogren syndrome. Brain Dev, 3(4):403–406
7. Zimmer C, Gosztonyi G, Cervos-Navarro J, von Moers A, Schröder JM (1992): Neuropathy with lysosomal changes in Marinesco-Sjögren syndrome: fine structural findings in skeletal muscle and conjunctiva. Neuropediatrics; 23: 329–335.
8. Müller-Felber W, Zafiriou D, Scheck R, et al. (1998): Marinesco Sjögren syndrome with rhabdomyolysis. A new subtyp of the disease. Neuropediatrics; 29: 97–101.
9. Merlini L, Gooding R, Lochmüller H, et al. (2002): Genetic identity of Marinesco-Sjögren/myoglobinuria and CCFDN syndromes. Neurology; 58(2): 231–236.
10. Tournev I, Kalaydjieva L, Youl B, Ishpekova B, Guergueltcheva V, et al. (1999): Congenital cataracts facial dysmorphism neuropathy syndrome, a novel complex genetic disease in Balkan gypsies: clinical and electrophysiological observations. Ann Neurol; 45(6): 742–750.

11. Angelicheva D, Turnev I, Dye D, Chandler D, Thomas PK, Kalaydjieva L (1999): Congenital cataracts facial dysmorphism neuropathy (CCFDN) syndrome: a novel developmental disorder in Gypsies maps to 18qter. Eur J Hum Genet; 7: 560–566.
12. Aguglia U, Annesi G, Pasquinelli G, et al. (2000): Vitamin E deficiency due to chylomicron retention disease in Marinesco-Sjögren syndrome. Ann Neurol; 47(2): 260–264.
13. Georgy BA, Snow RD, Brogdon BG, Wertelecki W (1998): Neuroradiologic findings in Marinesco-Sjögren syndrome. Am J Neuroradiol; 19: 281–283.
14. McLaughlin JF, Pagon RA, Weinberger E, Haas JE (1996): Marinesco-Sjögren syndrome: Clinical and magnetic resonance imaging features in three children. Dev Med Child Neurol; 38: 636–644.
15. Bromberg MB, Junck L, Gebarski SS, McLean MJ, Gilman S (1990): The Marinesco-Sjogren syndrome examined by computed tomography, magnetic resonance, and 18F-2-fluoro-2-deoxy-D-glucose and positron emission tomography. Arch Neurol; 47(11): 1239–1242.
16. Shimizu T, Matsuishi T, Yamashita Y, Koga Y (1997): Mariensco-Sjogren syndrome: can the diagnosis be made prior to cataract formation? Muscle and Nerve: 909–910.
17. Ishikawa T, Kitoh H, Awaya A, Nonaka I (1993): Rapid cataract formation in Marinesco-Sjögren syndrome. Pedriatr Neurol; 9: 407–408.
18. Ultmann MC, Siegel SF, Hirsch WL, Finegold DN, Foley TP (1993): Pituitary stalk and ectopic hyperintens T1 signal on magnetic resonance imaging: implications for anterior pituitary dysfunction. Am J Diseas Child; 147: 647–652.
19. Abrahams JJ, Trefelner E, Boulware SD (1991): Idiopathic growth hormone deficiency: MR findings in 35 patients. Am J Neuroradiol; 12: 155–160.
20. Farah S, Sabry MA, Khuraibet AJ, Anim JT, Quasrawi B, et al. (1997): Marinesco-Sjögren syndrome in a Bedouin family. Acto Neurol Scand; 96: 387–391.

Marinesco-Sjögren Syndrom in Kombination mit Pyruvat Dehydrogenase Defizienz

A. Blaschek, I. Harting, J. Smeitink, H.H. Göbel, F. Ebinger, N.I. Wolf, D. Rating

Zusammenfassung

Wir beschreiben die klinischen, histopathologischen und biochemischen Befunde eines jungen Patienten mit Marinesco-Sjögren Syndrom. Klinik und Bildgebung passen sehr gut zu den in der Literatur beschriebenen Fällen von Kindern mit Marinesco-Sjögren Syndrom. Auch in der neuropathologischen Beurteilung fanden sich typische autophagische Vakuolen und membranartige Strukturen in der Nähe des Zellkerns. Biochemisch konnten wir erstmals eine Beeinträchtigung des mitochondrialen Energiestoffwechsels mit einem Pyruvat-Dehydrogenase Defekt nachweisen.

Das Marinesco-Sjögren Syndrom ist eine seltene autosomal rezessiv vererbte Erkrankung, die sich in der frühen Kindheit mit zerebellärer Ataxie, einer Katarakt und verzögerter psychomotorischer Entwicklung manifestiert. Seltenerer wurden Hypogonadismus und Kleinwuchs beschrieben. Neben diesen Kardinalsymptomen scheint die Beteiligung des neuromuskulären Systems mit progressiver Muskelschwäche, Hypotonie und motorischer oder sensibler Neuropathie typisch.

Die Diagnose des Marinesco-Sjögren Syndroms fußt neben der klinischen Charakteristik auf der zerebralen Bildgebung sowie charakteristischen Veränderungen in der Muskulatur, die sich vor allem elektronenmikroskopisch dokumentieren lassen.

Der Patient ist ein mittlerweile $4^{6/12}$ Jahre alter Junge türkischer, konsanguiner (Cousin/Cousine) Eltern, der einen älteren gesunden Bruder hat. Die Familienanamnese ist leer bezüglich neuromuskulärer Erkrankungen.

Nach unkomplizierter Schwangerschaft wurde er bei Querlage mit primärer Sektio entbunden. Die Neugeborenenperiode verlief zunächst unauffällig, doch mit dem 6 Monat wurde das verzögerte Erreichen der kindlichen Meilensteine deutlich. Er konnte sich mit 2 Jahren drehen, freies Sitzen mit 3 Jahren und aktuell mit knapp 5 Jahren kann er nur gehalten Laufen. Auch die sprachliche Entwicklung deutlich retardiert, wobei das Sprachverständnis wesentlich besser ist als die expressive Sprache (10 Worte).

In der Untersuchung fällt neben einer progredienten Mikrocephalie, einem Kleinwuchs eine axial betonte Hyopotonie mit Rumpfataxie und schmächtigem Muskelrelief auf. Zugleich ein mäßiger Intentionstremor; auch die Augenfolgebewegungen zeigen eine Unterbrechung der Sakkaden.

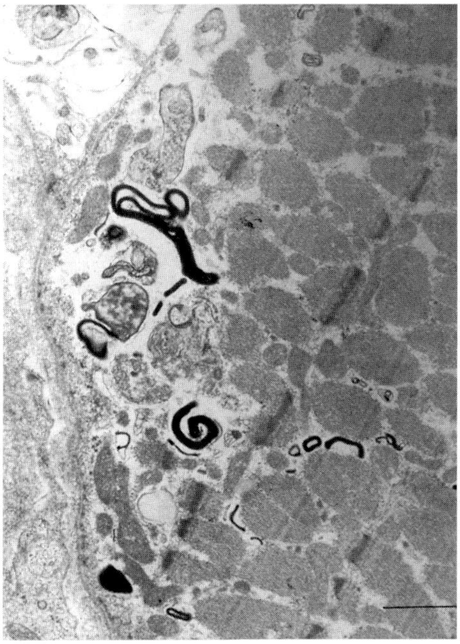

Abb. 3

Abb. 4

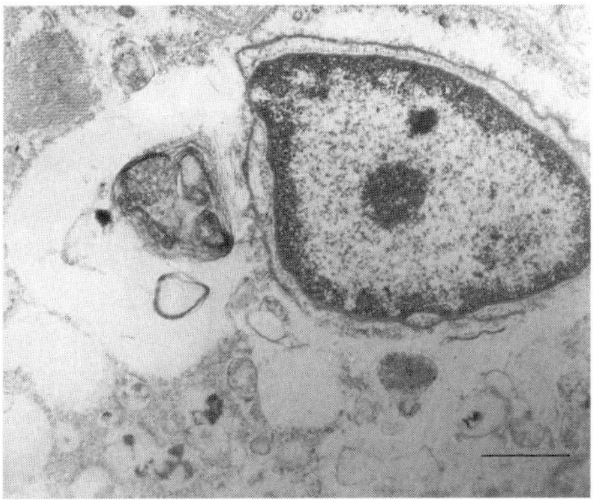

Die neurophysiologischen Untersuchungen zeigen ein myopathisches EMG mit niedrignormaler motorischer NLG. Ophthalmologisch eine geringe Katarakt beidseits. Laboruntersuchungen zeigen eine normale CK.

Das MRT zeigt primär eine generalisierte Kleinhirnvolumenminderung, die keine Progression aufweist (Abb. 1). Interessanterweise findet sich eine deutliche Signalsteigerung des cerebellären Cortex, ein Befund der bislang als charakteristisch für die neuroaxonale Dystrophie gilt, die bei unserem Patienten durch eine tiefe Hautbiopsie ausgeschlossen wurde (Abb. 2). Supratentoriell hingegen eine unauffällige Darstellung des Cortex und des Hirnparenchyms bei altersentsprechender Myelinisierungsstruktur.

Die für das Marinesco-Sjögren Syndrom typischen histopathologischen Veränderungen lassen sich bei dem Patienten erst auf der elektronenmikroskopischen Ebene darstellen. Besonders subsarcolemmal findet sich immer wieder eine Vakuolisierung des Sarcoplasmas, zum Teil mit myelinartigen Lamellen und anderen amorphen Einschlüssen (Abb. 3). Diese eine frühe Autophagozytose darstellenden Veränderungen sind unspezifischer Natur, doch ist die Differentialdiagnose im Kindesalter sehr begrenzt (Nemaline Myopathie, distale Myopathien, Einschlusskörperchenmyositis/-myopathie). Des weiteren ließ sich in unmittelbarer Nachbarschaft der Zellkerne eine schlingenartige Pseudomembranbildung darstellen (Abb. 4), die bislang nur beim Marinesco-Sjögren Syndrom beobachtet wurde. Die Natur dieser Membranen ist ungeklärt, doch scheinen sie zumindest bei diesem Patienten in Teilen von der Lamina externa des Zellkerns auszugehen.

Abb. 2

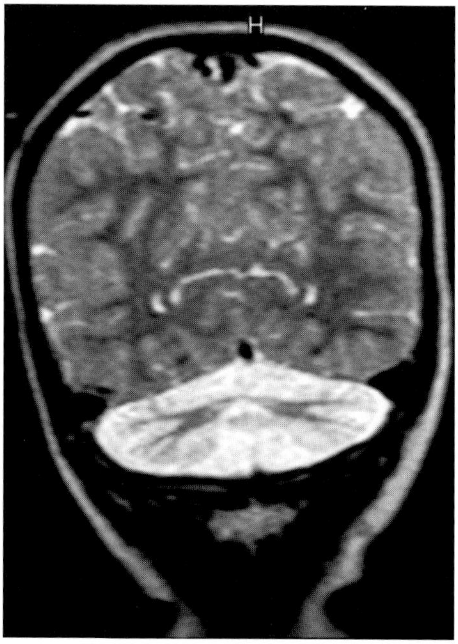

Abb. 1

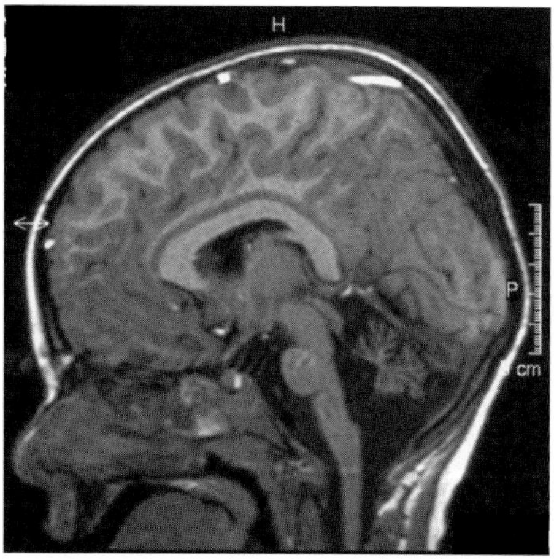

In tiefgefrorenem Muskel dieses Patienten konnten wir eine PDHc Defekt nachweisen, der bislang für Kinder mit Marinesco-Sjögren Syndrom nicht beschrieben ist (Tab. 1).

Das Marinesco-Sjögren Syndrom stellt bislang eine primär klinisch definierte Entität dar, die ein großes Spektrum an klinischen Symptomen aufweist. Eine nosologische Zuordnung ist nicht gelungen, auch wenn in der Literatur immer wieder Auffälligkeiten beschrieben finden, die zumindest eine mitochondriale Beteiligung nahe legen.

Klinisch gibt es Patienten mit Marinesco-Sjögren Syndrom, die ein Ptose oder progressive externe Ophthalmoplegie zeigen, beides Symptome die auch bei den klassischen mitochondrialen Erkrankungen als charakteristisch angesehen werden (1). Interessanterweise sind auch Patienten mit Ragged-Red Fibers oder disseminierten Cytochrom-c-Oxidase negativen Fasern in der Muskulatur beschrieben (2,3). Daneben finden sich Berichte mit elektronenmikroskopischen Veränderungen der Größe, Form und Binnenstruktur der Mitochondrien, die als charakteristisch für eine mitochondriale Erkrankung gelten (4).

Unser Patient zeigt die bislang noch nicht beschriebene Kombination eines Marinesco-Sjögren Syndroms mit PDHc Mangel, damit zum ersten Mal den direkten biochemische Nachweis einer mitochondrialen Energiestoffwechselstörung im Rahmen dieses Syndroms. Klassischerweise präsentieren sich Patienten mit PDHc Defekt entweder mit einem Leigh-artigen Krankheitsbild in der Neonatalperiode oder im Verlauf der Säuglingszeit. Demgegenüber ist eine sehr seltene Form des PDHc Defektes mit dem führenden Symptom einer episo-

Tab. 1:

	Patient		**Kontrolle**	
	mU/mg Protein	mU/U CS	mU/mg Protein	mU/U CS
NADH: Q1 Oxidoreduktase (CI)	5,4	103	5,3 – 19,6	84 – 273
Succinat:CytC Oxidoreduktase (CII+CIII)	9	161	4 – 28	40 – 285
Cytochrome C Oxidase (CIV)	53	1001	53 – 86	520 – 2080
Citrat Synthase (CS)	53		45 – 187	
Pyruvat Dehydrogenase (PDHc)	0,41	8	2,76 – 8,2	29 – 89
E3 Subunit des PDHc Komplexes	56,0	1061	68,6 – 136,9	700 – 1340

dischen Ataxie beschrieben, die zudem auch eine Myopathie oder Neuropathie haben können. Diese Entität zeigt zumindest Überlappungen im klinischen Bild mit dem Marinesco-Sjögren Syndrom.

Insgesamt passt das Krankheitsbild unseres Patient nicht zu den typischen Beschreibungen eines PDHc Mangels. Es könnte sich bei dem Jungen um eine bisher nicht beschriebene Erscheinungsform des PDHc Mangels oder aber um den ersten biochemischen Nachweis einer mitochondrialen Störung beim Marinesco-Sjögren Syndrom handeln.

Literatur

1. Berio A, Piazzi A (1996) Marinesco-Sjögren syndrome with chronic progressive ophthalmoplegia caused by presumed defective oxidative phosphorylation. *Pediatr Med Chir* 18(1):99–103
2. Torbergsen T, Stalberg E, Aasly J, Lindal S (1991) Myopathy in Marinesco-Sjögren syndrome: an electrophysiological study. *Acta Neurol Scand* 84(2):132–138
3. Kodama S, Kamatsu M, Mioshi M, Nakao H, Sakurai T. (1992) Marinesco-Sjögren syndrome with reduced cytochrome c oxidase in muscle. *Kobe J med Sci* (1992) 38(4): 245–254
4. Thorbergsen T, Aasly J, Borud O, Lindal S, Mellgren SI (1991) Mitochondrial myopathy in Marinesco-Sjögren syndrome. *J Ment Defic Res* (1991) 35(Pt2): 154–149

Schnelles Screening von Purin- und Pyrimidin-Stoffwechselerkrankungen im Urin mit Tandem Massen Spektrometrie (HPLC-MS/MS)

H. Korall, S. Wallner, M. Löffler

Zusammenfassung

Die Symptomatik von Purin- und Pyrimidinstoffwechselerkrankungen ist teilweise sehr uncharakteristisch. Wir haben unter Verwendung der HPLC und Tandem Massen Spektrometrie eine sehr schnelle analytische Methode zur Detektion der pathognomischen Metabolite aus dem Urin im MRM-Modus entwickelt. Diese Analytik ermöglicht einen hohen Probendurchsatz und eignet sich aufgrund der hohen Spezifität hervorragend für ein effektives Screening von Erkrankungen des Purin- und Pyrimidin-Stoffwechsels.

Hintergrund und Ziele

Die Klinik angeborener Erkrankungen des Purin- and Pyrimidin-Stoffwechsels ist mit Symptomen wie mentaler Retardierung, Anämie, Nierensteinen, Immundefekt, Wachstumsretardierung und Autismus sehr variabel und unspezifisch. Wir stellen eine neue Methode zum Screening der pathognomischen Metabolite dieser Stoffwechselstörungen im Urin vor.

Erkrankungen des Purin- und Pyrimidin-Stoffwechsels

A. Allgemeine klinische Symptome

- Mentale Retardierung
- Anämie
- Nierensteine
- Immundefekte
- Wachstumsretardierung
- Autismus

B. Defekte des Purin-/Pyrimidin-Stoffwechsels/Spezielle Klinik

I. PURINE

- *Hypoxanthin-Guanin Phosphoribosyltransferase Defekt (HPRT): Lesch-Nyhan Syndrom (LNS)*
  Mentale Retardierung, Choreoathetose, selbstzerstörerisches Beißen, Blut-

bildabnormalitäten (makrozytische Erythrozyten, abnormale Blutplättchen), Hyperurikämie

- *Adenin Phosporibosyltransferase Defekt (APRT)*
  Renale Koliken (Steinbildung), Harnwegsinfekte, Hämaturie
- *Adenosin Deaminase Defekt (ADA)*
  Immundefekt (zellulärer und hormoneller Immunfunktionen), Lymphopenie, erhöhte Infektionanfälligkeit
- *Xanthinurie (XDH)*
  Renale Koliken (Urolithiasis), Hämaturie, Arthritis
- *Purin Nucleosid Defekt (PNP)*
  Immundefekt (zellulläre Immunfunktionen), neurologische Abnormalitäten (verzögerte motorische Entwicklung, mentale Retardierung)

II. PYRIMIDINE

- *Dihydropyrimidin Dehydrogenase Defekt (DHPD)*
  Vergrößerte Leber, EEG-Abnormalitäten, mentale Retardierung, Nystagmus
- Dihydropyrimidinase Defekt (DHPA)
  Metabolische Azidose, Essstörungen, Krämpfe

Methode

Unter Verwendung der Flüssigkeitschromatographie und Tandem Massen Spektrometrie haben wir eine neue Methode zur Diagnose von Purin- and Pyrimidin-Stoffwechselerkrankungen im Urin entwickelt. Der Urin wurde auf einen Creatininwert von 5 mmol/L verdünnt. Nach Zugabe interner Standards wurden 35 µL des Ansatzes über eine C-18 Reversed Phase Säule (150 mm x 4.6 mm, 3 µm, Phenomenex) injiziert. Die Komponenten wurden mit 50 mM Ammoniumformat, das 38% Methanol enthielt, bei einer Flussrate von 0.9 mL/min eluiert. Das Eluat wurde mit einem PE-Sciex API 365 Tandem Massen Spektrometer unter Atmospheric Pressure Chemical Ionisation (Heated Nebulizer) analysiert. Im Multiple Reaction Monitoring (MRM) Modus wurden die MS/MS Spektren der charakteristischen Ionen erfasst (Abb. 1).

Ergebnisse

Die Analysenzeit pro Probe beträgt nur 6 Minuten und reduziert den Zeitfaktor um 5 im Vergleich zur konventionellen HPLC bei deutlich erhöhter Spezifität. Erfasst werden die für Purin-/Pyrimidin-Stoffwechselerkrankungen wegweisenden Metabolite: Uracil, Thymin, Uridin, Pseudouridin, Thymidin, 5-Hydroxymethyluracil, Xanthin, Hypoxanthin, Adenin, Adenosin, Inosin, Guanosin, Desoxyadenosin, Desoxyinosin und Desoxyguanosin. Alle erfassten

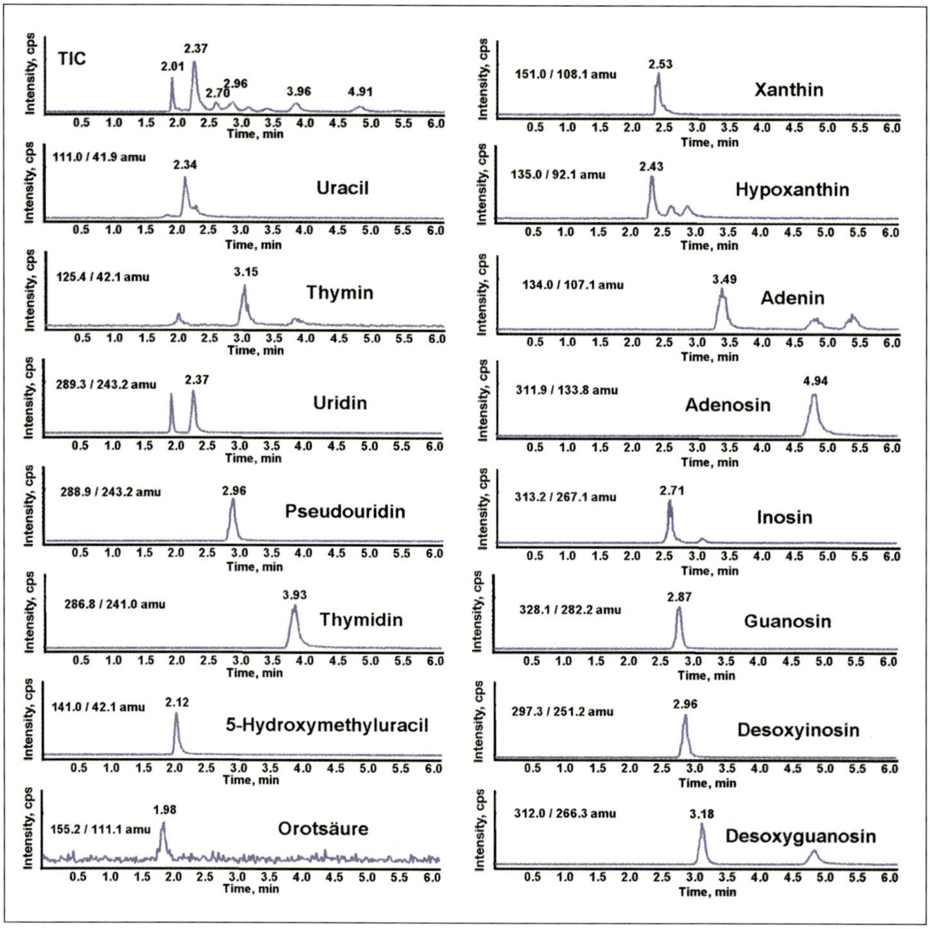

Abb. 1: HPLC-MS/MS Chromatogramme der Standardmischung von Purinen bzw. Pyrimidinen in pathologischen Konzentrationen unter Angabe der Transitions.

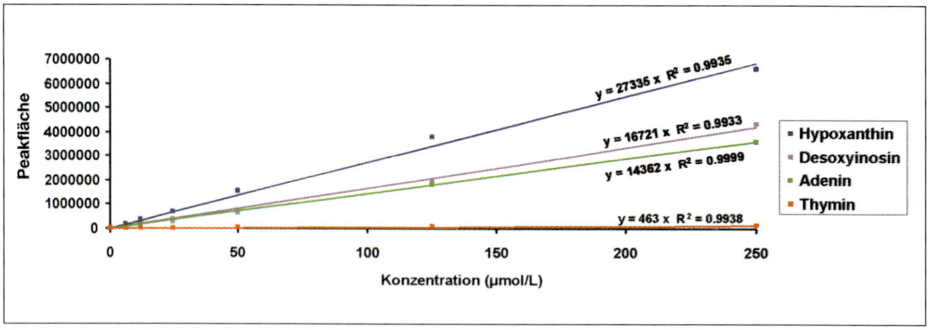

Abb. 2: Linearität der Kalibrationskurven von 4 exemplarischen Metaboliten bei 4 verschiedenen Erkrankungen.

Komponenten und deren Transitions zeigt Abb. 1. Im Urin von unauffälligen Patienten sind diese Metabolite nicht oder nur in Spuren nachweisbar. Alle Analyte zeigen eine ausgezeichnete Linearität zwischen 5 und 250 µmol/L (Abb. 2). Orotsäure ist zwar nachweisbar, zeigt aber eine schlechte Linearität bei einer unteren Nachweisgrenze von 20 µmol/L. Mit der oben gezeigten Einschränkung ist diese Methode von der Wiederfindungsrate, der Reproduzierbarkeit und Genauigkeit hervorragend für ein Massen-Screening geeignet.

Zusammenfassung

Die schnelle und leichte Probenaufbereitung sowie die hohe Spezifität der HPLC-MS/MS Detektion im MRM-Modus erlauben bei hohem Probendurchsatz ein effektives und schnelles Screening von Erkrankungen des Purin- und Pyrimidin-Stoffwechsels.

Neonatale Citrullinämie: Verbessertes Out-come durch Frühdiagnose im Neugeborenen-Screening

T. Lücke, S. Scholl, R. Heyer, M. Meder, J. Sander, A.M. Das

Zusammenfassung

Angeborene Harnstoffzyklus-Störungen wurden bislang meist erst im Rahmen einer lebensbedrohlichen Stoffwechselentgleisung mit Hyperammonämie diagnostiziert.

Wir berichten über 3 Patienten, bei denen eine neonatale Form der Citrullinämie durch das Neugeborenen-Screening mittels Tandem-Massenspektrometrie diagnostiziert wurde, bevor es zu einer metabolischen Entgleisung kam. Die psychomotorische Entwicklung der 3 Patienten verläuft dank einer frühzeitig begonnenen Therapie bislang normal. Wir halten eine Erweiterung des Screenings auf die neonatale Citrullinämie für indiziert. Eine Vorverlegung des Screeningzeitpunktes auf Tag 3 nach Geburt wird diskutiert.

Einleitung

Bei der Citrullinämie handelt es sich um eine autosomal-rezessiv vererbte Störung des Harnstoffzyklus. Aufgrund eines Defektes der Argininosuccinatsynthase kommt es zu einem Anstau des Citrullins und in Folge der mangelhaften Stickstoff-Elimination zu einer Hyperammonämie. Arginin und Harnstoff im Plasma sind häufig erniedrigt (Abb. 1) (1, 2).

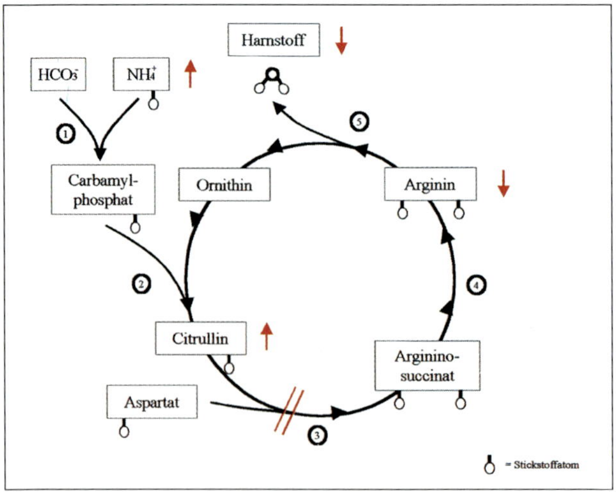

Abb. 1: Schematische Darstellung der Elimination des Stickstoffs (schwarze Anhängsel) durch den Harnstoffzyklus und biochemische Veränderungen bei einem Argininosuccinatsynthase-Mangel (rot).
Carbamylphosphat-Synthase (1), Ornithin-Carbamylphosphat-Transferase (2), Argininosuccinatsynthase (3), Argininosuccinat-Lyase (4), Arginase (5) (mit freundlicher Genehmigung von N. Albers).

Zwei Formen der Citrullinämie werden unterschieden: (1) bei der neonatalen, schwer verlaufenden Citrullinämie Typ I fehlt das Enzym in allen Körpergeweben; (2) bei der milderen Citrullinämie Typ II ist es nur in der Leber nicht nachweisbar. Den beiden Formen liegen Mutationen auf zwei unterschiedlichen Genen (Chromosom 9 bzw. 7) zugrunde (3).

Bei der *neonatalen Citrullinämie* (geschätzte Häufigkeit 1 : 57.000–250.000) entwickeln die zunächst unauffälligen Neugeborenen typischerweise in den ersten Lebenstagen eine Hyperammonämie (Plasma-Ammoniakkonzentration über 110 µmol/l) und zeigen im Verlauf eine schwere Enzephalopathie mit Verlust des normalen Reflexmusters, Hypothermie, Tachy- und Apnoen. Ohne Therapie werden die Patienten komatös und versterben häufig; bei Überleben ist mit schweren neurologischen Symptomen im Sinne eines Residualsyndroms zu rechnen (2, 3). Für die Langzeitprognose sind Dauer und Höhe der Hyperammonämie entscheidend.

Wir berichten über 3 Patienten, bei denen die Diagnose einer neonatalen Citrullinämie durch das Neugeborenenscreening mittels Tandem-Massenspektrometrie (TMS) vor oder mit Einsetzen klinischer Symptome gestellt wurde. Eine Therapie konnte rechtzeitig begonnen werden. Alle Patienten entwickeln sich normal. Befunde und Therapie der Patienten sind in Tabelle 1 zusammengefasst.

Tab. 1:

	Patient 1	**Patient 2**	**Patient 3**
Symptome (initial)	schlapp, trinkschwach tachydyspnoeisch	sepsis-ähnlich tachydyspnoeisch	schlapp, trinkschwach nie richtig wach
Screeningtermin	Tag 4	Tag 4	Tag 3
max. Ammoniak in µmol/l Norm: < 50	282	632	124
Glutamin in µmol/l Norm: < 800	1725	1776	594
Citrullin in µmol/l Norm: < 5	3496	4199	511
Diät (in 24 h)	0,8 g/kgKG nat. Protein 0,2 g/kgKG EAM 2	0,6 g/kgKG nat. Protein 0,3 g/kgKG EAM 1	1,0 g/kgKG nat. Protein 0,5 g/kgKG EAM 1
Therapie (in 24 h)	L-Arginin 140 mg/kgKG Phenylbutyrat 160 mg/kgKG	L-Arginin 340 mg/kgKG Phenylbutyrat 380 mg/kgKG	L-Arginin 63 mg/kgKG
Neurologischer Befund	**normal** (27 Monate)	**normal** (24 Monate)	**normal** (17 Monate)

Fall 1

Der männliche Patient ist das 1. Kind gesunder Eltern türkischer Herkunft. Die Eltern sind Cousin und Cousine 2. Grades. Die Mutter hatte drei Aborte. Der Junge wurde nach unauffälliger Schwangerschaft in der 41. Schwangerschaftswoche spontan geboren. Am 3. Lebenstag wurde das Neugeborene durch Trinkschwäche sowie eine Tachydyspnoe auffällig und wurde unter dem Verdacht auf eine Pneumonie antibiotisch behandelt. Im Neugeborenen-Screening konnte eine massiv erhöhte Citrullin-Konzentration nachgewiesen werden, so dass der Junge in unsere Klinik verlegt wurde. Bei Aufnahme bestand bereits eine Hyperammonämie (s. Tab.). Unter Eiweißrestriktion und einer intravenösen Therapie mit L-Arginin und Natrium-Benzoat kam es zu einem raschen Abfall der Ammoniak-Konzentration. Der Patient wurde in der 5. Lebenswoche entlassen und entwickelt sich bisher unauffällig.

Fall 2

Der männliche Patient ist das 2. Kind (2Para/4Gravida) nicht konsanguiner türkischer Eltern. Zwei Schwestern der Mutter seien im Alter von 2 und 4 Jahren an »Darminfektionen« verstorben, ein Bruder des Vaters sei mit 2 Jahren an einer »Blinddarm-Entzündung« verstorben. Die Geburt erfolgte nach vorzeitigem Blasensprung komplikationslos. Am 4. Lebenstag wurde der Patient mit einem sepsis-artigen Krankheitsbild bei Tachypnoe und sich verschlechternder Vigilanz zu uns verlegt. Im neonatalen Screening fand sich eine Citrullinämie. Zum Zeitpunkt der Diagnose bestanden bereits eine Hyperammonämie (s. Tabelle) sowie eine Tachydyspnoe. Dank der rasch begonnenen Therapie konnte das Ammoniak schnell gesenkt werden. Der Patient zeigt jetzt eine altersentsprechende Entwicklung.

Fall 3

Der männliche Patient ist das 2. Kind konsanguiner türkischer Eltern (Cousin und Cousine). Ein Onkel väterlicherseits ist im Alter von etwa 1 Jahr im Rahmen einer »infektiösen Erkrankung« verstorben. Schwangerschaft und Geburt waren unauffällig. Das Kind wurde primär wegen eines erhöhten Citrullins im Neugeborenenscreening (Tag 3) eingewiesen. Retrospektiv ergab sich, dass der Patient in den ersten Lebenstagen schlecht getrunken habe und nie richtig wach gewesen sei. Nach Diagnose-Sicherung konnte mit der Therapie begonnen werden, so dass es nicht zu einer neurologischen Symptomatik kam. Die Argininosuccinatsynthase-Aktivität in kultivierten Fibroblasten war mit 0,015 nmol/min pro mg Protein stark erniedrigt (Norm 0,15–0,75 nmol/min pro mg Protein). Der Patient entwickelt sich altersentsprechend.

Diskussion

Bei der neonatalen Form der Citrullinämie kommt es häufig im Rahmen der anfänglichen Katabolie schon innerhalb der ersten Lebenstage zu Stoffwechselentgleisungen mit Hyperammonämien, die zu schweren neurologischen Schäden oder gar zum Tode führen. Dauer und Höhe der Hyperammonämie sind entscheidend für die Langzeitprognose der betroffenen Patienten. Bislang wurde die Diagnose der neonatalen Citrullinämie häufig erst im Rahmen einer ersten Stoffwechselentgleisung oder nach gezielter Diagnostik (z.B. bei Index-Patienten in der Familie) gestellt. Die Citrullinämie, wie auch die übrigen Harnstoffzyklus-Störungen, gehört noch nicht zu den von der Arbeitsgemeinschaft für Pädiatrische Stoffwechselstörungen (APS) empfohlenen Neugeborenen-Screeninguntersuchungen (4, 5).

Seit Einführung der TMS ist allerdings ein erweitertes Neugeborenen-Screening möglich, das auch die Citrullinämie sowie einige weitere Harnstoffzyklusdefekte ohne wesentlichen zeitlichen oder finanziellen Mehraufwand erfasst (6). Es sollte jedoch zunächst die Methode der Tandem MS, wie beispielsweise im Rahmen eines Modellprojektes in Bayern bereits begonnen (7), weiter evaluiert werden. Im Rahmen des erweiterten Neugeborenen-Screenings werden sicherlich auch milde Formen gefunden, die möglicherweise überhaupt nicht entgleisen (wie z.B. unser Patient III). Bei diesen muss die Therapieindikation im Verlauf geprüft werden.

Der bisher übliche Screening-Zeitpunkt vom 4.–7. Lebenstag kann für Patienten mit Citrullinämie zu spät sein, da sich bei der neonatalen Form der Erkrankung bereits schon in den ersten Lebenstagen eine Hyperammonämie entwickeln kann. Deshalb wird empfohlen, den Zeitpunkt des Neugeborenen-Screenings nach Einführung der Tandem-Massenspektrometrie auf den 3. Lebenstag vorzuverlegen (5). Durch die Früh-Diagnose der Citrullinämie vor Auftreten einer bleibenden Hirnschädigung konnte in unseren Fällen bisher eine normale Entwicklung erreicht werden. Dies gibt Anlass zur Hoffnung, dass die Langzeitprognose auch bei der neonatalen Form durch Frühdiagnose und Frühtherapie verbessert werden kann.

Zusammenfassend zeigen wir, dass Citrullinämien im erweiterten Neugeborenen-Screening mittels Tandem-MS diagnostiziert werden können. Bei frühzeitiger Diagnosestellung und Therapie kann mit einer altersentsprechenden Entwicklung gerechnet werden. Da die schweren Formen der Citrullinämie bereits in den ersten Lebenstagen symptomatisch werden können, ist eine Durchführung des Neugeborenen-Screenings am 3. Lebenstag zu erwägen.

Literatur

1. Albers N, Schweitzer S, Byrd DJ, Offner G, Brodehl J (1996) Diagnostik und Therapie von Harnstoffzyklusdefekten. Monatsschr Kinderheilkd 144: 1078–1086
2. Bartlett K, Eaton SJ, Pourfarzam M (1997) New developments in neonatal screening. Arch Dis Child 77: F151–F154
3. Brusilow SW, Maestri NE (1996) Urea cycle disorders: diagnosis, pathophysiology, and therapy. Adv Pediatr 43: 127–170
4. Richtlinien zur Organisation und Durchführung des Neugeborenenscreenings auf angeborene Stoffwechselstörungen und Endokrinopathien in Deutschland (1997) Monatsschr Kinderheilkd 145: 770–772
5. Stellungnahme der ständigen Screening-Kommission der deutschen Gesellschaft für Kinderheilkunde und Jugendmedizin (1999) Verwendung der Tandem-Massenspektrometrie (TMS) für das Neugeborenen-Screening. Monatsschr Kinderheilkd 147: 310–311
6. Millington DS, Kodo N, Norwood DL, Roe CR (1990) Tandem mass spectrometry: a new method for acylcarnitine profiling with potential for neonatal screening for inborn errors of metabolism. J Inherit Metab Dis 13: 321–324
7. Roscher AA, Fingerhut R, Liebl B, Olgemöller B (2001) Erweiterung des Neugeborenenscreenings durch Tandemmassenspektrometrie. Monatsschr Kinderheilkd 149 : 1297–1303
8. Sander J, Janzen N, Sander S, Melchiors U, Steuerwald U (2000) Tandemmassenspektrometrie. Beitrag zum Neugeborenenscreening auf angeborene Störungen des Stoffwechsels. Monatsschr Kinderheilkd 148: 771–777

Seltene Ursache von präpubertärer Demenz und Gangstörung: Methylentetrahydrofolat-Reduktase-Mangel

T. Lücke, H. Langen, S. Illsinger, R. Heyer, A.M. Das

Zusammenfassung

Wir berichten über ein 13 Jahre altes Mädchen, das nach unauffälliger Vorgeschichte und einer normalen psychomotorischen Entwicklung im Alter von 11½ Jahren ein ataktisches Gangbild entwickelte und eine deutliche Abnahme der intellektuellen Leistungsfähigkeit mit Wortfindungsstörungen und Konzentrationsproblemen zeigte. Bei der klinischen Untersuchung fiel eine beginnende Paraspastik auf. Laborchemisch fand sich ein erhöhter Homocysteinwert im Blut bei niedrigen Methionin als Hinweis auf einen Methylentetrahydrofolat-Reduktase-Mangel. Unter Therapie mit Betain und Folinsäure trat sowohl klinisch als auch laborchemisch eine Besserung ein. Bei mentalem Abbau und Gangataxie sollte auch an den Methylentetrahydrofolat-Reduktase-Mangel gedacht werden, zumal therapeutische Optionen bestehen und ein Teil der Symptome reversibel ist.

Einleitung

5-Methylentetrahydrofolat ist Methylgruppendonator für die Vitamin B_{12}-abhängige Methionin-Synthase, die Homocystein zu Methionin remethyliert. Das entstehende Tetrahydrofolat wird über die Methylentetrahydrofolat-Reduktase (MTHFR) wieder zu 5-Methylentetrahydrofolat umgewandelt. Das gebildete Methionin wird mittels Methioninadenosyltransferase zu S-Adenosylmethionin umgewandelt, dem wichtigsten Methylgruppendonator im Zellstoffwechsel (Abb. 1).

Beim MTHFR-Mangel (MIM 236250) ist das Recycling des 5-Methylentetrahydrofolat gestört und es kommt zu einer Homocystein-Erhöhung bei niedrigen Methionin-Werten. Durch eine gesteigerte Sulfatbildung und eine Homocystin-Ausscheidung wird die Brand-Probe im Urin positiv.

Die klinischen Symptome eines MTHFR-Mangels zeigen sich zumeist im frühen Kindesalter. Bei der frühmanifesten Form kommt es zu schwerer psychomotorischer Entwicklungsretardierung, Mikrocephalie, Epilepsie und Apnoen. Bei der spätmanifesten Form stehen mentale Beeinträchtigung, Tremor, Ataxie, Gangstörungen, spastische Tetraplegie, schizophrenieähnliche Zustände, Myelinisierungsstörungen des Gehirns und cerebrovaskuläre Symptome mit Thrombembolien im Vordergrund. Es finden sich keine Blutbildveränderungen.

Die klinische Symptomatik ist variabel, der Erbgang autosomal rezessiv;

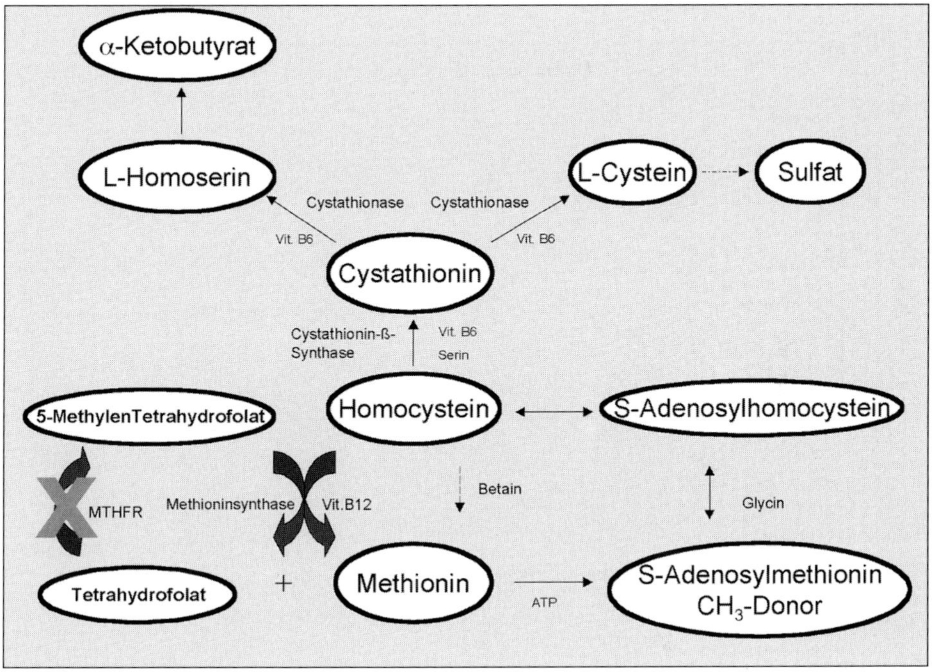

Abb. 1: Homocystein-Stoffwechsel.

unterschiedliche Mutationen im MTHFR-Gen auf Chromosom 1p36.3 sind bekannt (Goyette P et al, 1994).

Fall-Bericht

Wir berichten über ein jetzt 13 Jahre altes Mädchen, das nach unauffälliger Vorgeschichte und einer normalen psychomotorischen Entwicklung im Alter von 11½ Jahren ein ataktisches Gangbild entwickelte und eine deutliche Abnahme der intellektuellen Leistungsfähigkeit mit Wortfindungsstörungen und Konzentrationsproblemen zeigte. In der Schule kam es zu einem Leistungsabfall um 2 Schulnoten. Größe und Gewicht des Mädchens liegen über der 97. Perzentile, wobei mehrere Familienmitglieder einen Hochwuchs aufweisen.

Bei der klinischen Untersuchung fiel eine beginnende Paraspastik mit unsicherem Gangbild auf.

Laborchemisch fand sich im Blut ein erhöhtes Gesamthomocystein (217 µmol/l, NB: 5–15 µmol/l) und ein niedriges Methionin (9 µmol/l, NB: 9–40 µmol/l). Die organischen Säuren im Urin waren unauffällig, insbesondere fand sich keine Methylmalonsäureausscheidung. Das 5-MTHF im Liquor war mit 5,1 nmol/l deutlich erniedrigt (NB: 41–117 nmol/l). Im EEG fielen mittelgradige Allgemeinveränderungen und Zeichen einer umschrieben erhöhten zerebralen Anfallsbereitschaft links centro-temporo-parietal auf. Das craniale MRT zeigte eine Hirnatrophie ohne Marklager-Veränderungen. In der molekulargenetischen Untersuchung konnte ein Heterozygotenstatus für die häufige C677T-Mutation des MTHFR-Gens nachgewiesen werden.

Unter einer Therapie mit Betain (3 x 5 g/Tag) und Folinsäure (10 mg/Tag) besserte sich die Symptomatik deutlich; die schulischen Leistungen verbesserten sich, und das Gangbild wurde wieder flüssig. Laborchemisch sank das Gesamthomocystein auf Werte um 70 µmol/l (Abb. 2).

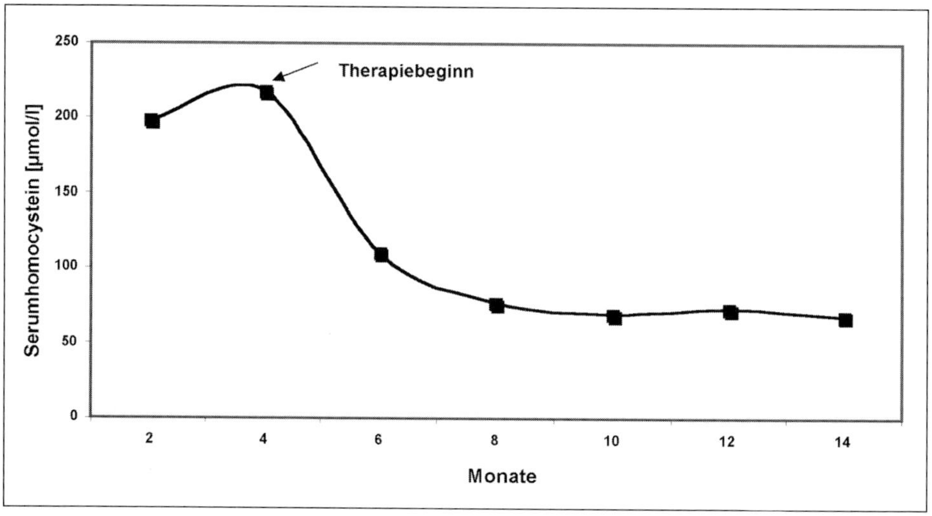

Abb. 2: Gesamthomocysteinspiegel unter Betain und Folinsäuresubstitution.

Diskussion

Im vorliegenden Fall musste aufgrund des mentalen Abbaus und des neurologischen Befundes an eine neurodegenerative Erkrankung gedacht werden. Richtungsweisend war ein erhöhtes Homocystein. Molekularbiologisch konnte eine Heterozygotie für die MTHFR-Mutation C677T gefunden werden. Wahrscheinlich liegt ein compound-Heterozygotenstatus vor, die zweite Mutation konnte bislang noch nicht identifiziert werden.

Die Pathophysiologie der Erkrankung ist bislang noch unklar. In der Literatur beschriebene Myelinisierungsstörungen werden durch einen intrazellulären Methionin- und S-Adenosylmethioninmangel erklärt (Surtees R, 1998). Zudem soll der 5-MTHF-Mangel eine Störung im Neurotransmitterstoffwechsel mit reduziertem 5-Hydroxytryptamin- und Dopamin-Umsatz bewirken (Surtees R et al, 1994). Die häufig beobachteten cerebrovasculären Veränderungen scheinen bedingt durch eine Homocystein-vermittelte Störung des Stickstoffmonoxid-Metabolismus. Dabei scheint das erhöht gemessene asymmetrische Dimethylarginin (ADMA) als endogener Inhibitor der Stickstoffmonoxid-Synthase bedeutsam (Böger RH et al, 2001). Die Erhöhung des Homocysteins scheint ferner zu neurotoxischen Effekten durch eine Überstimulation von bestimmten Glutamat-Rezeptoren, den N-Methyl-D-Aspartat (NMDA)-Rezeptoren, zu führen (Lipton SA et al., 1997).

Bei unserer Patientin konnten weder Veränderungen der Neurotransmitterkonzentrationen noch cerebrovaskuläre Veränderungen nachgewiesen werden, lediglich das 5-MTHF im Liquor war erniedrigt. Es muss also insgesamt von einer milderen Ausprägung der Erkrankung ausgegangen werden.

Ziel der Behandlung von Patienten mit MTHFR-Mangel ist die Vermeidung bzw. Verhinderung der Progredienz der Enzephalopathie, der Demenz sowie der

Gefäßkomplikationen durch Senkung der Homocysteinkonzentration im Blut. Bei der Behandlung der C677T-Mutation lässt sich in der Regel die Konzentration von Homocystein im Blut durch die Gabe von Folat wesentlich und dauerhaft senken. Zusätzlich kommt Trimethylglycin (Betain) zum Einsatz. Dieser Alternativweg der Remethylierung des Homocysteins erfolgt über die Betain-Homocystein-Methyltransferase, die in der Leber nachweisbar ist und im Gehirn fehlt. Die Wirkung im ZNS ist dann u.a. durch die mittels Therapie angehobenen S-Adenosylmethionin- und Methioninspiegel zu erklären (Neirich U & Sewell A, 1998).

Da die organischen Säuren im Urin keine Ausscheidung von Methylmalonsäure zeigten, wurde ein Therapieversuch mit Cobalamin (Vit. B_{12}), nicht durchgeführt. In unserem Fall konnte eine Reduktion der Homocystein-Konzentration im Blut, die mit einer deutlichen Besserung der klinischen Symptome einherging, durch den Einsatz von Betain und Folinsäure erzielt werden.

Konklusion

Bei mentalem Abbau und Gangataxie sollte auch an den Methylentetrahydrofolat-Reduktase-Mangel gedacht werden, zumal therapeutische Optionen bestehen und ein Teil der Symptome reversibel ist. Eine Messung des Homocysteins im Blut sollte bei diesen Patienten erfolgen. Die Tatsache, dass die MTHFR-Mutation in homozygoter Form bei ca. 5–15% der europäischen Bevölkerung vorliegen soll (Harmon DL et al., 1999), lässt vermuten, dass es sich beim MTHFR-Mangel um eine unterdiagnostizierte Erkrankung handelt .

Literatur

1. Böger RH, Lentz SR, Bode-Böger SM, Knapp HR & Haynes WG (2001) Elevation of asymmetrical dimethylarginine may mediate endothelial dysfunction during experimental hyperhomocyst(e)inaemia in humans. *Clin Sci,* 100, 161–167.
2. Goyette P, Summer JS, Milos R, Duncan AMV, Rosenblatt DS, Matthews RG & Rozen R (1994) Human methylentetrahydrofolatreduktase; isolation of cDNA, mapping, and mutation identification. *Nat Genet.,* 7, 195–200.
3. Harmon DL, Doyle RM, Meleady R, Doyle M, Shields DC, Barry RM, Coakley D, Graham IM & Whitehead AS (1999) Genetic Analysis of the thermolabile variant of 5, 10-Methylentetrahydrofolate Reductase as a risk factor for ischemic stroke. *Arterioscl, Thromb, and Vasc Biol,* 19, 208–211.
4. Lipton SA, Kim WK, Choi YB, Kumar S, D'Emilia DM, Rayudu PV, Arnelle DR & Stamler JS (1997) Neurotoxicity associated with dual actions of homocysteine at the N-methyl-D-aspartate receptor. *Neurobiol,* 94, 5923–5928.
5. Neirich U & Sewell A (1999) Methylentetrahydrofolsäure-Reduktase-Defizienz – Eine seltene Ursache progressiver Hirnatrophie. In: Bentele KHP, Kohlschütter A (Hrsg.) *Aktuelle Neuropädiatrie* 1998 Novartis Pharma Verlag, Nürnberg, 351–354.
6. Surtees R (1998) Demyelination and inborn errors of the single carcon transfer pathway. *Eur J Pediatr,* 157 (Suppl. 2), 118–121.
7. Surtees R, Heales S & Bowron A (1994) Association of cerebrospinal fluid deficiency of 5-methyltetrahydrofolat, but not S-adenosymethionine, with reduced concentrations of the acid metabolites of 5-hydroxytryptamine and dopamine. *Clin Sci,* 86, 697–702.

Zerebrovaskuläre Anomalien beim Menkes Syndrom

A. Merkenschlager, T. Pfluger, S. Springer, D. Reinhardt, A. Muntau-Heger

Zusammenfassung

Der Krankheitsverlauf und die neuroradiologischen Befunde bei einem Säugling mit genetisch gesichertem Menkes Syndrom werden dargestellt. Der klinische Verlauf nach anfänglich normaler Entwicklung war geprägt durch therapieresistente zerebrale Anfälle, Hypothermie und im Alter von einigen Monaten Entwicklungsstillstand und schließlich Regression. Die neuroradiologischen Befunde waren typisch für das Syndrom durch eine zerebrale Atrophie und mangelnde Myelinisierung, jedoch ungewöhnlich durch eine deutliche Erweiterung der venösen zerebralen Gefäße. Diese war sehr früh im Verlauf MR-angiographisch erkennbar und kann somit ein frühes neuroradiologisches Zeichen der Erkrankung darstellen.

Hintergrund

Das Menkes Syndrom ist eine neurodegenerative Erkrankung des Kupfer-Stoffwechsels (1). Gelegentlich wurde dabei eine auffällige Anatomie der zerebralen Arterien beschrieben (2). Anhand neuroradiologischer Verlaufsuntersuchungen soll dargestellt werden, dass zerebrovaskuläre Anomalien früh auftreten und auch das zerebral-venöse System betreffen können.

Material und Ergebnis

Wir berichten von einem Patienten mit einer ausgedehnten Deletion des ATP 7A Gens. Im Alter von *drei Monaten* traten zerebrale Anfälle auf, das Vollbild der Erkrankung war zu diesem Zeitpunkt noch nicht ausgebildet.

Die *Kernspintomographie* mit MRA zeigte eine Kleinhirnhypoplasie, zerebrale Atrophie und mangelnde Myelinisierung. Der auffälligste Befund bestand in einer erheblichen Erweiterung der venösen Sinus und der Vena Galeni (Abb. 1). Zum sicheren Ausschluss von arteriovenösen Fisteln wurde eine *konventionelle zerebrale Angiographie* durchgeführt.

Die zerebrale Angiographie bestätigte die venösen Anomalien, gleichzeitig wurden Elongation und Tortuositas der extra- und intrazerebralen Arterien dargestellt (Abb. 2).

Im Alter von 10 Monaten fand sich trotz Kupfer-Histidin-Therapie ein Progression der Befunde, darüberinaus hatten sich subdurale Hygrome entwickelt.

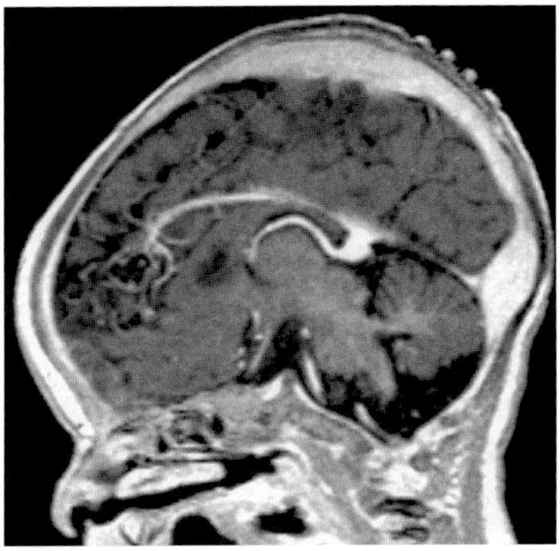

Abb. 1: MRT im Alter von 3 Monaten: zerebrale Atrophie, erhebliche Erweiterung der venösen Sinus und der Vena Galeni.

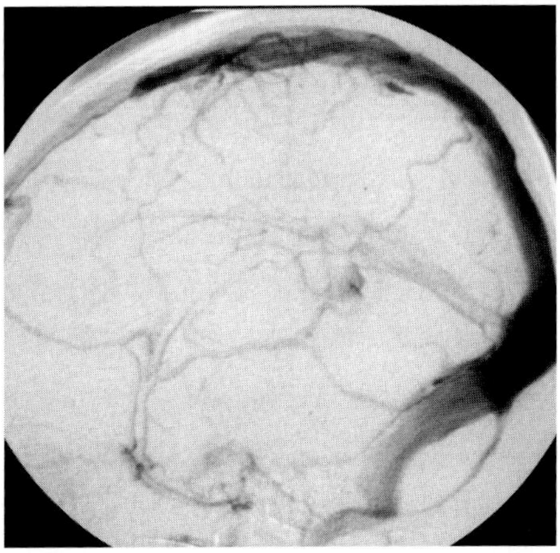

Abb. 2: Digitale zerebrale Substraktionsangiographie (Lateralansicht): Erweiterung der venösen zerebralen Gefäßen in Entsprechung zu den MR-tomographischen Befunden, Ausschluss einer arteriovenösen Fistel bzw. eines Vena Galeni-Aneurismas.

Schlussfolgerung

Beim Menkes Syndrom sind bereits früh (vor Ausprägung des klinischen Vollbildes) zerebrovaskuläre Anomalien möglich, sie können besonders das venöse System betreffen. Eine Beeinflussung der Progression durch Kupfer-Histidin scheint nicht möglich (3).

Literatur

1. Cizewski Culotta V, Gitlin JD (2001) Disorders of Copper Transport. In: Scriver CR et al. (Herausg.) The Metabolic and Molecular Basis of Inherited Disease, 8th edition. McGraw-Hill, New York.
2. Kim,OH, Suh,JH (1997) Intracranial and extracranial MR angiography in Menkes disease. Pediatr.Radiol. 27:782–784.
3. Waslen TA et al. (1995) Menkes' kinky-hair disease: radiological findings in a patient treated with copper histidinate. Can Assoc Radiol J; 46: 114–117.

Afghanische Variante einer spätinfantilen neuronalen Ceroidlipofuscinose?

V. Boda, A. Kohlschütter, S. Vlaho, M. Wesendahl, M. Kieslich

Zusammenfassung

Vorgestellt wird ein afghanischer Junge mit nachgewiesener neuronaler Ceroidlipofuscinose (NCL), dessen Befundkonstellation Schwierigkeiten bereitet ihn in eine der aktuell definierten Untergruppen der NCL einzuordnen. Am ehesten handelt es sich um eine CLN6-Variante der spätinfantilen NCL, möglicherweise jedoch um einen neuen Subtyp.

Einleitung

Die neuronale Ceroidlipofuscinose (NCL) wird z.Z. in vier Hauptgruppen eingeteilt, die nach Eintrittsalter der Erkrankung, klinischer Verlaufsform und elektronenmikroskopischem Befund verschiedener Gewebe eingeteilt werden. Zwischen diesen Hauptgruppen mit typischen Kriterien werden auch Kinder beschrieben mit überlappenden Befunden, die entsprechenden Subgruppen zugeordnet werden. In den letzten Jahren wurden für diese Gruppen jeweils zugrundeliegende Gendefekte postuliert und die Gene mit CLN1–8 bezeichnet. Von diesen Genloci konnten inzwischen sieben lokalisiert werden. Von deren Genprodukten sind sechs bekannt (1). In der Hauptgruppe der spätinfantilen NCL werden eine klassische Form (CLN 2) und 4 Varianten (CLN 1,5,6,7) unterschieden (2).

Fallvorstellung

1. Kind konsanguiner, afghanischer Eltern, unauffällige Schwangerschaft und Geburt, regelrechte Entwicklung im Säuglings- und Kleinkindalter. Ab dem Alter von 5 Jahren konsekutiv Sehstörungen, muskuläre Hypotonie, Ataxie, zunehmende psychomotorische Retardierung und schwer antikonvulsiv einzustellende fokale, sekundär generalisierende Krampfanfälle. Erworbene Mikrozephalie.

Weitere Untersuchungsbefunde: Retinitis pigmentosa-like Retinopathie, Riesenpotentiale in den SEP, deutlich verzögerte VEP, in der cMRT Signalanhebung im periventrikulären Marklager in der T2-Wichtung. Keine vakuolisierende Lymphozyten. Die Diagnose einer NCL erfolgte mit dem elektronenmikroskopischen Nachweis von kurvilinearen Profilen in Zytosomen von Schweißdrüsenzellen eines Hautbiopsates (Abb. 1, 2). Die Aktivitätsmessung des Genproduktes des CLN2-Genes (Tripeptidyl-Peptidase, TPP) wurde leicht oberhalb der Aktivität von Kontrollfibroblasten gemessen.

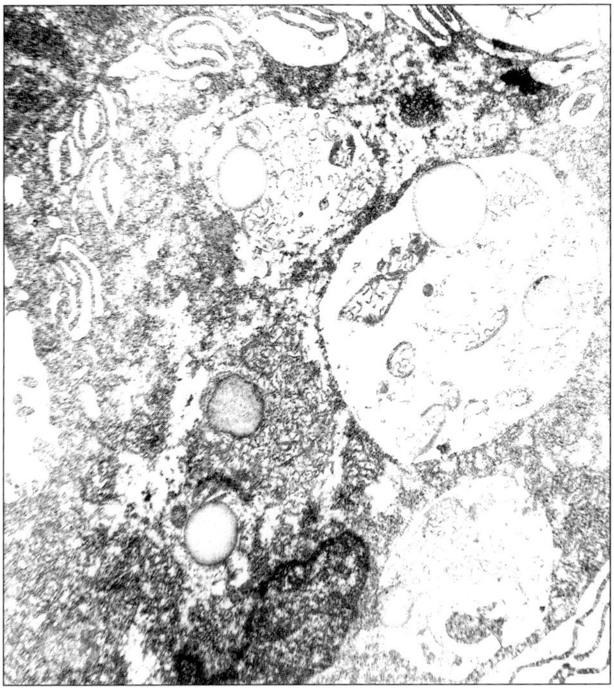

Abb. 1: Elektronenmikroskopische Darstellung von Zytosomen in Schweißdrüsenzellen eines Hautbiopsates. Nachweis von überwiegend kurvilinearen Profilen in multiplen Zytosomen.

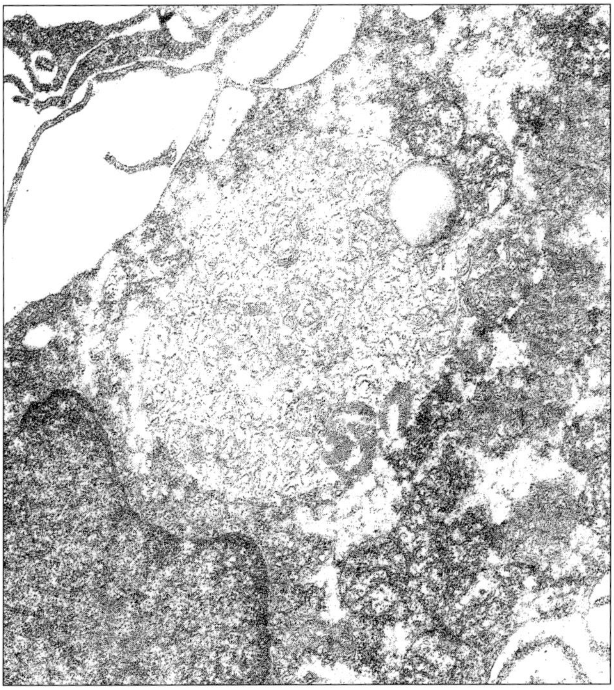

Abb. 2: In stärkerer Vergrößerung ein mit überwiegend kurvilinearen Profilen dichtgepacktes Zytosom.

Diskussion

Bei Zuordnung des Patienten in eine der NCL-Gruppen sind ausgeschlossen: 1. Eine Variante der infantilen NCL (CLN1), aufgrund des elektronenmikroskopischen Befundes (fehlende GRODs). 2. Eine klassische spätinfantile NCL (CLN2), aufgrund der nachweisbaren TPP-Aktivität. 3. Eine juvenile NCL (CLN3), aufgrund des rasch progredienten klinischen Verlaufes und fehlender vakuolisierender Lymphozyten. Die beschriebenen Varianten der spätinfantilen NCL Typ CLN5 und 7 stammen aus anderen, definierten Kulturkreisen (Finnen bzw. Türken). Die Befundkonstellation unseres Patienten deutet am ehesten auf eine Variante der spätinfantilen NCL Typ CLN6. Gegen einen Typ CLN6 spricht der elektronenmikroskopische Befund, bei der typischerweise curvilineare, rectilineare und finger-print Profile nebeneinander nachgewiesen werden. Die Gruppe des Typ CLN6 ist jedoch heterogen, was durch neue Erkenntnisse auf genetischer Ebene gestützt wird. Im erst kürzlich identifizierten verantwortliche CLN6-Gen auf Chromosom 15q21-23 (FLJ20561) wurden mindestens 6 unabhängige Mutationen bei Patienten verschiedener Kulturkreise nachgewiesen, die zu Veränderungen des kodierten transmembranären Proteins führen (3; 4). Die kulturelle Nähe unseres afghanische Patienten zu bereits beschriebenen pakistanischen und indischen Patienten mit CLN6 legt nahe, dass möglicherweise auch hier eine Form des Typ CLN6 vorliegt.

Schlussfolgerung

Der klinische Verlauf und der Großteil der Befundkonstellation unseres Patienten sprechen für das Vorliegen einer spätinfantilen NCL Typ CLN6. Untypisch ist der elektronenmikroskopische Befund. Die Untersuchung der erst kürzlich nachgewiesenen Mutationen im CLN6-Gen sollten hier eine weitere Zuordnung ermöglichen.

Literatur

1. Mole S (2002) Gene table: Neuronal ceroid lipofuscinoses. Eur J Paed Neurol 6: 129-30
2. Goebel HH, Mole SE, Lake BD (1999) Introduction. In: Goebel HH, Mole SE, Lake BD (Herausgeb.), IOS Press, 1–4
3. Gao H, Boustany RMN, Espinola JA, Cotman SL, Srinidhi L, Antonellis KA, Gillis T, Qin X, Liu S, Donahue LR, Bronson RT, Faust JR, Stout D, Haines JL, Lerner TJ, MacDonald ME (2002), Mutations in a novel CLN6-encoded transmembrane protein cause variant neuronal ceroid lipofuscinosis in man and mouse. Am J Hum Genet 70: 324–35
4. Wheeler RB, Sharp JD, Schultz RA, Joslin JM, Williams RE, Mole SE (2002) The gene mutated in variant late-infantile neuronal ceroid lipofuscinosis (CLN6) and in *nclf* mutant mice encodes a novel predicted transmembrane protein. Am J Hum Genet 70: 537–542

Niemann-Pick Typ C Krankheit assoziert mit peripherer Neuropathie

D.I. Zafeiriou, P. Triantafyllou, N. Gombakis, E. Vargiami, C. Tsantali, E. Michelakaki, M. Vanier

Zusammenfassung

Niemann-Pick Typ C (NP-C) Krankheit ist ein vererbtes neuroviszerales Leiden des Lipidakkumulationsstoffwechsels, die durch eine progressive Neurodegeneration charakterisiert ist. Wir berichten über einen 3.5 Jahre alten griechischen Patienten mit NP-C Krankheit, der mit einem langsam progredierten Verlauf im motorischen und kognitiven Bereich auffällig wurde. Die klinische Symptomatologie (Verhaltensstörungen, Ataxie, Dysarthrie, Stürze zu Boden, vertikale Blicklähmung) zusammen mit der persistierenden Hepatosplenomegalie, führte zum Verdacht einer NP-C Krankheit. Nerveleitgeschwindlichkeitsstudien demonstrierten eine milde demyelinierende periphere Neuropathie. Die Diagnose wurde mittels Cholesterolesterifications Studien gesichert.

Einleitung

Niemann-Pick Typ C (NP-C) Krankheit ist ein vererbtes neuroviszerales Leiden des Lipidakkumulationsstoffwechsels, das durch eine progressive Neurodegeneration charakterisiert ist (1). Die genetische und klinische Heterogenität der Krankheit führt zu einem erweiterten phenotypischen Spektrum je nach Manifestationsalter, Organomegalie und neurologischer Verschlechterung (2). Die wichtigsten klinischen Symptome sind frühe Hepatosplenomegalie und progrediente neurologische Krankheit. Der unterliegende zellulärer Defekt betrifft Protein NPC1 oder Protein HE1, welches zu einer intrazellulären Akkumulation des nicht-esterifiertes Cholesterols in Gehirn und anderen Organen führt (3–6). Wir berichten über einen 3.5 Jahre alten griechischen Patienten mit NP-C Krankheit, der mit einem langsam progredienten Verlauf im motorischen und kognitiven Bereich auffällig wurde.

Fallbericht

Schwangerschaft, Geburt und die neonatale Periode verliefen unauffällig. Im Alter von 2 Monaten fiel eine milde Gelbsucht mit Hepatosplenomegalie auf; extensive hämatologische, biochemische und metabolische Untersuchungen (NP-A und NP-B Testing inklusiv) führten zu diesem Zeitpunkt zu keiner definitiven Diagnose. 10 Monate vor der Aufnahme fielen progressive Verhaltensstörungen, Sprachschwierigkeiten und mehrmalige Stürze zu Boden auf. Die neurologische Untersuchung zeigte Ataxie, Dysarthrie und eine vertikale Blicklähmung

Die obengenannte Symptomatologie, zusammen mit der persistierenden Hepatosplenomegalie, führte zum Verdacht einer NP-C Krankheit. Die Knochenmarkbiopsie zeigte für eine Lipidose typische Zellen; MRI des Gehirns, sowie frühakustische, visuelle und somatosensorische evozierte Potentiale zeigten normale Befunde. Nerveleitgeschwindlichkeitsstudien demonstrierten eine milde demyelinierende periphere Neuropathie (motorische Nervenleitgeschwindlichkeit des N. peroneous 33.2 m/sec und des N. tibialis 32.0 m/sec; untere Normwerte 46.7 m/sec und 38.2 m/sec, respektiv). Die Diagnose wurde mittels Cholesterolesterifications-Studien gesichert; der Patient demonstrierte massive Akkumulation von nicht-esterifiertem Cholesterol und eine sehr niedrige intrazelluläre Esterifikation von exogenem Cholesterol (70 pmol/mg Protein; Normalwerte 2950+1000). Der Patient wurde in der NPC1 Komplementationgruppe klassifiziert, obwohl moleculare Studien für das NPC1 Gen (welches für 95% der Krankheit verantwortlich ist) negativ waren.

Diskussion

Nach unserer Kenntnis ist der beschriebene Patient einer der wenigen NP-C Fälle assoziert mit einer peripheren Neuropathie in Menschen (7–9). Die Kombination von Organomegalie und anderen progressiven neurologischen Symptomen (Demenz, Verhaltensstörungen, Ataxie, Dystonie, Stürze zu Boden), besonders eine vertikale Blicklähmung, sollte zum Verdacht einer NP-C Krankheit führen (1, 2). Die NP-C Krankheit sollte auch in der Differentiadiagnose von Patienten, die nur mit isolierter Hepatosplenomegalie und Gelbsucht auffallen, berücksichtigt werden (1). Die richtige Diagnose sollte bei der genaueren genetischen Beratung für zukünftige Schwangerschaften helfen.

Literatur

1. Kolodny EH (2000). Niemann-Pick disease.Curr Opin Hematol; 7: 48–52
2. Natowicz MR, Stoler JM, Prence EM, et al (1995). Marked heterogeneity in Niemann-Pick disease, type C. Clinical and ultrastructural findings. Clin Pediatr (Phila); 34: 190–7
3. Cruz JC, Sugii S, Yu C, et al (2000). Role of Niemann-Pick type C1 protein in intracellular trafficking of low-density lipoprotein-derived cholesterol. J Biol Chem; 275: 4013–21
4. Naureckiene S, Sleat DE, Lackland H, et al (2000). Identification of HE1 as the second gene of Niemann-Pick C disease. Science; 290: 2298–301
5. Millat G, Chikh K, Naureckiene S, et al (2001). Niemann-Pick disease type C: spectrum of HE1 mutations and genotype/phenotype correlations in the NPC2 group. Am J Hum Genet; 69: 1013–21
6. Ioannou YA (2000). The structure and function of the Niemann-Pick C1 protein. Mol Genet Metab; 71: 175–81
7. Veyron P, Mutin M, Touraine JL (1996). Transplantation of fetal liver cells corrects accumulation of lipids in tissues and prevents fatal neuropathy in cholesterol-storage disease BALB/c mice. Transplantation; 62: 1039-45
8. Hahn AF, Gilbert JJ, Kwarciak C, et al (1994). Nerve biopsy findings in Niemann-Pick type II (NP-C). Acta Neuropathol; 87: 149–154
9. Alvelious G, Hjalmarson O, Griffiths WJ, et al (2001). Identification of unusual 7-oxygenated bile acid sulfates in a patient with Niemann-Pick disease, type C. J Lipid Res; 42: 1571–7

Pontozerebellaere Hypoplasie Typ II: ein eigenartiges dyskinetisches Syndrom

D.I. Zafeiriou, E. Vargiami, E. Pavlou, A. Vardarinos, E. Giza, A. Christoforidis, P. Barth

Zusammenfassung

Die Pontozerebellare Hypoplasie (PCH) Typ 2 ist ein autosomal-rezessives Syndrom neuroradiologisch charakterisiert durch ein Kombination von zerebellärer und pontiner Hypoplasie, und klinisch durch eine ausgeprägte Bewegungsstörung mit Choreoathetose und/oder Dystonie, Mikrozephalie und schwere psychomotorische Retardierung. Wir berichten über 2 frühgeborene griechische Patienten mit PCH Typ 2 und schwerer Bewegungsstörung. Die MRI beider Patienten zeigten die pathognomonische pontozerebelläre Hypoplasie, sowie periventrikuläre Leukomalazie milden Grades. PCH Typ II sollte in der Differentialdiagnose von Säuglingen mit psychomotorischer Retardierung, Microzephalie und Choreoathetose/Dystonie berücksichtigt werden, auch wenn zusätzliche Risikofaktoren vorliegen.

Einleitung

Die Pontozerebellare Hypoplasie (PCH) Typ 2 ist ein autosomal-rezessives Syndrom neuroradiologisch sowie neuropathologisch charakterisiert durch eine Kombination von zerebellärer und pontiner Hypoplasie (1, 2). Vom klinischen Standpunkt leiden betroffene Patienten an ausgeprägter Choreoathetose und/oder Dystonie, Mikrozephalie und schwerer psychomotorischer Retardierung, die zum Tod in den ersten Lebensjahren führt. Wir berichten über 2 griechische Patienten mit PCH Typ 2 mit schwerer Bewegungsstörung.

Fallbericht

Beide Patienten waren Frühgeborene (24. und 26. Schwangerschaftswoche), wobei der erste Patient auch untergewichtig war (SGA). Die Frühgeburt wurde bei beiden Patienten durch bronchopulmonale Dysplasie (BPD), intraventriculäre Blutung II Grad (IVH), Neugeborenekrämpfe, sowie Frühgeburtsretinopathie beim ersten Patient kompliziert. Seit den ersten Lebensmonaten bis heute, im Alter von 2.5 und 4 Jahren, zeigen beide Patienten eine bizarre Bewegungsstörung mit Athetose, Dystonie und einigen Elementen von Ballismus und Parkinsonismus. Der Kopfumfang liegt unter der dritten Perzentile; keiner von beiden kann sich auf die Arme stützen, frei sitzen oder gezielt greifen. Es liegen auch ausgeprägte Ess- und Schluckschwierigkeiten vor. Die ophthalmologische Untersuchung demonstrierte Strabismus convergens und milde Vertikalblickparese beim zweiten Patienten; der erste ist praktisch blind aufgrund seiner schweren Retinopathie (fehlende ERG- und VEP Antworten). Die MRI zeigte die

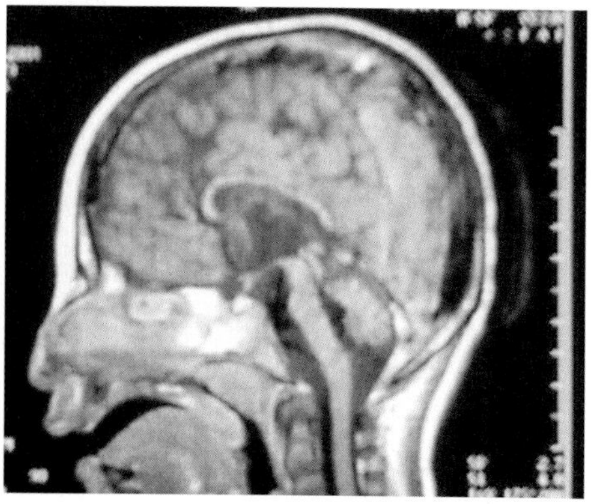

Abb. 1: Typische pontozerebellare Hypoplasie beim Patient 1. Zusätzliche Verdünnung des Corpus-Callosum.

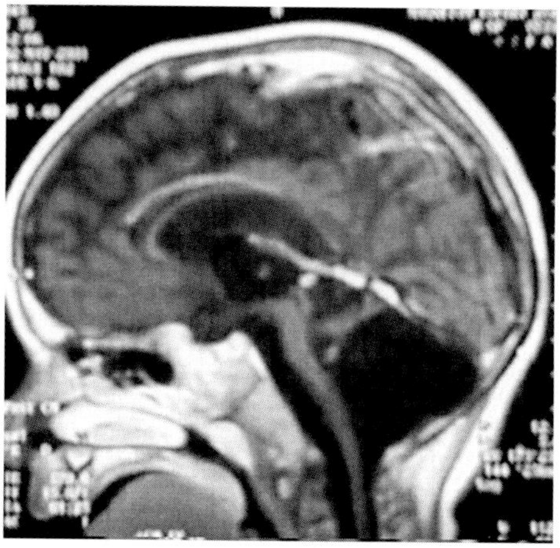

Abb. 2: Typische pontozerebellare Hypoplasie beim Patient 2. Zusätzliche Verdünnung des Corpus-Callosum.

pathognomonische pontozerebelläre Hypoplasie (Abb. 1 und Abb. 2), sowie eine periventrikuläre Leukomalazie milden Grades bei beiden Patienten. Die durchgeführte hämatologische und biochemische Diagnostik (mit besonderer Berücksichtigung von CPK, LDH, Aldolase, SGOT und SGPT), die metabolische Untersuchung (mit besonderer Berücksichtigung des Laktates, des Ammoniaks und der Aminosäuren im Serum und Urin, sowie des TBG-Tests) und das EMG, ergaben keine auffälligen Befunde.

Diskussion

Beide Patienten erfüllen die klinischen und radiologischen Kriterien einer PCH Typ II (1–5); ihre zusätzlichen Symptome war auf die Frühgeburtkomplikationen zurückzuführen. Alle anderen bisherigen beschriebenen Ursachen einer PCH (CDG Typ I-Syndrom, Merosin-negative kongenitale Muskel-Dystrophie, PCH Typ I-Syndrom mit infantiler spinaler Muskel-Atrophie, mitochondriale Enzephalomyopathie mit Störung des Pyruvatmetabolismus oder der respiratorischen Atemkette, Enzephalopathie bei Störung des Krebszyklus), könnten klinisch, biochemisch oder neurophysiologisch ausgeschlossen werden (6–8). Die PCH Typ II soll in der Differentialdiagnose bei Säuglingen mit psychomotorischer Retardierung, Microzephalie und Choreoathetose/Dystonie berücksichtigt werden, auch wenn zusätzliche Risikofaktoren vorliegen. Die Eltern solcher Patienten sollten über die infauste Prognose und den autosomal-rezessiven Erbgang frühzeitig informiert werden.

Literatur

1. Barth PG, Blennow G, Lennard HG, et al (1995). The syndrome of autosomal recessive pontocerebellar hypoplasia, microcephaly, and extrapyramidal dyskinesia (pontocerebellar hypoplasia type 2): Compiled data from 10 pedigrees. Neurology; 45: 311–317
2. Barth PG. Pontocerebellar hypoplasias. An overview of a group of inherited neurodegenerative disorders with fetal onset (1993). Brain Dev; 15: 411–422
3. Bardot C, Carneiro G, Melo J (1997). Pontocerebellar hypoplasia, microcephaly and dyskinesia: report of 2 cases. Dev Med Child Neurol; 39: 554–557
4. Coppola G, Muras I, Pascotto A (2000). Pontocerebellar hypoplasia type II (PCH2): report of 2 siblings. Brain Dev; 22: 188–192
5. Chaves-Vischer V, Pizzolato GP, Hanquinet S, et al (2000). Early fatal pontocerebellar hypoplasia in premature twin sisters. Eur J Pediatr Neurol; 4: 171–176
6. de Koning TJ, de Vries LS, Groenendaal F, et al (1999). Pontocerebellar hypoplasia associated with respiratory-chain defects. Neuropediatrics; 30: 93–95
7. Sans-Fito A, Campistol-Plana J, Mas-Salguero MJ, et al (2002). Pontocerebellar hypoplasia type 2 and Reye-like syndrome. J Child Neurol; 17: 132–134
8. Gardner RJ, Coleman LT, Mitchell LA, et al (2001). Near-total absence of the cerebellum. Neuropediatrics; 32: 62–68

11. Neurologie in Neonatologie und Intensivmedizin

Quantitative Hirndurchblutungsmessung mittels farbkodierter Duplexsonographie bei zerebral gesunden Früh- und Neugeborenen

M. Kehrer, R. Goelz, I. Krägeloh-Mann, M. Schöning

Zusammenfassung

Bei 67 zerebral gesunden Früh- und Neugeborenen wurde die Gesamthirndurchblutung (cerebral blood flow, CBF) mittels farbkodierter Duplexsonographie der extrakraniellen hirnversorgenden Halsarterien gemessen. Das CBF-Volumen stieg um durchschnittlich 6 ml/min pro Woche von durchschnittlich 33 ml/min bei einem aktuellen Gestationsalter (GA) von 34 Wochen auf 83 ml/min bei einem GA von 42 Wochen kontinuierlich an. Bei diesen Ergebnissen handelt es sich um die ersten Daten zur Gesamthirndurchblutung bei gesunden Früh- und Neugeborenen. Gegenüber anderen quantitativen Messverfahren ist die hier dargestellte Methode weder invasiv noch mit Strahlenbelastung verbunden sowie bettseitig durchführbar. Sie eignet sich somit gut zur klinischen Anwendung und zur Durchführung von Verlaufskontrollen.

Ausgangssituation und Ziel

Veränderungen der Gesamthirndurchblutung (CBF) spielen eine zentrale pathogenetische Rolle bei der Entstehung ischämischer Hirnschädigungen von Früh- und Neugeborenen (periventrikuläre Leukomalazie, hypoxisch-ischämische Enzephalopathie), die häufig zu Entwicklungsstörungen und spastischer Zerebralparese führen (Volpe 2001). Gegenwärtig kann CBF quantitativ (in *ml/100 g/min)* mit hochentwickelten nuklearmedizinischen Techniken gemessen werden, die aber gewöhnlich für die klinische Praxis nicht verfügbar sind. Die gebräuchlichste Methode, CBF bei Neugeborenen einzuschätzen, basiert auf der Messung von Blutfluss*geschwindigkeiten* in intrakraniellen Arterien mit Hilfe von dopplersonographischen Methoden. Eine signifikante Korrelation zwischen den Blutflussgeschwindigkeiten in den basalen Hirnarterien und CBF konnte von Greisen et al. (1984) nachgewiesen werden. Quantitative dopplersonographische Messungen von CBF-*Volumen* sind jedoch mit dieser Methode nicht möglich, da der Durchmesser der *intrakraniellen* Gefäße nicht bestimmt werden kann.

In der Vergangenheit konnten wir zeigen, dass CBF-Volumen (in *ml/min*) mittels Farbduplexsonographie der *extrakraniellen* hirnversorgenden Arterien bei Kindern und Erwachsenen gemessen werden kann (Schöning u. Hartig 1996, Scheel et al. 2000). Außerdem konnten wir zeigen, dass die Reproduzierbarkeit der Messergebnisse für CBF-Volumen zwischen unterschiedlichen Untersuchern (Korrelationskoeffizient $r = 0{,}90$, $p < 0{,}0001$; relative Test-Retest-Differenz $1{,}7 \pm 9{,}2\,\%$

(Schöning u. Scheel 1996)) gleichermaßen gut war wie die von CBF-Messungen mittels $H_2{}^{15}O$-PET ($r=0{,}83$, $p<0{,}001$; relative Test-Retest-Differenz $2{,}3 \pm 8{,}7\%$ (Matthew et al. 1993)). Darüber hinaus stimmten die erhobenen Normwerte mit denen, die zuvor mit invasiven Techniken erstellt worden waren, gut überein (Schöning u. Hartig 1996, Scheel et al. 2000).

Mittlerweile haben wir die Methode der quantitativen sonographischen CBF-Volumen-Messung an die kleinen Verhältnisse bei Früh- und Neugeborenen adaptiert. Ziel der gegenwärtigen Studie war es, das CBF-Volumen bei zerebral gesunden Früh- und Neugeborenen zu bestimmen und die Beziehung zum Gestationsalter zu untersuchen.

Methode

Bei 67 zerebral gesunden Früh- und Neugeborenen [35 m, 32 w, Gestationsalter bei Geburt 24+2 bis 41+6 Wochen (Mittelwert 36+1 Wochen); Gestationsalter zum Zeitpunkt der Untersuchung (GA) 34+1 bis 42+2 Wochen (Mittelwert 38+3 Wochen)] wurden die extrakraniellen hirnversorgenden Arterien farbduplexsonographisch untersucht. Alle Früh- und Neugeborenen waren am Tag der Untersuchung klinisch stabil; keines von ihnen war beatmet, benötigte Atemhilfe oder zusätzlichen Sauerstoff, keines hatte jemals im Verlauf neurologische Auffälligkeiten gezeigt. Die Schädelsonographie war in allen Fällen unauffällig. Alle Kinder waren zum Zeitpunkt der Untersuchung mindestens 24 Stunden alt (postnatales Alter 1–83 Tage (Mittelwert 17 Tage)). Von jeder GA-Woche zwischen 34 und 42 Wochen wurden mindestens 6 Kinder untersucht. Die CBF-Volumen-Messungen erfolgten an schlafenden Kindern. Die Dauer der Untersuchung beträgt 15–20 min.

Die extrakraniellen hirnversorgenden Arterien (A. carotis interna, A. vertebralis) beider Seiten wurden mit Hilfe eines 10.0-MHz-Linearschallkopfs (Apertur 26 mm) eines Computersonographiegerätes (Acuson 128 XP10) untersucht. Die winkelkorrigierte mittlere-gewichtete Flussgeschwindigkeit (TAV = time-averaged velocity) und der Durchmesser jedes Gefäßes wurden gemessen. Die intravaskulären Flussvolumina wurden als Produkt der TAV und der Gefäßquerschnittsfläche errechnet. Das CBF-Volumen wurde als Summe der Flussvolumina der inneren Karotiden und der Vertebralarterien beider Seiten ermittelt.

Ergebnisse

Von einem GA von 34 bis 42 Wochen stieg das CBF-Volumen um durchschnittlich 6 ml/min pro Woche linear an. Das mittlere CBF-Volumen bei einem GA von 42 Wochen (83 ml/min) war 2,5 mal höher als jenes bei einem GA von 34 Wochen (33 ml/min). Es fand sich eine signifikante Korrelation zwischen CBF-Volumen und GA ($r=0{,}82$; $p<0{,}0001$; Abb. 1), zwischen CBF-Volumen und Körpergewicht ($r=0{,}72$; $p<0{,}0001$) und zwischen CBF-Volumen und Kopf-

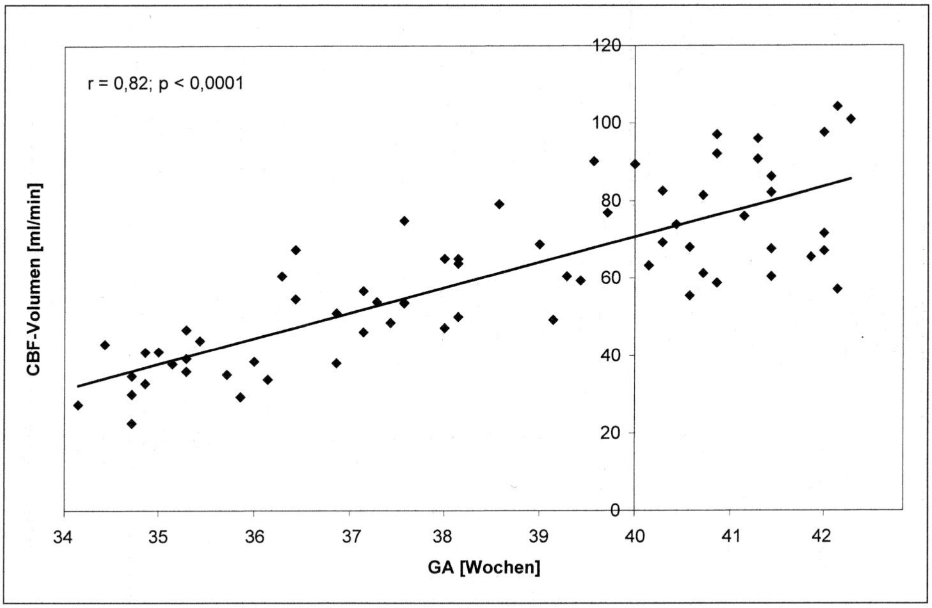

Abb. 1: Beziehung zwischen CBF-Volumen und dem Gestationsalter zum Zeitpunkt der Untersuchung (GA).

umfang (r=0,69; p<0,0001). Bei einem Reifealter von 40 Wochen betrug das CBF-Volumen durchschnittlich 70 ml/min. Ausgehend von einem normalen Gehirngewicht von 350 g bei reifen Neugeborenen beträgt die Gehirndurchblutungsrate somit 20 ml/100 g/min.

Diskussion

Die hier vorgestellten Ergebnisse stellen die ersten Werte für die Gesamthirndurchblutung bei gesunden Früh- und Neugeborenen dar. Aus ethischen Gründen sind Hirndurchblutungsmessungen mit nuklearmedizinischen Techniken nur bei Früh- und Neugeborenen mit bedeutsamen klinischen und neurologischen Problemen zur Anwendung gekommen. Altman et al. (1988) berichten über CBF-Messungen mittels $H_2{}^{15}O$-PET bei Neugeborenen, die postnatal neurologische Auffälligkeiten zeigten. Acht der untersuchten Neugeborenen erwiesen sich bei Verlaufskontrolluntersuchungen als neurologisch und/oder kognitiv normal; die CBF-Werte dieser Neugeborenen stimmen mit den Ergebnissen unserer Studie überein.

Da die hier dargestellte Methode nicht-invasiv, unschädlich und insbesondere nicht radioaktiv belastend ist, ist sie besonders geeignet für die Untersuchung von Früh- und Neugeborenen. Ferner ist die Methode bettseitig einsetzbar und für Verlaufsuntersuchungen der Gesamthirndurchblutung geeignet. Die weitreichende Verfügbarkeit der notwendigen technischen Ausrüstung erleichtert die

Einführung der sonographischen CBF-Volumen-Messmethode in die klinische Praxis. Zuverlässige Ergebnisse können jedoch nur erzielt werden, wenn eine exakte Untersuchungstechnik beachtet wird (Schöning und Scheel 1996). Dieser methodische Ansatz eröffnet neue Möglichkeiten, Veränderungen von CBF-Volumen unter pathologischen Umständen zu überwachen.

Danksagung

Die Studie wird durch die Reinhold-Beitlich-Stiftung gefördert.

Literatur

1. Altman DI, Powers WJ, Perlman JM, Herscovitch P, Volpe SL, Volpe JJ. (1988) Cerebral blood flow requirement for brain viability in newborn infants is lower than in adults. Ann Neurol 24: 218–226
2. Greisen G, Johansen K, Ellison PH, Fredriksen PS, Mali J, Friis-Hansen B. (1984) Cerebral blood flow in the newborn infant: comparison of Doppler ultrasound and 133-xenon clearance. J Pediatr 104: 411–418
3. Matthew E, Andreason P, Carson RE, Herscovitch P, Pettigrew K, Cohen R, King C, Johanson CE, Paul SM (1993) Reproducibility of resting cerebral blood flow measurements with $H_2{}^{15}O$ positron emission tomography in humans. J Cereb Blood Flow Metab 13: 748–754
4. Scheel P, Ruge C, Petruch UR, Schöning M. (2000) Color duplex measurement of cerebral blood flow volume in healthy adults. Stroke 31: 147–150
5. Schöning M, Hartig B. (1996) Age dependence of total cerebral blood flow volume from childhood to adulthood. J Cereb Blood Flow Metab 16: 827–833
6. Schöning M, Scheel P. (1996) Color duplex measurement of cerebral blood flow volume: intra- and interobserver reproducibility and habituation to serial measurements in normal subjects. J Cereb Blood Flow Metab 16: 523–531
7. Volpe JJ (2001) Neurology of the newborn, 4th ed. WB Saunders, Philadephia, PA, USA

Herzfrequenzvariabilität bei schwerstkranken Neugeborenen unter Extrakorporaler Membran Oxygenierung (ECMO) im Verlauf – 2 Kasuistiken

E. Longin, M. Teich, T. Schaible, S. Demirakca, St. König

Zusammenfassung

Schwere kardio-respiratorische Erkrankungen führen zu einer Einschränkung der Herzfrequenzvariabilität (HFV). Dies wird als eine durch Krankheit induzierte Imbalance im autonomen Nervensystem interpretiert. Im Zuge der Genesung scheinen diese Veränderungen reversibel. Ziel dieser Studie war die Analyse der HFV bei schwerstkranken Neugeborenen unter ECMO-Therapie und während Erholung. Wir zeichneten täglich während und nach ECMO-Therapie über jeweils 15 Minuten computergestützt die EKG- und Respirationskurven auf. Daraus berechneten wir sowohl statistische als auch spektralanalytische Parameter der HFV. Beide Kinder zeigten zu Beginn der Erkrankung eine erhebliche Einschränkung aller Parameter der HFV, im Verlauf kam es mit zunehmender klinischer Erholung zu einer Zunahme der HFV. Es bleibt zu klären, inwieweit diesen Veränderungen der HFV ein prognostischer Aussagewert zugewiesen werden kann.

Einleitung

Die Herzfrequenzvariabilität (HFV) wird definiert als die Schwankungen der Länge aufeinanderfolgender RR-(Zacken)-Intervalle. Diese physiologischen Oszillationen entstehen aufgrund modulierender Einflüsse wie Atmung (Respiratorische Sinusarrhythmie), Blutdruckschwankungen aufgrund des Barorezeptorreflex sowie thermoregulatorischer Einflüsse. Schwere kardiorespiratorische Erkrankungen führen zu einer Einschränkung der HFV, was eine Beeinträchtigung des autonomen Nervensystems widerspiegelt. Zwei Fallberichte demonstrieren den Verlauf der HFV bei schwerstkranken Neugeborenen unter ECMO-Therapie und während der Erholungsphase.

Methoden

Die Erfassung der HFV erfolgte während und nach ECMO-Therapie. Es wurden jeweils über 15 Minuten das EKG und die Respirationskurve aufgezeichnet. Daraus wurden folgende Parameter der HFV berechnet: Statistisch: Mittelwert, Standardabweichung, RMSSD (root mean square of successive differences), VK (Variationskoeffizient), E/I-Quotient (Expiratorisch/Inspiratorische-Quotient). Weiterhin wurden die Frequenzleistungs-Spektren folgender Frequenzbänder ermittelt: High Frequency (HF): 0,2–1 Hz, Low Frequency (MF): 0,05–0,2 Hz, Very Low Frequency (LF): 0,01–0,05 Hz u. TOTAL: 0,01–1 Hz.

Patient 1

Hierbei handelt es sich um ein weibliches Neugeborenes (GG: 3100 g; 39 SSW) mit linkseitiger konnataler Zwerchfellhernie. Veno-arterielle (VA)-ECMO-Therapie war ab dem 2. Lebenstag wegen kardio-respiratorischer Insuffizienz erforderlich.

Im Vergleich der Mittelwerte während (12 Messungen) und nach ECMO (5 Messungen) zeigt sich eine Zunahme für alle berechneten Parameter der HFV (Abb. 1 u. 2) .

Die Abbildungen 3 und 4 stellen die Einschränkung und Zunahme der HFV im Verlauf anhand des Tachogramms für eine typische Beispielmessung dar.

Auch innerhalb der Frequenzleistungsspektren (FFT) (Abb. 5 und 6) ist im Vergleich während u. nach ECMO eine Leistungszunahme sichtbar.

Patient 2

Männliches reifes Neugeborenes (GG: 3500 g; 37 SSW). VA-ECMO-Therapie seit dem 1. Lebenstag bei Mekoniumaspirationssyndrom. Auch bei diesem Patient zeigt sich im Vergleich der Mittelwerte während (10 Messungen.) und nach ECMO (8 Messungen) eine Zunahme für alle berechneten Parameter der HFV (Abb. 7 u. 8).

Auch die Poincare-Diagramme (Abb. 9 u. 10) zeigen am Beispiel jeweils einer Messung während und nach ECMO-Therapie eine Zunahme der HFV nach ECMO.

Diskussion

Beide Kinder zeigten zu Beginn der Erkrankung eine erhebliche Einschränkung der HFV, im Verlauf kam es mit zunehmender klinischer Erholung zu einem Anstieg der Parameter der HFV. Diese Zunahme entspricht jedoch weiterhin einer erheblichen Beeinträchtigung der HFV im Vergleich mit gesunden Neugeborenen. Es bleibt zu klären, inwieweit diesen Veränderungen der HFV ein prognostischer Aussagewert zugewiesen werden kann.

Literatur

1. Griffin M, Scollan D, Morrman J (1994) The Dynamic Range of Neonatal Heart Rate Variabiltiy. J Cardiovasc Electrophysiol 5: 112–124.
2. Rosenstock EG, Cassuto Y, Zmora E (1999) Heart rate variability in the neonate and infant: analytical methods. Physiological and clinical observations. Acta Paediatr 88:477–82
3. Jenkins JG, McC Reid M, McClure BG (1980) Study of heart rate variability in sick newborn infants. Acta Paediatr Scand 69:393–6

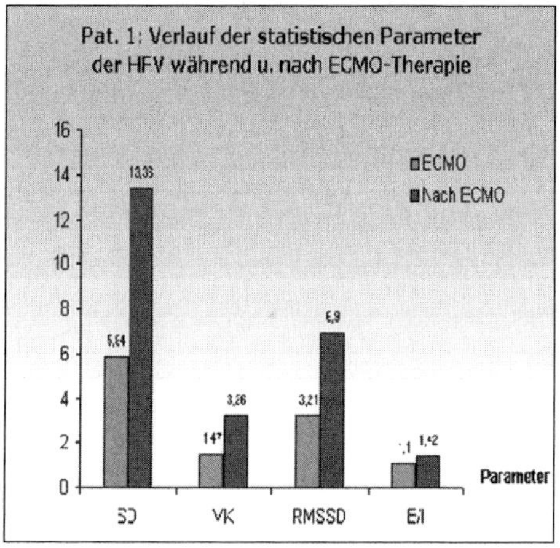

Abb. 1

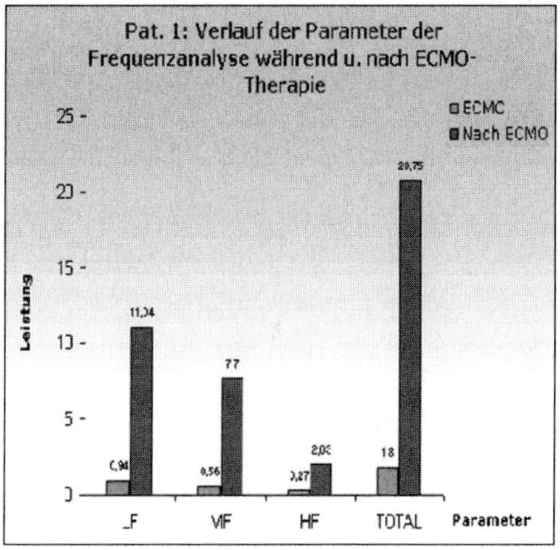

Abb. 2

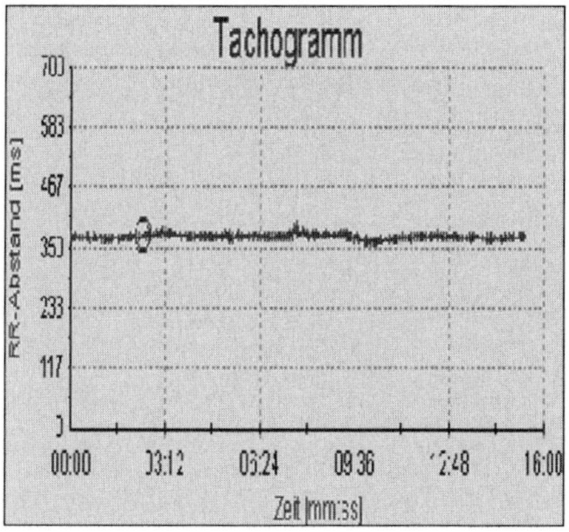

Abb. 3: Beispielmessung Patient 1: Tachogramm unter ECMO-Therapie.

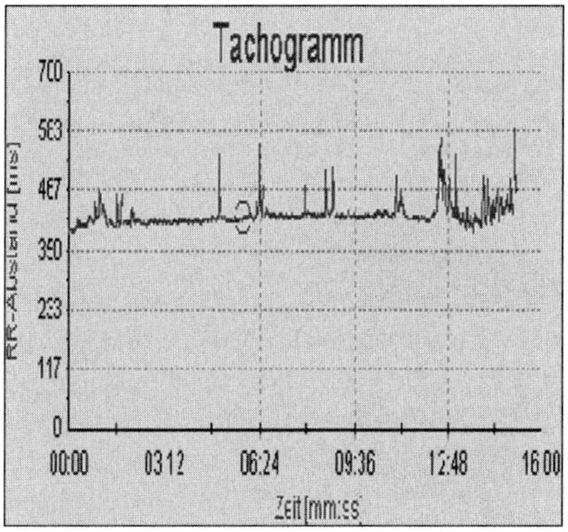

Abb. 4: Beispielmessung Patient 1: Tachogramm nach ECMO-Therapie.

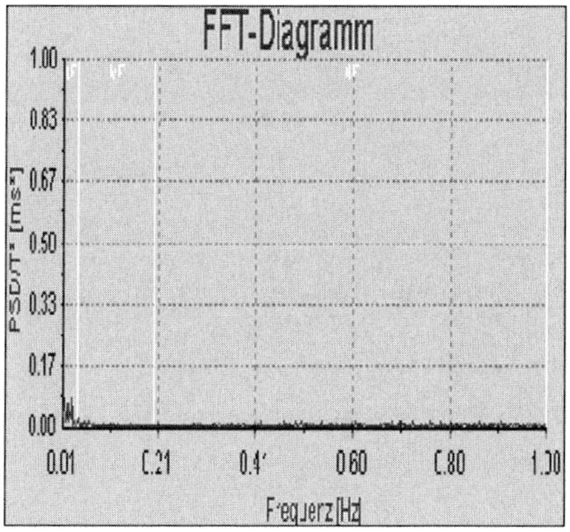

Abb. 5: Beispielmessung Patient 1: FFT-Analyse unter ECMO-Therapie.

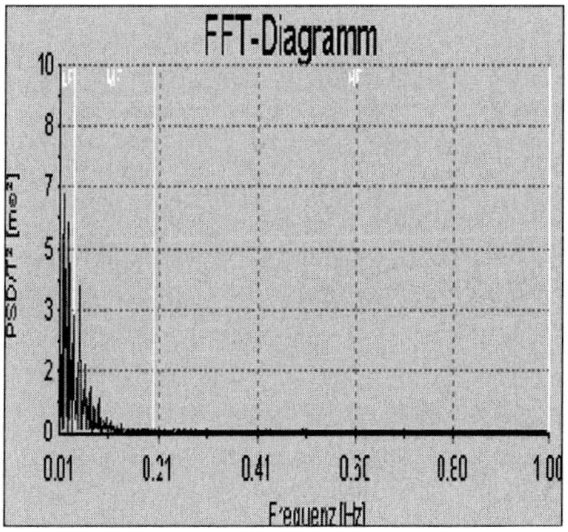

Abb. 6: Beispielmessung Patient 2: FFT-Analyse nach ECMO-Therapie.

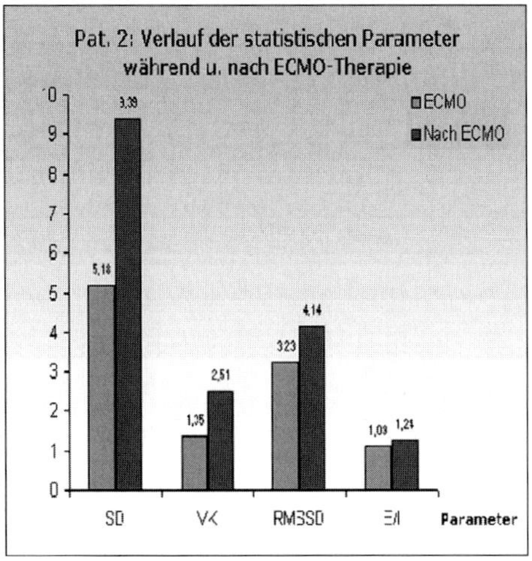

Abb. 7

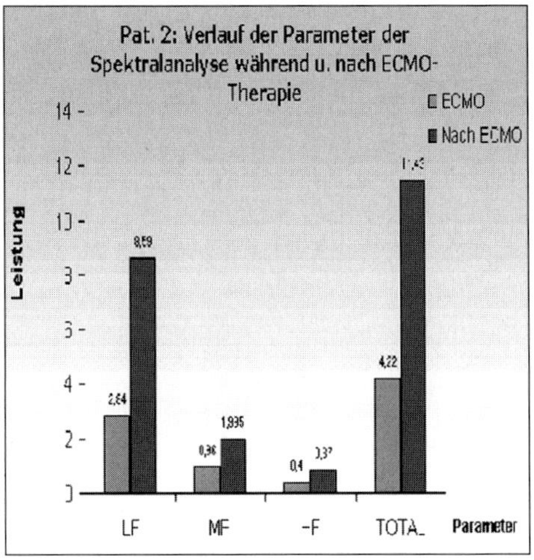

Abb. 8

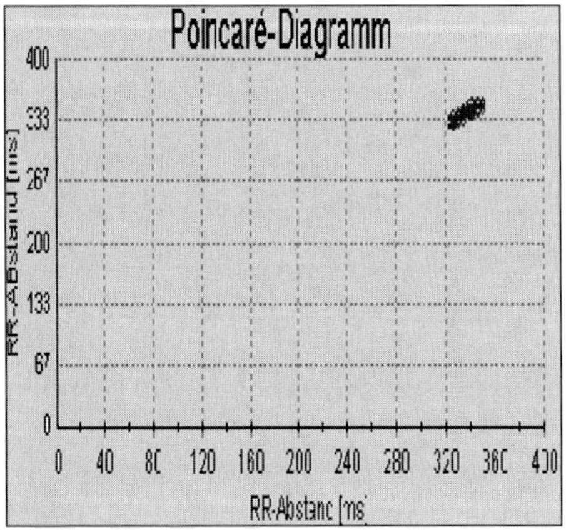

Abb. 9: Beispielmessung Patient 2: Poincaré-Diagramm unter ECMO-Therapie.

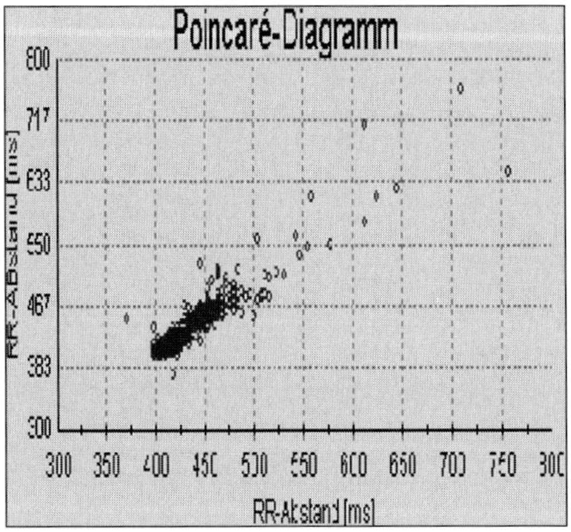

Abb. 10: Beispielmessung Patient 2: Poincaré-Diagramm nach ECMO-Therapie.

Epileptische Anfälle bei Frühgeborenen nach Gabe von Midazolam

B. v. Maydell, R. Korinthenberg, M. Krüger

Zusammenfassung

Wir stellen drei Frühgeborene vor, bei denen es nach intravenöser Einzelgabe von Midazolam zum Auftreten von Krampfanfällen kam. Basierend auf dieser klinischen Erfahrung und tierexperimentellen Daten plädieren wir für einen zurückhaltenden Einsatz von Benzodiazepin-, insbesondere Midazolam-Einzelgaben bei sehr kleinen Frühgeborenen.

Einleitung

Midazolam wird als kurzwirksames Benzodiazepin zur Sedierung in der Neonatologie verwendet. Midazolam hat in der Regel eine Halbwertszeit von ca. 2 Stunden, wobei diese bei Frühgeborenen aufgrund der funktionellen Unreife von Leber und Niere verlängert ist. Das Medikament ist wasserlöslich. Eine gefürchtete Komplikation stellt die Atemdepression dar. Zur Sedierung werden in der Regel Einzeldosen zwischen 0,05–0,2 mg / kg KG verwandt, bei beatmeten Patienten gegebenenfalls höhere Dosen. Einzelfälle sind beschrieben, in denen durch Midazolam bei Neugeborenen epileptische Anfälle ausgelöst wurden (1). Wir stellen drei Frühgeborene vor, bei denen es nach intravenöser Gabe von Midazolam zum Auftreten von Krampfanfällen kam.

Patienten

Die nachfolgende Tabelle fasst die klinischen Daten der Patienten zusammen. Die Anfälle ereigneten sich jeweils innerhalb von wenigen Minuten nach intravenöser Einzelgabe des Midazolams. Laborchemisch zeigten sich keine akuten metabolischen oder infektiologischen Ursachen für die Krampfanfälle. Alle drei Kinder hatten keine Anfälle in der Voranamnese und keine Anfälle im weiteren Verlauf, wobei Patient 2 vier Stunden nach dem ersten Anfall einen weiteren kurzen Anfall hatte, welcher im EEG dokumentiert wurde.

Zusammenfassung

Wir gehen davon aus, dass die Krampfanfälle bei diesen Frühgeborenen durch Midazolam ausgelöst worden sind, da sie sich kurz nach der i.v.-Gabe ereig-

Tab. 1:

	Patient 1 (JH)	Patient 2 (CE)	Patient 3 (JE)
Gestationsalter	22 + 6/7	24 + 5/7	25 + 3/7
Geburtsgewicht	540 g	530 g	1060 g
Voranamnese	Z.n. Amnioninfektionssyndrom, Z.n. Atemnotsyndrom, BPD II	Z.n. Atemnotsyndrom, BPD, offener Duktus. 2 Tage vor Anfall Diagnose einer Serratiensepsis.	Z.n. neonataler Sepsis, Z.n. Atemnotsyndrom, schwere BPD II-III, Apnoe-Bradykardie-Syndrom. Z.n. offenem Duktus mit Indometacin-Therapie
Neurologische Charakteristika	Konnatale nasale Enzephalozele mit nasaler Liquorrhoe, Deckung der Zele 4 Tage nach dem Anfall	Im weiteren Verlauf hyperexcitabel, allg. Hypotonie	Leichte muskuläre Hypotonie und Hyperexcitabilität
Vitalparameter	Zum Zeitpunkt des Anfalles kreislaufstabil und spontanatmend.	Zum Zeitpunkt des Anfalles intubiert und beatmet, jedoch kreislaufstabil.	Zum Zeitpunkt des Anfalles intubiert und beatmet. Kreislaufstabil bei geringem Katecholaminbedarf.
Bildgebung	CT/ MRT: frontale Enzephalozele Sono Schädel: IVH II und PVL rechts, IVH I links	Sono Schädel altersentsprechend normal	Sono Schädel: IVH I-II rechts, im Verlauf milde periventrikuläre Hyperechogenität bds.
Alter / Gewicht zum Zeitpunkt der Anfälle	90 Tage / 1820 g	36 Tage /680 g	29 Tage / 1200 g
Midazolam-Einzeldosis	0,15 mg/kg KG, (Sedierung für MRT)	0,15 mg/kg KG (Sedierung bei Unruhe unter Beatmung)	0,33 mg/kg KG (Sedierung bei Unruhe unter Beatmung)
Morphe und Dauer der Anfälle	Gen. klonisch (re>li.), 40 Minuten	Gen. klonisch, ca. 20 Min.	Kloni beider Arme, 3 Minuten
Therapie	22 mg/kg KG Phenobarbital, Sistieren erst nach 2 x 2 µg Flumazenil	23 mg/kg KG Phenobarbital	keine
EEG	EEG während des Anfalls mit generalisiertem Anfallsmuster	EEG 4 Stunden nach dem Anfall, dabei erneuter Anfall für 1 Min mit generalisiertem Anfallsmuster	EEGs eine Woche sowie 6 Wochen nach Anfall unauffällig.

neten. Zusätzlich wird diese Annahme dadurch gestützt, dass der Krampf beim ersten Patienten erst durch die Gabe des Benzodiazepinantagonisten Flumazenil beendet wurde. Diese Beobachtungen sind bemerkenswert, da Midazolam üblicherweise nicht eine prokonvulsive, sondern eine starke antikonvulsive Wirkung zugeschrieben wird.

Midazolam erhöht die Affinität des $GABA_A$-Rezeptors für GABA. Der $GABA_A$-Rezeptor stellt primär einen Kanal für Chloridionen dar. In Anwesenheit von $GABA_A$ öffnet sich der Chloridkanal, es entsteht ein inhibitorisches Potential. Benzodiazepine erhöhen die Frequenz der Öffnung des Chloridkanals und verstärken somit die $GABA_A$-Wirkung (2). Es muss vermutet werden, dass Midazolam bei jungen Frühgeborenen auf Neurotransmitter- oder Ionenkanalebene oder durch Änderung des zerebralen Blutflusses andere Nebenwirkungen hat als bei älteren Kindern. Dies steht in Übereinstimmung mit tierexperimentellen Untersuchungen, bei denen eine $GABA_A$-Aktivierung im neonatalen Rattenhirn aufgrund eines altersspezifisch umgekehrten Chloridgradienten zu einer Depolarisation führte, da bei neonatalen Neuronen intrazellulär eine höhere Chloridkonzentration besteht als extrazellulär (3).

Ein aktueller Cochrane-Review befasst sich kritisch mit der Sedierung von Neonaten auf der Intensivstation durch eine Midazolam-Dauerinfusion (4). Die Studie kam zu dem Schluss, dass eine Midazolam Dauerinfusion bei Frühgeborenen nicht befürwortet werden kann, da definitive Aussagen über die Effizienz und das Sicherheitsprofil nicht getroffen werden konnten.

Flumazenil ist ein kompetitiver Benzodiazepin-Antagonist, der parenteral appliziert werden muss. Die Wirkung setzt innerhalb von 1–3 Minuten ein. Da die Wirkdauer mit ca. 2 Stunden relativ kurz ist, besteht bei nachlassender Wirkung des Flumazenils die Möglichkeit einer Resedierung durch die zuvor gegebenen Benzodiazepine. Flumazenil weist als Nebenwirkung Übelkeit, Erbrechen, Unruhe, Angstsymptomatik und die Gefahr einer Benzodiazepin-Entzugssymptomatik bei vorheriger Benzodiazepin-Dauertherapie auf (5). Besteht der Verdacht, dass ein Krampfanfall durch Benzodiazepine ausgelöst wurde, sollte die Krampfunterbrechung mit Flumazenil versucht werden. Die Beendigung des Krampfes durch Flumazenil bei unserem ersten Patienten ist letztendlich nicht beweisend, jedoch ein starker Hinweis für die prokonvulsive Wirkung des Midazolams. Flumazenil wird in der Pädiatrie in einer Dosis von 0,01 mg/kg Kg eingesetzt (6). Bei unserem Patienten führte eine wesentlich geringere Dosis zum Sistieren des Anfalls.

Auffällig ist, dass die oben beschriebenen Anfälle alle bei Kindern mit extremer Frühgeburtlichkeit auftraten, auch wenn die Kinder bei Auftreten der Anfälle bereits zwischen 29–90 Tagen alt waren. Wir möchten zusammenfassend dafür plädieren, mit Einzelgaben von Midazolam bei jungen Frühgeborenen sehr restriktiv zu verfahren und eher auf andere Sedativa wie zum Beispiel Fentanyl zurückzugreifen.

Literatur

1. Montenegro MA, Guerriero MM, Caldas JPS, Moura-Ribeiro MVL, Guerriero CAM (2001). Epileptic manifestations induced by midazolam in the neonatal period. Arq Neuropsiquiatr; 59, (2A):242–243
2. Homan RW, Rosenberg HC (1996). Benzodiazepines. In: Wyllie E, The treatment of epilepsy: principles and practice. 2 Aufl.,Williams and Wilkins, Baltimore, 865–83
3. Owens DF, Boyce LH, Davis MBE, Kriegstein AR (1996). Excitatory GABA responses in embryonic and neonatal cortical slices demonstrated by gramicidin perforated-patch recordings and calcium imaging. The Journal of neuroscience,16(20):6414–6423
4. Ng E, Taddio A, Ohlsson A (2001). Intravenous midazolam infusion for sedation of infants in the neonatal intensive care unit (Cochrane review). In: The Cochrane Library, Issue 3, Oxford: Update Software.
5. Karow T, Lang R (1994). Allgemeine und spezielle Pharmakologie und Toxikologie, S. 261
6. Nicholson JF, Pesce MA. (1996). Laboratory testing and reference values in infants and children. In Behrman I, Richard E, Arvin AM (Herausg). Nelson textbook of pediatrics. 15. Auflage, W.B. Saunders, Philadelphia

Ischämischer Hirninfarkt bei einem Neugeborenen assoziiert mit Apolipoprotein(a) G121A Polymorphismus

C. Härtel, S. Schilling, U. Nowak-Göttl, J. Sperner

Einleitung

Der ischämische Hirninfarkt ist ein seltenes Ereignis im frühen Kindesalter mit einer Inzidenz von 1–13/100.000 pro Jahr. Die Hirninfarktlokalisation betrifft in erster Linie das Versorgungsgebiet der Arteria cerebri media, wobei unilaterale Hirninfarkte 4–5mal häufiger auftreten als bilaterale Hirninfarkte (1, 2).

Neben zerebrovaskulären Traumata, Infektionen, Gefäßanomalien und angeborenen Herzfehlern werden zunehmend prothrombotische Risikofaktoren (APC-Resistenz, Mangel an Protein C, S und Antithrombin, Homocysteinurie und auch erhöhte Werte für Lipoprotein (Lp) a (antifibrinolytische Aktivität) als Ursachen für ischämische Hirninfarkte im Kindesalter diskutiert (3). Lp (a) hat mit dem LDL (low density lipoprotein) den vergleichbar hohen Cholesterinanteil bzw. das Vorhandensein von einem Molekül Apolipoprotein B (apo) B gemeinsam. Zusätzlich enthält Lp (a) ein Proteinmolekül apo (a), das eine Proteasen-Domäne (Kringle V-like domain) enthält, die in ihrer Anzahl variieren kann (Kringle IV repeats) und strukturelle Homologien zum Plasminogen aufweist. Erhöhte Werte für Lp (a) sind genetisch festgelegt (plasmatische Ebene Kringle IV Repeats <28; genetisch Apolipoprotein (a) G121 A Polymorphismus) (4).

Der illustrative Fall eines Neugeborenen mit bilateralem ischämischem Hirninfarkt im Versorgungsgebiet beider Aa. cerebri mediae bei Apolipoprotein (a) G121 A Polymorphismus als thrombophilem Riskofaktor wird beschrieben.

Fallbericht

Ein weiblicher Säugling nicht-konsanguiner Eltern wurde uns im Alter von 4 Wochen mit Schreiattacken und Opisthotonus vorgestellt. Die Schwangerschaft wurde als unauffällig beschrieben, das Neugeborene war gut gediehen. Fieber, Trinkschwäche oder ein Trauma bestanden nicht. Der internistische Befund erwies sich als unauffällig, während neurologisch ein deutlicher Opisthotonus mit Hyperexzitabilität und gesteigerte Muskeleigenreflexe der unteren Extremität auffielen. In der schädelsonographischen Untersuchung zeigten sich bilaterale periventrikuläre Echoanreicherungen. Das MRT des Gehirns wies ausgedehnte Residualbefunde bilateraler Hirninfarkte im Versorgungsgebiet der Aa. cerebri mediae auf (Abb. 1). Das EEG zeigte bilateral frontotemporale epileptische Aktivität. Die klinisch-chemische Untersuchung einschließlich Liquordiagnostik, sowie die Echokardiographie, Duplexsonographie der Halsarterien, MR-Angiographie und die ophthalmologische Untersuchung waren unauffällig. Mittels molekularbiologischer Diagnostik prothrombotischer Mutationen wurde eine Heterozygotie des Apolipoprotein-(Lp)-A-Allels (G121A) gefunden. Die Serum-Lipoprotein-A-Konzentration betrug 1,3 mg/dl, wobei im Neugeborenenalter normalerweise

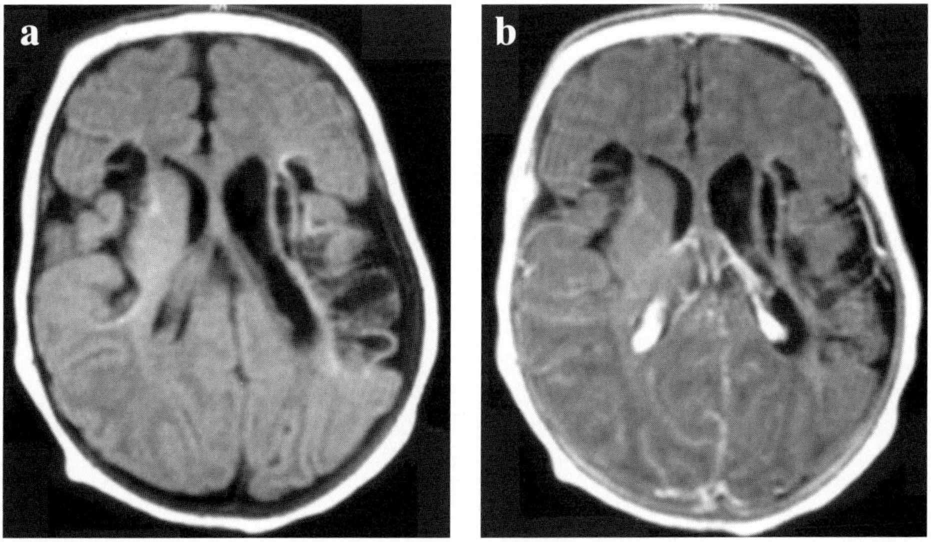

Abb. 1: MRT mit axialen Schichten mit Nachweis bilateraler Hirninfarkte (Residualstadium) im Versorgungsgebiet der Aa. cerebri mediae vor (a) und nach (b) Kontrastmittelgabe.

kein Lipoprotein A gebildet wird. Eine Antikoagulationsbehandlung wurde nicht begonnen. Trotz krankengymnastischer Übungsbehandlungen und Frühförderung zeigten sich im Laufe des ersten Lebensjahres eine deutliche statomotorische Entwicklungsverzögerung sowie die Ausbildung einer spastischen Tetraparese. Der Lipoprotein-A-Serumspiegel betrug im Alter von 12 Monaten 11,0 mg/dl (Ref. <30 mg/dl). Fokale Krampfanfälle wurden zum 18. Lebensmonat nicht beobachtet, ein erneuter ischämischer Hirninfarkt war bisher nicht aufgetreten.

Diskussion

Diese Fallbeschreibung unterstreicht die klinische Relevanz von prothrombotischen Polymorphismen für zerebrovaskuläre Erkrankungen im Kindesalter. Erhöhte Lp(a) Werte werden deshalb als Risikofaktor für thromboembolische Ereignisse diskutiert, weil Lp(a) die Bindung von Plasminogen sowie die Aktivierung von Plasminogen und tPA (tissue plasminogen activator) inhibiert (4). Interessanterweise ging im beschriebenen Fall der genetische Nachweis des Apolipoprotein (a) G121 A Polymorphismus zwar mit einer ungewöhnlichen Expression von Lp(a) im Neugeborenenalter, jedoch im weiteren Säuglingsalter ohne erhöhte Lp(a) Serumkonzentrationen einher. Daher sind weitere Untersuchungen im Fall-Kontroll-Ansatz erforderlich, um die Rolle einer isolierten G121A Mutation ohne gleichzeitige Erhöhung von Lp(a) als thrombophiler Risikofaktor zu evaluieren. Betont werden muss, dass neben den erwähnten kindlichen Risikofaktoren für ischämische Hirninfarkte im Neugeborenenalter weitere antenatale, perinatale (milde Asphyxie?) und auch maternale Faktoren eine Rolle spielen könnten. Ebenso existieren Hinweise, dass Autoimmunität bzw. Hyperkoagulabilität als Folge von früheren Aborten bzw. Plazentainfarkten einen kausalen Einfluss haben könnten (3).

Der Fallbericht, der die erheblichen funktionellen Auswirkungen eines ischämischen Hirninfarkts aufzeigt, legt ebenso nahe, dass multizentrische prospektive Langzeitstudien zur Analyse der motorischen und kognitiven Leistungsfähigkeit von kindlichen Infarktpatienten notwendig sind, um (a) die Auswirkungen in Korrelation zu Risikofaktoren, Diagnostik und Therapieschemata zu setzen und (b) frühzeitig individuell angepasste Förderungsmöglichkeiten zu veranlassen.

Literatur

1. Satoh S, Shirano R, Yoshimato T (1991). Clinical survey of ischemic cerebrovascular disease in children in a district of Japan. *Stroke* 122: 586–589.
2. Sreenan C, Bhargava R, Robertson CMT (2000). Cerebral infarction in the term newborn: Clinical presentation and long-term outcome. *J Pediatr* 137: 351–355.
3. Lynch JK, Hirtz DG, de Veber G, Nelson KB (2002). Report of the National Institute of neurological Disorders and Stroke Workshop on perinatal and childhood stroke. *Pediatrics* 109: 116–123.
4. Nowak-Göttl U, Junker R, Hartmeier M, Koch HG, Münchow N, Assmann G, von Eckardstein A (1999). Increased lipoprotein (a) is an important risk factor for venous thromboembolism in childhood. *Circulation* 100: 743–748.

Sind bei postnatal über die Muttermilch mit CMV-infizierten Frühgeborenen langfristig Auswirkungen auf Entwicklung und Hörvermögen zu erwarten?

B. Vollmer, K. Seibold-Weiger, C. Schmitz-Salue, K. Hamprecht, Ch.P. Speer, I. Krägeloh-Mann

Zusammenfassung

Durch Ernährung mit CMV positiver Muttermilch wird ein hoher Prozentsatz gestillter Frühgeborener postnatal mit CMV infiziert. Wir untersuchten die Folgen (motorische und sprachliche Entwicklung, neuromotorische Funktion, Hörvermögen) einer postnatalen CMV Infektion durch Muttermilch bei sehr kleinen Frühgeborenen durch Vergleich einer Gruppe von CMV positiven Frühgeborenen mit einer CMV negativen strukturgleichen Kontrollgruppe im Alter von 2,5–4 Jahren. Es ergeben sich bislang keine Hinweise für negative Auswirkungen einer früh postnatal durch Muttermilch übertragenen CMV Infektion bei unseren Patienten.

Hintergrund und Fragestellung

Cytomegalieviren sind die häufigsten Erreger *kongenitaler* Infektionen. Die Häufigkeit wird mit 0,4–2,3% aller Lebendgeborenen in den Industriestaaten angegeben (1). Die Mehrheit der Neugeborenen, die intrauterin infiziert werden, sind in der Neugeborenenzeit asymptomatisch. Es besteht jedoch für diese Kinder trotzdem ein erhöhtes Risiko für spätere Entwicklungsstörungen, neurologische Auffälligkeiten (neuromotorische Funktionsstörungen) und insbesondere Hörstörungen (2, 3). Cirka 5–10% der Kinder mit intrauteriner CMV Infektion zeigen Symptome in der Neonatalzeit. Diese Kinder haben ein deutlich höheres Risiko für Entwicklungsstörungen, als Kinder ohne neonatale Symptome. Innerhalb der Gruppe der in der Neonatalzeit symptomatischen Kinder haben Kinder mit neurologischen Symptomen wie z.B. Zeichen der Meningoencephalitis, Neugeborenenanfällen, intrakraniellen Verkalkungen, Mikrozephalie eine schlechtere Prognose als Kinder, die lediglich Zeichen einer systemischen Infektion ohne neurologische Symptomatik haben.

Wesentlich häufiger als eine intrauterine CMV Infektion sind *peri- und postnatale* CMV Infektionen, die entweder während der Geburt übertragen werden, postnatal durch Gabe CMV positiver Blutprodukte oder durch Ernährung mit CMV positiver Muttermilch. Die Häufigkeit der peri/postnatalen CMV Infektion wird mit 10–15% (4) angegeben.

In der Regel verläuft die peri/postnatale CMV Infektion bei Reifgeborenen in der Neugeborenenzeit asymptomatisch oder mit nur sehr milden Symptomen.

Bei Frühgeborenen ist häufiger ein symptomatischer Verlauf in der Neugeborenenzeit zu erwarten (5–7).

Muttermilch ist aufgrund ernährungsphysiologischer und immunologischer Vorteile die ideale Ernährung für Frühgeborene. Nachdem heutzutage fast ausschließlich CMV negative Blutprodukte verwendet werden, ist Muttermilch jedoch die Hauptinfektionsquelle für eine postnatale CMV Infektion bei Frühgeborenen, da es bei seropositiven Müttern während der Laktation zur Virusaktivierung und zur Ausscheidung des Virus in der Muttermilch kommen kann.

In einer Studie von Vochem et al. (8), die sich mit der CMV Transmission durch Muttermilch auf sehr kleine Frühgeborene (<32SSW/<1500 g GG) befasste, zeigte sich, dass 52% der Mütter seropositiv waren und dass es bei diesen Müttern in 85% zur Reaktivierung und Aussscheidung des Virus in die Muttermilch kam. Bei 60% der mit CMV positver Muttermilch ernährten, bei Geburt CMV negativen, Kindern, konnte in der Folge in den ersten Lebenswochen eine CMV Infektion nachgewiesen werden (Methoden siehe (8)). Bei 23% dieser infizierten Kinder traten innerhalb der ersten 3–8 Wochen Zeichen einer akuten CMV Infektion mit sepsis-ähnlichem Krankheitsbild auf.

Bezüglich langfristiger Folgen einer früh postnatal erworbenen CMV Infektion bei sehr kleinen Frühgeborenen gibt es nur wenig Informationen in der Literatur.

Wir untersuchten deshalb an einer gut definierten Gruppe von sehr kleinen früh postnatal über die Muttermilch CMV infizierten Frühgeborenen, die Frage, ob bei diesen Kindern im Vergleich zu einer CMV negativen strukturgleichen Kontrollgruppe, neurologische Auffälligkeiten, Entwicklungsstörungen und Störungen des Hörvermögens häufiger auftreten.

Patienten und Methoden

Wir untersuchten 22 sehr kleine Frühgeborene (Geburtsgewicht <1500 g oder geboren <32 Schwagerschaftswoche), die postnatal über die Muttermilch mit CMV infiziert worden waren (zum Nachweis der postnatalen Infektion siehe Vochem et al. (8)). Die Kontrollgruppe bildeten 22 CMV negative Frühgeborene, die bezüglich des Gestationsalters, Geburtsgewichtes, Geschlechts, Dauer der Beatmung und Ultraschallbefundes des Gehirns vergleichbar waren. Tabelle 1 zeigt die Charakteristika der Patienten- und Kontrollgruppe.

Tab. 1: Charakteristika der Patienten- und Kontrollgruppe

CMV	positiv	negativ
n	22 (4 w /18 m)	22 (6 w /16 m)
Geburtsgewicht (g)	1131 (600 – 1870)	1023 (490 – 1700)
Gestationsalter (SSW)	27,9 (23,9 – 30,7)	28,3 (23,6 – 31,7)
Beatmungsdauer (Tage)	7,2	7,6

Median (min-max)

Die Kinder wurden im Alter von 2,5–4 Jahren untersucht. Es wurde eine standardisierte neurologische Untersuchung durchgeführt. Bezüglich des neurologischen Befundes wurden 3 Kategorien gebildet:

- Normal: ein unauffälliger Befund, oder leichte muskuläre Hypotonie ohne funktionelle Einschränkung
- Suspekt: Asymmetrie, muskuläre Hypertonie, jedoch keine Spastik oder eine deutliche muskuläre Hypotonie
- Pathologisch: eindeutige spastische Hemi-, Di. oder Tetraparese.

Die Beurteilung der sprachlichen und motorischen Entwicklung erfolgte anhand des Konzepts der essentiellen Meilensteine (9) und die Entwicklung wurde als entweder normal oder verzögert eingestuft.

Es wurde eine pädaudiologische Untersuchung durchgeführt, die eine spielaudiometrische Bestimmung der Hörschwelle, eine seitengetrennte Bestimmung des Hörvermögens über Luft- und Knochenleitung sowie eine tympanometrische Untersuchung umfasste.

Ergebnisse

Tabelle 2 zeigt die Zusammenfassung der neurologischen Befunde. Bei 19 CMV positiven Kindern und bei 18 CMV negativen Kndern zeigte sich ein Normalbefund, bei je einem Kind in der Patienten- und Kontrollgruppe zeigte sich ein eindeutig pathologischer Befund. Das CMV positive Kind (GA 26 SSW) hatte eine armbetonte spastische Tetraparese nach Grad IV Hirnblutung, das CMV negative Kind (GA 31 SSW) eine leichte beinbetonte Tetraparese (normaler Ultraschallbefund des Gehirns).

Tab. 2: Neurologische Befunde der Patienten- und Kontrollgruppe

	CMV + (n = 22)	**CMV – (n = 22)**
Normal	19	18
Suspekt	2	3
Pathologisch	1	1

Tab. 3: Motorische und sprachliche Entwicklung

Motorische Entwicklung	**CMV + (n = 22)**	**CMV – (n = 22)**
normal	19	19
verzögert	3*	3*
*jeweils 1 Kind mit CP		
Sprachliche Entwicklung		
normal	14	14
verzögert	8	8

Es zeigte sich weder bei der motorischen noch bei der sprachlichen Entwicklung ein Unterschied zwischen den beiden Gruppen.

Bei keinem Kind wurde eine Schallempfindungsschwerhörigkeit diagnostiziert. 5 Kinder hatten eine eingeschränkte Trommelfellbeweglichkeit, ohne dass das Hörvermögen beeinträchtigt gewesen wäre. 12 Kinder zeigten bei der Erstuntersuchung eine Schallleitungsschwerhörigkeit bei Serotympanon.

Zusammenfassung und Schlussfolgerung

Neurologische Auffälligkeiten, motorische oder sprachliche Entwicklungsstörungen traten bei CMV infizierten Frühgeborenen bei der Nachuntersuchung im Alter von 2,5–4 Jahren nicht häufiger auf, als in der strukturgleichen Kontrollgruppe.

Sensorineurale Hörstörungen sind in unserem Kollektiv nicht aufgetreten. Es ergibt sich also bislang kein Anhalt für langfristige negative Auswirkungen der früh postnatal erworbenen CMV Infektion durch Muttermilch bei sehr kleinen Frühgeborenen.

Eine detaillierte neuropsychologische Beurteilung der Kinder im Vorschulbzw. Schulalter steht jedoch noch aus.

Literatur

1. Demmler GJ. Summary of a workshop on suveillance for congenital cytomegalovirus disease. *Rev Infect Dis* 2002;*13*:315–329.
2. Fowler KB, McCollister FP, Dahle AJ, Boppana S, Britt WJ, Pass RF. Progressive and fluctuating sensorineural hearing loss in children with asymptomatic congenital cytomegalovirus infection. *Journal of Pediatrics* 1997;*130(4)*:624–630.
3. Hicks T, Fowler KB, Richardson M, Dahle AJ, Adams L, Pass RF. Congenital cytomegalovirus infection and neonatal auditory screening. *Journal of Pediatrics* 1993;*123(5)*:779–782.
4. Volpe *J. Neurology of the Newborn.* Philadelphia: W.B. Saunders Company, 2001.
5. Ballard RA, Drew WL, Hufnagle KG, Riedel PA. Acquired cytomegalovirus infection in preterm infants. *Am J Dis Child* 1979;*133(5)*:482–485.
6. Paryani SG, Yeager AS, Hosford-Dunn H, et al. Sequelae of acquired cytomegalovirus infection in premature and sick term infants. *Journal of Pediatrics* 1985;*107*:451–456.
7. Stagno S. Significance of cytomegaloviral infections in pregnancy and early childhood. *The Pediatric Infectious Disease Journal* 1990;*9(10)*:763–764.
8. Vochem M, Hamprecht K, Jahn G, Speer CP. Transmission of cytomegalovirus to preterm infants through breast milk. *The Pediatric Infectious Disease Journal* 1998;*17*:53–58.
9. Michaelis R, Niemann G. *Entwicklungsneurologie und Neuropaediatrie: Grundlagen und diagnostische Strategien.* Stuttgart, New York: Thieme, 1999

Heparin-induzierte Thrombozytopenie Typ II bei einem Kind mit ausgedehnter Sinusvenenthrombose

T. Severin, U. Tacke, B. Zieger, M. Uhl, M. Nauck, J. Kühr, R. Korinthenberg, A. H. Sutor

Zusammenfassung

Die Heparin-induzierte Thrombozytopenie Typ II (HIT II) ist auch bei Kindern eine gefährliche Komplikation der Heparintherapie. Im Kindesalter sind bisher nur wenige Erfahrungen zu alternativer Antikoagulation mit Lepirudin nach Auftreten einer HIT II vorhanden. Berichtet wird über eine 8 Jahre alte Patientin, die eine ausgedehnte Sinusvenenthrombose mit gravierender neurologischer Symptomatik erlitten hatte. Unter Behandlung mit Heparin entwickelte das Mädchen eine Heparin-induzierte Thrombozytopenie Typ II. Hinweise hierfür waren ein Rückgang der Thrombozyten, ein steigender Heparin-Bedarf und anhaltendes Fieber. Mit dem Einsatz von Lepirudin gelang eine effektive Antikoagulation, eine schnelle Verbesserung des klinischen Zustandes der Patientin und ein problemloser Übergang auf orale Dauerantikoagulation.

Einleitung

Bei Vorliegen einer Sinusvenenthrombose werden die Patienten, sofern keine Kontraindikationen vorliegen, mit Heparin behandelt. Eine potentiell gefährliche Komplikation der Heparintherapie ist die Heparin-induzierte Thrombozytopenie Typ II (HIT II). Eine nicht-immunologische Interaktion zwischen Heparin und Thrombozyten kann die HIT Typ I hervorrufen, hier tritt innerhalb der ersten 5 Tage der Heparin-Behandlung eine reversible milde Thrombozytopenie auf. Der Verzicht auf Heparin und eine alternative Antikoagulation sind in diesem Fall nicht notwendig (1, 2). Die HIT Typ II stellt hingegen eine potentiell sehr bedrohliche Komplikation dar. Sie beinhaltet eine Immun-Reaktion gegen Komplexe aus Heparin und Plättchenfaktor IV (PF-4), die Aktivierung von Thrombozyten und Endothelzellen, die Freisetzung von prokoagulatorischen Mikropartikeln und die Bildung von Thrombin (1, 3, 4, 5). Eine Thrombozytopenie oder ein Rückgang der Thrombozyten tritt im allgemeinen ab dem 5. Tag der Heparin-Behandlung auf (früher nach vorheriger Heparin-Exposition). Thrombosen und Thromboembolien als Folge des HIT II Pathomechanismus können zu schwerwiegenden, potentiell lebensbedrohlichen Komplikationen führen. Weiterhin sind systemische Reaktionen (6), Haut-Läsionen (7, 8, 9) und auch ein Patient mit globaler Amnesie (10) beschrieben worden.

Bei Verdacht auf HIT II müssen die Heparin-Zufuhr beendet und weitere Kontakte mit Heparin (z.B. über mit Heparin beschichtete Katheter, Spritzen,

Plasmaprodukte) vermieden werden. Schon das Spülen von zentralen Venenkathetern mit Heparin kann zu einer erneuten HIT II führen (11).

Nach Absetzen von Heparin wird eine alternative Antikoagulation zur Vermeidung einer Thrombose durch den HIT II Pathomechanismus benötigt (2, 12). Bei erwachsenen Patienten werden hierfür in der Regel Danaparoid oder rekombinantes Hirudin (Lepirudin) verwendet (2, 12–17).

Das Auftreten einer HIT II bei pädiatrischen Patienten wurde in einer Untersuchung an Neugeborenen (18) und einigen Fallberichten beschrieben. Thrombotische Komplikationen treten wie bei Erwachsenen auf (19–36).

Im Gegensatz zu umfangreicheren Untersuchungen, auch prospektiven Studien, zur optimalen Behandlung einer HIT II bei Erwachsenen, sind im Kindesalter bisher nur wenige Erfahrungen zu alternativer Antikoagulation mit dem Thrombininhibitor Lepirudin vorhanden.

Kasuistik

Ein 8 Jahre altes Mädchen mit Ullrich-Turner Syndrom wurde seit drei Jahren mit Wachstumshormon behandelt. Die Patientin entwickelte plötzliche Kopfschmerzen, eine komplette Hemiparese links, cerebrale Krampfanfälle und Somnolenz. Die MRT-Angiographie zeigte eine ausgedehnte Thrombose des Sinus (S) sagittalis superior, des S. rectus und des S. transversus sowie der Vena cerebri magna beidseits (Abb. 1–3). Aufgrund des erhöhten Heparin-Bedarfs zur therapeutischen aPTT-Verlängerung wurde am 3. Tag der Heparintherapie ein HIT-Antikörpertest durchgeführt, der ein negatives Ergebnis ergab. Nach zunächst klinischer Besserung entwickelte das Mädchen eine Kathetersepsis. Trotz adäquater Antibiotika-Therapie bestand anhaltendes Fieber und ein schlechter Allgemeinzustand. Der Heparin-Bedarf stieg erneut leicht an (Abb. 4). Nach Rückgang der Thrombozyten von 342 G/l um 45% auf 190 G/l ergab ein zweiter HIT-Antikörper-Test, der 16-Tage nach Beginn der Heparin-Therapie durchgeführt wurde, ein positives Ergebnis (Abb. 4). Daher wurde zur weiteren Antikoagulation Heparin durch Lepirudin ersetzt (3 Tage). Nach der Einstellung mit Phenprocoumon konnte die Patientin in gutem Allgemeinzustand entlassen werden. Die MRT-Angiographie zeigte bereits unter Heparin eine teilweise Rekanalisierung der Sinus (Abb. 5 und 6).

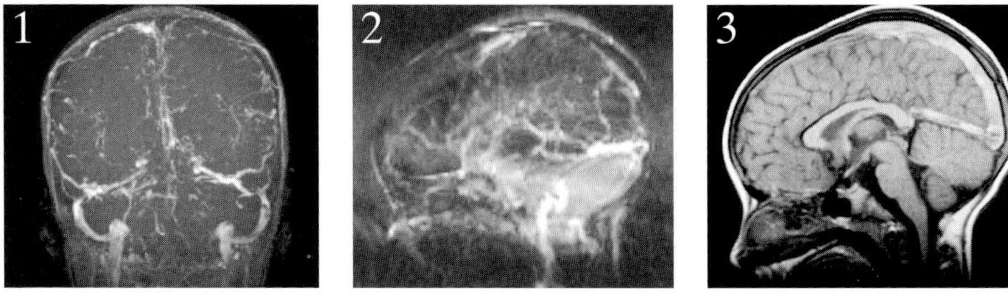

Abb. 1–3: MR-Angiographie: 2D coronar. Time of Flight (TOF) Angio (Abb. 1). Sagittal (Abb. 2). Spinecho, T1, sagittal (Abb. 3). Ausgedehnte Thrombose: Sinus sag. sup., S. rectus, S. transversus beidseits sowie Vena cerebri magna.

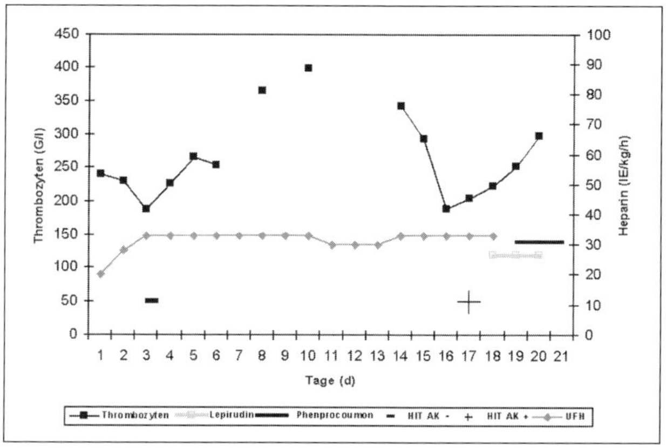

Abb. 4: Thrombozytenverlauf und Antikoagulation. Heparinbedarf maximal 33 IE/kg/h. Tag 18-20: Lepirudin 0,15–0,16 mg/kg/h. Ab Tag 19 orale Antikoagulation mit Phenprocoumon. HIT-Test Tag 3 negativ, Tag 17 positiv.

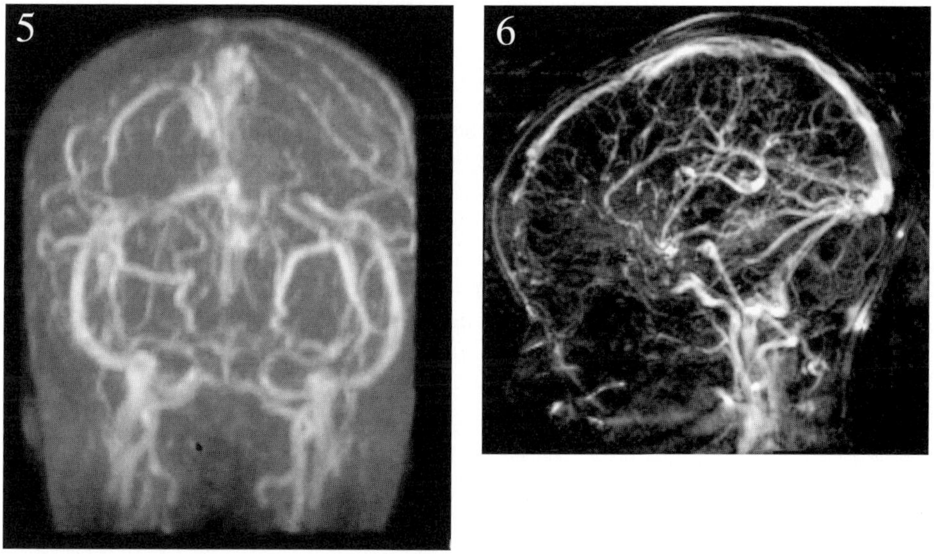

Abb. 5–6: MR-Angiographie Tag 13. 2D Coronar-Schnitt. TOF Angiographie. Partielle Rekanalisation. Restthrombus im Sinus confluens, S. sagittalis sup., S. transversus (Abb. 5). Tag 18. 2D Sagittal-Schnitt. TOF Angiographie. Weitere Rekanalisation (Abb. 6).

Diskussion

Nach Auftreten einer Sinusvenenthrombose beinhaltet die Behandlung die Gabe von Heparin (37). Die Heparin-induzierte Thrombozytopenie als mögliche Komplikation tritt auch im Kindes- und Jugendalter auf (22, 35). Eine Thrombozytopenie ist nicht obligat, auch ein Rückgang der Thrombozyten um 30–50%, wie bei der beschriebenen Patientin, erfüllt die Kriterien. Ein weiterer Hinweis kann ein steigender Heparin-Bedarf zur therapeutischen aPTT-Verlängerung sein.

Die Mehrzahl der in der Literatur beschriebenen pädiatrischen Patienten mit HIT II wurde mit Danaparoid behandelt (22, 35).

Bei Erwachsenen mit HIT II wurden prospektive Multicenter Studien mit dem Thrombin Inhibitor Lepirudin (rekombinantes Hirudin) durchgeführt. Diese zeigten eine effektive und sichere Antikoagulation, einen Wiederanstieg der Thrombozyten und eine reduzierte Inzidenz von HIT-Komplikationen (14, 16, 38, 39). Bisher wurde die Anwendung von Lepirudin als alternative Antikoagulation nur bei drei weiteren pädiatrischen Patienten (Alter 12, 13 und 15 Jahre) beschrieben (26, 28, 32). Bei zwei dieser Patienten wurde die Behandlung wegen vermuteter Kreuzreaktivität mit HIT-Antikörpern von Danaparoid auf rekombinantes Hirudin umgestellt (26, 28).

Während der Antikoagulation mit Lepirudin trat bei dieser kleinen Zahl pädiatrischer Patienten keine Zunahme der Thrombose oder eine neue Thrombose auf. Negative Begleiteffekte wurden nicht beschrieben. Bei Erwachsenen wird eine Bolusgabe von 0,4 mg/kg rekombinantes Hirudin gefolgt von einer Dauerinfusion von 0,15 mg/kg/h empfohlen (40). Unsere Patientin erhielt wegen des Zustandes nach Sinusvenenthrombose keine Bolusgabe und wurde nur mit einer Lepirudin-Dauerinfusion unter PTT- und Hirudinspiegelkontrolle behandelt.

Bei der beschriebenen Patientin mit ausgedehnter Sinusvenenthrombose, gravierender neurologischer Symptomatik und Komplikation der HIT II gelang durch den Einsatz von Lepirudin eine effektive Antikoagulation, eine schnelle Verbesserung des klinischen Zustandes der Patientin und ein problemloser Übergang auf orale Dauerantikoagulation.

Weitere Untersuchungen bei pädiatrischen Patienten mit HIT II werden die optimale Behandlungsform und den Stellenwert von rekombinantem Hirudin als therapeutische Option zeigen.

Literatur

1. Greinacher A (1999) Heparin-induzierte Thrombozytopenie – Pathogenese und Behandlung. Hämostaseologie 19:1–12.
2. Greinacher A. (1999) Treatment of heparin-induced thrombocytopenia. Thromb Haemost 82:457–467.
3. Visentin GP (1999) Heparin-induced thrombocytopenia: molecular pathogenesis. Thromb Haemost. 82:448–456.
4. Warkentin TE, Chong BH, Greinacher A (1998) Heparin-induced thrombocytopenia: towards consensus. Thromb Haemost 79:1–7.
5. Fabris F, Ahmad S, Cella G et al. (2000) Pathophysiology of heparin-induced thrombocytopenia. Arch Pathol Lab Med. 124:1657–1666.
6. Warkentin TE, Soutar RL, Panju A, Ginsberg JS (1992) Acute systemic reactions to intravenous bolus heparin therapy: characterization and relationship to heparin-induced thrombocytopenia. Blood;80:160a.
7. Ali O (2000) Images in Heparin-induced thrombocytopenia. J Thromb Thrombolys 10:S27–S33.
8. Warkentin TE (1996) Heparin-induced skin lesions. Br J Haematol 92:494–497.
9. Hartman AR, Hood RM, Anagnostopoulus CE (1988) Phenomenon of heparin-induced thrombocytopenia associated with skin necrosis. J Vasc Surg 7:781–784.
10. Warkentin TE, Hirte HW, Anderson DR, et al (1994) Transient global amnesia associated with acute heparin-induced thrombocytopenia. Am J Med 97:489–491.

11. Kadidal VV, Mayo DJ, Horne MK (1999) Heparin-induced thrombocytopenia (HIT) due to Heparin flushes: a report of three cases. J Intern Med 246:325–329.
12. Walenga JM, Lewis BE, Bakhos M (2000) Anticoagulant management of patients with heparin-induced thrombocytopenia. Turk J Haematol 17,3 (suppl.):68–77.
13. Magnani HN (1993) Heparin-induced thrombocytopenia (HIT): an overview of 230 patients treated with Orgaran. Thromb Haemost 70:554–561.
14. Chong BH, Magnani HN (2001) Danaparoid for the treatment of heparin-induced thrombocytopenia: In: Warkentin TE, Greinacher A: (Herausg.) Heparin-induced thrombocytopenia, Dekker, New York, p. 323–347.
15. Greinacher A (1999) Rekombinantes Hirudin zur weiteren Antikoagulation bei Heparin-induzierter Thrombozytopenie. Hämostaseologie 19:19–29.
16. Greinacher A, Völpel H, Janssens U, Hach-Wunderle V, Kemkes-Matthes B, Eichler P, Mueller-Velten HG, Pötzsch B (1999) Recombinant hirudin (Lepirudin) provides safe and effective anticoagulation in patients with heparin-induced thrombocytopenia. Circulation 99:73–80.
17. Greinacher A, Janssens U, Berg G, Böck M, Kwasny H, Kemkes-Matthes B, Eichler P, Völpel H, Pötzsch B, Luz M, and for the Heparin-associated Thrombocytopenia Study (HAT) investigators (1999) Lepirudin (recombinant hirudin) for parenteral anticoagulation in patients with heparin-induced thrombocytopenia. Circulation 100:587–593.
18. Spadone D, Clark F, James E, Laster J, Hoch J, Silver D (1992) Heparin-induced thrombocytopenia in the newborn. J Vasc Surg 15:306–312.
19. Laster J, Cikrit D, Walker N et al. (1987)The heparin-induced thrombocytopenia syndrome: an update. Surgery 102:763–770.
20. Boon DMS, Michiels JJ, Stibbe J, van Vliet HHDM, Kappers-Klunne MC (1994) Heparin-induced thrombocytopenia and antithrombotic therapy. Lancet 344:1296.
21. Butler TJ, Sodoma LJ, Doski JJ, Cheu HW, Berg ST, Stokes GN, Lancaster KJ (1997) Heparin-associated thrombocytopenia and thrombosis as the cause of a fatal thrombus on extracorporeal membrane oxygenation. J Ped Surg. 32:768–771.
22. Ranze O, Ranze P, Magnani HN, Greinacher A (1999) Heparin-induced thrombocytopenia in paediatric patients - a review of the literature and a new case treated with danaparoid sodium. Eur J Pediatr 158 [Suppl 3]: S130–S133.
23. Murdoch IA, Beattie RM, Silver DM (1993) Heparin-induced thrombocytopenia in children. Acta Paediatr 82:495–497.
24. Oriot D, Wolf M, Wood C, Brun P, Sidi D, Devictor D, Tchernia G, Huault G (1990) Severe thrombocytopenia induced by heparin in an infant with acute myocarditis. Arch Fr Pediatr 47:357–359. (MEDLINE)
25. Saxon BR, Black MD, Edgell D, Noel D, Leaker MT (1999). Pediatric heparin-induced thrombocytopenia: management with danaparoid (Orgaran). Ann Thorac Surg 68:1076–1078.
26. Zöhrer B, Zenz W, Rettenbacher A, Covi P, Kurnik K, Kroll H, Grubbauer HM, Muntean W (2001) Danaparoid sodium (Orgaran) in four children with heparin-induced thrombocytopenia type II. Acta Paediatr 90:765–71.
27. Neuhaus TJ, Goetschel P, Schmugge M, Leumann E (2000) Heparin-induced thrombocytopenia type II on hemodialysis: switch to danaparoid. Pediatr Nephrol 14:713–716.
28. Schiffmann H, Unterhalt M, Harms K, Figulla HR, Völpel H, Greinacher A (1997) Erfolgreiche Behandlung einer Heparin-induzierten Thrombozytopenie Typ II im Kindesalter mit rekombinantem Hirudin. Monatsschr Kinderheilkd 145:606–612.
29. Potter C, Gill JC, Scott JP, McFarland JG (1992) Heparin-induced thrombocytopenia in a child. J Pediatr 121:135–138.
30. Bocquet R, Blanot S, Dautzenberg MD et al. (1999) Antiphospholipid antibody syndrome in pediatric neurosurgery: a hemostasis problem. Ann Fr Anesth Reanim 18:991–995.
31. Wilhelm MJ, Schmid C, Kececioglu D, Möllhoff T, Ostermann H, Scheld HH (1996) Cardiopulmonary bypass in patients with heparin-induced thrombocytopenia using Org 10172. Ann Thorac Surg 61:920–924.

32. Severin T, Ensenauer R, Wiedensohler A, Fischer K-G, Zieger B, Greinacher A, Brandis M, Sutor AH (1999) HIT type II without thrombocytopenia in a 15-year-old boy with protein-S deficiency and recurrent deep vein thrombosis. In: Procceedings of the 30th Hemophilia Symposium Hamburg. Springer-Verlag Berlin Heidelberg New York:114–116.
33. Klement D, Rammos S, v. Kries R, Kirschke W, Kniemeyer H-W, Greinacher A (1996) Heparin as a cause of thrombus progression. Eur J Pediatr 155:11–14.
34. Sauer M, Gruhn B, Fuchs D, Altermann W, Zintl F (1998) Heparin-induzierte Thrombozytopenie Typ II im Rahmen einer Hochdosis-Chemotherapie mit anschließender Stammzellrescue. Klin. Pädiatr. 210:102–105.
35. Severin T, Sutor AH (2001) Heparin-induced thrombocytopenia in pediatrics. Sem Thromb Hemost 27: 293–299.
36. Weigel B, Lasky A, Krishnamurti L et al (1999) Danaparoid (orgaran) anticoagulation of pediatric patients with heparin-induced thrombocytopenia (HIT). J Pediatr Hematol Oncol 21:327.
37. deVeber G, Chan A, Monagle P, Marzinotto V, Armstrong D, Massicotte P, Leaker M, Andrew M. Anticoagulation therapy in pediatric patients with sinovenous thrombosis: a cohort study. Arch Neurol 1998;55:1533–7.
38. Lubenow N, Greinacher A (2000) Management of patients with heparin-induced thrombocytopenia: focus on recombinant hirudin. J Thromb Thrombolys 10: S47–S57.
39. Greinacher A, Lubenow N (2001) Recombinant hirudin in clinical practice. Circulation 103:1479–1484.
40. Product Information: Refludan. Aventis, Frankfurt, Germany.

Apallisches Syndrom nach Beinahe-Ertrinken: Unterschiedliches Outcome von 3 Geschwistern in Korrelation zu neuroradiologischen und elektrophysiologischen Befunden

J. Wänninger, C. Bäumel, M. Wruk, G. Kluger

Zusammenfassung

Wir verglichen den klinischen Verlauf, bildgebende und neurophysiologische Befunde dreier Geschwister im apallischen Syndrom nach Beinahe-Ertrinken über insgesamt 8 Jahre. Wie der klinische Verlauf zeigte, war eine Vorhersage über das definitive Outcome auch retrospektiv nicht möglich.

Einleitung

Das apallische Syndrom ist gekennzeichnet durch eine länger als 4 Wochen anhaltende Unfähigkeit, sich oder die Umwelt wahrzunehmen, Kontakt aufzunehmen oder zu reagieren. Dabei sind die hypothalamischen und autonomen Hirnstammfunktionen teilweise oder vollständig erhalten (1, 6).

Synonyme für das apallische Syndrom sind Schlaf-Wach-Niveau (SWN) und Persistierender Vegetativer Status (PVS) (7).

Die Diagnose eines apallischen Syndroms impliziert ein sehr schlechtes Outcome, das nach hypoxämischer Hirnschädigung noch schlechter ist als nach traumatischer (2, 8). In der Behandlung von Patienten mit dem Bild eines apallischen Syndroms werden v.a. ethische Aspekte diskutiert (3, 9).

Wir hatten die Möglichkeit den Verlauf dreier Geschwister über 8 Jahre zu beobachten, die alle das Bild eines apallischen Syndroms nach Beinahe-Ertrinken (BE) zeigten, jedoch ein unterschiedliches Outcome hatten. Dieses korrelierten wir mit dem klinischen Verlauf und Untersuchungsbefunden (CCT, MRT, VEP, AEP, EEG, PET und SPECT).

Kasuistik

1.) Anamnese

Die 3 Geschwister, ein Junge (M, Alter bei Beinahe-Ertrinken: 8 Jahre und 7 Monate) und 2 jüngere Schwestern (J, Alter bei Beinahe-Ertrinken: 5 Jahre und C, Alter bei Beinahe-Ertrinken: 2 Jahre 3 Monate) sind im Rahmen eines Verkehrsunfalls im Winter in einen Fluss gestürzt. Die Submersionszeiten lagen zwischen 15 und 20 Minuten. Sie wurden nacheinander geborgen, zuerst das jüngere Mädchen (C), dann das ältere Mädchen (J) und schließlich der Junge (M).

Tab. 1: Klinik und Befunde innerhalb der ersten 4 Wochen

	Jüngstes Mädchen (C)	**Mittleres Mädchen (J)**	**Ältester Junge (M)**
Beatmungszeit		7 Tage	
Klinik		Apallisches Syndrom, Tetraspastik, Unruhezustände	
EEG nach 4 Wochen		Schwere Allgemeinveränderungen, keine ETP's	
VEP		Schwere Funktionsstörung der Sehbahn	
Anfälle	keine	1x gen. ton klon.	keine
AEP	gering pathologisch	nicht durchgeführt	pathologisch

C (♀) **J (♀)** **M (♂)**

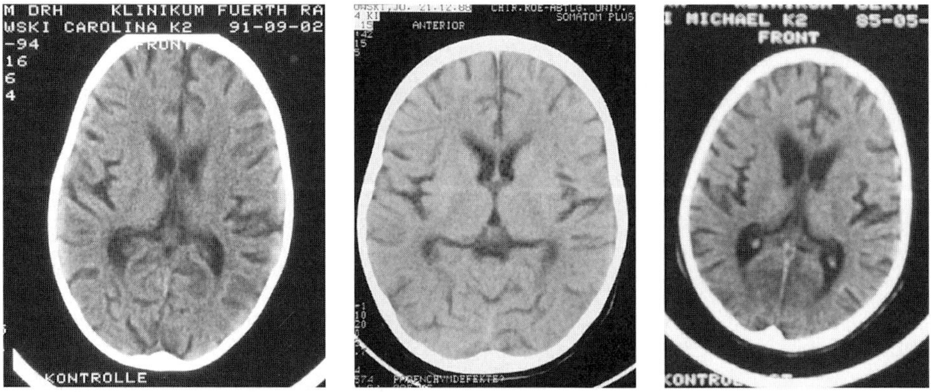

Abb. 1: natives CCT axial von 3 Geschwistern, 4 Wochen nach dem Ereignis.

2.) Verlauf und Befunde in den ersten 4 Wochen (siehe Tab. 1)
Nach der Reanimation am Unfallort wurden die Geschwister in verschiedenen Kliniken erstversorgt. Alle drei zeigten bei Klinikaufnahme keine sicheren Eigen- oder Fremdreflexe, hatten einen schlaffen Muskeltonus und erreichten auf der Glasgow Koma Skala 4 Punkte. Sie wurden 7 Tage beatmet.

Nach 4 Wochen boten die drei Geschwister klinisch das Bild eines apallischen Syndroms mit Tetraspastik und ausgeprägten Unruhezuständen. Im Elektroencephalogramm (EEG) imponierten schwere Allgemeinveränderungen, jedoch keine Epilepsie-typischen Potentiale. Die visuell evoziierten Potentiale (VEP) zeigten eine schwere Funktionsstörung der Sehbahn. Im CCT nach 4 Wochen imponierte jeweils eine Atrophie aller Hirnabschnitte (siehe Abb. 1).

Während bei J einmalig in der Akutphase ein generalisiert tonisch klonischer Anfall beobachtet wurde, hatten C und M zunächst keine Anfälle. Die AEP waren bei M eindeutig pathologisch. Bei C waren sie geringgradig pathologisch, bei J wurden sie in der Akutphase nicht durchgeführt.

3.) Weiterer Verlauf und Befunde (siehe Tab. 2)
C begann 5 Wochen und 6 Tage nach dem Ereignis zu fixieren. 4 Monate nach dem Unfall imitierte sie erste Worte und konnte nach 5 Monaten Mehrwortsätze sprechen.

Bei J wurde erstmals 6 Wochen und 6 Tage nach dem Ereignis ein Fixieren beobachtet. Sie begann 3 Monaten nach dem Unfall einzelne Silben zu sprechen und konnte nach 4 Monaten Mehrwortsätze bilden. Sie hat eine andauernde ataktische Dysarthrophonie.

Beide Mädchen konnten 4 Monate nach dem Unfall mit Hilfe und nach 5 Monaten frei gehen. Sie zeigten eine ataktisch-dystone Bewegungsstörung, die bei J stärker ausgeprägt war als bei C. 8 Jahre nach dem Unfall weist J noch eine mäßig ataktisch-dystone Bewegungsstörung auf, C nur eine diskrete Ataxie. Beide besuchen eine Regelschule.

Tab. 2: Weiterer Verlauf und Befunde

	C	J	M
Fixieren	5 Wochen	6 Wochen	–
Sprache	Nach 4 Monaten imitieren, nach 5 Monaten Mehrwortsätze, Dysarthrie	Nach 3 Monaten einzelne Silben, nach 4 Monaten Mehrwortsätze, Ataktische Dysartrophonie, Verlangsamung	–
Laufen	Beginn nach 4 Monaten, frei nach 5 Monaten, im Verlauf nur noch diskrete Ataxie	Beginn nach 4 Monaten, frei nach 5 Monaten, anhaltend mäßige ataktisch-dystone Bewegungsstörung	–
Epilepsie	1. Anfall 5 1/2 Wochen nach dem Unfall, unter VPA anfallsfrei, im Verlauf nach 2 Jahren abgesetzt	Keine	Therapie resistent, weiter viele tonische Anfälle
2002–8 Jahre nach BE	Regelschule	Regelschule	Apallisches Syndrom

C (♀) **J (♀)** **M (♂)**

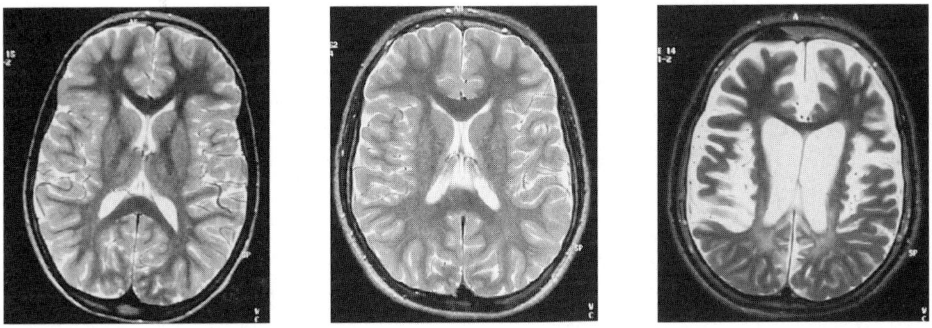

Abb. 2: MRT axial von 3 Geschwistern, T2 gewichtet, 7,5 Jahre nach BE.

C entwickelte eine posthypoxämische Epilepsie und war unter Valproinsäure (VPA) anfallsfrei. J hatte keine weiteren Anfälle. M zeigt anhaltend das Bild eines apallischen Syndroms. Er hat viele Anfälle, die sich im Verlauf als Therapie resistent erwiesen.

Sowohl die AEP als auch die VEP waren 9 Monate nach dem Ereignis bei C normal. Bei J zeigte sich eine diskrete Funktionsstörung beider EP und bei M eine schwere.

Im Single Photonen Emissions Computertomogramm *(SPECT)* 4 Monate nach dem Unfall zeigte C eine leichte frontale Hypoperfusion, J eine mäßige frontale und zentrale Hypoperfusion und M eine deutlich diffuse Hypoperfusion.

Im Photonen Emissionstomogramm *(PET)* 3-5 Monate nach Beinahe-Ertrinken waren bei allen drei Geschwistern unterschiedlich ausgeprägte Auffälligkeiten in den für Hypoxie besonders empfindlichen Strukturen (Cortex, Hippocampus/ Parahippocampalregion, Thalamus, Basalganglien) zu sehen.

Im craniellen *MRT*(siehe Abb. 2), das erstmals 7,5 Jahren nach Beinahe-Ertrinken durchgeführt wurde, zeigte sich bei C und J ein altersentsprechender Normalbefund. Eine Erklärung für die im CCT 4 Wochen nach dem Ereignis vorhandene Atrophie ist vermutlich eine Hirnödemprophylaxe mit Steroiden in der Akutphase.

Bei M zeigte sich im cMRT eine ausgeprägte Atrophie mit Erweiterung der inneren und äußeren Liquorräume, sowie Veränderungen im paraventrikulären Marklager.

Diskussion

Was wären mögliche *Gründe* für das unterschiedliche Outcome der 3 Geschwister?

1. *Alter:* es gibt Studien die zeigen, dass sich das jüngere Gehirn aufgrund seiner größeren Plastizität besser erholt als das Ältere (2, 3).
2. *Dauer der Hypoxämie:* die Submersionszeit zeigt eine positive Korrelation mit dem späteren Outcome (2).
3. *Erstversorgung:* C und M wurden kontrolliert beatmet, J kam zur Erwärmung an die Herz-Lungen Maschine.

Unserer Meinung nach begründet sich das unterschiedliche Outcome der Geschwister in der unterschiedlichen Dauer der primären Hypoxie.

Welche Befunde wären wegweisend für das unterschiedliche Outcome gewesen und wann hätte man es vorhersagen können?

1. *Klinische Beobachtung*
2. Atrophie im *MRT* im Verlauf
3. *SSEP* im Verlauf

Bisher gibt es nur Studien die anhand der Blutzuckerwerte, bildgebender Verfahren wie SPECT, PET und MRT das Outcome nach Beinahe-Ertrinken in neurologisch unauffällig, auffällig und apallischem Syndrom einteilen. Es existieren keine Studien, die Aussagen über die definitive Prognose nach dem apallischen Syndrom treffen (1, 10, 11, 12, 13).

Eine eigene Studie (5) belegt, dass eine Korrelation zwischen MRT innerhalb der ersten 4 Wochen nach Ertrinken und Outcome nicht möglich ist, jedoch eine gute Korrelation zwischen Outcome und MRT nach mehr als 8 Wochen besteht.

Neuere Studien zeigen, dass die somato-sensibel evoziierten Potentiale eine hohe prognostische Bedeutung für das Outcome von Patienten im apallischen Syndrom nach Hypoxieereignissen haben (2, 4).

Schlussfolgerung

Auch in der retrospektiven Zusammenschau des Verlaufes und der Befunde war das Outcome von den 3 Geschwistern mit dem Bild des sog. Apallischen Syndroms nach schwerem Beinahe-Ertrinkungsunfall in den ersten Wochen in diesem Fall nicht definitiv vorhersagbar.

Literatur

1. Dubowitz d, Bluml S, Arcinue E, Dietrich RB: MR of hypoxic encephalopathy in Children after near drowning: a correltaion with quantitative proton MR spectroscopy and clinical outcome, AJNR 1998 Oct;19 (9): 1617–27.
2. Hagel K, Rietz S: Prognostic of the apallic Syndrome. A literature Review, Anaesthesist 1998 Aug;47 (8): 677–82.
3. Celesia GG: Persistent vegetative state: Clinical and ethical issues, Theor Med 1997 Sep; 18 (3): 221–36.
4. Chen R, Bolton CF, Young B: Prediction of Outcome in patients with anoxic coma: a clinical and electrophysiological study. Crit Care Med 1996 Apr;24 (7): 672–8
5. Kluger G, Staudt M: Persistent vegetative State after Near-Drowning: Prognostic Value of late MR Imaging. European Journal of Pediatric Neurology 2001;5: A175.
6. The Multi-Society Task Force on PVS. Medical Aspects of the Persistent Vegetative State. N Engl J Med 1994; 330: 1499-1508 & 1572–1579
7. Romein E, Kluger G, Lütjen S, Holthausen H in Aksu F.(Hrsg) Aktuelle Neuropädiatrie 2001, Novartis Pharma Verlag 2001: 52-57.
8. Heindl u, Laub M: Outcome of Persistent Vegetative State Following Hypoxic or Traumatic Brain Injury in Children ans Adolescents. Neuropädiatrics 27 (1996) 94–100.
9. Shewmon DA, De Giorgio CM: Early prognosis in anoxic coma. Reliability and rationale. Neurol Clin 1989; 7: 823–843.
10. Biggart MJ, Bohn DJ: Effect of hypothermia and cardiac arrest on outcome of near-drowning accidents in children. J Pediatr 1990 Aug;117 (2 Pt 1): 179–83.
11. Aicardi J: Accidental and Nonaccidental Injuries by Physical Agents and Toxic Agents: Near-Drowning in Diseases of the Nervous System in Childhood, 2nd Edition, Mac Keith Press 1998: 476.
12. Lopez-Pison J, Pineda-Ortiz I, Oteiza C, Loureiro B, Abenia P, Melendo J: Supervivencia sin seculas tras casi-ahogamiento con muy malos signos prognosticos, incluida midriasis arreactiva bilateral persistente, REV NEUROL 1999;28 (4): 388–390.
13. Van der Lely N, Vreede WB: Drowning and near-drowning in children, Ned Tijdschr Geneeskd 1998 Oct 17; 142 (42): 2294–7.

12. Epilepsie 1: prächirurgische Befunde und chirurgische Behandlung

Bandheterotopien – Klinik, EEG, funktionelle Kernspintomografie (fMRI) und Genetik

P. Martin, J. Spreer, G. Uyanik, P. Burkart

Zusammenfassung

Als Bandheterotopien bezeichnet man eine Form der neuronalen Migrationsstörungen, bei der Nervenzellen unvollständig zum Cortex ausgewandert und beidseits im Großhirnmarklager, zwischen Ventrikelwand und Cortex, bandförmig gelegen sind. Diese Gehirnmalformation ist klinisch meist mit Intelligenzminderung unterschiedlicher Schwere sowie mit Epilepsien verbunden und wird dann als »double-cortex-Syndrom« bezeichnet. Bei Patienten mit Bandheterotopien, die meist weiblich sind, liegt häufig eine X-chromosomal dominante Störung vor mit einer Funktionsbeeinträchtigung des das Doublecortin-Protein kodierenden Doublecortin-Gens (DCX).

Anhand der Daten von 15 eigenen Patienten und weiteren in der Literatur publizierten Fällen mit Bandheterotopien werden die typischen klinischen – und EEG-Befunde beschrieben, neben eigenen molekulargenetischen Untersuchungsergebnissen mit mehreren neuen Mutationen und Nachweis einer männlichen Mosaikform. Funktionell-kernspintomografische Untersuchungen wurden bei 3 der eigenen Patienten ausgeführt und zeigen, dass die Neurone in Bandheterotopien, zumindest unter bestimmten Voraussetzungen, an der physiologischen Aktivität des Gehirns partizipieren.

Einleitung

Moderne bildgebende Diagnostik mit der Kernspintomografie (MRI) hat es ermöglicht, auch subtile Gehirnmalformationen bei Patienten in vivo zu diagnostizieren. Parallel zu einer zunehmenden Präzision in der strukturellen Charakterisierung der Fehlbildungen verdanken wir den sehr rasch anwachsenden molekulargenetischen Methoden die Möglichkeit, cerebrale Entwicklungsanomalien in ihrer Ursache aufzuklären, differenzierter zu klassifizieren und auch in ihrer Pathophysiologie genauer zu beschreiben.

Laminäre – oder Bandheterotopien kommen als seltene Gehirnentwicklungsstörung im Sinne einer Migrationsstörung vor, die durch bilaterale Bänder von Nervenzellen charakterisiert ist, welche vom Rindenband und von der Ventrikelwand jeweils durch weiße Substanz getrennt sind (Friede, 1989; Barkovich et al., 1994) (Abb. 1).

Die Seitenventrikel sind bei bilateralen Bandheterotopien häufig über die Altersnorm hinausgehend weit. In der Nachbarschaft zum heterotopen Neuronenband finden sich nicht selten, im Sinne von Pachygyrien, verbreiterte

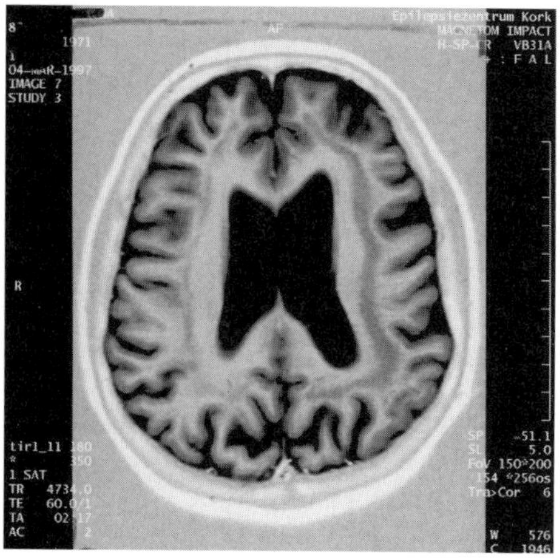

Abb. 1: Bilaterale Bandheterotopien, links betont.
Kernspintomografie (IR-Sequenzen in T1-Signalcharakteristik)

Windungen bzw. abgeflachte Sulci (Barkovich et al., 1994). Feingeweblich sind ungeordnete Pyramidenzellen in äußeren Abschnitten des Heterotopiebandes und eine säulenförmige Neuronenanordnung in ventrikelnäheren Teilen beschrieben (Harding, 1996). Benachbart ist meist ein normaler sechsschichtiger Cortex, der jedoch auch vierschichtig sein kann (Friede, 1989).

Klinische – und EEG-Befunde

In der Literatur finden sich überwiegend Beschreibungen kleinerer Patientenzahlen oder aus mehreren Zentren zusammengefasste Gruppen. In den vergangenen Jahren haben wir am Epilepsiezentrum Kork insgesamt 15 Patienten mit bilateralen Bandheterotopien gesehen und überwiegend über längere Zeit betreut (11 w, 4 m; 14–45 Jahre, M = 29,2 Jahre).

In Tabelle 1 sind die klinischen –, EEG- und MRI-Daten der von uns gesehenen Patienten zusammengefasst.

In Zusammenschau der eigenen und der in der Literatur publizierten Fälle zeigt sich, dass das Syndrom der bilateralen subkortikalen Bandheterotopien bzw. das »Double-cortex«-Syndrom klinisch aus einem Zusammentreffen von Intelligenzminderung unterschiedlicher Schwere, Epilepsie und einer häufig verzögerten statomotorischen bzw. sprachlichen Entwicklung besteht. Im Jugend- und Erwachsenenalter werden aber meist keine oder nur geringfügige neurologische Ausfälle bzw. Störungen (z.B. Ataxie oder Strabismus) gefunden.

Eine Analyse der Daten von insgesamt 79 eigenen und publizierten Fällen zeigt, dass Patienten mit bilateralen Bandheterotopien nur selten keine Epilepsie haben (Gleeson et al., 2000; Franzoni et al., 1995; Barkovich et al., 1994; Kirkham et al., 1994; Granata et al., 1994; Parmeggiani et al., 1994; Landy et al., 1993; Ianetti et al., 1993; Ricci et al., 1992; Palmini et al., 1991; Livingston et al., 1990). Dies könnte, zumindest teilweise, selektionsbedingt sein. Für das Alter bei Beginn der Epilepsie zeigt sich eine zweigipfelige Verteilung. Meist beginnt die Epilepsie in des Epilepsiezentrums Kork

	Alter	Geschl.	Alter bei Erstmanifestation	Anfallsarten	Neurologisch	Intelligenz (IQ)	EEG	MRI	Familienanamnese
B.O.	19	w	9 J	GTKA/KPA/AtA	–	79	Leichte AV / bisynchr. Theta-Delta-Paroxysmen mit Spikes (frontal li betont)	BHT li bet.	–
A.M.	25 J	w	13 J	GTKA/KPA/EPA (mot)	Strabismus div. conc. Amblyopie re	76-79	Mäßige AV / bisynchr. Theta-Delta-Paroxysmen mit sharp w. (front. li betont)	BHT li bet. / Macrogyrien li	–
R.N.	25 J	w	9 J	GTKA/KPA/EPA	–	86	Leichte AV / bisynchr. Irreg. spike wave (zentro-temp. li / parietal re herdförmig)	BHT symmetrisch	–
G.S.	30 J	w	7 Mo	KPA/TA/MA/AtA/A(?)	Strabismus div. conc. Ataxie	Mittelschwere Intelligenzmind.	Mäß. AV / bisynchr. Theta-Delta-Paroxysmen mit eingelag. sharp w., spikes	BHT symm. bilat., front. bet. / front. Pachygy.	–
G.A.	22 J	w	7. Lj.	GTKA/KPA/TA	–	91	Unregel., hochampl. Alpha-EEG (leichte AV) diskont. bilat. (unab.) spike w. temporo-occip. / sharp w. re zentro-temp.	BHT bilat. symm. – hint. Quadranten / posteriore Pachygyrien	–
Z.H.	35 J	w	7. Lj.	GTKA/A/KPA	–	Leichte Intelli-genzmind.	Leichte AV / bisynchr. front. bet. Theta-Delta-Paroxysmen / front. sharp w. u. spikes unter HV	BHT bilat. symm. sehr breit, frontopariet. bet. / unregelm. Windungsrelief + Pachygyrien. HS. re.	–
Z.J.	27 J	w	10. Lj.	GTKA, MA	–	Leichte Intelligenzmind.	Mäß. AV / bisynchr. Theta-Delta-Paroxysmen mit sharp w., z. T. re. bet., fok. Spikes (C4/P4)	BHT bilat. symm. / Pachygyrien	Tochter der Schwester mit Intell. mind.
J.R.	24 J	w	12 J	GTKA/KPA	–	85	Leichte AV / langs. u. steile Elemente re frontotemp.	BHT symm. (DVA re front.)	Cousine mit Epilepsie
K.H.	42 J	m	9 J	GTKA/KPA/TA/MA	Leichte Ataxie, kongen. Nyst.	76	Bisynchr. Theta-Delta-Paroxysmen / multifok. Spikes	BHT symm. / bilat. Pachygyrie	–
T.M.	32 J	m	2. Lj.	GTKA/KP/MA	–	75	Leichte AV / bisynchr. Theta-Delta-Paroxysmen mit Spitzen	BHT bifrontal / re. parietal bet.	Tante mit Epilepsie
D.F.	45 J	m	5. Lj.	GTKA/MA	–	ca. 55	Leichte AV / sharp w. frontotemp.	Bipost. BHT / Pachygyrien	–
K.V.	14 J	w	10. Lj.	GTKA, MA, A, TA	–	75	leichte AV, irregul. gen. Polyspike-wave, sharp-slow-w. re bet., Verlangs. bifront., Polyspikes li temp.-pariet./zentrotemp.	BHT symm., frontal betont / Seitenventrikelerweiterung	–
F.U.	45 J	w	5 J	GTKA/KPA/TA/TKPA/ AtA /A	Milde, re. betonte Tetraspastik (Amygdalotomie li mit 16 J)	Schwere Intelligenzminderung	Unregelm., verl. GA, bisynchr. Theta-Delta-Paroxysmen mit spikes u. sharp w.	BHT symm. posterior bet / (Stichkanal nach Amygdaloto-mie li)	
S.R.	30 J	m	6 Mo	GTKA/AtA/A/MA	Strabism. div. con. Paraspast. bei cervik. Syringomyelie	Schwere Intelligenzminderung	Leichte AV, li post. Theta-/Delta. Bisynchr. front. bet. Theta-Delta Paroxysmen mit sharp w., fokale sharp w. li temp.	BHT symm. bilat. sehr breit, frontal betont / Frontale Pachygyrien	–
T.A.	23 J	w	11 J	GTKA/MA/TA/TKPA/AtA/ Dämmerattacken	Hypakusis bds	Schwere Intelligenzminderung	Leichte AV, Verl. bifronto-temp. Bisynchron. Theta-Delta Paroxysmen fronto-zentro-pariet. bet. mit sharp w., z.T. sharp w. li bet.	BHT bilat. symm., sehr breit frontal bis parietal	–

GTKA = generalisiert tonisch-klonische Anfälle (mit/ohne fokalen Beginn) – KPA = komplex-partielle Anfälle – EPA = einfach-partielle Anfälle – MA = myoklonische Anfälle – TA = tonische Anfälle – A = Absencen / atypische Absencen – AtA = atonische Anfälle – TKPA = tonisch-psychomotorische Anfälle – BHT = Bandheterotopien – HS = Hippocampussklerose – DVA = developmental venous anomaly den ersten drei bis fünf Lebensjahren. Ein zweiter Altersgipfel findet sich um das zehnte Lebensjahr, wobei die Epilepsie in Einzelfällen noch in der Mitte der zweiten Lebensdekade beginnen kann.

Häufig kommen mehrere Anfallsarten bei einem Individuum gleichzeitig vor. In 78% der Fälle finden sich generalisiert tonisch-klonische Anfälle, häufig fokal beginnend. Einfach-partielle Anfälle kommen in 34%, Absencen und atypische Absencen in 30% vor. Bei 28% der Patienten mit bilateralen Bandheterotopien finden sich komplex-partielle –, bei 20% myoklonische – und bei 18% tonische Anfälle. Seltener werden BNS-Anfälle (6%) und Versiv-Anfälle (4%) berichtet.

Die Epilepsie nimmt häufig einen therapierefraktären Verlauf. In Einzelfällen kann jedoch Anfallfreiheit unter Medikation erreicht werden.

Das EEG zeigt in der überwiegenden Mehrzahl der Fälle abnorme, zum Teil durchaus charakteristische Befunde. In 81,5% der Fälle ist die Grundaktivität (meist leicht bis mäßig) verlangsamt. Generalisierte epilepsietypische Abläufe, wie spike-waves, slow-spike-waves, Polyspike-waves sowie paroxysmale frontal betonte Theta(-Delta)-Gruppen mit eingelagerten spikes und sharp waves werden in 29 von 30 Fällen (97%) gefunden. Die genannten paroxysmalen Theta (-Delta)-Gruppen mit eingelagerten epilepsietypischen Abläufen sind beim double-cortex-Syndrom besonders häufig und interindividuell recht gleichförmig. Generalisierte Abläufe sind nicht selten seitenbetont. Fokale und multifokale epilepsietypische Abläufe zeigten sich bei 16 von 30 Patienten (54%). Es kommen also häufig beim selben Patienten sowohl generalisierte wie auch fokale epilepsietypische EEG-Veränderungen vor.

Studien zur Funktion der heterotopen Neuronengruppen

Es ist wenig darüber bekannt, ob heterotope Neurone mit anderen Nervenzellen funktionell verbunden sind bzw. ob sie an physiologischer Gehirnaktivität teilhaben. Tiermodelle neuronaler Migrationsstörungen (Mäusemutanten/reeler-Mutation/Hld-Mutation) zeigen, dass heterotope Nervenzellen teilweise ihre physiologische Kontakte zu anderen Neuronen ausbilden und an der normalen Informationsverarbeitung beteiligt sind (Nowakowski, 1987).

Ableitungen mit Tiefenelektroden aus Bandheterotopien haben nachweisen können, dass diese eine normale, dem Cortex entsprechende elektrische Aktivität hervorbringen und es war auch eine organisierte epileptische Aktivität aus den Bandheterotopien ableitbar (Morell et al., 1992).

Studien mit der Positronen-Emissions-Tomografie (PET) zeigen einen Glucosestoffwechsel im heterotopen Band, der im Vergleich mit dem benachbarten Neocortex gleich oder erhöht war (Miura et al., 1993; De Volder et al., 1994).

Erste publizierte Untersuchungen bei einem Patienten mit der funktionellen Kernspintomografie (fMRI) haben die Aktivierung der Heterotopien bei physiologischer Gehirnaktivität erkennen lassen (Pinard et al., 2000). Dabei zeigt die Abbildung der Kernspintomografie bei diesem Patienten neben den Bandheterotopien auch abnorm breite Großhirnwindungen mit abgeflachten Windungstälern.

In einer eigen fMRI-Studie haben wir drei unserer Patienten (B. O., A. M., K. H.) untersucht. Die funktionelle Aktivierung erfolgte mit motorischen Aufgaben (Faustschluss) bei allen und mit visueller Stimulation bei zwei der Patienten. Während der bilateralen Handbewegungen konnte bei allen untersuchten Patienten ein aktivierungsabhängiger BOLD- (blood oxygen level dependent) Kontrast sowohl des (äußeren) Cortex als auch des heterotopen Neuronenbandes gefunden werden. Diese Aktivierung war am sichersten bzw. deutlichsten bei unserem männlichen Patienten, dessen Großhirnwindungsrelief Charakteristika der Pachygyrien aufwies. Unter visueller Stimulation sahen wir eine Aktivierung des Heterotopiebandes nur bei einem Patienten (Spreer et al., 2001).

Die Befunde zur metabolischen – bzw. funktionsabhängigen Aktivität der Bandheterotopien deuten darauf hin, dass diese, zumindest unter bestimmten Voraussetzungen, in neuronale Netze, die sie zusammen mit kortikalen Neuronen bilden, integriert sind und unter physiologischen Bedingungen aktiviert werden können. Möglicherweise ist dies besonders dann der Fall, wenn das angrenzende Großhirnwindungsrelief Abnormitäten im Sinne von verbreiterten Windungen (Pachygyrien) zeigt.

Molekulargenetische Befunde

Das double-cortex-Syndrom ist genetisch eine heterogene Erkrankung. Bisher sind zwei Gene bekannt, die mit dieser Gehirnfehlbildung assoziiert sind (Dobyns 1999). Durch genetische Kopplungsanalysen in Familien mit double-cortex-Syndrom und Lissenzephalien konnte das sog. Doublecortin-Gen (DCX-Gen) auf dem X-Chromosom (Xq22.3-q23) lokalisiert und schließlich identifiziert werden (des Portes et al., 1998; Gleeson et al. 1998). Dieses Gen codiert für ein Mikrotubulinassoziiertes Protein (Doublecortin), das an Aufbau- bzw. Umbau-vorgängen des Zytoskeletts maßgeblich beteiligt ist. Neurone ohne funktionierendes Doublecortin sind in ihrem Migrationsverhalten gestört und bleiben während der Gehirnentwicklung auf dem Weg von der subventrikulären Proliferationszone zur Gehirnoberfläche in der weißen Substanz hängen.

Während Mutationen in dem DCX-Gen bei weiblichen heterozygoten Anlageträgerinnen zum double-cortex-Syndrom führen, bewirken DCX-Mutationen bei männlichen hemizygoten Patienten eine Lissenzephalie. Dieser Unterschied ist dadurch zu erklären, dass Frauen mit zwei X-Chromosomen eines ihrer X-Chromosomen relativ früh in der Embryogenese abschalten. Diese Inaktivierung geschieht in der Regel zufällig (Lyon-Hypothese), d.h. bei ca. 50% der Zellen ist das eine, bei den anderen 50% das andere X-Chromosom aktiv. Bei heterozygoten weiblichen Patienten bedeutet dies, dass die Neurone mit dem Wildtyp-Allel ungestört zu ihrem Zielort migrieren und einen unauffälligen Cortex bilden können, während die Neurone mit dem mutierten Allel in der weißen Substanz unterhalb des Cortex verbleiben und zu dem Bild der subkortikalen laminären Bandheterotopie führen. Bei den hemizygoten männlichen Patienten mit Mutationen im DCX-Gen hingegen sind alle Neurone in ihren Migrationseigenschaften gestört, so dass sich eine Lissenzephalie ausbildet.

Dabei kann vereinfacht gesagt werden, dass dieser lissenzephale Cortex dem subkortikalen laminären Band der Patienten mit double-cortex Syndrom entspricht.

Nach Angaben in der Literatur ist es möglich, bei Patientinnen mit double-cortex-Syndrom in 70–80% der Fälle die zugrunde liegende Mutation durch Analyse des DCX-Gens zu identifizieren (Dobyns 1999). Wir haben in unserem Kollektiv von 11 Patientinnen, von denen 8 bereits untersucht sind, in 5 Fällen eine DCX-Mutation (62,5%) finden können. Dabei bestätigt der Nachweis von 4 bisher noch nicht identifizierten Mutationen die Notwendigkeit der Sequenzierung des gesamten DCX-Gens bei der molekulargenetischen Diagnostik.

Für Nachkommen einer Anlageträgerin einer DCX-Mutation besteht eine Wahrscheinlichkeit von 1/2, das mutierte DCX-Gen zu erben. Für weibliche heterozygote Anlageträgerinnen einer DCX-Mutation bedeutet dies, dass für Töchter dieser Patientin eine Wahrscheinlichkeit von 50% besteht, ebenfalls von einem double-cortex-Syndrom betroffen zu sein. Für Söhne beträgt die Wahrscheinlichkeit, von einer Lissenzephalie betroffen zu sein, 50%.

In seltenen Fällen können auch männliche Patienten von einem double-cortex-Syndrom betroffen sein, das auf Mutationen im DCX-Gen zurückgeführt werden kann (Pilz et al. 1999). Wir haben ebenfalls bei einem männlichen Patienten eine Missense-Mutation nachweisen können. Allerdings liegen hier die Mutationen meist, wie in unserem Fall, als somatische Mosaik-Mutationen vor, d.h. dass sie nur bei einem Teil der Körperzellen zu finden sind. Hierzu kann es kommen, wenn eine Mutation z.B. sehr früh in der Blastogenese in einer einzelnen Zellen als *de novo* Mutation entsteht und an deren Tochterzellen weitergegeben wird, während die übrigen Zellen und deren Tochterzellen die nicht mutierte Erbanlage besitzen. Prinzipiell können diese somatischen Mutationen auf die Keimblätter beschränkt bleiben, so dass nach Abschluss der Keimblattdifferenzierung die Mutationssuche im Blut durch Analyse der Lymphozyten-DNA erfolglos bleiben kann. In solchen Fällen stellt die Untersuchung anderer Gewebe wie z.B. Haarwurzelzellen (ektodermaler Ursprung) eine Alternative dar.

Das zweite Gen, das mit einem double-cortex-Syndrom assoziiert sein kann, ist das *LIS1*-Gen. Für gewöhnlich führen Mutationen des autosomalen LIS1-Genes (Chromosom 17p12) durch dominante Vererbung zu einer isolierten Lissenzephalie. Es sind bisher zwei Fälle von double-cortex-Syndrom beschrieben, bei denen eine LIS1-Mutation als ursächliche Veränderung angenommen wird. Wichtig ist zu erwähnen, dass diese Patienten nur eine inkomplette und dabei nur eine lokuläre subkortikale Bandheterotopie aufwiesen. In diesen Fällen wird von sogenannten »milden Mutationen« mit teilweise vorhandener Restfunktion ausgegangen, so dass es nicht zu einer voll ausgeprägten Lissenzephalie kommt.

Der Unterschied zwischen dem LIS1-Gen und dem DCX-Gen, die beide sowohl zu einem double-cortex Syndrom als auch zu einer Lissenzephalie führen können, liegt darin, dass Mutationen des DCX-Genes eher zu frontal betonten Malformationen führen, während Veränderungen des LIS1-Gens mehr occipital betonte Fehlbildungen bewirken (Dobyns et al. 1999; Pilz et al. 1998). Somit kann weniger beim double-cortex-Syndrom als vielmehr bei der Lissenzephalie unter Berücksichtigung der Lokalisation und Ausprägung der zerebralen Veränderungen eine Vorentscheidung bezüglich der weiteren molekular-genetischen Diagnostik getroffen werden (Leventer et al. 2000).

Literatur

1. Barkovich AJ, Guerrini R, Battaglia G, Kalifa G, N'Guyen T, Parmeggiani A et al. (1994) Band heterotopia: correlation of outcome with magnetic resonance imaging parameters. Ann Neurol 36: 609–617
2. De Volder A, Gadisseux JFA, Michel CJ, Maloteaux JMV, Bol AC, Grandin CB et al (1994) Brain glucose utilization in band heterotopia: synaptic activity of »double cortex«. Pediatr Neurol 11: 290–294
3. Des Portes V, Pinard JM, Billuart P, Vinet MC, Koulakoff A, Carrie A et al (1998) A novel CNS gene required for neuronal migration and involved in x-linked subcortical laminar heterotopia and lissencephaly syndrome. Cell 92: 51–61
4. Dobyns WB, Truwit CL, Ross ME, Matsumoto N, Pilz DT, Ledbetter DH, Gleeson JG, Walsh CA, Barkovich AJ (1999) Differences in the gyral pattern distinguish chromosome 17-linked and X-linked lissencephaly. Neurology 53:270–7
5. Dobyns WB (Updated 4 Oct 1999) Lissencephaly Overview. In: Geneclinics:Medical Genetics Knowledge Database [database online]. Copyright, University of Washington, Seattle. Available at *http://www.geneclinics.org/profiles/lis-overwiev/index.html*
6. Franzoni E, Bernardi B, Marchiani V, Crisanti AF, Marchi R, Fonda C (1995) Band brain heterotopia. Case report and literature review. Neuropediatrics 26: 37–40
7. Friede RL (1989) Developmental neuropathology. Berlin, Heidelberg, New York. Springer-Verlag: 333–334
8. Gleeson JG, Allen KM, Fox JW, Lamperti ED, Berkovic S, Scheffer I (1998) Doublecortin, a brain-specific gene mutated in human x-linked lissencephaly and double cortex syndrome, encodes a putative signaling protein. Cell 92: 63–72
9. Gleeson JG, Luo RF, Grant PE, Guerrini R, Huttenlocher PR, Berg MJ (2000) Genetic and neuroradiological heterogeneity of double cortex syndrome. Ann Neurol 47: 265–269
10. Granata T,Battaglia G, D'Incerti L, Franceschetti S, Zucca C, Savoiardo M, Avanzino G (1994) Double cortex syndrome: electroclinical study of three cases. Ital, J, Neurol Sci 15: 15–23
11. Harding B (1996) Gray matter heterotopia. Guerrini R et al. (Hg.) Dysplasias of cerebral cortex and epilepsy. Philadelphia, Raven-Lippincott: 81–88
12. Iannetti P, Raucci U, Basile LA, Spalice A, Di Biasi C, Trasimeni G, Gualdi GF (1993) Neuronal migrational disorders: diffuse cortical dysplasia or the »double cortex« syndrome. Acta Paediatr 82: 501–503
13. Kirkham FJ, Ebbing A (1994) Case summary: Kate. Seizure 3 (Suppl.A): 33–36
14. Landy HJ, Curless RG, Ramsay RE, Slater J, Ajmone-Marsan C, Quencer RM (1993) Corpus callosotomy for seizures associated with band heterotopia. Epilepsia 34: 79–83
15. Leventer RJ, Pilz DT, Matsumoto N, Ledbetter DH, Dobyns WB (2000) Lissencephaly and subcortical band heterotopia: molecular basis and diagnosis. Mol Med Today (6) 277–284
16. Livingston JH, Aicardi J (1990) Unusual MRI appearance of diffuse subcortical heterotopia or »double cortex« in two children. Journal Neurol Neurosurg Psychiatry 53: 617–620
17. Miura K, Watanabe K, Maeda N, Matsumoto A, Kumagai T, Ito K, Kato T (1993) Magnetic resonance imaging and positron emission tomography of band heterotopia. Brain Dev 15; 288–290
18. Morrell F, Whisler WW, Hoeppner TJ, Smith MC, Kanner AM, Pierre-Louis SJC, Chez MG, Hasegawa H (1992) Electrophysiology of heterotopic gray matter in the »double cortex« syndrome. Epilepsia 33 (Suppl. 3): 76.
19. Nowakowski RS (1987) Basic Concepts of CNS Development. Child Dev 58: 568–595

20. Palmini A, Andermann F, Aicardi J, Dulac O, Chaves F, Ponsot G (1991) Diffuse cortical dysplasia, or the »double cortex« syndrome: the clinical and epileptic spectrum in 10 patients. Neurology 41: 1656–1662
21. Parmeggiani A, Santucci M, Ambrosetto P, Amadi A, Baioni E, Giovanardi Rossi P(1994) Interictal EEG findings in two cases with »double cortex« syndrome. Brain and Development 16: 320–324
22. Pilz DT, Matsumoto N, Minnerath S, Mills P, Gleeson JG, Allen KA, Walsh CA, Barkovich AJ, Dobyns WB, Ledbetter DH, Ross ME (1998) LIS1 and XLIS (DCX) mutations cause most human classical lissencephaly, but different patterns of malformation. Hum Mol Genet 7:2029–37
23. Pilz DT, Kuc J, Matsumoto N, Bodurtha J, Bernadi B, Tassinari CA, Dobyns WB, Ledbetter DH (1999) Subcortical band heterotopia in rare affected males can be caused by missense mutations in DCX (XLIS) or LIS1. Hum Mol Genet 8:1757–60
24. Pinard JM, Feydy A, Carlier R, Perez N, Pierot L, Burnod Y (2000) Functional MRI in double cortex: functionality of heterotopia. Neurology 54: 1531–1533
25. Ricci S, Cusmai R, Fardello G, Fusco L, Vigevano F (1992) Double cortex. A neuronal migration anomaly as a possibile cause of Lennox-Gastaut Syndrome. Archives of Neurology 49: 61–64
26. Spreer J, Martin P, Greenlee M, Wohlfarth R, Hammen A, Arnold S, Schumacher M (2001) Functional MRI in patients with band heterotopia. NeuroImage 14: 357–365

Voxel-basierte 3D-MRT-Analyse zur Erkennung und Lokalisation fokaler kortikaler Dysplasien

H.-J. Huppertz, J. Kassubek, F. D. Juengling, J. Spreer, A. Schulze-Bonhage

Einleitung

Fokale kortikale Dysplasien, d.h. umschriebene Veränderungen der kortikalen Textur aufgrund einer Störung der Hirnrindenentwicklung, werden zunehmend häufiger als Ursache von medikamentös schwer behandelbaren Epilepsien erkannt (8). Dysplastische Läsionen können sich in kernspintomographischen Aufnahmen als abnorme Gyrierung oder Verdickung des Kortexbandes zeigen oder durch eine unscharfe Mark-Rinden-Grenze auffallen (4–7). Trotz der zunehmenden Anwendung hochauflösender Sequenzen in der Magnetresonanztomographie (MRT) ist die Erkennung diskreter Dysplasien bei der konventionellen visuellen Auswertung von MRT-Aufnahmen oft schwierig. Sie hängt sehr von der Expertise und Aufmerksamkeit des Untersuchers ab und unterliegt zudem dessen subjektiver Bewertung. Wir haben daher ein Verfahren zur automatischen und Untersucher-unabhängigen Auswertung von dreidimensionalen MRT-Datensätzen entwickelt, das die Erkennung und Lokalisation solcher Läsionen verbessern kann.

Methoden

Das Verfahren beruht auf Algorithmen der SPM99-Software (Statistical Parametric Mapping, Wellcome Department of Cognitive Neurology, London) (2, 3) und folgt den Prinzipien der Voxel-basierten Morphometrie (9). Ausgangspunkt der Untersuchung ist die Aufnahme eines dreidimensionalen, T1-gewichteten MRT-Datensatzes (MPRAGE-Sequenz, TR = 9,7 ms, TE = 4 ms, flip angle = 12°, 256 x 256 mm Matrix, 160–180 sagittale Schichten, Voxelgröße = 1 x 1 x 1 mm^3; 1,5 T Magnetom Vision, Siemens, Erlangen). Dieser Datensatz wird räumlich normalisiert durch Abbildung auf einen standardisierten stereotaktischen Raum, ähnlich dem bekannten Talairach-Tournoux-Atlas, wobei SPM99 hierfür das Standardhirn des Montreal Neurological Institute (MNI) verwendet. Die Normalisierung beinhaltet sowohl affine Transformationen wie auch nichtlineare Verformungen, korrigiert aber lediglich globale Abweichungen zum Standardhirn und nicht lokale, feinere Unterschiede der Gyrierung (1). Im weiteren Verlauf wird aus dem normalisierten MRT-Datensatz die graue Substanz automatisch segmentiert und mit Hilfe eines Gauss-Filters (6 mm Halbwertsbreite) geglättet. Die resultierenden 3D-Datensätze stellen »kortikale Dichte-Maps« dar, in denen die Grauwerte der einzelnen Voxel die Konzentra-

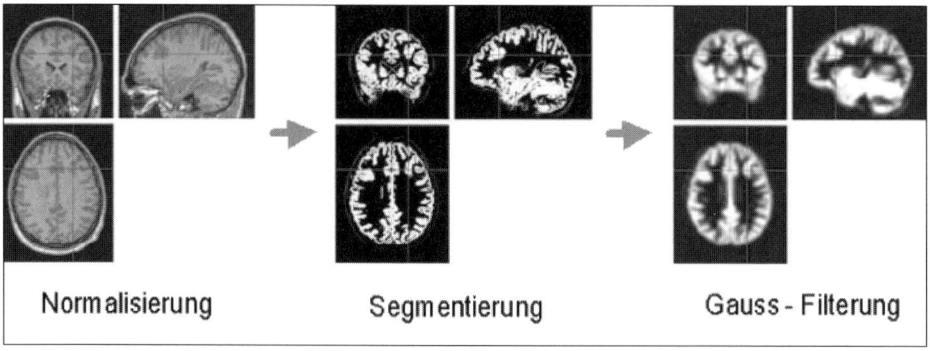

Abb. 1: Ergebnis der 3 Arbeitsschritte »Normalisierung«, »Segmentierung« und »Glättung mittels Gauss-Filter«.

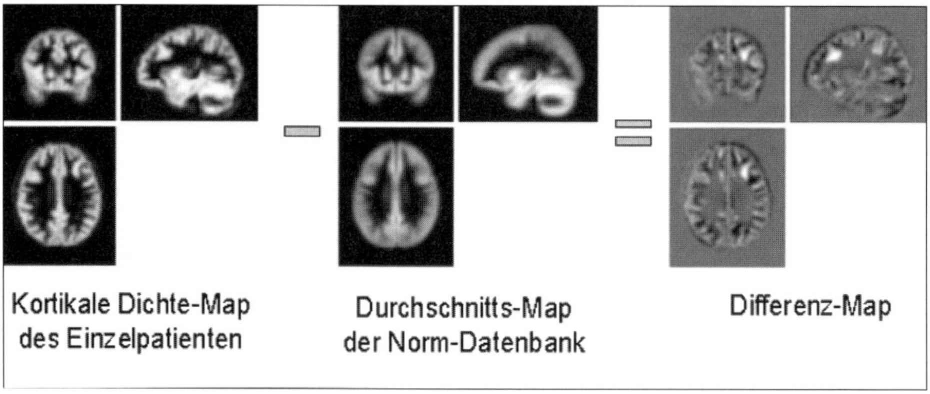

Abb 2: Berechnung der Differenz-Map durch voxel-weise Subtraktion.

tion der grauen Substanz an den entsprechenden Positionen im originalen strukturellen MRT-Datensatz kodieren (Abb. 1).

Zum Aufbau einer Norm-Datenbank wurden die oben beschriebenen Arbeitsschritte auf die MRT-Datensätze von 30 gesunden Probanden (17 m, 13 w, Alter: 15–52 Jahre) angewandt. Aus den resultierenden kortikalen Dichte-Maps wurde anschließend durch einfache Mittelung ein Durchschnittsdatensatz für die Norm-Datenbank berechnet.

Der MRT-Datensatz eines zu untersuchenden Patienten kann nun auf mögliche Dysplasien hin überprüft werden, indem von seiner kortikalen Dichte-Map der Durchschnittsdatensatz der Norm-Datenbank voxel-weise subtrahiert und der resultierende Differenz-Datensatz automatisch auf lokale und globale Maxima hin durchsucht wird. Diese Maxima repräsentieren dann Areale, an denen beispielsweise graue Substanz abnorm weit in das Marklager hineinreicht und sich dadurch von der durchschnittlichen Verteilung des kortikalen Gewebes in der Norm-Datenbank unterscheidet (Abb. 2). Als ein Maß für die Größe der Abweichung von der Norm-Datenbank wird jeweils bestimmt, um wieviel Standardabweichungen der Grauwert am Maximum der Differenz-Map den

Mittelwert der Grauwerte an der entsprechenden Position in der Norm-Datenbank übertrifft.

Bislang wurden insgesamt 12 Patienten (7 w + 5 m, Alter: 14–51 J.) mit fokaler Epilepsie, die sich in der Abteilung für Prächirurgische Epilepsiediagnostik des Universitätsklinikums Freiburg vorstellten, retrospektiv mit dieser Methode auf kortikale Dysplasien hin untersucht. Einschlusskriterien waren der Verdacht auf eine fokale kortikale Dysplasie in der konventionellen visuellen Auswertung der MRT-Daten sowie konkordante Befunde der prächirurgischen Epilepsiediagnostik (EEG, Anfallssemiologie, FDG-PET, ECD-SPECT etc.). Bei vier der Patienten wurde im Verlauf ein epilepsiechirurgischer Eingriff vorgenommen und das resezierte Gewebe histologisch untersucht. Die Diagnose einer kortikalen Dysplasie wurde dabei in drei Fällen bestätigt, in einem Fall war keine eindeutige histologische Klassifikation möglich.

Zu Kontrollzwecken wurden die einzelnen MRT-Datensätze der 30 Probanden in gleicher Weise untersucht wie die Patienten, d.h. für jeden Probanden wurde eine Differenz-Map erstellt, das Maximum in dieser bestimmt und die Größe der Abweichung von der Norm-Datenbank bestimmt.

Ergebnisse

Bei 9 von 12 Patienten stimmte das globale Maximum der Differenz-Map, d.h. der Ort der größten Differenz zwischen Patientendaten und Norm-Datenbank bezüglich der Konzentration von grauer Substanz, mit der Lokalisation der Dysplasie gemäß visueller MRT-Auswertung überein (Abb. 3). Dabei übertraf der jeweilige Grauwert am Maximum der Differenz-Map den Durchschnittswert der Norm-Datenbank an dieser Stelle um 3,3 bis 15,6 Standardabweichungen. Im Vergleich dazu wurden bei den gesunden Probanden am Ort der maximalen Abweichung zur Norm-Datenbank nur Werte zwischen 1,8 und 4,1 Standardabweichungen gefunden.

Ein Patient zeigte 2 dysplastische Läsionen bei 2 lokalen Maxima der Differenz-Map, während sich am Ort des globalen Maximums keine eindeutigen Zeichen einer Dysplasie fanden. Bei den übrigen beiden Patienten ergab sich keine Übereinstimmung zwischen den gefundenen Maxima und der visuellen Befundung der MRT-Aufnahmen.

Erwähnenswert ist, dass bei einem Patienten im Vorfeld bereits zwei MRT-Untersuchungen vorgenommen und als unauffällig befundet worden waren, bevor die hier durchgeführte 3D-MRT-Analyse den Verdacht auf eine frontal links gelegene Dysplasie ergab (Abb. 3: Patient SB). Bei konkordanten Befunden der prächirurgischen Diagnostik wurde die Läsion operativ entfernt. Die histologische Untersuchung betätigte hier wie auch bei einem weiteren der korrekt mittels 3D-MRT-Analyse erkannten Patienten die Diagnose einer kortikalen Dysplasie.

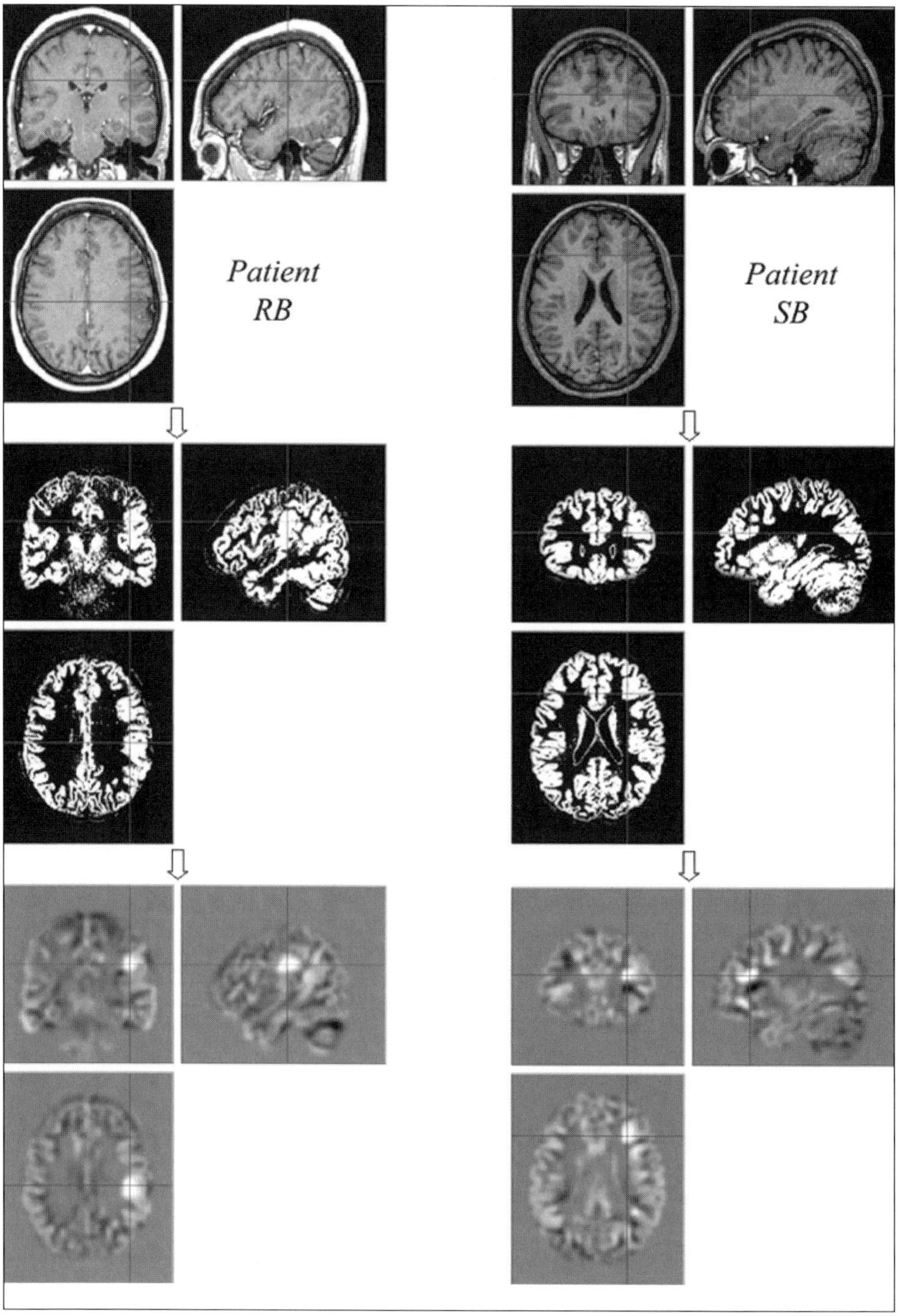

Abb. 3: Ergebnisse der 3D-MRT-Analyse bei 2 Patienten mit fokaler kortikaler Dysplasie parieto-okzipital (Patient RB) bzw. frontal links (Patient SB): Die Fadenkreuze markieren das jeweilige Maximum der Differenz-Map (Reihe 3) und die korrespondierenden Positionen im normalisierten 3D-MRT-Datensatz (Reihe 1) und der kortikalen Dichte-Map (Reihe 2).

Diskussion

Die hier vorgestellte Methode zur Erkennung und Lokalisation von kortikalen Dysplasien mittels 3D-Analyse von MRT-Datensätzen bietet eine Reihe von Vorteilen gegenüber der herkömmlichen visuellen Befundung. Die Auswertung ist komplett automatisiert und damit unabhängig von der Expertise und subjektiven Beurteilung des Untersuchers. Das Verfahren beinhaltet einen inhärenten Vergleich mit einer Norm-Datenbank, während bei der visuellen Auswertung meist nur die Patientenbilder zur Verfügung stehen, nicht aber Vergleichsdaten, die die Variabilität kortikaler Strukturen bei Gesunden widerspiegeln. Zudem erfolgt die 3D-Analyse automatisch in allen drei Raumrichtungen, wodurch Fehlbeurteilungen durch Anschnittphänomene vermieden werden. Schließlich ist die Methode leicht implementierbar, benötigt relativ wenig Zeit (ca. 20 min pro Patient) und kann auch von nicht-ärztlichem Personal durchgeführt werden.

Nachteilig ist, dass sich die Erkennung von Dysplasien bislang nur auf eine abnorme Gyrierung bzw. ein verdicktes Kortexband stützt. Das Kriterium einer unscharfen Mark-Rinden-Grenze wird vernachlässigt, und Dysplasien, die nicht über das normale Kortexband hinausgehen, werden übersehen. Dies erklärt auch, warum die Methode bei zwei der 10 untersuchten Patienten keine Dysplasie gefunden hat. Sensitivität und Spezifität des Verfahrens werden zur Zeit an einer größeren Zahl von Patienten untersucht. Schon jetzt lässt sich aber feststellen, dass die Methode eine wertvolle Hilfe bei der Erkennung und Lokalisation fokaler kortikaler Dysplasien darstellt und daher routinemäßig in unserer Abteilung zum Screening von MRT-Datensätzen von Patienten mit kryptogener Epilepsie eingesetzt wird.

Literatur

1. Ashburner J, Friston KJ. Nonlinear spatial normalization using basis functions. *Hum Brain Mapp* 1999; 7: 254–266
2. Ashburner J, Friston KJ. Voxel-based morphometry – the methods. *Neuroimage* 2000; 11: 805–821
3. Friston KJ, Holmes AP, Poline JB, Grasby PJ, Williams SC, Frackowiak RS, Turner R. Analysis of fMRI time-series revisited. *Neuroimage* 1995; 2 (1): 45–53
4. Gomez-Anson B, Thom M, Moran N, Stevens J, Scaravilli F. Imaging and radiological-pathological correlation in histologically proven cases of focal cortical dysplasia and other glial and neuronoglial malformative lesions in adults. *Neuroradiology* 2000; 42: 157–16
5. Kuzniecky R, Garcia JH, Faught E, Morawetz RB. Cortical dysplasia in temporal lobe epilepsy: magnetic resonance imaging correlations. *Ann Neurol* 1991; 29: 293–298
6. Raymond AA, Fish DR, Sisodiya SM, Alsanjari N, Stevens JM, Shorvon SD. Abnormalities of gyration, heterotypias, tuberous sclerosis, focal cortical dysplasia, microdysgenesis, dysembryoplastic neuroepithelial tumour and dysgenesis of the archicortex in epilepsy. *Brain* 1995; 118: 629–660
7. Sasaki K, Ohsawa Y, Sasaki M, Kaga M, Takashima S, Matsuda H. Cerebral cortical dysplasia: assessment by MRI and SPECT. *Pediatr Neurol* 2000; 23 (5): 410–415
8. Taylor DC, Falconer MA, Bruton CJ, Corsellis JA (1971) Focal dysplasia of the cerebral cortex in epilepsy. *J Neurol Neurosurg Psychiatry;* 34: 369–387
9. Woermann FG, Free SL, Koepp MJ, Ashburner J, Duncan JS. Voxel-by-voxel comparison of automatically segmented cerebral gray matter--A rater-independent comparison of structural MRI in patients with epilepsy. *Neuroimage* 1999; 10 (4): 373–384

EEG-Analyse invasiver Registrierungen bei Kindern mit fokalen Epilepsien mit Hilfe von Rangautokorrelation und Rekurrenzrate

**T. Maiwald, M. Winterhalder, H. U. Voss,
R. Aschenbrenner-Scheibe, J. Timmer, A. Schulze-Bonhage**

Zusammenfassung

Wir stellen zwei neue Verfahren vor, mit denen epileptische Anfälle automatisch aus EEG-Daten erkannt werden können. Eine Evaluation an intracraniellen EEG-Daten von sechs Kindern zeigt, dass die Sensitivität und Spezifität der Methoden ausreicht, um einen Experten in der Offline-EEG-Analyse zu unterstützen.

Einleitung

Im Rahmen des Langzeit-EEG-Monitorings bei Epilepsiepatienten fallen erhebliche Datenmengen an, die retrospektiv hinsichtlich des Auftretens von Anfallsmustern untersucht werden müssen. Im Folgenden stellen wir zwei neuentwickelte Methoden der Zeitreihenanalyse zur Anfallsdetektion vor und geben eine statistische Evaluation der beiden Verfahren. Es zeigt sich, dass die Methoden unterstützend in der Offline-EEG-Analyse eingesetzt werden können.

Die Daten

Insgesamt wurden in der vorliegenden Studie 45 Anfälle und 72 Stunden interiktale Phasen von sechs Kindern mit pharmakorefraktären fokalen Epilepsien untersucht. Die Daten wurden im Rahmen eines prächirurgischen Monitorings mit intracraniellen Elektroden und einer Samplingfrequenz von 256 Hz aufgenommen. Im Anschluss wurden die EEG-Signale zwischen 0,5 und 120 Hz bandpassgefiltert und durchliefen einen 50 Hz-Notchfilter.

Abbildung 1 zeigt exemplarisch einen Ausschnitt von 28 Sekunden einer EEG-Zeitreihe. Die vertikale Linie markiert den Beginn eines Anfalls.

Die Methoden RACe und VarRec

Eindimensionale Zeitreihen $x(t)$ der Länge N können mehrdimensional zu Vektoren $\vec{x}(t) = (x(t), x(t-\tau), \ldots, x(t-(m-1)\tau))$ eingebettet werden. Bei einer richti-

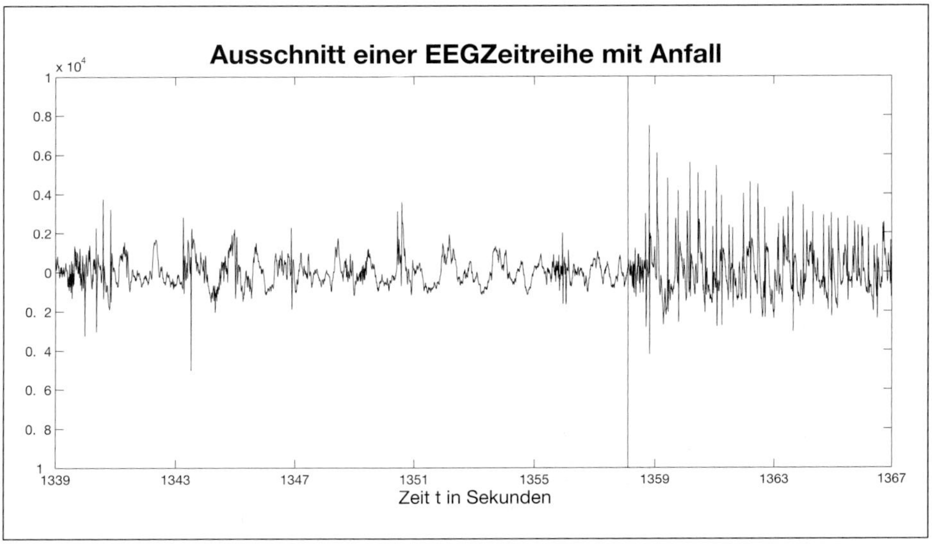

Abb. 1

gen Wahl der Einbettungsdimension m und des Delays τ liefern diese Einbettungsvektoren Informationen über das zugrundeliegende dynamische System (1).

Die Autokorrelationsfunktion $ACF(\tau)$ beschreibt zeitliche Korrelationen in einer Zeitreihe $x(t)$:

$$ACF(\tau') := \frac{1}{N} \sum_{t=1}^{N-\tau'} \frac{x(t)x(t+\tau')}{< x^2(t) >} \quad \textit{für} < x(t) >= 0$$

Betrachtet man den Zerfall der Autokorrelationsfunktion $ACF(\tau)$, so lässt sich das Delay τ bestimmen:

$$\tau = \min \arg\left(ACF(\tau') = \frac{1}{e} \right).$$

Um Robustheit gegenüber Ausreißern zu erreichen, werden die EEG-Signale vor der Analyse auf eine Gleichverteilung skaliert, also ein Ranking durchgeführt. Das so bestimmte Delay τ zeigt ein charakteristisch unterschiedliches Verhalten iktaler und interiktaler Phasen. Hierauf beruht der RACe-Algorithmus: *R*anking *A*utoCorrelation = 1/*e*.

Abbildung 2 zeigt beispielhaft Ergebnisse des Algorithmus RACe für je eine Stunde ohne Anfall (oben) und mit Anfall (unten). Die beiden vertikalen Linien markieren den Anfallsbeginn bzw. das Ende des Anfalls. Deutlich erkennbar sind signifikante Unterschiede der Werte des Algorithmus zwischen iktaler und interiktaler Aktivität.

Für den Algorithmus VarRec werden *Va*rianzen der EEG-Zeitreihe für Zeitfenster von je einer Sekunde, also 256 Datenpunkte, berechnet. Die so erhaltene neue Zeitreihe $\sigma(t)$ wird mehrdimensional zu $\vec{\sigma}(t)$ eingebettet. Hiervon wird eine

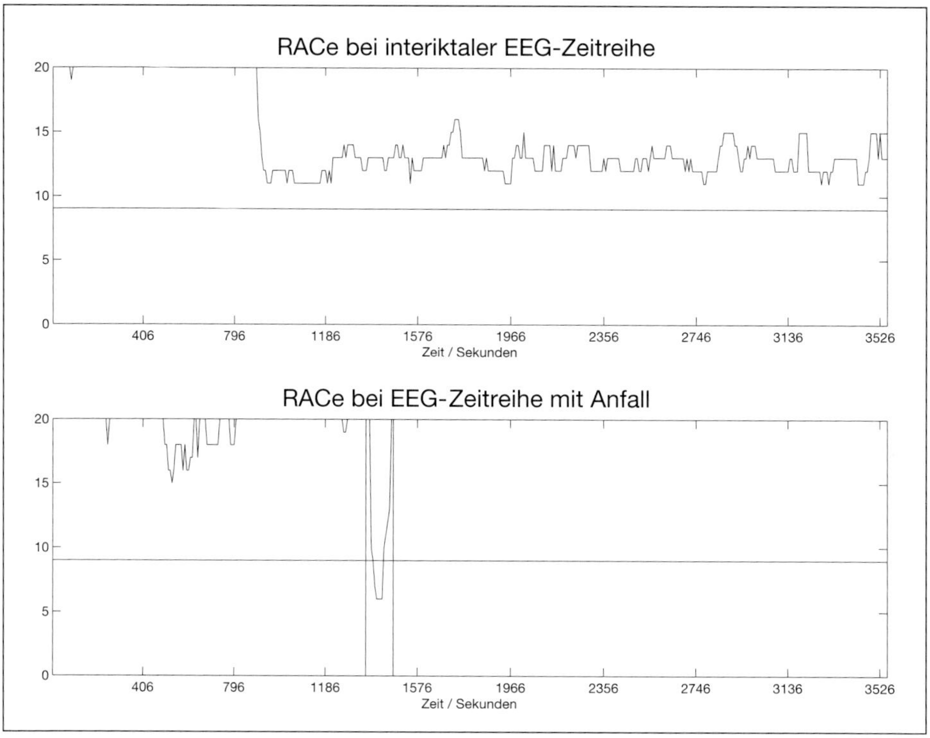

Abb. 2

*Rec*urrence-Rate berechnet, die ein Maß für die Wiederkehr gleicher Muster ist (2):

$$R_\varepsilon(t) := \frac{1}{N}\sum_{t'=1}^{N}\Theta\left(\varepsilon - \left\|\vec{\sigma}(t) - \vec{\sigma}(t')\right\|\right)$$

mit der Heaviside-Sprungfunktion

$$\Theta(x) = \begin{cases} 1 & \textit{für} \quad x \geq 0 \\ 0 & \textit{für} \quad x < 0 \end{cases}$$

Wird zuvor wiederum ein Ranking der Varianz-Zeitreihe $\sigma(t)$ durchgeführt und der Parameter ε=0,1 (entspricht 10% des größten Abstands der Varianz-Zeitreihe) gewählt, zeigen sich deutliche Unterschiede der so berechneten Rekurrenzrate zwischen iktalen und interiktalen Phasen.

Abbildung 3 verdeutlicht dies anhand einer Stunde ohne Anfall (oben) und einer Stunde mit Anfall (unten). Der Anfallsbeginn und das Ende des Anfalls sind wiederum durch die vertikalen Linien gekennzeichnet. Iktal zeigt die Methode VarRec signifikant höhere Werte als in der interiktalen Phase.

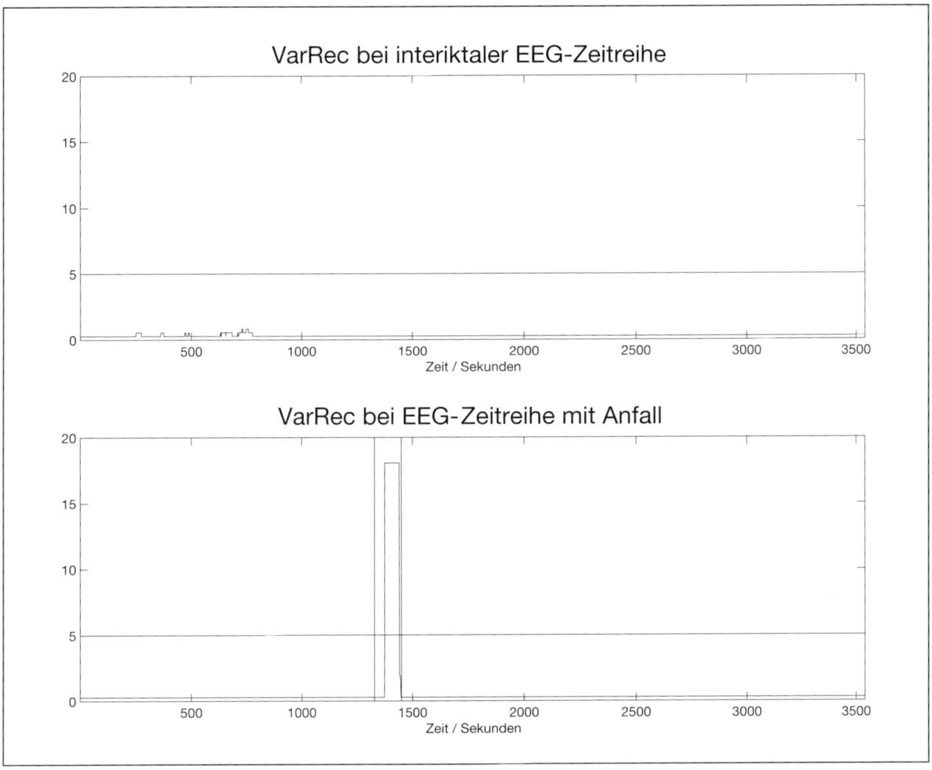

Abb. 3

Statistische Auswertung

Zur Quantifizierung der Sensitivität und der Rate falsch positiver Detektionen der beiden Verfahren müssen patientenadaptiert Schwellen gesetzt werden. In den Abbildungen 2 und 3 sind mögliche Werte für den Schwellen-Parameter durch die horizontalen Linien angedeutet. Ein Unterschreiten (beim Algorithmus RACe) bzw. Überschreiten (beim Algorithmus VarRec) führt zur Detektion eines Anfalls.

Um ein Optimum zwischen Sensitivität und der Rate falsch positiver Detektionen zu erhalten, wurden alle Daten für einen weiten Bereich des Schwellen-Parameters analysiert. Da die Anzahl der Anfälle pro Patient meist auf fünf beschränkt war, konnte keine Out-of-Sample Untersuchung durch Aufteilen in Lern- und Testdatensatz durchgeführt werden.

Ergebnisse

Die Studie ergab folgende Ergebnisse:

	RAC		VarRec	
Patient	**Sensitivität in Prozent**	**falsch Positive pro Stunde**	**Sensitivität in Prozent**	**falsch Positive pro Stunde**
1	0%	0,00	40%	0,07
2	80%	0,15	100%	0,00
3	50%	1,54	50%	0,15
4	33%	0,22	17%	0,00
5	67%	0,00	46%	0,09
6	100%	0,00	100%	0,00
Gesamt	**55%**	**0,32**	**59%**	**0,05**

Im Schnitt sind RACe und VarRec in der Lage, 55% bzw. 59% der Anfälle zu detektieren. Dabei passiert alle drei bzw. 20 Stunden eine falsche Detektion. Bei einer Kombination beider Verfahren erhöht sich die Sensitivität auf 65% bei einer Rate falsch positiver Detektionen von 0,07 pro Stunde.

Schlussfolgerung

Die Verfahren liefern Werte für Sensitivität und der Rate falsch positiver Detektionen, deren Güte stark zwischen den Patienten variiert. Dies deutet auf ein prinzipielles Problem hin, Algorithmen zu entwickeln, die auf alle Patienten anwendbar sind. Die Gründe hierfür sind Gegenstand weiterer Untersuchungen. Jedoch bereits zum jetzigen Zeitpunkt können die Verfahren einen Experten in der Offline-EEG-Analyse unterstützen.

Literatur

1. Takens F (1981) Detecting strange attractors in turbulence. In: D.A. Rand and L.S. Young (editors) Dynamical Systems and Turbulence, volume 898 of Lecture Notes in Mathematics, pages 366–381, Springer, Berlin.
2. Casdagli M.C. (1997) Recurrence plots revisited. Physica D 108:12–44.

Ergebnisse epilepsiechirurgischer Eingriffe bei Kindern mit fokalen corticalen Dysplasien

H. Carmona, A. Schulze-Bonhage, K. Strobl, J. P. Ernst, R. Keimer, T. Bast, D. Rating, S. Rona, J. Honegger, R. Korinthenberg, J. Zentner

Zusammenfassung

Die unvollständige Resektion der epileptogenen Zone basierend auf der Ausdehnung der kernspintomographisch sichtbaren Dysplasie wahrscheinlich die häufigste Ursache für das schlechtere operative Outcome der pharmakorefraktärer Epilepsien aufgrund fokaler corticaler Dysplasie. In der vorliegenden Studie wurde untersucht, ob das postoperative Outcome verbessert ist nach epilepsiechirurgischer Resektion fokaler corticaler Dysplasien durch Verwendung hochauflösender MR-Tomographien und zusätzlicher Elektrocorticographie zur vollständigen Entfernung des epileptogenen dysplastischen Areals. 19 Kinder im Alter von 2–16 Jahren mit histologisch gesicherter fokaler corticaler Dysplasie und pharmakorefraktärer Epilepsie wurden in Freiburg epilepsiechirurgisch behandelt. 17/19 (90%) Patienten erzielen ein Outcome gemäß Engel-Klasse I, die übrigen 2/19 (10%) Patienten erzielten eine Reduktion der Anfallfrequenz um mehr als 75% (Engel III). Unsere gegenwärtigen Daten zeigen, dass bei pharmakorefraktären Epilepsien von Kindern, auch wenn Sie durch fokale corticale Dysplasien verursacht sind, eine ausgezeichnete Anfallskontrolle durch einen epilepsiechirurgischen Eingriff erreicht werden kann.

Fokale corticale Dysplasie, pharmakorefraktärer Epilepsie, Anfallsoutcome

Einleitung

Verläßliche Daten über die Inzidenz und Prävalenz fokaler corticaler Dysplasien liegen bislang nicht vor (1, 2), Dysplasien werden jedoch immer häufiger als Ursache von Epilepsien und Entwicklungsstörungen von Kindern und Erwachsenen erkannt und stellen bei bis zu 25% der Patienten die Ursache pharmakorefraktärer fokaler Epilepsien dar (3). Mehr als die Hälfte der Kinder, die Epilepsiezentren aufgrund pharmakorefraktärer Epilepsien zugewiesen werden, haben eine zugrunde liegende Entwicklungsstörung des Cortex (2), bis zu 76% hiervon sind pharmakorefraktär (4, 5) und somit Kandidaten für eine operative Epilepsietherapie.

Frühere chirurgische Serien zeigten ein schlechteres postoperatives Outcome bei corticalen Dysplasien verglichen mit Patienten mit symptomatischen Epilepsien aufgrund von Tumoren oder mesialer Temporallappenepilepsie (6, 7). Anfallsfreiheit wurde bei 43–57% der operativ behandelten Kinder erzielt (3, 7,

8, 9). Die Vollständigkeit der Entfernung der Läsion wurde als wichtigster prognostischer Faktor für das Erzielen einer guten Anfallskontrolle nachgewiesen (10, 11, 12). Die Abgrenzung fokaler corticaler Dysplasien von intaktem Cortex anhand kernspintomographischer Untersuchungen ist trotz der Fortschritte der Bildgebung weiterhin problematisch (3, 13, 14, 15); entsprechend ist bislang eine unvollständige Resektion der epileptogenen Zone basierend auf der Ausdehnung der kernspintomographisch sichtbaren Dysplasie wahrscheinlich die häufigste Ursache für das gegenüber anderen Ätiologien schlechtere operative Outcome.

Die Sensitivität der in der prächirurgischen Epilepsiediagnostik eingesetzten Verfahren zur Detektion und Abgrenzung dysplastischen Hirngewebes von normalem Cortex wurde in den letzten Jahren verbessert (16, 17, 18, 19). In der vorliegenden Studie wird untersucht, ob sich die verfeinerte Diagnostik unter Einschluss von Analysen von kernspintomographischen 1 mm T1-3D-Datensätzen, multimodalem Imaging und Elektrocorticographie in einem erhöhten Anteil postoperativ anfallsfreier Patienten niederschlägt.

Patienten und Methodik

Im Zeitraum von 1998–2001 wurden insgesamt 19 Patienten im Alter von 2–16 Jahren (Mittel: 11 J, 9 weiblich und 10 männlich) mit histologisch gesicherter fokaler corticaler Dysplasie und pharmakorefraktärer Epilepsie in Freiburg operiert. Die Erstmanifestation der Epilepsie lag zwischen 1 Monat und 7 Jahren (im Mittel: 3,2 J). Die Dauer der Epilepsie betrug zwischen 2 und 15 Jahre (im Mittel: 8,5 J). Die präoperative Anfallsfrequenz lag zwischen 3 Anfällen/Monat und 70 Anfällen/die.

Die prächirurgische Epilepsiediagnostik umfasste bei allen Patienten eine eingehende Erhebung der Anamnese, Video-EEG-Langzeitmonitoring, hochauflösende kerspintomographische (Magnetom Vision Siemens 1.5 Tesla: T1, T2, FLAIR, MPRAGE) und neuropsychologische Untersuchungen. Bei unzureichender Evidenz für den Anfallsursprung wurde zusätzlich eine funktionelle Bildgebung (FDG-PET, interiktales und iktales ECD-SPECT, Iomazenil-SPECT) durchgeführt. Bei 8/19 Patienten wurde ausschließlich anhand eines non-invasiven Video-EEG-Langzeitmonitorings die Zone des Anfallsursrpunges identifiziert, bei 6 Patienten wurde ein invasives Video-EEG-Langzeitmonitoring unter Verwendung von Tiefelektroden, subduralen Streifen- und/oder Gitterelektroden – auch zur Abgrenzung eloquenter Hirnareale – durchgeführt, und bei weiteren 6 Patienten wurde der exakte Umfang der Resektion durch intraoperative Elektrocorticographie festgelegt.

Das Outcome der Kinder mit fokaler corticaler Dysplasie wurde anhand klinischer Verlaufsuntersuchungen 3–31 Monate (im Mittel: 10 Monate) postoperativ untersucht und entsprechend einer modifizierten Klassifikation nach Engel eingeteilt (Klasse I: anfallsfrei (inklusive Auren) nach dem Eingriff, hiervon Klasse Ia: Anfallsfrei ohne Auren, Klasse II: Seltene Anfälle (>90% Anfallsreduktion), Klasse III: Reduktion der Anfallsfrequenz >75%, Klasse IV: Reduktion der Anfallsfrequenz <75%.

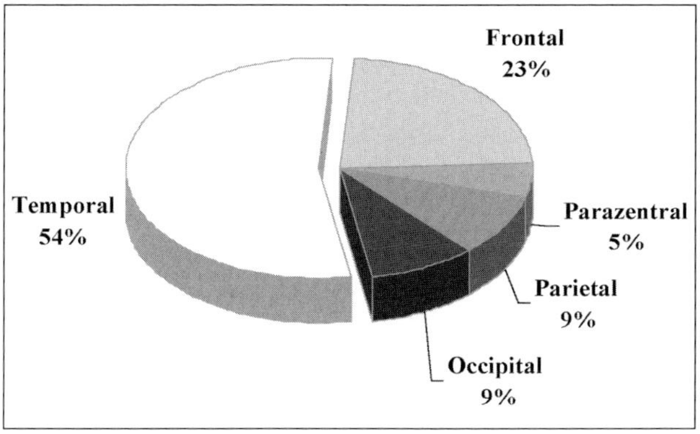

Abb. 1: Lokalisation der fokalen corticalen Dysplasie (2 Patienten hatten eine multilobäre fokale corticale Dysplasie).

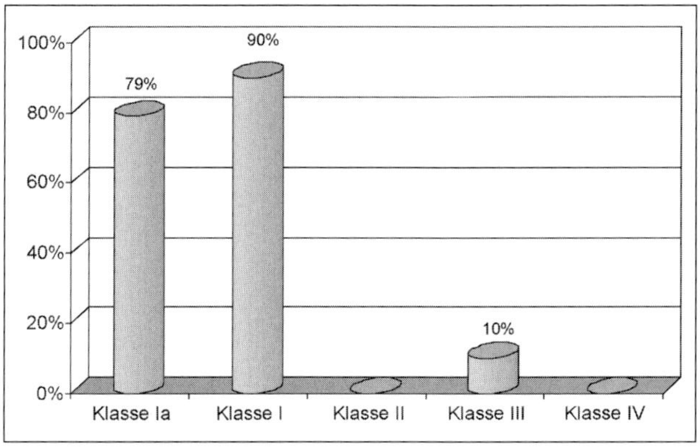

Abb. 2: Anfallsoutcome gemäß Klassifikation nach Engel.
* = Unvollständige Resektion der Dysplasie sowie multiple subpiale Transektionen.

Ergebnisse

8 Patienten hatten zusätzlich zur corticalen Dysplasie eine Hippocampussklerose, 2 Patienten eine fokale Heterotopie. Die Lokalisation der Dysplasie war bei 54% der Patienten temporal, bei 46% extratemporal, bei je einem Patienten temporo-occipital bzw. temporoparietooccipital (vgl. Abb. 1).

Insgesamt waren 15/19 Patienten (79%) nach einem mittleren Follow-up von 10 Monaten vollständig anfallsfrei (Engel Ia), weitere 2 Patienten hatten lediglich noch isolierte Auren. Somit erzielten 17/19 (90%) Patienten ein Outcome gemäß Engel-Klasse I. 2/19 (10%) Patienten erzielten lediglich eine Reduktion der Anfallfrequenz um mehr als 75% (Engel III), dies waren die einzigen Patienten, bei denen die Resektionen entsprechend der durchgeführten Untersuchungen nicht vollständig durchgeführt werden konnten, da die Dysplasien eloquente Cortexareale mit umfassten; bei ihnen wurden zusätzliche multiple subpiale Transektionen in nicht resezierten Dysplasieanteilen durchgeführt. Anfallsrezidive nach initialer Anfallsfreiheit traten im dem beobachteten Zeitraum nicht auf (vgl. Abb. 2).

Als transiente Komplikationen traten bei zwei Patienten hirnorganische Psychosyndrome und in einem Fall eine Durchtrennung des Temporalmuskelansatzes auf. Bleibende Schädigungen waren zwei Quadrantenanopsien bei Entfernung des posterioren Hippocampus und zwei inkomplette Hemiparesen (10,5%) bei Teilresektionen des motorischen Cortex; diese unter Berücksichtigung eines elektrophysiologischen Mappings der Motorcortex erwarteten postoperativen Defizite waren mit den Patienten und ihren Eltern zuvor ausgiebig diskutiert und in Abwägung der Schwere der Epilepsie in Kauf genommen worden.

Schlussfolgerungen

Die Daten der vorgelegten Studie zeigen, dass pharmakorefraktäre Epilepsien von Kindern, auch wenn Sie durch fokale corticale Dysplasien verursacht sind, erfolgreich durch einen epilepsiechirurgischen Eingriff behandelt werden können. Eine umfassende elektrophysiologische und MR-tomographische präoperative Untersuchung für die Lokalisation des Anfallsursprungs und der epileptogenen Zone sowie die funktionelle Abgrenzung der dysplastischen Läsion sind obligatorisch. Die vollständige Entfernung des epileptogenen dysplastischen Gewebes ermöglichte in dieser Serie eine ausgezeichnete Anfallskontrolle.

Literatur

1. Dobyns WB, Kuzniecky RI. (1996) Normal Development and Malformations of the Cortex. In: Wyllie E (ed) The Treatment of Epilepsy: Principles and Practice. pp 93-105. Baltimore, Williams & Wilkins.
2. Whiting S, Duchowny M. (1999) Clinical Spectrum of Cortical Dysplasia in Childhood: Diagnosis and treatment issues. J. Child Neurol. 14: 759–771
3. Kuzniecky R, Murro A, King D, Morawetz R, Smith J, Powers R, Yaghmai F, Faught E, Gallagher B, Snead OC. (1993) Magnetic resonance imaging in childhood intractable parcial epilepsies: pathologic correlations. Neurology 43: 681–687
4. Stephen LJ, Kwan P, Brodie MJ. (2001) Does the cause of localisation-related epilepsy influence the response to antiepileptic drug treatment? Epilepsia 42:357–62
5. Semah F, Picot MC, Adam C, Broglin D, Arzimanoglou A, Bazin B, Cavalcanti D, Baulac M. (1998) Is the underlying cause of epilepsy a major prognostic factor for recurrence? Neurology 51:1256–62.
6. Palmini A. (2000) Disorders of cortical development. Curr Opin Neurol. 13:183–92.
7. Sisodiya SM. (2000) Surgery for malformations of cortical development causing epilepsy. Brain 123: 1075–1091
8. Edwards JC, Wyllie E, Ruggeri PM, Bingaman W, Lüders H, Kotagal P, Dinner DS, Morris HH, Prayson RA, Comair YG. (2000) Seizure outcome after surgery for epilepsy due to malformation of cortical development. Neurology 55: 1110–1114
9. Hong SC, Kang KS, Seo DW, Hong SB, Lee M, Nam DH, Lee JI, Kim JS, Shin HJ, Park K, Eoh W, Suh YL, Kim JH. (2000) Surgical treatment of intractable epilepsy accompanying cortical dysplasia. J. Neurosurg 93: 766–773
10. Palmini A, Andermann F, Olivier A, Tampieri D, Robitaille Y. (1991) Focal neuronal migration disorders and intractable partial epilepsy: results of surgical treatment. Ann Neurol. 30:750–7.

11. Palmini A, Gambardella A, Andermann F, Dubeau F, da Costa JC, Olivier A, Tampieri D, Robitaille Y, Paglioli E, Paglioli Neto E, et al. (1994) Operative strategies for patients with cortical dysplastic lesions and intractable epilepsy. Epilepsia 35 Suppl 6:S57–71.
12. Palmini A, Gambardella A, Andermann F, Dubeau F, da Costa JC, Olivier A, Tampieri D, Gloor P, Quesney F, Andermann E, et al. (1995) Intrinsic epileptogenicity of human dysplastic cortex as suggested by corticography and surgical results. Ann Neurol. 37:476–87
13. Kuzniecky R, Garcia JH, Faught E, Morawetz RB. (1991) Cortical Dysplasia in temporal lobe epilepsy: magnetic resonance imaging correlations. Ann. Neurol. 29:293–298
14. Hwang SI, Kim JH, Park SW, Han MH, Yu IK, Lee SH, Lee DS, Lee SK, Chung CK, Chang KH. (2001) Comparative analysis of MR imaging, positron emission tomography, and ictal single-photon emission CT in patients with neocortical epilepsy. Am J Neuroradiol. 22(5):937–46
15. Janota I, Polkey CE (1992) Cortical dysplasia in epilepsy: a study of material from surgical resections for intractable epilepsy. In: Pedley TA, Meldrum BS (eds) Recent Advances in Epilepsy, pp 37–49. Edinburgh: Churchill Livingstone.
16. Bastos AC, Comeau RM, Andermann F, Melanson D, Cendes F, Dubeau F, Fontaine S, Tampieri D, Olivier A. (1999) Diagnosis of subtle focal dysplastic lesions: curvilinear reformatting from three-dimensional magnetic resonance imaging. Ann Neurol. 46(1):88–94
17. Schulze-Bonhage AH, Huppertz HJ, Comeau RM, Honegger JB, Spreer JM, Zentner JK. (2002) Visualization of Subdural Strip and Grid Electrodes Using Curvilinear Reformatting of 3D MR Imaging Data Sets. Am J Neuroradiol 23(3):400–03
18. Kassubek J, Huppertz HJ, Jüngling FD, Spreer J, Schulze-Bonhage A. (2002) Detection and localization of focal cortical dysplasia by voxel-based 3D MRI Analysis. Epilepsia, 43: 596–602
19. Carmona H, Talazko Z, Huppertz HJ, Martin P, Moser E, Zentner J, Schulze-Bonhage A. (2002) Relevanz der Ausdehnung hypometaboler Areale im FDG-PET für das Outcome von Resektionen bei Patienten mit fokaler corticaler Dysplasie. Epileptologie, Z Epileptol 15: 55–56

Neurochirurgische Resektion eines Hypothalamus-Hamartoms

H. M. Straßburg, R. Kiene, J. V. Rosenfeld

Zusammenfassung

Hypothalamus-Hamartome sind eine zwar seltene, aber wichtige Differentialdiagnose bei therapieresistenten Epilepsien, vor allem in Verbindung mit Lachanfällen und tiefgreifenden Entwicklungsstörungen. Entgegen den bisherigen Erfahrungen mit der operativen Resektion erlaubt die transkallosale Operationstechnik durch einen sehr erfahrenen Neurochirurgen offensichtlich eine wesentliche Verbesserung der Prognose.

Einleitung

Hamartome sind komplexe, fokale Fehlbildungen mit überzähligen reifen Nervenzellen, die makroskopisch einem Tumor ähneln und prinzipiell ubiquitär im ZNS vorkommen können. Nach der WHO-Klassifikation der ZNS-Tumore gehören sie zu den »Tumor-ähnlichen Läsionen«, im Bereich des Hypothalamus sind sie vor allem im Tuber cinerum, das zum limbischen System gehört, lokalisiert (5).

Die klinische Symptomatik kann sich einerseits in einer Pubertas präcox, andererseits in einer Epilepsie mit gelastischen Anfällen sowie z.T. schweren Entwicklungs- und Verhaltensstörungen mit autistischen Symptomen äußern. In Verbindung mit einer bifiden Epiglottis und einer Polydaktylie tritt ein Hypothalamus-Hamartom als Pallister-Hall-Syndrom spontan oder mit autosomal-dominanter Vererbung auf.

Während sich polypöse Hamartome in der Regel operativ gut resezieren lassen, ist das therapeutische Vorgehen bei diffus-breitbasigen Formen wegen der Verbindung zum limbischen System sowohl medikamentös als auch operativ umstritten und schwierig (1–4).

Kasuistik

Bei dem jetzt 10jährigen J.K. bestand nach primär altersentsprechender Entwicklung seit dem 3. Lebensjahr eine rasch progrediente Epilepsie mit komplex-fokalen, myoklonisch-astatischen und gelastischen Anfällen. Die kognitive und emotionale Entwicklung stagnierte auf dem Niveau einer mittelschweren Intelligenzminderung, er zeigte zunehmend autistische Verhaltens- und Schlafstörungen. Das EEG wies initial eine Allgemeinveränderung mit schwerer, seitenwechselnd betonter Dysrhythmie und irregulären sharp-waves auf, im MRT konnte eine 0,8 cm messende, nicht Kontrastmittel-aufnehmende Verdickung im rechten Tuber

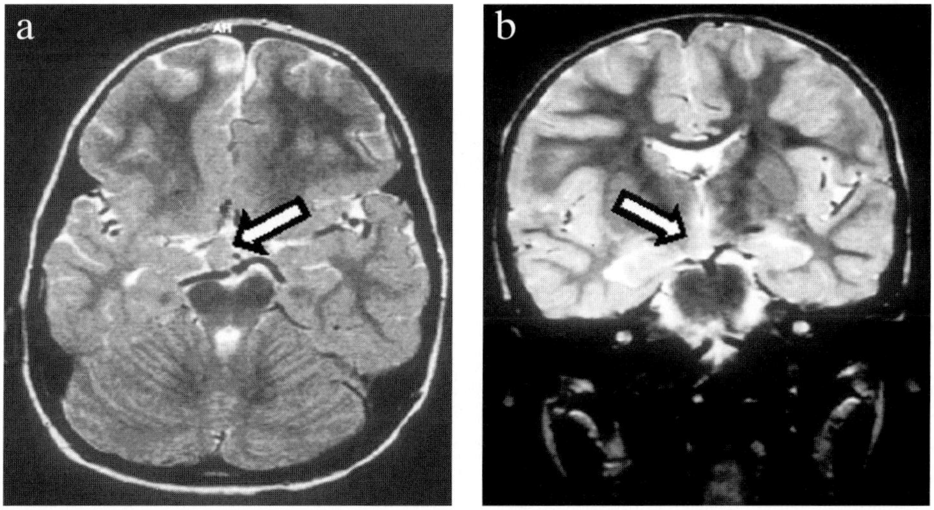

Abb. 1 a und b: MRT mit Darstellung einer nicht Kontrastmittel aufnehmenden Verdickung des Tuber cinerum rechts.

cinerum ohne Größenprogredienz bei Kontroll-Untersuchung nachgewiesen werden (Abb. 1a und b). Endokrinologisch bestanden keine Auffälligkeiten.

Die zerebralen Anfälle waren trotz hochdosierter antikonvulsiver Therapie, u.a. mit Carbamazepin, Sultiam, Vigabatrim, Valproat und Lamotrigen nicht zu beherrschen.

Mehrere konsultierte Neurochirurgen im In- und Ausland lehnten eine operative Vorgehensweise aus Furcht vor zunehmenden Verhaltensstörungen postoperativ ab.

Die Eltern nahmen von sich aus Kontakt mit J.V.R. vom Royal Children's Hospital, Melborne, Australien, auf, der im Jan. 2001 in »Neurosurgery« (6) über eine neue Technik der transkallosalen Resektion von Hypothalamus-Tumoren mit gelastischer Epilepsie berichtet hatte.

Im Juli 2001 wurde J. als 20. Patient in Folge mittels mikrochirurgischer Technik mit einem speziellen Ultraschall-Cusor und rahmenfreier Stereotaxie in Melborne operiert. Postoperativ kam es zu einem kurzzeitigen Diabetes insipidus sowie zu einer Appetitsteigerung, die zerebralen Anfälle sistierten bereits am 2. postoperativen Tag, das EEG war deutlich stabilisiert und blieb auch in der Folgezeit ohne HSA (Abb. 2 und 3), 10 Monate nach der Operation zeigte J. kontinuierliche Entwicklungsfortschritte, einen zunehmend besseren Sozialkontakt, machte Lernfortschritte (befolgt einfache Aufforderungen, legt Puzzle über 30 Teile) und hat keine Schlafstörungen mehr.

Diskussion

Die klinische Symptomatik von Hamartomen im Tuber cinerum kann sehr unterschiedlich sein, – neben nur diskreten Entwicklungsauffälligkeiten mit und ohne Pubertas präcox können wie in unserem Fall schwerste Epilepsien mit komplex-fokalen und gelastischen Anfällen sowie schwere, überwiegend mental-kognitive Entwicklungs- und Verhaltensstörungen mit autistischen Symptomen vorliegen. In der Regel ist bei diesen Kindern mit medikamentöser Antikonvulsiva-Behandlung nur eine kurzfristige Stabilisierung der Epilepsie ohne wesent-

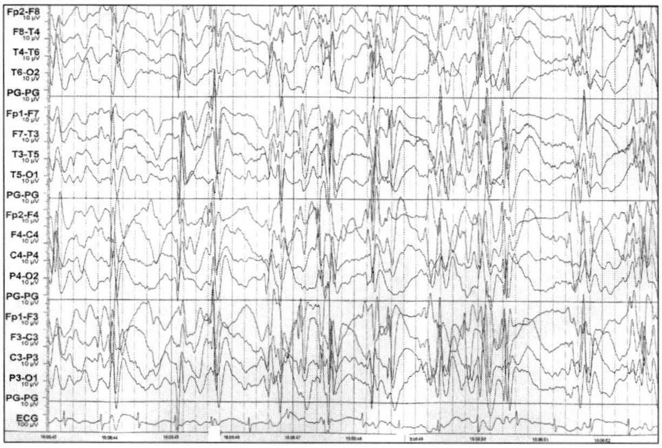

Abb. 2: EEG unmittelbar vor der Operation im Juli 2001.

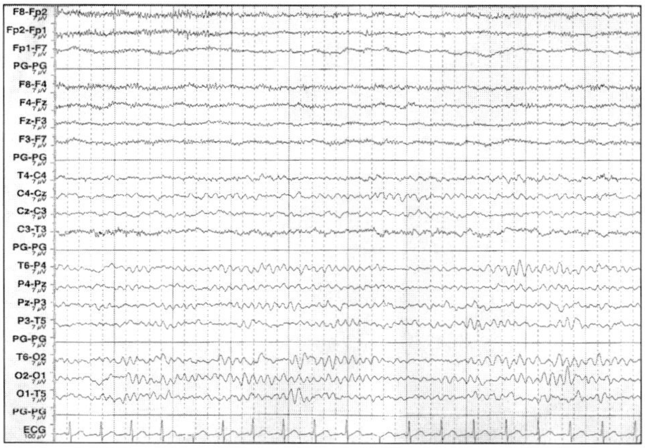

Abb. 3: EEG 10 Tage nach der Operation.

liche Verbesserung der sozio-emotionalen und kognitiven Symptome möglich. Andererseits wurde wiederholt über deutliche Befundverschlechterungen, z.T. mit vermehrter Aggressivität und pathologischer Steigerung des Essverhaltens nach operativer Resektion über einen subtemporalen Zugang berichtet. Unseres Wissens ist unser Patient der erste in Europa, der bei dieser Krankheit mit der neuen, von J. V. Rosenfeld entwickelten Technik operiert wurde und sich so eindrucksvoll sowohl in seiner klinischen Symptomatik als auch vom EEG her verbessert hat. Soweit bekannt, haben sich alle mit dieser Methode operierten Patienten deutlich gebessert, unser Patient ist aber ein besonders positives Beispiel. In Zukunft kann diese Operationstechnik auch in Deutschland von sehr erfahrenen Neurochirurgen eingesetzt werden, die Behandlung mit anderen, z.B. auch radiologischen Methoden, muss in jedem Einzelfall kritisch diskutiert werden.

Literatur

1. Berkovic SF, Kuzniecky RI et al. (1997): Human epileptogenesis and hypothalamic hamartomas: new lessons from experiments of nature. Epilepsia 38, 1–3
2. Deonna T, Ziegler AL (2000):Hypothalamic hamartoma, precocius puberty and gelastic seizures: a special model of »epileptic« developmental disorder. Epileptic Disord 2, 33–37
3. Dammann O, Commentz JC et al. (1991): Gelastische Epilepsie und Pubertas praecox beim Hamartom des Hypothalamus. Klin Pädiatr 203, 439–447
4. Frattali CM, Liow K et al. (2001): Cognitive deficits in children with gelastic seizures and hypothalamic hamartoma. Neurology 57, 43–46
5. Kleihues P, Burger PC, Scheithauer BW(1993):The new WHO classification of brain tumors. Brain Pathology 3, 255–268
6. Rosenfeld JV, Harvey AS et al. (2001): Transcallosal resection of hypothalamic hamartomas, with control of seizures, in children with gelastic epilepsy. Neurosurgery 48, 108–118

Stereotaktische ^{125}J-Seed-Implantation als Therapieoption pharmakorefraktärer Epilepsien bei hypothalamischen Hamartomen

V. Homberg, A. Schulze-Bonhage, R. Keimer, D. Cyron, P.C. Warnke, Ch. Ostertag

Einleitung

Hypothalamische Hamartome sind eine häufig Ursache besonders pharmakorefraktärer fokaler Epilepsien, die sich meist schon im frühen Kleinkindesalter in Form gelastischer Anfälle manifestieren und im Laufe der weiteren Entwicklung mit vielfältigen anderen fokalen, meist auch sekundär generalisierten Anfallstypen oder reinen Sturzanfällen kombiniert auftreten können (1, 6, 7). Aufgrund der Lage im Bereich des Tuber cinereum und der damit verbundenen räumlichen Beziehung zu Hypothalamus und Hypophyse, besteht eine häufige Assoziation mit hormonellen Störungen v.a. in Form der Pubertas präcox (1, 2, 12). Darüber hinaus wird im Zusammenhang mit hypothalamischen Hamartomen über Verhaltensauffälligkeiten bis hin zu schweren Lernbehinderungen berichtet, auch anlagebedingte Knochenmissbildungen, typischerweise in Form von Syn- und Polydaktylien, können begleitend auftreten (1, 4, 11). Histologisch handelt es sich um sog. non-neoplastische kongenitale Malformationen mit geringer oder fehlender Wachstumstendenz, die der grauen Substanz des zentralen Nervensystems ähneln und teilweise eingelagerte hyperplastische Neurone und gliale Zellen aufweisen (13).

Die anatomische Lage dieser Hamartome erklärt die Schwierigkeiten und Risiken jeglicher interventioneller Therapie bei Versagen der antikonvulsiven Medikation. Insbesondere die chirurgische Resektion birgt aufgrund möglicher Verletzungen der hypothalamischen-hypophysären Achse das Risiko der Entwicklung eines Diabetes insipidus, einer Hyperphagie oder eines Hypopituitarismus. Eine Verletzung der Corpora mamillaria kann zum Korsakoff-Syndrom führen und, je nach Zugangsweg, werden zentrale Paresen beschrieben (2, 5). Als schonendere interventionelle Behandlungsmethoden kommen zunehmend radiochirurgische Verfahren wie Gamma Knife bzw. LINAC zum Einsatz. In Einzelfällen wurden auch Behandlungsversuche mittels stereotaktischer Thermokoagulation unternommen (3, 8).

Im Nachfolgenden möchten wir die interstitielle Radiochirurgie mittels ^{125}J-Seed als eine weitere gut verträgliche Therapieoption pharmakorefraktärer Epilepsien bei 6 Patienten mit hypothalamischen Hamartomen vorstellen. In der Behandlung niedriggradiger Gliome ist die Seedimplantation bereits als effektive und mit niedrigen Komplikationsraten verbundene Therapie etabliert, im Langzeit-Follow-Up konnte ein gutes Outcome bestätigt werden (10).

Tab. 1: Demographische Daten und antikonvulsive Medikation

Name	Geschl.	Geb.-Datum	Epilepsie-Beginn	Pubertas präcox	bisherige Medikation	Medikation bei station. Aufnahme	aktuelle Medikation
O. L.	m	01.08.68	1971	keine	CBZ, VPA, LTG PHT, PRM	LTG: 450 mg/die CBZ: 800 mg/die	LTG: 400 mg/die
C. L.	m	03.05.84	1994	mit 7 Jahren	VGB, CBZ, LTG VPA	CBZ: 1700 mg/die LTG: 350 mg/die	LTG: 1150 mg/die
M. H.	m	02.01.91	1992	keine	STH, CBZ, VPA PHT, CLB	TPM: 100 mg/die LEV: 2000 mg/die CLB: 20 mg/die	TPM: 100 mg/die LEV: 2000 mg/die
T. S.	m	29.05.87	1987	mit 9 Jahren	VPA, LTG, LEV OXC, CBZ, CLB PRM, Brom	LTG: 300 mg/die LEV: 3000 mg/die	LTG: 300 mg/die LEV: 3000 mg/die
D. F.	w	16.01.77	1977	keine	VPA, LTG, CBZ VGB, PB, PRM ESM, CLB, TGB	CBZ: 1200 mg/die GBP: 2400 mg/die CLB: 10 mg/die	OXC: 1800 mg/die LEV: 4000 mg/die
M. K.	m	07.02.91	1993	keine	VPA, LTG, TPM VGB	LTG: 350 mg/die CBZ: 1000 mg/die	LTG: 350 mg/die CBZ: 800 mg/die

Methoden

In Freiburg wurden bislang 6 Patienten (w=1, m=5) behandelt, deren Alter zum Zeitpunkt des Eingriffes zwischen 9 und 32 Jahren lag. Die gelastischen Anfälle hatten bei 3 Patienten in den ersten Lebensmonaten, bei den anderen 3 Patienten zwischen dem 2. und 8. Lebensjahr eingesetzt. Es konnte somit ein durchschnittlicher Erkrankungsverlauf von 17,3 Jahren überblickt werden, während dem eindeutige Pharmakorefraktärität, auch in Mehrfachkombinationen der antikonvulsiven Medikation nachgewiesen wurde (siehe Tab. 1). Alle Patienten hatten neben den rein gelastischen Anfällen, die teilweise mit, teilweise ohne Veränderungen des Bewusstseins einher gingen, zusätzlich einfach- und komplex-fokale Anfälle anderer, meist frontaler oder temporaler Semiologie; 3 Patienten litten zusätzlich unter sekundär generalisierten tonisch-klonischen Anfällen. Die Anfallsfrequenz unter Medikation lag bei 10 bis >100 Anfällen pro Monat unterschiedlicher Semiologie. Neben der Epilepsie zeigten 4/6 Patienten erhebliche neuropsychologische Defizite und Verhaltensauffälligkeiten mit Konsequenzen im Schul- und Berufsalltag, 2/6 Patienten hatten in der Vorgeschichte eine Pubertas präcox, 1 Patient eine inzwischen chirurgisch korrigierte Polydaktylie beider Hände.

Mittels Kernspintomographie wurde zunächst die Diagnose eines hypothalamischen Tumors gesichert (siehe Abb. 1). Nach den Klassifikationskriterien von Valdueza et al. handelte es sich um nicht gestielte Typ IIa- oder IIb-Hamartome. Alle Patienten erhielten präoperativ ein mehrtägiges non-invasives Video-EEG-Monitoring, welches bei 5/6 Patienten durch ein invasives Video-EEG-Monitoring mittels stereotaktisch implantierter Tiefenelektroden ergänzt wurde.

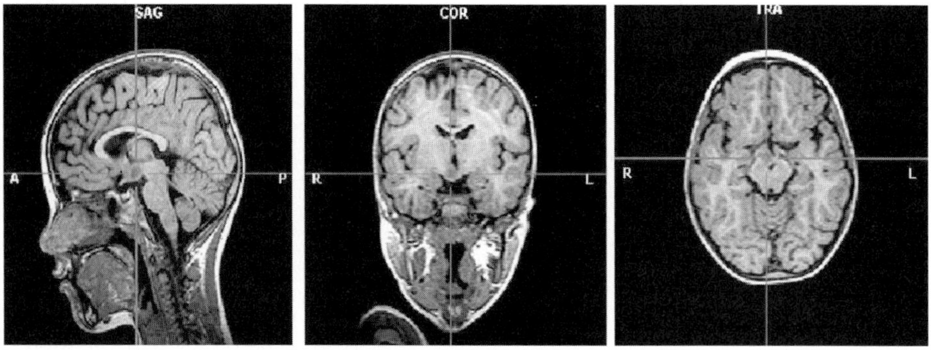

Abb. 1: Hypothalamisches Hamartom in typischer Lokalisation.

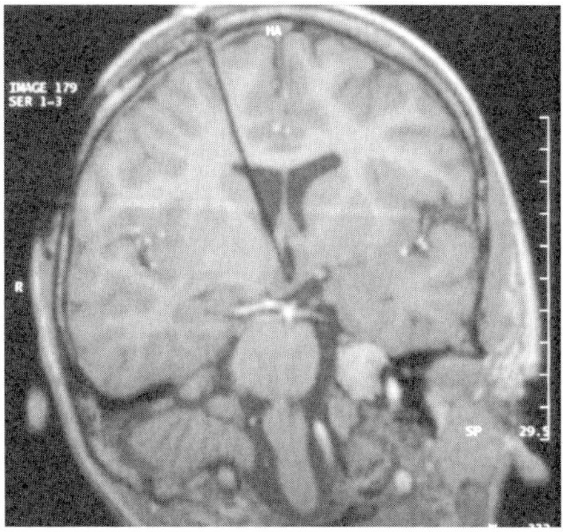

Abb. 2: Elektrodenlage im Hamartom (MRT coronar).

Die Ausarbeitung des Implantationsschema erfolgte hierbei in Abhängigkeit von den interiktal und iktal erhobenen EEG-Befunden aus der Oberflächen-EEG-Ableitung, insbesondere jedoch in Abhängigkeit des jeweiligen abgeleiteten EEG-Anfallsbeginns. So wurden neben einer 6-kontaktigen Tiefenelektroden direkt im Hamartom selbst (siehe Abb. 2), meist zusätzliche temporale Tiefenelektroden und bei einem Patienten auch temporo-basale und fronto-basale Streifenelektroden implantiert. Im Anschluss an die Diagnostik erfolgte bei allen 6 Patienten die stereotaktische Implantation eines ^{125}J-Seeds direkt in das Hamartom, bei 2 Patienten in Lokalanästhesie, bei 4 Patienten in Intubationsnarkose. Die mittlere Verweildauer des Seeds betrug bei einem durchschnittlichen Hamartomvolumen von 0,56 ml 26 Tage. Die Referenzdosis wurde hierbei auf 60 Gy berechnet, die mittlere Strahlenaktivität lag bei 2,04 mCi und die mittlere Energiedosisleistung bei 10,1 cGy/h. Im Rahmen der Seedimplantation wurde bei einem Teil der Patienten Hamartomgewebe zur histologischen Aufbereitung gewonnen und damit die kernspintomographische Verdachtsdiagnose bestätigt.

Ergebnisse

– *Klinische Befunde und Outcome*

Die interstitielle Radiochirurgie mittels ^{125}J-Seed konnte in geplanter Weise bei 5/6 Patienten durchgeführt werden. Bei 1 Patienten war trotz mehrfachen Versuche eine zentrale Plazierung des Seeds im Hamartom aufgrund einer derben Konsistenz des Hamartomgewebes nicht möglich mit daraus resultuierendem Behandlungsmisserfolg. Von den 5 Patienten, bei denen der Eingriff wie vorgesehen erfolgte, waren 2 Patienten über eine Follow-up-Periode von 12–15 Monate anfallsfrei. 1 Patient hatten über den bisherigen Beobachtungszeitraum von 9 Monaten eine >50%iger Reduktion der Anfallsfrequenz und Anfallsschwere mit nur noch einzelnen einfach- und komplex-fokalen Anfälle pro Monat bei zuvor bis zu 5 Anfällen pro Tag und mehreren sekundär generalisierten tonisch-klonischen Anfällen pro Monat. Gelastische Anfälle traten bei ihm bislang nicht mehr auf. 1 weiterer Patient hatte zumindest über 6 Monate eine >50%ige Reduktion der Anfallsfrequenz, entwickelte jedoch in den Folgemonaten wieder vermehrte, u.a. auch erneut gelastische Anfälle. Nach 12 Monaten führten wir daher eine zweite ^{125}J-Seedimplantation mit höherer Strahlenaktivität (2,7 mCi) und Energiedosisleistung (9,8 cGy/h) durch. Der Patient ist inzwischen über 6 Monate anfallsfrei. Neben dem o.g. Patienten profitierte ein zweiter Patient, in diesem Fall trotz korrekter Seedlage im Hamartom nicht von der Therapie. Dieser Patient wurde ebenfalls zum zweiten Mal implantiert, das Follow-up ist allerdings zur Beurteilung des Verlaufes noch nicht ausreichend. Die mittlere Follow-up-Periode der genannten Patienten liegt bei 10 Monaten.

Bei 3/6 Patienten kam es nach erfolgter Radiochirurgie zu erheblichen Verbesserungen der schulischen und beruflichen Leistungsfähigkeit, bei insgesamt 4/6 zu einer Verbesserung des Sozialverhaltens, wobei sich besonders die aggressiven Verhaltensweisen besserten. Unabhängig hiervon konnten allerdings bei 4/6 Patienten testpsychologisch diskrete Verschlechterungen von Teilgedächtnisleistungen nachgewiesen werden, die jedoch weder subjektiv den einzelnen Patienten noch ihrem Umfeld aufgefallen waren und offensichtlich ohne Alltagsrelevanz blieben. Neurologische oder hormonelle Störungen traten im Rahmen dieses radiochirurgischen Verfahrens bislang nicht auf.

– *EEG-Befunde*

Die zunächst durchgeführten Oberflächen-EEG-Ableitungen zeigten häufig multifokale Verlangsamungen. Die Sharp-wave-Aktivität war zwar meistens unilateral und konstant über einem Fokus nachzuweisen mit jedoch sehr weitem Feld und ohne sichere Übereinstimmung mit dem EEG-Anfallsbeginn. Der EEG-Anfallsbeginn zeigte sich bei 4/6 Patienten seitenwechselnd über den temporalen oder fronto-temporalen Ableitungen, bei den anderen zwei Patienten jeweils rechts temporo-anterior bzw. rechts frontal. Anhand der invasiven EEG-Ableitung über die im Hamartom plazierte Tiefenelektrode konnte eine Beteiligung des Hamartoms an der interiktalen und iktalen epileptischen Aktivität nachgewiesen werden.

Die post operationem durchgeführten Kontrollen des Oberflächen-EEGs zeigten bei den 4 Patienten, die von der Therapie profitiert hatten, bereits nach 3 Monaten eine Beschleunigung der Hintergrundaktivität um mindestens 1–2 Hz und eine signifikante Abnahme der interiktalen epilepsietypischen Potentiale. Bei den beiden Therapieversagern blieben die postoperativen EEG-Befunde annähernd unverändert.

Schlussfolgerung

In der hier vorgestellten Serie konnten wir nachweisen, dass die interstitielle Radiochirurgie mittels ^{125}J-Seed eine wirksame und relativ schonende Behandlungsoption einer pharmakorefraktären Epilepsie bei hypothalamischen Hamartomen darstellt. Insbesondere die kleinen und nicht gestielten breitbasigen Typ II Hamartome (nach Valdueza et al., 13) bieten sich für ein radiochirurgisches Verfahren an (9), da sie einem offenen chirurgischen Vorgehen nur schlecht zugängig sind und ein Eingriff in dieser Lokalisation mit erheblichen Nebenwirkungen und teilweise nicht reversiblen Folgeerkrankungen einher gehen kann (5, 9). Die Option einer offenen chirurgischen Therapie sollte daher nur Fällen vorbehalten sein, bei denen ein radiochirurgisches Verfahren ohne Effekt bleibt (13). Ein weiterer Vorteil zur offenen Chirurgie ergibt sich aus der Möglichkeit, die Implantation bei älteren und kooperativen Kindern in Lokalanästhesie durchzuführen.

Im Vergleich zu anderen radiochirurgischen Therapien wie z.B. dem Gamma Knife bietet die interstitielle Therapie mittels ^{125}J-Seed die Möglichkeit einer Lagekorrektur der Strahlenquelle, bevor die endgültige Strahlendosis am Zielort erreicht ist. Offensichtlich ist eine zentrale Lage des Seeds im Hamartom wichtig für den weiteren Therapieerfolg. Auch scheint eine zweite Seedimplantation bei nicht ausreichendem Therapieeffekt unproblematisch möglich zu sein. Bei einer erneuten Implantation kann die Strahlendosis neu gewählt und entsprechend angepasst werden.

Literatur

1. Berkovic S F, Andermann F et al. (1988) Hypothalamic hamartomas and ictal laughter: evolution of a characteristic epileptic syndrome and diagnostic value of magnetic resonance imaging. Ann Neurol 23: 429–439
2. Breningstall G N (1985) Gelastic seizures, precocious puberty and hypothalamic hamartoma. Neurology 35: 1180–1183
3. Fukuda M, Kameyama S et al. (1999) Stereotaxy for hypothalamic hamartoma with intractable gelastic seizures: technical case report. Neurosurgery 44: 1347–1350
4. Katayama H, Miyao M et al. (1993) A case of hypothalamic hamartoma with gelastic seizures, precocious puberty, poly- and syndactyly [in Japanese]. No To Hattatsu 25(4): 341–346
5. Kuzniecky R, Guthrie B et al. (1997) Intrinsic epileptogenesis of hypothalamic hamartomas in gelastic epilepsy. Ann Neurol 42: 60–67

6. Nishio S, Morioka T et al. (1994) Surgical treatment of intractable seizures due to hypothalamic hamartoma. Epilepsia 35(3): 514–519
7. Pallini R, Bozzini V et al. (1993) Callosotomy for generalized seizures associated with hypothalamic hamartoma. Neurol Res 15: 139–141
8. Parrent A G (1999) Stereotactic radiofrequency ablation for the treatment of gelastic seizures associated with hypothalamic hamartoma. J Neurosurg 91: 881–884
9. Régis J, Bartolomei F et al. (2000) Gamma knife surgery for epilepsy related to hypothalamic hamartomas. Neurosurgery 47: 1343–1352
10. Schätz Ch R, Kreth F W et al. (1994) Interstitial 125-iodine radiosurgery of low-grade gliomas of the insula of reil. Acta Neurochir 130: 80–89
11. Tsugu H, Fukushima T et al. (1998) Hypothalamic hamartoma associated with multiple congenital abnormalities. Pediatr Neurosurg 29: 290–296
12. Unger F, Schröttner O et al. (2000) Gamma knife radiosurgery for hypothalamic hamartomas in patients with medically intractable epilepsy and precocious puberty. J Neurosurg 92: 726–731
13. Valdueza J M, Cristante L et al. (1994) Hypothalamic hamartomas: with special reference to gelastic epilepsy and surgery. Neurosurgery 34: 949–958

Vagusnerv-Stimulation bei Kindern zur Therapie pharmakoresistenter Epilepsien

J. Sperner, B. Altmann, P. Borusiak, C. Bussmann, M. Feucht, S. Gannam, B. Haffner, H. Holthausen, S. König, B. Kruse, S. Kuczaty, T. Pieper, B. Püst, S. Rinnert, A. Sälke-Kellermann, R. Sassen, H.-L. Spohr, K. Stollhoff, I. Tuxhorn, W. Wittmann, G. Wohlrab

Zusammenfassung

Die Vagusnerv-Stimulation ist auch bei Kindern und Jugendlichen mit pharmakorefraktärer Epilepsie eine sichere und effektive Behandlungsalternative. Bei zunehmendem positivem Langzeiteffekt erfahren bis zu 50% der betroffenen, häufig mehrfach behinderten Patienten eine signifikante Anfallsreduktion mit mindestens einer Halbierung der Anfälle. Zusätzliche positive psychische Nebenwirkungen auf Vigilanz und Kognition werden von Eltern und Betreuern bei bis zu 80% der Patienten nach zwei Jahren berichtet. Zusätzlich wird die aktive Möglichkeit, im Bedarfsfall selbst durch zusätzliche Stimulationen mit einem Magneten Anfälle zu beeinflussen, von 42% als erfolgreich bewertet.

Einleitung

Das erste antiepileptische Medikament ist bei 40% aller Patienten mit Epilepsie nicht erfolgreich, d.h. es muss durch andere antikonvulsive Medikamente ersetzt oder ergänzt werden. Nach dem dritten Antikonvulsivum ist die Chance, anfallsfrei zu werden, kleiner als 5% (3). Therapeutische Alternativen sind dringend erforderlich und die Epilepsiechirurgie wird hier in zunehmendem Maße erfolgreich eingesetzt. Jedoch bleiben nicht alle pharmakoresistenten Epilepsiepatienten nach einem chirurgischen Eingriff anfallsfrei, und ein großer Teil ist a priori nicht operabel. So bleiben nach vorsichtigen Schätzungen im deutschsprachigen Raum etwa 8000 Kinder und Jugendliche mit pharmakorefraktären Epilepsien, die durch Antikonvulsiva und Operation nicht befriedigend behandelt werden können. Bei diesen Kindern ist die Epilepsie häufig mit einer Entwicklungsretardierung verbunden und durch Begriff »catastrophic epilepsy« charakterisiert. Hier stellt die Vagusnervstimulation (VNS) auch bei kleinen Kindern eine sinnvolle Therapiealternative dar. Die VNS ist seit 1996 in Europa zugelassen und wurde 1998 erstmals bei Kindern im deutschsprachigen Raum eingesetzt.

Methoden

An einer Anwendungsbeobachtung beteiligen sich bisher 15 Epilepsiezentren aus Deutschland, Österreich und der Schweiz. Die Indikation zur VNS-Implantation wird nach erfolgloser Pharmakotherapie von jedem behandelnden Arzt individuell gestellt. Pharmakoresistenz und erfolglose epilepsiechirurgische Operation oder die Unmöglichkeit eines erfolgreichen epilepsiechirurgischen Eingriffs sind eindeutige Indikationen für die VNS. Zur Vergleichbarkeit der Daten mit dem Internationalen Patientenregisters für VNS wurden die entsprechenden Fragebogenprotokolle benutzt und durch ein deutschsprachiges Protokoll mit weiteren Fragen zur Ätiologie, dem EEG und zu Nebenwirkungen erweitert. Datensätze wurden vor der VNS-Implantation, und nach 3, 6, 12, 18 und 24 Monaten erhoben. Zusätzlich wurde ein Lebensqualitäts-Fragebogen eingesetzt, der vorher, sowie nach 6, 12 und 24 Monaten erhoben wurde (Auswertung Tuxhorn).

Bei einer Stimulationsdauer von 30 sec wurde die Stimulationsstärke des VNS-System durch einfache externe Programmierung vom behandelnden Arzt in 7–14tägigen Intervallen jeweils um 0,25 mA gesteigert, bis ein befriedigender Effekt zu erkennen ist. In der Regel wurden Stromstärken von 2,5 mA nicht überschritten, in Einzelfällen wurden auch bei höheren Stromstärken bis 3,5 mA noch positive Effekte ohne Nebenwirkungen gesehen. Wenn dadurch keine Anfallsreduktion erreicht wurde, konnte das Pausenintervall zwischen den Stimulationen von 5 auf 3 oder 1,8 Min verkürzt werden oder ein rascher Zyklus mit 7 sec Stimulation und 30 sec Pausenintervall gewählt werden.

Ergebnisse

Seit 1999 werden Kinder und Jugendliche im deutschsprachigen Raum mit der VNS behandelt. Bis April 2002 wurden 120 Patienten in die Studie aufgenommen, der Beobachtungszeitraum erstreckte sich für 13 Pat. über 2 Jahre, 27 Pat. über 18 Monate, 49 Pat. über 12 Monate, 67 Pat. über 6 Monate und 84 Pat. über 3 Monate. 77% der Patienten waren psychomotorisch retardiert, 64% wurden vor der VNS-Implantation epilepsiechirurgisch evaluiert und 19% waren bereits vor der VNS epilepsiechirurgisch voroperiert. Das mittlere Alter zum Zeitpunkt der VNS-Implantation betrug 10 Jahre (Bereich 2,8 bis 21 Jahre), nur 3 Pat. mit Lennox Gastaut-Syndrom waren älter als 18 Jahre. Die mittlere Anfallsdauer bis zur VNS-Implantation betrug 8 Jahre (1,7–18). Der Epilepsiebeginn lag im Median bei 1,7 Jahren (0–11).

Epilepsien fokaler Genese lagen in über 92% der Fälle vor (davon 19% mit Lennox-Gastaut-Syndrom), primär generalisierte Epilepsien nur in 8%. Die Ätiologie der Epilepsien verteilte sich auf 26% mit erworbenen Läsionen, 43% epileptische Syndrome (incl. Migrationsstörungen), 7% genetische Syndrome (Chromosomopathien, Rett, Angelman, Tuberöse Hirnsklerose) und bei 24% war keine Zuordnung möglich.

Die Anfallsreduktion wurde nach 3, 6, 12, 18 und 24 Monaten mit der Ausgangssituation der Anzahl der Anfälle für einzelne Anfallstypen im Monat vor

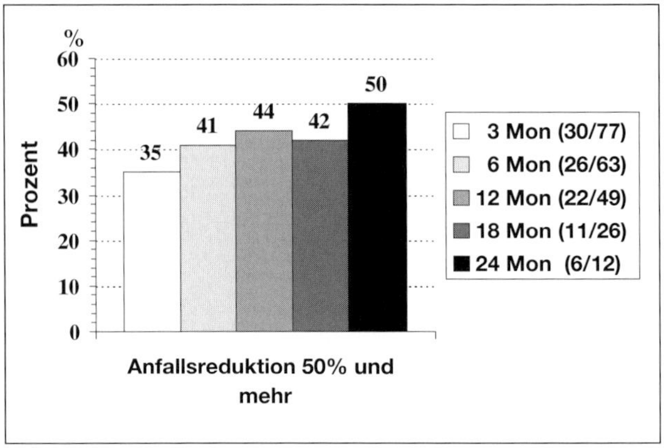

Abb. 1: Prozentsatz aller Patienten, die unter VNS eine Anfallsreduktion von mindestens 50% erfahren haben, die zunehmende Wirkung der VNS bei einer Therapiedauer bis zu 2 Jahren ist erkennbar.

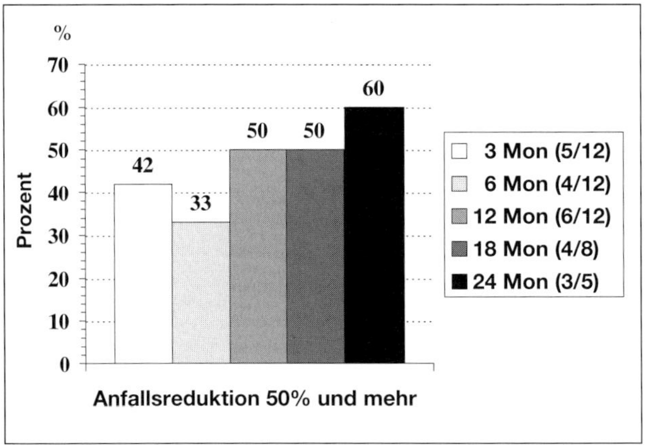

Abb. 2: Ergebnisse der Anfallsverbesserung bei Patienten mit Lennox-Gastaut-Syndrom, die ein besseres Ansprechen auf VNS zeigen als das Gesamtkollektiv.

VNS-Implantation verglichen. Kein Anfallstyp konnte durch die VNS signifkant besser beherrscht werden. Als Besserung wurde nur gewertet, wenn eine Anfallsreduktion um mindestens 50% erreicht wurde. Dies trat nach 3 Monaten bei 35% aller Patienten ein, nach 6 Monaten bei 41%, nach 12 Monaten bei 44%, nach 18 Monaten bei 42% und nach 24 Monaten bei 50%. Dauerhaft anfallsfrei für mehr als 18 Monate wurde kein Patient, vorübergehend anfallsfrei bis zu einer Dauer von 18 Monaten wurden 5 Patienten.

Die Situation der 20 Patienten mit Lennox-Gastaut-Syndrom besserte sich insgesamt deutlicher als beim Gesamt-Kollektiv, eine Anfallsverbesserung erreichten bereits 50% nach 6 Monaten, die sich nach 2 Jahren auf 69% (3 von 5 Pat.) verbesserte. Auch bei Patienten ohne signifikante Anfallsreduktion waren häufig die Anfälle gemildert, weniger Notfallmedikation und weniger Krankenhausaufenthalte waren erforderlich, kürzere postiktale Erholungsphasen wurden berichtet. Insgesamt profitierten von positiven psychischen Nebenwirkungen sehr deutlich auch solche Patienten, bei denen keine Anfallsreduktion erreicht werden konnte. So wurde über eine verbesserte Vigilanz schon nach 3 Monaten bei 60% der Patienten berichtet, was sich mit zunehmender VNS-Dauer auf 80%

(8 von10 Pat.) nach 2 Jahren steigerte. Positive Effekte wurden auch in Bezug auf Kognition, Schulleistungen und Grundstimmung berichtet, wenngleich in geringerem Ausmaß.

Eine positive Beeinflussung während oder nach einem Anfall durch die Bedarfstimulation mit dem Handmagneten durch Eltern, Betreuer oder den Patienten selbst wurde von 42% der Betroffenen gemeldet, in vielen Fällen konnten der Anfallsablauf erheblich abgekürzt und abgeschwächt werden.

Es ergaben sich keine signifikanten Unterschiede in der Anfallsreduktion in Bezug auf die Dauer der Epilepsie (kürzer oder länger als 5 Jahre), die Ätiologie (erworbene Läsionen versus Epilepsie-Syndrome) oder spezifische EEG-Charakteristika (fokale versus multifokale epilepsietypische Muster). Überraschend erfolgreich war die VNS-Therapie bei 16 Patienten mit einem vorangegangenem epilepsiechirurgischen Eingriff (Lobektomie): hier zeigten 8 von 12 Patienten (66%) nach 6 Monaten eine Anfallsreduktion 75% und mehr. Ein Patient war anfallsfrei geworden.

Diskussion

In Anbetracht der sehr selektionierten Patienten mit überwiegend schwerer körperlicher und geistiger Retardierung sind die vorläufigen Ergebnisse der VNS-Therapie bei Kindern sehr ermutigend. Im Vergleich zu den bisher publizierten Behandlungserfolgen bei Kindern sind die Ergebnisse aus dem deutschsprachigen Raum ebenbürtig (1,2,4–8). Aufgrund der bisherigen Daten sprechen Kinder und Jugendliche jedoch nicht besser als Erwachsene auf diese Therapie an. In unserem Kollektiv hatten das Alter der Patienten, die Epilepsiedauer, die Ätiologie der Anfälle oder EEG-Kriterien keinen Einfluss auf den Therapieerfolg der VNS. Weltweit ist es bis jetzt noch nicht gelungen, Patienten prospektiv zu identifizieren, die von der VNS mit Sicherheit profitieren. Neue Untersuchungsergebnisse zeigen jedoch, dass eine Epilepsiedauer von weniger als 5 Jahren und nicht mehr als vier antikonvulsive Medikamente vor Beginn der VNS einen größeren Therapieerfolg (15% versus 5% Anfallsfreiheit nach 3 Monaten) versprechen (9).

Literatur

1. Frost M, Gates J, Helmers SL, Wheless JW, Levisohn P, Tardo C, Conry J A, (2001) Vagus Nerve Stimulation in Children with Refractory Seizures Associated with Lennox- Gastaut Syndrome. Epilepsia 42; 9: 1148–1152
2. Hornig GW, Murphy JV, Schallert G, Tilton C, (1997) Left Vagus Nerve Stimulation in Children With Refractory Epilepsy. Journal of the Southern Medical Association 90; 5: 484–488
3. Kwan P, Brodie M (2000) Early identification of refractory epilepsy. New Engl J Med 342:314–319
4. Labar D, (2000) Vagus nerve stimulation for intractable epilepsy in children. Developmental Medicine & Child Neurology 42: 496–499
5. Lundgren J, Åmark P, Blennow G, Strömblad L G, Wallstedt L, (1998) Vagus Nerve Stimulation in 16 Children with Refractory Epilepsy. Epilepsia 39; 8: 809–813
6. Murphy J V, Pediatric VNS Study Group (1999) Left vagal nerve stimulation in children with medically refractory epilepsy. J Pediatr 134: 563–566
7. Parker A P J, Polkey C E, Binnie C D, Madigan C, Ferry C D, Robinson R O (1999) Vagal Nerve Stimulation in Epileptic Encephalopathies. Pediatrics 103: 778–782
8. Patwardhan RV, Stong B, Bebin EM, Mathisen J, Grabb PA, (2000) Efficacy of Vagal Nerve Stimulation in Children with Medically Refractory Epilepsy. Neurosurgery 47: 1353–1358
9. Wheless J (2002) Interim results of a prospective study of early adjunctive vagus nerve stimulation (VNS) theapy. Neurology58 (Suppl.3): A53

13. Epilepsie 2: Pathophysiologie, Verlauf, Differentialdiagnose

Epilepsie bei Patienten mit congenitaler Hemiplegie: Korrelation zwischen EEG und neuroradiologischen Befunden, prognostische Faktoren

C. Panteliadis, G. Jacobi, M. Tzitiridu, G. Arsos, A. Covanis

Einführung

Die kongenitale Hemiplegie (CH) ist die halbseitige Form einer motorischen Lähmung bei einer cerebralen Parese (CP). Sie kommt am häufigsten bei termingerechten Neugeborenen vor. In den letzten Jahren hat ihr Auftreten bei Frühgeborenen mit sehr niedrigem Geburtsgewicht zugenommen. In über 2/3 der Fälle reifer Neugeborener mit CH ist die Ursache eine cerebrale Hämorrhagie oder ein Infarkt (meist einseitig) im Bereich der Arteria cerebri media (ACM) (11, 12, 21).

Die Häufigkeit der CH wird auf 0.41–0.79 lebend Geborener geschätzt. Die Ursachen sind heterogen und in den meisten Fällen dominieren pränatale vor perinatalen Faktoren (zusammen: 70–90%). Bei 25–30% bleibt die Ursache unklar (5, 12, 19, 22, 24, 25). Die Semiologie wird gewöhnlich von den Eltern im Alter von 6–9 Monaten bemerkt, nur selten früher von einem erfahrenen Pädiater.

Die Häufigkeit einer Epilepsie bei Kindern mit CH variiert zwischen 27% und 47%, während andere Probleme wie mentale Retardierung (20–45%), Skoliose (10–15%), Sehstörungen (10–25%), Hörverluste (3–5%) oder Sprachstörungen (20%) seltener vorkommen (7, 18, 25).

Das Auftreten einer Epilepsie hängt vom Schweregrad der Hemiplegie ab und von anderen additiven Defiziten einschließlich Verhaltensstörungen. Das Vorkommen epileptischer Anfälle hängt jedoch in den meisten Fällen direkt von der Intensität des motorischen Handicaps ab (5, 15, 21). Die Ausdehnung der neuroradiologischen Befunde korrespondiert häufig mit einer Epilepsie. Es wird berichtet, dass Patienten mit corticalen und subcorticalen Läsionen häufiger an epileptischen Anfällen leiden als Patienten mit einer einseitigen Erweiterung des Seitenventrikels (SV) (3, 17).

Unsere Studie stützt sich auf eine große Zahl von Patienten mit einer CH (N: 203) und konzentriert sich auf den Zusammenhang zwischen EEG-Veränderungen, Häufigkeit und dem Typ der Epilepsie. Weiterhin wird eine Korrelation zwischen der Schwere der Parese, dem Grad der EEG-Veränderungen und den neuroradiologischen Befunden untersucht.

Patienten und Methoden

Wir untersuchten prospektiv und retrospektiv 203 Kinder mit CH (112 Jungen, 91 Mädchen) im Alter von 3 Monaten bis zu 12 Jahren. Die Überweisungsgründe waren: bei 91 Patienten Verdacht auf Anfälle, bei 92 die motorische Behinderung sowie bei 20 andere, nicht-neurologische Probleme. 79 wurden in der Universitäts-Kinderklinik Thessaloniki, 83 in der Abteilung für Pädiatrische Neurologie in Frankfurt/Main und 41 im Kinderkrankenhaus »Agia Sophia« in Athen vorgestellt. Alle Kinder wurden eingehend allgemeinpädiatrisch, neurologisch und auf ihre Entwicklung hin untersucht. Es wurden mehrere EEG's gemacht. CCT und MRT-Aufnahmen wurden bei 150 Patienten durchgeführt. Die Kindern wurden regelmäßig alle 6 Monate etwa drei Jahre lang von einem Neuropädiater/in wieder beurteilt. Hierzu wurde ein ausführliches Protokoll mit Daten aus der Schwangerschaft, der Perinatalperiode und der Neugeborenenzeit verwendet.

Die CH wurde gemäß der Klassifikation von INGRAM in 3 Grade unterteilt (13):
a) leichte Form mit diskretem Seitenunterschied, einseitiger Reflexsteigerung bzw. Tonuserhöhung,
b) mittelschwere Form mit deutlichem Seitenunterschied, Umfangsdifferenz der betroffenen Extremität, typischen Bewegungsmustern, positiven Pyramidenzeichen, und
c) schwere Form mit ausgeprägter Hemiatrophie, erheblicher Spastik, Pyramidenzeichen und Unfähigkeit, die obere Extremität im Alltag zu benutzen. Als Epilepsie definierten wird 2 oder mehr afebrile Anfälle: Neonatale und febrile Konvulsionen (FK) wurden daher ausgeschlossen. Die Anfallsklassifizierung erfolgte nach den Kriterien der ILAE von 1981 (6).

Die Patienten wurden nach dem Alter bei Anfallsbeginn in 4 Gruppen unterteilt:
a) 1–12 Monate
b) 1–5 Jahre
c) 6–10 Jahre und d) >10 Jahre.

Die EEG-Befunde wurden in 4 Gruppen eingeordnet:
a) normal,
b) leichte einseitige Abnormalität wie fokale Dysrhythmie, Schlafspindelreduktion, lokale Spannungsminderung,
c) deutliche einseitige/fokale Veränderungen, mässige Allgemeinveränderungen (AV), fokaler Spike-Wave-Fokus, und
d) schwere AV, Hypsarhythmie, Spike-Slow-Wave-Fokus (Variantenmuster), gemischter Spike-Slow-Wave-Fokus.

Die CT- MRT-Befunde wurden in 5 Gruppen eingeteilt:
a) normal,
b) symmetrische Ventrikelerweiterung,
c) einseitige/seitenbetonte Ventrikelerweiterung,
d) kombinierte cortical/ subcorticale Läsion und
e) Malformation.
Für die statistische Analyse wurde der Chi-squared und der Mann-Whitney-Test verwendet (2).

Ergebnisse

Das Alter der Patienten lag zwischen 3 Monaten und 12 Jahren. Bei 82/203 Patienten (40.4%) wurde eine pränatale Hirnschädigung angenommen. Bei 58/203 (28.5%) hatte es perinatale Komplikationen gegeben: bei 38 (18.7%) lag eine postnatale Ursache vor, bei 25 Kindern (12.3%) konnte kein eindeutiger Grund eruiert werden; ein Teil dieser Kinder dürfte denen mit pränatalen Ursachen zuzuordnen sein, ebenso ist nicht auszuschließen, dass Kinder mit perinatalen Komplikationen auch eine pränatale Schädigung erlitten hatte, die dann ihrerseits auch Anlass zu einer erschwerten bzw. lagewidrigen Geburt gegeben hatte.

Eine leichte Hemiparese wurde bei 30.5% der Patienten diagnostiziert, eine mittelschwere Hemiplegie bei 47.8% und eine schwere bei 21.7%. Bei 54.4% war die rechte Seite betroffen, von diesen 110 Kindern hatten wiederum 70 (64%) epileptische Anfälle; Epilepsie wurde insgesamt bei 79/203 (38.9%) der Kinder diagnostiziert. Anfälle begannen bei 26.5% der Kinder im 1. Lebensjahr (LJ), bei 36.7% im 2.–5. LJ, bei 24% zwischen dem 6. und 10. LJ sowie bei 12.6% erst nach dem 10. LJ. Bei 7/79 Kinder lag in der Familie Epilepsie vor (ohne FK).

Die Anfallsfreguenz differierte deutlich zwischen der Gruppe der Patienten mit unterschiedlicher Schwere der CH ($X^2=25.857$, $p<0.0001$). Insbesondere war die Häufigkeit von Anfällen bei Kindern mit leichter CH (12/62, 19.4%) deutlich niedriger als bei Kinder mit mittelgradiger und schwerer Hemiplegie (67/141, 47.5%, $X^2=13.208$, $p<0.0001$), Tabelle 1.

Tab. 1: Korrelation zwischen Schweregrad der congen. Hemiplegie und Anfallsfrequenz

Schweregrad CH	N	Zahl der Patienten mit Epilepsie (%)
Leichte	62	12/62 (19.4)*
Mittelschwere	97	37/97 (38.1)
Schwere	44	30/44 (68.2)
Total	203	79/203

*x2, $p<0.0001$

Das EEG war bei 49 (24.1%) Kindern normal. 154mal (75.9%) wurden Pathologica registriert: bei 36/154 (23.3%) eine einseitige leichtgradige fokale Dysrhythmie, bei 73/154 (47.4%) eine ausgeprägte fokale Dysrhythmie, evt. mit Allgemeinveränderungen (AV), bei 45 (29.2%) ein massiver Detawellenfokus, ein SW-Fokus oder eine Hypsarhythmie. Von den 154 Kindern mit pathologischem EEG entwickelten nur 79 (=51.3%) epileptische Anfälle: am häufigsten komplexe Partialanfälle (26/79), gefolgt von generalisierten tonisch-klonischen Anfällen (16/79), myoklonisch-astatischen Anfällen (12/79), einfachen Partialanfällen (10/79), einem West-Syndrom (6/79), komplexen Partialanfällen mit sekundärer Generalisierung (6/79) und einfachen Partialanfällen und Generaliserung (3/79). Der Grad der EEG-Veränderung verlief parallel zur Häufigkeit epileptischer Anfälle (Mann-Whitney, $p=0.014$). Kein Kind mit einem normalem EEG bekam eine Epilepsie. Die Patienten mit den schwerwiegendsten EEG-Veränderungen hatten in >80% Anfälle (s. Tab. 2).

Tab. 2: Korrelation zwischen Grad der EEG Veränderungen und Anfallsfrequenz

EEG-Befunde	N	Zahl der Patienten mit Epilepsie (%)
Normal	49	0/49(00.0)
leichte Abnormalität	36	9/36 (25.0)
deutliche Abnormalität	73	32/73 (43.9)
Schwere Verdänderungen	45	38/45(84.4)
Total	**203**	**79/203**

Mann – Whitney, p = 0.014

Ein kraniales CT oder MRT wurde bei 150 Kindern mit CH durchgeführt: CT: 69, MRT: 81. Bei 14/150 dieser Kinder war der Befund normal. Eine leichte symmetrische Ventrikelerweiterung hatten 6/150, eine einseitige deutliche Ventrikeldilatation 48/150. In 68/150 Fällen wurden kombiniert cortical/subcorticale Läsionen gesehen, bei 14/150 Malformationen. Keines der Kinder mit schwerer CH hatte ein normales oder nur leicht abnormes CT/MRT. 88% der Kinder mit kombiniert cortical/subcorticalen Läsionen hatten mittlere und schwere Hemiplegien. Der Umfang des neuroradiologischen Befundes korrespondiert gut mit der Häufigkeit einer Epilepsie (s. Tab. 3, Mann-Whitney, p<0.01).

Tab. 3: Korrelation zwischen CT/MRT-Befunde und Anfallsfrequenz

CT/MRT Befunde	N	Zahl der Patienten mit Epilepsie (%)
Normal oder leichte symmetrische Ventrikelerweiterung	20	3/20 (15.0)
einsetige Ventrikelerweiterung	48	15/48 (31.3)
kombinierte cortical/ subcortical/Läsion	68	32/68 (47.1)
Malformation	14	11/14 (78.6)
Total	**150**	**61/150**

Mann – Whitney, p<0.01

Diskussion

Das Auftreten einer Epilepsie bei Kindern mit CP variiert zwischen 30% und 60%, was mit der Heterogenie der CP zusammenhängt (1, 7, 10, 16, 18, 20).

Spastische Formen einer CP sind häufig mit Epilepsie verbunden. Bei CH bewegt sich die Inzidenz zwischen 22% und 47%. Dies hängt u.a. von der Definition der Epilepsie und von der Auswahl des Krankenguts ab (9). Goutieres et al. berichten, dass 44% ihrer hemiplegischen Kinder eine Epilepsie entwickelten, wobei aber FK und ein einmaliges Anfallsgeschehen eingeschlossen wurden (23). Wir hatten als Ausschlusskriterien: keine neonatalen Konvulsionen, keine FK, 2 oder mehr afebrile Episoden, sodass die nur 38% in unserem Krankengut nicht überraschen.

Das Ausmaß der EEG-Veränderungen korreliert mit der Häufigkeit von epileptischen Anfällen und der Inzidenz einer Epilepsie im gesamten Krankengut. Dazu ist anzumerken, dass nicht alle Kinder mit leichten oder mässig ausgeprägten EEG-Befunden klinische Anfälle bekamen. Epileptische Anfälle kommen aber nur selten bei Kindern vor, die einen Normalbefund im EEG haben, bei 2% nach Peterson und Eeg-Olofsson (23). Andererseits werden mässige Herdbefunde und fokale Spikes nicht selten bei Kindern mit einer CH nachgewiesen, die keine Epilepsie haben (9,18). Es wird angenommen, dass diese Kinder mögliche Kandidaten für ein späteres Auftreten epileptischer Anfälle sind.

Wegen des z.T. retrospektiven Charakters der Studie war es bisweilen schwer, den Beginn der Anfälle und die initiale Semiologie exakt festzulegen. Wir müssen dabei vor allem annehmen, dass einige Patienten eine sekundäre Generalisation hatten, die aber einer Beobachtung entging. Uvebrand (25) berichtet gemäß ILAE-Klassifikation von 1981, hatten 31% seiner Patienten mit CH komplex-partiale Anfälle, 23% generalisierte tonische-klonische und 11% einfache Partialanfälle. BNS-Anfälle kommen häufiger bei Kindern mit Diplegie oder Quadriplegie vor (9,20), bei unseren hemiplegischen Kindern nur bei 6/79. Unsere Studie zeigt, dass der häufigste Anfallstyp bei CH complex Partialanfälle (33%) sind, gefolgt von generalisierten Anfällen (20%).

Bei 64% unserer Kinder war die rechte Seite, bei 36% die linke betroffen; Diese Daten zeigen, dass Läsionen der primär sprachdominanten (linken) Hemisphäre häufiger als rechtshemisphärische mit dem Krankheitsmerkmal Epilepsie verbunden sind; ähnliches ist nach offenen Hirnverletzungen zu beobachten. Nach Dean et al. (1997) generiert die linke Hemisphäre häufiger als die rechte fokale Anfälle, dies ergibt sich aber aus einem Gesamtkrankengut kindlicher Epilepsiepatienten. Radiologische Studien (4) weisen auf die Möglichkeit hin, dass sich eine solche Prädisposition der linken Hempshäre sich erst nach dem 1. LJ entwickelt. Unsere Studie dagegen lässt einen relativen Gipfel des Anfallsbeginns bei Kindern mit CH um das 1. LJ erkennen, was auf eine genetische und gegen eine rein lokalisatorische Bedingung dieser linkshemisphärischen Prävalenz hinweist. Je ausgedehnter der neuroradiologische Befund ist, umso früher manifestitiert sich bei einer CP eine Epilepsie: bei quadriplegischen Kindern früher als bei Patienten mit einer CH (9, 22).

Familiäres Vorkommen von Epilepsie bei Anfalls-Kindern mit CH wird auch von anderen Autoren berichtet (16, 24). Andererseits ist es auch wahrscheinlich, dass auch SW-Tätigkeit bei Kindern mit symptomatischen Krampfanfällen auf einen hereditären Co-Faktor hinweist, sodass sich das Bedingungsgefüge: genetische Merkmale und das Ausmaß einer Hirnschädigung für das Zustandekommen einer Epilepsie bei Kindern mit CH ergibt.

In früheren Studien (14, 17, 21) wurde versucht, den neuroradiologischen Befund im Verhältnis zum klinischen Bild zu evaluieren; in unserer Studie gehen das Ausmaß pathologischer Befunde im Neuro-Imaging und der klinische Schweregrad der motorischen Behinderung weitgehend parallel: Kinder mit normalem neuroradiologischen Befund hatten ein nur leichtes motorisches Defizit; das Resultat des Neuroimaging kann also als wichtiger prognostischer Aussagefaktor gelten.

Umgekehrt korreliert wiederum der Schweregrad der motorischen Behinderung mit der Inzidenz einer Epilepsie (5, 7). Es besteht also eine positive Korrelation zwischen: Grad einer motorischen Behinderung – Ausmaß des neuroradiologischen Befundes-Inzidenz und Verlaufscharakteristika (früher Beginn, höhere Anfallsfrequenz) einer beigeordneten Epilepsie. Insgesamt war die Häufigkeit einer Epilepsie am größten bei Kindern mit einem kombiniertem cortical-subcorticalen Defekt (s.a. 3, 5, 21); hierbei ist im Neuro-Imaging bei der angewandten Technik eine sichere Läsion hippokampaler Strukturen nur schwer oder überhaupt nicht auszumachen; es kann daher auch keine Aussage darüber getroffen werden, ob nicht bei wenigstens einem Teil der Kinder mit CH und Epilepsie eine duale Pathologie eine Rolle spielt.

Zusammenfassung

Die Mehrheit der Patienten mit einer CH hat EEG-Veränderungen, etwas mehr als 1/3 dieser Patienten entwickelt eine Epilepsie. Der Schweregrad der motorischen Behinderung, der Grad der EEG-Veränderungen und die Häufigkeit einer Epilepsie hängen voneinander ab. Der Umfang eines im Neuro-Imaging nachgewiesen Hirnsubstanzverlustes wiederum muss parallel betrachtet werden zu den 3 vorgenannten Variablen. Dies gilt besonders für die große Gruppe von Kindern mit cortical-subcorticalen Defekten bei CH.

Literatur

1. Aksu F (1990). Nature and prognosis of seizures in patients with cerebral palsy. Dev Med Child Neurol 32: 661–668
2. Altman DG (1991). Practical statistics for medical research, Chapman & Hall, London
3. Andermann F (2000). Cortical dysplasias and epilepsy: a review of the architectonic, clinical, and seizure patterns. Adv Neurol 84: 479–496
4. Chiron C, Jambaque I, Nabbout R, Lounes P, Syrota A, Dulac O (1997). The right brain hemisphere is dominant in human infants. Brain 120: 1057–1065
5. Cioni G, Sales B, Paolicelli PB, Petacchi E, Scusa R, Canapicchi FM (1999). MRI and Clinical Characteristics of Children with Hemiplegic Cerebral Palsy. Neuropediatrics 30:249–255
6. Commission on Classification and terminology of the international league against epilepsy: Proposal for revised classification of epilepsies and epileptic syndromes (1981). Epilepsia 22: 489–501
7. Curatolo P, Arpino C, Stazi MA, Medda E (1995). Risk factors for the co-occurrence of partial epilepsy, cerebral palsy and mental retardation. Dev Med Child Neurol 37: 776–782
8. Dean AC, Solomon G, Harden C, Papakostas G, Labar DR (1997). Left hemispheric dominance of epileptiform discharges. Epilepsia 38: 503–505
9. Goutieres F, Challamel MJ (1972). Les hemiplegies coongenitales: semiologie, etiologie et prognostic. Archives Francaises de Pediatric 29: 839–851
10. Hadjipanayis A, Hadjichristodouiou C, Youroukos S (1997). Epilepsy in patients with cerebral palsy. Dev Med Child Neurol 39: 659–663

11. Hagberg B, Hagberg G, Glow I (1984). The changing panorama of cerebral palsy in Sweden. IV. Epedemiological trends 1959-78, Acta Pediatr Scand 73: 433–440
12. Hagberg B, Hagberg G, Glow I (1996). The changing panorama of cerebral palsy in Sweden. VII. Prevalence and origin in the birth year period 1987-90. Acta Peadiatr 85: 954–960
13. Ingram TT (1964). Pediatric Aspects of Cerebral Palsy Livingston, London 1964
14. Jacobs KM, Kharazia VN, Prince DA (1999). Mechanisms underlying epileptogenesis in cortical malformations. Epilepsy Res 36: 165–188
15. Kotlarek F, Rodewig R, Brull D (1981). Computer tomographic findings in congential hemiparesis in childhood and their relation to etiology and prognosis. Neuropediatrics 12: 101–108
16. Kwong KL, Wong SN, So KT (1998). Epilepsy in children with cerebral palsy. Pediatr Neurol 19: 31–36
17. MacLennan A (1999). A template for defining a causal relation between acute intrapartum events and cerebral palsy: international consensus statement. BMJ 319: 1054–1059
18. Mercuri E, Spano M, Bruccini F, Frisone M, Trombetta J, Blandino A (1996). Visual Outcome in Cliildren with Congenital Hemiplegia: Correlation with MRI Findings. Neuropediatrics 27: 184–188
19. Michaelis R, Rooschotz B, Dopfer R (1980). Prenatal origin of congenital spastic hemiparesis. Early Hum Dev 4: 243–255
20. Okumura A, Hayakawa F, Kato T, Kuno K, Watanabe K (1999). Epilepsy in patients with spastic cerebral palsy: correlation with MRI findings at 5 years of age. Brain Dev 21: 540–543
21. Panteliadis C, Fiedler A, Jacobi G (1992). Kongenitale Hemiplegie: Klinik, neuroradiologische Befunde und Grad der mentalen Behinderung. In: Lischka A, Bernert G, eds. Aktuelle Neuropädiatrie. Wehr: Giba-Geigy Verlag, 387–390
22. Panteliadis Chr (1999). Cerebral palsy. In: Panteliadis C and Darras B eds. Encyclopedia of Pediatric neurology. Theory and Practice, 2nd ed. Thessloniki, Greece Giahoudi-Giapouli, 322–363
23. Petersen I, Eeg-Olofsson O, Sellden U (1968). Paroxysmal activity in EEG of normal children, In: Kellaway P, Petersen I, eds. Clinical Electroencephalography of Children. Almquist and Wiksell, Stockholm, 167–188
24. Steinlin M, Good M, Martin E, Baenziger O, Largo R.H, Boltshauser E (1993). Congenital Hemiplegia: Morphology of Cerebral Lesions and Pathogenetic Aspects from MRI. Neuropediatrics 24: 224–229
25. Uvebrant P (1988). Hemiplegic cerebral palsy: aetiology and outcome. Acta Pediatr Scand 345:1–100

Interhemisphären Differenzen visuell evozierter Potentiale (VEP) bei Kindern mit Rolando Epilepsie

D. Dralle, A. Portisch, J. Töller

Zusammenfassung

8 von 10 Kindern mit Rolando Epilepsie zeigten auf Lichtreize gesteigerte neuronale Erregbarkeit im Temporallappen. Der Nachweis wurde mit der VEP Differenz-Mapping Methode geführt.

Einleitung

In einer früheren Untersuchung von Kindern mit Hirntumoren und Epilepsie konnte gezeigt werden, dass über dem Temporallappen ipsilateral zum Tumor gesteigerte neuronale Aktivität auf Lichtreize auftrat. Die Latenz der temporalen Reizantwort war abhängig von der Schwere der Epilepsie, sie betrug nach längerer Anfallsfreiheit 200 ms (N200). Kinder der Kontrollgruppe zeigten nicht diese zusätzliche Reaktion auf Licht (Dralle 2000). Es entstand daraus die Frage, ob eine Übererregbarkeit auf Lichtreize auch bei Patienten mit Epilepsie ohne strukturelle Hirnläsionen über der Temporalregion nachweisbar sei, und ob diese ebenfalls abhängig wäre von der Schwere der Erkrankung. Es wurden deswegen Kinder mit Rolando Epilepsie untersucht. Bei benignem Verlauf der Erkrankung war eine Reaktion nach 200 ms (N200) zu erwarten.

Patienten

Untersucht wurden 10 Kinder mit Rolando Epilepsie im Alter zwischen 7 und 15 Jahren, davon 3 Mädchen und 7 Knaben. Sie erfüllten die klinischen und elektroencephalographischen Kriterien der Rolando Epilepsie. Zur Zeit der Untersuchung war bei 6 Kindern das EEG bereits saniert, bei 3 Patienten gebessert und bei einem Patienten erfolgte die Untersuchung vor Beginn der antikonvulsiven Therapie mit ausgeprägten Rolando spikes im EEG. Die Anfallsfreiheit lag zwischen wenigen Tagen und 5 Jahren. Von 5 Kindern lagen MRT Befunde vor, die nur in einem Fall diskrete periventrikuläre Infarkte links aufwiesen. Keines der Kinder war photosensibel.

Methode

VEP wurden bei wachem Kind mit geschlossenen Augen aus einer Entfernung von 12–15 cm mit weißem Blitzlicht (0,3 Joule) durchgeführt. Gereizt wurde sowohl binoculär als auch monoculär rechts und links. Die Reizfrequenz betrug 0,9 Hz. Abgeleitet wurde das digitalisierte EEG über 19 Elektroden nach dem 10–20 System mit einer Referenz aus dem Summenpotential. Grenzfrequenzen betrugen 0,5 und 100 Hz. Es wurden 100 Reizantworten verrechnet, von denen im Postprozessing artefaktbehaftete Anteile nach visueller Bewertung jeder einzelnen Epoche eliminiert wurden. Die Samplingrate betrug pro Kanal für die VEP 1250/s und für das synchron abgeleitete EEG 256/s. Ein Amplitudenmapping der VEP erfolgte durch lineare Interpolation zwischen den 19 Elektroden in 2 ms Intervallen über eine Dauer von 400 ms. Für das Differenz Mapping wurden die Differenzwerte der Amplituden zwischen zwei korrespondierenden Elektoden beider Hemisphären berechnet. So wurden z.B. die Amplituden über T3 substrahiert von denen über T4 und entsprechend die Werte über T4 substrahiert von T3. Die beiden daraus resultierenden Differenzen unterschieden sich somit in ihrem Vorzeichen. Amplituden der mittelständigen Elektroden wurden von sich selbst auf Null substrahiert. Danach erfolgte wiederum ein Mapping zwischen den 19 Elektroden wie oben beschrieben.

Ergebnisse

Die Latenzen der N70 und P100 wurden sowohl für die binoculären als auch für die monoculären Ableitungen bestimmt. Sie waren bei allen Kindern seitengleich und bei 9 Patienten im Normbereich gelegen. Das Kind mit frisch diagnostizierter Epilepsie bot Latenzverzögerungen (Tab. 1).

4 Patienten zeigten im konventionellen Mapping eine negative Reizantwort über der rechten Temporalregion von mindestens 60 ms Dauer nach einer Latenz von etwa 200 ms = N200 (Abb. 1: Die Aufzeichnung beginnt 20 ms nach dem Reiz und schreitet dann in 12 ms Intervallen in horizontaler Richtung fort. Der letzte Kopf in der zweiten Reihe zeigt die Ergebnisse nach 200 ms. Jeder einzelne Kopf ist frontal nach oben, occipital nach unten, rechts nach rechts und links nach links ausgerichtet. Die blaue Farbe steht für positive, die rote Farbe für negative

Tab. 1: VEP Latenzen und Amplituden.
BA: beide Augen gereizt, RA: rechtes – LA: linkes Auge gereizt. A: Amplitude

	N_{70}(ms)	P_{100}(ms)	A_{01}(uV)	A_{02}(uV)
BA n = 10	77,5 (49–105)	123,5 (84–155)	3,7 (2,4–6,8)	4,0 (1,8–9,4)
RA n = 7	73 (57–90)	123 (99–137)	2,8 (1,2–3,8)	3,2 (1,1–8,0)
LA n = 7	70 (58–85)	127 (99–134)	1,6 (0,8–5,0)	2,2 (0,9–5,8)

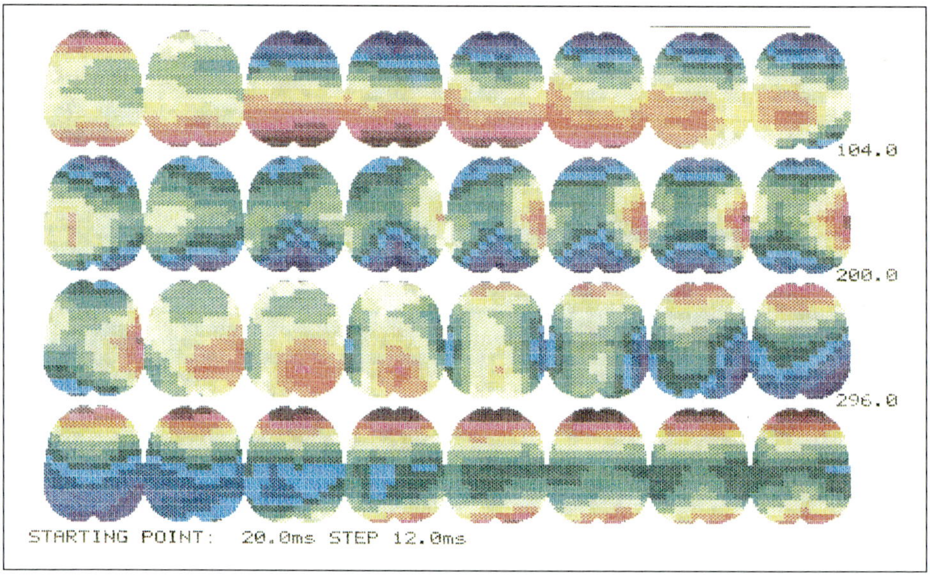

Abb. 1: VEP-Mapping (n = 4).

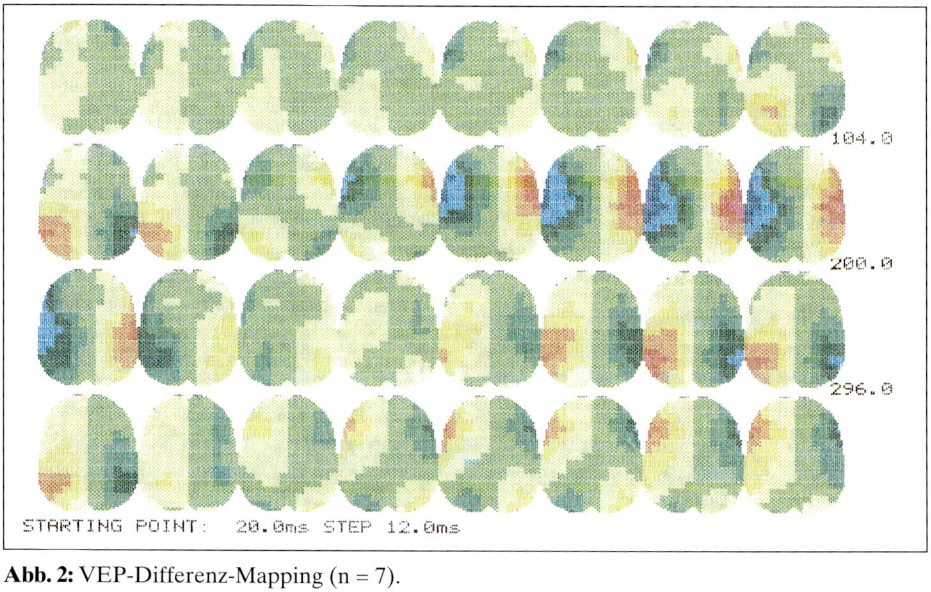

Abb. 2: VEP-Differenz-Mapping (n = 7).

Amplitudenwerte). Von diesen 4 Kindern waren zwei erst seit 3 Monaten anfallsfrei, nur bei einem Patienten wies das synchron abgeleitete EEG noch hypersynchrone Aktivität auf und ein Patient hatte im MRT diskrete periventrikuläre Infarkte links.

Mit der Differenz-Mapping Methode konnte bei 8 Kindern eine temporale N200 nachgewiesen werden, 7 mal auf der rechten Seite. Alle 8 Patienten boten

80–100 ms später eine weitere negative Reizantwort über der kontralateralen Temporalregion (Abb. 2). Bei den restlichen 2 Kindern konnte auch im Differen-Mapping keine neuronale Übererregbarkeit im Temporallappen nachgewiesen werden. Eines dieser beiden Kinder war von allen am längsten anfallsfrei.

Diskussion

Bei Patienten mit Rolando Epilepsie sind strukturelle Hirnläsionen nicht ursächlich anzunehmen. Die Art der fokalen Anfälle und der Nachweis centrotemporaler spikes lassen auf eine funktionelle Störung im Bereich sensomotorischer Areale schließen. Gesteigerte Erregbarkeit dieser Regionen kann mit »extremely high-amplitude somatosensory evoked potentials (SEP)« nachgewiesen werden, die in Bezug zu Rolando spikes stehen (Manganotti et al. 2000).

Vermehrte Erregbarkeit auf visuelle Reize wurde bislang bei Rolando Epilepsie nicht beschrieben.

Die visuelle Reizverarbeitung erfolgt nicht nur in der primären occipitalen Sehrinde, der V1 Region, sie findet unter anderm auch im inferioren und im mesialen Temporallappen, der MT/V5 Region statt. Räumliche visuelle Wahrnehmung wird im Hippocampus verarbeitet, einer Region, die bei Epilepsie eine nicht unerhebliche Rolle spielt (Pack et al. 2001, Pascual-Leone et al. 2001, Wang et al. 2000). Durch Licht induzierte komplex fokale Anfälle sind auch ohne Beteiligung der primären occipitalen Sehrinde im mesialen Temporallappen nachgewiesen worden (Benbadis et al. 1996, Isnard et al. 1998). In einer früheren Untersuchung konnte gesteigerte neuronale Aktivität auf Lichtreiz bei Kindern mit supratentoriellen Hirntumoren und Epilepsie im ipsilateral zum Tumor gelegenen Temporallappen beobachtet werden. Die gesteigerte Reizantwort war in der Latenz abhängig vom Verlauf der Epilepsie, sie betrug bei längerer Anfallsfreiheit 200 ms und wurde als N200 bezeichnet (Dralle 2000).

In der vorliegenden Untersuchung wurde der Frage nachgegangen, ob Patienten mit Rolando Epilepsie, die im Gegensatz zu Kindern mit Hirntumoren keine strukturelle Hirnläsion aufweisen, überschießende neuronale Reaktionen nicht nur der SEP sondern auch auf visuelle Reize haben. Bei benigner Krankheit wurde in Analogie zu Patienten mit Hirntumoren eine negativ gepolte Reaktion nach 200 ms (N200) im Temporallappen vermutet. Tatsächlich ließ sich bei 4 der 10 Kinder mit Rolando Epilepsie im konventionellen VEP Mapping nach 200 ms eine gesteigerte neuronale Aktivität in der Temporalregion rechts nachweisen. Die Methode des Differenz-Mappings ermöglicht eine genauere Analyse von Seitendifferenzen, da physiologische, seitengleiche Reizantworten heraussubstrahiert werden. Mit Hilfe dieser Methode zeigten 8 der 10 Kinder eine N200 über dem Temporallappen, 7 von ihnen auf der rechten Seite. Eine weitere Reaktion war 80–100 ms später kontralateral nachweisbar, die bei negativer Polung ebenfalls auf Übererregbarkeit hinwies. Damit muss davon ausgegangen werden, dass Patienten mit Rolando Epilepsie nicht nur im sensomotorischen sondern auch im visuellen Bereich gesteigerte neuronale Erregbarkeit auf Reize aufweisen. Bisherige Befunde im VEP Mapping an Patienten mit Epilepsie bei

Hirntumoren als auch bei Kindern mit Rolando Epilepsie deuten auf Zusammenhänge zwischen dem Krankheitsverlauf und der Latenz der lichtinduzierten Reaktionen im Temporallappen hin.

Literatur

1. Benbadis SR, Gerson WA, Harvey JH, Luders HO (1996) Photosensitive temporal lobe epilepsy. Neurology 46: 1540–1542
2. Dralle D (2000) Follow up of visually evoked potentials in children with brain tumor and fokal seizures. Brain Topology 12: 300
3. Isnard J, Guenot M, Fischer C, Mertens P, Sindou M, Mauguiere F (1998) A stereo-electroencephalographic (SEEG) study of light-induced mesiotemporal epileptic seizures. Epilepsia 39: 1098–1103
4. Manganotti P, Zanette G (2000) Contribution of motor cortex in generation of evoked spikes in patients with benign rolandic epilepsy. Clin. Neurophysiol. 111: 964–974
5. Pack CC, Berezovskii VK, Born RT (2001) Dynamic properties of neurons in cortical area MT in alert and anaesthetized macaque monkeys. Nature 414: 905–908
6. Pascaul-Leone A, Walsh V (2001) Fast backprojections from the motion to the primary visual area necessary for visual avareness. Science 292: 510–512
7. Wang Y, Fujita I, Murayama Y (2000) Neural mechanisms of selectivity for object features revealed by blocking inhibition in inferotemporal cortex. Nature Neurosci. 3: 807–813

Entwicklungsstörungen und subklinische Entladungen im EEG – Therapie ja oder nein? Fallberichte über drei Brüder.

G. Skirl, Ch. Bravidor, A. Eichhorn, T. Rating, U. Brandl

Zusammenfassung

Es werden die Fallberichte von drei Brüdern vorgestellt, die als Gemeinsamkeiten Entwicklungsstörungen und multifokale epilepsietypische Veränderungen im EEG aufweisen, unterschiedlich sind jedoch klinischer Verlauf und das Ansprechen auf eine antiepileptische Behandlung. Während der mit einem Anfall erkrankte Junge neben einer Anfallsfreiheit auch mental von der Therapie zu profitieren scheint, zeigen sich bei seinen Brüdern weder im EEG noch in der psychologischen Testung Verbesserungen.

Diese unterschiedlichen Ausgänge zeigen das Problem auf, dass es bisher keine sicheren Kriterien gibt, die eine Therapieindikation bei der Kombination von Entwicklungsstörungen und subklinischen Entladungen begründen lassen. Hier sind weitere Studien notwendig.

Problemstellung

Die Indikationsstellung einer Therapie mit Antiepileptika bei der Kombination von Entwicklungsstörungen und subklinischen Entladungen im EEG wird kontrovers diskutiert.

Es besteht die klinische Erfahrung, dass einzelne Kinder von einer solchen Therapie – neben adäquaten medizinischen und anderen Fördermaßnahmen – profitieren können, jedoch fehlen noch immer allgemein anerkannte Kriterien, die bei der Entscheidungsfindung hilfreich sein können.

Die Fallberichte über drei Brüder sollen ein mögliches Vorgehen illustrieren.

Patientenvorstellung

Index-Patient ist *Leo* (* 28.10.1994), der am 01.08.2001 mit einem Anfall akut erkrankt, die Anfallsbeschreibung ist unscharf, es werden Zittern am ganzen Körper, Blausucht und anhaltende Bewusstseinstrübung berichtet.

L. ist der zweite von vier Jungen, nach unauffälliger Schwangerschaft und Geburt sei die frühkindliche Entwicklung normal verlaufen, es wird über zweimalige Fieberkrämpfe berichtet.

Er besucht die 1. Klasse der Grundschule, wegen Problemen im Anfangsunterricht ist die Umsetzung in eine Diagnose-Förderklasse vorgesehen.

Nach dem akuten Ereignis klinisch-neurologisch unauffälliger Befund, es bestehen aber Lautvertauschungen, die Sprache ist gering dysgrammatisch.

Die initiale Labordiagnostik (einschließlich Stoffwechsel-Untersuchungen) erbrachte keine abweichenden Befunde, das postparoxysmal abgeleitete EEG zeigte mäßig schwer ausgeprägte Allgemeinveränderungen. Die zerebrale MRT war unauffällig.

Die Kontrolle des EEG im Schlaf zeigte mehrere voneinander unabhängige Foci, wobei der fronto-zentro-temporal links gelegene die stärkste Aktivität aufwies.

Psychologische Untersuchungen

Bei Untersuchungen im August 2001 mit der K-ABC fanden sich signifikante Differenzen zwischen dem SED: SW=56 und dem SGD: SW=76 bei einem SIF: SW=67, im HAWIVA wurde ein IQ_V von 90 und ein IQ_H von 105 ermittelt, die Kontrollen im Februar 2002 zeigten in der K-ABC eine deutliche Besserung mit SED: SW=75, SGD: SW=83 und SIF: SW=80, im HAWIK-R wurden bei einem Gesamt-IQ von 73 im sprachgebundenen Teil ein IQ_V von 72 und im handlungsbezogenen Teil ein IQ_H von 83 erreicht, wobei durch den Verfahrenswechsel keine direkte Vergleichsmöglichkeit gegeben ist. Kommentar: Belastbarkeit und Konzentrationsfähigkeit deutlich gesteigert, das Sprechen ist z.T. noch dysgrammatisch mit Ungenauigkeiten in der Artikulation, noch einzeln Wortfindungsstörungen, Fehler sind bei Aufmerksamkeit zu korrigieren, insgesamt deutliche Besserung der intellektuellen Leistungsfähigkeiten.

Unter Berücksichtigung des ausgeprägten EEG-Befundes und den Ergebnissen der psychologischen Untersuchung wurde nach einem einmaligen Anfall die Indikation zu einer Therapie mit Sultiam gestellt, es trat bisher kein erneuter Anfall auf, zweimalige Schlafentzugs-Schlaf-EEG zeigten eine deutliche Verringerung der Spitzenpotentiale. Die Tagesdosis von 200 mg Sultiam wird gut toleriert.

Familienanamnestisch sind zu berichten

Die Mutter hat eine multiple Dyslalie, die seit ihrer Kindheit bestehen würde, der Vater ist wegen einer Herzerkrankung erwerbsunfähig.

Von drei Geschwistern zeigten zwei eine Entwicklungsstörung, wegen der anzunehmenden Familiarität wurde empfohlen, diese beiden Jungen ebenfalls vorzustellen.

Frank ist am 12.05.1992 geboren und der Älteste der vier Jungen. Schwangerschaft und Geburt seien unauffällig gewesen, auch die motorische Entwicklung verlief normal, die Sprachentwicklung aber verzögert. Epileptische Anfälle sind bei ihm bisher nicht aufgetreten. *F.* besucht eine Schule für Lernbehinderte.

Klinisch-neurologisch gestörte Feinmotorik, im Sprachstatus fallen eine partielle Dyslalie sowie eine Einschränkungen des Wortschatzes auf, weiter besteht ein Dysgrammatismus.

Im Schlafentzugs-Schlaf-EEG vom 06.10.2001 zeigten sich bei *F.* drei voneinander unabhängig aktive Herde.

Psychologische Untersuchungen

Hier liegen Untersuchungen vom 12.10.2001 und vom 08.02.2002 vor. In der K-ABC erreichte F. die Werte SED: SW=61 bzw. 59, SGD: SW=61 bzw. 58, SIF: SW=62 bzw. 59, im HAWIK-R IQ_{Ges}=52 bzw. 50, IQ_V=60 bzw. 57, IQ_H=55 bzw. 55. Kommentar: Schwierigkeiten im Aufgabenverständnis, hoher Zeitbedarf für alle Aufgaben, mitunter haftendes Denken, teilweise ungenau und dysgrammatisch artikuliert, spricht in einfachen spärlichen Sätzen, unsichere Feinmotorik, keine Entwicklungsfortschritte, eher Entwicklungsstagnation, aber kein Hinweis für Abbau intellektueller Leistungen.

Nach der psychologischen Diagnostik erfolgte die probatorische Einstellung auf Sultiam, die Kontrolle des Schlafentzugs-Schlaf-EEG am 23.11.2001 zeigte eine geringere Ausprägung der epileptischen Foci, die Tagesdosis von 200 mg Sultiam wurde zunächst gut vertragen, kurz vor Kontrolle im Februar sei aber vermehrt Müdigkeit aufgetreten. Das Schlafentzugs-Schlaf-EEG vom 09.02.2002 zeigte unverändert die epileptischen Foci. Aktuell wird eine probatorische Therapie mit Valproat eingesetzt.

Martin ist am 18.09.1997 geboren, nach unauffälliger Schwangerschaft und Geburt verzögerte motorische Entwicklung und in der Sprache, so wird Laufen erst nach dem 18. Lebensmonat berichtet, erste sprachliche Äußerungen nach dem 2. Geburtstag. *M.* besucht eine integrative Kindertagesstätte und wird logopädisch betreut, epileptische Anfälle sind bei ihm bisher nicht aufgetreten. Der Sprachentwicklungsstand entspricht dem eines 2jährigen Kindes.

Sowohl im Schlaf- als auch im Wach-EEG Anfang Oktober 2001 finden sich multifokale voneinander unabhängige Foci, wobei der occipito-temporal rechts in seiner Aktivität am stärksten ausgeprägt ist.

Psychologische Untersuchungen

Sie erfolgten am 05.10.2001 und am 08.02.2002 mit der Münchner Funktionellen Entwicklungsdiagnostik bei 36 bzw. 41 Lebensmonaten und ergaben nachstehende Werte:

Laufen 31/33, Handgeschicklichkeit 31/31, Perzeption 25/25, Sprechen 23/23, Sprachverständnis 26/26, Sozial 19/19, Selbständigkeit 23/23 (jeweils Lebensmonate), jeweils nur 08.02.2002 durchgeführt K-ABC: SED: SW = 65, SGD: SW = 63, SIF: SW = 64 und KRAMER IQ = 56. Kommentar: Äußert sich in Ein- und Zweiwortsätzen mit undeutlicher Artikulation, Beeinträchtigungen in der Feinmotorik, Früh-Förderung dringend weiter indiziert, kein Entwicklungsfortschritt, eher Stagnation.

Auch hier wird nach der Leistungsdiagnostik eine probatorische Einstellung auf Sultiam empfohlen, die Kontrolle am 23.11.2001 zeigt keine Verminderung des Spitzenpotentialanteils, die bis dahin gegebene Tagesdosis von 100 mg Sultiam wird auf 150 mg erhöht, diese Dosis wird vertragen, auch hier wird aber kurz vor der Kontrolle im Februar 2002 über Müdigkeit, zusätzlich aber über Schlafstörungen berichtet. Das Schlafentzugs-Schlaf-EEG vom 08.02.2002 zeigt einen unverändert pathologischen Befund. Auch hier wurde die Therapie auf Valproat umgesetzt.

Diskussion

Sharp wave foci sind als genetisches Merkmal bei 3,5% der Kinder zu finden. Eine unbekannte Anzahl, vermutlich die Mehrheit davon ist asymptomatisch, auch bei intensiver Befragung sind keine Hinweise für Anfälle, Teilleistungsstörungen, insbesondere im Sprachbereich oder Verhaltensstörungen zu ermitteln.

Weiter werden sie aber bei Neugeborenen- und Fieberkrämpfen, idiopathischen fokalen Epilepsien und kognitiven Störungen gesehen.

Die epileptische Aktivität ist regelhaft in Schlafableitungen zu aktivieren, gleichartige Veränderungen werden bei 30% der Geschwister beobachtet. Weiter finden sich bei Kindern mit Teilleistungsstörungen bei 15 bis 30% der betroffenen Kinder identische Veränderungen.

Ausgehend vom Index-Fall Leo und der anamnestisch bekannten Entwicklungsprobleme bei Frank und Martin war der pathologische EEG-Befund bei beiden eigentlich keine Überraschung.

Bei allen drei Kindern besteht eine Erkrankung aus dem Formenkreis der idiopathischen fokalen Epilepsien, bei der Mutter ist eine überbleibende Sprachbehinderung auf der gleichen Grundlage zu vermuten. Die Erkrankung präsentiert sich klinisch in unterschiedlicher Weise, verschieden ist auch das Ansprechen auf die Medikation mit Sultiam.

Während Leo frei von Anfällen ist, deutlich bessere Testergebnisse bei der Leistungsdiagnostik zeigt und auch im Schlaf-EEG eine verringerte Aktivität der epileptischen Foci aufweist, zeigen sich weder bei Frank noch bei Martin Veränderungen in den Ergebnissen der Leistungsdiagnostik oder im Schlaf-EEG, beide haben unverändert keine Anfälle, über den Effekt der Umsetzung auf Valproat kann bislang keine sichere Aussage getroffen werden.

Bei Leo ist ein Zusammenhang zwischen dem Zurückdrängen der epileptischen Aktivität und der Verbesserung in der Leistungssituation anzunehmen, hier ist die Tendenz mehr zu den typischen Formen der idiopathischen fokalen Epilepsien zu sehen.

Für Frank und Martin muss diese Frage derzeit noch offen bleiben, es überwiegen allein durch das Fehlen von Anfällen Merkmale der atypischen Formen. Auf der einen Seite kann ein Zusammenhang zwischen der Spike-Aktivität und den Leistungsprobleme diskutiert, die mangelnde Besserung dem fehlendem Ansprechen auf Sultiam angelastet werden. Auf der anderen Seite ist es denkbar, dass eine zu Grunde liegende Enzephalopathie per se für das mentale Defizit verantwortlich ist und keine direkten Beziehung zwischen der Ausprägung der epileptischen Aktivität und der Leistungssituation besteht.

Die Verläufe bei Frank, Leo und Martin illustrieren die klinische und elektroenzephalographische Kenntnis, dass idiopathische fokale Epilepsien bei autosomaldominanter Vererbung eine variable Expressivität aufweisen und das Spektrum mehr im Sinne eines Kontinuums mit vielfältigen Überlappungen von den asymptomatischen Sharp-Wave-Foci über die typischen Formen mit zentro-temporalen und occipitalen Entladungen bis zu den atypischen Formen als Pseudo-LENNOX-, LANDAU-KLEFFNER- oder CSWS-Syndrom reicht (DOOSE 1998).

Auf LAUB geht das Modell der »Indikationswaage« zurück, die uns mahnt bei jeder Epilepsie vor der Einleitung einer antiepileptischen Langzeittherapie Nutzen und Schaden der Therapie gegen die Nicht-Therapie abzuwägen.

Die Effektivität von Sultiam bei guter Verträglichkeit ist für die benigne fokale Epilepsie mit zentro-temporalen spikes (BECT) belegt (RATING et al. 2000), ebenso der Ausgang ohne Beeinträchtigung der kognitiven Funktionen (DEONNA et al. 2000), die Behandlungsindikation kann hier sehr zurückhaltend gestellt werden, da vom natürlichen Verlauf keine Schädigung zu erwarten ist.

Bei schweren Verläufen einer BECT oder der Entwicklung zu einer atypischen Form zeichnet sich ein anderes Bild ab, hier führen prolongierte Verlangsamungsherde und die starke Aktivierung der nächtlichen spike und wave zu einem kognitiven Abbau und Störungen der Aufmerksamkeit, hier kann ein aktiver epileptischer Fokus mit der normalen Reifung der kognitiven Funktionen interferieren (SAINT-MARTIN et al. 2001).

MASSA et al. (2001) beschreiben an Hand einer Studie bei 35 Kindern mit BECT interiktale EEG-Kriterien, die prädiktiv für einen komplizierenden Verlauf sind: intermittierende Verlangsamungsherde, multiple asynchrone spike-wave-Herde, lange Cluster von spike-wave, generalisierte 3/sec. »Absence-ähnliche« spike-wave Entladungen, Verbindung von interiktalen Paroxysmen mit negativen oder positiven Myoklonien und das reichliche Vorkommen interiktaler Abnormalitäten im Wachen und Schlafen. Sie schlussfolgern, dass die unterschiedliche Kombination von wenigstens drei der sechs interiktalen EEG-Muster und deren Persistieren für mehr als 6 Monate die Patienten kennzeichnet, für die ein Risiko einer neuropsychologischen Beeinträchtigung besteht.

Hier sind Schäden durch die Anfälle zu erwarten, die Indikation für die Therapie ist damit zu stellen. Gleichwohl ist bekannt, dass die atypischen Formen schwer zu behandeln sind.

Sultiam ist bei einem Teil der Patienten wirksam, eine sichere Validierung der Wirksamkeit auf kognitive Störungen ähnlich dem antikonvulsiven Effekt bei BECT steht für Sultiam bislang aber aus.

Für Carbamazepin wird die Förderung eines CSWS diskutiert, im Weiteren sind für unterschiedliche Kombinationen von Valproat, Benzodiazepinen und Succinimiden einzelne Erfolge, aber auch Toleranzentwicklungen beschrieben. Im therapeutischen Arsenal werden weiter Steroide und Immunglobuline angeführt. Zu den neueren Antiepileptika gibt es bisher keine sichere Datenlage. Letztlich wird in einzelnen Fällen auch die Epilepsiechirurgie diskutiert (RATING 2001).

Bei Fehlen von Anfällen muss die Wirksamkeit der Therapie durch regelmäßige psychologische Re-Tests und Schlaf-EEG-Ableitungen (ggf. mit Video-Monitoring) validiert werden.

Die unterschiedliche Methodik allein im Einsatz neuropsychologischer Testverfahren, aber auch bei den Schlafableitungen lässt nur schwer Vergleiche einzelner Therapien ziehen.

Die Frage der Wirksamkeit einer antikonvulsiven Therapie auch auf kognitive Defekte im Rahmen der idiopathischen fokalen Epilepsien wird sich nur in einem multizentrischen Ansatz beantworten lassen, diese Untersuchung steht bisher aus.

Literatur

1. Deonna T, Zesiger P, Davidoff V, Maeder M, Mayor C; Roulet E (2000) Benign partial epilepsy of childhood: a longitudinal neuropsychological and EEG study of cognitive function. Dev-Med-Child-Neurol. 2000 Sep; 42(9): 595–603
2. Doose H (1998) Epilepsien im Kindes- und Jugendalter, 11. revidierte und erweiterte Auflage, Desitin Hamburg, 1998
3. Laub CM (1996) Indikation zur antiepileptischen Langzeittherapie bei Kindern. In: Besser R, Gross-Selbeck G (Herausg.) Epilepsiesyndrome – Therapiestrategien. 2. überarb. und erweit. Aufl, Thieme Stuttgart
4. Massa R, Saint-Martin AD, Carcangiu R, Rudolf G, Seegmuller C, Kleitz C, Metz-Lutz MN, Hirsch E, Marescaux C (2001) EEG criteria predictive of complicated evolution in idiopathic rolandic epilepsy. Neurology. 2001 Sep 25; 57(6): 1071–1079
5. Rating D, Wolf C, Bast T (2000) Sulthiame as monotherapy in children with benign childhood epilepsy with centrotemporal spikes: a 6-month randomized, double-blind, placebo-controlled study. Sulthiame Study Group. Epilepsia 2000 Oct; 41(10): 1284–1288
6. Rating D (2001) Treatment in typical and atypical rolandic epilepsy. Epileptic-Disord. 2000; 2 Suppl 1: S69–72
7. Saint-Martin AD, Seegmuller C, Carcangiu R, Kleitz C, Hirsch E, Marescaux C, Metz-Lutz M-N (2001) Cognitive consequences of Rolandic Epilepsy. Epileptic-Disord. 2001 Jul; Spec issue 2: 59–66

Visuell betonte kognitive Funktionsstörung bei kryptogener fokaler Epilepsie: Ein Fallbericht

S. Keßler, S. Rinnert, G. v. Ondarza, U. Stephani

Präsentiert wird eine 11 Jahre alte Patientin mit Schulproblemen, kryptogener fokaler Epilepsie und visueller Verarbeitungs- und Merkfähigkeitsstörung.

Kasuistik

Erste epileptische Anfälle mit 10 Jahren (atypische Absencen, Myoklonien, komplex-partielle und tonische) assoziiert mit Schulproblemen.

Neuropsychologische Untersuchung (z.T. mit EEG):

Subnormales Gesamtniveau (Lernbehinderung; Abb. 1). *Visuelle Verarbeitung und räumlich-konstruktive Leistung: schwer reduziert.* Visuelle Exploration: Übersehen / Verkennung von Zielreizen: z.B. beim Figurenlegen (Pferd)

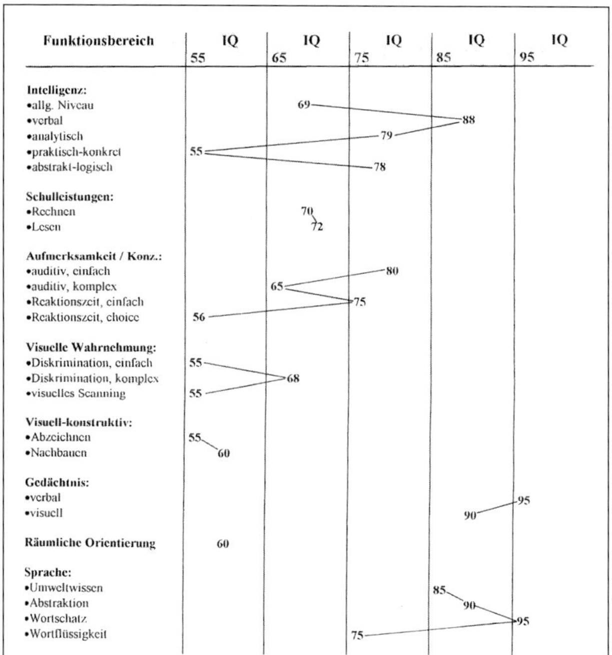

Abb. 1: Neuropsychologische Befunde.

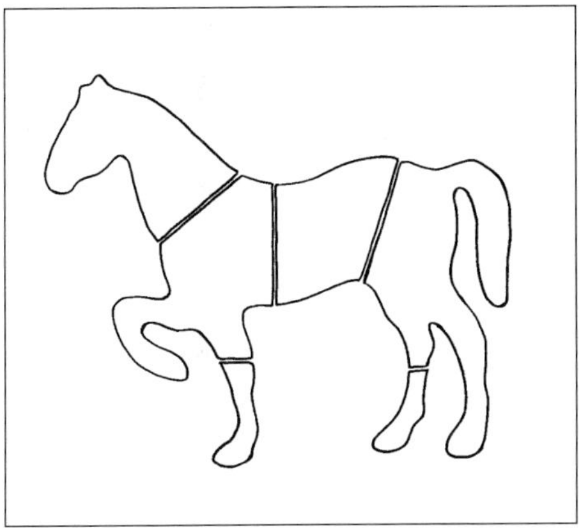

Abb. 2: HAWIK III, Untertest Figurenlegen.

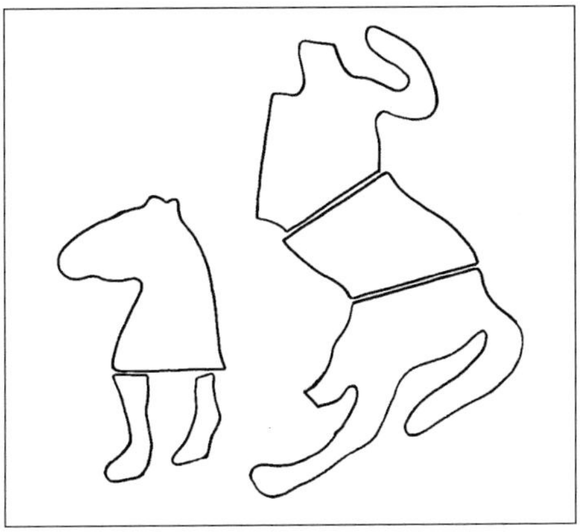

Abb. 3: Bizarre Legung: »2 tanzende Mädchen ohne Kopf«.

bizarre Legung durch Patientin. Sie konnte markanten Umriss des Pferdekopfes nicht als solchen deuten und baute ihn in eigenes Wahrnehmungsraster ein. (Abb. 2 und 3). Schwächen bei Analyse räumlicher Beziehungen, Einschätzung von Winkeln und Proportionen erschwerten Orientierung im Raum. Komplexe sprachliche Anforderungen: Probleme bei der Umsetzung. Ausgeprägte Rechts-Links-Unsicherheit und komplette Uhrzeit-Agnosie.

Im Wach-*EEG* (während Testung): Verlangsamung Grundaktivität, unabhängige Spike- und Sharp-waves occipital beidseits, rechts betont (Generalisierung alle 20–30 Sek., Dauer: 1–5 Sek). (Abb. 4.) Unter Photostimulation Aktivierung hypersynchroner Aktivität mit stimulationssynchronem Auftreten von Ketten von Spikes, Photosensibilität 1°. Im Schlaf-EEG keine Aktivierung. Wach-EEG von Eltern und Bruder o.p.B.. Unauffälliges cerebrales MRT.

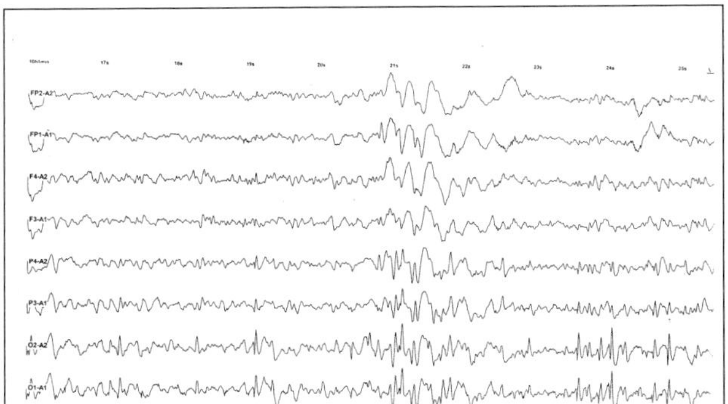

Abb. 4: Wach-EEG.

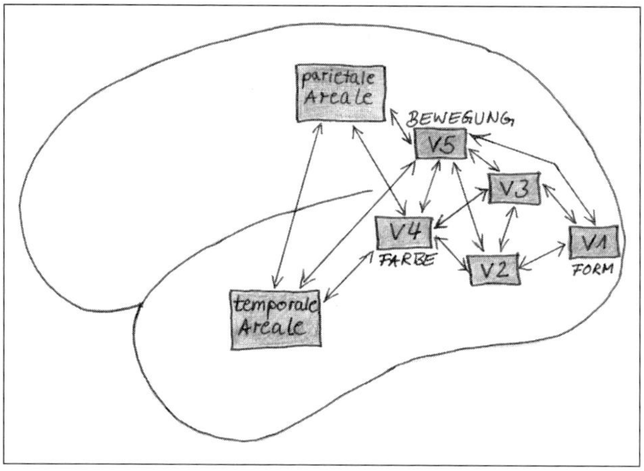

Abb. 5: Merkmalsverarbeitung.

Diagnose

Kryptogene fokale Epilepsie bei gleichzeitig bestehender genetischer Disposition in Form der Photosensibilität. Aufgrund der neuropsychologischen Testergebnisse, die während der EEG-Ableitung erhoben wurden, deuteten wir die *visuell betonten Wahrnehmungsprobleme als iktogenes Geschehen im Sinne einer nicht-transitorischen kognitiven Funktionsstörung.*

Beim Sehen trifft die visuelle Information occipital auf die primäre Sehrinde. Von dort wird die Objektinformation zur Verarbeitung und Erkennung spezieller Objektmerkmale in andere Hirnregionen weitergeleitet. Abhängig vom Objektmerkmal findet die Informationsverarbeitung in speziellen Neuronenverbänden (Assemblies) unterschiedlicher Hirnregionen statt. (Abb. 5.) Um einzelne Objekte von anderen unterscheiden zu können, müssen zusammengehörene Bildbereich und deren Merkmale abgegrenzt werden. Die Grundlage dieser Abgrenzung (Segmentierung) ist die Merkmalsbindung. Diese findet vermutlich dadurch statt, dass einzelne Objekte durch Verbände von synchron aktivierten Neuronen (Assembly) repräsentiert werden. Dabei repräsentiert die zeitliche Korrelation die Zusammengehörigkeit der Merkmale eines Objektes. (Engel, A., Singer W. 1997) (Abb. 6.) Wenn durch kontinuierliche occipitale Entladungen die Aufnahme und synchronisierte Weiterleitung von Information

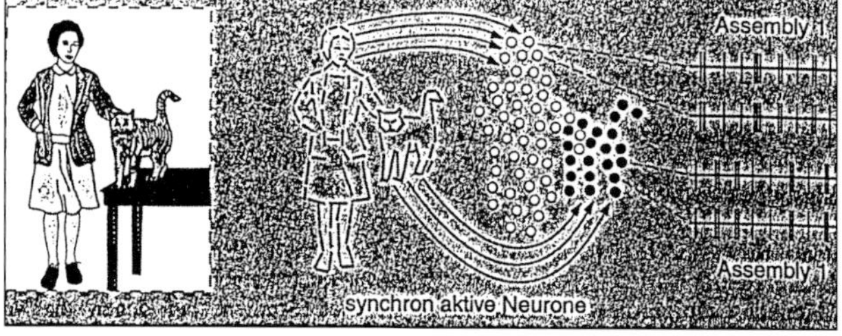

Abb. 6: Merkmalsbindung durch Synchronisation (übernommen aus Engel, A., Singer, W. »Neuronale Gestaltwahrnehmung« Spektrum der Wissenschaft, Dossier 4. 1997).

gestört ist, gehen zur Objekterkennung wichtige Inhalte verloren und die visuelle Wahrnehmung ist konsekutiv gestört. Zusätzlich können generalisierte Entladungen die Merkfähigkeit reduzieren, die Reaktionszeit verlängern und die Konsolidierung von Lerninhalten stören. (Binnie, C. D. 1990, Aldenkamp, A.P. 1990).

Frustrane *Behandlungs*versuche mit: STM, VPA, LTG, ESM, CBZ und OXC in Mono- und Kombinationstherapie. Weiterhin Anfälle: Myoklonien rechter lateraler Augenwinkel, Zusammenkneifen rechtes Auge, Abwesenheitszustände. Die Unterdrückung der hypersynchronen Aktivität im EEG und damit erwartete Verbesserung der kognitiven Leistungen (bes. visuell) ist weiterhin oberstes Therapieziel.

Literatur

1. Binnie, C.D. »Learning Disabilities in Epilepsy« Epilepsia Vol.31, Suppl.4, 1990
2. Aldenkamp, A.P. »Neuropsychological Aspects of Learning Disabilities in Epilepsy« Epilepsia Vol. 31, Suppl. 4, 1990
3. Engel, A., Singer W. »Neuronale Gestaltwahrnehmung« Spektrum der Wissenschaft, Dossier 4, 1997

Neuronenspezifische Enolase bei Kindern mit Fieberkrämpfen – Kinetik und prädiktiver Wert

P. Borusiak, S. Herbold

Zusammenfassung

Die Ergebnisse über Erhöhungen der neuronenspezifischen Enolase (NSE) im Serum und Liquor bei erwachsenen Patienten und Kindern mit epileptischen Anfällen werden kontrovers diskutiert. In unserer Studie haben wir den zeitlichen Verlauf der NSE-Werte im Serum bei Kindern nach Fieberkrämpfen (FK) bestimmt. Ferner wurde der prädiktive Wert der NSE für weitere FK oder die zukünftige Entwicklung einer Epilepsie untersucht. NSE-Werte im Serum wurden zu folgenden Zeiten bestimmt: (1) 0–2 h, (2) 6–8 h und (3) 20–24 h nach einem ersten oder zweiten FK. Ausschlusskriterien waren manifeste Epilepsien oder andere neurologische Erkrankungen. Das Follow-up betrug zwischen 14 und 28 Monate. Es erfolgte eine Analyse der Gesamtgruppe und eine Subgruppenanalyse der Kinder, die während des Follow-up weitere FK oder eine Epilepsie entwickelten. Untersucht wurden 82 Kinder (35 w, 47 m) im Alter von vier Monaten bis 5;7 Jahren. Weder in der Gesamtgruppe noch in den Subgruppenanalysen zeigten sich statistisch signifikante Unterschiede. Die Kinetik der NSE-Werte erbrachte ebenfalls keine signifikanten Unterschiede zu den verschiedenen Zeitpunkten. Bei Kindern mit FK ist die NSE als Marker zur Diagnostik und als prädiktiver Wert für weitere Anfälle bzw. die Entwicklung einer Epilepsie nicht geeignet. Die Ergebnisse nach einzelnen Anfällen oder einem Status epilepticus bei Erwachsenen lassen sich für unsere untersuchte Gruppe nicht bestätigen.

Fieberkrämpfe, mesiale temporale Sklerose und Temporallappenepilepsie

Über die Zusammenhänge zwischen prolongierten oder komplizierten Fieberkrämpfen und der späteren Entwicklung einer Temporallappenepilepsie auf der Basis einer mesialen temporalen Sklerose gibt es seit Jahrzehnten kontroverse Diskussionen. Hauptsächlich werden drei Hypothesen diskutiert: (1) Die Fieberkrämpfe führen zu einer Schädigung der mesialen temporalen Strukturen mit konsekutiver Ammonshornsklerose, die dann ihrerseits für die Entstehung der Temporallappenanfälle verantwortlich ist. (2) Fieberkrämpfe und Temporallappenepilepsie existieren unabhängig voneinander. (3) Ein prädisponierender Faktor führt sowohl zu prolongierten bzw. komplizierten Fieberkrämpfen und ist auch für die Entstehung der mesialen temporalen Sklerose mit den dort generierten Anfällen verantwortlich. Die bisher vorhandenen Daten sind teilweise widersprüchlich und lassen keine eindeutigen Schlussfolgerungen zu (Übersicht bei Holthausen 1994).

Neuronenspezifische Enolase (NSE)

Die Enolase ist ein Enzym der Glycolyse und besteht aus drei immunologisch unterscheidbaren Untereinheiten (α, β, γ), die fünf verschiedene Isoenzyme ($\alpha\alpha$, $\beta\beta$, $\gamma\gamma$, $\alpha\beta$, $\alpha\gamma$) bilden, von denen Gliazellen lediglich $\alpha\alpha$-Enolase und Neurone $\gamma\gamma$-Enolase (neuronen-spezifische Enolase = NSE) enthalten. In den übrigen Organen kommt NSE nur in Spuren vor.

Die NSE im Serum (sNSE) hat sich im Tierversuch und bei Erwachsenen als Marker für eine Zellschädigung (Ischämie oder Nekrose) im Gehirn erwiesen (Hay et al. 1984; Persson et al. 1987; Taylor et al. 1983). Es handelt sich um eine spezifische neuronale Schädigung und zusätzliches oder alleiniges Absterben von Gliazellen ist ohne Einfluss auf die Höhe der sNSE (Schmechel et al. 1978; Lafon-Cazal et al. 1992). Eine Zellnekrose ist nicht zwingend, lediglich eine (auch reversible) Schädigung. Als Parameter hat sich die sNSE bei cerebrovaskulären Erkrankungen bewährt, wobei die prädiktive Wertigkeit bei hypoxisch-ischämischen Ereignissen besser war, als bei hämorrhagischen (Schaarschmidt et al. 1994).

Berichte über NSE im Serum bzw. Liquor bei erwachsenen Patienten mit Epilepsien liegen vor. Rabinowicz et al. (1995) beobachteten bei zwei Patienten nach einem non-konvulsiven Status einen Anstieg der NSE. DeGiorgio et al. (1995) fand signifikante Unterschiede der sNSE-Werte von 19 Patienten mit Status epilepticus verglichen mit 18 gesunden Kontrollpersonen und 13 Patienten mit einer Epilepsie, die mehr als 7 Tage anfallsfrei waren. Die gleiche Untersuchungsgruppe stellte 1996 acht Patienten mit einem komplex-fokalen Status vor, die ebenfalls signifikant höhere Werte der sNSE aufwiesen. Die Ergebnisse dieser Untersuchungsgruppe konnten von Palmio et al. (2001) bisher nicht bestätigt werden. Bei 22 Patienten mit tonisch-klonischen Anfällen ließ sich keine NSE-Erhöhung nachweisen. Bei Kindern untersuchten Ko et al. (1990) NSE-Werte bei unterschiedlichen neurologischen Erkrankungen. Hierbei finden sich enge Korrelationen zwischen den Werten der sNSE und den entsprechenden Liquorwerten. Kinder mit epileptischen Anfällen wiesen signifikant höhere sNSE-Werte auf, als eine Vergleichsgruppe, wobei die angegebenen Daten als unzureichend zu bezeichnen sind (u.a. fehlen Angaben zu Alter der Kinder und Art und Häufigkeit der Anfälle). Rodriguez-Nunez et al. (2000) und Tanabe et al. (2001) fanden im Serum bzw. Liquor von 90 bzw. 53 Patienten mit Fieberkrämpfen keine signifikante Erhöhung bei Abnahme unmittelbar nach dem Anfall. Tierexperimentell ließ sich ein zeitabhängiger Anstieg der NSE nach einem Trauma bei Ratten mit einem Maximum der Werte nach 6 Stunden nachweisen (Woertgen et al. 2000).

Fragestellungen

Unter Berücksichtigung der bisherigen Ergebnisse war die Frage, inwieweit sich die bei Erwachsenen nachgewiesenen Erhöhungen der NSE auf Kinder mit Fieberkrämpfen übertragen lassen, und somit Hinweise für die Einordnung als epileptisch oder nicht bzw. eine neuronale Schädigung geben. Ferner sollten über eine Differenzierung des Abstandes der Blutabnahme zum Anfall Aufschlüsse über mögliche Änderungen über die Zeit gewonnen werden. Sollte sich eine Erhöhung der NSE-Werte ergeben, wäre die Frage einer Korrelation der sNSE-Werte mit den bekannten Risikofaktoren für die Entwicklung einer späteren Epilepsie zu evaluieren.

Methode

Die Blutabnahme fand zu drei Zeitpunkten (0–2 h, 6–8 h und 20–24 h) nach einem ersten oder zweiten Fieberkrampf statt. Anschließend erfolgte eine Zentrifugation und Einfrieren des Serums bei –20°C bis zur Bestimmung der sNSE mittels EIA (monoklonale Antikörper gegen die γ-Einheit, Referenzbereich bis 13 µg/l). Patienten mit progredienten neurologischen Erkrankungen, manifesten Epilepsien und Tumorerkrankungen wurden ebenso ausgeschlossen, wie hämolytische Proben. Die statistische Auswertung erfolgte mittels Mittelwertbildung mit entsprechenden statistischen Variablen, t-Tests für verbundene Stichproben bzw. U-Tests nach Wilcoxon, Mann und Whitney für unverbundene Stichproben.

Patienten

- 82 Kinder (47 m, 35 w)
- Alter 4–67 Monate (Ø 27,6 ± 14,6 Mo.)
- 71 generalisierte, 7 fokale Anfälle, 4 nicht eindeutig zuzuordnen
- Dauer der Anfälle 1–50 min (Ø 6,4 ± 7,2 min)
- Bei 13 Kindern Verabreichung von Diazepam durch Eltern bzw. Notarzt
- Temperatur bei Aufnahme Ø 39,3 ± 0,7 °C
- 17 Kinder mit positiver Familienanmnese bzgl. FK
- 11 Kinder mit positiver Familienanamnese bzgl. Epilepsien

Ergebnisse

Die sNSE-Werte lagen nach 0–2 h bei 9,7 µg/l (± 3,5 µg/l; Range 2,5 µg/l bis 22,5 µg/l; 63 Patienten), nach 6–8 h bei 10,0 µg/l (± 4,2 µg/l; Range 2,9 µg/l bis 25,8 µg/l; 36 Patienten) und nach 20–24 h bei 9,8 µg/l (± 4,0 µg/l; Range 3,8 µg/l bis 16,9 µg/l; 17 Patienten). Es ergab sich keine signifikante Erhöhung der Werte für die Gesamtgruppe der Kinder mit einem ersten bzw. zweiten Fieberkrampf. Die Werte zu den verschiedenen Abnahmezeitpunkten unterschieden sich ebenfalls nicht signifikant. Es gab zwar Veränderungen der Werte bei einzelnen Patienten zu den verschiedenen Abnahmezeitpunkten, wobei sich jedoch keine einheitliche Tendenz ablesen ließ. Bei einigen Patienten kam es zu einer leichten Erhöhung der Werte im Verlauf, bei anderen eher zu einer Abnahme. Eine Korrelation der sNSE-Werte mit bekannten Risikofaktoren für die spätere

Entwicklung einer (Temporallappen-)Epilepsie ließ sich nicht feststellen. Auch die Werte der 13 Kinder, die während des Follow-up von 14 bis 28 Monaten weitere Fieberkrämpfe hatten unterschieden sich nicht von der Gruppe ohne weitere fiebergebundene Anfälle. Fünf Kinder aus der ursprünglich untersuchten Gruppe haben während des Follow-up wiederholt afebrile Anfälle und somit definitionsgemäß eine Epilepsie entwickelt (einmal Absencenepilepsie, einmal symptomatische fokale Epilepsie, dreimal kryptogene fokale Epilepsie). Die sNSE-Werte dieser Kinder wiesen keinen signifikanten Unterschied im Vergleich mit der Gesamtgruppe auf.

Diskussion

Die von der Arbeitsgruppe um DeGiorgio und Rabinowicz vorgestellten Daten zur NSE bei Erwachsenen mit einzelnen Anfällen und Epilepsien sind zwar eindrücklich, allerdings handelte es sich entweder um Einzelbeschreibungen oder um Untersuchungen an kleinen Gruppen, die teilweise auch methodische Schwächen aufweisen und von anderen Untersuchern bisher nicht bestätigt wurden. Wir haben nun versucht, die Ergebnisse auf ein möglichst homogenes Patientenkollektiv im Kindesalter zu übertragen. Die Auswahl »Patienten mit Fieberkrämpfen« lag nahe, da es sich zwar um die häufigste Art epileptischer (Gelegenheits-)Anfälle handelt, häufig aber auch Kinder mit nicht eindeutigen fiebergebundenen Ereignissen beim Arzt vorgestellt werden. Da sich in mehreren Untersuchungen gute intraindividuelle Korrelationen der Serum- und Liquorwerte zeigen (Tanabe et al. 2001, Ko et al. 1990) verzichteten wir auf eine grundsätzliche Bestimmung der Liquorwerte.

Die bisherigen Versuche Serummarker wie beispielsweise Prolactin zur Klärung der Zustände zu finden, sind mit Unsicherheiten behaftet. Aufgrund der amerikanischen Ergebnisse wäre auch eine deutliche Erhöhung der sNSE zu erwarten gewesen, die sich jedoch in unserer Untersuchung nicht zeigte. Die sNSE ist somit als Marker zur Unterscheidung, inwieweit es sich um ein epileptisches oder nicht-epileptisches fiebergebundenen Ereignis handelt, nicht geeignet. Wir können somit die Ergebnisse von Rodriguez-Nunez et al. (2000), Dorta-Contreras et al. (1998) und Tanabe et al. (2001) bestätigen, die ebenfalls keine Erhöhung der NSE im Serum und/oder Liquor fanden. Im Unterschied zu diesen Untersuchungen hatten wir bei unseren Patienten nicht nur eine Abnahme unmittelbar nach dem Anfall durchgeführt. Hierbei besteht zumindest auf Grund der tierexperimentellen Daten von Woertgen et al. (2000) die Gefahr, einen verzögerten Anstieg der NSE nicht zu erfassen. Nach traumatischer Schädigung von Neuronen bei Wistar-Ratten zeigte sich eine zeitabhängige Freisetzung der NSE mit einem Maximum nach 6 Stunden.

Die zweite Fragestellung betraf die Wertigkeit als prognostischer Marker. Auch wenn Fieberkrämpfe in der Regel als ungefährlich eingeordnet werden können, gibt es doch die Koinzidenz von prolongierten Fieberkrämpfen im Kindesalter und einer späteren Temporallappenepilepsie auf dem Boden einer mesialen temporalen Sklerose – auch wenn kausale Zusammenhänge kontrovers diskutiert werden. Die Ergebnisse der Arbeitsgruppe um DeGiorgio lassen eine neuronale Schädigung bei einzelnen Anfällen vermuten. Hierbei muss es nicht zwingend zu einem Nervenzelluntergang kommen, da bereits eine reversible Schädigung ausreicht, um eine Anstieg der sNSE zu bewirken. Unter der Vorstellung, dass der Fieberkrampf eine solche Schädigung mit der Folge einer mesialen temporalen Sklerose (Hypothese 1 bei der Spekulation über die Entstehung von Temporallappenepilepsien) verursacht, wäre eine Erhöhung der sNSE zu erwarten gewesen. Wir konnten diese jedoch nicht nachweisen, was Schädigungen im Einzelfall nicht ausschließt, die prinzipielle Einschätzung eines Fieberkrampfes als ungefährlich jedoch bestätigt.

Schlussfolgerung

Wir konnten bei unserer untersuchten Gruppe von Kindern mit Fieberkrämpfen keine Erhöhung der NSE im Serum nachweisen. Die NSE ist als Marker zur Unterscheidung von epileptischen und nicht-epileptischen Geschehen nicht geeignet. Auch als prädiktiver Parameter für das weitere Auftreten von Fieberkrämpfen oder einer Epilepsie eignet sich dieser Wert nicht.

Literatur

1. DeGiorgio CM, Correale JD, Gott PS, Ginsburg DL, Bracht KA, Smith T, Boutros R, Loskota WJ, Rabinowicz AL (1995) Serum neuron-specific enolase in human status epilepticus. Neurology 45:1134–1137
2. Dorta-Contreras AJ, Tabio-Valdes E, Tabio-Valdes A, Delgado-Fernandez C, Reiber H (1998) Non increased neuron-specific enolase concentration in cerebrospinal fluid during first febrile seizures and a year follow-up in pediatric patients. Arq Neuropsiquiatr 56:540–4
3. Hay E, Royds JA, Davies-Jones GA, Lewtas NA, Timperley WR, Taylor CB (1984) Cerebrospinal fluid enolase in stroke. J Neurol Neurosurg Psychiatry 47:724–729
4. Holthausen H (1994) Febrile convulsions, mesial temporal sclerosis and temporal lobe epilepsy. In: Wolf P. (Ed.) : Epileptic seizures and syndromes. S. 449-469; John Libbey & Co.; London
5. Ko F, Chiang C, Wu C, Wu L (1990) Studies of neuron-specific enolase levels in serum and cerebrospinal fluid of children with neurological diseases. Kaohsiung J Med Sci 6:137–143
6. Lafon-Cazal M, Bougault I, Steinberg R, Pin JP, Bockaert J (1992) Measurement of gamma-enolase release, a new method for selective quantification of neurotoxicity indepenently from glial lysis. Brain Res 593:63–68
7. Palmio J, Peltola J, Vuorinen P, Laine S, Suhonen J, Keranen T (2001) Normal CSF neuron-specific enolase and S-100 protein levels in patients with recent non-complicated tonic-clonic seizures. J Neurol Sci 15:27–31
8. Persson L, Hardemark HG, Gustafsson J, Rundstrom G, Mendel-Hartvig/I, Esscher T, Pahlman S (1987) S-100 protein and neuron-specific enolase in cerebrospinal fluid and serum: markers of cell damage in human central nervous system. Stroke 18:911–918
9. Rabinowicz AL, Correale JD, Bracht KA, Smith TD, DeGiorgio CM (1995) Neuron-specific enolase is increased after nonconvulsive status epilepticus. Epilepsia 36:475–479
10. Rodriguez-Nunez A, Cid E, Rodriguez-Garcia J, Camina F, Rodriguez-Segade S, Castro-Gago M (2000) Cerebrospinal fluid purine metabolite and neuron-specific enolase concentrations after febrile seizures. Brain Dev 22:427–31

11. Schaarschmidt H, Prange HW, Reiber H (1994) Neuron-specific enolase concentrations in blood as prognostic parameter in cerebrovascular diseases. Stroke 25:558–565
12. Schmechel D, Marangos PJ, Zis AP, Brightman M, Goodwin FK (1978) Brain enolases as specific markers of neuronal and glial cells. Science 199:313–315
13. Tanabe T, Suzuki S, Hara K, Shimakawa S, Wakamiya E, Tamai H (2001) Cerebrospinal fluid and serum neuron-specific enolase levels after febrile seizures. Epilepsia 42:504–507
14. Taylor CB, Royds JA, Parsons MA, Timperley WR (1983) Diagnostic aspects of enolase isoenzymes. Isozymes Curr Top Biol Med Res 11:95–119
15. Woertgen C, Rothoerl RD, Brawanski A (2000) Time profile of neuron specific enolase serum levels after experimental brain injury in rat. Acta Neurochir Suppl 76:371–3

Reflexepilepsie bei Down Syndrom

S. Springer, R. Gillessen, C. Mühe, K. Kugler, A. Enders, A. Merkenschlager

Einleitung

Echte Reflexepilepsien (darunter am häufigsten die photogene Epilepsie) sind mit einem Anteil von ca. 2% aller kindlichen Epilepsien relativ selten. Sie treten meist im präpubertären Alter auf und sind oft therapirefraktär. Patienten mit einer Trisomie 21 sollen, möglicherweise wegen einer gestörten kortikalen Inhibition, häufiger an Epilepsien erkranken (1). In der Literatur findet man Hinweise, dass diese Patientengruppe im Verlauf ihrer Epilepsie gehäuft (in bis zu 20% der Fälle) Reflexanfälle zeigen kann (1). Antikonvulsiva der ersten Wahl sind Valproat aber auch Carbamazepin (2).

Fallbeschreibung

Wir berichten den Fall eines 7jährigen Jungen mit Trisomie 21, welcher als erstes Symptom seiner beginnenden Epilepsie tonische Reflexanfälle auf Schreckreize hin entwickelt hat. Der Patient zeigte bisher ein vollkommen unauffälliges Wach- und Schlaf-EEG. Nur mit Hilfe eines Video-Langzeit-EEG konnten die Spitzenpotentiale während des Anfalls nachgewiesen werden. Analog zum Vorgehen bei der Photoepilepsie wurde der Patient zunächst mit Valproat (bis 20 mg/kg/d) behandelt. Darunter änderte sich die Symptomatik nicht. Daraufhin wurde Valproat gegen Carbamazepin in der selben Dosierung ausgetauscht. Darunter wurde unser Patient anfallsfrei. Das interiktale EEG war und blieb unauffällig.

Diskussion

Wir möchten mit dieser Fallbeschreibung auf ein möglicherweise unterschätztes Begleitphänomen bei Patienten mit Trisomie 21 hinweisen, die ohnehin häufiger an Epilepsien erkranken. Die häufigen Reflexanfälle können nicht nur Teil, sondern auch der Beginn der Epilepsie sein.

Ungewöhnlich bei unserem Patienten ist, dass die Reflexanfälle die bisher einzige Anfallsform geblieben sind, und dass der Patient nicht mit einem typischen generalisierten tonisch-klonischen Anfall, sondern mit einem tonischen Sturz auf externe Stimuli reagiert.

Dieser Fall zeigt weiterhin in Übereinstimmung mit der Literatur, dass Valproat und Carbamazepin gleichermaßen Therapeutika der ersten Wahl sind (2).

Schlussfolgerung

Es muss nicht nur bei nicht erklärbaren motorischen Phänomenen (Wadenkrämpfe, Stürze) bei Patienten mit Trisomie 21 auch an die Möglichkeit einer Reflexepilepsie gedacht werden. Es muss auch bedacht werden, dass die Diagnose einer Epilepsie bei atypischer Symptomatik letztlich nur durch ein iktales Video-EEG gestellt und zum Beispiel von einer Hyperekplexie unterschieden werden kann (2).

Literatur

1. Guerrini R et al. Reflex seizures are frequent in patients with Down syndrome and epilepsy. Epilepsia 1990; 31(4): 406–417
2. Pueschel SM et al. Reflex seizures in Down syndrome. Childs Nerv Syst 1993 ; 9(1) : 23–24

Einfache fokale Anfälle bei ungewöhnlichen, komplexen Anomalien des Aortenbogens, der Halsgefäße und der intrakraniellen Gefäße bei Fallotscher Tetralogie

D. Dundurs, P. Zinn, H. Friedburg, U. Meyer, G. Rupprath

Einleitung

Zerebrale Komplikationen bei angeborenen Herzfehlern können mit transitorischen ischämischen Attacken, ischämischen Infarkten und zerebralen Anfällen einhergehen.

Fallbeschreibung

Bei einem fast 14 Jahre alten, bisher beschwerdefreien Mädchen kam es wiederholt in Abständen von wenigen Tagen über wenige Minuten zum Auftreten von Parästhesien und Kloni der rechten Hand mit begleitender Sprechhemmung bei erhaltenem Bewusstsein und interiktaler Symptomfreiheit. Initial geklagte rechtsseitige Stirnkopfschmerzen sistierten rasch, eine Anisokorie blieb bestehen.

Bei acyanotischer Fallotscher Tetralogie mit linkem Aortenbogen, valvulärer und infundibulärer Pulmonalstenose war die Patientin uns im Alter von 2 Jahren zur Herzkatheteruntersuchung vorgestellt worden. In der Untersuchung sahen wir über das echokardiographisch diagnostizierte Vitium cordis hinaus eine ungewöhnliche spiralige Doppelwindung der Aorta im Aortenbogenbereich mit getrenntem Abgang der Halsgefäße. Im Verlauf bestand Wohlbefinden ohne wesentliche Einschränkung der körperlichen Leistungsfähigkeit. In der medikamentösen Prophylaxe hypoxämischer Anfälle wurde Propranolol eingesetzt. Die operative Korrektur mit Infundibulumresektion und Kommissurotomie der valvulären Pulmonalstenose wurde ohne Komplikationen mit gutem Spätergebnis bei geringer Restpulmonalstenose und kleinem Rest-Ventrikelseptumdefekt im Alter von 5 Jahren durchgeführt.

Die aktuelle Diagnostik der neurologischen Symptomatik ergab im EEG einen auffälligen Befund bei Spitzenaktivität links präcentral, central und temporal. Bei anhaltender Anisokorie wurden in der Untersuchung des Augenhintergrundes Auffälligkeiten nicht beschrieben. In den entsprechenden Laboruntersuchungen konnten pathologische Ergebnisse nicht erhoben werden.

In der weiterführenden bildgebenden Diagnostik führten wir eine Magnetresonanztomographie des Schädels und eine Magnetresonanzangiographie der intrakraniellen Gefäße, der Halsgefäße und der thorakalen Aorta durch.

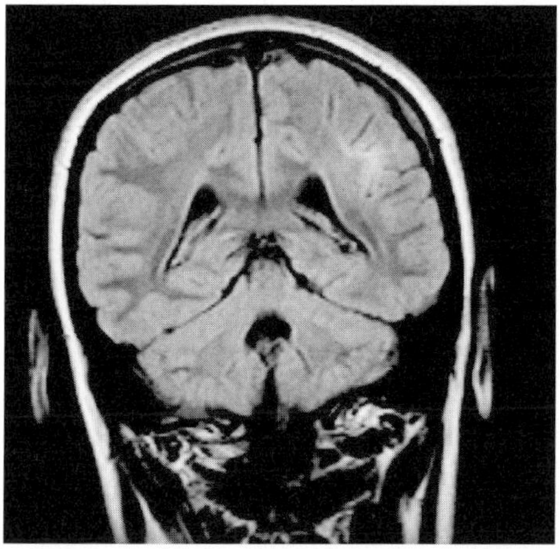

Abb. 1: Links hochparietal occipitopolar subkortikale Läsion nach ischämischem Infarkt im Media-Stromgebiet (FLAIR-Sequenz mit Liquorsignalunterdrückung).

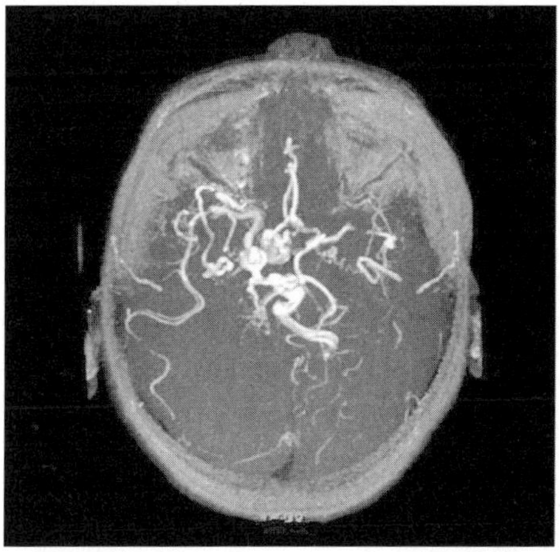

Abb. 2: Atypisches Bild der intrakraniellen Gefäße mit kräftiglumiger A. basilaris, die rechte und linke A. cerebri media über kräftig entwickelte Aa. communicantes posteriores versorgt, wobei die linke A. cerebri media im mittleren Segment eine hochgradige Stenosierung zeigt und die A. carotis interna sich beidseits in multiplen kleinen Gefäßen im Sinne von Kollateralsystemen darstellt, die Anschluss an die intrakraniellen Gefäße finden (TDF-MRA intrakraniell/arteriell/3D-Sequenz).

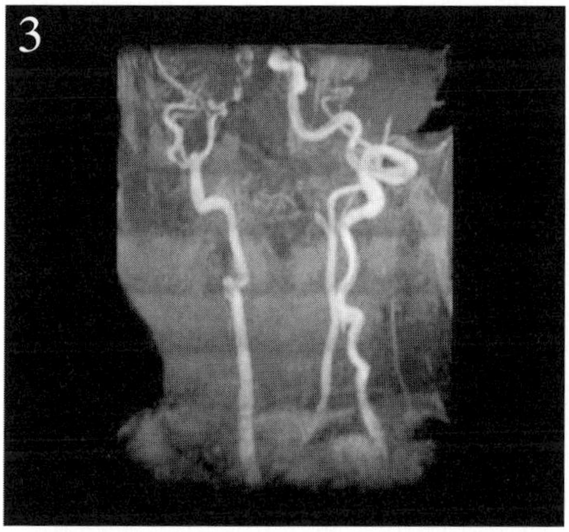

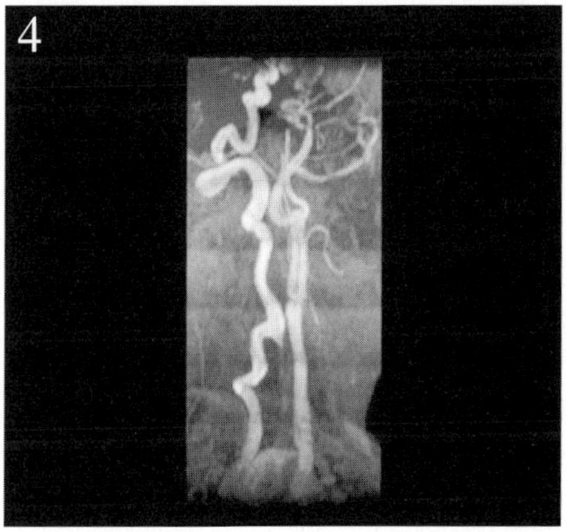

Abb. 3 und 4: Im Bereich der Halsregion stellen sich drei arterielle Gefäße dar, wobei die ersten im Aortenverlauf abgehenden Gefäße den Carotiden entsprechen, die bis zur Schädelbasis mit kräftigen Lumina zur Darstellung kommen. Das dritte distal des Aortenbogens abgehende Gefäß entspricht der linksseitigen A. vertebralis, die sich in eine ebenfalls kräftige A. basilaris fortsetzt. (TDF-MRA cervikal/arteriell/3D-Sequenz).

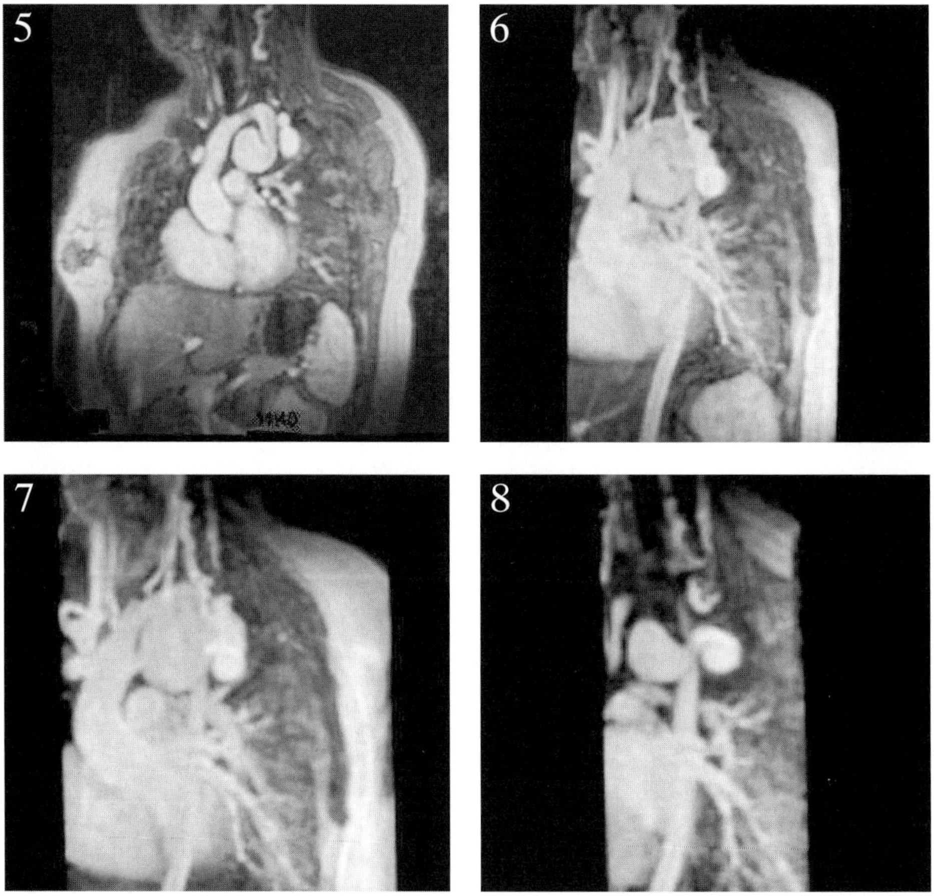

Abb. 5, 6, 7 und 8: Nach Abgang der linken A. carotis communis stellt sich der Aortenbogen mit Bildung einer größeren vollständigen Schleife und einer kleineren rudimentär angelegten Schleife mit Fortsetzung in die Aorta descendens dar. (CE-MRA/3D-Sequenz/Kontrastmittel-unterstützte MRA der thorakalen Gefäße/Subtraktion/ MIP).

In der arteriellen MR-Angiographie der Halsgefäße und der thorakalen Aorta fanden sich Fehlbildungen mit ungewöhnlicher und bisher nicht publizierter spiraliger Doppelwindung der Aorta descendens mit isolierter A. vertebralis sinistra und korkenzieherartig gewundener A. basilaris.

Ausgehend von der Diagnose symptomatischer einfacher fokaler Anfälle begannen wir eine antikonvulsive Behandlung mit Oxcarbazepin. Seitdem besteht Anfallsfreiheit. Bei Thrombozytenaggregationshemmung mit Acetylsalicylsäure werden im Verlauf weiterhin Parästhesien, dazu Schwindel und eine leichte Hemiparese geklagt.

Schlussfolgerung

Ungewöhnliche intrakranielle Gefäßanomalien können über lange Zeit symptomlos bleiben. Bei komplexen Anomalien des Aortenbogens und der Halsgefäße sollte bei Auftreten diskreter neurologischer Symptome hiernach gezielt gesucht werden.

Literatur

1. Fisher M, Bogousslavsky J (1998) Further evolution toward effective therapy for acute ischemic stroke, JAMA, 279:1298
2. Martin PJ, Enevoldson TP, Humphrey PRD (1997) Causes of ischaemic stroke in the young, Postgrad Med J, 73:855
3. Riela AR, Roach ES (1993) Etiology of stroke in children, Journal of Child Neurology, 8. 201–220
4. Smith CD, Baumann RJ (1991) Clinical features and magnetic resonance imaging in congenital and childhood stroke, J Child Neurol, 6:263–272
5. Wisnitzer M, Masaryk TJ (1991) Cerebrovascular abnormalities in pediatric stroke: Assessment using parenchymal and angiographic magnetic resonance imaging, Ann Neurol, 29:585–589

Alternierende Hemiplegie des Kindesalters – Falldarstellung

I. Treiss, St. Karch, Th. Bast, St. König

Einleitung

Die alternierende Hemiplegie des Kindesalters, erstmals 1971 von Verret und Steele beschrieben, ist eine seltene Erkrankung mit wechselseitigen Hemiplegien, abnormen Augenbewegungen, dystonen Episoden sowie Zeichen autonomer Dysfunktion. Die Erkrankung beginnt im Kleinkindesalter und geht in aller Regel mit einer deutlichen psychomotorischen Entwicklungsretardierung und bleibenden neurologischen Defiziten einher.

Die Genese der Erkrankung ist unklar. Initial wurde die alternierende Hemiplegie des Kindesalters als eine Variante der Migräne angesehen. Auch genetische Faktoren wurden in Betracht gezogen, es liegt jedoch nur eine Fallbeschreibung einer autosomal dominanten Form der Erkrankung mit fünf betroffenen Familienmitgliedern in drei Generationen vor (3).

Falldarstellung

Wir berichten über den Krankheitsverlauf eines 5,5 Jahre alten Mädchens, das als zweites Kind gesunder, nicht miteinander verwandter Eltern nach unauffälliger Schwangerschaft geboren wurde. Im Alter von zwei Monaten traten erstmals Zustände mit Blickdeviation, Kloni einer Körperhälfte und Bewusstseinstrübung auf, eine medikamentöse Theapie erfolgte zunächst mit Phenobarbital, später in Kombination mit Carbamazepin.

Ab dem zweiten Lebensjahr wurden wechselseitige Hemiplegien zum führenden Symptom. Das Mädchen zeigte ein Vorgefühl im Arm, es trat eine Blickdeviation auf, gleichzeitig eine dystone Armbewegung. Die in Folge auftretende Hemiplegie war begleitet von einer deutlichen Verlangsamung mit leiser Sprache und Speichelfluss. Auslösemechanismen waren Schreck oder Freude, durch Schlaf konnte jeweils eine Remission erzielt werden.

Die psychomotorische Entwicklung des Mädchens verlief deutlich verzögert, freies Laufen wurde mit 3 Jahren erlernt.

Die im Rahmen der Diagnostik durchgeführten Untersuchungen (MRT, Blut-, Liquoruntersuchungen, Stoffwechseluntersuchungen, Muskelbiopsie) ergaben keine pathologischen Befunde.

Die interiktalen EEG-Untersuchungen zeigten eine Allgemeinveränderung mit nicht altersgemäßer Grundaktivität ohne sichere epilepsietypischen Potentiale. Während einer Hemiplegie trat mehrfach eine Akzentuierung der Theta/Deltaaktivität rechts temporo-parietal auf, ebenfalls ohne sichere epilepsietypischen Potentiale. Diese Befunde konnten auch im Langzeit-Video EEG bestätigt werden. Gesicherte Krampfanfälle traten als Status epilepticus mit notwendiger Beatmung nach Absetzen der antikonvulsiven Medikation auf. Ein weiterer generalisierter tonisch klonischer Krampfanfall ereignete sich mit 5,5 Jahren unter Valproatmedikation.

Aufgrund der typischen klinischen Symptomatik stellten wir bei unserer Patientin – zusätzlich zur Epilepsie – die Diagnose einer alternierenden Hemiplegie des Kindesalters und führten Flunarizin in die Therapie ein. Dies reduzierte zeitweilig die Dauer, die Häufigkeit und die Schwere der Hemiplegien. Therapeutische Versuche mit Acetylsalizylsäure, Propranolol und Magnesium zeigten keinen Erfolg. Chloralhydrat – im Anfall verabreicht – vermag die Dauer der Hemiplegien zu verkürzen.

Diskussion

Die alternierende Hemiplegie des Kindesalters ist aufgrund des klinischen Erscheinungsbildes differentialdiagnostisch von einer Epilepsie abzugrenzen. Insbesondere in der ersten Phase der Erkrankung, in welcher abnorme Augenbewegungen und Kloni das klinische Bild prägen, ist die Abgrenzung gegenüber epileptischen Anfällen oft schwer. Zudem treten – wie bei unserer Patientin – in etwa 20% der Betroffenen Krampfanfälle neben den Hemiplegien auf (4). Die im weiteren Verlauf hinzukommenden Hemiplegien sichern in aller Regel die Diagnose.

Seltene Differentialdiagnosen sind die hemiplegische Migräne, metabolische Erkrankungen (MELAS-Syndrom), und paroxysmale Dyskinesien, in deren Rahmen es auch zu hemiplegischen Episoden kommen kann.

Als Mittel der Wahl in der Therapie der alternierenden Hemiplegie hat sich Flunarizin, ein Kalziumkanal-Blocker, bewährt. Berichte über ein therapeutisches Ansprechen liegen auch für Benzodiazepine, Verapamil und Memantine

Tab. 1: Klinische Hauptmerkmale der alternierenden Hemiplegie des Kindesalters in 44 berichteten Fällen (4)

Merkmal	%
Hemiplegie	100
Episoden mit Tetraplegie	93
Abnorme Augenbewegungen	100
Dystonie	95
Entwicklungsretardierung	91
Autonome Phänomene	78
Dysarthrie	65
Choreoathetose	50
Krampfanfälle	19

(2) vor. Flunarizin erzielte in ca 70% der Fälle einen günstigen Effekt auf Häufigkeit und Schwere der Hemiplegien (4,5). Inwiefern Flunarizin neben einem Kurzzeiteffekt auch einen Einfluss auf die Langzeitprognose hat, ist nicht gesichert.

Ein Großteil der Betroffenen zeigt im weiteren Verlauf einen Rückgang der hemiplegischen Attacken. Neurologische Auffälligkeiten, insbesondere Dyskinesien und Sprachstörungen als auch eine mentale Retardierung bleiben jedoch bestehen.

Literatur

1. Bourgeois M, Aicardi J, Goutieres F (1993) Alternating hemiplegia of childhood. J Pediatr 122:673–9
2. Korinthenberg R. (1996) Is infantile alternating hemiplegia mediated by glutamate toxycity and can it be treated with memantine? Neuropediatrics 27:277–8
3. Mikati MA, Maguire MD, Barlow CF, et al. (1992) A syndrome of autosomal dominant alternating hemiplegia: Clinical presentation mimicking intractable epilepsy; chromosomal studies and physiologic investigations. Neurology 42:2251–7
4. Mikati MA, Kramer U, Zupanc ML, Shanahan R (2000) Alternating hemiplegia of childhood: Clinical manifestations and long-term outcome. Pediatr Neurol 23:134–141
5. Sasaki M, Sakuragawa N, Osawa M. (2001) Long-term effect of flunarizin on patients with alternating hemiplegia of childhood in Japan. Brain-Dev.23:303–5
6. Verret S, Steele JC. (1971) Alternating hemiplegia in childhood: a report of eight patients with complicated migraine beginning in infancy. Pediatrics 47:675–680

Frühmanifestation einer Alternierenden Hemiplegie des Kindesalters – eine Kasuistik

S. Schilling, C. Härtel, J. Sperner

Die Alternierende Hemiplegie des Kindesalters (AHC) ist eine sehr seltene Erkrankung mit unspezifischem Beginn in der Säuglingszeit, die zuerst von Steele und Verret beschrieben wurde (1). Seitdem gibt es eine wachsende Anzahl von Einzelfallbeschreibungen und nur wenige systematische Studien (2). Bis zur Diagnosestellung vergehen meist viele Monate, währenddessen die Patienten, in der Annahme einer Epilepsie antikonvulsiv behandelt werden. Bei Verwandten ersten Grades tritt gehäuft Migräne auf (4), weshalb von vielen Autoren eine ätiologische Ähnlichkeit mit der hemiplegischen Migräne vermutet wird. Molekulargenetische Untersuchungen des CACNA-1a-Gen auf dem Chromosom 19, das einen zerebralen Kalzium-Kanaldefekt bei der hemiplegischen Migräne kodiert, konnten jedoch für die AHC keinen Defekt aufzeigen (4), auch andere Kandidatengene konnten jedoch bisher nicht identifiziert werden. In einer Familie konnte ein autosomal dominanter Vererbungsmodus nachgewiesen werden (3).

Kasuistik

Der Patient wurde als erstes Kind nicht verwandter, gesunder Eltern nach problemloser Schwangerschaft und Spontangeburt geboren (APGAR 8/9/10). Ab dem zweiten Lebenstag traten wiederholt hemilaterale, tonische Überstreckungen mit tonischer Adversivbewegung des Kopfes auf, mit vertikalem einseitigem Nystagmus und Blickdeviation. Diese motorischen Phänomene dauerten bis zu 20 Min, dabei war das Neugeborene nicht sicher wach und reaktionsfähig, es zeigten sich keine motorischen Stereotypien oder weitere Anfallskorrelate. Unter dem Verdacht fokaler Anfälle erfolgte die Verlegung in eine Kinderklinik. Dort traten die beschriebenen hemilateralen Dystonien seitenwechselnd und die abnormen Augenbewegungen, trotz antikonvulsiver Therapie mit Benzodiazepinen, Phenobarbital und Phenytoin, unbeeinträchtigt bis zu 60 min lang auf. Ab der dritten LWO kam ein down beat Nystagmus hinzu, der auch unabhängig von den Dystonien auftrat. Nach drei Wochen wurde das Kind entlassen, ohne eine komplette »Anfallsfreiheit« erreicht zu haben.

Die motorische Entwicklung war unter hochdosiertem Phenobarbital verzögert. An motorischen Meilensteinen wurde mit 6 Monate die Körperdrehung über beide Seiten erreicht.

Mit drei Monaten wurde eine Behandlung mit Valproat begonnen, die infolge vorübergehende Erfolge bei intravenöser Anfallsunterbrechung in hoher Dosierung über vier Monate fortgesetzt wurde. Mit vier Monaten zeigte Finn erstmals nach einer dystonen Episode mit protrahierter Dauer von 90 Minuten eine linksseitige Hemiparese, die 24 Stunden anhielt. Nach dieser Episode wiederholten sich diese Lähmungsbilder mit seitenwechselnder Lokalisation. Eine zunehmende Entwicklungsretadierung wurde erkennbar.

Mit jetzt 15 Monaten haben sich unter einer Medikation mit Flunarizin die Frequenz und die Intensität der hemiplegischen Episoden deutlich reduzieren lassen.

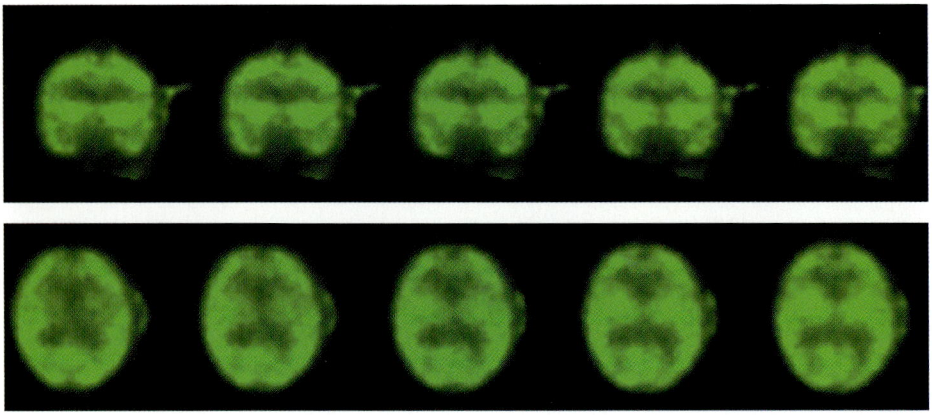

Abb. 1: Normales iktuales ECD-SPECT während einer Episode mit Dystonien und pathologischer Okulomotorik im Alter von 6 Monaten.

Diagnostik

Die Routineserum- und Stoffwechseluntersuchungen ergaben Normalbefunde. Auch die Liquor- und die Urindiagnostik war immer unauffällig.

Die radiologische Bildgebung vom Kopf mit wiederholten MRTs und iktalem SPECT waren, wie in Abbildung 1 zu sehen, ohne pathologischen Befund.

Alle neurophysiologischen Untersuchungen, eingeschlossen iktuale Wach-EEGs , Schlaf-EEG, Langzeit-EEG, NLG, SSEP, AEP und VEP waren unauffällig (Abb. 2).

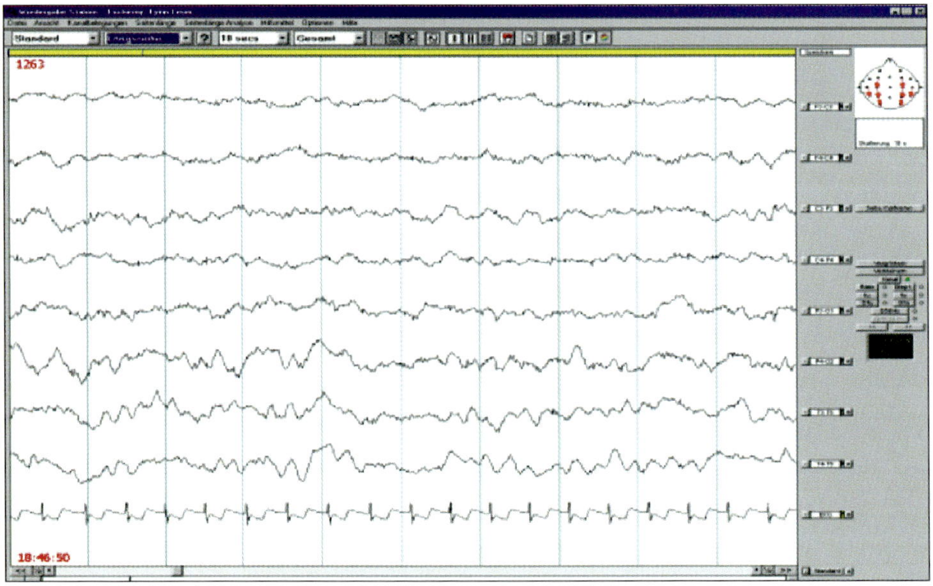

Abb. 2: Iktuales EEG.

Verlauf

Die alternierenden Hemiplegien konnten mit Antikonvulsiva (PB, OCBZ, STM, DZM, PHT) weder in der Frequenz noch der Dauer der Attacken beeinflusst werden. Ausschließlich kontinuierlich hochdosiertes Valproat zeigte einen Einfluss auf die interiktualen Phasen und einen verkürzenden Effekt auf die Dystonien und den Nystagmus. Während akuter Attacken wurde deshalb noch zusätzlich intravenös Valproat mit reproduzierbar positivem Effekt injiziert. Wiederholte Absetzversuche mündeten sofort in progrediente Anfälle. Mit Alkohol angereichertes Chloralhydrat erbrachte trotz ermutigender Einzelfallberichte keinen Effekt (6). Im Schlaf sistierten die Dystonien und der Nystagmus komplett. Aufgrund erhöhter Nebenwirkunkungen von Valproat führten wir eine Umstellung auf Flunarizin über 4 Monate durch. Seit 3 Monaten besteht eine reproduzierbare Rhythmik des klinischen Verlaufes zwischen gutem (10 Tage) – , befriedigendem (3 Tage) und schlechten Allgemeinzustand. In den schlechten Phasen treten Nystagmus und Dystonien wiederholt in Phasen von bis zu 20 Minuten auf, der Muskeltonus ist hypoton, die Vigilanz herabgesetzt und eine Hemiparese vorhanden. Insgesamt ist die psychomotorische Entwicklung nun wieder langsam fortschreitend und hat das Niveau eines 6 Monate alten Kindes erreicht.

Diskussion

Entsprechend der Verlaufsstudie von Mikati (5) bei 44 Kindern mit AHC findet sich auch bei unserem Patienten ein 3-Stufen-Verlauf. Die erste Krankheitsphase wird geprägt durch Nystagmen mit Blickdeviation und Dystonien. Verglichen mit den Beschreibungen von Mikati, tritt die Erstmanifestation unseres Patienten mit 2 Lebenstagen ungewöhnlich früh auf. Erst in der zweiten Phase treten die pathognomischen alternierenden, episodischen hemilateralen Paresen und ein deutlich regressiver psychomotorischer Entwicklungsverlauf auf. Auch bei unserem Fall wurde erst zu diesem Zeitpunkt die richtige Diagnose gestellt. Die protrahierte Diagnosestellung deckt sich leider mit den publizierten Fallvorstellungen. In der Studie von Mikati zeigt sich, dass eine sehr frühe Manifestation mit einem schlechteren Entwicklungsverlauf belegt ist. In unserem Fall erschien unter intravenösem Valproat eine Unterbrechung der akuten Hemiplegien möglich und unter Flunarizin als Monotherapie ist eine leicht voranschreitende Entwicklung erkennbar. Die gute Wirksamkeit von Valproat, u.a. als Akutmedikament ist bei einem angenommenen Kalzium-Kanal-Defekt pathophysiologisch nicht zu erklären und stellt in Frage, ob die AHC mit einem Kalzium-Kanal-Defekt ausschließlich zu erklären ist.

Zusammenfassung

Die AHC ist eine seltene, meist verzögerte diagnostizierte Erkrankung, die als Differenzialdiagnose bei frühkindlichen Episoden mit Dystonien und pathologischer Okulomotororik besteht. Insbesondere soll an die AHC gedacht werden, wenn alle diagnostischen Bemühungen (MRT, EEG, SPECT) ohne pathologisches Korrelat und ohne Hinweis für eine Epilepsie bleiben.

Literatur

1. Verret S, Steele JC (1971) Alternating hemiplgia in childhood: a report of 8 patients with complicated migraine beginning in infancy. Pediatrics 47: 675–80
2. Bourgeois M Aicardi J (1993) Alternating hemiplegia of childhood. J Pediatr 122: 673–679
3. Mikati M A et al (1992), A syndrome of autosomal dominant alternating hemiplegia Neurology; 42:2251–2257
4. Rho J M, Chugani M T, (1998) Alternating hemiplegia of childhood: Insigts into its pathophysiology J Child Neurol 13:39–45
5. Mikati M A (2000) Alternating hemiplegia in childhood: Clinical manifestation and long-term outcome. Pediatr Neurol 23:134–141
6. Siemes H, Casaer P (1996) Alternierende Hemiplegie im Kindesalter. Monatsschr Kinderheilkd 27:227–278

14. Epilepsie 3: medikamentöse und diätetische Behandlung

Einleitung der ketogenen Diät im Säuglingsalter

J. Klepper, B. Leiendecker, Th. Voit

Zusammenfassung

Die ketogene Diät ist Therapie der Wahl bei Pyruvat-Dehydrogenase-Defekt und Glukosetransporter(GLUT1)-Defekt. Beide Erkrankungen werden zunehmend im Säuglingsalter diagnostiziert, es gibt jedoch keine Erfahrung mit der ketogenen Diät in dieser Altersgruppe. Wir berichten über die komplikationslose, erfolgreiche Einleitung der ketogenen Diät bei vier Säuglingen mit V.a. GLUT1-Defekt.

Einleitung

Die ketogene Diät (KD) ist eine sehr fettreiche, kohlenhydratarme Diät zur Behandlung schwer einstellbarer Epilepsien und einiger seltener Stoffwechselerkrankungen. Sie ist eine individuell berechnete und einseitige Ernährung, die verschiedene Nahrungssupplemente erforderlich macht und nur unter ärztlicher Anleitung durchgeführt werden darf. Die KD imitiert den metabolischen Zustand des Fastens, in dem sie aus Nahrungsfett – anstelle von körpereigenem Fett – eine Ketose erzeugt. Die Ketonkörper dienen dem Körper, insbesondere dem Gehirn, als alternative Energiequelle. Der genaue antikonvulsive Wirkmechanismus der ketogenen Diät, ob direkt über die Ketonkörper oder indirekt durch hervorgerufene Veränderungen des zerebralen Milieus, ist letztlich unbekannt. Diskutiert werden Veränderungen im Energiestoffwechsel, der Zusammensetzung der Zellmembranen, sowie des pH-, Wasser- und Elektrolythaushaltes (1).

Anerkannte Einsatzgebiete der KD im Kindesalter sind therapieresistente Epilepsien, der GLUT1-Defekt, sowie der Pyruvat-Dehydrogenase-Defekt (2). Mit Ausnahme einer aktuellen retrospektiven Studie gibt es keine Daten zur Anwendung der KD bei Kindern unter einem Jahr (3). Zum Einen ist es schwierig, in dieser Altersgruppe eine adäquate Ketose zu erreichen, des Weiteren sind Säuglinge durch eine nutritiv einschneidende Diät besonders gefährdet. Das Bekanntwerden des GLUT1-Defektes und zunehmende Patientenzahlen mit unklar erniedrigtem Liquorzucker (Hypoglykorrhachie) eröffnen jedoch die Möglichkeit einer frühen Diagnose und Therapie – dadurch bietet sich die Chance, zu einem frühen Zeitpunkt zu intervenieren und damit möglicherweise eine therapieresistente Epilepsie und irreversible Entwicklungsschäden zu vermeiden.

Tab. 1: Symptome, Liquor-/Blutglukose-Quotient und Alter zu Beginn der ketogenen Diät in vier Patienten mit V.a. GLUT1-Defekt. Die erniedrigten Glukosequotienten aus initialen Lumbalpunktionen (grau unterlegt) wurden jeweils durch eine elektive Nüchtern-Lumbalpunktion bestätigt (fett gedruckt).

	Patient 1 **m**	**Patient 2** **w**	**Patient 3** **w**	**Patient 4** **m**
1. Anfall	14 Wo	4 Wo	5 Mo	2 Wo
Hypotonie	+	–	+	+
Glukose-Quotient	0,26			
(Liquor/Blut)	0,43	0,38	0,36	0,33
< 0,4	**0,37**	**0,37**	**0,36**	**0,34**
Ketogene Diät ab:	17 Wo	6 Wo	7 Mo	6 Wo

Patientengut, Zusammensetzung und Einleitung der KD

Bei zwei männlichen und zwei weiblichen Säuglingen wurde aufgrund von zerebralen Krampfanfällen und isoliert niedrigem Liquorzucker der Verdacht auf GLUT1-Defekt gestellt. Die Hypoglykorrhachie wurde jeweils durch eine kontrollierte Nüchtern-Lumbalpunktion bestätigt und die KD eingeleitet (Tab. 1). Die Diät wurde im Verhältnis 3:1 berechnet und als Flaschennahrung aus emulgierten langkettigen Triglyzeriden (Calogen, Fa. SHS), sowie kohlenhydratfreier Säuglingsnahrung (basic-ch, Fa. Milupa) angeboten. Erlaubte »Rest«-Kohlenhydrate wurden in Form von Stärke (Malto-Dextrin19, Fa. SHS) zugesetzt. Nach Erreichen einer stabilen Ketose wurden zur Deckung des individuellen Bedarfs Vitamine, Spurenelemente und Mineralstoffe supplementiert.

Da zum Zeitpunkt der Einleitung der KD in Patient 4 emulgierte langkettige Triglyzeride auf dem europäischen Markt noch nicht verfügbar waren, wurde die KD initial mit mittelkettigen Triglyzeriden begonnen (Liquigen, Fa. SHS). Nach Entwicklung einer ausgeprägten Gedeihstörung wurden emulgierte langkettige Triglyzeride aus den USA importiert und eingesetzt (Microlipid, Fa. Mead-Johnson, USA).

Die Patienten wurden stationär gemäß den Empfehlungen des 1. Workshops KD 2000 voruntersucht und die KD nach Ausschluss von Kontraindikationen eingeleitet (4). Gleichzeitig begann die Schulung der Eltern in der Zubereitung und Durchführung der KD. Durch initiales Fasten ohne Flüssigkeitsrestriktion wurde eine ketotische Stoffwechsellage erreicht und mittels kapillären Blutzucker- und 3-Hydroxy-Butyrat-Messungen am Patientenbett überwacht. Die ketogene Flaschennahrung wurde nach Erreichen der Ketose zunächst in halber Menge angeboten und je nach Verträglichkeit auf die endgültige Menge gesteigert.

Ergebnisse

Alle Patienten entwickelten innerhalb von 18 Stunden eine signifikante Ketose ohne Flüssigkeits- oder Elektrolytverschiebungen, Azidose, Erbrechen, oder

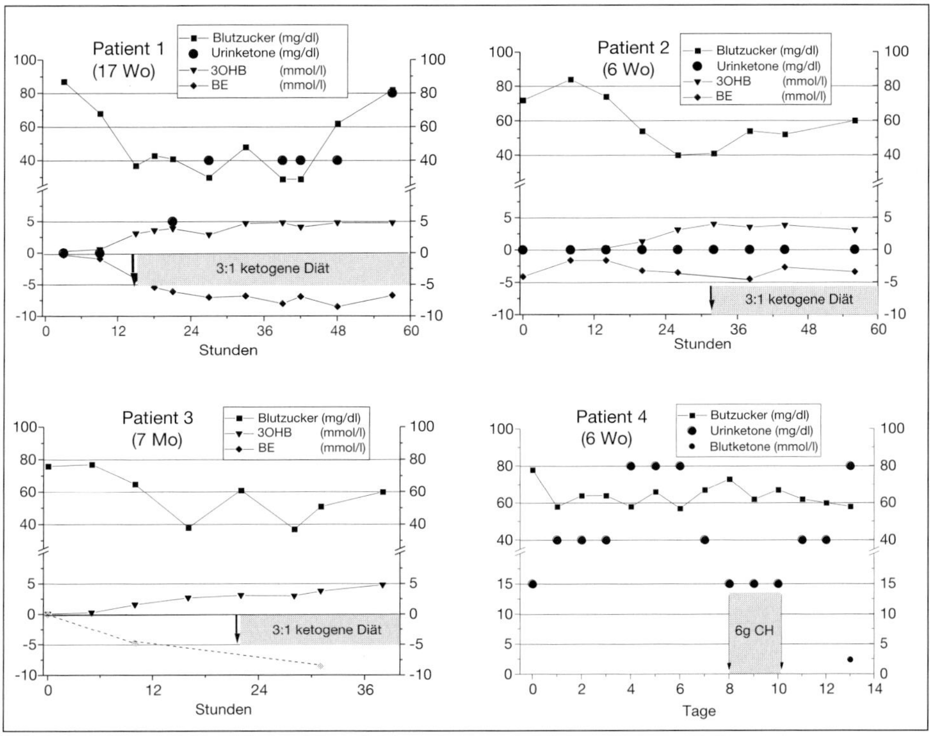

Abb. 1: Verlauf von Blutzucker, Urinketonen, 3-Hydroxy-Butyrat und Basenüberschuss während der initalen Fastenphase. Der Beginn der KD ist durch einen Pfeil gekennzeichnet (↓). Die letzte Teilabbildung (Patient 4) zeigt den Verlust der Ketose nach Ergänzung der Diät durch 6 g Kohlenhydrate.

eine klinisch manifeste Hypoglykämie. Die Konzentration von 3-Hydroxy-Butyrat im Plasma korrelierte invers mit dem negativen Base-Excess. Der Nachweis von Ketonen im Urin war abhängig von der Miktion des Patienten, im Vergleich zur Plasmaketose verzögert und in Patient 3 trotz signifikanter Plasmaketose nicht führbar (Abb. 1).

Die Einleitung der KD nach 15 bis 32 Stunden Fasten wurde von allen Säuglingen gut toleriert. Erbrechen und Obstipation als bekannte Nebenwirkungen der Einführung der KD blieben aus. Das Anlernen von Eltern und Pflegepersonal im Umgang mit der Diät war ebenfalls unproblematisch. Alle vier Patienten wurden mit Erreichen der Ketose anfallsfrei und blieben dies in einem Beobachtungszeitraum von minimal drei Monaten (Patient 2) bis maximal 2,5 Jahren (Patient 4). Mit Ausnahme von Nierensteinen (Patient 4) zeigten sich im genannten Nachbeobachtungszeitraum keine weiteren Nebenwirkungen der KD.

Patient 4 zeigte unter einer 3:1 KD mit mittelkettigen Triglyzeriden eine ausgeprägte Gedeihstörung, die jedoch nach Verwendung von langkettigen Triglyzeriden (Microlipid) reversibel war (Abb. 2).

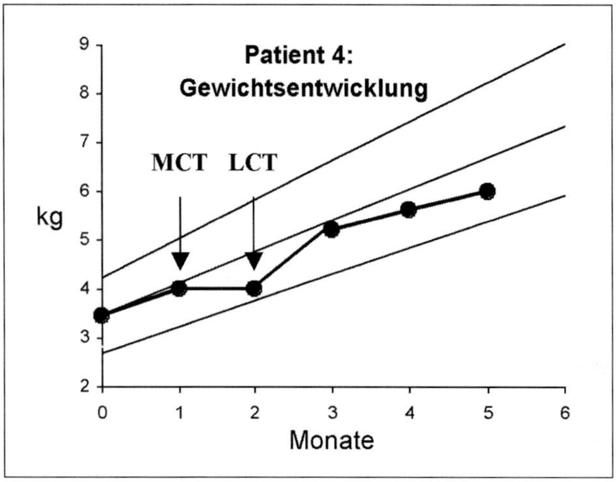

Abb. 2: Gewichtsentwicklung von Patient 4 unter Verwendung von mittelkettigen Triglyzeriden (MCT) und langkettigen Triglyzeriden (LCT).

Schlussfolgerung

Eine KD im Verhältnis 3:1 lässt sich unter Verwendung von langkettigen Triglyzeriden und kohlenhydratfreier Säuglingsnahrung im Säuglingsalter erfolgreich etablieren. Alle vier Säuglinge wurden anhaltend anfallsfrei. Niedrige Blutzuckerwerte während der initialen Fastenphase blieben asymptomatisch, da zeitgleich eine beginnende Ketose nachweisbar war. Die Entwicklung einer Ketose bei Säuglingen ließ sich deutlich präziser im Blut als im Urin nachweisen. Daher ist die kapilläre Bestimmung von Blutzucker und Plasmaketonen am Krankenbett Voraussetzung für eine sichere Einleitung der KD in dieser Altersgruppe. Eine Diät mit mittelkettigen Triglyzeriden erscheint im Säuglingsalter aufgrund der bei Patient 4 beobachteten reversiblen Gedeihstörung nicht angezeigt. Obwohl die beobachteten Nebenwirkungen gering waren, sind die längerfristigen Auswirkungen einer KD mit Beginn im frühen Säuglingsalter noch ungeklärt.

Literatur

1. Schwartzkroin PA (1999) Mechanisms underlying the anti-epileptic efficacy of the ketogenic diet. *Epilepsy Res 37:*171–80.
2. Nordli DR Jr, De Vivo DC (1997) The ketogenic diet revisited: back to the future. *Epilepsia 38:*743–9.
3. Nordli DR JR, Kuroda MM, Carroll J, Koenigsberger DY, Hirsch LJ, Bruner HJ, Seidel WT, De Vivo DC (2001) Experience with the ketogenic diet in infants. *Pediatrics 108:*129–33.
4. Klepper J, Ecker D, Burkart P, Leiendecker B, Voit T, Baumeister FAM (2001) Indikation und Anwendung der ketogenen Diät im Kindesalter. 1. Workshop ketogene Diät am 15. Dezember 2000 in Essen. *Monatsschr Kinderheilk 149:*1383–1390.

^{1}H-MR-Spektroskopie detektiert Ketonkörper im Gehirn von Kindern unter ketogener Diät unabhängig vom klinischen Ansprechen

M. Wilke, F.A.M. Baumeister, S. Wolf, J. Egger, D. Auer

Zusammenfassung

In dieser Pilotstudie wurden 3 Kinder unter ketogener Diät mittels lokalisierter ^{1}H-MRS untersucht. In allen Fällen konnten die natürlichen Ketonkörper Aceton und β-Hydroxy-Butyrat nachgewiesen werden, obwohl die Diät nur in einem Fall eine positiven Effekt hatte. Wir folgern, dass Ketonkörper alleine nicht das Wirkprinzip der Diät darstellen und dass die ^{1}H-MRS eine nützliche Methode sein könnte, den unklaren Wirkmechanismus der Diät aufzuklären.

Einführung

Die ketogene Diät wird insbesondere im Kindesalter erfolgreich zur Therapie zerebraler Anfälle eingesetzt. Sie imitiert den biochemischen Zustand des Hungerns, indem sie den Großteil der Kalorien in Form von Fett bereit stellt (1). In den letzten Jahren wurde die ketogene Diät als nützliche und wirksame Behandlung des therapieresistenten Anfallsleidens wiederentdeckt, insbesondere für Kinder (1). Obwohl die ketogene Diät seit vielen Jahrzehnten eingesetzt wird, ist der exakte Wirkmechanismus weiterhin unbekannt (2).

In einer Pilotstudie von Seymour *et al.* (3) wurden Patienten, die bereits unter Therapie mit ketogener Diät standen, mittels Protonen-Magnet-Resonanz-Spektroskopie (^{1}H-MRS) untersucht. In unserer Studie wollten wir die metabolischen Umstellungsprozesse während der Einstellung auf die Diät darstellen. Insbesondere sollten das Auftreten der natürlichen Ketonkörper Azeton (ACE), Azeto-Azetat (ACAC) und β-Hydroxy-Butyrat (BHB) nicht-invasiv *in vivo* mittels lokalisierter ^{1}H-MRS untersucht werden.

Patienten und Methoden

In dieser Pilotstudie konnten wir 3 Patienten zu jeweils drei Zeitpunkten untersuchen (am ersten Tag des Fastens vor dem Beginn der Diät, nach einer sowie nach 4 Wochen unter Diät). Die MR-Untersuchung wurde jeweils morgens zwischen 9.30 und 11.00 Uhr durchgeführt. Die Studie wurde von der zuständigen Ethikkommission genehmigt, und alle Eltern gaben ihr schriftliches Einverständnis. Schlaf während der Untersuchung wurde durch vorherigen Schlafentzug,

Tab. 1: Klinische Daten aller Patienten

	Geschlecht, Alter	Anti-epileptische Medikation	Diagnose
Patient 1	männlich, 6,5 J.	Valproat, Phenobarbital, Ethosuximid	? Epilepsie-Dysmorphie Syndrom; Niereninsuffizienz (transplantiert)
Patient 2	männlich, 8 Wochen	Vigabatrin, Phenobarbital, Vitamin B6	? peroxisomale Störung
Patient 3	weiblich, 1,5 J.	Valproat, Diazepam bei Bedarf	schwere peripartale Asphyxie

direkt vorhergehende Fütterung und niedrige Dosen von rektalem Chloralhydrat erreicht. In einem Fall wurde zusätzlich Kindermusik über ein MR-kompatibles Audio-System zur Beruhigung eingesetzt. Alle Patienten wurden kontinuierlich von einem qualifizierten Kinderarzt überwacht. Zu klinischen Daten siehe auch Tabelle 1.

Die MR-Untersuchung wurde an einem klinischen 1.5T MR-Scanner durchgeführt (GE Signa Horizon Echospeed, General Electric, Milwaukee, WI). Wir verwendeten eine PRESS-Sequenz mit kurzer Echozeit (TE=35 ms, TR=2000 ms, Voxel-Volumen: 8 ml) um parietalen Kortex zu untersuchen, da diese Region eine gut reproduzierbare Voxelplazierung erlaubt und vorwiegend graue Substanz enthält. Zur Plazierung der Spektroskopie-Voxel wurden zusätzliche, axiale T2-gewichtete Bilder angefertigt (Abb. 1). Die MR-Daten wurden mithilfe einer LCModel-Software (4) analysiert, die absolute Metaboliten-Quantifizierungen (in »institutional units«, basierend auf lokal untersuchten Modell-Lösungen) erlaubt. Um den Nachweis der natürlichen Ketonkörper ACE, ACAC und BHB zu ermöglichen, wurden zusätzliche Modell-Lösungen angefertigt und in die Metaboliten-Bibliothek der Software integriert. Die MR-Spektren wurden automatisch mithilfe der neu-integrierten Referenz-Spektren ausgewertet (Abb. 2). Metabolitenmessungen mit einer unzureichenden Fit-Genauigkeit (>35%) wurden nicht in die Auswertungen einbezogen.

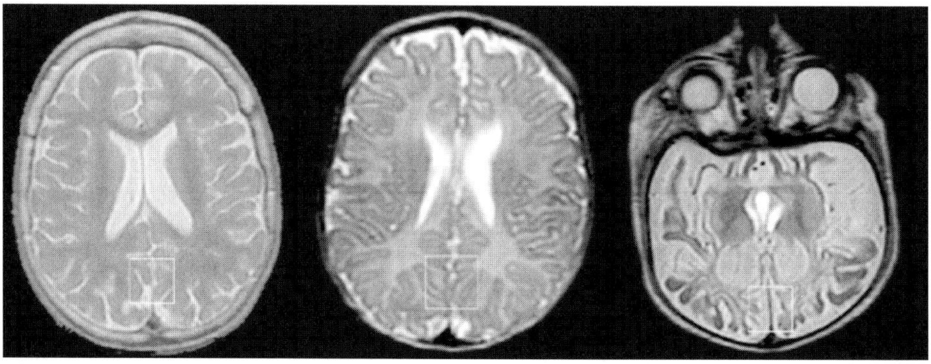

Abb. 1: Plazierung der MR-Voxel in allen Patienten.

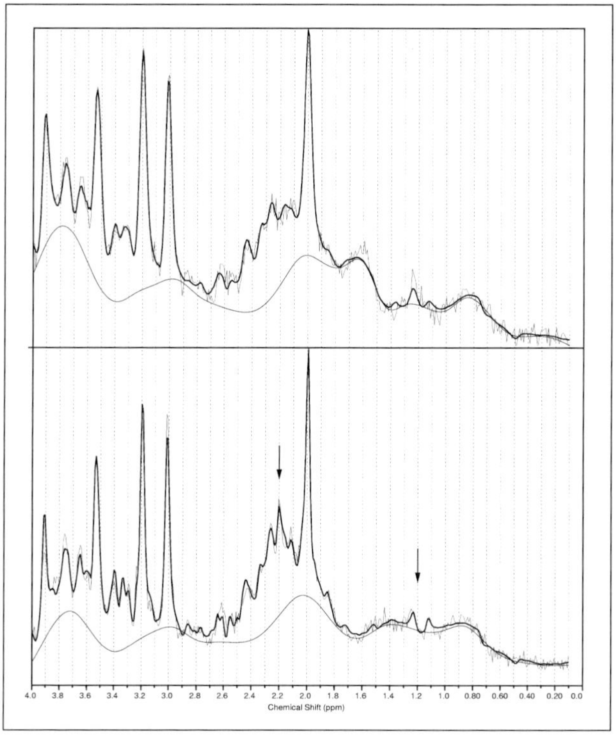

Abb. 2: ^{1}H-MR-Spektren, Patient 2. Oben: vor, unten: nach einer Woche ketogener Diät. Neue Resonanz bei ca. 2.2 ppm (ACE) und betontes Doublet bei ca. 1.2 ppm (BHB) (Pfeile).

Ergebnisse

Alle Patienten litten unter schweren, therapierefraktären zerebralen Krampfanfällen (Tab. 1). Ein befriedigender Effekt auf die Krampfanfälle konnte nur in Patient 2 erreicht werden, wohingegen bei Patient 1 und 3 nur eine minimale Abnahme von Krampfaktivität und/oder -frequenz erreicht werden konnte. Patient 1 hatte zum Zeitpunkt der dritten Untersuchung (nach 4 Wochen) eine Infektion, die seinen ketotischen Status durchbrach. Morphologisch konnte bei allen Patienten eine kombinierte Erweiterung der Liquorräume nachgewiesen werden, die bei Patient 3 am stärksten ausgeprägt war (Abb. 1).

Ketonkörper konnten in allen Patienten wenigstens einmal nachgewiesen werden (Tab. 2). ACAC konnte in keiner Untersuchung nachgewiesen werden.

Zusammenfassung und Ausblick

Mittels ^{1}H-MRS können Veränderungen der zerebralen Biochemie nachgewiesen werden, die durch die Diät hervorgerufen werden. Wie bereits *in vitro* gezeigt sind Ketonkörper alleine nicht ausreichend, um den anti-epileptischen

Tab. 2: Konzentration der Ketonkörper in allen Patienten: absolute Konzentrationen (IU) und Fit-Genauigkeit

	Zeitpunkt 1	Zeitpunkt 2	Zeitpunkt 3
Patient 1			
ACE	0	0.245 (34%)	0
BHB	0	0	0
ACAC	0	0	0
Patient 2			
ACE	0	0.387 (15%)	0.191 (29%)
BHB	0	0.522 (31%)	0.444 (28%)
ACAC	0	0	0
Patient 3			
ACE	0	0.187 (27%)	0.272 (25%)
BHB	0	0	0
ACAC	0	0	0

Effekt der KD zu erklären (5). Die ^{1}H-MRS könnte ein wertvolles Instrument in der weiteren Erforschung des unklaren Wirkungs-Mechanismus der Diät sein, insbesondere vor dem Hintergrund der möglichen Beeinflussungen von Neurotransmittern (6).

Literatur

1. Vining EP, Freeman JM, Ballaban-Gil K, Camfield CS, Camfield PR, Holmes GL, Shinnar S, Shuman R, Trevathan E, Wheless JW (1998): A multicenter study of the efficacy of the ketogenic diet. Arch Neurol 55: 1433–11437
2. Schwartzkroin PA (1999): Mechanisms underlying the anti-epileptic efficacy of the ketogenic diet. Epilepsy Res 37: 171–180
3. Seymour KJ, Bluml S, Sutherling J, Sutherling W, Ross BD (1999): Identification of cerebral acetone by 1H-MRS in patients with epilepsy controlled by ketogenic diet. MAGMA 8: 33–42
4. Provencher SW (1993): Estimation of metabolite concentrations from localized in vivo proton NMR spectra. Magn Reson Med 30: 672–679
5. Thio LL, Wong M, Yamada KA (2000): Ketone bodies do not directly alter excitatory or inhibitory hippocampal synaptic transmission. Neurology 54: 325–331
6. Yudkoff M, Daikhin Y, Nissim I, Lazarow A, Nissim I (2001): Ketogenic diet, amino acid metabolism, and seizure control. J Neurosci Res 66: 931–940

Effektivität der ketogenen Diät zur Behandlung therapierefraktärer Epilepsien im Kindesalter

F. A. M. Baumeister, G. M. Liebhaber, E. Riemann

Zusammenfassung

Während sich die ketogene Diät in anglo-amerikanischen Ländern als effektiv zur Behandlung therapierefraktärer Epilepsien erwiesen hat, zeigte ein Evaluationsversuch im deutschen Sprachraum (Workshop ketogene Diät, 2000) einen schlechten Therapieerfolg. Von 32 erfassten Patienten mit therapierefraktärer Epilepsie wurde keiner anfallsfrei, eine Anfallsreduktion >50% erreichten nur 16% der Patienten.

Anhand des eigenen Patientengutes, welches in die Evaluation des Workshops nicht eingegangen war, wurde retrospektiv die Effektivität der ketogenen Diät bei therapierefraktären Epilepsien ausgewertet.

24 Kinder mit therapierefraktärer Epilepsie wurden zwischen Februar 1997 und Januar 2002 mit ketogener Diät behandelt. Bei zwei Patienten wurde bereits bei Initiierung der Ketose wegen Nebenwirkungen (Erbrechen, Somnolenz) die ketogene Diät abgebrochen. Bei den übrigen 22 Patienten wurde durch die ketogene Diät eine Anfallsreduktion >50% bei 59% der Patienten erreicht. Unter ketogener Diät kam es bei 2/22Patienten (9%) zur Anfallsfreiheit (seit 22 Monaten bzw. 3,8 Jahren), eine Anfallsreduktion >90% erreichten weitere 5/22 Patienten (23%) und eine Anfallsreduktion um 50-90% weitere 6/22 Patienten (27%).

Wir können die Ergebnisse der angloamerikanischen Studien bestätigen, die ketogene Diät ist eine effektive Behandlungsmöglichkeit therapierefraktärer Epilepsien im Kindesalter.

Hintergrund

Seit der Antike ist bekannt, dass Fasten bei Patienten mit Epilepsien zum Sistieren der Anfälle führen kann (9, 13, 14). Aus dem Bestreben, die positiven Effekte der metabolischen Veränderungen im Hungerzustand auf das Anfallsgeschehen zu nutzen, entstand um 1920 die ketogene Diät (15). Die ketogene Diät ist eine fettreiche, an Kohlenhydraten reduzierte Ernährungsform mit ausreichendem Eiweiß- und Energiegehalt und führt zu einer anhaltenden Ketose. Die ketogene Diät wurde Bestandteil der Epilepsietherapie zu einer Zeit, als für die Behandlung der Epilepsien neben Brom nur Phenobarbital zur Verfügung stand. Mit der Entwicklung weiterer Antikonvulsiva geriet die ketogene Diät in Vergessenheit (14). In den letzten Jahren erlebt die ketogene Diät im angloameriksanischen Sprachraum eine Renaissance, wenn in der Behandlung von schwer verlaufenden Epilepsien die konventionellen und neuen Antiepileptika versagt haben und eine operative Therapie nicht in Frage kommt (1, 2, 6, 9, 10, 12, 13).

Der Versuch einer Standortbestimmung im deutschen Sprachraum (Workshop »ketogene Diät 2000« in Essen) ergab im Unterschied zur anglo-amerikanischen Literatur nur eine extrem geringe Effektivität der ketogenen Diät bei therapierefraktären Epilepsien. Von 32 Patienten mit therapierefraktärer Epilepsie wurde keiner anfallsfrei, eine Anfallsreduktion >50% erreichten nur 16% der Patienten (8).

In diese Evaluation gingen die von uns betreuten Patienten nicht ein. Wir berichten daher über die Effektivität der ketogenen Diät bei therapierefraktären Epilepsien an Hand unseres eigenen Patientengutes.

Patienten

24 Patienten mit therapierefraktärer Epilepsie wurden zwischen Februar 1997 und Januar 2002 mit ketogener Diät behandelt. Bei Beginn der ketogenen Diät betrug im Median (Streubreite) das Alter 6,0 Jahre (0,8–13,2), die Anzahl der bisher eingesetzten Antikonvulsiva 7 (3–13), die Epilepsiedauer 53 Monate (5–159). 13 Kinder hatten eine symptomatische, 8 Patienten eine kryptogene und 3 eine idiopathische Epilepsie. Die Patienten wiesen unterschiedlichste Anfallsformen auf, 50% myoklonisch, 42% tonisch-klonisch generalisiert, 50% tonisch, 38% atonisch und 29% atypische Absencen. Die Anfallsfrequenz betrug 140/Wo (250 Myokloni/Tag bis 1 Status epilepticus/Monat). Patienten mit Stoffwechseldefekten, insbesondere mit Glukosetransporterdefekt, Pyruvatdehydrogenase-Mangel und Atmungskettendefekten wurden für die Auswertung nicht berücksichtigt. 5 Patienten waren auswärts auf die ketogene Diät eingestellt worden.

Vor Beginn der ketogenen Diät erfolgte stets der Ausschluss von Kontraindikationen, insbesondere Störungen der β-Oxidation, Ketogenese und Ketolyse sowie von Kardiomyopathien.

Die Durchführung der ketogenen Diät erfolgte entsprechend dem Protokoll des »John Hopkins Pediatric Epilepsy Center« (3). Um eine gute Compliance und Akzeptanz zu erreichen, erfolgte ergänzend zur ärztlichen Betreuung eine intensive Schulung und engmaschige ambulante, sowie telephonische Betreuung der Familien durch eine spezialisierte Diätassistentin. Bei ausbleibendem Therapieerfolg (Anfallsreduktion < 50%) in den ersten Monaten nach Beginn rieten wir zu einem Abbruch der ketogenen Diät.

Ergebnisse

Die ketogene Diät wurde bei Initiierung der Ketose bei zwei Patienten bereits in der ersten Behandlungswoche wegen Nebenwirkungen abgebrochen. Die Nebenwirkungen, rezidivierendes Erbrechen und Somnolenz, beruhten nicht auf einer metabolischen Entgleisung und klangen mit Rückbildung der Ketose vollständig ab.

Bei 13 der restlichen 22 Patienten (59%) erreichte die ketogene Diät eine Anfallsreduktion >50%.

Anfallsfreiheit erreichten unter ketogener Diät 2/22 Patienten (9%). Der eine Patient erhält seit 4,3 Jahren ketogene Diät und ist seit 3,8 Jahren ohne medikamentöse Therapie anfallsfrei, der andere Patient erhält seit 24 Monaten ketogene Diät und ist seit 22 Monaten anfallsfrei.

Eine Anfallsreduktion >90% trat bei weiteren 5/22 Patienten (23%) ein. Unter den Respondern mit einer Anfallsreduktion >90% (5/22) befinden sich zwei Patienten, bei denen es unter ketogener Diät initial zur Anfallsfreiheit für 14 und 15 Monate kam bis Anfallsrezidive mit einer Frequenz <10% im Vergleich mit dem Ausgangspunkt vor ketogener Diät auftraten.

Eine Anfallsreduktion um 50–90% trat bei weiteren 6/22 Patienten (27%) ein.

Die Responder mit einer Anfallsreduktion >50% waren zum Zeitpunkt der Auswertung für 116 Wochen (13–221) unter ketogener Diät. Zu Beginn der ketogenen Diät betrug ihr Alter 5 Jahre (0,8–12,4), die Epilepsiedauer 50 Monate (6–144) und die Anzahl der vor ketogener Diät eingesetzten Antikonvulsiva 7,5 (3–13). Die Non-Responder (Anfallsreduktion <50%) unterschieden sich nicht signifikant. Zu Beginn der ketogenen Diät betrug ihr Alter 6,6 Jahre (1,5–13,4), die Epilepsiedauer 56 Monate (5–159) und die Anzahl der vor ketogener Diät eingesetzten Antikonvulsiva 7 (4–11). Es bestand auch kein signifikanter Unterschied hinsichtlich der Anfallsformen.

Die Patienten mit einer Anfallsreduktion <50% waren mit Ausnahme eines Patienten im Median nur 10,1 Wochen (5–16) unter ketogener Diät. Bei dem einen Patienten war es für 7 Monate zu einer Anfallsreduktion um 60% gekommen. Bei erneuter Zunahme der Anfallsfrequenz wurde die ketogene Diät nach 34 Wochen abgebrochen.

Fünf Patienten waren auswärts auf die ketogene Diät eingestellt worden. Davon waren einer anfallsfrei, zwei zeigten eine Anfallsreduktion >90% und zwei eine Anfallsreduktion um 50–90% unter ketogener Diät.

Werden für die Auswertung nur die in unserer Abteilung auf ketogene Diät eingestellten Patienten berücksichtigt, so erreichten unter ketogener Diät bei 8/17 Patienten (47%) eine Anfallsreduktion um >50%. Anfallsfrei wurde ein Patient (6%) eine Anfallsreduktion >90% zeigten weitere 3/17 Patienten (18%) und eine Anfallsreduktion um 50–90% weitere 4/17 Patienten (24%).

Diskussion

Zur Behandlung therapierefraktärer Epilepsien fand die ketogene Diät vor allem in den anglo-amerikanischen Ländern Verbreitung. Eine systematische Metaanalyse, welche Studien bis 1998 umfasst und die Effektivität der ketogenen Diät bei therapierefraktären Epilepsien analysierte, zeigte Anfallsfreiheit in 16%, Anfallsreduktion >90% in 32% und eine Anfallsreduktion >50% in 56% der Patienten (9). Zwischenzeitlich demonstrierten weitere Studien aus USA und Kanada die Effektivität der ketogenen Diät bei der Behandlung therapieresistenter Epilepsien, mit Anfallsfreiheit bei 12 bis 19% und einer Anfallsreduktion von >50% bei 55 bis 71% der Patienten (5, 7, 11). Bemerkenswert sind die Ergebnisse von Hemingway et al. (6) welche 150 Kinder einer prospektiven Studie mit therapieresistenter Epilepsie 3 bis 6 Jahre nach Initiierung der ketogenen Diät untersuchten. 12 Monate nach Beginn der ketogenen Diät waren von den 150 Kindern 7% anfallsfrei, 27% hatten eine Anfallsreduktion >90% und 49% eine Anfallsreduktion >50%. 83 Kinder (55%) führten die ketogene Diät im Mittel für 2,3 Jahre durch. 3–6 Jahre nach Beginn der ketogenen Diät waren von den ursprünglich 150 Patienten 13% anfallsfrei, 27% hatten eine Anfallsreduktion >90% und 44% eine Anfallsreduktion >50% (6).

Angesichts der Effektivität der ketogenen Diät bei therapierefraktären Epilepsien in den anglo-amerikanischen Studien überrascht das Ergebnis des Evaluationsversuches im deutschsprachigen Raum im Rahmen des »Workshop ketogene Diät 2000« in Essen (8). Keiner der erfassten Patient mit therapierefraktärer Epilepsie wurde unter ketogener Diät anfallsfrei. Nur 16% von 32 Patienten hatten eine Reduktion der Anfälle um >50% (8).

Dieses Ergebnis ist wahrscheinlich nicht repräsentativ. Die Daten der von uns behandelten Patienten gingen nicht in die Auswertung des »Workshop ketogene Diät« ein und zeigen eine bessere Effektivität der ketogenen Diät bei therapierefraktären Epilepsien, mit einer Reduktion der Anfallsfrequenz >50% bei 59% der Patienten und einer Anfallsreduktion >90% bei 32% (7/22). Anfallsfreiheit erreichten 9% (2/22) der Patienten.

Insgesamt entsprechen die Ergebnisse des von uns betreuten Patientenkollektives den anglo-amerikanischen Studien, wobei wir uns in der Durchführung der ketogenen Diät an das Protokoll des »John Hopkins Pediatric Epilepsy Center's halten (3).

Einen besonderen Stellenwert in der Betreuung der Familien besitzt für uns die regelmäßige und intensive Schulung durch die Diätassistentin in 3–4 monatigen Abständen sowie die Möglichkeit zur kurzfristigen telephonischen Beratung.

Ketogene Diät und medikamentöse antikonvulsive Therapie sind keine konkurrierenden Behandlungsstrategien, vielmehr stellen sie in der Behandlung der therapieresistenten Epilepsien eine wechselseitige effektive Ergänzung dar. Obwohl wir unter ketogener Diät bei 32% der Patienten eine Anfallsreduktion >90% beobachteten, wurde nur bei einem Patienten die antikonvulsive Medikation vollständig ausgeschlichen. Andere Zentren sind forcierter in der Reduktion der antikonvulsiven Medikamente. Hemingway et al. beschreiben in ihrer prospektiven Studie, dass von 83 Kindern die über 12 Monate die ketogene Diät erhielten 54% keine Antikonvulsiva mehr bekamen (6). Von diesen 83 Kindern hatten 49% eine Anfallsreduktion >90% (6). Die Reduktion von Antikonvulsiva ist ein Nebeneffekt und sollte kein Therapieziel der ketogenen Diät darstellen.

Die ketogene Diät ist eine effektive Therapie in der Behandlung therapierefraktärer Epilepsien, sie hat jedoch in gut einem Drittel der Patienten keinen wesentlichen Einfluss auf das Anfallsgeschehen (9).

Nach unserer Auffassung ist es wichtig, das Drittel der Patienten mit therapierefraktärer Epilepsie, die unter ketogener Diät eine Anfallsreduktion >90%

aufweisen, herauszufinden. Das von uns verfolgte Konzept ist es daher, relativ frühzeitig nach ca. zweijähriger Epilepsiedauer und dem fachkundigen Einsatz von mindestens drei Antikonvulsiva die ketogene Diät anzubieten, jedoch bei fehlendem Ansprechen in der Testphase auch wieder rasch abzusetzen.

Zu Beginn der ketogenen Diät wird die antikonvulsive Therapie belassen und in der Anfangs/Testphase nicht verändert, um die Effektivität der ketogenen Diät beurteilen zu können. Bei ausbleibendem oder geringem Therapieerfolg in den ersten Monaten raten wir zu einem Absetzen der ketogenen Diät, wodurch die Dauer der ketogenen Diät bei Patienten mit einer Anfallsreduktion <50% in dem von uns betreuten Patientengut mit im Median 10 Wochen sehr kurz ist. Dieses Vorgehen wird durch die Erfahrungen aus anderen Studien gestützt. Nach 3 Monaten ist nur noch selten mit einem Ansprechen auf die ketogene Diät zu rechnen (4, 7) und Patienten mit einer Anfallsreduktion <50% beenden in über 80% im Verlauf eines Jahres die ketogene Diät (4). Andererseits zeigt die prospektive Studie von Freeman et al. (4), an der 150 Kinder teilnahmen, sowie unsere eigenen Erfahrungen, dass eine Anfallsreduktion >50% dazu führt, dass die ketogene Diät über mehrere Jahre durchführbar ist.

Der positive Effekt der ketogenen Diät auf das Anfallsgeschehen bleibt bei der Mehrheit der Patienten mit einer Anfallsreduktion >90% auch nach Abschluss der Behandlung mit ketogener Diät bestehen (6).

Die ketogene Diät ist somit eine effektive, ergänzende therapeutische Option für schwer zu behandelnde Epilepsien, die sich medikamentös nicht beherrschen lassen und für die eine epilepsiechirurgische Behandlung nicht in Frage kommt.

Literatur

1. Bainbridge JL, Gidal BE, Ryan M (1999) The ketogenic diet. Pharmacotherapy 19:782-786
2. Ben-Menachem E (2000) New antiepileptic drugs and non-pharmacological treatments. Curr Opin Neurol 13:165–170
3. Freeman JM, Kelly MJ, Freeman JB (1996) The epilepsy diet treatment: An Introduction to the ketogenic diet. Demos Publications, New York
4. Freeman JM, Vining EPG, Pillas DJ, Pyzik PL, Casey JC, Kelly MT (1998) The efficacy of the ketogenic diet-1998: A prospective Evaluation of intervention in 150 children. Pediatrics 102:1358–1363
5. Hassan AM, Keene DL, Whiting ShE, Jacob PJ, Champagne JR, Humphreys P (1999) Ketogenic diet in the treatment of refractory epilepsy in childhood. Pediatr Neurol 21:548-552
6. Hemingway C, Freeman JM, Pillas DJ, Pyzik PL (2001) The ketogenic Diet: A 3- to 6- year follow-up of 150 children enrolled prospectively. Pediatrics 108:898–905
7. Katyal NG, Koehler AN, McGhee B, Foley CM, Crumrine PK (2000) The ketogenic diet in refractory epilepsy: The experience of children's hospital of pittsburgh. Clin Pediatr 39:153–159
8. Klepper J, Burkart P, Ecker D, Brockmann K; Baumeister FAM (2001) Indikation und Anwendung der ketogenen Diät im Kindesalter. 1. Workshop Ketogene Diät, 14.-15. Dezember 2000 in Essen. Monatsschr Kinderheilkd 149:1383–1390
9. Lefevre F, Aronson N (2000) Ketogenic diet for the treatment of refractory epilepsy in children: A systematic review of efficacy. Pediatrics 105:1–7
10. Nordli DR, De Vivo DC (1997) The ketogenic diet revisited: Back to the future. Epilepsia 38: 743–749

11. Nordli DR, Kuroda MM, Carroll J, Koenigsberger DY, Hirsch LJ, Bruner HJ, Seidel WT, De Vivo DC (2001) Experience with the ketogenic diet in infants. Pediatrics 108:129–133
12. Schmidt D, Bourgeois B (2000) A risk-benefit assessment of therapies for Lennox-Gastaut Syndrome. Drug Safety 22:467–477
13. Wheless JW, Ashwal S (1999) The ketogenic diet. In: Swaiman KF, Ashwal S (Hrsg) Pediatric Neurology: Principles & Practice, Mosby, St. Louis, S719–728
14. Wheless JW (2001) Vagus nerve stimulation and the ketogenic diet. Neurologic Clinics 19:371–407
15. Wilder RM (1921) The effect of ketonemia on the course of epilepsy. Bull Mayo Clin 2:307–308

Wirksamkeit der ketogenen Diät: Evidenz aus Fall-Serien zur Behandlung schwerer Epilepsien bei Kindern

T. Reckert, D. Ecker, R. Madeleyn

Abstract

Einleitung: Ketogene Diät enthält zu 80% Fett, die notwendigen Proteine und kaum Kohlenhydrate. Sie wurde in den 20er Jahren entwickelt, um Effekte des Fastens auf die Anfallskontrolle zu imitieren und führt wie das Fasten durch einen Kohlenhydratmangel zur Ketonkörperbildung. Ketonkörper werden dann zur überwiegenden Energiequelle des Gehirns. Hierdurch vermindern sich häufig Anfälle. *Frage:* Wieviel Prozent der Kinder mit einer auch gegen neuere Antiepileptika therapieresistenten Epilepsie erreichen a.) Anfallsfreiheit, b.) eine >90%ige Anfallsreduktion oder c.) eine >50%ige Anfallsreduktion? *Einschlusskriterien:* Studien wurden eingeschlossen, wenn sie 1/1990–11/2001 publiziert waren, und für obige Frage relevante Ergebnisse aus kompletten Fall-Serien von Patienten mit therapieresistenter Epilepsie berichteten. *Ergebnisse:* Wir konnten 10 Fallserien mit insg. 569 Kindern einschließen. Durch die ketogene Diät konnte a.) Anfallsfreiheit in 11% b.) eine >90%ige Anfallsreduktion in 27% und c.) eine >50%ige Anfallsreduktion in 50% der Kinder erreicht werden. Bei 50% der Kinder wurde die ketogene Diät als nicht erfolgreich angesehen, da keine Anfallsreduktion >50% auftrat oder die Diät vorzeitig abgebrochen werden musste. *Schlussfolgerung:* Bei einem Viertel bis zur Hälfte der in Fallserien publizierten Patienten scheint es zu durchgreifenden Besserungen der Anfälle zu kommen. Diese Patienten und ihre Eltern sind motiviert, die schwierige Diät beizubehalten.

Einleitung

Zwischen dem 1.–15. Lj. tritt Epilepsie mit einer Inzidenz von ca. 38–45/100.000 auf (1). Sie hat häufig eine gute Prognose. Die Epilepsien von 10–30% der Kinder sind jedoch auch heute noch mit einer konventionellen Pharmakotherapie nicht ausreichend zu kontrollieren. Neben der Epilepsiechirurgie und neuerdings dem Vagusnervstimulator bietet die ketogene Diät eine radikale aber gut erprobte ergänzende Alternative für die Patientengruppe mit konventionell-pharmakologisch schlecht einstellbaren Epilepsien. Diese Alternative wird jedoch in Deutschland selber noch kaum angewandt (2), und war hier (im Gegensatz zu den Erfahrungen vor allem aus den USA) in der Behandlung therapierefraktärer Epilepsien bisher noch nicht in breitem Maße erfolgreich. Lediglich eine Arbeitsgruppe aus München um Herrn PD Dr. Baumeister publizierte vergleichbar gute Ergebnisse bei ihren 23 mit ketogener Diät behandelten Patienten mit therapierefraktärer Epilepsie (3).

Nach Brom (1857) und Phenobarbital (1910) wurde die klassische ketogene Diät erstmals 1921 gezielt als damals dritte antikonvulsive Therapieoption eingeführt (4). Man hatte beobachtet, dass Hungern bei vielen Patienten günstig auf die Anfallssituation wirkt und versuchte, den Zustand des Kohlenhydratmangels beim Hungern mit genügender Kalorien- und Proteinzufuhr zu kombinieren. Proteine können teilweise und Fette nur zu geringem Teil zu Glucose umgebaut werden. Im Hungerzustand bildet der Körper aus seinen Fettreserven vielmehr Ketonkörper, mit denen unter anderem das Gehirn bei Glucoseunterversorgung seinen Energiebedarf effizient auf alternative Weise deckt (5). In der ketogenen Diät deckt der Patient seinen Energiebedarf über die Ketose nicht aus Körperfett wie beim Hungern sondern aus Nahrungsfett. Man kann korrelieren, dass bei guter Ketose die ketogene Diät besser antikonvulsiv wirkt (6,7), weiss aber letztlich nicht, warum die ketogene Diät wirkt (8).

Für eine ketogene Diät wird der Energiebedarf (30–80 kcal/kg je nach Alter und Energieumsatz) und der Proteinbedarf (0,7–2 g/kg je nach Alter) sorgfältig berechnet und dann die sog. »ketogene Ratio« (typischerweise 3–4,5:1) festgelegt. Die ketogene Ratio bestimmt das Gewichtsverhältnis von Fett zu Kohlenhydraten + Proteinen. Eine ketogene Ratio von 4:1 bedeutet also, dass die Nahrung zu 80% Gewichtsanteilen aus Fetten bestehen muss. In den restlichen 20% Gewichtsanteilen muss eine den Bedarf deckende Proteinmenge untergebracht werden. Dementsprechend dürfen Kohlenhydrate nur in minimalen Mengen gegessen werden, um eine wirksame Ketose aufrechtzuerhalten. Zum Beispiel bekäme ein 4,5-jähriger, mit 18,4 kg normalgewichtiger Junge eine 1300 kcal – 4:1 – Diät bestehend aus 24,5 g Protein, 8 g Kohlenhydraten und 130 g Fett täglich (9). Eine Ketose infolge eines willkürlich herbeigeführten Kohlenhydratmangels wird durch die Zufuhr geringer überzähliger Kohlenhydratmengen innerhalb kürzester Zeit durchbrochen (10), was prompt wieder zu vermehrten Anfällen führen kann (6, 9). Dieses strenge Diätregime erfordert eine sorgfältige Indikationsstellung, erhebliche Detailkenntnisse und eine enge Zusammenarbeit mit Patienten, ihren Eltern und deren Umfeld (9, 11, 12).

Um die Durchführbarkeit zu vereinfachen, wurde 1971 erstmals versucht, die klassische Diät durch mittelkettige Triglyceride (MCT-Öl) so zu verbessern, dass mehr Kohlenhydrate möglich werden (13). Diese modifizierte Diät schien vergleichbar effektiv zu sein. Das MCT-Öl selbst schmeckte jedoch im Vergleich schlechter und verursachte mehr Magen-Darm-Beschwerden (14).

Die ketogene Diät fand trotz ihrer schwierigen Durchführbarkeit mangels Alternativen in der ersten Hälfte des letzten Jahrhunderts vor allem in den USA Verbreitung als erfolgreiche Behandlungsmöglichkeit kindlicher Epilepsien (15). Als neue Antiepileptika eine bessere und einfachere pharmakologische Anfallskontrolle auch bei bis dahin schwierig zu kontrollierenden Epilepsiesyndromen wie dem Lennox-Gastaut-Syndrom versprachen, geriet die ketogene Diät weitgehend in Vergessenheit und wurde von erfahrenen Teams nur noch in wenigen Zentren und selten durchgeführt. Da jedoch trotz ständig fortschreitender Neuentwicklungen bei antikonvulsiven Medikamenten nach wie vor eine Untergruppe von Kindern verbleibt, denen auch diese Medikamente nur wenig helfen, bekommt die ketogene Diät seit den 90er Jahren wieder ein wachsendes Interesse in Fach- und Laienkreisen (15, 16). Dies führte zu einer größeren Anzahl durchgeführter Effektivitätsstudien in Kollektiven, die auch unter heutigen Bedingungen mit der üblichen Pharmakotherapie nicht gut behandelbar sind. Die Ergebnisse dieser neueren Studien sollen hier zusammengefasst werden. Eine ähnliche Metaanalyse wurde 2000 veröffentlicht, sie beinhaltete 11 Studien von 1970–1998 (17), drei der auch dort berücksichtigten Studien werden auch hier mitenthalten sein.

Fragestellung

Wieviel Prozent der Kinder mit einer auch gegen neuere Antiepileptika therapieresistenten Epilepsie erreichen in neueren Studien mit ketogener Diät a.) Anfallsfreiheit, b.) eine >90%ige Anfallsreduktion oder c.) eine >50%ige Anfallsreduktion? Welche Nebenwirkungen berichten diese Studien? Wie lange wird die Diät durchgehalten? Welches Setting erscheint dafür notwendig?

Methode

Es wurde eine Volltextsuche in MEDLINE 1/1990-11/2001 mit den Stichworten »(ketogen* diet) AND (epilep* OR seizure* OR convuls*)« vorgenommen. In den Literaturverzeichnissen relevanter Artikel wurde nach weiteren Quellen gesucht.

Studien wurden eingeschlossen, wenn sie 01/1990–11/2001 publiziert waren, und für obige Fragen relevante Ergebnisse aus kompletten Fall-Serien konsekutiv behandelter pädiatrischer Patienten mit definierter therapieresistenter Epilepsie berichteten. Zur Therapieresistenz musste als Mindestdefinition die fachkundige aber erfolglose Vorbehandlung mit ≥2 Antiepileptika erkennbar sein. Die Studien konnten prospektiv oder retrospektiv angelegt sein. Die Methoden und Ergebnisse wie epidemiologisches Setting, Ein- und Ausschlusskriterien, Erhebung der Anfallsfrequenz zu Beginn und im Verlauf, Art der Diätdurchführung, Begleittherapien, Dauer des Follow-up mussten ausreichend nachvollziehbar beschrieben sein. Daher wurden bloße Abstracts ausgeschlossen.

Die Ergebnisse werden in Tabellenform für die einzelnen Studien und wo möglich in metaanalytischer Übersicht im Text zusammengefasst.

Ergebnisse

Die oben beschriebene Medline-Suche erbrachte 127 Zitate. 84 erwiesen sich nach Lektüre der Überschrift und evt. des Abstracts als eindeutig irrelevant für die Fragestellung. 43 Arbeiten wurden im Volltext incl. Literaturverzeichnis näher studiert. 14 in vollständigen Texten publizierte Arbeiten beinhalteten Original-

Tab. 1: Übersicht über die eingeschlossenen Studien. (NB: nicht berichtet; KD: ketogene Diät; AED: Antiepileptikum).

Erstautor Jg. **(Quelle)** **(Ort, Staat)**	**Studien-Design, epidemiologisches Setting**	**n**	**Alter: Bereich Mittel**	**Anfälle/ Monat vor KD**	**AED vor KD**	**Diätdauer: ≤3 Monate >12Monate**	**Anfallsfrei**	**>90% weniger Anfälle**	**>50% weniger Anfälle**
Freeman 1998 (22) (Baltimore, USA)	prospekt. Studie aller von 8/94-8/96 im Johns-Hopkins Hospital mit KD behandelten Kinder	150	1-16 5,3	410	6,24	25/150 83/150	3. Mon.: 4/150 (3%) 6. Mon.: 5/150 (3%) 12. Mon.: 11/150 (7%)	3. Mon.: 50/150 (33%) 6. Mon.: 48/150 (32%) 12. Mon.: 41/150 (27%)	3. Mon.: 89/150 (60%) 6. Mon.: 77/150 (51%) 12. Mon.: 75/150 (50%)
Hassan 1999 (23) (Ottawa, Kanada)	retrosp. Studie zu allen Kindern, die am Childrens-Hospital of Eastern Ontario KD bekamen.	52	2-9 5,5	NB	NB	32/52 7/52.	»while on diet«: 6/52 (12%) (kurzer Zeitraum?).	NB	»while on diet«: 35/52 (67%) (kurzer Zeitraum?)
Katyal 2000 (24) (Pittsburgh, USA)	9/94-1/98 begannen am Childr. Hosp. of Pittsburgh 56 Kinder KD. 48 Eltern beantworteten Fragebogen.	48	1-14 NB	NB	NB	NB 22/48;	3/48 konnten nach 2 Jahren KD entwöhnt werden.	16/48 (33%) nach 45 Tagen	30/48 (63%) nach 45 Tagen
Kinsman 1992 (25) (Baltimore, USA)	retrosp. Studie aller von 1/80-1/85 im Johns Hopkins Hospital mit KD behandelten Kinder.	58	1 – 19 5	NB	4,9	NB NB	NB	17/58 (29%) »virtually complete seizure control«	39/58 (67%)
MacCracken 1999 (26) (Eugene, USA)	prosp. Studie aller Kinder, bei denen 1/95-3/98 im Sacred Heart Medical Center KD begonnen wurde.	11	1 – 12,5 4,8	NB	NB	5/11 3/11	2/11 nach 2–28,5 Monaten	3/11 nach 2–28,5 Monaten	4/11 nach 2–28,5 Monaten
Mak 1999 (27) (Taichung, Taiwan)	wahrsch. retrospekt. Studie: Kinder, die 9/97-8/98 im Taichung Veterans General Hospital KD bekamen.	13	3–13 NB	NB	3,9	7/13 NB	Fastenzeit: 3/13 1 Monat: 0/13 3 Monate nach Diät oder am Ende der Studie: 0/13	Fastenzeit: NB 1. Monat: NB 3 Monate nach Diät oder am Ende der Studie: 5/13	Fastenzeit: 5/13 1. Monat: 10/13 3 Monate nach Diät oder am Ende der Studie: 8/13
Maydell 2001 (28) (Cleveland, USA)	retrosp. Studie aller Kinder, bei denen 1/95-9/99 an der Cleveland Clinic Foundation KD begonnen wurde.	143	4/12–29; 7,5	600	NB	(durchschn. 14,7 Monate).	3. Monat: 21/143 (15%) 6. Monat: 24/143 (17%) 12. Monat: 23/143 (16%)	3. Monat: 43/143 (31%) 6. Monat: 41/143 (29%) 12. Monat: 38/143 (27%)	3. Monat: 59/143 (41%) 6. Monat: 60/143 (42%) 12. Monat: 54/143 (38%)
Moreno-Villares 2001 (29) (Madrid, Spanien)	retrosp. Studie zu Kindern, bei denen am Hospital 12 de Octubre eine KD begonnen wurde.	12	1 6/12–9 3,5.	490	4,8	NB 9/12	3. Monat: 1/12 6. Monat: 2/12 12. Monat: 1/12	3. Monat: 2/12 6. Monat: 4/12 12. Monat2/12	3. Monat: 9/12 6. Monat: 6/12 12. Monat: 3/12
Nordli 2001 (30) (Chicago, USA)	retrosp. Studie: Kinder <2Lj, die 10/83-6/97 im Columbia Presbyterian Medical Center KD bekamen.	31	13,8 ± 5,7 Monate	NB	NB	3/31 NB	6/31, darunter 6/17 mit infantilen Spasmen	NB	17/31
Vining 1998 (31) (Baltimore, USA)	prosp. Multicenterstudie 1/94-12/95 an 7 Institutionen nach einheitlichem Protokoll	51	1,3-8,6 4,7	230	7	6/51 24/51	3. Monat: 6/51 (12%) ? ?	3. Monat: 13/51 (25%) 6. Monat: 15/51 (29%) 12. Monat: 11/51 (22%)	3. Monat: 28/51 (55%) 6. Monat 27/51 (53%) 12. Monat: 20/5 (39%)

studien, die die obigen Fragen berührten. Das Studium der Literaturverzeichnisse erbrachte keine weitere relevante Originalstudie, es sei denn in Abstraktform. Von den ursprünglich lokalisierten 14 Arbeiten mussten vier ausgeschlossen werden: Eine Studie wurde ausgeschlossen, weil die dort eingeschlossenen Kinder durchschnittlich nur <2 Antiepileptika vor der KD bekommen hatten (18), eine Studien wurden ausgeschlossen, weil die Anfallsverbesserung nur vage angegeben war (»besser, nicht besser«) (19). Eine weitere Studie (beschrieben in einer Doppelpublikation (20, 21) mit dem selben Kollektiv) musste ausgeschlossen werden, weil »intractable epilepsy« für diese Studie schon vorlag, wenn nur ein Medikament der ersten Wahl in therapeutischer Serumkonzentration versagt hatte. Die ausgeschlossenen Studien berichteten überdurchschnittlich gute Ergebnisse.

Es fanden sich keine kontrollierten Studien, aber drei prospektive und sieben retrospektive Fallsammlungen mit konsekutiven Patientenkollektiven, die mit KD behandelt waren (siehe Tab. 1) (22–31). Sieben Studien kamen aus den USA, neun der zehn Studien erschienen 1998 oder später. Sechs Studien geben an, dass ihre Patienten ab 1994 behandelt wurden (siehe Tab. 1).

In den 11 Studien wurden insgesamt die Ergebnisse bei 569 Kindern publiziert. Die Altersspanne reichte vom Säuglings- bis zum jungen Erwachsenenalter und hat ihren Schwerpunkt im späten Kindergartenalter. Alle Anfallsformen und -ätiologien waren vertreten, wobei besonders oft Patienten mit Anfallsmischbildern (z.B. Lennox-Gastaut-Syndrom), multifokalen und verschiedenen generalisierten Anfallsformen behandelt wurden. Bei 356 Patienten war die Anfallsfrequenz vor Diätbeginn erwähnt und lag durchschnittlich bei ca. 460 Anfällen im Monat. Bei 284 Patienten war die vorherige (erfolglose) Medikation erwähnt und lag bei durchschnittlich 5,9 Antiepileptika. 75% von 449 Patienten hatten eine kognitive Entwicklungsstörung.

Ganz wesentlich überwog die Anwendung der klassischen 4:1-Diät nach dem Johns-Hopkins-Protokoll gegenüber einer MCT-Diät, die nur in zwei kleinen Studien mit insg. 25 Patienten durchgeführt wurde. Die Studien stammen alle aus Epilepsiezentren und neuropädiatrischen Abteilungen zumeist von Universitätskliniken. Im Behandlungsteam war immer ein Neuropädiater, eine speziell ausgebildete Diätassistentin und meistens eine spezialisierte Krankenschwester beteiligt. Gelegentlich arbeitete noch ein Psychologe im Team mit. Die Diät wurde immer in einem mindestens 5-tägigen stationären Aufenthalt unter Fasten eingeleitet. Dem voraus gingen in der Regel ein bis zwei ausführliche Ambulanztermine, in denen die Indikation sorgfältig gestellt wurde und die Eltern erste Informationen bekamen. Ausführliche Schulungsprogramme für die Eltern waren immer Bestandteil des Settings und wurden durchweg als maßgeblich für den Erfolg angesehen. Nach Entlassung war immer ein enger Telephonkontakt (z.B. durchschnittlich 40 h im ersten Jahr pro Patient (9)) und ein mehr oder weniger enges Netz an ambulanten Verlaufsuntersuchungen vorgesehen.

Die Art, wie über den Zeitpunkt und die Ursache von Diätabbrüchen berichtet wird, variiert: Ein oft verwendetes Maß ist die Anzahl der Patienten, die vor dem 3. Monat abbrachen, und derjenigen, die die Diät über ein Jahr durchführten: Wo dies erwähnt war, brachen 74 von 308 Patienten (24%) vor dem

3. Monat ab und führten 148 von 324 Patienten (46%) die Diät länger als 12 Monate fort. Vorzeitige Diätabbrüche kamen vor allem dann vor, wenn die Diät nicht ausreichend wirkte und erst in zweiter Linie, wenn sie zu restriktiv war oder nicht vertragen wurde. Die erhöhte Wahrscheinlichkeit, die Diät über ein Jahr fortzuführen, hängt ganz wesentlich von ihrem Erfolg in den ersten drei Monaten ab, wie in mehreren Studien eindrucksvoll demonstriert werden konnte (u.a. (22, 25, 31)). Dies gilt um so mehr, je erfahrener das Team ist, das die KD betreut. Ist die ketogene Diät erfolgreich, wird versucht, sie über 2–3 Jahre beizubehalten, und sie dann langsam auszuschleichen (9, 37).

Die Maße »Anfallsfreiheit«, »>90%ige Anfallsreduktion« und »>50%ige Anfallsreduktion« häufig nach 3, 6 und 12 Monaten wurden in den meisten neueren Studien als Erfolgsmaßstab genommen. Bewertet wurde in der Regel der elterliche Anfallskalender. Sind Anfallsreduktionen für verschiedene Zeitpunkte differenziert angegeben, so wird hier der letzte Zeitpunkt verwertet. Therapieabbrüche vor diesem Zeitpunkt wurden dann als Therapieversager gewertet. Es werden stets kumulative Prozentangaben gemacht, die anfallsfreien Patienten also in die Gruppe derjenigen mit >90%iger oder >50%iger Anfallsreduktion mit hereingerechnet usw.: Anfallsfrei nach 2–12 Monaten waren 58 von 511 Patienten (11%). Eine >90%ige Anfallsreduktion nach 1–12 Monaten hatten 133 von 468 Patienten (28%). Eine >50%ige Anfallsreduktion nach 1–12 Monaten hatten 285 von 558 (50%) der Patienten. In vier Studien mit insgesamt 359 Kindern (22, 28, 29, 31) wurden die Therapieresultate nach 3, 6 und 12 Monaten angegeben (siehe Diagramm 1): Die Zusammenfassung dieser Daten zeigt, dass die Erfolgswahrscheinlichkeit innerhalb des ersten Jahres leicht abnimmt.

Als Komplikationen gab es in nahezu jeder Serie Einzelfälle von Nierensteinen (insgesamt zu ca. 3–4%). Diese ließen sich oft durch vermehrte Flüssigkeitsgabe, Alkalisieren des Urins und Gabe von Kaliumcitrat auflösen und mussten nur ganz vereinzelt mit Stoßwellen zertrümmert oder operiert werden. Sie waren meistens kein Grund, die Diät abzubrechen. Ein generelles Screening auf Nierensteine unter der Diät (z.B. wöchentliche Untersuchung auf Blut im Urin per Stix) erscheint sinnvoll (32). Unter den gastrointestinalen Nebenwirkungen

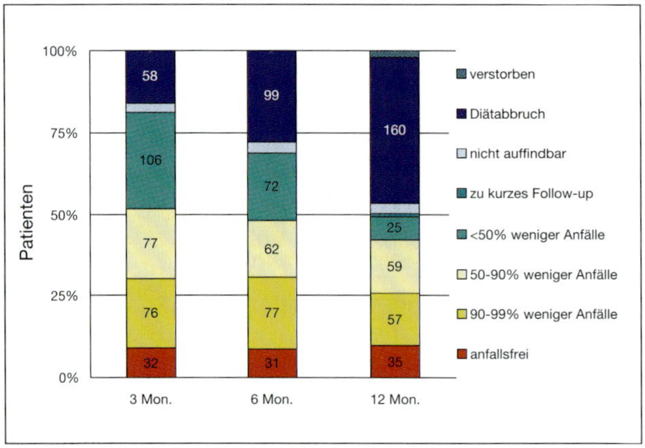

Diagramm 1: Therapieverläufe bei 359 Patienten aus 4 Studien (22, 28, 29, 31).

dominierte die Obstipation, die (wenn berichtet) in 30–40% der Fälle auftrat und beherrschbar ist. Ferner wurde von Azidose und Erbrechen, Hunger oder Appetitlosigkeit und Lethargie vor allem in der Anfangsphase und vereinzelt über rezidivierende Infekte, Verhaltensprobleme, Gallensteine, Herzrhythmusstörungen (hier spielt insbesondere das Manifestwerden eines Long-QT-Syndroms eine Rolle (33), weswegen ein EKG-Screening vor Einleitung einer ketogenen Diät empfohlen wird) und Ataxie berichtet. Es fanden sich in den berücksichtigten Studien insgesamt 7 Todesfälle unter ketogener Diät, die nicht der Diät selber sondern den oft schweren Grunderkrankungen der behandelten Kinder zugeordnet wurden (28).

Die ketogene Diät wurde breit bei vielen unterschiedlichen Anfallsformen, Epilepsieätiologien und Altersbereichen angewandt. Es ist nicht klar herauszufiltern, welche Patientenuntergruppen besonders profitieren, bei welchen die ketogene Diät besonders schwer durchzuführen ist oder welche Patientengruppen besonders komplikationsanfällig sind. Einzelne Tendenzen sind in verschiedenen Studien dennoch erkennbar: So scheinen generalisierte Anfälle etwas besser anzusprechen als fokale Anfälle (28) (gute Ergebnisse gab es beim therapierefraktären West-Syndrom (30)); die ketogene Diät scheint jenseits des 8.-12. Lebensjahres an Wirksamkeit zu verlieren und schwieriger durchführbar zu sein (22,28), ist aber bei Säuglingen unter einem Jahr ebenso erfolgreich anzuwenden, wie jenseits des ersten Lebensjahres (30).

Diskussion

Die Anzahl an Outcome-Studien zur ketogenen Diät hat in den letzten vier Jahren sprunghaft zugenommen. Neuere Arbeiten orientieren sich zunehmend methodisch an der zur Zeit wichtigsten prospektiven Kohortenstudie von Freeman et al. (1998) (22), die in der Evaluationsforschung zu der ketogenen Diät Standards gesetzt hat. Diese Studie, und diejenigen von Vining et al. (31) und Kinsman et al. (25) sind in einer älteren systematischen Übersichtsarbeit (17) zu den von 1970–1998 erschienenen Evaluationsstudien mitenthalten. Sie werden dort als die bisher qualitativ besten Studien bewertet.

Diese ältere Übersichtsarbeit (17) konnte ebenfalls 11 Studien mit insgesamt 483 Kinder einschließen und erbrachte etwas bessere Ergebnisse: 15,8% (95%-Konfidenzintervall: 11–21,7%) der mit ketogener Diät behandelten Kinder wurden anfallsfrei, 32,2% (95%-Konfidenzintervall: 25,3–39,8%) hatten eine >90%ige Anfallsreduktion und 55,8% (95% Konfidenzintervall: 41,2–69,7%) hatten eine >50%ige Anfallsreduktion. Dort wurde schon ausgeführt, dass diese Ergebnisse nicht durch den Spontanverlauf (vergleiche dazu (34)) und nicht durch einen sogenannten Placeboeffekt erklärbar seien. (In den bei (35) zusammengefassten Studien zu den neueren Antiepileptika: hatten nur 9,8% der Patienten eine über 50%ige Besserung der Anfälle auf Placebogabe hin). Ferner sind die zur ketogenen Diät publizierten Ergebnisse bei therapierefraktärer Epilepsie im Kindesalter vielfach besser als die Ergebnisse einer Add-on Therapie eines neueren Antiepileptikums (17).

Dennoch sollen einige methodenkritische Anmerkungen gemacht werden: Es gab bisher keine Studien mit Kontrollgruppen irgendwelcher Art. Alle Studien machen einen Vorher-Nachher Vergleich. Dies kann prinzipiell problematisch sein, weil Epilepsien Erkrankungen mit schubweisem Spontanverlauf (aus häufig unerkennbaren Gründen schwankender Anfallsfrequenz und -schwere) sind. Die Entscheidung zu einer so eingreifenden Therapie wie der ketogenen Diät wird man möglicherweise leichter dann fällen, wenn die Anfälle gerade besonders ausgeprägt sind. Insofern dies der Fall ist, gibt es eine gute Chance der Besserung durch oder eben trotz Diät (regression to the mean). Die Protokolle der prospektiven Studien von Freeman (22) und Vining (31) sehen vor, dass die Anfallsfrequenz des Monats vor Diätbeginn (base-line) mit der Anfallsfrequenz jeweils in den Monaten vor dem Kontrolltermin (also vor dem Monat 3, 6 und 12 nach Diätbeginn) verglichen wird. Gemessen an der Erkrankungsdauer und den dort häufig vorkommenden Schwankungen mag jeweils ein herausgegriffener Monat kurz erscheinen. Möglichkeiten, in diesem Punkt die Studienmethodik zu verbessern, werden bei Kiene 2001 S. 41 ff. diskutiert (36): Je besser und vollständiger man die Vorher-Nachher-Zeitverhältnisse der Anfallsfrequenzen im Zusammenhang mit der Durchführung der ketogenen Diät darstellen kann, um so überzeugender wird man am Einzelfall die Therapiewirkung als eine »phänomenologisch-kausale« Wirkung beurteilen können. Solche Einzelfallbeurteilungen können in prospektiven Kohortenstudien dann zu gut dokumentierten Fallserien zusammengestellt werden, mit der man die Gesamteffektivität des Therapieverfahrens evaluieren kann.

Längerfristige Studien mit geeigneten Kontrollgruppen wären wünschenswert. Eine Studie mit komplexen Interventions-Wirkungs-Kurzzeitverläufen und einem gut durchdachten placebokontrollierten randomisierten Cross-Over-Design planen Freeman et al. (1999) durchzuführen (6). Ob allerdings Kontrollgruppen für längerfristig angelegte Interventionsstudien durch Randomisation vergleichbar gemacht werden können, erscheint fraglich, da die ketogene Diät eine starke Patientenmitarbeit und -motivation erfordert und andererseits einem motivierten Patienten wegen der doch schon gut belegten und bekannten Wirksamkeit kaum willkürlich vorenthalten werden kann. Die nötige, vertrauensvolle und vom therapeutischen Willen geprägte Arzt-Patienten-Beziehung würde durch Studienprotokolle potentiell gestört, was sich direkt auf die Therapie selber auswirken kann. Insofern ist die häufig geäußerte Forderung nach randomisierten Studien nicht selbstverständlich gerechtfertigt. Solche Studien müssen in der Beurteilung sorgfältig auf Quellen für einen false-negative-bias abgeklopft werden (36).

Oft angemahnte Langzeitergebnisse liegen unterdessen auch aus neuerer Zeit vor. Die Kohorte von Freeman et al. ist 3–6 Jahre nachbeobachtet mit weiterhin guten Ergebnissen (37). Ferner ist eine Auswertung zur Lebensqualität und zur verbesserten kindlichen Entwicklung unter ketogener Diät aus dem selben Kollektiv erschienen (38).

In den USA ist man sich unterdessen weitgehend einig, dass die Frage: »The ketogenic diet: Fa(c)t or Fiction?« (16) unfruchtbar und nicht mehr zeitgemäß ist und es vielmehr darauf ankomme, in die Zukuft zu schauen (»The ketogenic diet revisited: Back to the future« (39)). Hierzu müsse gefragt werden, warum die ketogene Diät wirkt, bei wem sie wirkt, wie man sie komfortabler und sicherer machen, wie man ihren Effekt optimieren kann und ob sie nur antikonvulsiv oder in einigen Fällen sogar antiepileptogen, also kausal wirke. Schließlich erhofft man sich durch die genauere Erforschung der ketogenen Diät wesentliche grundlegende Einblicke für das genauere Verständnis der ja immer noch rätselhaften Epilepsien überhaupt (9). Im Gegensatz hierzu war die ketogene Diät in Deutschland nie etabliert und gilt immer noch vielen Epileptologen als eine Außenseitermethode die vor allem weitere Beschränkungen in der Lebensqualität der sowieso schon beeinträchtigten Patienten mit sich bringe. Breitere positive Erfahrungen mit der ketogenen Diät fehlen dem gegenüber hierzulande bisher (2): Eine Umfrage erbrachte, dass in Deutschland in 11 Kliniken bis zum Jahr 2000 52 Patienten mit ketogener Diät behandelt wurden, von denen 36 eine therapieresistente Epilepsie hatten (17 dieser Patienten kamen aus der Kinderabteilung der Filderklinik, 15 aus der Epilepsieklinik in Kehl-Kork). Weitere 7 Patienten hatten einen PDH-Mangel, 9 Patienten hatten einen Glucosetransporterdefekt. Bei nur 3/36 Patienten mit therapieresistenter Epilepsie zeigte sich ein gutes Ansprechen und bei 14/36 Patienten ein mäßiges Ansprechen auf die ketogene Diät. Nicht in diese Umfrageergebnisse eingeschlossen waren jedoch 23 Patienten aus München, von denen Ergebnisse berichtet werden konnten, die den amerikanischen Erfahrungen vergleichbar sind (3).

Amerikanische Konzepte vor allem für den praktischen Bereich (Kochrezepte, Schulungsprogramme, Betreuungsstrukturen) sind nicht 1:1 nach Deutschland übertragbar. Die deutschsprachige Literatur zum Thema für medizinisches Personal und Eltern ist spärlich. Es gibt ein Buch mit Rezeptvorschlägen (40); eine allgemeiner gehaltene Patientenbroschüre wurde kürzlich veröffentlicht (41). Ob es gelingen wird, die international guten Erfahrungen zum Nutzen einer unserer am schwierigsten zu behandelnden Patientengruppe auch breiter erfolgreich zu nutzen, wird die Zukunft zeigen. Hierfür wird wichtig sein, dass sich eine vernünftig große Zahl an Kliniken der ketogenen Diät widmet, und diese in einem gegenseitigen Austausch steht. Ein weiterer Schritt auf diesem Weg ist der zweite Workshop ketogene Diät in Essen 12/02.

Literatur

1. Camfield CS, Camfield PR, Gordon K, Wirrell E, Dooley JM (1996) Incidence of Epilepsy in Childhood and Adolescence: A Population-Based Study in Nova Scotia from 1977 to 1985. Epilepsia 37:19–23
2. Klepper J, Ecker D, Burkart P, Leiendecker B, Voit T, Baumeister FAM (2000) Indikation und Anwendung der ketogenen Diät im Kindesalter 1. Workshop ketogene Diät am 15. Dezember 2000 in Essen. Monatsschr Kinderheilk 149:1383–90
3. Baumeister FAM, Liebhaber GM, Riemann E (2002) Efficacy of the Ketogenic Diet for the Treatment of Refractory Epilepsy in Children. Neuropediatrics 33:A23.
4. Wilder RM (1921) Effects of ketonuria on the course of epilepsy. Mayo Clin Bull 2:307-8
5. Cahill GF jr (1982) Starvation. Trans Am Clin Climatol Assoc 94:1–21
6. Freeman JM, Vining EPG (1999) Seizures decrease rapidly after fasting – Preliminary studies of the ketogenic diet. Arch Pediatr Adolesc Med 153:946–9

7. Gilbert DL, Pyzik PL, Freeman JM (2000) The ketogenic diet: seizure control correlates better with serum beta-hydroxybutyrate than with urine ketones. J Child Neurol 15:787-90
8. Schwartzkroin PA (1999) Mechanisms underlying the anti-epileptic efficacy of the ketogenic diet. Epilepsy Res 37:171–180
9. Freeman JM, Freeman JB, Kelly MT (2000) The ketogenic diet. A treatment for epilepsy. 3. Aufl., Demos Medical Publishing, New York.
10. Sankar R, Sotero de Menezes M (1999) Metabolic and endocrine aspects of the ketogenic diet. Epilepsy Res 37:191–201.
11. Batchelor L, Nance J, Short B (1997) An interdisciplinary team approach to implementing the ketogenic diet for the treatment of seizures. Pediatr Nurs 23:465–71
12. Casey JC, McGrogan J, Pillas D, Pyzik P, Freeman J, Vining EP (1999) The implementation and maintenance of the Ketogenic Diet in children. J Neurosci Nurs 31:294–302
13. Huttenlocher PR, Wilbourn AJ, Signore JM (1971) Medium-chain triglycerides as a therapy for intractable childhood epilepsy. Neurology 21:1097–103
14. Schwartz RH, Eaton J, Bower BD, Aynsley-Green, A (1989) Ketogenic diets in the treatment of epilepsy: short-term clinical effects. Dev Med Child Neurol 31:145–51
15. Swink TD, Vining EP, Freeman JM (1997) The ketogenic diet: 1997. Adv Pediatr 44:297-329
16. Wheless JW (1995) The ketogenic diet: Fa(c)t or Fiction? J child neurol 10:419–23
17. Lefevre F, Aronson N (2000) Ketogenic diet for the treatment of refractory epilepsy in children: A systematic review of efficacy. Pediatrics 105:E46. Volltext frei erhältlich unter: www.pediatrics.org/cgi/content/full/105/4/e46
18. Caraballo R, Tripoli J, Escobal L, Cersosimo R, Tenembaum S, Palacios C, Fejerman N (1998) Dieta cetogenica: eficacia y tolerabilidad en epilepsia refractaria en pediatria. Rev Neurol 26:61–4
19. Edelstein SF, Chrisholm M (1996) Managment of intractable childhood seizures using the non-MCT oil ketogenic diet in 20 patients. J Am Diet Assoc 96:1181–82
20. Panico LR, Demartini MG, Rios VG, Carniello MA (2000) Dieta cetogenica en la epilepsia refractaria infantil: respuesta electroclinica, complicaciones y efectos secundarios. Rev Neurol 31:212–20
21. Panico, LR; Rios, VG; Demartini, MG; Carniello, MA: »Evolucion electroencefalografica de un grupo de pacientes en dieta cetogenica.« Rev Neurol. 2000 Jan 1-15; 30(1): 8–15
22. Freeman JM, Vining EPG, Pillas DJ, Pyzik PL, Casey JC, Kelly LM (1998) The efficacy of the ketogenic diet-1998: a prospective evaluation of intervention in 150 children. Pediatrics 102:1358–63
23. Hassan AM, Keene DL, Whiting SE, Jacob PJ Champagne JR, Humphreys P (1999) Ketogenic diet in the treatment of refractory epilepsy in childhood. Pediatr Neurol 21:548–52
24. Katyal NG, Koehler AN, McGhee B, Foley CM, Crumrine PK (2000) The ketogenic diet in refractory epilepsy: the experience of Children's Hospital of Pittsburgh. Clin Pediatr (Phila) 39:153–9
25. Kinsman SL, Vining EP, Quaskey SA, Mellits D, Freeman JM (1992) Efficacy of the ketogenic diet for intractable seizure disorders: review of 58 cases. Epilepsia 33:1132-6
26. MacCracken KA, Scalisi JC (1999) Development and evaluation of a ketogenic diet program. J Am Diet Assoc 99:1554–8
27. Mak SC, Chi CS, Wan CJ (1999) Clinical experience of ketogenic diet on children with refractory epilepsy. Acta Paediatr Taiwan 40:97–100
28. Maydell BV, Wyllie E, Akhtar N, Kotagal P, Powaski K, Cook K, Weinstock A, Rothner AD (2001) Efficacy of the ketogenic diet in focal versus generalized seizures. Pediatr Neurol 25:208–12
29. Moreno-Villares JM, Oliveros-Leal L, Simón-Heras R, Mateos-Beato F (2001) La vuelta a la dieta cetogénica. Qué papel desempeña en el tratamiento de las convulsiones infantiles refractarias? Rev Neurol 32:1115–9
30. Nordli DR, Kuroda MM, Carroll J, Koenigsberger DY, Hirsch LJ, Bruner HJ, Seidel WT, De Vivo DC (2001) Experience with the ketogenic diet in infants. Pediatrics 108:129–33

31. Vining EP, Freeman JM, Ballaban-Gil K, Camfield CS, Camfield PR, Holmes GL, Shinnar S, Shuman R, Trevathan E, Wheless JW (1998) A multicenter study of the efficacy of the ketogenic diet. Arch Neurol 55:1433–7
32. Furth SL, Casey JC, Pyzik PL, Neu AM, Docimo SG, Vining EP, Freeman JM, Fivush BA (2000) Risk factors for urolithiasis in children on the ketogenic diet. Pediatr Nephrol 15:125-8
33. Best TH, Franz DN, Gilbert DL, Nelson DP, Epstein MR (2000) Cardiac complications in pediatric patients on the ketogenic diet. Neurology 54:2328–30
34. Huttenlocher PR, Hapke RJ (1990) A Follow-up study of intractable seizures in childhood. Ann Neurol 28:699–705
35. Marson AG, Kadir ZA Hutton JL et al. (1997) The new antiepileptic drugs: A systematic review of their efficacy and tolerability. Epilepsia 38:859–80
36. Kiene H (2001) Komplementäre Methodenlehre der klinischen Forschung – Cognition-based Medicine. Springer, Berlin, Heidelberg, New York.
37. Hemingway C, Freeman JM, Pillas DJ, Pyzik PL (2001) The ketogenic diet: A 3- to 6-year follow-up of 150 children enrolled prospectively. Pediatrics 108:898–905
38. Pulsifer MB, Gordon JM, Brandt J, Vining EP, Freeman JM (2001): Effects of ketogenic diet on development and behavior: Preliminary report of a prospective study. Dev Med Child Neurol 43: 301–6
39. Nordli DR, De Vivo DC (1997) The ketogenic diet revisited: Back to the future. Epilepsia 38:743–9
40. Reidelbach S (2000) Die ketogene Diät. Ketogene Rezepte für eine Diätbehandlung bei Epilepsien im Kindesalter und Glukosetransporterdefekt. Reha-Verlag GmbH, Remagen. ISBN 3-88239-229-0 (auch direkt über die Verfasserin zu beziehen: Susanne Reidelbach, Diät und Ernährungsberatung, Tel: 0177–3393488)
41. Klepper J, Leiendecker B, Szcerbak B, Mallm C (2002) Die Ketogene Diät – Grundlagen, Einsatzgebiete, Berechung und Anwendung – Ein Ratgeber mit praktischen Anleitungen. Zu beziehen über Milupa GmbH, Tel: 06172–99–1187

Ketogene Diät bei Rett-Syndrom: Ein Fallbericht

G. M. Liebhaber, E. Riemann, F. A. M. Baumeister

Zusammenfassung

Bisher gibt es in der Literatur nur eine Arbeit über die Behandlung des Rett-Syndroms mit Ketogener Diät. Haas et al. beschrieben 1986 die positiven Effekte der Ketogenen Diät auf Anfallsfrequenz und Verhalten bei Patientinnen mit Rett-Syndrom (4).

Wir berichten über eine Patientin mit Rett-Syndrom, die wegen ihrer therapierefraktären Epilepsie mit Ketogener Diät behandelt wurde. Die Ketogene Diät wurde im Alter von 8 Jahren begonnen und führte zu einer Anfallsreduktion um 70%, sowie zu Verbesserungen in den Bereichen Sprache und Verhalten.

Die Diagnose Rett-Syndrom wurde molekulargenetisch gesichert. Die nachgewiesene Mutation im MECP2-Gen (Ser134Cys) wurde bisher nur bei Patientinnen mit klassischem Rett-Syndrom beschrieben (2, 5, 9).

Dieser Fallbericht stützt die von Haas et al. beschriebene Beobachtung, dass eine Ketogene Diät bei Patientinnen mit Rett-Syndrom einen positiven Einfluss auf Anfallsfrequenz und Verhalten besitzt.

Hintergrund

Das Rett-Syndrom (6) ist eine häufige Ursache für geistige Behinderung bei Mädchen, mit einer geschätzten Häufigkeit von 1:10–15 000 (1). Molekulargenetisch beruht das Rett-Syndrom auf einer Mutation im MeCP2-Gen auf dem Genlocus Xp28 (1), welche sich bei 70–80% der Mädchen mit Rett-Syndrom nachweisen lässt (2, 5, 9).

Klinisch ist das Rett-Syndrom charakterisiert durch Verlust von erlernten sinnvollen Handfunktionen, Regression des Verhaltens, schwere Sprachstörung, schwere psychomotorische Retardierung, stereotype Handbewegungen, Ataxie und Apraxie nach unauffälliger Pränatal- und Perinatalperiode und unauffälliger psychomotorischer Entwicklung in den ersten 6 Monaten. Desweiteren kommt es bei normalem Kopfumfang bei Geburt zur Verlangsamung des Kopfwachstums. (8). Weitere unterstützende Diagnosekriterien sind Atemstörungen, pathologisches EEG, Krampfanfälle und Kleinwuchs (8). Patientinnen mit Rett-Syndrom zeigen eine progressive Verschlechterung ihrer motorischen, geistigen und sozialen Fähigkeiten.

Bisher gibt es nur eine Arbeit, welche die Effekte der Ketogenen Diät bei Patientinnen mit Rett-Syndrom beschreibt. 1986 berichteten Haas et al. über positive Effekte einer Ketogenen Diät auf Anfallsfrequenz und Verhalten bei Mädchen mit Rett-Syndrom und therapierefraktärer Epilepsie (4). Von 5 Mädchen unter Ketogener Diät wurde eines anfallsfrei, eines zeigte eine Anfallsreduktion um 75%, zwei weitere um 50%. Bei allen Patientinnen konnten positive Veränderungen im Verhalten festgestellt werden (4).

Die Ketogene Diät ist eine Ernährungsform mit sehr hohem Fett-, ausreichendem Protein- und sehr geringem Kohlenhydratanteil. Sie wurde von Wilder 1921 entwickelt, um eine ketogene Stoffwechsellage ähnlich wie im Hungerzustand herbeizuführen mit dem Ziel, hierdurch über längere Zeit den antikonvulsiven Effekt des Fastens zu imitieren (7). Nachdem die Ketogene Diät beinahe in Vergessenheit geraten war, erlebte sie in den letzten Jahren eine Renaissance in der Behandlung therapierefraktärer Epilepsien (3, 7, 10). Der folgende Fallbericht beschreibt den Verlauf einer Patientin mit Rett-Syndrom, die auf die Behandlung mit Ketogener Diät angesprochen hat.

Fallbereicht

Die 12-jährige Patientin wurde termingerecht und komplikationslos als erstes Kind ihrer gesunden Eltern geboren.

Im ersten Lebensjahr fiel sie durch vermehrte Unruhe, Schlafstörungen, Schreien, Trinkschwäche und schließlich durch verzögerte statomotorische Entwicklung auf. Sie erlernte mit 12 Monaten zu krabbeln und mit 21 Monaten frei zu laufen. Die Sprachentwicklung setzte zeitgerecht ein, blieb jedoch auf niedrigem Niveau stehen. Sie sprach nur kurze, einzelne Sätze und verfügte über einen sehr geringen Wortschatz.

Im Alter von 4 Jahren traten atypische Absencen und Myoklonien auf. Das EEG zeigte parallel zu den Anfällen hypersynchrone Muster. Die Anfälle traten statusartig in einer Frequenz von bis zu 40 Ereignissen/Stunde auf. Valproinsäure, Vigabatrin und Clobazam blieben erfolglos, Carbamazepin, Mesosuximid und Phenytoin wurden nicht vertragen. Letzlich führte die Kombination von Phenobarbital und Sultiam zu einer Reduktion der Anfälle auf 20–30 pro Tag.

Neben der Anfallsproblematik traten zunehmend eine geistige Retardierung, Abbau kognitiver Funktionen, autistische Verhaltenszüge und ein Kleinwuchs in Erscheinung.

Wegen der therapieresistenten Anfälle wurde im Alter von 8 Jahren eine klassische Ketogene Diät (4:1) nach dem Protokoll der John-Hopkins-Universität (3,7) begonnen, während die antikonvulsive Therapie mit Phenobarbital und Sultiam unverändert fortgeführt wurde. Die Ketogene Diät führte zu einer Anfallsreduktion auf 10 Anfälle/Tag. Mutter und Lehrerin berichten von einer deutlichen Besserung von Aufnahmefähigkeit, Kontaktfreudigkeit, Verhalten und Sprache. Augenblicklich spricht die Patientin in längeren, zusammenhängenden Sätzen, hat einen deutlich größeren Wortschatz, spricht mehr und klarer.

Ein Ersatz von Phenobarbital durch Lamotrigen brachte eine weitere Reduktion der absenceartigen Zustände auf 5/Tag. Bei akzidentellen Auslassversuchen (Diätfehlern), die mit verminderter Ketonurie verbunden waren, kam es vermehrt zu Anfällen.

Die letzten EEG-Untersuchungen zeigten außer einer retardierten Grundaktivität keine pathologischen Befunde. Als Nebenwirkung der Ketogenen Diät kam es bei der Patientin zu einer Obstipation, welche sich durch Magnesiumgabe gut behandeln ließ. Desweiteren fand sich im EKG eine QT-Zeit an der oberen Norm.

Im Alter von 11 Jahren fielen erstmals Handstereotypien und Hyperventilation auf. Die Diagnose eines Rett-Syndrom wurde durch den Nachweis einer Mutation im MeCP2-Gen bestätigt.

Diskussion

Die beschriebene Patientin zeigt für ein Mädchen mit Rett-Syndrom einen außerordentlich milden Verlauf mit deutlicher Anfallsreduktion und deutlicher Verhaltensverbesserung unter Ketogener Diät. Die bei der Patientin nachgewiesene Mutation ist bisher nur bei Patientinnen mit klassischem Rett-Syndrom beschrieben, welche einen klinisch schwereren Verlauf zeigten (2, 5, 9).

Bereits Haas beschrieb, dass bei 4 von 5 Mädchen mit Rett-Syndrom, die er wegen therapierefraktärer Epilepsie mit Ketogener Diät behandelte, eine Rückgang der Anfallsfrequenz um 50–100% erreicht werden konnte. Außerdem führte die Ketogene Diät bei allen 5 Mädchen – in unterschiedlichem Ausmaß – zu Verbesserung des sozialen Verhaltens und der motorischen Funktionen (4).

Dieser Fallbericht stützt die von Haas et al. beschriebene Beobachtung des positven Einflusses einer Ketogenen Diät auf Epilepsie und Verhalten bei Patientinnen mit Rett-Syndrom.

Literatur

1. Amir RE, Van den Veyver IB, Wan M, Tran CQ, Francke U, Zoghbi HY (1999) Rett syndrome is caused by mutations in X-linked MECP2, encoding methyl-CpG-binding protein 2. Nature Genet 23: 185–188
2. Cheadle JP, Gill H, Fleming N, Maynard J, Kerr A, Leonard H, Krawczak M, Cooper DN, Lynch S, Thomas N, Hughes H, Hultén M, Ravine D, Sampson JR, Clarke A (2000) Long-read sequence analysis of the MECP2 gene in Rett syndrome patients: correlation of disease severity with mutation type and location. Hum Mol Genet 9: 11119–1129
3. Freeman JM, Kelly MT, Freeman JB (1996) The epilepsy diet treatment – An introduction to the ketogenic diet. 2. Aufl. Demos Vermande, New York
4. Haas RH, Rice MA, Trauner DA, Merritt T (1986) Therapeutic effects of a ketogenic diet in Rett syndrome. Am J Med Genet Suppl. 1: 225–246
5. Huppke P, Laccone F, Kramer N, Engel W, Hanefeld F (2000) Rett syndrome: analysis of MECP2 and clinical characterization of 31 patients. Hum Mol Genet 9: 1369–1375
6. Rett A (1966) Über ein eigenartiges hirnatrophisches Syndrom bei Hyperammonämie im Kindesalter. Wien Med Wochenschr 116: 723–726
7. Swink TT, Vining EPG, Fremann JM (1997) The Ketogenic diet: 1997. Chapter 9 in: Advances in Pediatrics. St. Louis, Mosby-Year Book Inc. Vol 44, pp. 297–329
8. The Rett Syndrome Diagnostic Criteria Work Group (1988) Diagnostic criteria for Rett syndrome. Ann Neurol 23: 425–428
9. Vacca M, Filippini F, Budillon A, Rossi V, Mercadante G, Manzati E, Gualandi F, Bigoni S, Trabanelli C, Pini, G, Calzori E, Ferlini A, Meloni I, Hayek G, Zappella M, Renieri A, D'Urso M, D'Esposito M, MacDonald F, Kerr A, Dhanjal S, Hultén M (2001) Mutation analysis of the MECP2 gene in British and Italian Rett syndrome females. J Mol Med 78: 648–655
10. Wheless JW, Baumgartner J, Ghanbari C (2001) Vagus nerve stimulation and the ketogenic diet. Neurol Clin 19: 371–407

Erfahrungen mit Topiramat-Plasmaspiegel-bestimungen bei Kindern mit Epilepsie

S. Vlaho, E. Solem, V. Boda, M. Wesendahl, H. Böhles, M. Kieslich

Einleitung

Die Bedeutung von Topiramat(TPM)-Plasmaspiegelbestimungen wird kontrovers diskutiert. Insbesondere zu therapeutischen Grenzwerten bei Kindern bezüglich Nebenwirkungen, Dosis- und Altersabhängigkeit gibt es bislang wenig Daten.

Das Monitoring der antiepileptischen Therapie über Spiegelbestimmung ist ein allgemein akzeptiertes Vorgehen in der klinischen Praxis. Zur Regelung eines sinnvollen Einsatzes hat die International League Against Epilepsy eine Richtlinie zum antikonvulsiven Therapiemonitoring verabschiedet:

Pharmakologsiche Eigenschaften welche ein therapeutisches Monitoring eines bestimmten Antikonvulsiva potentiell sinnvoll erscheinen lassen, sind: 1. Nachgewiesene verstärkte interindividuelle pharmakokinetische Variabilität. 2. Intraindividuelle Schwankung in der Kinetik (bezogen auf pharnakokinetische Medikamenteninteraktion, Zweiterkrankung oder Altersabhängigkeit). 3. Nachgewiesene Korrelation zwischen der Medikamentenkonzentration und seines therapeutischen oder toxischen Effekts. 4. Enge therapeutische Breite (1; 2; 3).

Die genaue Beziehung zwischen klinischen Zeichen der Toxizität und Plasma-TPM-Spiegeln ist gegenwärtig nicht gesichert. Der große interindividuelle Unterschied in der TPM-Clearancerate, die mögliche Aufklärung eventueller klinischer Interaktioen, sowie die Informationsgewinnung bei eingeschränkter Compliance, lassen das therapeutische Monitoring von TPM wünschenswert erscheinen.

TPM ist ein Antikonvulsiva, welches über eine Verstärkung der GABA-Rezeptorenaktivität, der Blockade der spannungsabhängigen Na-Kanäle, sowie über die Antagonisierung der Kainate/AMPA-Glutamat-Rezeptoren wirkt. TPM wird oral aufgenommen, schnell absorbiert und minimal verstoffwechselt. Peak-dose Plasmakonzentrationen werden ca. 2–3 Stunden nach Einnahme erreicht. Steady-state Plasmakonzentrationen nehmen annähernd linear mit der verabreichten Dosis zu. Die Plasmaproteinbindung ist gering (in der Regel weniger als 15%). Die Elimination erfolgt vorwiegend über die Niere mit einer Elimiationshalbwertszeit von 20–30 Stunden. Plasma-TPM-Spiegel liegen in den bisher veröffenlichten Studien zwischen 2–5 mg/l. in der Regel wurde eine Anfallskontrolle mit TPM-Plasmaspiegeln zwischen 3,4–5,2 mg/l erreicht (4; 5).

Tab. 1: Deskriptive Patientendaten

	Altersgruppen in Jahren 0–7 Jahre	> 7 Jahre	Gesamt
Messungen (n)	31	35	66
Patienten (n)	13	8	24
Alter (Jahr, Monat)			
Mittelwert	4,26	12,59	8,7
Range	0,75–6,92	7,08–20,67	0,75–20,67
Geschlecht (m/w) %	46/54	61/39	54/46
Epilepsietyp	Symptomatische therapieresistente Epilepsien		
Messungen (n): *TPM–Monotherapie*	1	2	3
TPM–Add on bei *Einfachtherapie*	17	19	36
(Mit VPA /Induktoren)	(6/11)	(4/15)	(10/26)
TPM–Add on bei *Zweifachtherapie*	10	9	19
(Mit VPA /Induktoren)	(2/8)	(8/1)	(10/9)
TPM–Add on bei *Mehrfachtherapie*	3	5	8
(Mit VPA /Induktoren)	(2/1)	(5/0)	(7/1)

Methode

Die quantitative Bestimmung von TPM erfolgte in heparinisiertem Plasma über ein Fluoreszens-Polarisations-Immunoassay (INNOFLOUR® TOPIRAMATE Assay System, OXIS International Inc.) mittels TDxFLx® Analyser (6). Dieses System erbrachte in verschiedenen Studien exakte Bestimmungen für heparinisierte Plasmauntersuchungen mit Variationskoeffizienten (Inter- und Intraanalyse) von <4% (7; 8). Die Blutentnahme erfolgte vor Einnahme der Morgendosis (Talkonzentration).

Ergebnisse

Insgesamt wurden in einem Zeitraum von 15 Monaten 66 TPM-Plasmaspiegelbestimmungen von 24 Patienten (11 weiblich und 13 männlich) analysiert. Es wurden keine schwerwiegenden Nebenwirkungen registriert. Bei allen Patienten handelte es sich um therapierefraktäre, meist symptomatische Epilepsien, wobei TPM sowohl als Monotherapie, wie auch als Add-on Medikation in 2- bis 4fach-Therapie gegeben wurde (Tab. 1).

Das durchschnittliche Alter betrug 8,7 Jahre (Range 0,75–20,67 J.). Die bei einem durchschnittlichen Gewicht von 27,6 kg (Range 6,0–56,0 kg) applizierte

Tab. 2: TPM-Dosis-Plasmaspiegelbeziehungen

	Altersgruppen in Jahren **0–7 Jahre**	**> 7 Jahre**	**Gesamt**
Gewicht (kg)			
Mittelwert	15,96	37,94	27,6
Range	6,0–25,6	19–56	6,0–56,0
Tägliche Dosierung TPM (mg/kgKG)			
Mittelwert	5,19	4,36	4,75
Range	0,93–8,48	0,55–7,15	0,55–8,65
Plasmaspiegelbestimmung (µg/ml)			
Mittelwert	2,52	3,70	3,15
Range	0,31–9,7	0,49–11,1	0,8–11,1

TPM-Dosis betrug im Mittel 4,75 mg/kgKG/d (Range 0,55–8,65). Der mittlere TPM-Plasmaspiegel lag bei 3,15 µg/ml (Range 0,8-11,1 µg/ml) (Tab. 2).

In einer Subgruppe mit Patienten von 0–7 Jahren (Abb. 2) lagen die täglichen TPM-Dosierungen mit durchschnittlich 5,1 mg/kgKG/d (Range 0,93–8,48 mg/kgKG/d) höher als in der Subgruppe mit Patienten >7 Jahre (Abb. 3) (mit durchschnittlich 4,36 mg/kgKG/d (Range 0,55–7,15 mg/kgKG/d). TPM in Comedikation mit Enzyminduktoren ergab in unseren Untersuchungen niedrigere TPM-Plasmaspiegel (Abb. 4) mit der Folge der Höherdosierung zur Erzielung des

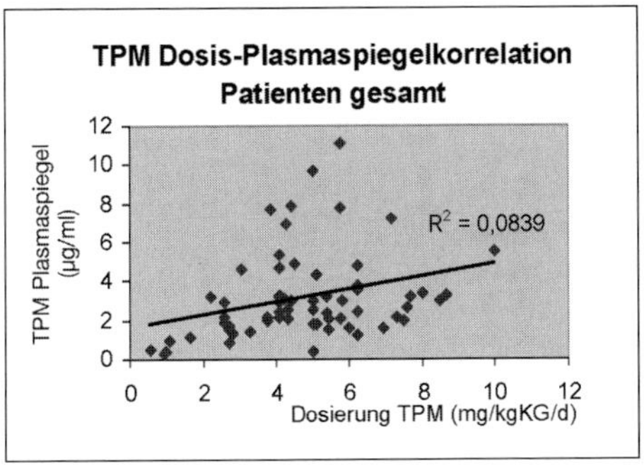

Abb. 1

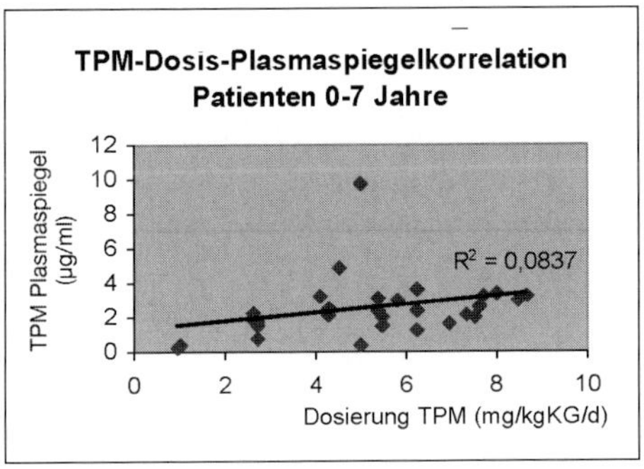

Abb. 2

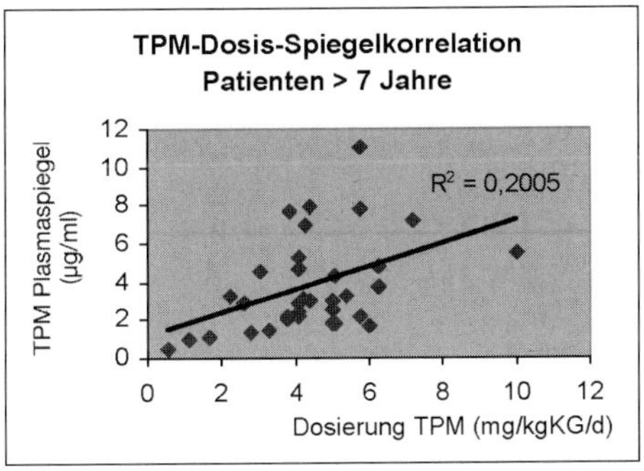

Abb. 3

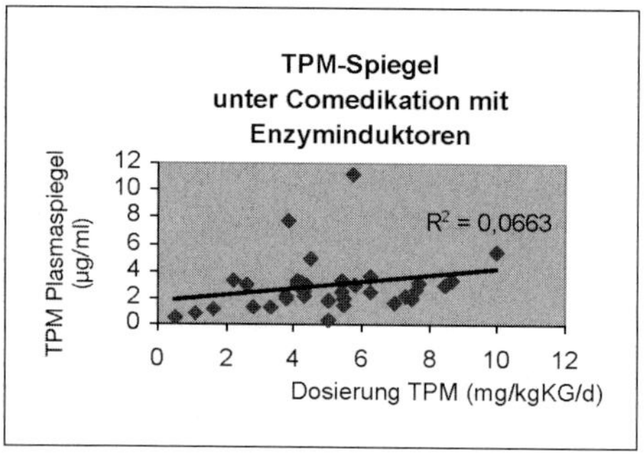

Abb. 4

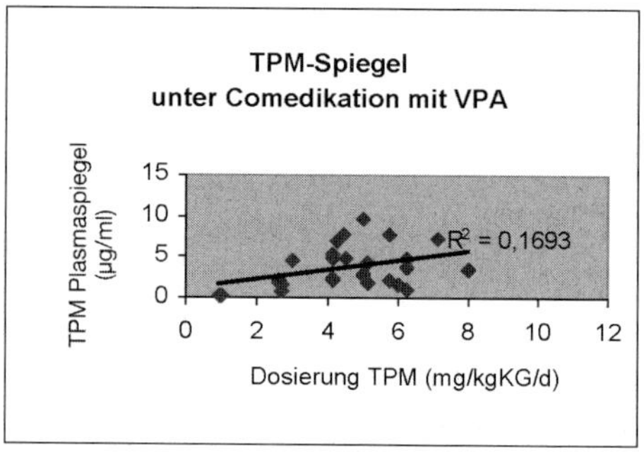

Abb. 5

gleichen therapeutischen Effekts. Dagegen zeigte sich bei TPM in Comedikation zu VPA (Abb. 5) erhöhte TPM-Plasmaspiegel mit der Folge der Dosisreduktion zur Erzielung des gleichen therapeutischen Effektes.

Diskussion

Die an einem pädiatrischen Patientengut gemessenen Dosis-Spiegel-Verhältnisse sind vergleichbar mit den in der Literatur publizierten Daten.

Demnach steigt die TPM-Plasmakonzentration bei Kindern wie Erwachsenen linear und proportional mit der applizierten Dosis. Die Plasmaclearance liegt jedoch bei Kindern durchschnittlich 55% höher als bei Erwachsenen. Somit können die bei gleicher oraler Dosis im Kindesalter um ca. 33% niedrigeren TPM-Plasmakonzentrationen erklärt werden. Insbesondere bei Kleinkindern kommt dies verstärkt zum Ausdruck. Kinder unter 7 Jahren benötigten höhere Dosierungen zum Erreichen vergleichbarer Plasmaspiegel.

Wenn TPM in Comedikation zu enzyminduzierenden Antiepileptika gegeben wird, reduziert sich die Plasmaeliminationshalbertszeit auf 12–15 h (in Abwesenheit von Enzyminduktoren beträt diese bei gesunden Erwachsenen ca. 19–23 h) (9). Dies hat bei gleicher Dosierung niedrigere TPM-Plasmaspiegel zur Folge. TPM führt zu einem moderaten Abfall der VPA-Plasmakonzentration über die Induktion der β-Oxidation. Bei gleicher Dosierung hat dies höhere TPM-Plasmaspiegel zur Folge. Die niedrige Proteinbindung macht Proteinbindungsinteraktionen unwahrscheinlich.

Bisher gibt es keinen etablierten Plasmaspiegel-Zielbereich für TPM, dafür fehlt es bislang an ausreichenden Studien zu Konzentrations-Effekt-Korrelationen. In dieser Untersuchung traten bei Plasmaspiegeln bis zu 11,1 µg/ml keine kritischen Nebenwirkungen auf. Die Dosierung sollte anhand therapeutischen Effektes erfolgen. Aufgrund des Fehlens von gundlegenden, verbindlichen Angaben zu Zielspiegeln der neueren Antikonvulsiva (z.B.: Lamotrigin, Topiramat, Tiagabin), kann die routinemäßige Bestimmung der Serumplasmaspiegel nicht empfohlen werden. Unabhängig davon sind aber Plasmaspiegelbestimmungen bei ausgewählten Patienten nützlich, besonders bei jenen

Patienten, bei welchen durch Zweiterkrankung oder Gabe von zusätzlichen Medikamenten pharmakokinetische Änderungen verursacht werden können, bei Patienten mit erwarteter niedriger Therapiecompliance, sowie bei Verdacht auf Intoxikation. Ein Therapiemonitoring kann prinzipiell empfohlen werden bei Langzeittherapie eines potentiell toxischen Medikamentes um eine mögliche Überexposition zu vermeiden und somit eine Reduktion des Risikos einer chronischen Nebenwirkung zu ermöglichen.

Schlussfolgerungen

- Patienten <7 Jahre brauchen höhere TPM-Dosierungen um gleiche Plasmaspiegel zu erreichen.
- Bei TPM in Comedikation zu VPA ergeben sich höhere TPM-Plasmakonzentrationen
- Bei TPM in Comedikation zu Enzyminduktoren ergeben sich niedrigere TPM-Plasmakonzentrationen
- Bei Plasmaspiegeln bis zu 11,1 µg/ml traten keine kritischen Nebenwirkungen auf.
- Therapeutisches Monitoring von TPM ist in bestimmten ausgewählten Fällen begründet (z.B.: V.a. Intoxikation, Complianceschwierigkeiten), eine generelle Empfehlung zur Spiegelbestimmung kann zum gegenwärtigen Zeitpunk nicht gegeben werden.

Literatur

1. Tomson T, Johannessen SI. Therapeutic monitoring of the new antiepileptic drugs. Eur J Clin Pharmacol 2000; 55(10):697–705.
2. International League Against Epilepsy. Guidelines for therapeutic monitoring on antiepileptic drugs. Commission on Antiepileptic Drugs, International League Against Epilepsy. Epilepsia 1993; 34(4):585–587.
3. International League Against Epilepsy. Guidelines for clinical evaluation of antiepileptic drugs. Commission on Antiepileptic Drugs of the International League Against Epilepsy. Epilepsia 1989; 30(4):400–408.
4. Reife R, Pleger G, Doose D, Lim P, Ward C. Topiramate PK/PD analysis. Epilepsia 1995; 36:152.
5. Perucca E, Bialer M. The clinical pharmacokinetics of the newer antiepileptic drugs. Focus on topiramate, zonisamide and tigabine. Clin Pharmacokinet 1996; 31:29–46.
6. Oxis International Inc. InnoFlour(R) Topiramate Assay System. 1997. Portland, OR, Oxis International, Inc.
7. Masucci JA, Ortegon ME, Jones WJ, Shank RP, Caldwell GW. In vivo microdialysis and liquid chromatography/thermospray mass spectrometry of the novel anticonvulsant 2,3:4,5-bis-O-(1- methylethylidene)-beta-D-fructopyranose sulfamate (topiramate) in rat brain fluid. J Mass Spectrom 1998; 33(1):85–88.
8. Berry DJ, Patsalos PN. Comparison of topiramate concentrations in plasma and serum by fluorescence polarization immunoassay. Ther Drug Monit 2000; 22(4):460–464.
9. Mozayani A, Carter J, Nix R. Distribution of topiramate in a medical examiner's case. J Anal Toxicol 1999; 23(6):556–558.

Levetiracetam: Wirkung und Nebenwirkung im Kindes- und Jugendalter

A. Wiemer-Kruel, H. Schneble

Zusammenfassung

Retrospektiv wurden 101 Kinder, Jugendliche und junge Erwachsene der Kinderklinik des Epilepsiezentrums Kork mit schweren, therapieresistenten Epilepsien untersucht, die in der Zeit von Juni 2000 bis November 2001 mit Levetiracetam behandelt wurden.

Einleitung

Levetiracetam (LEV) ist ein neues Antiepilepticum, das seit dem 1.11.2000 zur Behandlung fokaler Epilepsien bei Patienten ab 16 Jahren in Deutschland offiziell zugelassen ist. Bei jüngeren Kindern kann es vorerst nur im Rahmen eines individuellen Heilversuchs eingesetzt werden. Der spezifische Wirkungsmechanismus ist bis jetzt nicht bekannt. Nebenwirkungen werden als gering eingeschätzt, insbesondere sind toxische Erscheinungen bisher nicht berichtet worden. Bei den bisher bekannt gewordenen Nebenwirkungen handelt es sich vor allem um Schwindel, Müdigkeit, allgemeine Schwäche und Begünstigung von Infektionen.

Methode/Untersuchungsgruppe

Seit Juni 2000 wurden insgesamt 101 meist mehrfachbehinderte Kinder, Jugendliche (n=80) und junge Erwachsene (n=21) des Epilepsiezentrums Kork aus Ambulanz, Klinik oder Langzeitbereich mit schwer einstellbaren, therapieresistenten Epilepsien (n=65 weiblich, n=36 männlich) mit LEV behandelt und retrospektiv untersucht. Die Altersstruktur unserer Patienten war relativ breit gefächert (siehe Tab. 1), 2 Patienten waren jünger als 1 Jahr. Die Anzahl der vor

Tab. 1: Alter der Patienten

Jahre	**<5**	**5–10**	**11–15**	**16–20**	**>20**
n	7	22	28	23	21

Tab. 2: Anzahl der zuvor verwendeten Antiepileptika

AED	**<5**	**5–10**	**11–15**	**>15**
n	3	35	48	15

Tab. 3: Epilepsiedauer bis zum Einsatz von LEV

Jahre	≤5	6–10	11–15	>15
n	21	23	26	31

Tab. 4: Behandlungsdauer der Patienten, die noch unter LEV-Therapie stehen (n=53)

Monate	≤3	4–6	7–9	10–12	13–15	>15
n	8	15	15	10	2	3

LEV verabreichten Antiepileptika war in unserem Kollektiv hoch (siehe Tab. 2), d.h. LEV war immer Mittel fernerer Wahl; dementsprechend war auch die Epilepsiedauer bis zum Einsatz von LEV hoch (siehe Tab. 3). 19 Patienten hatten eine generalisierte, 11 eine nicht klassifizierbare, 8 eine kryptogen fokale und 63 eine symptomatisch fokale Epilepsie. Die Dosis von LEV richtete sich nach der klinischen Wirksamkeit; die Initialdosis lag bei 20–30 mg/kg/die, die mittlere Enddosis bei 30–60 mg/kg/die, wobei in Einzelfällen Dosierungen bis 100 mg/kg/die eingesetzt und auch gut vertragen wurden.

Von den insgesamt 101 Patienten hatten 48 (47,5%) die Behandlung zum Zeitpunkt der retrospektiven Überprüfung bereits wieder abgebrochen (siehe auch Tab. 6). Bei 8 (8/48=16,7%) Kindern war die Behandlungszeit kürzer als 1 Monat, bei 34 betrug die Therapiedauer 1–6 Monate (34/48=70,8%) und 6 brachen zwischen dem 7.–12. Monat die Therapie ab (6/48=12,5%). Eine Übersicht über die jeweilige Therapiedauer bei den 53 Patienten, die zum Zeitpunkt der Erhebung noch unter Therapie mit LEV standen, gibt Tabelle 4. Die maximale Behandlungsdauer mit LEV betrug bei 2 Patienten 17 Monate.

Ergebnisse

Von unseren 101 Patienten zeigten zum Zeitpunkt der Untersuchung 7 eine mehr als 50%ige Anfallsreduktion, die auf den Einsatz von LEV zurückgeführt werden konnte; dabei konnte kein Zusammenhang zwischen einer bestimmten Epilepsieform und dem Therapieerfolg hergestellt werden. Eine solche Beziehung fand sich auch nicht bei Patienten mit einer Anfallsreduktion zwischen 25–50% und < 25% (siehe Tab. 5; die Prozentangaben sollen Tendenzen aufzeigen und sind nicht im statistischen Sinne zu betrachten;). Kein langfristiger Effekt fand sich etwas vermehrt bei den generalisierten Epilepsien (n=12/19, entsprechend 63,2%). Bemerkenswert ist, dass wir bei unseren Patienten auffällig häufig eine Anfallsprovokation beim Eindosieren des Levetiracetams beobachteten (10 von 101 Patienten (9,9%)). Eine Anfallsprovokation sahen wir allerdings in vereinzelten Fällen auch beim Abdosieren des LEV, selbst dann, wenn die LEV-Therapie zuvor keinen Einfluss auf die Anfallsfrequenz gehabt hatte und deshalb wieder beendet worden war (siehe Tab. 6) – immerhin bei 5/48 Patienten (10,4%). Auch konnten Anfallsserien, meist tonischer Art, vermehrt auftreten, wobei diese aber grundsätzlich in der Vorgeschichte der Patienten bekannt waren, jedoch in

Tab. 5: Ergebnisse der LEV-Behandlung bei den einzelnen Epilepsieformen

Epilepsieform	**Anfallsreduktion > 50%**	**Anfallsreduktion 25–50%**	**Anfallsreduktion < 25%**	**kein Effekt**	**Anfallsprovokation bei Eindosierung**	**keine Rückmeldung**
kryptogen fokal (n=8)	1 (12,5%)	1 (12,5%)	1 (12,5%)	3 (37,5%)	2 (25%)	0
sympto. fokal (n=63)	1 (1,6%)	15 (23,8%)	16 (25,4%)	26 (41,3%)	5 (7,9%)	0
idiopath. gen. (n=19)	3 (15,8%)	2 (10,5%)	1 (5,3%)	12 (63,2%)	1 (5,3%)	0
fokal und/oder gen. (n=11)	2 (18,4%)	0	1 (9,1%)	5 (45,5%)	2 (18,2%)	1 (9,1%)
insgesamt (n=101)	**7 (6,9%)**	**18 (17,8%)**	**19 (18,8%)**	**46 (45,6%)**	**10 (9,9%)**	**1 (0,99%)**

Tab. 6: Weitere Effekte von LEV

Epilepsieform	**Initialeffekt**	**Abbruch der Therapie**	**Anfallsprovokation beim Absetzen**	**Provokation von Anfallsserien**
kryptogen fokal (n=8)	1/8 (12,5%)	4/8 (50%)	2/4 (50%)	0
symptomatisch fokal (n=63)	22/63 (34,9%)	28/63 (44,4%)	2/28 (7,1%)	5/63 (7,9%)
idiopathisch generalisiert (n=19)	8/19 (42,1%)	11/19 (57,9%)	0	0
fokal und/oder generalisiert (n=11)	1/11 (9,1%)	5/11 (45,5%)	1/5 (20%)	1/11 (9,1%)
insgesamt (n = 101)	**32/101 (31,7%)**	**48/101 (47,5%)**	**5/48 (10,4%)**	**6/101 (5,9%)**

der letzten Zeit nicht im Vordergrund gestanden hatten (Tab. 6). Einen Wirkungsverlust sahen wir vor allem in den ersten 3–6 Monaten der Therapie (Tab. 6). Ein Initialeffekt mit Anfallsreduktion um mehr als 50% und dann folgenden Wirkungsverlust wurde besonders bei den generalisierten Epilepsien (8/19 Pat. = 42,1%) beobachtet.

Nebenwirkungen traten bei 44 Patienten (43%) auf. Im einzelnen (Doppelnennungen sind möglich) zeigten sich 10x Provokation isolierter Anfälle (Tab. 6), 9x Aggressivität, je 8x Müdigkeit und Schlafstörungen, 6x Provokation von Anfallsserien (bei u.U. gleicher Anfallsfrequenz, Tab. 6), 5x Anfallsprovokation in der Absetzphase (Tab. 6), 3x Aggravierung von Verhaltensauffälligkeiten, je 2x Gewichtsverlust, Getriebenheit, Sprachstörungen, Hautprobleme (davon 1x eine allergisch-toxische Reaktion im Sinne einer ausgeprägten Akne vulgaris conglobata, nachgewiesen im Lymphozytenstimulationstest), je 1x Infektanfälligkeit, Tremorzunahme und 1x eine psychische Befindlichkeitsverbesserung.

Eine eindeutige Korrelation zwischen *Blutspiegel* und Dosis/kg Körpergewicht konnte nicht hergestellt werden; auch schwankten die Werte der Plasmakonzentrationen innerhalb eines Tagesprofils erheblich.

Die *Therapiekombinationen* mit LEV waren vielfältig, insgesamt 51 verschiedene, u.a. mitverursacht durch die hohe Anzahl der Polytherapien (28x eine 3-er- und 14x eine 4-er-Therapie) entsprechend unserem sehr therapieschwierigen Patientenklientel. Die häufigste Therapiekombination war VPA/LEV (10x). Beeinflussungen der Blutspiegel der Komedikamente durch die Add-on-Therapie mit LEV konnten nicht verifiziert werden.

Schlussfolgerung

Unsere Ergebnisse in der Kinderklinik Kork bezüglich der Effektivität von Levetiracetam sind nicht so positiv wie die der großen amerikanischen und europäischen Doppelblind-Studien, die eine mehr als 50%ige Anfallsreduktion bei 32–40% der Patienten belegen. Dies mag an unserem Patientenkollektiv mit sehr schweren Epilepsien und einer häufig desolaten Anfallssituation liegen.

Bezogen auf unser Patientenkollektiv kann LEV nicht nur eine Effektivität bei fokalen, sondern insbesondere auch bei generalisierten Epilepsien mit Myoklonien aufweisen. Leider ist jedoch gerade bei dieser Epilepsieform bei einer hohen Anzahl von Patienten eine Toleranzentwicklung bzw. ein Wirkungsverlust zu verzeichnen.

Die Nebenwirkungen von LEV waren gering, nur in einem Fall allergisch-toxischer Natur unter dem Bild einer Akne vulgaris conglobata; wichtig zu erwähnen ist allerdings die mögliche Anfallsprovokation, sowohl beim Ein- wie beim Abdosieren, auch die Provokation von u.U. dramatischen, überwiegend tonischen Anfallsserien.

Trotz des nur selten anhaltenden Therapieerfolgs (bei allerdings problemhaften Epilepsien) und trotz der Nebenwirkungen (insbesondere Anfallsprovokation) stellt LEV für uns bei Kindern und Jugendlichen mit behandlungsschwierigen Epilepsien durchaus eine lohnende Therapieoption dar.

Literatur

1. Bauer, J., Oehring, R.D., Elger, C.E.: Generalisiertes Exanthem bei Komedikation mit Levetiracetam. Z Epileptol 14:23–24, 2001
2. Ben-Menachem, E., Falter, U.: Efficacy and Tolerability of Levetiracetam 3000 mg/d in Patients with Refractory Partial Seizures: A Multicenter, Double-Blind, Responder-Selected Study Evaluating Monotherapy. Epilepsia 41(10): 1276–1283, 2000
3. Betts, T., Waegemans, T., Crawford, P.: A multicentre, double-blind, randomized, parallel group study to evaluate the tolerability and efficacy of two oral doses of levetiracetam, 2000 mg daily and 4000 mg daily, without titration in patients with refractory epilepsy. Seizure 9: 80–87, 2000

4. Dooley, M., Plosker, G.L.: Levetiracetam, A Review of its Adjunctive Use in the Management of Partial Onset Seizures. Drugs 60(4): 871–893, 2000
5. Grant, R., Shorvon, S.D.: Efficacy and tolerability of 1000-4000 mg per day of levetiracetam as add-on therapy in patients with refractory epilepsy. Epilepsy Research 42: 89–95, 2000
6. Shorvon, S.D., Löwenthal, A., Janz, D., Bielen, D., Loiseau, P.: Multicenter Double-Blind, Randomized, Placebo-Controlled Trial of Levetiracetam as Add-On Therapy in Patients with Refractory Partial Seizures. Epilepsia 41(9): 1179–1186, 2000

Klinisch relevante Interaktion von Levetiracetam und Phenytoin

S. Springer, R. Gillessen, C. Mühe, K. Kugler, A. Enders, A. Merkenschlager

Einleitung

Eine Interaktion von Levetiracetam und Phenytoin ist laut Hersteller unwahrscheinlich und in der Literatur bisher nicht beschrieben. Nicolas (1) schließt aufgrund in vitro Untersuchungen eine Interaktion mit Phenytoin (sowie Carbamazepin und Valproat) aus, ebenso Browne (2) nach in vivo Untersuchungen. Obwohl es theoretisch keine Interferenz der Stoffwechselwege geben soll, sind Interaktionen zwischen Levetiracetam und anderen Antikonvulsiva in der Dauertherapie aber nicht vollständig auszuschließen.

Wir berichten den Fall eines drei Jahre alten Patienten mit sekundär generalisierenden Anfällen, welcher unter einer Kombinationstherapie von Valproat, Phenytoin und Levetiracetam einen (um ein Drittel) rückläufigen Phenytoin-Bedarf bei steigender Levetiracetam-Dosierung im Laufe eines halben Jahres zeigte. Diskutiert werden muss, ob diese relevante Wechselwirkung durch die Pharmakologie von Levetiracetam, durch das niedrige Alter oder durch die Polytherapie zu erklären ist.

Fallbeschreibung

Unser kleiner Patient leidet seit dem Alter von neun Monaten an sekundär generalisierenden, subklinisch beginnenden, komplex fokalen, wiederholt prolongierten Anfällen. Diese waren über 15 Monate weder mit Phenobarbital, Vitamin B6 oder Valproat noch mit Tavor, Clobazam, Oxcarbazepin oder Topiramat suffizient zu kontrollieren. Auch die Kombinationstherapie von zuletzt Valproat, Phenytoin und Topiramat war nicht ausreichend, sodass einschleichend dosiert von 10 auf 60 mg/kg/d Levetiracetam gegen Topiramat ausgetauscht wurde (Bei Behandlung mit konstant 90 mg/kg/d Valproat – Spiegel 50–60 µg/ml – wurde Levetiracetam einschleichend dosiert von 10 auf 60 mg/kg/d bis zu einem maximalen Spiegel von zuletzt 11,1 mg/l. Es reduzierte sich gleichzeitig der Bedarf von Phenytoin von 11,7 auf 8,7 mg/kg/d bei weitgehend konstantem Spiegel um 14 µg/ml). Der Verlauf wurde regelmäßig mindestens 2-wöchentlich dokumentiert, weil Phenytoin bis an die klinische und laborchemische Nebenwirkungsgrenze ausdosiert werden musste, um eine erstmals halbjährige Anfallsfreiheit zu erzielen. Nach der hier dokumentierten Behandlungsphase traten zunächst mehrere prolongierte Anfälle im Rahmen einer infektbedingten Unterdosierung auf. Schließlich entwickelten sich innerhalb weniger Tage eine Thrombopenie bis minimal 35.000/µl, ein Anstieg der Leberenzyme und eine

Hyperammonämie bis maximal 133 µmol/l. Die Behandlung mit Valproat und Phenytoin musste daher sofort unter Intensivüberwachung beendet werden. Die Levetiracetam-Dosis konnte währenddessen unverändert beibehalten werden. Die deutliche klinisch relevante Wechselwirkung zwischen Phenytoin und Levetiracetam war bereits zu Beginn der Behandlung bei einer Dosis von 20 mg/kg/d mit Intoxikationszeichen und einem Phenytoinspiegel von 21 µg/ml aufgefallen.

Diskussion

Da Levetiracetam weitgehend unverändert ausgeschieden wird, ist der Einfluss anderer Antikonvulsiva auf Levetiracetam als gering zu erwarten. Der Einfluss von Levetiracetam auf die anderen Medikamente ist ebenfalls wahrscheinlich gering, da in vitro kein (beispielsweise kompetitiver) Einfluss auf die häufigsten metabolisch relevanten Leberenzyme nachgewiesen werden konnte (1). Obwohl in der Literatur eine Interaktion von Levetiracetam mit anderen Antikonvulsiva ausgeschlossen wird, beobachteten wir während einer Therapiephase, in der außer der Behandlung mit Levetiracetam keine Änderungen vorgenommen worden waren, eine signifikante Veränderung des Phenytoinspiegels. Da der Patient in dieser Phase eine Dreifachtherapie mit Valproat, Phenytoin und Levetiracetam erhielt, gibt es für das beobachtete Phänomen mehrere Erklärungsmöglichkeiten:

- entweder es gibt eine nicht nachgewiesene Interaktion von Levetiracetam und Phenytoin, die möglicherweise erst bei einer länger dauernden Kombinationstherapie erkennbar wird,
- oder aufgrund der Polytherapie bis an die Nebenwirkungsgrenze führt das Einführen von Levetiracetam als neue Substanz zur Destabilisierung des erreichten Gleichgewichts, obwohl die Substanzen nicht um die selben Enzyme konkurrieren
- oder Levetiracetam zeigt hochdosiert mit 60 mg/kg/d andere pharmakokinetische Eigenschaften als in niedrigerer Dosierung.

Wie bei allen anderen neuen Antikonvulsiva auch sollten deshalb unbedingt regelmäßige Kontrollen der Nebenwirkungen und Medikamentenspiegel bei einer Kombinationstherapie mit Levetiracetam durchgeführt werden, um bisher unbekannte Interaktionen nicht zu übersehen.

Literatur

1. Nicolas JN et al. Drug Metabol Dispos 1999; 27: 250-4
2. Browne TR, J Clin Pharmacol 2000; 40: 590–5

Add-on Therapie von Levetiracetam und Topiramat bei pharmakoresistenten kindlichen Epilepsien

C. Bäumel, G. Kluger, M. Wruk, J. Wänninger, V. Drudik, H. Holthausen

Fragestellung

Wirksamkeit, Verträglichkeit und Wirkverlust von Topiramat (TPM) und Levetiracetam (LEV) bei Patienten mit pharmakoresistenten kindlichen Epilepsien.

Methodik

Nach Markteinführung wurden 41 Patienten mit TPM und 50 Patienten mit LEV als Add-on Therapie behandelt und mindestens 6 Monate nachbeobachtet.

Patienten	**TPM**	**LEV**
Anzahl Patienten	41	50
Alter (Jahre)	1 bis 38 (Mittel 9 Jahre)	1 bis 38 (Mittel 10 Jahre)
Epilepsien (Anzahl Patienten) (nur symptomatische und wahrscheinlich symptomatische (»kryptogene«) Epilepsien)		
– fokale Epilepsien	30	32
– generalisierte Epilepsien	6	12
– nicht sicher klassifizierbare Epilepsie	5	6
zusätzliche Antiepileptika (Anzahl Patienten)		
ein Antiepileptikum	19	17
zwei Antiepileptika	20	22
drei Antiepileptika	2	11
Häufigste Begleitmedikamente (Anzahl Patienten)		
Valproinsäure	20	18
Oxcarbazepin	6	12
Lamotrigin	6	7
Aufdosierungszeit	2 bis 4 Monate	2 bis 4 Wochen
Zieldosis	5–7 mg/kg KG/Tag (max 10)	40–50 mg/kgKG/Tag (max. 70)

Ergebnisse I

		TPM	LEV
»Responder«*)	Responder mit Nebenwirkungen	8/41 Patienten (20%) 3/8	13/50 Patienten (26%) 2/13
	Anfallsfreiheit	1 Patient (Absetzen wegen Wesensveränderung und schwerer Essstörung)	1 Patient (nach 7 Monaten Anfallsrezidiv)
	Non- Responder – mit Nebenwirkungen	33/41 Patienten (80%) 19/33	37/50 Patienten (74%) 16/37

*) Definition: Patienten mit Reduktion der Anfallsfrequenz in den letzten 4 Wochen um mehr als 50% laut Anfallskalender der Eltern 6 Monate nach Erreichen der Zieldosis im Vergleich zu der Anfallsfrequenz in den letzten 4 Wochen vor Beginn der Therapie.

Ergebnisse II

		TPM 21/41 (54%)	LEV 18/50 (36%)
Nebenwirkungen*)	Symptome (Anzahl Patienten)		
	– Verhaltensstörungen	25	5
	– Appetitstörungen	9	0
	– Müdigkeit	4	15
	– Anfallsverschlechterung	1	7
	– Gewichtsabnahme	3	0
	– Verdauungsprobleme	1	3
	– Gedächtnisprobleme	2	0
	– Schlafstörungen	0	2
	– Kopfschmerzen	1	0
	– Apnoen	0	1

*) Mehrfachnennungen möglich, Elternangaben

Es handelte sich jeweils um pharmakoresistente Epilepsien mit Beginn vor dem 10. Lebensjahr, die erfolglos mit mindestens 4 Antiepileptika (im Mittel 7) vorbehandelt worden waren.

Ergebnisse III

Wirkverlust

Bisher kein Wirkverlust unter TPM beobachtet.

Bei 2/13 Respondern unter LEV trat bisher während der Nachbeobachtung ein Wirkverlust auf. Darunter befand sich ein Patient, der nach 6 Monaten anfallsfrei war, bei dem aber nach 7 Monaten Anfallsrezidive auftraten. Eine Dosissteigerung führte bei ihm erneut zur Anfallsreduktion, nicht aber wieder zur

Anfallsfreiheit. Bei 5/37 Non-Respondern unter LEV trat nach anfänglicher Anfallsreduktion bereits nach 6-8 Wochen ein Wirkverlust ein.

Zusammenfassung

In der klinischen Anwendung bei 2 Gruppen von Patienten mit schwer behandelbaren kindlichen Epilepsien zeigten sich TPM und LEV in der Add-on Therapie als ähnlich wirksam mit einer Responderrate von 20% und 26%. Unterschiede fanden sich bei einer Aufdosierungsgeschwindigkeit von 2–4 Monaten bei TPM und 2–4 Wochen bei LEV in der Häufigkeit des Auftretens von Nebenwirkungen: 54% unter TPM und 36% unter LEV. An Nebenwirkungen traten unter TPM vor allem Verhaltensauffälligkeiten und Essstörungen, unter LEV Müdigkeit auf. Unter TPM konnten wir bisher keinen Wirkverlust beobachten. Dagegen zeigte sich unter LEV ein früher Wirkverlust nach 6–8 Wochen bei 5 Patienten, die dann zu den 37 Non-Respondern zählten und ein später Wirkverlust nach 7 Monaten bei bisher 2 von 13 Respondern.

Levetiracetam und kontinuierliche Spike Wave-Aktivität im Schlaf (CSWS)

Th. Hoppen, T. Sandrieser und M. Rister

Zusammenfassung

Levetiracetam ist ein hocheffektives neues Antiepileptikum mit ausgezeichnetem pharmakologischen Profil und guter Verträglichkeit. Im Erwachsenenalter ist seine Wirksamkeit belegt. Für das Kindesalter liegen bislang jedoch nur wenige Mitteilungen vor. Es wird ein früher Bericht einer erfolgreichen Zusatztherapie mit Levetiracetam bei einem fünfjährigen Jungen mit atypischer benigner Partialepilepsie oder Pseudo-Lennox-Syndrom vorgestellt. Neun verschiedene Antiepileptika kamen bei diesem Patienten in hohen Tagesdosen und unterschiedlichen Kombinationen zum Einsatz. Hierunter wurde Anfallsfreiheit, jedoch keine Modifikation der kontinuierlichen generalisierten spike wave-Aktivität im ruhigen Schlaf erreicht. Auch eine Bolustherapie mit i.v.-Steroiden (25 mg/kgKG/Tag Prednisolon), appliziert an drei aufeinanderfolgenden Tagen einer Woche über einen Zeitraum von zehn Wochen, hatte keinen therapeutischen Effekt. Die Einführung von Levetiracetam (50 mg/kgKG/Tag) zur bestehenden Kombinationstherapie mit Topiramat, Gabapentin und Valproinsäure zeigte eine rasche und anhaltende Besserung des EEG-Musters im Schlaf. Der EEG-Befund blieb auch nach Beendigung der Medikation mit Topiramat und Gabapentin konstant. 15 Monate nach Beginn der Zusatztherapie mit Levetiracetam haben sich Verhalten und intellektuelle Leistungsfähigkeit des Patienten erheblich verbessert. Mit Levetiracetam steht möglicherweise ein brauchbares und effektives Dauermedikament bei pharmakoresistentem CSWS zur Verfügung.

Abkürzungen

ABPE	atypische benigne Partialepilepsie
AE	Antiepileptika
CSWS	kontinuierliche spike wave-Aktivität im ruhigen Schlaf
EEG	Elektroenzephalogramm
LEV	Levetiracetam
PLS	Pseudo-Lennox-Syndrom

Einleitung

Spektrum und klinischer Verlauf von ABPE/PLS zeigen eine große Variabilität. Einzelne Patienten mit wenigen Anfällen und unbeeinträchtigter mentaler

Entwicklung kontrastieren zu anderen mit langer Epilepsiedauer, charakterisiert durch unterschiedliche Anfallssemiologie, massive epileptiforme Aktivität im EEG und persistierende Behinderung nach Remission der Epilepsie (1, 6, 7). Die pharmakologische Therapie bei ABPE/PLS ist oftmals unbefriedigend (10). Kontrollierte Studien zum Einsatz alter und neuer AE fehlen bislang. Nachfolgend wird über den positiven Effekt einer Komedikation mit LEV bei einem Kind mit pharmakoresistentem CSWS bei ABPE/PLS berichtet.

Kasuistik

Nach Spontanentbindung in der 35. Schwangerschaftswoche bei vorzeitigen Blasensprung (Apgar 7-8-9) entwickelte der eutrophe Patient eine ätiologisch unklare niedriggradige intraventrikuläre Hirnblutung (Grad II links, Grad I rechts) und zeigte konsekutive Neugeborenenanfälle in der ersten Lebenswoche. Bei raschem Kopfwachstum und sonographisch nachweisbarem posthämorrhagischen Hydrozephalus erfolgte eine ventrikuloperitoneale Shuntanlage. In der sechsten Lebenswoche ereignete sich eine erneute intra-/periventrikuläre Hirnblutung linkshemisphäriell, es traten rechtsseitige tonisch-klonische Krampfanfälle auf. Während der folgenden Jahre wurde insgesamt viermal eine Shuntrevision aufgrund von Infektionen und Fehlfunktionen erforderlich. Im Alter von vier Jahren und elf Monaten wurde der Patient erstmals in unserer Klinik vorgestellt. Zur stationären Aufnahme führten neben Koordinationsdefiziten bei rechtsseitiger Hemiparese ein initial bestehendes rezidivierendes Erbrechen bei nonkonvulsivem Status epileptikus (Bewusstseinsminderung, Konfusion, Konzentrationsbeeinträchtigung und schlechte Grundstimmung). Zusätzlich traten während der ersten stationären Tage zwei je drei Minuten dauernde generalisierte tonisch-klonische Krampfanfälle und gehäuft generalisierte kleine Anfälle (atonische Anfälle, atypische Absencen) auf. Die zerebrale Kernspintomographie ergab eine bihemisphärische periventrikuläre Leukomalazie und Occipitallappenatrophie. Im EEG fanden sich multifokale sharp waves mit links-frontozentrotemporaler Dominanz. Im ruhigen Schlaf kam es zur massiven Aktivierung der epileptiformen Aktivität in Form eines bioelektrischen Status mit einem kontinuierlichen irregulären spike/sharp slow wave Muster (Abb. 1).

Neun verschiedene AE kamen in Mono- und Kombinationstherapie zum Einsatz. Hierunter wurde Anfallsfreiheit, jedoch keine Modifikation der CSWS erreicht. Im Einzelnen wurden Phenobarbital und Chloralhydrat (Einzelgaben initial), Sultiam (maximale Tagesdosis: 9,3 mg/kgKG), Clobazam (0,4 mg/kgKG), Topiramat (11 mg/kgKG), Valproinsäure (67 mg/kgKG), Gabapentin (89 mg/kgKG) und Oxcarbazepin (67 mg/kgKG) innerhalb eines Zeitraumes von vier Monaten verabreicht. Additiv erfolgte eine Kortison-Bolustherapie: Prednisolon (25 mg/kgKG/Tag) wurde an drei aufeinanderfolgenden Tagen einer Woche über insgesamt zehn Wochen (anschließend zwei Zyklen mit prolongiertem Intervall) ohne therapeutischen Effekt appliziert. Die Bolustherapie wurde nebenwirkungsfrei toleriert. Die Einführung von LEV (50 mg/kgKG/Tag), acht Monate nach Beginn der antiepileptischen Therapie, zur bestehenden Kombinationstherapie mit Topiramat, Gabapentin und Valproinsäure zeigte eine rasche und anhaltende Besserung des EEG-Musters im Schlaf. Erstmals seit Beginn der AE-Therapie konnte eine Modifikation der CSWS dokumentiert werden. Ein Tag vor Beginn der add-on-Therapie mit LEV fand sich im EEG persistierende CSWS, in der ersten darauffolgenden EEG-Ableitung acht Tage später, dokumentierte sich nur partielle epileptiforme Aktivität im Schlaf. Derzeit besteht im Wachen fokale sharp wave-Aktivität über der linken Frontozentrotemporalregion. Im Schlaf kommt es zur partiellen Aktivierung über der linken Hemisphäre, zusätzlich tritt fokale sharp wave-Aktivität frontozentrotemporal rechts auf (Abb. 2 und 3). Der EEG-Befund blieb auch nach Beendigung der Medikation mit Topiramat und Gabapentin konstant. Aktuell wird die Therapie mit LEV (56 mg/kgKG/Tag) und Valproinsäure (25 mg/kgKG/Tag) fortgeführt. 15 Monate nach Beginn der Zusatztherapie mit LEV haben sich Verhalten und intellektuelle Leistungsfähigkeit des Patienten erheblich verbessert.

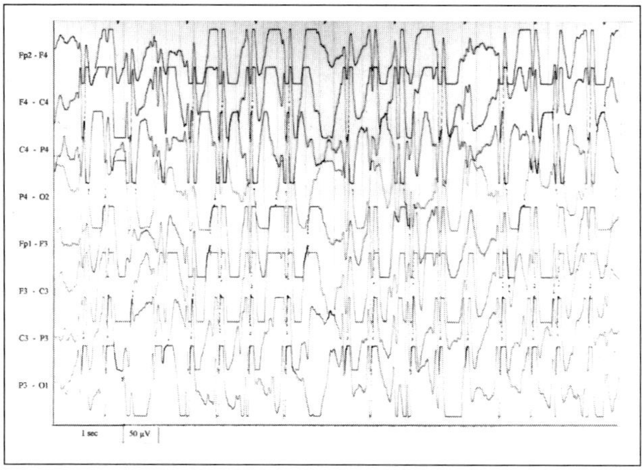

Abb. 1: 4 Jahre 11 Monate. Kontinuierliche generalisierte irreguläre spike/sharp slow wave-Aktivität im ruhigen Schlaf.

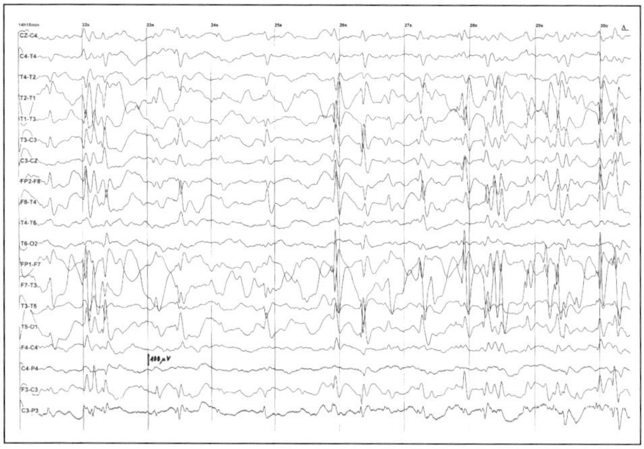

Abb. 2: 6 Jahre 7 Monate. Sharp waves linkshemisphäriell und frontozentrotemporal rechts im ruhigen Schlaf.

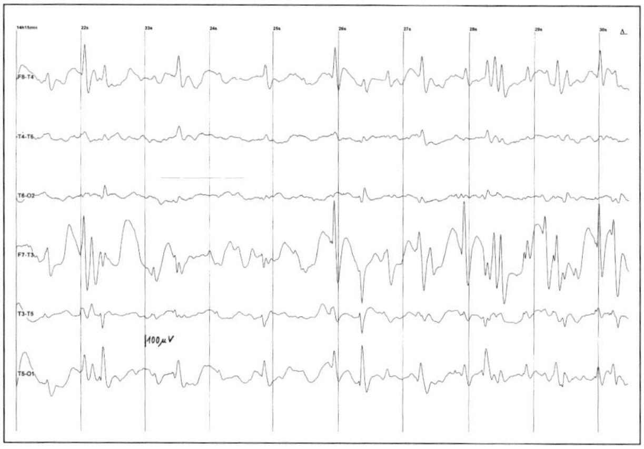

Abb. 3: Detailbild aus Abb. 2.

Diskussion

Im Management von ABPE/PLS ist die differenzierte Betrachtung von Anfällen, EEG-Phänomenen (CSWS) und klinischen Symptomen, insbesondere sprachlicher Auffälligkeiten, von Bedeutung (10). Die Therapie der Epilepsie stellt selten das Hauptproblem bei ABPE/PLS dar. Ziel der Pharmakotherapie ist es vielmehr den Patienten vor einer fortschreitenden neuropsychologischen Beeinträchtigung zu schützen (6, 7). Sultiam und Clobazam – evtl. in Kombination mit anderen AE können effektiv sein (3, 5, 11). Eine Pharmakoresistenz führt oft zum Einsatz von Steroiden (7). Eine Glucokortikoid-Bolustherapie scheint bei geringeren Nebenwirkungen gleichermaßen wirksam zu sein wie eine kontinuierliche Kortisongabe (3, 10). In Einzelfällen können eine intravenöse Immunglobulingabe, multiple subpiale Transsektionen oder eine Vagusnerv-Stimulator-Implantation erwogen werden (10). Bei dem vorgestellten Patienten mit ABPE/PLS führte der Einsatz verschiedener herkömmlicher und neuer AE nicht zu einem therapeutischen Erfolg. Erst durch die zusätzliche Gabe von LEV zur bestehenden Kombinationstherapie konnte die CSWS terminiert werden. Deutliche klinische Fortschritte und ein stabiles EEG charakterisieren den Verlauf seit Beginn der add-on-Therapie mit LEV.

Das neue Antiepileptikum LEV hat einen hohen therapeutischen Index (2, 9). Ergebnisse klinischer Studien bei partiellen und generalisierten Anfällen bei Erwachsenen haben seine Wirksamkeit nachgewiesen (12, 13). Die Pharmakokinetik von LEV ist günstig, die Neben- und Wechselwirkungsrate mit anderen Medikamenten sind gering (2, 9). Bislang liegen nur wenige Berichte über eine Anwendung im Kindesalter vor (4, 8). Der günstige therapeutische Effekt bei unserem Patienten unterstützt die Annahme, dass LEV eine effektive und gut verträgliche Therapie bei unkontrollierter CSWS bei ABPL/PLS darstellt.

Literatur

1. Aicardi J (2000) Atypical semiology of rolandic epilepsy in some related syndromes. Epileptic Disord 2 (Suppl 1): S5–S9
2. Dooley M, Plosker GL (2000) Levetiracetam. A review of its adjunctive use in the management of partial onset seizures. Drugs 60: 871–893
3. Ebinger F, Bast T, Pietz J, Benninger C, Rating D (2000) Glucocorticoid bolus therapy of epilepsies. Neuropediatrics 31: A6
4. Glauser T, Bebin M, Ritter F, Nohria V, Jensen C (1999) Open-label efficacy and safety of levetiracetam in pediatric patients with partial onset seizures. Epilepsia 40 (Suppl 7): S161–162
5. Groß-Selbeck G (1995) Treatment of benign partial epilepsy of childhood, including atypical forms. Neuropediatrics 26: 45–50
6. Hahn A (2000) Atypical benign partial epilepsy / pseudo-Lennox syndrome. Epileptic Disord 2 (Suppl 1): S11–S17
7. Hahn A, Pistohl J, Neubauer BA, Stephani U (2001) Atypical benign partial epilepsy or pseudo-Lennox syndrome. Part I: Symptomatology and long-term prognosis. Neuropediatrics 32: 1–8
8. Hoppen Th, Sandrieser T, Rister M (2001) Levetiracetam im Kindesalter. Z Epileptol 14: 56

9. Patsalos PN (2000) Pharmacokinetic profile of levetiracetam: toward ideal characteristics. Pharmacol Ther 85: 77–85
10. Rating D (2000) Treatment in typical and atypical rolandic epilepsy. Epileptic Disord 2 (Suppl 1): S69–S72
11. Rating D, Wolf Ch, Bast T (2000) Sulthiame as monotherapy in children with benign childhood epilepsy with centro-temporal spikes: a six-month randomised, double-blind, placebo-controlled study. Epilepsia 41: 1284–1288
12. Shorvon SD (2001) Pyrrolidone derivatives. Lancet 358: 1885–1892
13. Shorvon SD, Lowenthal A, Janz D, Bielen E, Loiseau P (2000) Multicenter double-blind, randomised, placebo-controlled trial of levetiracetam add-on therapy in patients with refractory partial seizures. European levetiracetam study group. Epilepsia 41: 1179–1186

Schwerwiegende Blutungskomplikationen mit Thrombozytopenie unter Valproat

St. König, M. Teich, I. Treiss, W. Koelfen, E. Longin

Zusammenfassung

Thrombozytopenien sind ein häufiger, in der Regel nicht klinisch bedeutsamer Nebenbefund bei Patienten, die mit Valproinsäure (VPA) behandelt werden. Andererseits können auch schwerwiegende Blutungskomplikationen vorkommen. Innerhalb von weniger als zwei Jahren zeigten 5 VPA-behandelte Patienten unserer Klinik schwerwiegende Blutungen. In der Literatur sind 37 Patienten publiziert. Die Thrombozytenzahl lag meist unter 30.000/µL, bei 9 Patienten darüber. Neun Patienten waren 11 Jahre oder älter, 15 Kinder waren 5–10 Jahre alt, 8 Patienten waren <2 J. Erwachsene waren nur in Einzelfällen betroffen. Eine bestimmte Begleitmedikation war nicht entscheidend, vielmehr ein hoher Blutspiegel von VPA. Bei den 5 eigenen Kindern zeigte sich, dass weitere Auffälligkeiten der Gerinnung bei manifesten Blutungen regelhaft vorkommen. Vier der fünf Patienten hatten eine reduzierte Faktor XIII-Aktivität u./o. ein von Willebrand-Jürgens-Syndrom. Bei Patienten mit Blutungskomplikationen unter VPA muss umgehend nicht nur die Thrombozytenzahl kontrolliert werden, sondern außerdem der Faktor XIII, der v. Willebrand-Jürgens- und der Ristocitin-Co-Faktor. Patienten mit deutlich reduzierten Thrombozyten müssen über diesen Befund aufgeklärt werden, ggf. sollte eine Dosisreduktion diskutiert werden. Präoperativ sind bei VPA-behandelten Patienten differenzierte Gerinnungsanalysen unumgänglich.

Einleitung

Thrombozytopenien im Zusammenhang mit einer Valproat-(VPA)-Therapie sind häufig und werden bei 10–40% aller Patienten gefunden. Die weitaus meisten Patienten sind asymptomatisch, bei deutlich unter 100.000 Thrombozyten/µL abgefallenen Werten steigt die Thrombozytenzahl nach einer geringen Dosis-Reduktion wieder an. Der Normbereich der Thrombozytenzahl wird zwischen 140.000 und 350.000 Thrombozyten/µL angegeben. In der Literatur sind 37 Patienten mit schwerwiegenden Blutungen unter VPA berichtet, von denen drei verstorben sind (Tab. 1).

Wir berichten über fünf Patienten, die in einem Zeitraum von 1,5 Jahren an unserer Klinik schwerwiegende Blutungskomplikationen unter VPA entwickelten (Tab. 2). Diese Patienten werden mit den in der Literatur publizierten zusammen analysiert und ausgewertet.

Tab.1: Literaturübersicht Valproat-assoziierte Thrombozytopenie mit Blutungssymptomatik

Patienten	Komedikation	Symptome	Thrombozytenzahl (/µl)	Therapie	Literatur
w, 10 j.	-	Hämatome	< 100.000	Absetzen von VPA mit Normalisierung von Thrombozyten-zahl und Klinik	Sutor et al.
w, 30 j.	-	kutane Ekkchymosen fatale pulmonale Hämorrhagie	15.000	trotz Thrombozytentransfusion im Lungenversagen verstorben	Sleiman et al.
»pädiatrischer Patient«	-	Petechien, Hämatome	17.000	Absetzen von VPA mit Normalisierung von Thrombozytenzahl und Klinik	Cheng et al.
m, 6 j.	-	massive Hämatome	24.000	Umsetzen auf Phenytoin mit Normalisierung von Thrombozytenzahl und Klinik	Sandler et al.
w, 9 m.	Acetazolamid	Petechien, KM-Suppression	6.000	Umsetzen auf Phenytoin mit Normalisierung von Thrombozytenzahl und Klinik	Kishi et al.
w, 19 j.	-	massive Epistaxis, großflächige Purpura, KM-Suppression	62.000	Absetzen von VPA mit Normalisierung von Thrombozytenzahl und Klinik	Smith et al.
m, 3 m.	-	Petechien	7.000	Absetzen von VPA mit Normalisierung von Thrombozytenzahl und Klinik	Stahl et al.
m, 14 j.	-	Purpura	10.000	Umsetzen auf Pheno-barbital mit Normalisierung von Thrombozytenzahl und Klinik	Brichard et al.
w, 15 j.	-	gingivale und Schleimhautblutungen	5.000	TK-Transfusion und Dosisreduktion von VPA mit Normalisierung von Thrombozytenzahl und Klinik	Ganick et al.
w, 13 m.	-	Purpura	20.000	Absetzen von VPA mit Normalisierung von Thrombozytenzahl und Klinik	Ware et al.
m, 6 j.	Primidon	Subarachnoidal-blutung	stark erniedrigt	TK-Transfusion, im Rahmen einer Pneumonie verstorben	
8 Patienten (1-18 j)	?	diffuse Petechien, Hämatome, Epistaxis	19.000 – 68.000	Absetzen oder Reduktion von VPA mit Normalisierung von Thrombozytenzahl und Klinik	Delgado et al.
18 Patienten (1 m – 12 j)	Phenobarbital (1x) Cotrimoxazol (1x)	Petechien, Hämatome, Ekkchymosen, Epistaxis, Gingivablutungen, Schleimhautblutungen (1x), Hämaturie (1x)	1.000 – 80.000	Absetzen, Reduktion (1x) von VPA mit Normalisierung von Thrombozytenzahl und Klinik 1 Pat. im Rahmen einer Pneumonie verstorben	Monnet et al.

Tab.2: Eigene Patienten mit valproat-assoziierter Thrombozytopenie und Blutungssymptomatik; vWF = von Willebrand-Faktor, Rcof = Ristocitin-Cofaktor

Patient	Komedikation	Symptome	Thrombozytenzahl (/µl) und weitere pathologische Gerinnungsparameter	Therapie
m, 8 j. ICP mit refraktären fokalen und generalisierten Anfällen	Vigabatrin, Ceftazidim, Gentamicin	Petechien, Suffusionen, Rektalblutung	23.000 F XIII 67%	Absetzen von VPA mit Normalisierung der Thrombozytenwerte und Klinik
m, 4 j. FG der 33. SSW mit generalisierten tonisch-klonischen Anfällen	Phenobarbital	Schleimhautblutungen, Petechien	12.000	Absetzen von VPA mit Normalisierung der Thrombozytenwerte und Klinik
w, 10 j. Hirnstammenzephalitis mit generalisierten Anfällen	Phenobarbital, Carbamazepin, Cefotaxim, Aciclovir	Epistaxis	46.000 F XIII 18%	Absetzen von VPA mit Normalisierung der Werte und Klinik
w, 18 j. ICP, generalisierte Anfälle	Flunitrazepam, Colecalciferol	Suggilationen, Petechien	51.000 vWF 41%, Rcof 28%	Absetzen von VPA mit Normalisierung der Werte und Klinik
w, 9 j. Lennox-Gastaut-Syndrom		Hämatome	87.000 Fibrinogen 78 mg/dL vWF 58%, Rcof 28% F XIII 55%	Reduktion von VPA mit Normalisierung der Werte und Klinik

Ergebnisse

Blutungskomplikationen traten überwiegend im Kindesalter auf, lediglich ein Patient war >20 Jahre alt, 2 Patienten lagen zwischen 15 und 19 Jahren. Kleine Kinder <2 Jahre waren mit 20% nicht überrepräsentiert, die am häufigsten betroffene Gruppe waren die 5–10-Jährigen mit insgesamt 45% der Gesamtgruppe (Abb. 1).

Die klinisch beobachteten Blutungskomplikationen waren Petechien, Suffusionen, Rektal- oder Nasenblutungen, massive Hämatome und bei zwei der drei verstorbenen Patienten einmal eine zerebrale Blutung (Ware et al., 1980), einmal eine Lungeneinblutung (Sleimann et al., 2000).

Es bestand ein deutlicher Zusammenhang mit hohen Blutspiegeln über 100 mg/L VPA. Lediglich zwei Patienten zeigten Blutungen bei niedrigeren Werten, wobei zusätzliche Faktoren im Sinne einer individuellen Disposition eine Rolle gespielt haben mögen (Brichard et al, 1994; Stahl et al, 1997). Es bestand kein systematischer Zusammenhang mit einer bestimmten Ko-Medikation, neben anderen Antiepileptika wurden gelegentlich Antibiotika gegeben. Dabei scheint eher der Infekt an sich von Bedeutung zu sein als die Antibiotika. Bei einzelnen

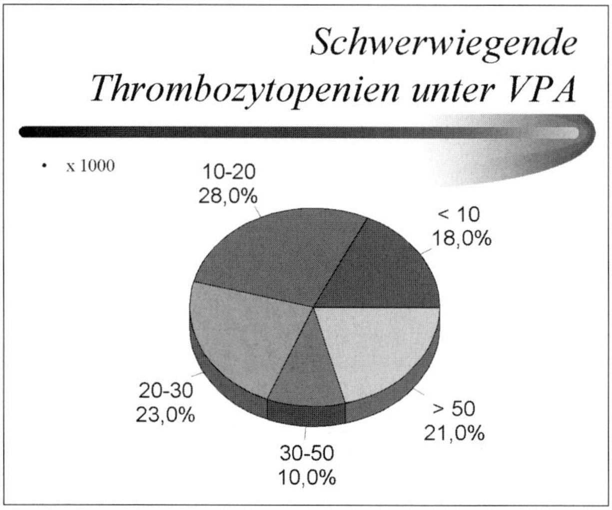

Abb. 1: Thrombozytenzahl/µL bei 39 Patienten mit klinisch relevanten Blutungen unter VPA (x 1000, in Prozent der Gesamtzahl angegeben).

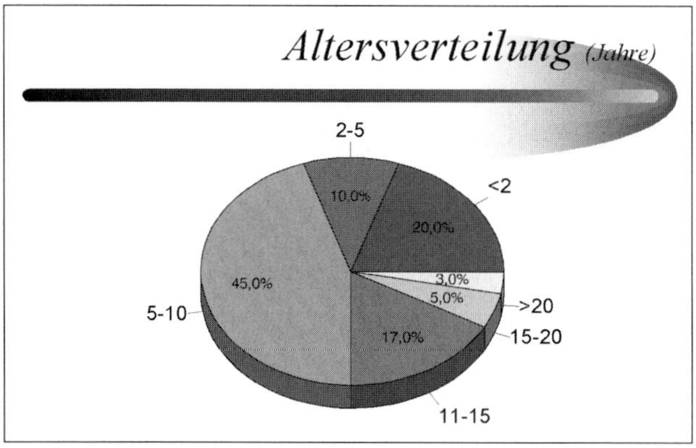

Abb. 2: Altersverteilung bei 39 Patienten mit schwerwiegenden Blutungskomplikationen unter VPA (Angabe in Prozent bezogen auf das Alter in Jahren).

der eigenen Patienten erholte sich die Thrombozytopenie unter fortgeführter Antibiose nach dem Absetzen des VPA.

Analysiert man die Thrombozytenanzahl so fällt auf, dass lediglich 18% der Patienten Thrombozytenwerte unter 10.000/µL aufwiesen, dagegen aber 21% bei Werten über 50.000/µL Blutungen entwickelten (Abb. 2). Dies weist darauf hin, dass die Thrombozytenanzahl nicht der alleine ausschlaggebende Faktor sein kann.

Die detaillierte Analyse der Gerinnung zeigte schließlich bei den eigenen fünf Patienten (Tab. 2), warum bei so verschiedenen Thrombozytenzahlen klinisch Blutungen auftreten können. Entscheidend sind häufig zusätzlich auftretende Auffälligkeiten der Gerinnung. Lediglich ein Patient hatte eine isolierte Thrombozytopenie von 11.000/µL. Ein weiteres Kind zeigte lediglich eine minimal erniedrigte Aktivität des Faktors XIII, dessen Mangel bei einem weiteren Kind mit 18% als wesentlich für die Blutungsneigung angesehen werden muss. Schließlich fanden wir bei zwei Kindern kombiniert reduzierte Aktivitäten des von-Willebrand-Jürgens-Faktors und des Ristocitin-Co-Faktors, bei einem der beiden Kinder außerdem in Kombination mit einem Faktor XIII-Mangel (Tab. 2).

Diskussion

Aufgrund der detaillierten Gerinnungsanalyse der eigenen Patienten ist anzunehmen, dass auch bei den in der Literatur berichteten Erfahrungen begleitende zusätzliche Gerinnungsstörungen eine entscheidende Rolle gespielt haben. Die Thrombozytopenie ist der einzige der relevanten Parameter, der mit einem einfachen Routine-Blutbild entdeckt wird und deshalb in seiner Bedeutung für die individuelle Blutungsneigung überschätzt wird. Wichtig sind auch Wechselbeziehungen zwischen den untersuchten Gerinnungsparametern, so wird zum Beispiel der Faktor XIII teilweise in den Thrombozyten synthetisiert, kann aber auch isoliert bei nur mäßig erniedrigten Gesamt-Thrombozyten deutlich in seiner Aktivität reduziert sein.

Wenn ein Patient also eine Thrombozytopenie mit klinisch relevanter Blutungsneigung unter einer VPA-Therapie zeigt, sollten also auch der von-Willebrand-Jürgens-Faktor, der Ristocitin-Co-Faktor und der Faktor XIII mit analysiert werden. Bei nicht bedrohlicher Klinik kann zunächst die VPA-Dosis reduziert werden. Bereits eine Zurücknahme der Dosis um 25% wird bei vielen Patienten zu einer erheblichen Besserung der Gerinnung führen. Bei schwerwiegenden Blutungen sollte VPA rasch ganz abgesetzt werden, eine spezifische Therapie wie in Tabelle 3 angedeutet kann durchgeführt werden. Diese Therapiemaßnahmen können auch bei Patienten mit Gerinnungsauffälligkeiten unter VPA genutzt werden, die unter VPA operiert werden sollen. Ein Absetzen des VPA ist so zu vermeiden, verbunden mit einer kontinuierlichen und stabilen Epilepsie-Behandlung.

Desmopressin kann insbesondere bei wiederholten Gaben zu einer Hyponatriämie führen, die Hyponatriämie wiederum zu zerebralen Krampfanfällen. In einer stationären und/oder perioperativen Situation können jedoch problemlos

Therapie VPA-assoz. Gerinnungsstörungen

• V.Willebrand-Jürgens Faktor-Mangel	• Desmopressin (0,4µg/kg KG i.v.)
• Ristocitin-Co-Faktor-Mangel	• Desmopressin (0,4 µg/kg KG i.v.)
• F XIII Mangel	• F XIII-Substitution
• (Vit-K-abh.Faktoren erniedrigt)	• (Vitamin-K-Gabe)

Tab. 3: Therapiemöglichkeiten VPA-assoziierter Gerinnungsstörungen.

entsprechende Elektrolyt-Kontrollen gewährleistet werden. Einen Beweis für eine eigenständige pro-konvulsive Wirkung des Desmopressins gibt es nicht. Zu beachten ist außerdem, dass die Desmopressin-Gaben, die den v. Willebrand-Jürgens und den Ristocitin-Co-Faktor aus dem Endothel freisetzen, in einzelnen Fällen keinen ausreichenden Anstieg der Aktivität bewirken. In diesem Fall – oder auch bei langen und komplizierten Operationen mit einem hohen Nachblutungsrisiko – kann auch direkt der Faktor substituiert werden (Haemate HS). Auch der Mangel an Faktor XIII ist durch die Substitution des Faktors korrigierbar (Fibrogammin).

Ein generelles Screening aller klinisch unauffälligen Patienten unter VPA auf pathologische Gerinnungswerte erscheint nicht erforderlich und unbezahlbar. Bei klinischen Auffälligkeiten und vor geplanten Operationen ist die detaillierte Diagnostik jedoch zwingend.

Durch ein besseres Verständnis der Vielzahl der VPA-induzierten Gerinnungsstörungen ist wie bei der Problematik des VPA-assoziierten Leberversagens ein erheblich sicherer Umgang mit der VPA-Therapie zu erreichen. Das prä-operative Absetzen von VPA, das nicht selten zu einer erheblichen Anfallszunahme bis hin zu Status epilepticus führen kann, ist durch die genannten Vorsichtsmaßnahmen zu vermeiden. Eine optimierte Epilepsie-Therapie ist so auch in solchen Situationen kontinuierlich durchführbar.

Literatur

1. Brichard B, Vermylen C, Scheiff JM, Ninane J, Cornu G (1994) Haematological disturbances during long-term valproate therapy. Eur J Pediatr 153:378–380
2. Cheng RD, Kohrman MH, Kerr SL, Duffner PK, Cohen ME (1989) Thrombocytopenia associated with valproic acid that requires platelet transfusion. Ann Neurol 26:457–458
3. Delgado MR, Riela AR, Mills J, Browne R, Roach ES (1994) Thrombocytopenia secondary to high valproate levels in children with epilepsy. J Child Neurol 9:311–314
4. Ganick DJ, Sunder T, Finley JL (1990) Severe hematologic toxicity of valproic acid. A report of four patients. Am J Pediatr Hematol Oncol 12:80–85
5. Kishi T, Fujita N, Kawaguchi H, Ishimae M, Watanabe K, Tanaka T (1994) Bone marrow suppression induced by high dose valproic acid. Arch Dis Child 71:153–155
6. Kreuz W, Linde R, Funk M, Meyer-Schrod R, Foll E, Nowak-Gottl U, Jacobi G, Vigh Z, Scharrer I (1992) Valproate therapy induces von Willebrand disease type I. Epilepsia 33: 178–184
7. Monnet P, David M, Philippe N, Dechavanne M, Floret D, Renaud H, Trezeciak MC, Brazier JL, Bourdillon D (1979) Altérations de l'hemostase lors des traitements au dipropylacetate de sodium (Depakine). Pédiatrie 34: 603–620
8. Sandler RM, Emberson C, Roberts GE, Voak D, Darnborough J, Heeley AF (1978) IgM platelet auto-antibody due to sodium valproate. Br Med J 2:1683–1684
9. Sleiman C, Raffy O, Roue C, Mal H (2000) Fatal pulmonary hemorrhage during high-dose valproate monotherapy. Chest 117: 613
10. Smith FR, Boots M. Sodium valproate and bone marrow suppression (1980) Ann Neurol 8:197–199
11. Stahl MMS, Neiderud J, Vinge E (1997) Thrombocytopenic purpura and anemia in a breast-fed infant whose mother was treated with valproic acid. J Pediatr 130:1001–1003
12. Sutor AH; Jesdinsky-Buscher (1975) Veränderungen der Hämostase bei Epilepsie-Behandlung mit Dipropylessigsäure. Fortschr Med 6: 411–414
13. Ware S, Millward-Sadler GH (1980) Acute liver disease associated with sodium valproate Lancet 22: 1110–1113

Faktor XIII Mangel unter Valproattherapie

M. Teich, E. Longin, C.E. Dempfle, St. König

Zusammenfassung

Die Beeinflussung der Hämostase ist eine häufige Nebenwirkung von Valproat (VPA). Eine Erniedrigung von Faktor XIII mit Blutungssymptomatik wurde bisher noch nicht beschrieben. Wir berichten von zwei pädiatrischen Patienten, die in engem zeitlichen Zusammenhang mit Beginn bzw. Änderung der VPA-Medikation einen Faktor XIII-Mangel entwickelten.

Einleitung

Hämostatische Nebenwirkungen einer Therapie mit Valproat (VPA) wie Thrombozytopenie oder von Willebrand-Syndrom Typ I sind in der Vergangenheit immer wieder berichtet worden. Insbesondere unter hohen Dosierungen mit therapeutisch durchaus erwünschten Blutserumspiegeln >100 mg/l treten diese hämostaseologisch relevanten Wirkungen von VPA gehäuft auf.

Wir berichten von zwei pädiatrischen Patienten, die unter hochdosierter VPA-Therapie unter anderem einen bisher nicht beschrieben Mangel an Faktor XIII mit einer Blutungssymptomatik entwickelten.

Patienten

Patientin 1: nach zunächst unauffälligen Gerinnungsparametern trat nach intravenöser VPA-Schnellaufsättigung bei einem 10jährigen Mädchen (Hirnstammenzephalitis mit generalisierten zerebralen Krampfanfällen) eine Epistaxis auf (Faktor XIII 18%, Thrombozyten 46.000/µl, VPA-Spiegel 100 mg/l). Die übrigen Gerinnungsparameter (Quick, PTT, PTZ, Fibrinogen, von Willebrand Faktor, Vitamin K-abhängige Faktoren) lagen im Normbereich. Nach sofortigem Absetzen von VPA normalisierten sich Klinik und Gerinnungsparameter rasch.

Patient 2: ein 9jähriger Junge mit atypischen Absencen (VPA und Lamotrigin seit 2 Jahren, VPA-Spiegel 110 mg/l) entwickelte eine rezidivierende Epistaxis. Neben Faktor XIII (49%) war auch der von Willebrand Faktor erniedrigt (47%). Nach schrittweiser Reduktion der VPA-Dosis normalisierten sich Klinik und Gerinnungsparameter innerhalb von 9 Tagen.

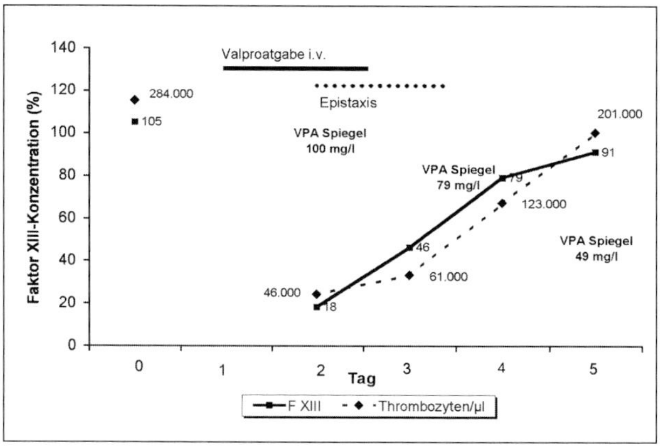

Abb. 1: Verlauf von Klinik und Gerinnungsparametern bei Patientin 1.

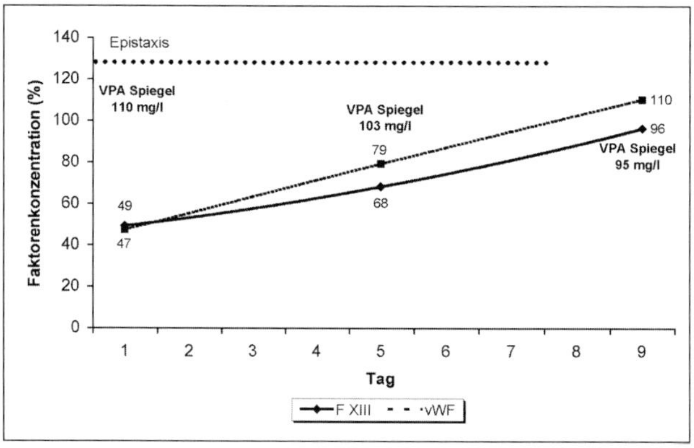

Abb. 2: Verlauf von Klinik und Gerinnungsparametern bei Patient 2.

Therapie

Wie auch bei anderen VPA-induzierten Gerinnungsstörung war die Beendigung bzw. Reduktion der VPA-Therapie allein ausreichend, um sowohl die klinischen Symptome als auch die veränderten Laborparameter zu normalisieren. Zusätzliche Maßnahmen wie Substitution der fehlenden Faktoren waren bei fehlender vitaler Indikation nicht notwendig.

Diskussion

Bei beiden Patienten bestand ein auffälliger zeitlicher Zusammenhang zwischen Änderung der Faktor XIII-Aktivität und der VPA-Medikation. Die Beeinflussung von Synthese und/oder Freisetzung von Faktor XIII in der Leber erscheint plausibel, da der hepatische Metabolismus bekanntermassen dem Einfluss von VPA unterliegt.

Da Faktor XIII auch in Megakaryozyten nachgewiesen werden kann, ist ein Faktorenmangel möglicherweise auch als Epiphänomen einer VPA-induzierten

Thrombozytopenie zu deuten: der suppressive Effekt von VPA auf Megakaryozytenzahl und -metabolismus wurde mehrfach beschrieben (1).

Über die (Mit-) Verantwortlichkeit der Faktor XIII-Erniedrigung für die Blutungssymptomatik kann in unseren Fällen allerdings nur spekuliert werden, da der Mangel bei beiden Patienten nicht isoliert auftrat.

Eine Faktor XIII-Konzentration >10% der Norm führt im Alltag zu keiner wesentlichen Blutungsneigung (2). Wahrscheinlich ist die bei unseren Patienten aufgetretenen Blutung also eher auf die anderen erniedrigten Gerinnungsparameter zurückzuführen. Unter Umständen kann sich der Faktorenmangel aber verstärkend auf die Blutungssymptomatik auswirken.

Nach chirurgischen Eingriffen kann aber bereits eine Serumkonzentration 10–40% (2) zu (lebens-) bedrohlichen Blutungen führen (3).

In der präoperativen »Routine«-Gerinnungsdiagnostik (Quick, PTT, PTZ) wird aber ein Faktor XIII-Mangel nicht erfasst, so dass es postoperativ zu eventuell erheblichen Blutungskomplikationen kommen kann.

Die Messung der Blutungszeit (einfacher und schneller als eine Faktor XIII-Bestimmung) mag zwar Hinweise auf einen Faktor XIII-Mangel geben, da aber VPA-induzierte Störungen der Hämostase meist in Kombination (s.o.) auftreten, bleibt die spezifische Aussagekraft der Blutungszeit eingeschränkt.

Die in der Literatur beschrieben, z.T. letal verlaufenden Blutungskomplikationen unter VPA-Therapie (4) erwähnen nicht die Faktor XIII-Konzentration, die vermutlich nicht bestimmt wurden. Man kann spekulieren, ob ein unerkannter Faktorenmangel eine Rolle bei dem dramatischen Verlauf der Blutung spielte.

Fazit

Neben den bereits bekannten Wirkungen auf die Hämostase scheint VPA auch die Faktor XIII-Konzentration zu beeinflussen.

Insbesondere bei operativen Eingriffen unter VPA-Therapie kann ihm klinische Bedeutung zukommen, da er der Routinediagnostik entgeht und ernste postoperative Blutungen auslösen kann.

Literatur

1. Watts RG, Emanuel PD, Zuckerman KS, Howard TH (1990) Valproic acid-induced cytopenias: evidence for a dose related suppression of hematopoiesis. J Pediatr 117:495–9
2. Fickenscher K (1998) Faktor XIII. In: Thomas L (Herausg.) Labor und Diagnose. TH-Books Verlagsgesellschaft, 5. Auflage, Frankfurt/Main
3. Heene DL, Matthias FR (1993) Koagulopathien. In: Begemann H, Rastetter J (Herausg.) Klinische Hämatologie. Thieme Verlag, Stuttgart
4. Sleiman C, Raffy O, Roué C, Mal H (2000) Fatal pulmonary hemorrhage during high-dose valproate monotherapy. Chest 117:613

15. Verschiedenes

Outcome von 22 Medulloblastom-Patienten Retrospektive Untersuchung von 1976–2001

E. Noser, U. Heiniger, M. Weissert, J. Greiner

Zusammenfassung

Die Untersuchung bezweckte die Erfassung der körperlichen sowie kognitiven Langzeitfolgen und die Beurteilung der Lebensqualität von Medulloblastom-Patienten. Informationen aus den Krankenakten sowie klinische und neuropsychologische Nachuntersuchungen wurden ausgewertet. Die Jugendlichen wurden gemäß des Freiburger Persönlichkeitsinventars (FPI) über ihre Lebensqualität befragt. Das Verhalten der Kinder wurde durch die Eltern mittels der Child Behavior Checklist (CBCL) erfasst. Die Ergebnisse der Untersuchungen zeigen, dass der Operationserfolg und die Überlebensraten in engem Zusammenhang stehen, und dass die Folgen der Behandlung eine langfristige psychologische Betreuung für die Entwicklung und berufliche Integration der Kinder erfordern.

Einführung

In den letzten zwanzig Jahren haben sich die Therapieformen des Medulloblastomes stark gewandelt. Dies hat dazu geführt, dass die Langzeitüberlebenschance im Vergleich zu früher deutlich zugenommen hat. Es besteht aber der Eindruck, dass die Lebensqualität gegenüber der Normalpopulation beeinträchtigt ist.

Ziel

Die retrospektive Untersuchung diente einerseits der Erfassung der körperlichen und kognitiven Langzeitfolgen, andererseits der Lebensqualität dieser Kinder und Jugendlichen.

Methoden

Aus den Krankengeschichten wurden Angaben über die Erstsymptome, die Zeit bis zur Diagnosestellung und das Alter bei Diagnose sowie die jeweilige Therapieform entnommen. Zusätzlich erfolgte eine klinische und neuropsychologische Nachuntersuchung zur Überprüfung der kognitiven Funktionen und der affektiven Situation. Zudem wurden die Jugendlichen über ihre Lebensqualität

(FPI = Freiburger Persönlichkeitsinventar) befragt, während die Eltern einen Fragebogen (CBCL = Child Behavior Checklist) zur Einschätzung ihrer Kinder bezüglich Verhaltensauffälligkeiten zu beantworten hatten.

Ergebnisse

Insgesamt wurden die Krankenakten von 22 Patienten (16 m, 6 f) mit Medulloblastom aus den Jahren 1978–2001 retrospektiv untersucht. Das Alter bei Diagnose lag zwischen $1^{7}/_{12}$ – $13^{0}/_{12}$ Jahren (Median $7^{10}/_{12}$ Jahre) wobei 73% der Kinder bei Diagnosestellung jünger als 10 Jahre waren. Als Erstsymptome traten auf: Kopfschmerzen, Erbrechen, Gangunsicherheit und vermehrte Müdigkeit. Bei 7 Kindern war präoperativ eine Liquorpassage-Störung nachweisbar. Die Diagnose wurde mit einer Verzögerung von 1–2 Monaten gestellt. Die Operation erfolgte bei 10 Kindern total und bei 10 subtotal. Ein Mädchen verstarb perioperativ (p.v.) an einer intracraniellen Blutung und bei einem Knaben wurde keine Operation durchgeführt (inoperabel). Überlebenszeit seit der Diagnose bei lebenden und verstorbenen Medulloblastom-Patienten (Abb. 1).

Entsprechend der sich verändernden Therapieformen liegen für jedes Kind individuelle Therapiekombinationen vor. Postoperative Bestrahlung und Chemotherapie erfolgten bei 68% der Kinder. Die verschiedenen Überlebensraten in Abhängigkeit der Operationserfolge und Chemotherapien sind in Abbildung 2 und 3 ersichtlich.

In der klinischen Untersuchung zeigte sich, dass viele Patienten an körperlichen Folgen der Therapie leiden (Abb. 4).

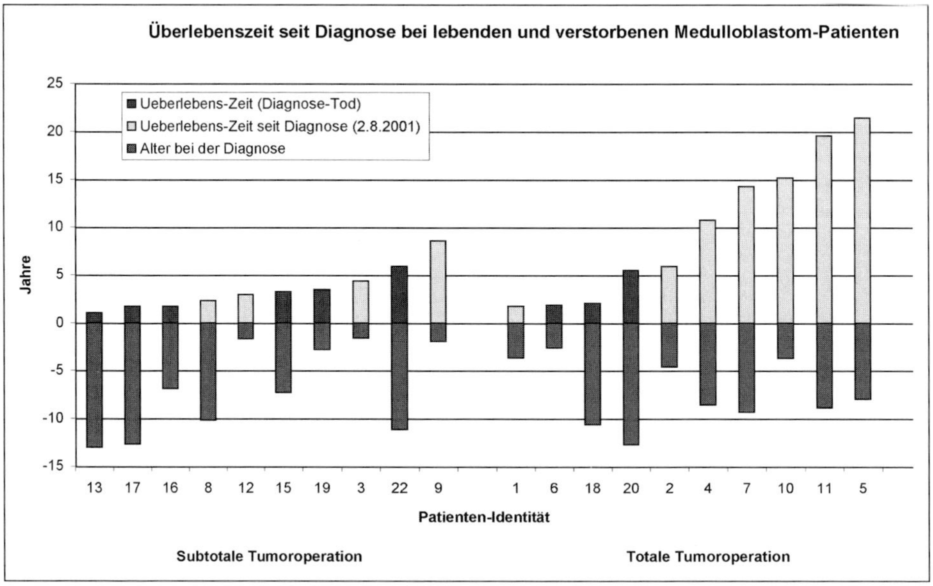

Abb. 1

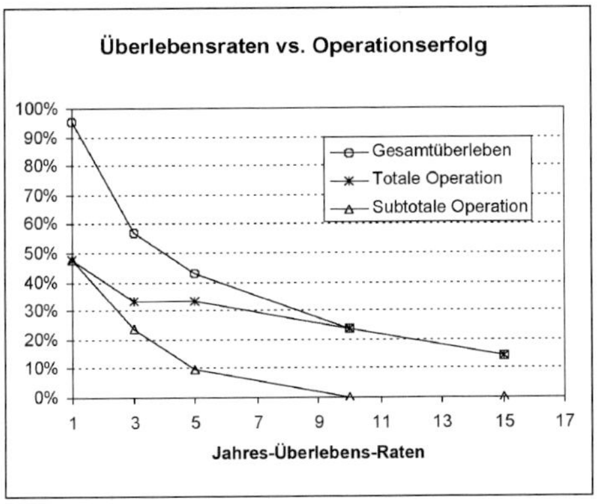

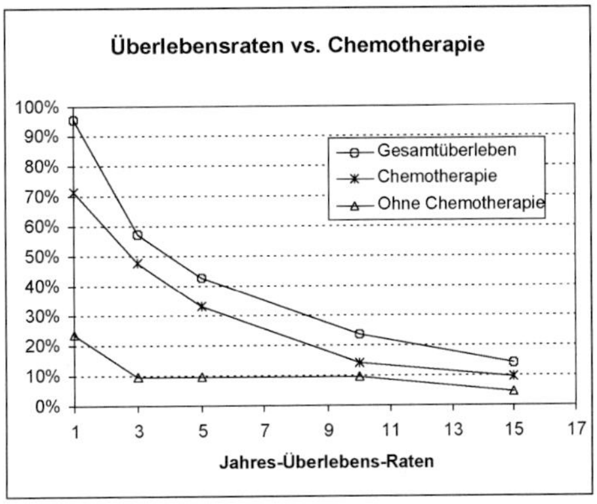

Abb. 2

Abb. 3

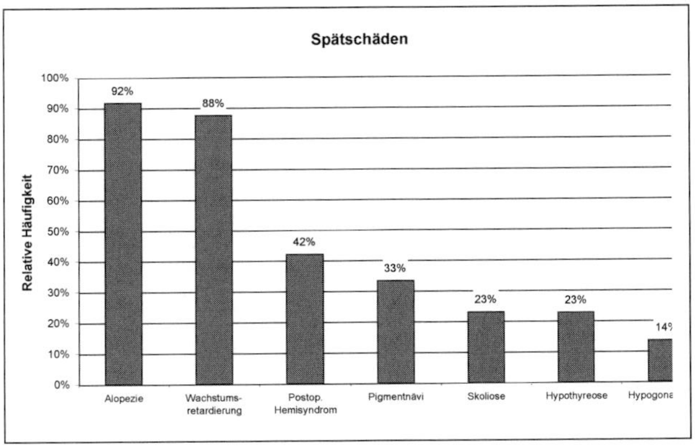

Abb. 4

Die Auswertung der Fragebogen (FPI, CBCL) ergab, dass Lebenszufriedenheit, Wohlbefinden und die weitere Entwicklung der Persönlichkeit gefährdet sind. Bei sechs Patienten konnte eine neuropsychologische Nachuntersuchung durchgeführt werden. Die gemessenen Intelligenzquotienten sind sehr unterschiedlich und nur ein Kind befindet sich im Normbereich (Abb. 5).

Zusätzliche Tests ergaben Schwächen im Lernen und Gedächtnis (Abb. 6).

Schlussfolgerungen

Unsere Untersuchungsergebnisse zeigen im Vergleich mit der Literatur (1) eine weitgehende Übereinstimmung. Die Resultate stützen die Forderung nach Konzepten für neue Behandlungsstrategien nicht nur quad vitam, sondern auch für die Lebensqualität (2). Hierzu wäre u.a. eine längerfristige stützende psychologische Betreuung der betroffenen Familien und der Patienten im privaten wie auch beruflichen Alltag sinnvoll. Zu empfehlen sind eine standardisierte Erfassung der Lebensqualität mit spezifischen Fragebogen sowie die neuropsychologische Untersuchung (3, 4) der Kinder im Schulalter. Damit werden frühzeitig

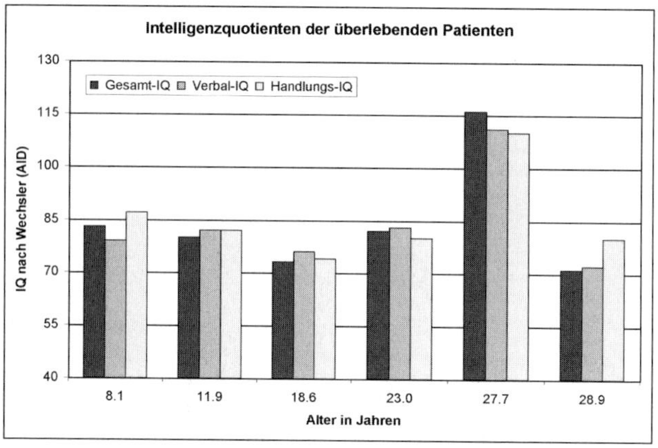

Abb. 5

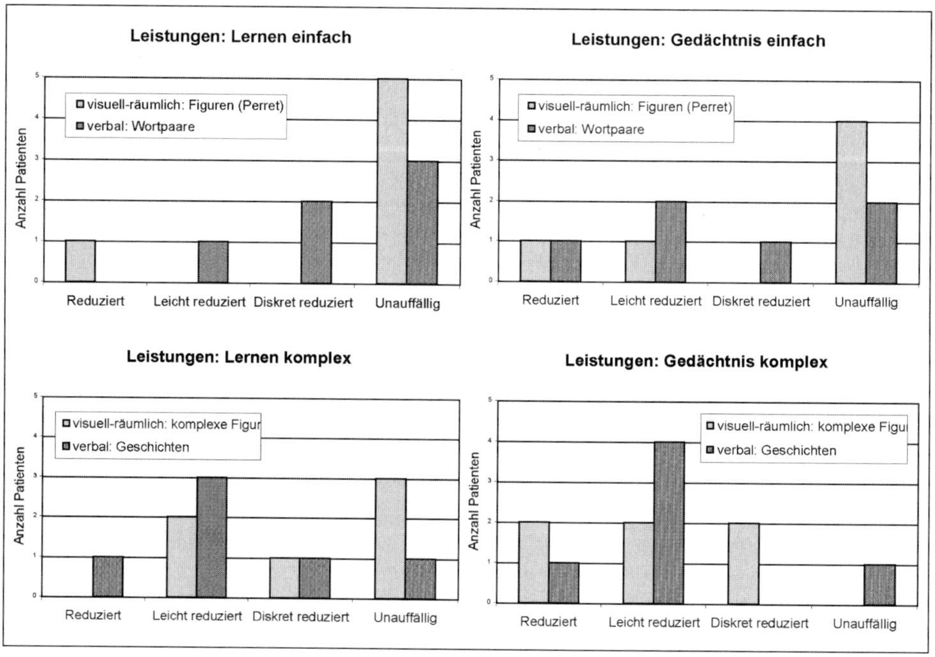

Abb. 6

kognitive Leistungsdefizite erkannt und die Kinder können gezielt gefördert sowie in ihrer Berufsfindung und beruflichen Integration unterstüzt werden.

Literatur

1. Modha A., Vassilyadi M. (2000), Medulloblastoma in children; Childs Nerv Syst; 16 (6): 341-50: Helseth E., Due-Tonnessen B. (1999), Posterior fossa medulloblastoma in children and young adults; survival and performance; Childs Nerv Syst; 15(9): 451–5:

2. In: King C. R., Hinds P. S.; Lebensqualität; Theorie, Forschung, Praxis; 1. Auflage 2001; Verlag Hans Huber
3. In: Heubrock D., Petermann F.; Lehrbuch der klinischen Kinderneuropsychologie; Grundlagen, Syndrome, Diagnostik und Intervention; 1. Auflage 2000, Hogrefe-Verlag
4. In: Lösslein H., Deike-Beth C.; Hirnfunktionsstörungen bei Kindern und Jugendlichen; Neuropsychologische Untersuchungen für die Praxis; 3. überarbeitete und erweiterte Auflage 2000, Deutscher Ärzte-Verlag

Ein isoliert kortikales unilaterales Hirnödem als neurologische Komplikation einer Coxsackievirus B Infektion

C. Härtel, S. Schilling, S. Gottschalk, J. Sperner

Abstrakt

Wir beschreiben das Auftreten eines isoliert kortikalen Hirnödems in Zusammenhang mit einer Coxsackievirus B Infektion. Ein 10jähriges Mädchen wurde mit einer Hemiparese rechts und komplex-partiellen Krampfanfällen vorgestellt. Die kranielle MRT-Untersuchung zeigte ein ungewöhnliches Muster eines isoliert kortikalen linksseitigen Hirnödems, welches die weiße Substanz aussparte, aber eine intravaskuläre Gadolinium-Anreicherung der linkshemisphärischen sulcalen Venen erkennen ließ. Nach antikonvulsiver Therapie erholte sich die Patientin rasch, auch die MRT-Veränderungen hatten sich zwei Monate später vollständig zurückgebildet. Im EEG zeigte sich jedoch auch nach 5 Monaten noch eine linkshemisphärische Verlangsamung.

Fallbericht

Ein 10 Jahre altes Mädchen, deren Schulleistungen im unteren Normbereich liegen, wurde in unserer Notfallambulanz mit eingeschränktem Bewusstsein, Husten, Fieber und Bauchschmerzen vorgestellt. Die frühere Anamnese ergab 3 Fieberkrämpfe im Alter von 2 Jahren, wobei die damaligen EEG-, CCT- und MRT-Untersuchungen einen unauffälligen Befund erbrachten.

Bei der Aufnahmeuntersuchung bestanden ein Wert von 12 auf der Glasgow-Coma-Scale, eine Hemiparese rechts mit Schwäche des Nervus facialis rechts, nicht auslösbare Muskeleigenreflexe an der oberen rechten Extremität und vermindert auslösbare Muskeleigenreflexe an der unteren rechten Extremität. Ein unmittelbar durchgeführtes CCT ergab einen unauffälligen Befund, die Liquoruntersuchung zeigte ebenfalls keinen pathologischen Befund (2 Leukozyten /µl, Protein 0,32 g/l, Glukose 0,6 g/l).

Im Laufe der folgenden 4 Tage nach stationärer Aufnahme zeigte die Patientin 4 komplex-fokale Krampfanfälle mit Blickdeviation nach rechts, die bis zu 20 Minuten andauerten. Nach erfolgloser Diazepam- und Clonazepamtherapie wurden die Krampfanfälle mit Phenytoin i.v. (300 mg = 12 mg/kg Körpergewicht) effektiv behandelt. Eine kranielle MRT-Untersuchung, die 48 Stunden nach dem letzten Krampfanfall durchgeführt wurde, zeigte eine erhöhte T-2-gewichtete Signalintensität der gesamten linkshemisphärischen kortikalen grauen Substanz mit einer isolierten Verdickung des kortikalen Bandes. Die subkortikale weiße Substanz zeigte keinen pathologischen Befund, ebenso war die Mark-Rinden-

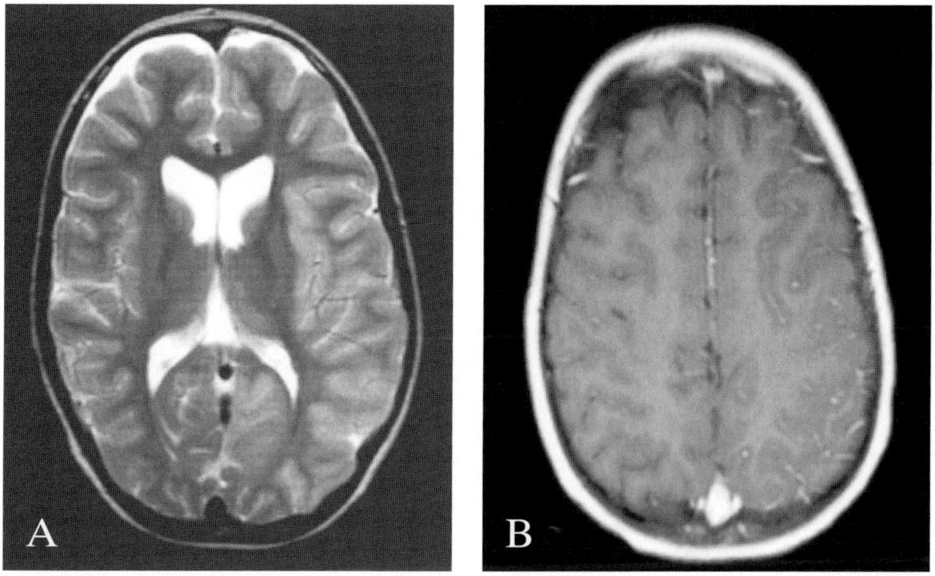

Abb. 1: MRT Veränderungen; T2 gewichtete Axialschnittbilder des Gehirns zeigen ein kortikales Ödem der gesamten links hemisphärischen grauen Substanz mit Verbreiterung und Signalsteigerung im Bereich des kortikalen Bandes (A). T1-Aufnahmen zeigen eine Anreicherung im Bereich der sulkalen Venen der linken Hemisphäre. Eine Blut-Hirn-Schranken-Störung war nach Gadolinium i.v. nicht zu erkennen (B).

Grenze nicht beeinträchtigt (Abb. 1A). Auf T-1-gewichteten Aufnahmen war eine intravaskuläre Gadolinium-Anreicherung der sulkalen Venen der linken Hemisphäre zu erkennen (Abb. 1B). Mehrfache EEG-Aufzeichnungen zeigten eine generalisierte pathologische Deltawellen-Verlangsamung über der gesamten linken Hemisphäre, wobei die EEG-Aktivität der rechten Hemisphäre als normal befundet wurde. Ein iktales EEG zeigte während eines komplexen Anfalls linksfrontale Sharp-wave-Komplexe mit ipsilateraler Ausbreitung.

Die molekularbiologische sowie serologische Diagnostik zum Nachweis neurotroper Organismen im Serum und Liquor zeigte bis auf eine Serumantikörperproduktion gegen Coxsackie-Virus B 1 bis 6 (1:320, positiv wenn größer 1:80) keinen pathologischen Befund.

Unter antiepileptischer Dauertherapie mit Oxcarbacepin (30 mg/kg Körpergewicht/Tag) ereigneten sich keine weiteren Krampfanfälle. Zwei Wochen später war lediglich eine leichte Schwäche der rechten Hand als einziges Residualsymptom nachweisbar, während die links-hemisphärische Verlangsamung im EEG weiterhin auffällig war.

In der Verlaufskontrolle 4 Wochen später war die klinisch-neurologische Symptomatik komplett zurückgebildet, ebenso waren die auffälligen MRT-Veränderungen nicht mehr nachweisbar und der Coxsackie-B-1- bis -6-Antikörpertiter auf 1:20 abgefallen. Im EEG war jedoch auch 5 Monate nach dem Ereignis weiterhin eine links-hemisphärische Verlangsamung mit vermehrten Deltawellen nachweisbar.

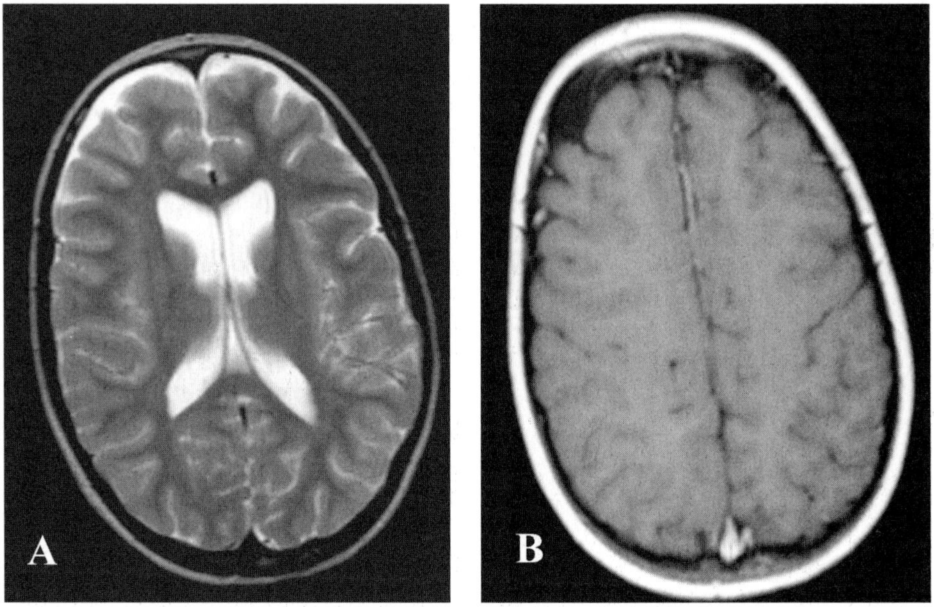

Abb. 2: Verlaufskontrolle nach 4 Wochen: T1 nach Gadolinium i.v. (B) und T2 gewichtete Bilder (A) zeigten einen unauffälligen Befund.

Diskussion

Enterovirale Infektionen treten in der Kindheit gehäuft auf und verbreiten sich von Person zu Person auf dem fäkal-oralen bzw. oral-oralen Übertragungsweg. Die Infektion ist häufig asymptomatisch (bis zu 95% der infizierten Individuen), jedoch können Enteroviren auch verschiedene neurologische Komplikationen wie z.B. eine aseptische Meningitis, eine Encephalitis sowie eine akute schlaffe Lähmung in 0,01 bis 2,8 Fällen pro 1.000 Kinder pro Jahr hervorrufen (1). Der ätiologische Nachweis wird durch serologische Bestimmungen (Antikörpertiter) geführt, selten können Coxsackie-Viren aus Liquorflüssigkeit isoliert werden. Wir beschreiben hier erstmalig den Nachweis eines transienten, isoliert kortikalen, unilateralen Hirnödems als parainfektiöses Phänomen einer enteroviralen Infektion.

Ein unilaterales Hirnödem könnte differentialdiagnostisch durch Diffusionsveränderungen bei einem Partialstatus epilepticus auftreten (2,3). In diesem Falle wären die MRT-Signalveränderungen als Resultat einer Hyperperfusion in der epileptogenen Region zu interpretieren, wobei diese nicht initial, sondern mehrere Tage nach dem Status epilepticus nachweisbar sind und generell sowohl die weiße als auch die graue Substanz betreffen. Bei unserer Patientin, die keinen Status epilepticus erlitten hatte, zeigten serielle EEG-Aufnahmen eine langanhaltende Delta-Verlangsamung der gesamten linken Hemisphäre mit frontaler epileptischer Aktivität während eines komplexen partialen Anfalls. Es bestand keine enge Zeitkorrelation zwischen den MRT-Veränderungen und der epileptischen Aktivität, so dass eine Assoziation des isoliert kortikalen unilateralen Hirnödems zur enteroviralen Enzephalitis wahrscheinlicher ist als zu den komplex-partiellen Krampfanfällen. Im Gegensatz zu früheren Publikationen bezüglich struktureller Auswirkungen des Partialstatus epilepticus im MRT zeigten sich die MRT-Veränderungen bei unserer Patientin als isoliert auf den Kortex bezogen und nicht die weiße Substanz betreffend. Das Hirnödem bildete sich komplett zurück und zeigte keine kortikale Atrophie wie bei anderen Erkrankungen (3, 4). Weiterhin könnte ein unilaterales Hirnödem bei ischämischem Hirninfarkt im Kindesalter als Ausdruck eines zytotoxischen oder vasogenen Ödems nachweisbar sein, wobei sich in unserem Fall sowohl klinisch als auch kernspintomografisch kein Anhalt ergab. Im Gegensatz zur Arbeitsgruppe von Meaney et al. (5), welche ein transientes unilaterales Hirnödem in Assoziation mit einer hemiplegischen Migräne berichtete, war bei unserer Patientin die Hemiparese rechts für einen Zeitraum von 5 Tagen nachweisbar, und die EEG-Veränderungen erwiesen sich für mehrere Monate als pathologisch. Ebenso hatte unsere Patientin nie über vormalige Kopfschmerzen berichtet, auch ergab sich kein Hinweis für Migräne aus der Familienanamnese. Des weiteren konnte die Rasmussen-Enzephalitis (6), eine chronisch unilaterale Enzephalitis einer Hemisphäre mit fokalen Krampfanfällen, Hemiparese, mentaler Regression und unilateraler frontaler Atrophie ausgeschlossen werden, da in unserem Fall sich eine komplette radiologische und klinische Remission parallel zur Normalisierung der Antikörpertiter für Coxsackie-Viren zeigte.

Dieser Fallbereicht zeigt die große Variabilität der klinischen und neuroradiologischen Manifestation von enteroviralen Infektionen, wobei das Auftreten eines isoliert kortikalen unilateralen Ödems in diesem Zusammenhang in der bisherigen Literatur noch nicht beschrieben wurde.

Literatur

1. Koskiniemi M, Rautonen J, Lehtokoski-Lehtiniemi E, Vaheri A (1991). Epidemiology of encephalitis in children: A 20-year survey. Ann Neurol 29: 492–497.
2. Lazeyras F, Blanke O, Zimine I, Delavelle J, Perrig SH, Seeck M (2000). MRI, H-MRS, and functional MRI during and after prolonged nonconvulsive seizure activity. Neurology 55: 1677–82.
3. Wieshmann UC, Symms MR, Shorvon SD (1997). Diffusion changes in status epilepticus. Lancet 350: 493–494.
4. Meierkord H, Wieshmann UC, Niehaus L, Lehmann R (1997). Structural consequences of status epilepticus demonstrated with serial magnetic resonance imaging. Acta Neurol Scand 96: 127–32.
5. Meaney, JF, Williams, CE, Humphrey PR (1996). Case report: transient unilateral cerebral oedema in hemiplegic migraine: MR imaging and angiography. Clin Radiol 51: 72–76.
6. Sener RN (2000). Rasmussen's encephalitis: proton MR spectroscopy and diffusion MR findings. J Neuroradiol 27: 179–84.

Polio-ähnliche Myelitis durch Coxsackie-Virus B 3 – Verlauf unter Pleconaril-Behandlung

N. Utzig, B. Friedrich, Ch. Burtzlaff, H. Lauffer

Einleitung

Myelitiden treten mit einem Häufigkeitsgipfel der Erkrankung zwischen dem 10. und 20. Lebensjahr auf. Sie sind überwiegend viral bedingt. Häufigste Erreger sind die Enteroviren (Poliomyelitisviren und Non-Polio-Enteroviren = NPEV), aber auch Herpes-, Arbo-, Zytomegalieviren, HIV und Hepatitis A-Viren. Die Gruppe der NPEV umfasst Coxsackieviren der Gruppe A und B, ECHO-Viren sowie Enteroviren der Serotypen 68–71. Diese Erreger können ein breites Spektrum von Enzephalitiden und Myelitiden mit vorrangigem Befall der motorischen Vorderhornzellen hervorrufen (3). Die Prognose der Erkrankungen ist sehr different, es werden überwiegend günstige Verläufe mit Besserung innerhalb von wenigen Wochen bis Monaten beschrieben, häufig verbleibt jedoch eine neurologische Restsymptomatik. Schwere, teilweise tödliche Verläufe können bei Coxsackievirus B 3 und B 6, Echovirus 2, 9, 17, und 25 sowie Enterovirus 71 auftreten (1, 2).

Mit dem Wirkstoff Pleconaril® (VP-63843) wurde jetzt ein Virustatikum mit breiter Aktivität gegen Picornaviren, insbesondere gegen Entero- und Rhinoviren entwickelt. Es zeichnet sich durch eine gute orale Bioverfügbarkeit, eine geringe Nebenwirkungsrate sowie eine in klinischen Studien des Kindes- und Erwachsenenalters belegte Wirksamkeit aus (4). Pleconaril® befindet sich derzeit noch in klinischer Erprobung.

Fallbericht

Vorgeschichte:

Die Aufnahme des 14-jährigen leicht mental retardierten, zuvor sonst gesunden Mädchens erfolgte wegen einer rasch progredienten Parese des linken Beines wenige Stunden nach einem Sturz auf den Rücken. Innerhalb von drei Tagen entwickelte sich ein polio-ähnliches Krankheitsbild mit linksbetonter Paraparese sowie Blasenentleerungsstörung und Überlaufinkontinenz.

Befunde:

Anfänglich bestand der Verdacht auf eine rein traumatische Genese, konventionelles Röntgen, spinales CT, zerebrale und spinale MRT (initial und nach 4 Wochen) wiesen jedoch keine Auffälligkeiten auf. Nach kortikaler elektromagnetischer Stimulation ließen sich keine motorischen Antworten an den Beinen ableiten, während periphere motorische sowie periphere und zentrale sensible Nervenleitung intakt waren. Das EMG zeigte eine vollständige Parese der Ober- und Unterschenkelmuskulatur links sowie eine erhebliche Polyphasie rechts.

Im Liquor fanden sich Zeichen einer aktiven Virusinfektion, mittels Serologie und PCR ließ sich eine Infektion durch Coxsackievirus Typ B 3 sichern (Liquor, Blut, Stuhl und Urin).

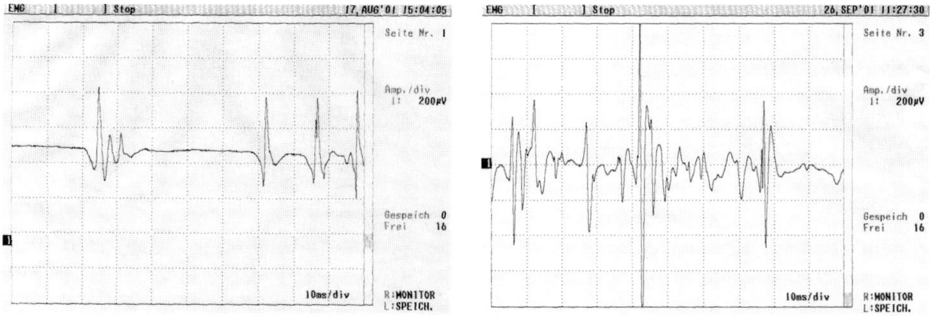

a b

Abb. 1: EMG a) nach 3 Wochen beginnende Willkürmotorik, polyphasische MAP, spontane Fibrillationen b) nach 10 Wochen gute Willkürmotorik, Polyphasie, keine Fibrillationen.

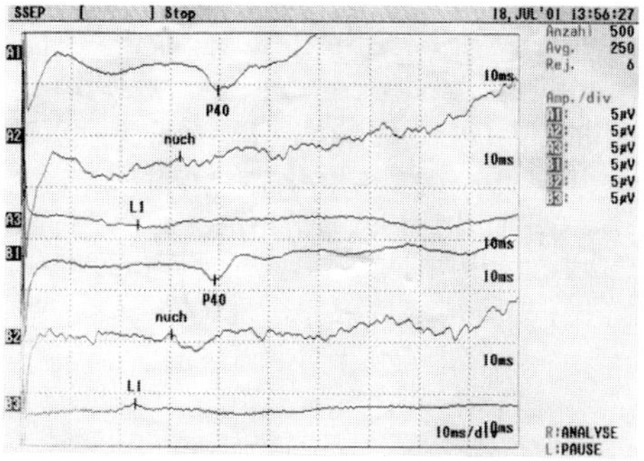

Abb. 2: Tibialis-SEP nach 2 Wochen: beidseits regelrechte periphere und zentrale Leitzeiten.

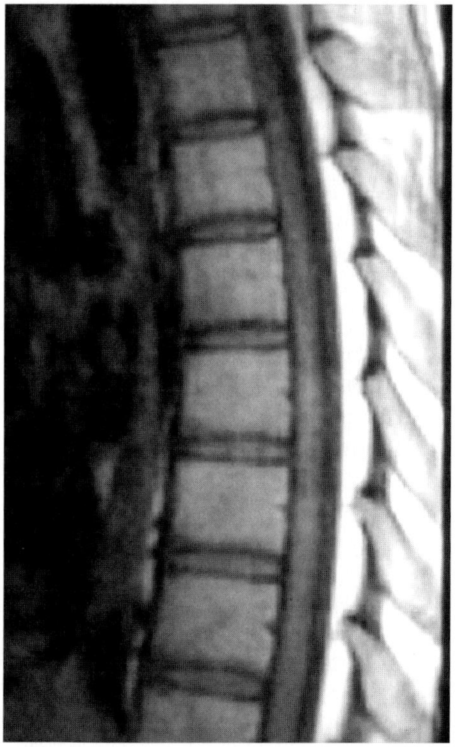

Abb. 3: Spinale MRT: Initial sowie im Verlauf kein Nachweis von Strukturveränderungen.

Verlauf:

Zwei Wochen symptomatischer Behandlung erbrachten zunächst keine klinische Besserung. Die Liquorkontrolle im Verlauf ließ eine zunehmende Pleozytose (bis max. 24 Leuko/µl) mit lymphozytär-reaktivem Zytogramm und Zeichen der intrathekalen Immunglobulinsynthese erkennen.

Wir behandelten die Patientin nun nach Eingang der virologischen Befunde über 7 Tage mit dem Virustatikum Pleconaril® (entspr. Studienprotokoll der Fa. ViroPharma mit 5 mg/kg KG/d). Nach Therapie-Ende waren die entzündlichen Liquorveränderungen deutlich rückläufig, durch PCR ließen sich keine Viren mehr nachweisen. Auch klinisch trat die Erkrankung in eine konstante Besserungsphase ein. Durch EMG konnte zunächst geringe Willkürmotorik mit kleinen polyphasischen Potenzialen, im weiteren Verlauf dann gute Willküraktivität mit höheramplitudigen, weiterhin polyphasischen Potenzialen bis 2 mV nachgewiesen werden.

Die Harnkontinenz erlangte die Patientin zurück, freies Laufen war innerhalb eines Zeitraumes von 10 Wochen ohne Gehhilfen möglich.

Diskussion

Akute Paresen stellen im Kindesalter immer eine Notfallsituation dar. Neben Enzephalitiden bzw. Myelitiden sind differenzialdiagnostisch v.a. das Guillain-Barré-Syndrom sowie myasthene Syndrome zu beachten. Myelitiden mit vorrangigem Befall der motorischen Vorderhornzellen wie im vorliegenden Fallbeispiel sind in Deutschland aufgrund der Polioimpfung selten und sollten immer an eine NPEV-Infektion denken lassen. Mit der Entwicklung neuer antiviraler Substanzen haben sich im Bereich der Neuropädiatrie erweiterte Behandlungsmöglichkeiten ergeben. Enteroviren als häufigste Erreger infektiöser ZNS-Erkrankungen können ein sehr differenziertes Spektrum klinischer Krankheitsbilder hervorrufen. Die Verläufe sind dabei oft mild bzw. asymptomatisch. Es können jedoch auch sehr schwere, lebensbedrohende Erkrankungen resultieren. Mit dem neuen Wirkstoff Pleconaril® steht eine kausale Therapieoption zur Verfügung. Ob und in welchem Ausmaß der vorgestellte Krankheitsverlauf durch die Gabe von Pleconaril® beeinflusst wurde, kann letztlich nicht gesagt werden. Virustyp und anfänglicher klinischer und paraklinischer Verlauf wiesen auf eine ungünstige Prognose hin, dennoch erlangte die Patientin relativ rasch eine gute motorische Funktionsfähigkeit beider Beine zurück.

Richtlinien der Indikationsstellung zur Behandlung lassen sich im Ergebnis der laufenden Studien erwarten.

Literatur

1. Behrmann, RE et al.: Nelson Textbook of Pediatrics – 16. Aufl.; Saunders Verlag 2000
2. Chen, C-Y et al.: Acute flaccid paralysis in infants and young children with enterovirus 71 infection – Amer. J. of Neurorad., Jan. 2001, 22:200–205
3. Kapoor, A et al.: Non-polio enteroviruses in acute flaccid paralysis – Indian J. of Pediatrics, Oct. 2001, 68 (10):927–9
4. Pevear, DC et al.: Activity of Pleconaril against enteroviruses – Antimicrobial Agents and Chemotherapy, Sept. 1999:2109–2115

Langzeitbeobachtung einer Interferon β 1b Therapie bei einem 15jährigen Patienten mit sekundär chronischer Multipler Sklerose

S. Schilling, C. Härtel, J. Sperner

Einleitung

Die Multiple Sklerose (MS) oder auch Enzephalitis disseminata ist die häufigste chronische demyelinisierende Erkrankung und tritt mit einer Häufigkeit von 3% der Erstmanifestationen vergleichsweise selten vor dem 17. Lebensjahr auf. Als Ätiologie der MS werden genetische, infektiologische und autoimmunologische Mechanismen diskutiert. Bei Erstmanifestation tritt im Kindesalter häufiger eine bulbäre Symptomatik als bei Erwachsenen auf. Die MS wird differenziert in einen schubförmigen Verlauf, der mit 95% hauptsächlich vorkommt, sowie den primär und sekundär chronisch progredienten Verlauf. Bei 1% der Erkrankten tritt eine primäre chronische Form auf und nur 3% hat einen sekundär chronischen Verlauf und damit auch die schlechteste Langzeitprognose.

In der Behandlung der MS werden verschiedene Immunmodulatoren eingesetzt. Zur akuten Entzündungshemmung gilt die hochdosierte kurzeitige Steroidtherapie als internationaler Standard. Für die Langzeittherapie gibt es in der Literatur die meisten kontrollierten prospektiven Studien bei Erwachsenen zu kontinuierlichen Interferon β Gabe, wobei die Effektivität für Interferon β 1b (Betaferon) und Interferon β 1a (Avonex, Rebif) je nach Verlaufstyp sich nicht im wesentlichen unterscheidet. Weitere gute klinische Wirksamkeit zeigte die intermittierende Therapie mit Immunglobulinen und eine Dauertherapie mit Glatirameracetat (Copaxone).

Die Empfehlungen zur dauerhaften immunmodulierenden Therapie für Jugendliche unter 17 Jahre, sind aufgrund der tendenziell besseren Prognose, verglichen mit erwachsenen Erkrankten, sehr zurückhaltend. Zusätzlich sind die Nebenwirkungen der zur Verfügung stehenden Immunmodulatoren für das präpubertäre Alter unzureichend bekannt. Im Kindes- und Jugendalter gibt es außer wenigen publizierten Einzelfallberichten nur zwei kürzlich veröffentlichte Langzeitstudien zu der Interferon β -Therapie bei Patienten unter 16 Jahren mit schubförmiger MS (1, 2).

Kasuistik

Wir berichten über einen 16jährigen Patienten mit einer sekundär chronischen MS. Die Erkrankung manifestierte sich erstmals im Alter von 11 Jahren mit Gangunsicherheit, Spastik und Kraftverlust in den unteren Extremitäten. Visuelle oder bulbäre Symptome fanden sich nicht.

Die pathologischen Untersuchungsbefunde beinhalteten disseminierte leukodystrophische Herde im zerebralen MRT (siehe Abb.1), oligoklonale Banden und verzögerte Latenzen

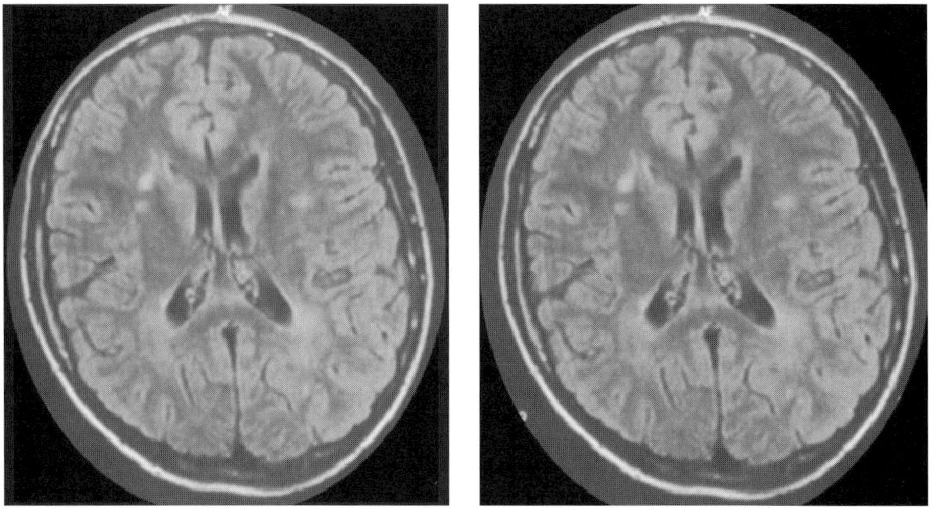

Abb. 1: Cerebrales MRT zum Zeitpunkt der Erstmanifestation.

für P100 im VEP. Nach einer Steroidpulstherapie folgte eine komplette Remission der neurologischen Symptomatik. Nach 7 und 24 Monaten traten weitere Schübe auf, die jeweils sehr gut auf Steroide ansprachen. Drei Jahre nach Erstmanifestation verschlechterte sich die neurologische Symptomatik kontinuierlich und besserte sich auch nicht nach wiederholt durchgeführten Hochdosis-Steroidtherapien. Nach einem dritten verlängerten Steroid-Block erreichte der Patient nur noch ein Expanded Disability Status Score von 5 (5). Die Gehstrecke ohne Pause betrug noch maximal 100 m und die Lebensqualität (ADL) war progredient reduziert. Psychisch wurden erstmals medikamentöse Interventionsmaßnahmen erwogen.

Zu diesem Zeitpunkt wurde in Absprache mit den Eltern und dem Patienten nach Aufklärung aller bekannten Risiken ein individueller Heilversuch mit Interferon β 1b (Betaferon) begonnen. Das Präparat wurde aufgrund der bis dahin einzigen repräsentativen Therapiestudie der European Study Group für die sekundär chronische MS ausgewählt (4). Die Kriterien zur immunmodulatorischen Dauertherapie erfolgten nach den internationalen Standards.

Methode

Die Therapie mit Betaferon wurde nach einer Erhebung des Status quo von Klinik, Serumleberwerte und hämatologischem Blutbild, zerebralem und spinalem MRT und Neurophysiologie begonnen. In der ersten Woche wurde Interferon mit 4 MIU alle zwei Tage s. c. eindosiert. Nach 14 Tagen wurde die Dosierung gesteigert auf Betaferon 18 MIU zweitäglich s.c.. Nach Tag 7, Woche 4, Monat 3 und weiter in halbjährlichem Abstand wurden klinische Untersuchungen mit dem Kurtzke EDSS und einem internistischen Status, serologischen Kontrollen der Leber- und Nierenwerte, des Blutbildes und der anamnestische Befragung auf etwaige Nebenwirkungen von dem gleichen Untersucher durchgeführt.

Der Patient wurde ambulant für weitere 3 Monate in der Applikationsform geschult und konnte dann die Injektion selbstständig durchführen. Insgesamt beträgt der Beobachtungszeitraum mittlerweile 19 Monate, die Therapie wird weitergeführt.

Ergebnisse

Die Nebenwirkungen beschränkten sich auf episodische erkältungsähnliche Symptome mit Fieber und Myalgie, die gut auf Ibuprofen ansprachen. Neben den kurzzeitigen postpunktionellen lokalen Hautrötungen gab es keine erwähnenswerte dermale Reaktion.

Es gab keine pathologische Veränderung des Blutbildes, der Leber- und Nierenserumwerte. Unser Patient nahm nach einer Therapiezeit von 12 Monaten akut 4 kg Körpergewicht ab, trotz gleichbleibender Kalorienzufuhr. Wiederholte Kontrollen der Stuhlausnutzung, der Schilddrüsenhormone, und das Blutzuckertagesprofil ergaben Normalbefunde. Durch ein deutliche Anhebung der Kalorienzufuhr konnte das Körpergewicht stabil gehalten werden.

Die Pubertätsentwicklung, das Körperwachstum und die Knochenentwicklung waren altersentsprechend.

Tab. 1:

Initialsymptomatik	Alter bei Erstmanifestation	Alter bei Therapiebeginn	Erkrankungsdauer vor Therapie	EDSS vor Therapie	EDSS nach 15 Monaten	Therapiedauer
Zerebrale Herde	11 Jahre	14 Jahre	3 Jahre	5	4	19 Monate

Diskussion

In der Literatur gibt es leider keine vergleichbaren Daten zur Wirksamkeit einer Interferon β 1b Therapie bei Patienten unter 16 Jahren mit sekundär chronischer MS.

Es kann aber für unseren Patienten festgestellt werden, dass es unter Therapie zu einer deutlichen klinischen Stabilisierung der neurologischen Defizite gekommen ist, orientiert am EDSS sogar zu einer Besserung des Scores. Nach internationalem Standard ist dies ein Indikator zur Therapiefortführung. Die beiden einzigen existierenden Studien von Mikaeloff et al. und Waubant et al. zur Interferon β-Therapie sind ausschließlich bei Patienten mit einem schubförmigen Verlauf durchgeführt worden. Somit lassen sich die Daten zur Wirksamkeit nicht mit unserer Kasuistik vergleichen.

Vergleichbar sind aber die Daten bezgl. Nebenwirkungen. Bei unserem Patienten traten an bekannten Symptomen die erkältungsähnlichen Symptome auf, die gut therapierbar waren. Der erhöhte Grundumsatz bei unserem Patienten ist bislang bei Kindern eine nicht beschriebene Nebenwirkung. Bei Patienten mit Diabetes ist ein höherer Insulinbedarf beschrieben. Ein okkulter Insulinmangel konnte bei unserem Patienten bislang ausgeschlossen werden. Durch eine

Ernährungsmodifikation normalisierte sich das Körpergewicht. Schwerwiegende Nebenwirkungen wie Hautnekrosen und schwere Infektionen traten nicht auf.

Zusammenfassung

Bei dem vorliegenden Langzeitverlauf kann für den jugendlichen Patienten eine gute Verträglichkeit der Betaferon-Therapie festgestellt werden. Die hohe Effektivität für die sekundär chronische progrediente MS kann in unserer Kasuistik bestätigt werden.

Literatur

1. Mikaeloff, J et al. (2001) Interferon β treatment in patients with childhood-onset multiple sclerosis. Pediatrics; 139(3)
2. Waubant, J et al. (2001) Interferon β 1a in children with MS is well tolerated. Neuropediatrics; 32:211–213
3. Poser, CM, et al. (1983) New diagnostic criteria for multiple sclerosis: Guidelines for research protocols. Ann Neurol, 13(4):227–230
4. European Study Group on Interferon β1b in secondary progressive MS (1998) Placebo-controlled multicenter study. Lancet;352:1491–1497
5. Kurtzke JF. (1983) Rating neurologic impairment: Expanded disability status score. Neurology, 33;1444–52

Zweiterkrankung nach Herpes-Simplex-Encephalitis: Virusreaktivierung oder (Auto-)Immunreaktion?

A. Brockhaus, S. Lütjen, M. Granel, G. Kluger, H. Holthausen

Zusammenfassung

Eine Zweiterkrankung nach Herpes-Simplex-Encephalitis (HSE) ist relativ selten. Der Pathomechanismus ist unklar.

Es werden die Krankheitsverläufe von 5 Patienten – insbesondere im Hinblick auf die MRT-Befunde und den zeitlichen Verlauf der Zweiterkrankung – geschildert.

Zum Zeitpunkt der Erstinfektion und bei Zweiterkrankung lagen bei 3 Patienten für eine HSE typische MRT-Befunde vor. Bei einem Patienten mit Erkrankung im Neugeborenenalter war der MRT-Befund primär unauffällig, bei der Zweiterkrankung zeigte sich ein untypischer Befund mit Befall beider Occipitallappen. Bei einem weiteren Patienten lag bereits bei Erstinfektion ein untypischer Befund mit Befall einer gesamten Hemisphäre vor, der sich im Verlauf weiter ausbreitete.

Der Virusgenomnachweis im Liquor bei Zweiterkrankung gelang nur in einem Fall.

Bei den drei Patienten mit typischem MRT-Befund kam es jeweils nach 4 Wochen zur Zweiterkrankung (»Frührezidiv«).

Aufgrund der unterschiedlichen MRT-Befunde und zeitlichen Krankheitsverläufe gehen wir bei unseren Patienten von verschiedenen Pathomechanismen als Ursache für die Zweiterkrankung aus. Auch bei fehlendem Virusgenomnachweis kann der MRT-Befund und der Zeitpunkt der Zweiterkankung zur ätiologischen Klärung der Zweiterkrankung beitragen.

Hintergrund

In der Literatur wird in einzelnen Kasuistiken über eine Zweiterkrankung (»Relapse«) nach einer Herpes-Simplex-Encephalitis (HSE) berichtet (1, 4, 5, 8). Dabei wird diskutiert, ob es sich um ein echtes Rezidiv mit nachgewiesener Virusreaktivierung oder um eine auto-immunologische Zweiterkrankung ähnlich einer akuten disseminierten Encephalomyelitis (ADEM) handelt (9). Der Pathomechanismus ist unklar.

Anhand von 5 eigenen Patienten, die uns zur neuropädiatrischen Rehabilitation zugewiesen wurden, werden die Verläufe einer Zweiterkrankung nach HSE geschildert. Besonderes Augenmerk wird auf die MRT-Befunde und den Zeitpunkt der Zweiterkrankung gelegt, mit der Frage, ob sich dadurch Hinweise auf verschiedene Ätiologien ergeben.

Tab. 1: Patientenübersicht. Fall 1–4: HSV-1, Fall 5: HSV-2.

Pat.	Alter bei Erstinfektion (Jahre) / Geschlecht	Intervall Erstinfektion/ Zweiterkrankung (Wochen)	HSV-DNA-Nachweis im Liquor		Therapie		Neurologisches Outcome
			bei Erstinfektion	bei Zweiterkrankung	bei Erstinfektion	bei Zweiterkrankung	
1	1 9/12 m	4	–	–	Zovirax (2 Wochen), beta-Interferon	Zovirax (3 Wochen), beta-Interferon	Hemiparese, akust. Agnosie, Schluckstörung, Epilepsie
2	1 1/12 w	4	+	–	Zovirax (3 Wochen)	Steroide, Immunglobuline	Mässige allgemeine Entwicklungsverzögerung, Aphasie, Epilepsie
3	5 1/12 w	4	–	–	Zovirax (2 Wochen), Steroide, Immunglobuline	Zovirax (4 Wochen), Steroide, Immunglobuline	Hemiparese, Ataxie, Sprachstörung, Epilepsie
4	5 Tage w	24	+	+	Zovirax (3 Wochen)	Zovirax (3 Wochen)	Schwere allgemeine Entwicklungsverzögerung, Tetraprese, Dystonie, Epilepsie
5	4 3/12 m	12	+	–	Zovirax (3 Wochen)	Steroide, Immunglobuline	Schwere kognitive Defizite, Tetraparese, Aphasie, Epilepsie

Kasuistiken

A. Patienten (vgl. Tab. 1)

Wir berichten über 5 Patienten, die sich in den Jahren 1992 bis 2001 wegen einer Zweiterkrankung nach einer primären HSE in unserer stationären Behandlung befanden. In vier Fällen lag primär eine HSV-1-Infektion, in einem Fall eine HSV-2-Infektion vor.

Das Alter bei Erstinfektion, die Zeitdauer zwischen Erstinfektion und Zweiterkrankung, die jeweilige medikamentöse Therapie sowie das neurologische Outcome sind in Tabelle 1 dargestellt.

Die Diagnose einer Herpes-Simplex-Encephalitis wurde zunächst bei 3 Patienten durch den positiven Nachweis von HSV-DNA mittels PCR im Liquor gestellt (Patient 2, 4 und 5).

Bei zwei Patienten (Patient 1 und 3) erfolgte die Diagnosestellung anhand des Nachweises von HSV-spezifischen Antikörpern in Liquor und Serum bzw. durch einen HSE-typischen MRT-Befund, d.h. Ödem bzw. Befall der Inselregion/Temporallappen (6).

Die ätiologische Zuordnung der Zweiterkrankung allein anhand virologischer Befunde war schwierig.

Die Diagnose »echtes Rezidiv« wurde in drei Fällen aufgrund eines Wiederanstieges der HSV-spezifischen Antikörper bzw. Nachweises von HSV-DNA im Liquor sowie aufgrund HSE-typischer MRT-Befunde gestellt (Pat. 1-4). In einem Fall (Pat. 5) blieb aufgrund fehlender bzw. nicht eindeutiger virologischer Befunde und ungewöhnlicher MRT-Befunde die Diagnose unklar.

Tab. 2: Betroffene Hirnregionen im MRT zum Zeitpunkt der Erst-/ Zweiterkrankung, Früh-/Spätrezidiv

	Frontal-lappen		Insel-region		Temporal-lappen		Parietal-lappen		Occipital-lappen		Kleinhirn		Pons		Rezidiv	
	1	2	1	2	1	2	1	2	1	2	1	2	1	2	früh	spät
Pat. 1		++	+	++	+	++		++							+	
Pat. 2			+	+	+	+		+							+	
Pat. 3		++	+	+	+	+		+		+					+	
Pat. 4	*	(+)	*		*	(+)	*	++	*	++						+
Pat. 5	+	++	+	++	+	++	+	++	+	++		+		+		+

Erläuterungen:
1 Zum Zeitpunkt der Erstinfektion
2 Zum Zeitpunkt der Zweiterkrankung
Frührezidiv: innerhalb 4 Wochen nach Beginn der Erstinfektion
Spätrezidiv: mehr als 4 Wochen nach Beginn der Erstinfektion
*bei Erstinfektion unauffälliges MRT
+ einseitig ++ beidseitig

B. MRT-Befunde (vgl. Tab. 2, Abb. 1 und 2)

Wie in Tabelle 2 ersichtlich ist, zeigten sich bei der Erstinfektion in drei Fällen (Pat. 1–3) für eine HSE typische Befunde mit einem Befall im Bereich der Inselregion und des Temporallappens (6). Bei Patient 4 und 5 lagen untypische Befunde vor: bei Patient 5 war primär die gesamte Hemisphäre betroffen, bei Patient 4 war der MRT-Befund initial unauffällig.

Im Rahmen der Zweiterkrankung kam es zu unterschiedlichen MRT-Befunden, wobei diese jedoch bei Patient 1, 3 und 5 weiterhin als typisch für HSE einzuordnen waren.

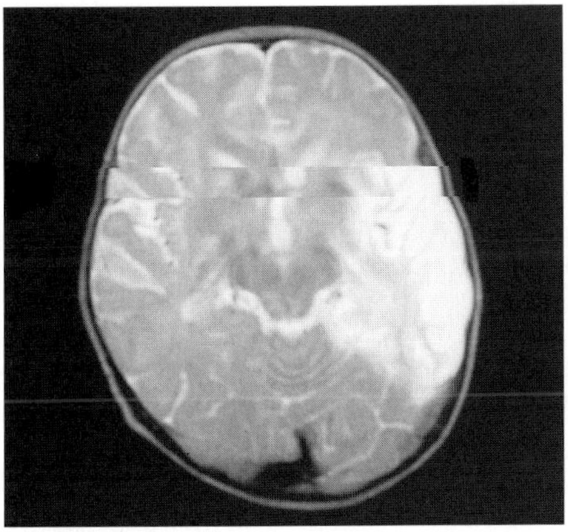

Abb. 1A: (T2, axial)

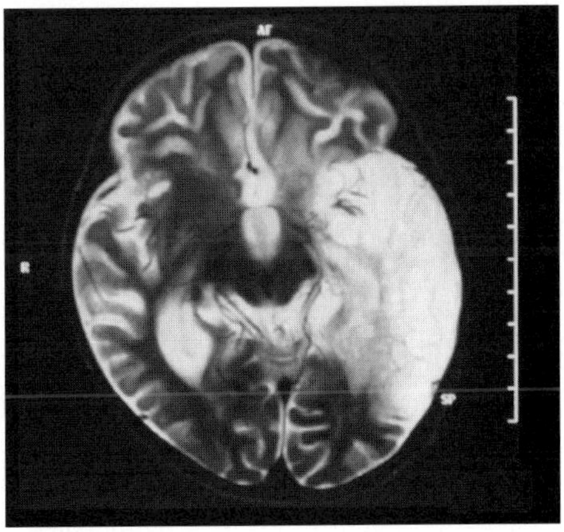

Abb. 1B: (T2, axial)

Abb. 1A + B: Patient 2: Frührezidiv. Klinik siehe Tab. 1. HSE-typischer MRT-Befund: bei Zweiterkrankung Befall der Inselregion/ Temporallappen.

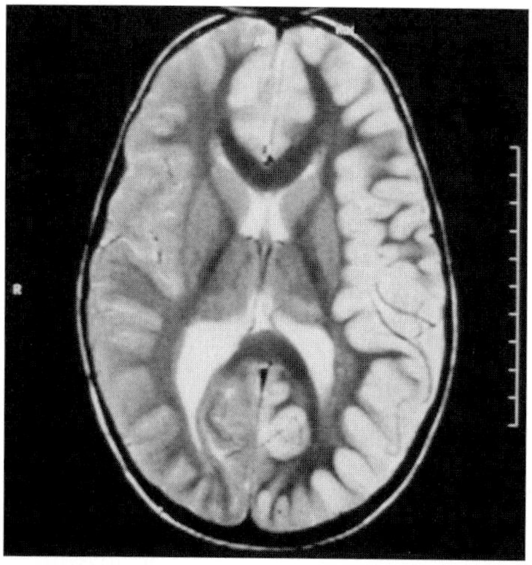

Abb. 2A: (T2, axial)

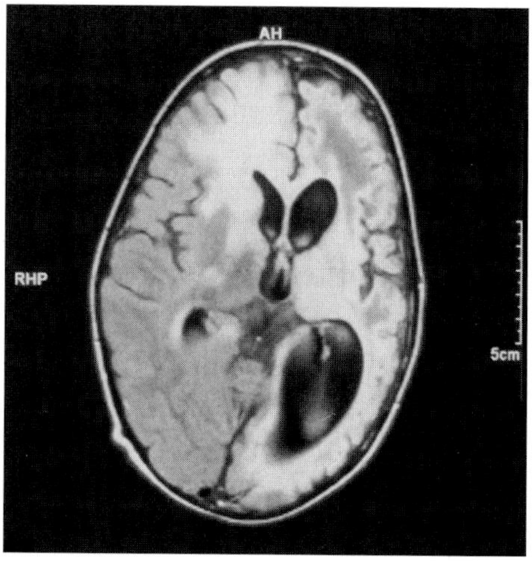

Abb. 2B: (T1, axial)

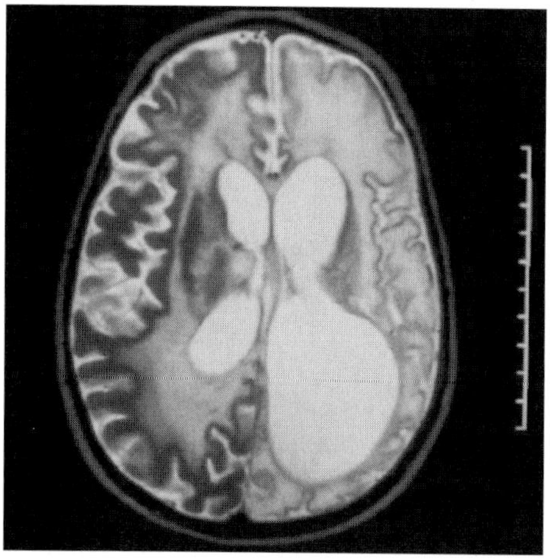

Abb. 2C: (T2, axial)

Abb. 2A–C: Paticnt 5: Spätrezidiv. Klinik siehe Tab. 1. HSE-untypische MRT-Befunde: zum Zeitpunkt der Erstinfektion (A), bei Zweiterkrankung (B) und im Verlauf (C); primärer Befall des gesamten Cortex einer Hemisphäre mit Ausbreitung auf die Gegenseite.

Diskussion

Erregernachweis

In der Literatur wird vereinzelt ein fehlender HSV-DNA-Nachweis bei Zweiterkrankung nach HSE beschrieben, wobei eine zu geringe Virusgenommenge oder das nur zeitlich begrenzte Wiederauftreten des Virus im Liquor diskutiert wird (5, 7). Bei unseren Patienten gelang der HSV-DNA-Nachweis nur in einem Fall (Patient 4). Diesen Fall möchten wir als »echtes« Rezidiv einordnen.

MRT-Befunde

Bei drei Patienten zeigten sich zum Zeitpunkt der Primärinfektion und bei Zweiterkankung für HSE typische MRT-Befunde. Bei den beiden Patienten mit untypischen MRT-Befunden handelt es sich um ein Mädchen mit Erkrankung im *Neugeborenenalter* mit Befall v.a. beider *Occipitallappen* bei Zweiterkankung sowie um einen Jungen mit *HSV-2*-Infektion, bei dem primär der gesamte Kortex einer Hemisphäre betroffen war.

Früh-/Spätrezidiv

Ein Frührezidiv (Zweiterkrankung innerhalb von 4 Wochen) lag nur bei den drei Patienten mit HSE-typischen MRT-Befunden vor.

Schlussfolgerung

Als Ursache der Zweiterkankung nach HSE lagen bei unseren Patienten sowohl eine Virusreaktivierung als auch ein Autoimmunprozess vor.

Neben dem Virusgenomnachweis können der Zeitpunkt der Zweiterkankung (Früh-/Spätrezidiv) und der MRT-Befund zur ätiologischen Klärung beitragen: ein Frührezidiv (innerhalb 4 Wochen) und ein HSE-typischer MRT-Befund machen eine Virusreaktivierung – auch ohne Virusgenomnachweis – wahrscheinlich.

Bei Zweiterkrankung nach einer HSE sollte frühzeitig – auch ohne eindeutige ätiologische Zuordnung – sowohl an eine virostatische als auch an eine immunmodulierende Therapie gedacht werden.

Literatur

1. Barthez M A, Billard C, Santini J J (1987) Relapse of Herpes Simplex Encephalitis. Neuropediatrics 18: 3–7
2. Dennett C, Klapper P E, Cleator G M (1996) Polymerase chain reaction in the investigation of »relapse« following herpes simplex encephalitis. J Med Virol 48 (2): 129–132
3. Fodor P A, Levin M J, Weinberg A, Sandberg E, Sylman J, Tyler K L (1998) Atypical herpes simplex virus encephalitis diagnosed by PCR amplification of viral DNA from CSF. Neurology 51: 554–559
4. Ito Y, Kimura H, Yabuta Y, Ando Y, Murakami T, Shiomi M, Morishima T (2000) Exacerbation of Herpes Simplex Encephalitis after Successful Treatment with Acyclovir. Clin Infect Dis 30: 185–187
5. Kimura H, Aso K, Kuzushima K, Hanada N, Shibata M, Morishima T (1992) Relapse of Herpes Simplex Encephalitis in Children. Pediatrics 89 (5): 891–894
6. Kluger G, Kloss S, Pieper T, Tuxhorn I, Holthausen H (1999) Spätfolgen nach Herpesenzephalitis: neurorradiologische, neurologische und neuropsychologische Befunde bei 20 Kindern. In: Millner M (Hrsg.) Aktuelle Neuropädiatrie 1999. Novartis Pharma Verlag, Nürnberg
7. Lellouch-Tubiana A, fohlen M, Robain O, Rozenberg F (2000) Immunocytochemical characterization of long-term persistent immune activation in human brain after herpes simplex encephalitis. Neuropathology and Applied Neurobiology 26: 285–294
8. Mandyla H, Anagnostakis D, Koutsovitis P, Siahanidou T, Youroukos S (2001) Late recurrence of herpes simplex virus meningoencephalitis in two infants. Eur J of Pediatrics 160: 732–735
9. Schwarz S, Knauth M, Mohr A, Wildemann B, Sommer C, Storch-Hagenlocher B (2001) Akute disseminierte Enzephalomyelitis (ADEM). Nervenarzt 72: 241–254

Idiopathische Säuglingsasymmetrie – Präsentation eines standardisierten Bewertungsscore

H. Philippi, T. Jung, H. Bergmann, A. Schleupen, B. Pabst

Zusammenfassung

Als Grundlage für Therapiestudien wurde eine standardisierte Bewertung der idiopathischen Säuglingsasymmetrie erarbeitet. Von 50 symmetrischen und asymmetrischen, ansonst gesunden Säuglingen in einem Reifealter von 6 bis 16 Wochen wurden spontane und induzierte Bewegungsmuster, Reaktionsantworten und Längenunterschiede gefilmt. Fünf verschiedene Bewegungskriterien wurden von 5 unabhängigen Untersuchern bewertet. Eine Bewertung erfolgte unter Benutzung von 3–8 Punkte-Skalen. Die Spontanmotorik und die Motorik bei aktiver Blickwendung nach rechts und links in Bauch- und Rückenlage waren die einzigen Bewegungen, die sich verlässlich videokumentieren ließen. *Rumpfkonvexität* und *HWS-Rotationsdefizit* stellten sich als repräsentative und hinreichende Bewertungskriterien für den Ausprägungsgrad der Asymmetrie heraus. Das Spektrum von asymmetrisch bis symmetrisch ließ sich am besten in einer 6-Punkte Skala abbilden. Der Gesamtscore umfasst 4–24 Punkte. Stabilität und Konsistenz des Scores sind gut (Intraclasskoeffizient 91,5%, Cronbach's Alpha 0,84).

Einleitung

Die idiopathische Säuglingsskoliose wurde 1954 von James definiert und ist häufig begleitet von weiteren asymmetrischen Befunden wie Plagiocephalus, Gesichtsasymmetrie, Strabismus, Torticollis, unilaterale Hüftdysplasie, Rippenkyphose und unilateraler Fußdeformität (Binder 1986, Canale 1982, Cheng 1994, James 1975, Lloyds-Roberts 1965, Mau 1979, McMaster 1983, Rosegger 1992, Walsh 1998, Wynne-Davies 1968 und 1975). Einige Autoren schlagen deshalb vor, diesen Symptomenkomplex als »Siebener Syndrom«, »Konnatales Prädilektionssyndrom« oder »Moulded baby syndrome« zu bezeichnen (Cheng 1994, James 1975, Lloyds-Roberts 1965, Lübbe 1979, Mau 1968, Pschyrembel 1998). Von unserer Arbeitsgruppe wird der Begriff Säuglingsasymmetrie verwendet.

Für die Ätiologie wird ein Zusammenspiel von endogenen und exogenen Faktoren postuliert. Endogen scheinen eine positive Familienanamnese für Skoliose, rasches Körperwachstum, Bewegungsarmut und ein reduzierter Muskeltonus die Entwicklung der Säuglingsasymmetrie zu begünstigen (Mau 1979, McMaster 1983, Wynne-Davies 1968 und 1975). Als exogene Faktoren gelten eine intrauterine asymmetrische Zwangshaltung, eine traumatische Geburt und eine einseitige postnatale Lagerung (Cheng 1994, Davids 1993,

Lloyds-Roberts 1965, Lübbe 1979, Rosegger 1992, Wynne-Davies 1975). Die Pathogenese wird unterhalten über einen Kreislauf aus fibrösen Schrumpfungskontrakturen, Wachstums- und Gewichtsdeformitäten und erneuten Schrumpfungskontrakturen (Mau 1979, Wynne-Davies 1975).

Die Prognose der Säuglingsasymmetrie wird anhand von retrospektiven Studien auf ein 10 bis 50%iges Risiko für eine spätere Skoliose geschätzt (Binder 1986, Canale 1982, Wynne-Davies 1968 und 1975, Ferreira 1972, James 1975, Lloyds-Roberts 1965, McMaster 1983, Rüppell 1977, Thompson 1980). Entsprechend uneinheitlich und nur empirisch gestützt werden die Therapiemaßnahmen gehandhabt. Sie reichen von Lagerungstechniken, Dehnungsübungen, über spezielle Physiotherapie, Osteopathie, Craniosacraltherapie bis hin zur Manualtherapie. Vielfach werden die Selbstregulationsmöglichkeiten des Säuglings als ausreichend eingeschätzt.

Um den Effekt von Therapiemaßnahmen evaluieren zu können, bedarf es einer möglichst objektiven, klinischen Bewertungsmethode der Säuglingsasymmetrie, die bisher nicht zur Verfügung steht. Bei der Erarbeitung eines solchen Messinstrumentes war es unser Ziel, die Bewertung anhand von klinischen Parametern unter Verzicht auf Röntgenstrahlen zu ermöglichen. Die Untersuchung sollte einfach durchzuführen und mit einer Videoaufzeichnung abzubilden sein. Die Bewertung aktiver Bewegungseinschränkungen sollte der Vorzug vor der Dokumentation von passiven Bewegungsdefiziten gegeben werden.

Methoden

Probanden: In den Jahren 1999 bis 2000 wurden 30 gesunde Säuglinge (16 weiblich, 14 männlich) mit einem Reifealter von 6 bis 15 Wochen (Median 10 Wochen) aus der Umgebung von Mainz rekrutiert. Das klinische Bewegungsmuster dieser Säuglinge repräsentierte das Spektrum von asymmetrisch bis symmetrisch und diente zur Entwicklung des Bewertungsscores für die Säuglingsasymmetrie. Im Jahr 2001 wurden weitere 20 Säuglinge (9 weiblich, 11 männlich) mit einem Reifealter von 9 Wochen (6 bis 16 Wochen) und dem gleichen klinischen Bild zur statistischen Evaluierung des optimierten Asymmetriescores rekrutiert.

Score: Folgende Items einer neurologischen Untersuchung des Säuglings wurden für die Evaluierung ausgewählt:

a) aktive Items: Spontanmotorik in Rücken- und Bauchlage, Motorik bei Kopfwendung nach rechts und links in Rücken- und Bauchlage, Landau-, Galant- und Abhangreaktion

b) passive Items: Seitendifferenz der Beinlänge und des Beckenstandes.

Für die Videoaufnahmen wurden die Säuglinge jeweils in Rücken- und Bauchlage auf eine vorgewärmte Matte auf den Boden gelegt und die Videokamera in 2 Meter Abstand direkt vertikal über die Säuglinge positioniert. Nur für die Aufnahme der Abhangreaktion wurde der Säugling auf der Untersucherliege mit horizontaler Kameraposition gefilmt. Untersucher und Eltern standen direkt hinter der Kamera. Licht- und Umgebungsverhältnisse wurden gleichförmig gehalten. Es wurde gewartet bis der Säugling sich in einem ruhigen Wachzustand befand (Prechtl 1974). Die Kopfwendung wurde durch die Präsentation von optischen und akustischen Reizen erreicht.

Die aktiven Items wurden bewertet nach *»Rumpfkonvexität, HWS-Rotationsdefizit, HWS-Neigung, Kopfvorzugsrotation und Schräglagentendenz«*. Die Bewertung wurde von 5 unabhängigen Beobachtern vorgenommen. Gemäß den Empfehlungen von Streiner und Norman (2001) wurden 3- bis 8-Punkte-Skalen untersucht. Schließlich wurden Bewertungsschwierigkeiten und Abweichungen in den Bewertungen analysiert und der Asymmetriescore in Aufbau, Durchführung und Bewertung entsprechend revidiert und optimiert.

Ergebnisse

Von den untersuchten Items ließen sich die Spontanmotorik und die Motorik bei induzierter Kopfwendung nach rechts und links auf einem Videofilm standardisiert abbilden und bewerten. Die dreidimensionalen raschen Bewegungsantworten bei der Galant-, Landau- und Abhangreaktion eigneten sich dafür nicht. Die Bewertung der Seitendifferenz der Beinlänge und des Beckenstandes waren vor allem deshalb nicht aussagekräftig, weil der maximale Seitenunterschied nur 1,5 cm betrug. Eine Unterteilung in Millimetereinheiten zur Graduierung von Asymmetrieunterschieden ging in der Messungenauigkeit, bedingt durch die Bewegung des Säuglings und die altersbedingt noch unvollständige Gelenkextension (Knie und Hüfte), unter.

Von den 5 zu bewertenden Bewegungsmustern der Spontanmotorik und der Motorik bei Seitwendung des Kopfes *(Rumpfkonvexität, HWS-Rotationsdefizit, HWS-vorzugsneigung, Kopfvorzugsrotation und Schräglagentendenz)* stellten sich die *Rumpfkonvexität* und das *HWS-Rotationsdefizit* als repräsentative und verlässliche Parameter heraus. Die Schräglagentendenz war deshalb nicht geeignet, weil sie nur bei 30% der asymmetrischen Säuglinge vorlag. Die HWS-Neigung zeigte sich als ein variables Muster, das offensichtlich je nach Blickrichtung und Liegeposition zur Kompensation von HWS-Rotationsdefiziten verändert wird. Die Kopfvorzugsrotation stimmte in 85% der Fälle mit einem Defizit in der HWS-Rotation überein, so dass dem klinisch relevanteren Kriterium des *HWS-Rotationsdefizits* der Vorzug gegeben wurde.

Die Frage, in wie viele Kategorien die Asymmetrieskala zu unterteilen ist, wurde mit 6 Kategorien beantwortet. Die Analyse der Asymmetriebewertung unter Benutzung von 3 bis 8-Punkte-Skalen zeigte, dass Skalen mit weniger als 6 Punkten nicht vollständig das klinische Spektrum der Säuglingsasymmetrie abbilden konnten. Skalen mit 7 oder 8 Punkten überstiegen die Unterscheidungsmöglichkeiten der Untersucher. Für jedes der beiden Items *(Rumpfkonvexität und HWS-Rotationsdefizit)* wurden die jeweiligen 6 Kategorien genau definiert (Abb. 1) und Schulungsvideos erstellt. Die Piktogramme der Abbildung 1 beziehen sich jeweils auf die Bewegungsmuster bei maximal möglicher Blickwendung nach rechts und links im Seitenvergleich. Zur Veranschaulichung

Kategorien		Wirbelsäulen-Piktogramm
1 Punkt	Keine oder seitengleiche Rumpfkonvexität.	oder
2 Punkte	Kaum erkennbarer Seitenunterschied in der Rumpfkonvexität.	
3 Punkte	Deutlich erkennbarer Seitenunterschied in der Rumpfkonvexität.	
4 Punkte	Die Rumpfkonvexität kann nur bis zu einer Geraden aufgelöst werden.	
5 Punkte	Die Rumpfkonvexität kann nur verbessert, nicht aufgelöst werden.	
6 Punkte	Die Rumpfkonvexität kann gar nicht aufgelöst werden.	

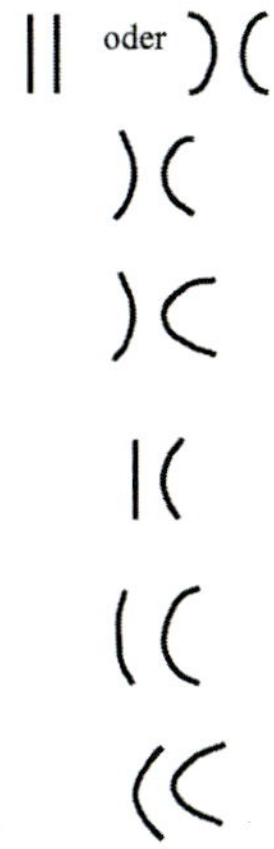

Abb. 1a: Definition der 6 Kategorien der Rumpfkonvexität. Die Rumpfkonvexität wird im Seitenvergleich bei maximaler Kopfwendung nach rechts und links bewertet.

Kategorien		Rotations-Piktogramm
1 Punkt	Freie Kopfrotation.	
2 Punkte	Gerade eben erkennbares Kopfrotationsdefizit.	
3 Punkte	Deutliches endgradiges Kopfrotationsdefizit, deutliche Kopfvorzugsrotation.	
4 Punkte	Eingeschränkte Kopfrotation bis zur grünen Linie, die kurzzeitig überschritten werden kann; Arbeitszone = grüner Pfeil.	
5 Punkte	Eingeschränkte Kopfrotation bis zur grünen Linie, die kurzzeitig überschritten werden kann, meistens entlang dem grünen Pfeil = Arbeitszone, selten entlang dem rotgepunkteten Pfeil.	
6 Punkte	Eingeschränkte Kopfrotation bis zur grünen Linie, die so gut wie nicht überschritten werden kann; Arbeitszone = grüner Pfeil.	

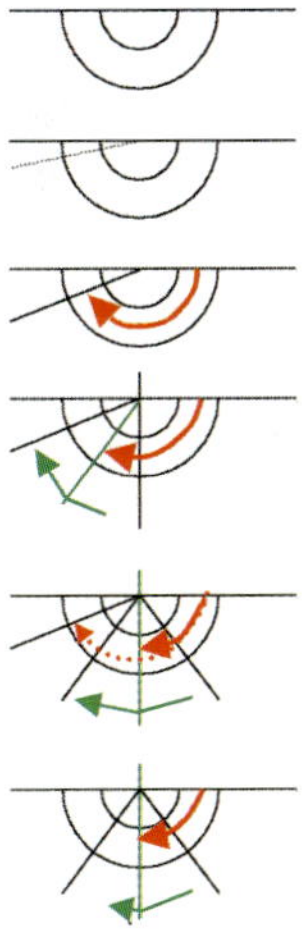

Abb. 1b: Definition der 6 Kategorien des HWS-Rotationsdefizites. Das HWS-Rotationsdefizit wird anhand der maximaler Kopfrotation nach rechts und links im Seitenvergleich von bewertet.

sind in Abbildung 2 ein HWS-Rotationsdefizit der Kategorie 6 in Rückenlage und eine Rumpfkonvexität der Kategorie 5 in Bauchlage dargestellt.

Der optimierte Asymmetriescore setzt sich aus der Summe von vier Items: *Rumpfkonvexität in Rückenlage, HWS-Rotationsdefizit in Rückenlage, Rumpfkonvexität in Bauchlage und HWS-Rotationsdefizit in Bauchlage* zusammen. Für jedes Item können 1–6 Punkte vergeben werden, so dass ein Score von 4 Punk-

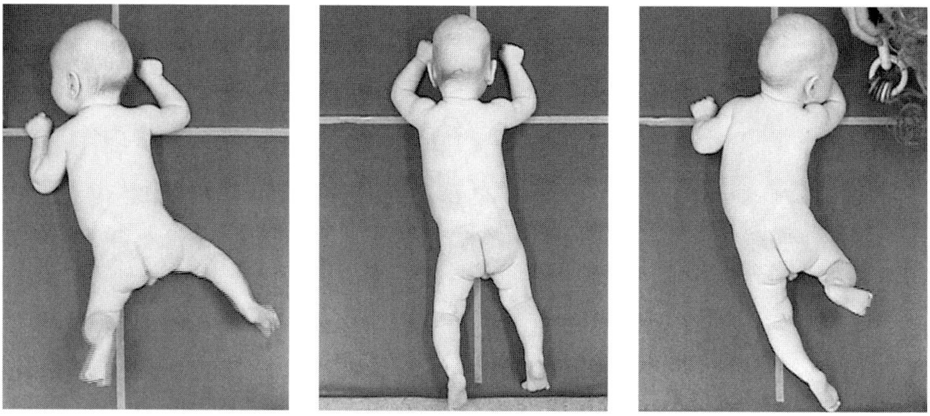

Abb. 2a: Bildreihe eines Säuglings mit Rumpfkonvexität der Kategorie 5 in Bauchlage.

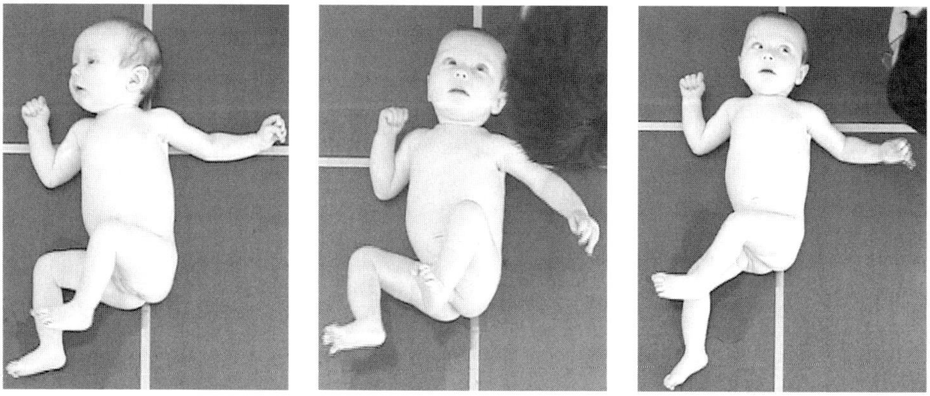

Abb. 2b: Bildreihe eines Säuglings mit HWS-Rotationsdefizit der Kategorie 6 in Rückenlage.

Abb. 3: Optimierter Bewertungsscore für die Säuglings-asymmetrie (Reifealter 6–16 Wochen).

Bauchlage	
Rumpfkonvexität	1– 6 Punkte
HWS-Rotationsdefizit	1– 6 Punkte
Rückenlage	
Rumpfkonvexität	1– 6 Punkte
HWS-Rotationsdefizit	1– 6 Punkte
Gesamtscore	4–24 Punkte
symmetrisch – asymmetrisch	

ten das »symmetrische« Ende und ein Score von 24 Punkten das »asymmetrische« Ende der Scala darstellt (Abb. 3). Aufgrund unserer klinischen Einschätzung haben wir eine Änderung von mindestens 3 Punkten auf der Skala als klinisch relevant eingestuft.

Der optimierte Asymmetriescore wurde anhand von 20 Videos von 20 Säuglingen aus dem Spektrum von *»symmetrisch«* bis *»asymmetrisch«*, die von 5 unabhängigen Untersuchern bewertet wurden, auf seine Konsistenz und Stabilität hin überprüft. Der Intraclasskoeffizient für den Beitrag der Patienten an der Gesamtvarianz des Scores liegt mit 91,5% bei einem 95%igen Konfidenzintervall von 86–97% in einem hohen Bereich. Entsprechend niedrig liegt mit 0,6% bei einem 95%igen Konfidenzintervall von 0,0–2,0% der Beitrag der Untersucher an der Gesamtvarianz des Scores. Das Cronbach's Alpha von 0,84 als Maß für die Konsistenz der Items liegt in einem verlässlichen Bereich (DeVellis 1991). Der Asymmetriescore ist damit als stabil und konsistent zu bewerten.

Diskussion

Unser Ziel war es, eine klinisch funktionelle Bewertungsmethode für die Säuglingsasymmetrie zu entwickeln. Dabei haben wir auf die Beurteilung von Bewegungsmustern zurückgegriffen. Durch den raschen Reifungsprozess sensomotorischer Funktionen im ersten Lebensjahr war es daher notwendig, sich auf einen kleinen Altersbereich zu konzentrieren, um eine standardisierte Bewertung zu ermöglichen. Wir haben uns aus drei Gründen für ein Reifealter zwischen 6 und 16 Wochen entschieden. In Anbetracht der Daten aus retrospektiven Untersuchungen, die dafür sprechen, dass ein früher Behandlungsbeginn mit einer guten Prognose einhergeht, haben wir uns auf die ersten Lebensmonate konzentriert (Binder 1986, James 1975, Rüppel 1977). Die ersten 6 Wochen wurden herausgenommen, weil es sinnvoll ist, in Anbetracht einer hohen Spontanremission, in dieser Zeit zunächst die Selbstregulationsmöglichkeiten des Säuglings abzuwarten (Lloyds-Roberts 1965, Mau 1968). Jenseits von 16 Wochen entwickeln die Säuglinge die Fähigkeit sich in die Seitenlage zu drehen, so dass beispielsweise eine blockierte Kopfdrehung durch eine Ganzkörperdrehung kaschiert werden kann.

Die Dokumentation der Bewegungsmuster in Rücken- und Bauchlage erfolgte über Videoaufnahmen. Dies ermöglicht neben einem hohen Maß an Objektivität auch die Möglichkeit neben den Kriterien des Scores *(Rumpfkonvexität und HWS-Rotationsdefizit)* andere morphologische und funktionelle Aspekte wie Plagiocephalus, Gesichtsasymmetrie, Thoraxasymmetrie, asymmetrische Bein- oder Fußposition, HWS-Neigung und Schräglage auszuwerten.

Die statistische Auswertung zeigt eine gute Konsistenz und Stabilität des Scores. Da es bisher keine vergleichbare Methode gibt, kann die Validität des Scores nur darüber abgeschätzt werden, ob vom Aspekt her der Asymmetriescore die wesentlichen Faktoren, die die Asymmetrie bestimmen, enthalten sind. Berücksichtigt man, dass die Säuglingsasymmetrie bevorzugt als Säuglingsskoliose bezeichnet und über eine Winkelmessung an einer Röntgenaufnahme der Wirbelsäule vorgenommen wird, so erscheint das Scorekriterium *»Rumpfkonvexität«* als guter Stellvertreter (Davids 1993, Metha 1972). Ebenso wird mit dem Scorekriterium *»aktives HWS-Rotationsdefizit«* eine Bewegungseinschränkung erfasst, die bei Kindern mit Torticollis bei einer Ausprägung von passiv mehr als 30° als prognostisch ungünstig eingeschätzt wird (Canale 1982, Cheng 1994).

Damit erscheint die Validität des Scores zunächst als ausreichend, kann aber letztlich erst durch die Anwendung in prospektiven Langzeitstudien verlässlich evaluiert werden.

Der Bewertungsscore ermöglicht eine einfache und verlässliche klinische Beurteilung asymmetrischer sonst gesunder Säuglinge in einem Reifealter von 6 bis 16 Wochen. Damit können zum einen kurzzeitige Therapieeffekte auf die idiopathische Säuglingsasymmetrie standardisiert evaluiert und zum anderen ein verlässlicher Ausgangsbefund für Langzeitstudien erhoben werden.

Literatur

1. Binder H, Eng GD, Gaiser JF, Koch B. (1987) Congenital muscular torticollis: results of conservative management with long-term follow-up in 85 cases. *Arch Phys Med Rehabil* 68: 222–5.
2. Canale ST, Griffin DW, Hubbard CN. (1982) Congenital muscular torticollis. A long-term follow-up. *J Bone Joint Surg* Am 64: 810–6.
3. Cheng JC, Au AW. (1994) Infantile torticollis: a review of 624 cases. *J Pediatr Orthop* 14: 802–8.
4. Davids JR, Wenger DR, Mubarak SJ. (1993) Congenital muscular torticollis: a sequela of intrauterine or perinatal compartment syndrome. *J Pediatr Orthop* 13: 141–7.
5. DeVellis, R.F. (1991): Scale Development: Theory and Applications. Sage, Newbury Park.
6. Ferreira JH, James JIP. (1972) Progressive and resolving infantile idiopathic scoliosis : The differential diagnosis. *J Bone Joint Surg Am* 54-B, 648–55.
7. James JIP. (1954) Idiopathic Scoliosis: the prognosis, diagnosis, and operative indications related to curve pattern and the age at onset. *J Bone Joint Surg Am* 36-B, 36–49.
8. James JIP. (1975) The management of infants with scoliosis. *J Bone Joint Surg Am* 57-B, 422–9.
9. Lloyds-Roberts, Pilcher MF. (1965) Structural idiopathic scoliosis in infancy: A study of the natural history of 100 patients. *J Bone Joint Surg Am* 47-B, 520–3.
10. Lübbe C. (1979) Eine neue Situation für die Säuglingsskoliose. *MMW* 121: 167–170.
11. Mau H. (1968) Ist die sogenannte Säuglingsskoliose behandlungsbedürftig? Dtsch Med Wochenschr 43: 2051–3.
12. Mau H. (1979) Zur Ätiopathogenese von Skoliose, Hüftdysplasie und Schiefhals im Säuglingsalter. *Z Orthop* 117: 784–9.
13. McMaster MJ. (1983) Infantile idiopathic scoliosis: can it be prevented? *J Bone Joint Surg Am* 65-B, 612–7.
14. Metha MH. (1972) The rib-vertebra angle in the early diagnosis between resolving and progressive infantile scoliosis. *J Bone Joint Surg Am* 54-B, 230–43.
15. Prechtl HFR. (1974) The behavioural states of the newborn infant (a review). *Brain Research* 76: 185–212.
16. Rosegger H, Steinwendner G. (1992) Transverse fetal position syndrome- a combination of congenital skeletal deformities in the newborn infant. *Paediatr Paediol* 27: 125–7.
17. Rüppell F, Dahmen G, Horst M, Michaelis M (1977). Wertung der Behandlungsergebnisse der Säuglingsskoliose. *Med Monatsschr* 31: 493–6.
18. Streiner DL, Norman GR, editors (2001) Health measurement scales: a practical guide to their development and use. Oxford: Oxford University Press.
19. Thompson SK. (1980) Prognosis in infantile idiopathic scoliosis. *J Bone Joint Surg Am* 62-B, 151–4.
20. Walsh JJ, Morrissy RT. (1998) Torticollis and hip dislocation. *J Pediatr Orthop* 18: 219–21.
21. Wynne-Davies R. (1968) Familial (idiopathic) scoliosis: a family survey. *J Bone Joint Surg Am* 50-B: 24–30.
22. Wynne-Davies R. (1975) Infantile idiopathic scoliosis: causative factors, particularly in the first six months of life. *J Bone Joint Surg Am* 57-B: 138–41.

Temporallappenhypoplasie – ein Risiko für subdurale Effusionen nach Bagatelltrauma

E. Boltshauser, A. Capone Mori, J. Schneider, St. Altermatt

Zusammenfassung

Wir berichten über 4 Schulkinder, bei denen es nach sportlichem Bagatelltrauma im Rahmen einer zuvor nicht bekannten Temporallappenhypoplasie (TLH) zu einer ipsilateralen subduralen Effusion kam. Die Beschwerden bestanden in protrahierten Kopfschmerzen und Ermüdbarkeit, der Neurostatus war normal. In der initialen Computertomographie wurde die Effusion bei 2 Kindern nicht erfasst. Bei persistierenden posttraumatischen Kopfschmerzen ist eine TLH ein Warnzeichen einer subduralen Effusion, die mit Magnetresonanzimaging zuverlässig nachgewiesen werden kann.

Einleitung

In der Literatur ist die Nomenklatur liquorgefüllter Kompartimente der mittleren Schädelgrube nicht einheitlich: gewisse Autoren sprechen von Temporallappenhypoplasie (bzw. -agenesie) (5), andere von Arachnoidalzysten der mittleren Schädelgrube (1). Man gewinnt den Eindruck, dass die Begriffe weitgehend synonym verstanden und gebraucht werden können (7). Auf die unterschiedlichen Ansichten zur möglichen Pathogenese wollen wir in diesem Zusammenhang nicht eintreten (2). Nach Angaben der Literatur ist eine TLH fast immer unilateral (Memo: bei bilateralem Befund ist eine Glutarsäurekrankheit zu erwägen), bevorzugt auf der linken Seite und beim männlichen Geschlecht vorkommend (8). In den meisten Fällen einer TLH handelt es sich um einen (asymptomatischen) Zufallsbefund, der oft bei Abklärung von Kopfschmerzen oder Anfällen eruiert wird (5). Ausnahmsweise kommt es zu einer Größenzunahme der Arachnoidalzyste und klinischen Symptomen (6).

Als seltene spontan oder nach Trauma vorkommende Komplikation einer TLH sind intrazystische Blutungen und ipsilaterale Subduralhämatome bekannt; diese können computertomographisch unter Umständen – je nach Signalverhalten der Blutbeimengung – »maskiert« d.h. verpasst werden (3, 4, 7).

Im folgenden beschreiben wir 4 Kinder mit subduralen Effusionen im Rahmen einer TLH nach einem Bagatelltrauma.

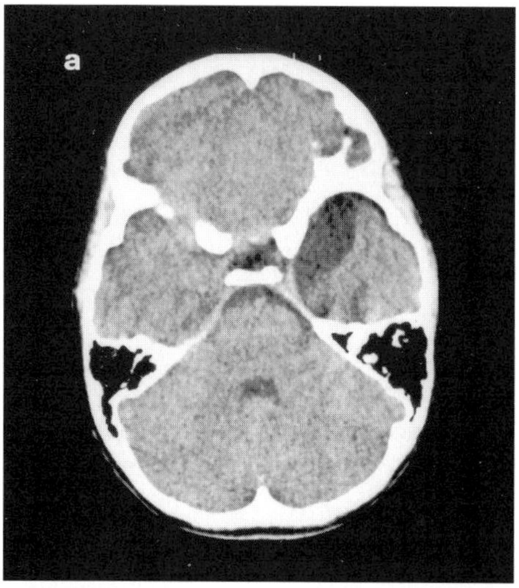

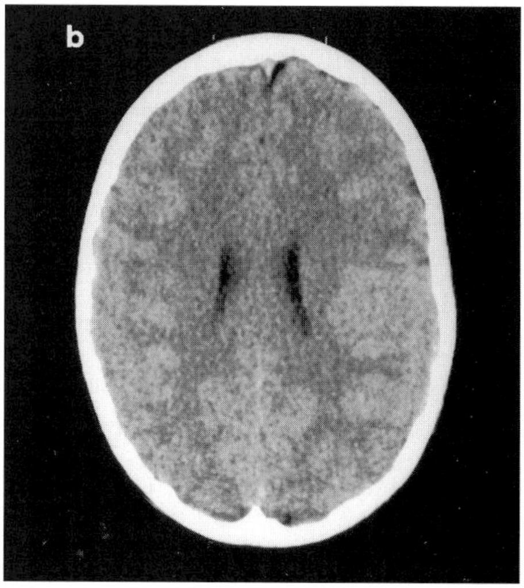

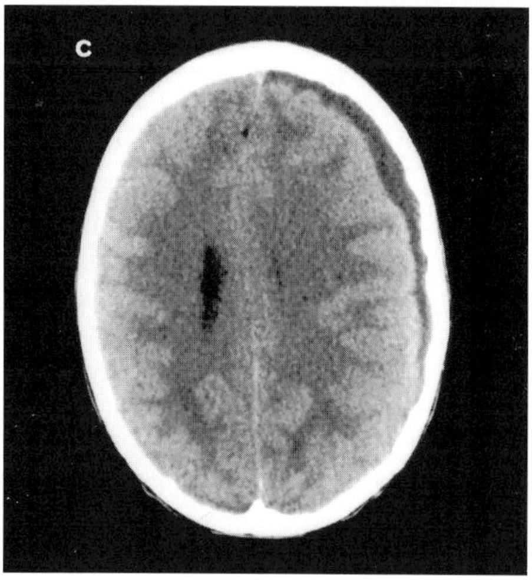

Abb. 1: (Patient 1):
a) CT 12 Tage nach Bagatelltrauma zeigt Temporallappenhypoplasie und (im »Retrospektroskop«)
b) diskrete Flüssigkeitsansammlung interhemisphärisch frontal.
c) CT 8 Wochen später: deutliche Effusion.

Kasuistik

Im Zeitraum 1995–2001 haben wir die Konstellation »subdurale Effusion bei TLH« bei 4 Schulkindern (Alter 9–11 Jahre) nach einem Bagatelltrauma ohne Bewusstseinsverlust bei sportlicher Aktivität (Sturz bei Fußball bzw. beim Skifahren, 2x Sprung ins Wasser) betreut. Nach einem freien Intervall von Stunden bis 6 Wochen wurden als Beschwerden insbesondere Kopfschmerzen und erhöhte Ermüdbarkeit angegeben, bei einem Knaben kam es nach 2 Wochen zu intermittierender Diplopie. Anamnestische »Ablenker«, die wohl zur verzögerten Diagnosestellung beigetragen haben, waren vorbestehende Kopfschmerzen, posttraumatische Rückenbeschwerden und (2x) Zeckenbiss. Der Neurostatus war bei der initialen Vorstellung unauffällig, insbesondere bestand kein Papillenödem. Die Bildgebung ergab jeweils eine Temporallappenhypoplasie, die aber als bedeutungslos eingestuft wurde. Bei 2 Knaben wurde die Computertomographie 12 Tage bzw. 6 Wochen nach dem Unfall als normal interpretiert; die Wiederholung der Bildgebung, aufgrund Persistenz klinischer Befunde, ergab 2 bzw. 8 Wochen

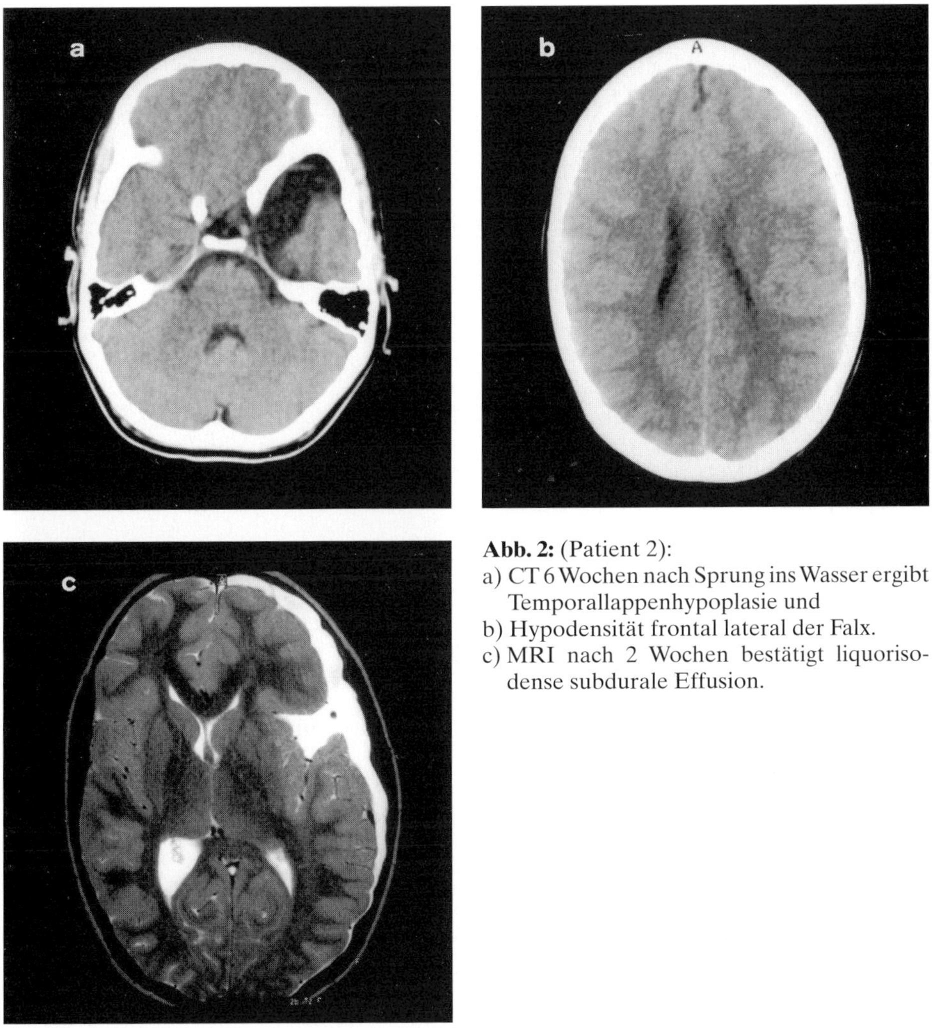

Abb. 2: (Patient 2):
a) CT 6 Wochen nach Sprung ins Wasser ergibt Temporallappenhypoplasie und
b) Hypodensität frontal lateral der Falx.
c) MRI nach 2 Wochen bestätigt liquorisodense subdurale Effusion.

später das Vorliegen subduraler Effusionen (Abb. 1 und 2). Bei einem Kind fiel 10 Tage nach Unfall das MRI diagnostisch (für Effusion) aus (Abb. 3).

Das Signalverhalten der Effusionen entsprach Liquor, entsprach also nicht einem Subduralhämatom. Therapeutisch brachte die externe Drainage über ein Bohrloch bei 3 Patienten rasche und bleibende Symptomfreiheit; bei einem Patienten musste bei Persistenz der Effusion eine interne (peritoneale) Drainage angelegt werden.

Diskussion und Schlussfolgerung

Eine Temporallappenhypoplasie stellt ein Risiko für eine subdurale Effusion nach einem Bagatelltrauma dar. Verantwortlich dafür ist eine vermehrte Beweglichkeit des Gehirns.

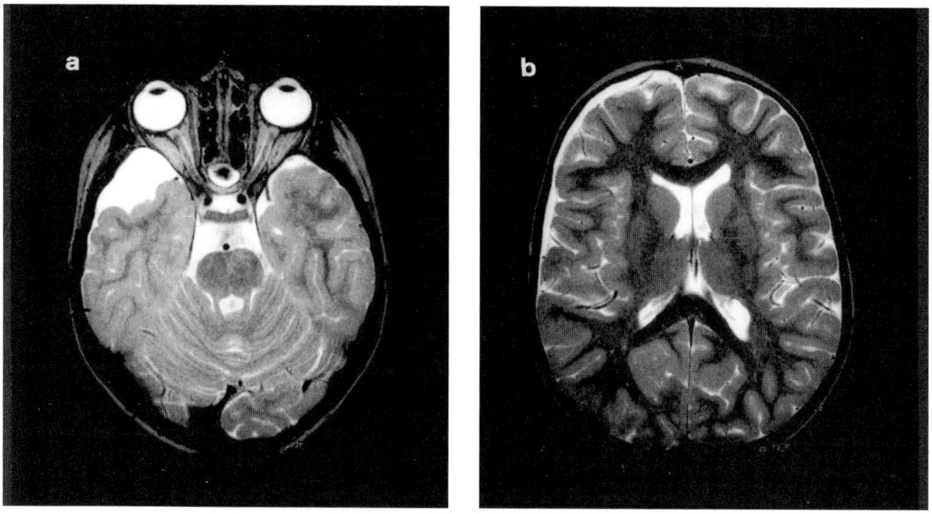

Abb. 3: (Patient 3):
a, b) MRI 10 Tage nach Bagatelltrauma (Sturz beim Skifahren) zeigt Temporallappenhypoplasie und ipsilaterale liquorisodense Effusion.

Die Diagnose ist klinisch nicht zu stellen, der Neurostatus fällt normal aus, daher ist bei entsprechender Anamnese eine großzügige Indikation zur Bildgebung gerechtfertigt.

In der Computertomographie wird die Effusion initial oft nicht erkannt. Bei Temporallappenhypoplasie im CT und entsprechenden Beschwerden ist daher eine MRI-Untersuchung zu erwägen.

Die Effusionen zeigten bei unseren Patienten ein Signalverhalten wie Liquor, es ist also – im Gegensatz zu Publikationen – kein subdurales »Hämatom« zu erwarten.

Literatur

1. Barkovich AJ (Ed.) (2000) Pediatric Neuroimaging, 3rd Ed. Raven Press, New York
2. Friede RL (1989) Developmental Neuropathology, 2nd Ed. Springer-Verlag, Berlin, Heidelberg, New York, London, Paris, Tokyo
3. Lund E, Buhl M, Miletic T, Knudsen V (1987) Kyste arachnoïdien isodense et hématome sous-dural de l'étage moyen: un problème diagnostique à la TDM. J Neuroradiology 14; 89–93
4. Page A, Paxton RM, Mohan D (1987) A reappraisal of the relationship between arachnoid cysts of the middle fossa and chronic subdural haematoma. J Neurol Neurosurg Psychiatry 50;1001–1007
5. Robertson SJ, Wolpert SM, Runge VM (1989) MRimaging of middle cranial fossa arachnoid cysts: temporal lobe agenesis syndrome revisited. AJNR 10;1007–1010
6. van der Meché FGA, Braakman R (1983) Arachnoid cysts in the middle cranial fossa: cause and treatment of progressive and non-progressive symptoms. J Neurol Neurosurg Psychiatry 46;1102–1107

7. Varma TRK, Sedzimir CB, Miles JB (1981) Post-traumatic complications of arachnoid cysts and temporal lobe agenesis. J Neurol Neurosurg Psychiatry 44;29–34
8. Wester K (1992) Gender distribution and sidedness of middle fossa arachnoid cysts: a review of cases diagnosed with computed imaging. Neurosurgery 31;940–944

Wie häufig sind postpunktionelle Kopfschmerzen bei Kindern und Jugendlichen?

F. Ebinger, Ch. Kosel, L. Memmert, D. Rating

Zusammenfassung

Nach Lumbalpunktionen können Kopf- und Rückenschmerzen die Patienten zum Teil deutlich belasten. Wir untersuchten die Häufigkeit solcher Beschwerden bei Kindern und Jugendlichen. Es zeigte sich, dass die typischen lageabhängigen postpunktionellen Kopfschmerzen in diesem Alter extrem selten sind. Sonstige Beschwerden traten mit einer Inzidenz von 46% auf. Es fand sich eine eindeutige Zunahme der Beschwerderate mit dem Alter. Bei Mädchen und bei Patienten mit onkologischen Erkrankungen fanden sich ebenfalls vermehrt Beschwerden.

Einleitung

Eine Lumbalpunktion ist unter anderem in der Diagnostik von Entzündungen des ZNS und seiner Häute sowie von neurometabolischen Erkrankungen und in der Diagnostik und Therapie von onkologischen Erkrankungen notwendig (1). Nach einer Lumbalpunktion kann es zu zum Teil heftigen Kopfschmerzen (2, 3) sowie weiteren postpunktionellen Beschwerden wie Rückenschmerzen oder Übelkeit kommen, die zum Teil zu einer Verlängerung des Klinikaufenthaltes führen.

Im Erwachsenenalter treten postpunktionelle Kopfschmerzen meist 24 bis 48 Stunden nach der Punktion auf und dauern in der Regel zwischen 4 und 7 Tagen, können aber auch wesentlich länger anhalten. Sie werden als dumpf, ziehend, seltener als pochend beschrieben. Meist sind sie occipital, oft aber auch frontal lokalisiert. Charakteristischerweise werden sie nach Einnahme einer aufrechten Körperhaltung stärker und bessern sich nach dem Hinliegen wieder (2, 3). Diese Lageabhängigkeit wird in der Kopfschmerz-Klassifikation der International Headache Classification für die Diagnose »postpunktioneller Kopfschmerz« gefordert (4). Schwindel, Übelkeit, Nackensteifigkeit und Rückenschmerzen gelten demgegenüber als Begleitsymptome.

Die Angaben zur Häufigkeit von Kopfschmerzen nach einer Lumbalpunktion sind extrem unterschiedlich. Bei Patienten im Alter von 30 bis 40 Jahren werden Inzidenzraten bis zu knapp 70% berichtet. Bei älteren Patienten sind sie deutlich seltener. Bei Frauen treten sie tendenziell häufiger auf, nur in einem Teil der Untersuchungen war diese Differenz signifikant. Eine Metaanalyse verschiedener Studien zeigte im Erwachsenenalter einen eindeutigen Zusammenhang der Inzidenzrate mit der Dicke der Punktionsnadel: 15–19G: 26%, 20–22G: 17%, 24–26G: 4%, 27–32G: 2%. (2,3) In mehreren Studien bei Erwachsenen zeigte sich, dass eine prophylaktische feste Bettruhe die Häufigkeit des Auftretens postpunktioneller Beschwerden nicht zu reduzieren vermag (5, 6).

Die Häufigkeit solcher Beschwerden bei Kindern und Jugendlichen gilt als wesentlich niedriger als bei Erwachsenen. Hierzu liegen jedoch nur wenige publizierte Daten vor (7, 8, 9), die sich alle auf onkologische Patienten beziehen. In den meisten Kinderkliniken wird eine prophylaktische strenge Bettruhe von 24 Stunden eingehalten. Oft werden Patienten nur deswegen stationär aufgenommen.

Probanden und Methode

In einer zweiteiligen Studie beobachteten wir zunächst bei den in unserem Hause durchgeführten Lumbalpunktionen prospektiv die Inzidenz von Kopfschmerzen oder Rückenschmerzen sowie sonstiger postpunktioneller Beschwerden unter dem bei uns üblichen Vorgehen einer verordneten festen Bettruhe von 24 Stunden. Dabei wurden als »relevant« angegebene Beschwerden berücksichtigt, ohne eine Skalierung der Schmerzen durchzuführen. Wir notierten neben den personenbezogenen Daten u.a. die Indikation zur Punktion, die Dicke der Punktionskanüle (immer Quincke-Schliff), die Menge des gewonnenen Liquors. Über die Befunde dieser prospektiven Beobachtung berichten wir hier. Im zweiten Teil der Untersuchung vergleichen wir gegenwärtig die Häufigkeit von Beschwerden bei fester Bettruhe und bei Mobilisation ad libitum.

Ergebnisse

Im Zeitraum von November 2000 bis Mai 2001 haben wir insgesamt 76 Lumbalpunktionen bei 63 Patienten im Alter zwischen 1 und 17 Jahren erfasst.

Insgesamt wurde nach 35 Punktionen (46%) postpunktionelle Beschwerden angegeben. Kopfschmerzen fanden sich jedoch nur bei 8 (11%), bei 16 zeigten sich Übelkeit und Erbrechen (21%), bei 24 Rückenschmerzen (32%). In 19 Fällen wurde Paracetamol oder Metamizol gegeben (25%). Bei den Kopfschmerzen war nur bei zwei Patienten eine Lageabhängigkeit zu erkennen, die jedoch nicht streng den Kriterien der International Headache Society entsprach.

Dauer:

Die Beschwerden dauerten bis zu 4 Tagen an.

Alter:

Nach den 25 Lumbalpunktionen bei Kindern unter 5 Jahren wurde in 6 Fällen (24%) überhaupt Beschwerden, in 1 Fall Kopfschmerzen (4%), 5 Rückenschmerzen (20%) und 4 Übelkeit und Erbrechen (16%) angegeben, bei den 37 Punktionen im Alter zwischen 5 und 11 Jahren 19 Beschwerden (51%), 5 Kopfschmerzen (14%), 11 Rückenschmerzen (30%), 8 Übelkeit und Erbrechen (22%), bei den 14 Punktionen von Jugendlichen ab 12 Jahren 10 Beschwerden (71%), 2 Kopfschmerzen (14%), 8 Rückenschmerzen (57%), 4 Übelkeit und

Erbrechen (29%). Die Unterschied zwischen den Altersgruppen waren für die Beschwerden insgesamt signifikant (Chi-Quadrat-Test nach Pearson: p=0,01), für die Rückenschmerzen an der Signifikanzgrenze (p=0,054).

Geschlecht:

Auffällig war ein Unterschied zwischen den Geschlechtern: Nach den 39 an Mädchen durchgeführten Punktionen fanden sich in 22 Fällen überhaupt Beschwerden (56%), in 6 Kopfschmerzen (15%), in 12 Rückenschmerzen (31%) und in 10 Übelkeit und Erbrechen (26%), während nach den 37 Punktionen von Jungen sich bei 13 überhaupt Beschwerden fanden (35%), bei 2 Kopfschmerzen (5%), bei 12 Rückenschmerzen (32%) und bei 6 Übelkeit und Erbrechen (16%). Die Unterschiede bei den Beschwerden insgesamt lagen knapp oberhalb der Signifikanzgrenze (p=0,06). Betrachtet man nur die Patienten ab dem 5. Lebensjahr, so ist der Unterschied zwischen Mädchen und Jungen für die Beschwerden insgesamt signifikant (p=0,02), für die Kopfschmerzen liegt p bei 0,08.

Nadeldicke:

Bei der Dicke der Punktionskanüle lässt sich zwischen den vorwiegend verwendeten 20G- und 22G-Kanülen kein Unterschied erkennen: 22G-Kanüle (36): 18 Beschwerden (50%), 3 Kopfschmerzen (8%), 12 Rückenschmerzen (33%), 9 Übelkeit und Erbrechen; 20G-Kanüle (37): 15 Beschwerden (40%), 5 Kopfschmerzen (14%), 10 Rückenschmerzen (27%), 6 Übelkeit und Erbrechen (16%). Von den nur drei Patienten, die mit der dicksten verwendeten Kanüle (19G) punktiert wurden, hatten zwei Rückenschmerzen.

Liquormenge:

Bei den 36 Punktionen mit einer Punktionsmenge bis 6 ml ergaben sich in 14 Fällen Beschwerden (39%), in 5 Kopfschmerzen (14%), in 8 Rückenschmerzen (22%) und in 8 Übelkeit und Erbrechen, bei den 40 Punktionen mit Punktionsmengen über 6 ml 21 Beschwerden (53%), 3 Kopfschmerzen (8%), 16 Rückenschmerzen (40%), 8 Übelkeit und Erbrechen (20%). Der Unterschied bei den Rückenschmerzen ist mit p=0,096 nicht signifikant.

Zahl der Punktionsversuche:

Es fanden sich keine relevanten Unterschiede zwischen Patienten, bei denen die erste Punktion erfolgreich war, und denjenigen, bei denen mehrere Punktionsversuche nötig waren.

Diagnosen:

Während sich Patienten mit Meningitis nicht wesentlich von solchen unterschieden, die z.B. zur Abklärung einer Stoffwechselerkrankung punktiert wurden, gaben Patienten mit einer Leukämie signifikant weniger Beschwerden an: 53% (28) gegenüber 26% (6), p=0,02. Die Unterschiede in den Einzelsymptomen waren nicht signifikant, zeigten aber dieselbe Tendenz: Kopfschmerzen 13% (7) vs. 4% (1), Rückenschmerzen 38% (20) vs. 17% (4), Übelkeit und Erbrechen 25% (13) vs. 13% (3).

Wertet man die onkologischen und die nicht-onkologischen Patienten getrennt aus, bleiben die Zusammenhänge zwischen dem Alter und der Häufigkeit von postpunktionellen Beschwerden erhalten (für die nicht-onkologischen Patienten mit $p=0{,}02$ signifikant); bei den Patienten ab 5 Jahren auch die größere Häufigkeit von Beschwerden bei Mädchen (nicht signifikant).

Logistische Regression:
Berücksichtigt man alle genannten Einflussgrößen (Alter, Geschlecht, Nadeldicke, Liquormenge, Punktionszahl, Diagnosen) als unabhängige Variablen bei einer logistischen Regressionsrechnung für die Häufigkeit von Beschwerden überhaupt, so werden bei den unter 5-Jährigen keine Variablen als signifikant einbezogen, bei den Älteren jedoch die Variablen Geschlecht und Alter.

Diskussion

Die dargestellten Häufigkeiten von Kopfschmerzen beziehen sich auf alle nicht vorbestehenden Kopfschmerzen, die nach einer Punktion beobachtet wurden. Nur bei den wenigsten Patienten konnte die klare Lageabhängigkeit festgestellt werden. Die Häufigkeit von postpunktionellen Kopfschmerzen im Sinne der Klassifikation der Internationalen Kopfschmerzgesellschaft ist also bei Kindern und Jugendlichen äußerst gering. Bei vielen Studien zum Kopfschmerz nach Lumbalpunktion im Erwachsenenalter wurde auf die Lageabhängigkeit nicht dezidiert geachtet. Die meist nur als »Begleitsymptome« referierten Beschwerden wie Rückenschmerzen oder Übelkeit und Erbrechen tragen wesentlich zur Morbidität bei.

Die geringere Zahl von Beschwerden bei Kindern im Vorschulalter entspricht unseren klinischen Beobachtungen. Auch die wenigen existierenden Studien zur Häufigkeit von postpunktionellen Kopfschmerzen bei Kindern zeigen eine klare Zunahme mit dem Alter (7, 8, 9). Diese drei Studien wurden an onkologischen Patienten durchgeführt und ergaben Häufigkeiten für lageabhängige postpunktionelle Kopfschmerzen bei Jugendlichen zwischen 20% und über 70%. Bei uns hatten die onkologischen Patienten häufiger Beschwerden, bei weitem nicht so häufig wie in den zitierten Studien. Sonstige Beschwerden wurden in diesen Arbeiten nicht berücksichtigt.

Die von uns beobachtete Differenz zwischen den Geschlechtern wird ab dem Schulalter deutlicher und wurde in einem Teil der Erwachsenenstudien ebenfalls beobachtet. Sie wird meist mit unterschiedlicher Beschaffenheit des Bindegewebes erklärt.

Zwischen den Kanülendicken 20G und 22G fand sich bezüglich der Häufigkeit von Beschwerden kein sicherer Unterschied. Eine deutliche Abnahme der Häufigkeit von Beschwerden wurde bei Erwachsenen bei noch dünneren Kanülen gefunden. Die Menge des gewonnenen Liquors hatte keinen eindeutigen Einfluss auf die Häufigkeit von Kopfschmerzen. Je mehr Liquor gewonnen werden muss, umso länger dauert in der Regel eine Lumbalpunktion. Dies könnte die von uns beobachtete größere Häufigkeit von Rückenschmerzen bei größerer Liquormenge erklären.

Im zweiten Teil der Studie untersuchen wir, ob die in vielen Kinderkliniken übliche prophylaktische Bettruhe das Auftreten postpunktioneller Beschwerden verhindern kann. Eine erste Zwischenauswertung deutet daraufhin, dass möglicherweise auch bei Kindern und Jugendlichen die Ergebnisse im Erwachsenenalter bestätigt werden, dass dies nicht der Fall ist (5, 6).

Literatur

1. Plaut TF (1968) Lumbar puncture in children: its value and risk. Clin Ped 7: 130-133
2. Diener HC, Bendig M, Hempel V (1985) Der postpunktionelle Kopfschmerz. Fortschr Neurol Psychiatr 53: 344–349
3. Schwarz U, Schwan C, Strumpf M, Witscher K, Zenz M (1999) Postpunktioneller Kopfschmerz. Schmerz 13: 332–340
4. Headache classification committee of the International Headache Society (1988) Classification and diagnostic criteria for headache disorders, cranial neuralgias and facial pain. Cephalalgia 8, Suppl. 7: 1–96
5. Thornberry EA, Thomas TA (1968) Posture and post-spinal headache. Br J Anaesth 60: 195–197
6. Vimala J, Peter JV, Jeyaseelan L, Prabhakar S, Cherian AM (1998) Postlumbar puncture headache: Is bed rest essential? J Assoc Phys India 46: 930–932
7. Bolder PM (1986) Postlumbar puncture headache in pediatric oncology patients. Anesthesiology 65: 696–698
8. Scher C, Amar D, Ginsburg I, Reinsel R, McDowall R, Barst S (1992) Post dural puncture headache in children with cancer. Anesthesiology 77: 1183
9. Wee LH, Lam F, Cranston AJ (1996) The incidence of post dural puncture headache in children. Anaesthesia 51: 1164–1166

Standardisierte Analyse visuell-räumlicher Wahrnehmung bei Kindern

M. Blankenburg, G. Schubert, F. Aksu

Einleitung:

Visuell-räumliche Wahrnehmungsstörungen kommen bei vielen neuropädiatrischen Erkrankungen vor und führen im Alltag z. B. zu Schwierigkeiten beim Ankleiden oder bei der Körperorientierung, beim Wiederfinden von Wegen, Abzeichnen von Objekten, bei der räumlichen Anordnung von Wörtern, beim Ablesen der Urzeit und beim Lesen, Schreiben, Rechnen. Die Ursache einer visuellen Raumwahrnehmungsstörung ist oft schwer zu erfassen, weil Raumorientierung aus unterschiedlichen Wahrnehmungs- und Verarbeitungsprozessen zusammengesetzt ist. Die subjektiven visuellen Hauptraumachsen (Horizontale, Vertikale und Mitte) sind unser zentrales Bezugssystem, mit dem wir uns durch Richtungs-, Entfernungs-, Ausdehnungs- und Tiefenwahrnehmung mit den räumlichen Eigenschaften unserer Umwelt in Beziehung setzen. Jede Störung eines dieser Parameter kann zu einer Wahrnehmungsstörung räumlicher Relationen zwischen Objekten führen. Davon zu unterscheiden ist eine Störung der inneren Repräsentation des visuellen Raumes (visuellen Raumagnosie) und eine Störung der Raumintegration (konstruktive Apraxie) bei der Objekte bezüglich der räumlichen Zuordnung ihrer Teile nicht konstruiert oder gezeichnet werden können. Scheinbar komplexe Störungen der Raumwahrnehmung können durch entsprechende Tests oft auf elementare Wahrnemungsdefizite zurückgeführt werden, die gesucht und getrennt voneinander untersucht werden müssen. Das ist durch die herkömmlichen Bleistift- und global visuell-konstruktiven Tests (Mosaik-, Benton-, Frostigtest) nicht möglich, da gleichzeitig motorische und planerische Fähigkeiten erfasst werden. Mittels eines spezifischen neuropsychologischen Testprogramms haben wir relevante Basisleistungen der visuellen Raumwahrnehmung unter Ausschluss möglicher Interaktionen zwischen motorischen und perzeptiven Faktoren untersucht.

Patienten und Methoden

Die quantitative Erfassung elementarer visuell-räumlicher Wahrnehmungsleistungen erfolgte bei 20 gesunden Kindern (6–9 Jahre) und Erwachsenen mit einem standardisierten computergestützten neuropsychologischen Testverfahren (»VS«, Kerkhoff und Marquardt, 1993 und 1994). Die subjektiven visuellen Hauptraumachsen (Horizontale, Vertikale, Mitte), die Winkel-, Abstands-, Distanz-, Entfernungs-, Längen-, Form-, und Positionsschätzung wurden nach dem klassischen Grenzverfahren untersucht. Auf einem Bildschirm wird neben einem Standardreiz ein sich deutlich unterscheidender Vergleichsreiz dargestellt. Er wird dem Standardreiz langsam angeglichen und der Bereich ermittelt, in dem beide identisch erscheinen. Dieses Verfahren wurde pro Testaufgabe 5mal wiederholt. Anfang und Ende des Bereiches, in dem Vergleichs- und Standardreiz identisch erscheinen, wird als Unsicherheitsbereich definiert und gibt den Bereich an, in dem 2 Reize gleich wahrgenommen werden. Der Median dieses Wertebereiches wird als Punkt subjektiver Gleichheit bezeichnet. Aus dem Bereich, in dem Vergleichs- und Standardreiz gerade different erscheinen, wird die Unterschiedsschwelle berechnet, die als Hälfte des Unsicherheitsbereiches definiert ist. Der konstante Fehler gibt die Differenz zwischen Punkt subjektiver Gleichheit und objektiv richtigem Wert an. Somit informieren Punkt subjektiver Gleichheit und konstanter Fehler über die mittlere Einstellung bzw. den mittleren Fehler und Unsicherheitsbereich und Unterschiedsschwelle über die Genauigkeit bzw. Unschärfe der Einstellung des Probanden.

Ergebnisse

Bei allen untersuchten Basisleistungen der visuellen Raumwahrnehmung unterschieden sich Kinder von Erwachsenen nicht in Bezug auf Mittelwerte und konstanten Fehler, aber durch eine geringere Genauigkeit in Form einer größeren Streubreite. Der mittlere Unsicherheitsbereich und die Unterschiedsschwelle waren bei Kindern aller Altersgruppen signifikant größere als bei Erwachsenen ($p<0,05$). Bei jüngeren Kindern zwischen 6–7 Jahren fanden sich im Vergleich zu älteren Kindern zwischen 8–9 Jahren größere Unsicherheitsbereiche und Unterschiedsschwellen bei der subjektiven Mitte, der Längen- und horizontalen Distanzschätzung ($p<0,05$), bei der subjektive visuelle Horizontalen und Vertikalen, der Winkel-, vertikalen Distanz-, Positions- und Formschätzung statistisch nur der Tendenz ($p<0,1$) nach.

Zusammenfassend zeigen Kinder im Vergleich zu Erwachsenen bei Basisfunktionen der visuellen Raumwahrnehmung keine systematischen Abweichungen, aber eine erhöhte Unsicherheit in Form einer größeren Standardabweichung in Abhängigkeit vom Alter.

Literatur

1. Kerkhoff G, Marquardt C. Standardisierte Analyse visuell-räumlicher Wahrnehmungsleistungen (VS). Konstruktion des Verfahrens und Anwendungen.Nervenarzt 1993b;64: 511–516.
2. Kerkhoff G, Marquardt C. Standardisierte Analyse visuell-räumlicher Wahrnehmungsleistungen (VS). Untersuchungen zur Objektivität, Reliabilität und Validität. Nervenarzt 1994; 65:689–695.

Verdacht auf neurodegenerative Erkrankung entpuppt sich als chronische Quecksilberintoxikation

C.G. Lipinski, J. Weisser, B. Schweisthal, R. Voll, R. Knapp

Zusammenfassung

Bei akut auftretenden zentralnervösen Symptomen im Kindesalter wird immer an die Möglichkeit einer Vergiftung gedacht. Bei chronisch-progredienter Symptomatik des ZNS sollte auch an Vergiftungen gedacht werden. Der damals 13-jährige Junge bot Verhaltens- und Lernstörungen, fiel in den Bereich der Lernbehinderung ab und bot nach 2½ J. das Bild einer geistigen Behinderung. Nach der notwendigen Internatsunterbringung besserte sich die Symptomatik, sodass an eine Intoxikation gedacht wurde. Hg-Spiegel im Blut und Urin waren stark erhöht ebenso wie die Messwerte der elterlichen Wohnung.

Der Junge gab an, vor 2–3 Jahren Quecksilber in der Wohnung verschüttet zu haben. Unter der Therapie mit DMPS und nach Wohnungssanierung erreichte der Junge wieder das Hauptschulniveau innerhalb von 1½ J.

Auch Langzeitintoxikation mit Hg-Dämpfen kann im Kindesalter mit weitgehender Reversibilität nach entsprechender Behandlung einhergehen.

Einleitung

Akzidentelle Vergiftungen im Kindesalter sind häufig, chronische dagegen selten, weshalb die differential-diagnostische Möglichkeit einer chronischen Intoxikation meist in den Hintergrund tritt. Die rechtzeitige Entdeckung einer Langzeitvergiftung ist wichtig, um entgiftende Maßnahmen zur Vermeidung von Dauerschäden einzuleiten.

Kasuistik

Torsten V., geb. 04/1985 – Vorgeschichte: Vater Frührentner, 2 ältere Schwestern, wovon eine außerhalb wohnt.

Unauffällige frühkindliche Entwicklung, Einschulung und Besuch der Hauptschule bis 1998. Danach entwickelte der 13-jährige Junge Gedächtnisstörungen, Leistungsabfall im Unterricht und Abwesenheitszustände. 1999 erfolgte stationäre Untersuchung in der Kinderpsychiatrie ohne diagnostisches Resultat. Danach wegen Zunahme eines Intentionstremors und Dysarthrie weitere Abklärung in der Kinderneurologie. Es wurde der Verdacht auf eine neurodegenerative Erkrankung ausgesprochen. Zur Ausschöpfung der weiteren Fördermöglichkeiten – der Junge war inzwischen wegen einer zunehmenden Lernbehinderung in die Förderstufe gekommen – erfolgte 2000 stationäre Aufnahme in unsere Klinik zur Schulabklärung und zur neuropsychologischen Testung.

Tab. 1: Quecksilber-Richtwerte

• UBA (Umweltbundesamt)	
– bei lebenslanger Dauerexposition von 0,035 µg/m³ = kein Risiko	
– bei Überschreitung von 0,35 µg/m³ = mögliches Risiko, Intervention	
• WHO	
– LOAEL (lowest observed adverse effect level)	
– Kinder und Schwangere	1,0 µg/m³
– Allgemeinbevölkerung	3,0 µg/m³
– Industrieller Schwellenwert (bei 40 h/Woche Exposition)	25,0 µg/m³
– Nephrotoxizität (bei 40 h/Woche Exposition)	50,0 µg/m³
– Klinisch-neurologische Symptome (bei 40 h/Woche Exposition)	100,0 µg/m³

Aufnahmebefund

Freundlicher, fahriger, leptosomer 15-jähriger Patient. Läufer. Torsten hat Mühe flüssig zu sprechen und verhaspelt sich ständig. Deutliche Koordinationsstörung in allen Bereichen, wechselnd ausgeprägter Intentionstremor, unregelmässige Schrift. Apraktische Störungen beim Anziehen, räumliche Orientierungsstörung auf Station, mangelnde Handlungsplanung. Taktile Wahrnehmungsstörung. Auf Station sozial gut integriert. EEG mit Verlangsamung im Theta-Bereich.

Neuropsychologische Testung

Es finden sich Einschränkungen im nonverbalen logischen Denken (T=23) und sprachlogischen Denken (T=27), verbalen, assoziativen Gedächtnis (T=23) und Leistungen der konstruktiven Praxie (T=29). Starke Störung der selektiven Aufmerksamkeit.

Insgesamt liegt Torstens kognitives Leistungsvermögen inzwischen im Bereich der Geistigen Behinderung.

Weitere Förderung ist nur in einem Lebensvorbereitenden Jahr möglich.

Verlauf

Es erfolgte Aufnahme in die Körperbehinderten-Schule (SHS) in Neckargemünd im Bereich Lebensvorbereitung mit gleichzeitiger Internatsunterbringung von Montag bis Freitag ab September 2000. Auffälligerweise bot Torsten danach eine stetige Verbesserung seiner Leistungen, sodass er im März 2001 in den Lernbehinderten Bereich wechseln konnte. Die Sprechstörung und der Tremor nahmen ständig ab.

Die rasche Reversibilität der Symptome ließ den Gedanken an eine chronische Intoxikation aufkommen, z.B. mit Schwermetallen? Handelte es sich um einen tremor mercurialis?

Laborwerte

Hg im Blut	9,2 ug/l normal –7.2 ug/l
Hg im 24h-Urin	39,0 ug/l normal 5–20 ug/l
Hg im Urin nach Gabe von 900 mg DMPS	1107,0 ug/l normal 5–25 ug/l

s.a.Tab.1.
Urin-Befund o.B.

Messwerte

Hg-Werte der elterlichen Wohnung Abb.1.

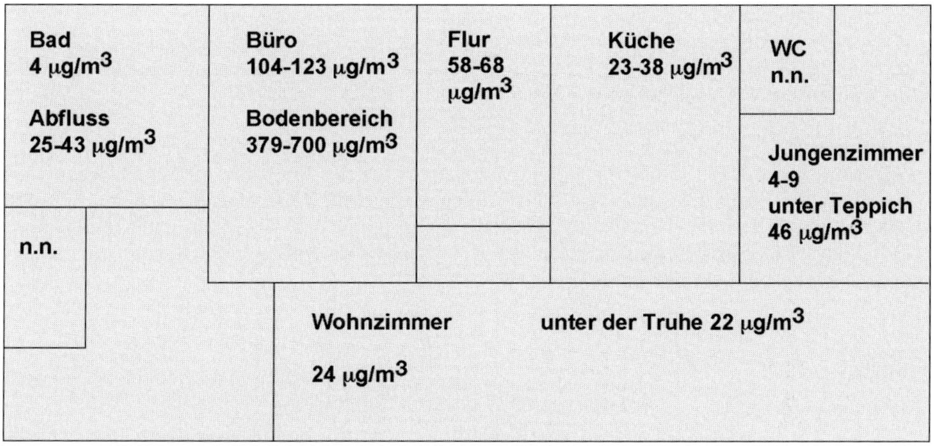

Abb. 1: Elterliche Wohnung des Patienten, Hg-Messwerte.

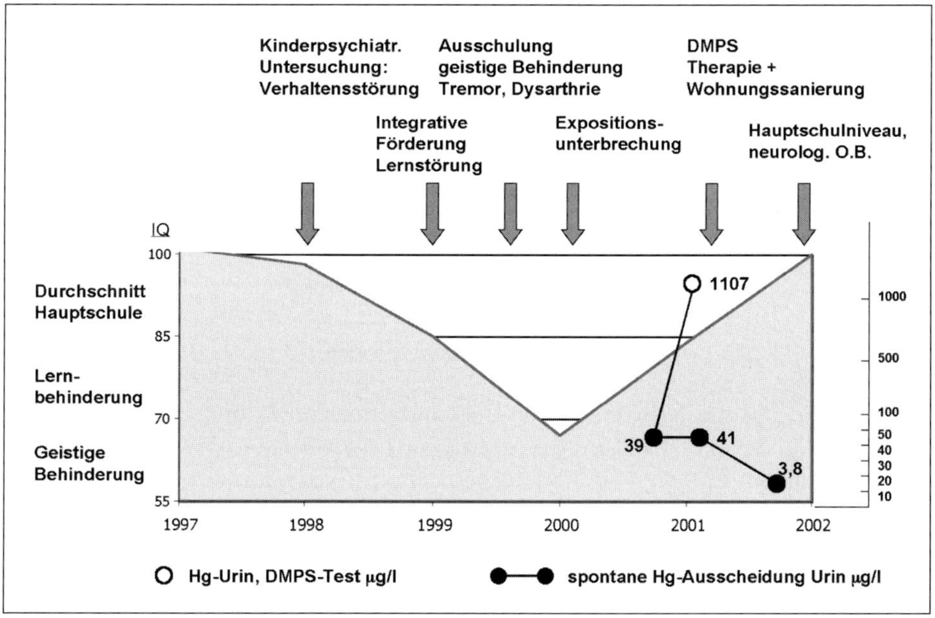

Abb. 2: Schulische und neurophysiologische Entwicklung über 5 Jahre vor und nach Expositionsstopp.

Diagnose
Chronische Quecksilbervergiftung Abb.2.

Ursache

Torsten berichtet, er habe mit seiner Schwester mit einer Dose Quecksilber im BÜRO gespielt, so etwa 1998, und dabei etwas verschüttet, das sich nicht wieder wegkehren ließ. Das BÜRO war sein Schlafzimmer.

Weitere Maßnahmen

Umgebungsuntersuchung von Vater und Schwester, sowie Einleitung einer DMPS-Therapie der 3 Betroffenen. Es erfolgte sofortige Wohnungssanierung und Entsorgung des Quecksilbers aus der väterlichen Werkstatt.

Katamnese

Rasche weitere Besserung der kognitiven Leistungen des Jungen und Normalisierung des neurologischen Befundes sowie des Schriftbildes. Auch das EEG normalisierte sich in einen flacheren Alpharhythmus. Nachtestung 2002 mit dem Ergebnis des Wiedererreichens des Hauptschulniveaus. Mit dem erfolgreichen Hauptschulabschluss im Rahmen des Berufsvorbereitenden Jahres wird jetzt gerechnet.

Conclusion

Quecksilber-Intoxikationen ereignen sich auch heute noch auf enteralem oder pulmonalem Weg (2). Führende Symptome sind Tremor, Verhaltensstörung, Sprechstörungen, Stomatitis, Proteinurie und allgemeiner Abbau der kognitiven Funktionen im Sinne einer Enzephalopathie. Das EEG zeigt eine mäßige Verlangsamung.

Elementares Hg wird im Körper zu Hg-Ionen oxydiert, die nach Bindung an SH-Gruppen als Eiweisgifte wirken. Die biologische Halbwertszeit für den (erwachsenen) Gesamtorganismus liegt bei ca. 60 Tagen, für das Gehirn bei mehreren Jahren (1). Um so bemerkenswerter ist die Reversibilität der Symptomatik in unserem Falle alleine durch partielle Expositionsunterbrechung – nämlich die Wohnheimunterbringung von Montag bis Freitag. Es genügten also jeweils 5 Tage Expositionsunterbrechung pro Woche, um die Hg-Bilanz zu negativieren.

Die Hg-Werte der elterlichen Wohnung überschritten die MAK-Werte um ein Vielfaches.

Wichtig sind die Richtlinien des Umweltbundesamtes und der WHO, siehe Tab. 1. und besonders die Kenntnis der *Lowest Observed Adverse Effect Levels.* Durch Amalgamfüllungen ist keine chronische Intoxikation zu erwarten, wenngleich bei Kindern sorgfältig zu prüfen ist, ob eine Amalgamtherapie notwendig ist (3).

Expositionsschutz und Behandlung mit Dimercaptopropansulfonsäure (DMPS) sind bei nachgewiesener Intoxikation sofort einzuleiten.

Literatur

1. AWMF-Leitlinien-Register Nr. 002/003 (1999)
2. Böse S, Drasch G, Eife R, Laub MC (1993) Chronische Metallintoxikationen als Ursache neuropädiatrischer Erkrankungen. Pädiatrische Praxis 45: 183–197
3. Harhammer R, (2001) Zur Risikobewertung des Zahnärztlichen Füllungswerkstoffes Amalgam. Bundesgesundheitsbl-Gesundheitsforsch-Gesundheitsschutz 44: 149–154

Neurologische Spätfolgen einer Interferon-Alpha-Therapie bei bedrohlichen Hämangiomen in den ersten drei Lebensjahren

U. Gruber-Sedlmayr, M. Brunner-Krainz, H. Lackner, A. Pfleger, B. Resch

Abstract

Alpha-Interferon wird bei bedrohlichen Hämangiomen des Säuglings- und Kleinkindesalter in zunehmender Häufigkeit therapeutisch eingesetzt. Neben den üblichen akuten Nebenwirkungen, die meist gut beherrschbar sind, besteht in dieser sehr jungen Patientengruppe die Gefahr von persistierenden neurologischen Spätfolgen im Sinne von spastischen Diplegien.

In einer Nachuntersuchung an der Univ.-Klinik für Kinder- und Jugendheilkunde in Graz von 10 Kindern, welche innerhalb der ersten drei Lebensjahre wegen lebens- oder organbedrohenden Hämangiomen Interferon Alpha bekommen hatten, fanden sich Hinweise, dass das Auftreten von neurologischen Spätschäden in erster Linie mit der maximalen Tagesdosierung korreliert.

Einleitung

Interferone sind Botenstoffe, die den Stoffwechsel von homologen Zellen derart verändern, dass diese gegen Virusinfektionen resistenter werden. Man teilt heute die verschiedenen Interferone nach ihren Hauptbildungszellen ein. Das Wirkungsspektrum ist großteils überlappend. Alpha-Interferone werden einerseits zur Therapie chronischer Virusinfektionen, wie der Hepatitis C eingesetzt, andererseits haben sie einen Einfluss auf Zellwachstum, Zellteilung und Zelldifferenzierung und finden daher auch bei vielen onkologischen Erkrankungen, wie z.B. der Haarzell-Leukämie oder auch dem Nierenzellkarzinom, Verwendung.

1989 wurde erstmals ein 12-jähriger Knabe mit pulmonaler Hämangiomatose erfolgreich mit Interferon behandelt (1). Im Jahr darauf erfolgte ebenfalls von White die Beschreibung von 5 Kindern mit verschiedenen angiomatösen Erkrankungen, welche großteils auf Interferon-Alpha gut ansprachen (2).

Seit der Arbeit von Ezekowitz et al. 1992, in welcher die großteils erfolgreiche Interferon-Alpha-Therapie bei 20 Kindern mit lebensbedrohenden Hämangiomen beschrieben worden war, findet diese Therapieform breite Anwendung (3).

Nebenwirkungen der Interferon-Alpha-Therapie

Die akuten Nebenwirkungen, wie grippeähnliche Symptome, Transaminasenerhöhungen, Blutbildveränderungen sowie gastrointestinale Symptome, sind im Allgemeinen gut beherrschbar.

An neurologischen Nebenwirkungen werden bei Erwachsenen reversible Störungen der Vigilanz sowie Gedächtnisverlust, Depression und Parästhesien beschrieben. 1991 ist allerdings in Neurology eine Arbeit erschienen, in welcher von 14 erwachsenen Patienten mit persistierender Neurotoxizität im Sinne von Demenz, Depression und Parkinsonismus nach Interferon-Alpha-Therapie berichtet wird (4).

Über neurologische Spätschäden bei Kindern im Sinne von spastischen Diplegien gibt es seit 1989 mehrere Einzelfallberichte (5, 6, 7). In einer prospektiven Studie, bei welcher 53 Kinder, welche in den ersten drei Lebensjahren Interferon-Alpha erhielten regelmäßig bezüglich Nebenwirkungen untersucht wurden, wurden 43 dieser Kinder auch neuropädiatrisch nachuntersucht. 10 davon wurden als neurologisch auffallend beschrieben, mit z.B. auffallend lebhaften Reflexen und auch einem positiven Babinski-Phänomen. Eines dieser Kinder entwickelt eine persistierende spastische Diplegie. Die Dosierung von Interferon wurde in dieser Studie beim Auftreten von Nebenwirkungen reduziert und die Dosis war im 1. Lebensjahr durchwegs niedriger, als die von Ezekowitz empfohlene Dosierung von 3 Mio. Einheiten/m^2 Körpergewicht/Tag (8).

Neuropädiatrische Untersuchung von 10 Kindern nach Interferon-Alpha-Therapie an der Univ.-Klinik für Kinder- und Jugendheilkunde Graz

10 Kinder waren in den Jahren 1992–1998 wegen lebensbedrohenden, oder organbedrohenden Hämangiomen an der Univ.-Klinik für Kinder- und Jugendheilkunde in Graz mit Alpha-Interferon behandelt worden. 8 Kinder davon hatten Hämangiome im Gesichts- und Halsbereich, teilweise mit Atemnotsymptomatik, bzw. Hämangiome der Orbita. Ein Kind hatte ein Riesenhämangiom der rechten Flanke mit Kasabach-Merritt-Syndrom und eines ein Hämangiom der Leber mit multiplen kutanen Hämangiomen. Der Beginn der Interferon-Therapie lag zwischen dem 1. Lebenstag und dem Alter von 15 Monaten, die Dauer der Therapie differierte zwischen 5–25 Monaten, und 9 der 10 Kinder sprachen auf die Therapie gut an.

Die neuropädiatrische Untersuchung fand bei 8 der 10 Kinder nach bereits beendeter Interferon-Alpha-Therapie statt, bei 2 Kindern waren neurologische Auffälligkeiten die Ursache für das Absetzen des Interferon.

Bei 4 der 10 Kinder fanden sich typische Zeichen einer spastischen Diplegie, 3 dieser Kinder haben eine unauffällige zerebrale MRT, ein schwer betroffener Bub hat eine Dysplasie der rechten Kleinhirnhemisphäre mit Aplasie des Unterwurms.

In der Gruppe der Kinder ohne spastische Diplegie hatte ein Mädchen einen intracraniellen Hämangiomanteil, dieses Kind benötigte kurzfristig eine extracorporale Membranoxygenierung wegen einer Pneumocystis carinii Infektion unter Cortisontherapie. Dieses Mädchen hat eine leichte allgemeine Entwicklungsverzögerung ohne Zeichen einer Spastizität.

In unserer Untersuchung betrug die kumulative Dosierung bei den Patienten mit den Zeichen einer spastischen Diplegie im Durchschnitt 1036 Mio IE/m^2 und

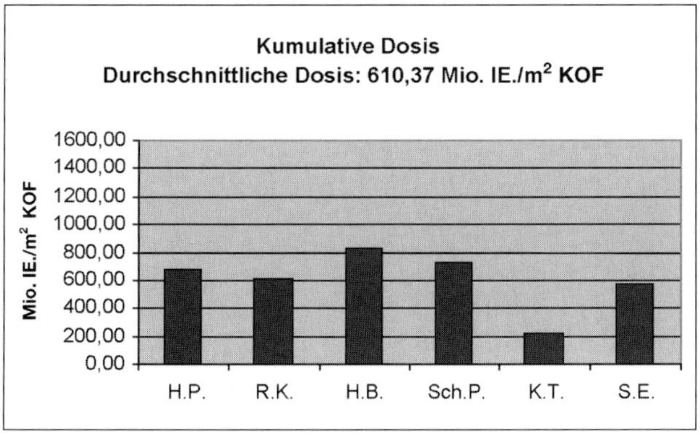

Abb. 1: Kumulative Dosis bei Patienten ohne Zeichen einer Cerebralparese.

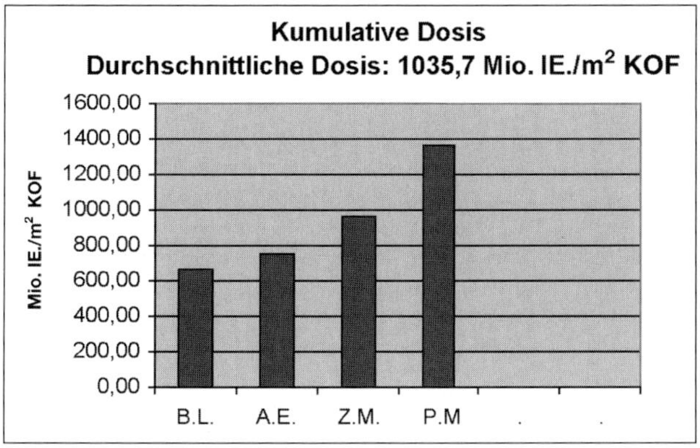

Abb. 2: Kumulative Dosis bei Patienten mit Zeichen einer Cerebralparese.

bei den Patienten ohne Zeichen einer Spastizität im Durchschnitt 610 Mio. IE/m^2. In beiden Patientengruppen gab es Kinder, die zeitweise Interferon alternierend, oder zwei- bis dreimal pro Woche erhielten.

In einem ähnlichem Verhältnis liegt der Vergleich der maximalen Tagesdosierungen. Die Patienten mit Cerebralparese erhielten im Durchschnitt 5,79 Mio. IE/m^2 als maximale Tagesdosierung, die ohne Cerebralparese im Durchschnitt 3,12 Mio. IE/m^2.

Die maximale Therapiedauer betrug bei den Patienten ohne neurologische Nebenwirkungen durchschnittlich 408 Tage, bei den Patienten mit Cerebralparese 308 Tage, was vermutlich darauf zurückzuführen ist, dass bei 2 Patienten die Interferon-Alpha-Therapie wegen der neurologischen Auffälligkeiten abgebrochen wurde.

Zusammenfassung

Eine persistierende spastische Diplegie ist eine häufige Komplikation einer Interferon-Alpha-Therapie im Säuglings- und Kleinkindesalter und es bestehen Hinweise für eine Dosisabhängigkeit dieser Nebenwirkung. Somit sollte eine

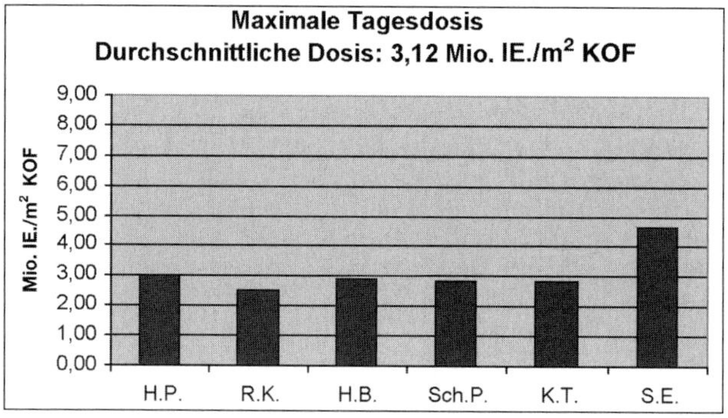

Abb. 3: Maximale Tagesdosierung der Patienten ohne Zeichen einer Cerebralparese.

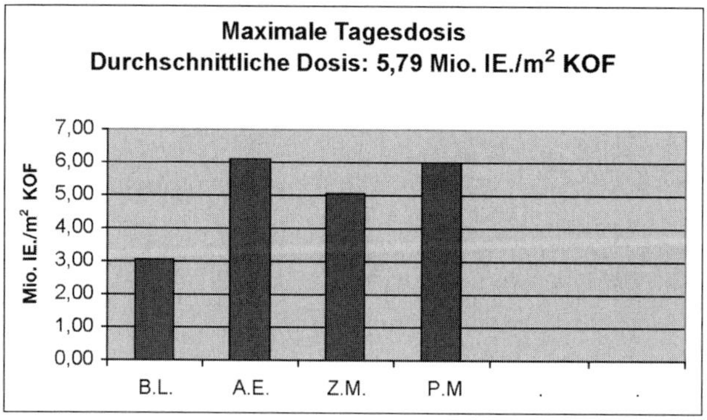

Abb. 4: Maximale Tagesdosierung der Patienten mit Zeichen einer Cerebralparese.

derartige Therapie bei Hämangiomen in den ersten drei Lebensjahren nur bei ungenügendem Ansprechen auf andere Therapien bei bedrohlichen Hämangiomen und mit der niedrigst möglichen Dosierung, sowie unter regelmäßiger neuropädiatrischer Kontrolle durchgeführt werden.

Literatur

1. White et al (1989) Treatment of pulmonary hemangiomatosis with recombinant interferon alfa-2a. N Engl J Med Vol. 320: 1197–200
2. White et al (1991) Treatment of childhood angiomatous diseases with recombinant interferon alfa-2a. J Pediatr Vol. 118, No. 1: 59–66
3. Ezekowitz R et al (1992) Interferon alfa-2a therapy for life-threatening hemangiomas of infancy. N Engl J Med Vol. 326, No. 22: 1456–1463
4. Meyers Ch et al (1991) Persistent neurotoxicity of systemically administered interferon-alpha. Neurology 41: 672–676
5. Wörle H et al (1999) Interferon alpha-2a therapy in haemangiomas of infancy: spastic diplegia as a severe complication. Europ J Pediatr 158(4): 344
6. Vesikari T et al (1988) Neurologic sequelae following interferon therapy of juvenile laryngeal papilloma. Acta Paediatr Scand 77: 619–622
7. Barlow CF et al (1998) Spastic diplegia as a complication of interferon alfa-2a treatment of hemangiomas of infancy. J Pediatr 132: 527–30
8. Dubois J et al (1999) Toxicity profile of interferon alfa-2b in children: A prospective evaluation. J Pediatr Vol. 135, No. 6: 782–785

Dorsaler Proboscis als Zeichen einer Spina bifida occulta mit Lipomyelocele und Dorsalfixierung des Filum terminale

M. Wesendahl, R. Gerlach, W. Galow, V. v. Loewenich, V. Boda, St. Vlaho, M. Kieslich

Zusammenfassung

Es wird die Kasuistik eines unbeeinträchtigten Neugeborenen dargestellt, bei dem ein seltenes dorsales Hautanhängsel auf eine Spina bifida occulta mit Lipomyelocele und Dorsalfixierung des Filum terminale hinwies.

Einleitung

Eine Spina bifida occulta ist in der Neugeborenenphase schwer zu erkennen und wird oft erst dann diagnostiziert, wenn die Kinder im Rahmen des Tethered cord-Syndroms paraplegische Symptome aufweisen. Wegweisend sind bereits postpartal vorliegende kutane Veränderungen.

Kasuistik

Spontanpartus nach unauffälliger Schwangerschaft in der 40. SSW. Geburtsgewicht 4100 g, Länge 59 cm, KU 37 cm, APGAR 9/10/10, NA-pH 7,28.

Bereits im Rahmen der U1 fiel ein medial gelegenes, lumbosakrales, 5 cm langes, wurmförmiges, weiches, sich akral verjüngendes Hautanhängsel auf. Der übrige internorganische Untersuchungsbefund war unauffällig. Auch neurologisch fanden sich keine Auffälligkeiten, insbesondere bestanden keine paraplegischen Symptome.

Während in der betreuenden Frauenklinik bereits diskutiert wurde, das Anhängsel abzubinden, veranlasste der konsiliarisch tätige Pädiater die weitere Diagnostik.

Der spinalsonographische Befund war verdächtig auf eine Konusdysplasie mit dorsaler Fixation. Kernspintomographisch kam eine Lipomyelocele mit Konustiefstand und dorsaler Fixation (Tethered cord-Konstellation) im lumbosakralen Übergangsbereich zur Darstellung. Schädel- und Nephrosonographie waren unauffällig.

Im 2. Lebensmonat erfolgte die neurochirurgische Abtagung des Hautanhängsel. Intraoperativ zeigte sich eine bindegewebige Fortsetzung des Proboscis bis in die Dura mit Übergang in ein intradural gelegenes Lipom, welches mit der Dura verwachsen war und teilreseziert werden konnte. Histologisch handelte es sich um eine epidermal-lipomatöse Fehlbildung mit einzelnen Nervenfaszikeln ohne sicheren Anhalt für zentralnervöses Gewebe. Es bestand kein Anhalt für Malignität.

Postoperativ unkomplizierter Verlauf. Klinisch-neurologische Verlaufskontrollen im Alter von 6 und 9 Monaten zeigten weiterhin keine paraplegischen Symptome.

Diskussion

Bei reifen Neugeborenen findet man in 4,8% angeborene dorsale Hautveränderungen (8). Hierbei handelt es sich in der überwiegenden Zahl um dorsale Grübchen (74%), seltener um Hämangiome, abnorme Pigmentierung, Behaarung, Lipome oder Hautanhängsel (8). Während bei kleinen Grübchen eine spinale Dysraphie unwahrscheinlich ist, ist bei den anderen lokalen Veränderungen in bis zu 50% mit einer Spina bifida occulta zu rechnen. Kriss et al. gehen sogar von einem 100%igen Dysraphie-Risiko aus, wenn die Hautläsion um mehr als 5 mm von der Hautoberfläche abweicht (8). In diesen Fällen ist die weiterführende Diagnostik mittels Sonographie und MRT indiziert (9). Gefahndet werden sollte nach dem Vorliegen einer Tethered cord-Konstellation, bei der es durch ein intradural gelegenes Lipom, Dermoid, Gliose, fibröses Bänder oder Bindegewebe zu einem Tiefstand mit Dorsalfixation des Conus medullaris gekommen ist (4). Auch bei zunächst klinisch asymptomatischen Kindern kann es im weiteren Verlauf aufgrund mechanischer oder ischämischer Irritationen zu zunehmenden neurologischen Ausfällen kommen. Neben Beinschmerzen, motorischen und sensiblen Ausfällen kommt es häufig zur Blasen- und Mastdarmlähmung (6, 5). Durch die frühzeitige neurochirurgische Intervention mit Entfesselung des Rückenmarks mit Lösen pathologischer Fixationen und Reduk-

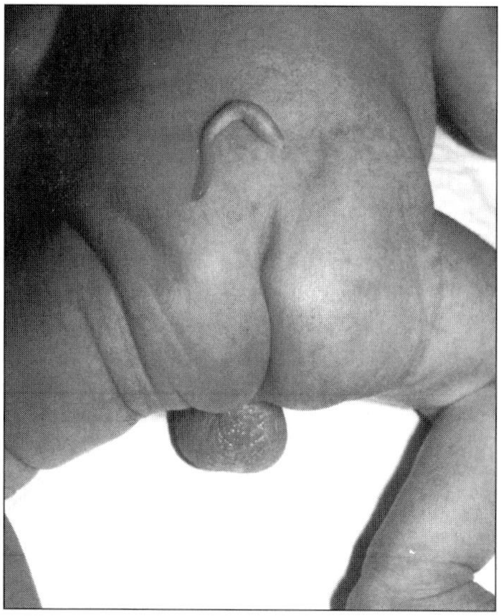

Abb. 1

tion raumfordernder Gewebsmassen kann das Auftreten dieser Symptome verhindert oder zumindest das Risiko einer solchen Verschlechterung deutlich reduziert werden (5, 7, 10).

Dorsale schwanz- oder rüsselartige Hautanhängsel wurden vereinzelt beschrieben (1, 2, 3, 8, 11, 12). In allen Fällen waren sie mit einer spinalen Dysraphie assoziiert.

In dem von uns beschriebenen Fall lag ein 5 cm langes, dorsales Hautanhängsel vor. Die bildgebende Diagnostik bestätigte den Verdacht auf eine Spina bifida occulta und zeigte eine Lipomyelocele mit Tiefstand und dorsaler Fixation des Conus medullaris. Es bestand somit eine Tethered cord-Konstellation. Zur Prävention einer späteren neurologischen Verschlechterung wurde die Indikation zur neurochirurgischen Intervention gestellt.

Schlussfolgerung

Dorsale Proboscen sind extrem selten. Wichtig ist es auch bei asymptomatischen Neugeborenen mit seltenen dorsalen Hautveränderungen die weiterführende Dysraphie-Diagnostik einzuleiten. Eine frühe neurochirurgische Intervention soll der Tethered cord-Syndrom-Entwicklung vorbeugen.

Literatur

1. Aso M, Kawaguchi T, Mihara M, Shimao S, Morimato K, Sakinaga Y (1987) Pseudotail associated with spinal dysraphism. Dermatologica 174 (1): 45–8
2. Belzberg AJ, Myles ST, Trevenen CL (1991) The human tail and spinal dysraphism. J Pediatr Surg 26 (10): 1243–5
3. Chakrabortty S, Oi s, yoshida Y, Yamada H, Yamaguchi M, Tamaki N, Matsumoto S (1993) Myelomenigocele and thick filum terminale with tethered cord appearing as a human tail. Case report. J Neurosurg 78 (6): 966–9
4. Jacobi G, Preisler B, Kieslich M (1998) Zentrales Nervensystem – Tethered Cord, Klinik und Diagnostik. In: Michael T (Hrsg.): Spina bifida, interdisziplinäre Diagnostik, Therapie und Beratung; de Gruyter, Berlin, New York
5. Kaplan Jo, Quencer RM (1980) The occult tethered conus syndrome in the adult. Radiology 137: 387–91
6. Kaplan WE, McLone DG, Richards I (1988) Theo urological manifestations of the tethered spinal cord. J Urol. 140: 1285–88
7. Krauß J (1998) Zentrales Nervensystem – Tethered Cord, Operative Therapie. In: Michael T (Hrsg.): Spina bifida, interdisziplinäre Diagnostik, Therapie und Beratung; de Gruyter, Berlin, New York
8. Kriss VM, Desai NS (1998) Occult spinal dysraphism in neonates: assessment of high risk cutaneous stigmata on sonography. AJR 171: 1687–92
9. Santiago Medina L, Crone K, Kuntz KM (2001) Newborns with suspected occult spinal dysraphism: a cost-effectiveness analysis of diagnostic strategies. Pediatrics 108 (6): 101–9
10. Satar N, Bauer SB, Shefner J, Kelly ND, Darbey NM (1995) The effects of delayed diagnosis and treatment in patients with an occult spinal dysraphism. J Urol. 154: 754–8
11. Tavafoghi V, Ghandchi A, Hambrick GW Jr., Udverhelyi GB (1978) Cutaneous signs of spinal dysrapism. Arch Dermatol. 114: 573–7
12. Yamada S, Mandybur GT, Thompson JR (1996) Dorsal midline proboscis associated with diastematomyelia and tethered cord syndrom. Case report. J Neurosurg 85 (4): 709–12

16. Stellungnahmen der Gesellschaft für Neuropädiatrie zu Therapieverfahren

Orofaziale Regulationstherapie nach Castillo Morales

Stellungnahme der Gesellschaft für Neuropädiatrie
Kommission zu Behandlungsverfahren bei Entwicklungsstörungen und zerebralen Bewegungsstörungen

D. Karch, G. Groß-Selbeck, J. Pietz, H-G. Schlack

Einleitung

Mitte des letzten Jahrhunderts wurden von verschiedenen Arbeitsgruppen die Grundlagen der Rehabilitation bei entwicklungsgestörten und behinderten Kindern neu überdacht und neue Therapiekonzepte entwickelt. Die Regulationstherapie wurde von Castillo Morales aus der persönlichen Erfahrung, den damals bestehenden Vorstellungen zur Entwicklungsneurologie und den Kontakten mit anderen wie B. und K. Bobath, V. Vojta u.a. als eigenes Behandlungskonzept entwickelt. Er bezeichnete sie als neuromotorische Entwicklungstherapie bzw. bei mundmotorischen Störungen als orofaziale Regulationstherapie. Die orofaziale Regulationstherapie wird seit langem als das wichtigste Behandlungskonzept angesehen und extensiv eingesetzt.

Konzeptionelle Voraussetzungen

Die Behandlung soll sich an der Funktion orientieren. Ziel der Regulation soll es sein, ein harmonisches Zusammenspiel und ein Gleichgewicht zwischen den verschiedenen Komponenten des orofazialen Komplexes untereinander und mit den übrigen Organsystemen des Körpers sowie zwischen Mensch und Kosmos zu erreichen (Castillo Morales 1991). Die Form diene nicht nur der Funktion, sondern werde auch durch diese geprägt, so dass sich jedes Organ durch eine harmonische Funktion selbst forme. So sei die Form des Gaumens einerseits wichtig für die Funktion der Zunge, werde andererseits aber auch von der Funktion der Zunge geformt.

Zum Verständnis der Funktionen des orofazialen Systems: Nahrungsaufnahme, Mimik, Atmung, und Phonation sei die genaue Kenntnis der muskuloskeletären Verhältnisse im Sinne der funktionellen Anatomie erforderlich. Wesentlich für das Konzept der orofazialen Regulation ist die Annahme, dass das orofaziale System eng verbunden sei mit dem gesamten Körper vom Schädel ausgehend über die Wirbelsäule bis zu den Füßen. Eine Veränderung der Beckenhaltung z.B. wirke sich ebenso auf die Mundmotorik aus wie umgekehrt eine Veränderung im orofazialen Bereich auf die Schultermuskulatur.

Castillo Morales schöpfte seine Vorstellungen auch aus seinen Beobachtungen der Lebensgewohnheiten von Ureinwohnern Lateinamerikas, insbesondere ihren Umgang mit Säuglingen und Kleinkindern. Seiner Meinung nach stellt der sehr enge Körperkontakt eine wesentliche Grundlage für eine gute sensomotorische und psychische Entwicklung der Kinder dar. Die intuitive Unterstützung der Kopfkontrolle durch eine Hand am Hinterhaupt sei dabei eine grundsätzliche sensomotorische Erfahrung für die Kinder.

Die physiologischen Abläufe beim Saugen, Kauen und Schlucken werden nach Castillo Morales beeinflusst von einem multisensorischen Integrationsprozess, in dem das vestibuläre, propriozeptive und taktile System besonders wichtig sind und von exakt abgestimmten funktionellen Abläufen gekennzeichnet seien. Die Einteilung des physiologischen Kaumechanismus in: Annäherungsphase, Greifphase, Abbeißphase und Zerkleinerungsphase entspricht ebenso den anerkannten physiologischen Vorstellungen wie die Tatsache, dass jede Phase durch feinabgestimmte Funktionsabläufe der Weichteile und des Kieferskeletts gewährleistet werden und der Kau- und Schluckmechanismus willkürlich, die Rachenphase dagegen rein reflektorisch gesteuert werden.

Die Befundaufnahme beim Patienten

Zur Analyse der mundmotorischen Funktionen wird eine detaillierte Beobachtung gefordert, die sich auf Lippen, Zunge, Gaumen, Gaumensegel und schließlich die gesamte orofaziale Funktion beziehen müsse. Bei der Beobachtung der Zungenfunktion könne man nicht nur krankheitsspezifische Störungen erkennen wie z.B. Athetosen, Tremor oder Faszikulationen, sondern auch unwillkürliche athetoide Bewegungen (sog. »primäre Zungenbewegungen«), die von Castillo Morales bei gesunden Kindern bis zum Alter von 5 Jahren und auch bei älteren Kindern mit geistiger Behinderung und ausgeprägter Muskelhypotonie oder mit zerebralen Bewegungsstörungen beschrieben werden. Es seien symmetrische Wellen, die an der Zungenwurzel begännen und sich allmählich zur Zungenspitze hin verlören. Wenn diese für Kleinkinder normalen Bewegungen persistierten, könne sich keine normale Zungenfunktion ausbilden (Castillo Morales et al. 1995).

Bei der Befunderhebung müsse auch auf Kompensationsmechanismen geachtet werden. Oft werde von den Patienten der Kopf rekliniert, verbunden mit einer Schulterprotraktion, um die mechanischen Voraussetzung dafür zu schaffen, dass die Nahrung trotz des insuffizienten Schluckaktes in den Ösophagus gelangen kann. So entwickelten Kinder mit generalisierter Muskelhypotonie, wie z.B. bei M. Down, eine zunehmende Fehlstellung der Kiefer (Progenie), eine schmale Oberlippe und einen schmalen Gaumen, infolge der konstanten Reklination und der hypotonen Zungenmuskulatur. Dadurch werden Nasenatmung, Nahrungsaufnahme bzw. das Schlucken und die Artikulation beeinträchtigt.

Bei Kindern mit zerebralen Bewegungsstörungen träten unterschiedliche Funktionsstörungen auf in Abhängigkeit davon, ob eine spastische oder eine dyskinetische Symptomatik besteht. Meist wiesen Kinder mit spastischen Bewegungsstörungen eine verstärkte Beißreaktion auf, kauten und schluckten unkoordiniert, nicht selten aspirierten sie und versuchten ihre Probleme durch Fehlhaltungen von Körper und Kopf sowie eine abnorme Atemregulation zu kompensieren.

Behandlungstechniken sind die manuelle Kopf- und Kieferkontrolle, die entsprechend der Grunderkrankung bzw. Symptomatik variiert werden muss, und die sensorische Stimulation durch Berühren, Streichen, Zug, Druck und Vibration der mimischen Muskulatur sowie der äußeren Mundmuskulatur und der oberen und unteren Zungenbeinmuskulatur. Hinzu kommen Massage von Zahnfleisch und Gaumen, Manipulationen an der Zunge oder die Stimulation des Saugens. Eine weiteres Behandlungsziel ist die »motorische Ruhe«.

Bei der *Kopf- und Kieferkontrolle,* die u.a. nach dem Bobath-Konzept entwickelt wurde, wird das Kind bei guter Körperhaltung mit einer Hand am Hinterkopf und Nacken stabilisiert, mit der anderen Hand wird der Unterkiefer umfasst und je nach vorliegender Pathologie mit Daumen und Fingern (an Mundboden, entlang der Mandibula, im Kinnbereich) stimuliert und kontrolliert. Dabei werden unterschiedliche taktile und propriozeptive Reize genutzt: Berühren, Streichen, Zug, Druck und vor allem Vibration. Ziel dieser manuellen Techniken sei es, »normale Bewegungsmuster anzubahnen« (Castillo Morales 1991, S. 112). Die Stabilisierung von Kopf- und Körperhaltung schafft dabei die notwendigen Voraussetzungen, die »motorische Ruhe«, u.a. durch die Einflussnahme auf abnorme Nacken- oder Labyrinthreaktionen, wie sie bei Kinder mit zerebralen Bewegungsstörungen bestehen (Castillo Morales 1991, S. 118). Dadurch würden die Körperhaltung verbessert, die Koordinierung der Atmung und die Bahnung von Hand-Hand, Hand-Mund und Hand-Fuß-Mund-Kontakt gefördert.

Castillo Morales (2000) geht davon aus, dass durch die *»motorische Ruhe«* und die damit verbundene bessere Aufmerksamkeit und Kommunikation mit dem Kind nicht nur ein besserer Zugang ermöglicht wird, der sich positiv auf die therapeutische Arbeit auswirkt.

Bei den *Basisübungen* werden Ausgangsstellungen für den Patienten geschaffen, um aus der Rückenlage oder im Sitzen gezielte Übungen durchführen zu können. Dabei müssen individuell angepasste Ausgangspositionen gefunden werden. Der gestörte Muskeltonus soll positiv beeinflusst werden, und es soll überprüft werden, ob sich bestehende Kompensationen funktionell günstig oder ungünstig auswirken. Muskeln und Bindegewebe werden durch diese Behandlungstechniken »modelliert« (ebda. S. 126), um z.B. eine hypomobile und hochgezogene Oberlippe zu lockern oder den verspannten Mundboden zu mobilisieren.

Spezielle Übungen dienen dem Vorverlagern der Mandibula, der aktiven Kieferöffnung, Aktivierung der Muskulatur des Zungenbeins, der Oberlippen, des Kinns oder der Wangen.

Durch die Stimulation bestimmter motorischer Zonen im Gesicht sollen spezifische Reaktionen und Funktionen ausgelöst werden.

Übungen im Mund haben zum Ziel, mundmotorische Störungen zu beeinflussen. Hierzu zählen die Zahnfleischmassage zur Verbesserung der Speichelflusskontrolle und zur Fazilitation des Schluckens, die Gaumenmassage zur Verminderung des Würgereflexes sowie die Elevation der Zungenspitze, die

Aktivierung lateraler Zungenbewegungen und Vibration der Zunge zur Verbesserung des Schluckens.

Bei den *Übungen zur Stimulation des Saugens* werden die genannten Techniken eingesetzt mit dem Ziel, die Bewegungsfolgen des normalen Saugens Schritt für Schritt anzuregen und zu unterstützen.

Kieferorthopädische Hilfsmittel

Zur Behandlung von Störungen der Zungen- und Schluckmotorik werden von Castillo Morales auch mechanische Hilfsmittel eingesetzt. Zur Förderung des Mundschlusses sollen dazu Geräte verwendet werden, die entweder als »Monoblock« oder als offenes System konstruiert sind. Zur Aktivierung der Zungenfunktion dienen Hilfsmittel wie kieferorthopädische Platten die mit unterschiedlichen Aufsätzen versehen sind wie Knöpfen, Rillen, Perlen u.a. Die Apparate bestehen aus Kunststoff und werden mit Metallklammern gehalten. Sie müssen individuell angepasst werden. Besonders häufig werden diese Gaumenplatten bei Kindern mit M. Down eingesetzt, bei denen die Zungenmuskulatur sehr hypoton ist und oft eine Diastase besteht. Ziel ist es, die Zunge zur Kontraktion nach hinten und oben anzuregen, die Oberlippe zu aktivieren und durch veränderte Zungenstellung und Lippenkontakt nicht nur die Nasenatmung zu erleichtern, sondern auch das Saug- und Schluckmuster zu verbessern. Die Anpassung von Hilfsmitteln erfordert viel Erfahrung, da es eine Reihe von Fehlermöglichkeiten gibt (Castillo Morales 1991, S.187). Von Limbrock et al. (1987) wurde darüberhinaus eine Mundvorhofspange entwickelt, durch die Impulse zwischen Zunge, Lippen und Wangen gesetzt werden mit dem Ziel, einen »reaktiven« Mundschluss zu erreichen.

Indikationen für die Orofaziale Regulationstherapie

Von Castillo Morales und anderen Autoren (Haberstock 1992) wurde eine Vielzahl von Krankheitsbildern oder Symptomenkomplexen angegeben, bei denen die Behandlung erfolgen sollte:

- Säuglinge mit Saug- und Schluckstörungen,
- Mundmotorische Störungen bei M. Down, Pierre-Robin Sequenz, Moebius Syndrom, zerebralen Bewegungsstöungen, Dyspraxien u.a.
- Lippen-Kiefer-Gaumenspalten oder nach Operationen im Gesichtsbereich
- Facialisparese
- Insuffizienter Mundschluss mit geringer Speichelflusskontrolle
- Artikulationsstörungen und Dysphonie

Auch eine präventive Behandlung bei Frühgeborenen wird empfohlen.

Stellungnahme zu dem Konzept

Das Konzept wurde entwickelt aus den Vorstellungen der 50er und 60er Jahre über die Entwicklung des zentralen Nervensystems sowie Kontrolle und Steuerung der Motorik in den ersten Lebensmonaten und -jahren. In Anlehnung an die theoretischen Vorstellungen von B. und K. Bobath wird unterstellt, dass durch Inhibition abnormer Haltungs- und Bewegungsmuster und Facilitation besserer Bewegungsabläufe Einfluss auf die zentralen Kontroll- und Steuerungsprogramme genommen und somit therapeutische Effekte erzielt werden können. Die Behandlung sollte daher in das Konzept der Krankengymnastik auf neurophysiologischer Grundlage nach Bobath (Castillo Morales 1991) bzw. Vojta (Ohrt und Block 1987) eingebunden werden. Die theoretischen Vorstellungen von Castillo Morales zu der herausragenden Bedeutung der Funktion bei der Beurteilung und Behandlung stimmen wenig überein mit den pragmatisch orientierten Vorgehensweisen der orofazialen Regulationstherapie.

Alle selbstkritischen Einwände, die in den letzten Jahren gegenüber den früheren Vorgehensweisen bei der Bobaththerapie geäußert worden sind, gelten insofern auch für das Konzept der orofazialen Regulationstherapie (Ohrt 1999). Entsprechend den neueren Konzepten zur motorischen Kontrolle und ihrer Entwicklung in den ersten Lebensmonaten sowie zum motorischen Lernen wird in der Bobaththerapie sehr viel Wert auf die Fähigkeit zur Selbstregulation des zentralen Nervensystems gelegt. Daher wird vor allem die Eigenaktivität der Kinder unterstützt und durch eine sinnvolle Aufgabenstellung, strukturierte Handlungskontexte, adäquate Ausgangspositionen sowie Beachtung der psychischen Befindlichkeit herausgefordert. In den letzten Jahren wurden diese Vorstellungen auch in den Ausbildungskursen zur orofazialen Regulationsterapie berücksichtigt und haben zu entsprechender Modifikation geführt. Immer mehr wird über sensorische Einflüsse von anderen Körperregionen Einfluss auf die orofaziale Funktion genommen.

Es ist zu bezweifeln, dass durch Techniken der manuellen Medizin, wie sie in der orofazialen Regulationstherapie verwendet werden, der Muskeltonus z.B. bei Kindern mit einer spastischen zerebralen Bewegungsstörung nachhaltig beeinflusst und dadurch wesentlich geschicktere Bewegungsabläufe erreicht werden. Der Einfluss der automatischen Körperstell- und Gleichgewichtsreaktionen auf die gesamte Mundmotorik insbesondere bei motorisch gestörten Patienten ist allerdings evident und durch videofluoroskopische Untersuchungen nachweisbar (Larnert und Ekberg 1995). Die Bemühungen bei der Physiotherapie nach dem Bobathkonzept, durch Inhibition von pathologischen Reaktionen und durch Facilitation möglichst normaler Bewegungsabläufe eine Verbesserung der aktiven zielgerichteten Bewegungen und Handlungen erreichen zu wollen, führen nur zu begrenzten Erfolgen. Auch die Vorstellung, dass durch spezifische physiotherapeutische Übungsbehandlungen wesentliche Symptome der zerebralen Bewegungsstörungen deutlich verringert werden könnten, hat sich nicht bewahrheitet (Bower et al. 2001). Ebensowenig lassen sich spezifische Effekte der krankengymnastischen Behandlung auf neurophysiologischer Grundlage nach dem Bobathkonzept (Butler u. Darrah 2001) bis heute verlässlich nachweisen.

Bei Kindern mit ausgeprägter Muskelhypotonie, ohne zerebrale Bewegungsstörung im eigentlichen Sinne, wie z.B. bei M. Down, kann dagegen durch die Stimulation von unterschiedlichen Muskeln bzw. Muskelgruppen durchaus eine Zunahme der Muskelkraft infolge aktiver Muskelarbeit erwartet werden. Es ist allerdings nicht zu erwarten, dass sich auch die Koordination der Bewegung »automatisch« verbessert und damit auch die Saug- Kau- und Schluckfunktionen oder die Artikulationsfähigkeit.

In einer Studie an Erwachsenen mit spastischen Zerebralparesen wiesen Barlow und Abbs (1984) nach, dass der Einfluss hyperaktiver (monosynaptischer) Muskelspindel-Reflexe auf die Mundmotorik unbedeutend ist. Sie untersuchten die Fähigkeit der Mundmuskulatur differenziert die Kraft zu kontrollieren. Bei der Lippen- und Zungenmuskulatur, die keine bzw. nur wenige Muskelspindeln besitzen, war die Koordinationsfähigkeit ebenso eingeschränkt wie bei der Kiefergelenkmuskulatur, die über sehr viele Muskelspindeln verfügt. Diese Studie weist außerdem auf die neurophysiologischen Unterschiede der mimischen, Zungen- und Kaumuskulatur hin, die für die Regulationstherapie von Bedeutung sind, da Vibrationsreize bei Muskeln ohne Muskelspindeln weniger effektiv sein können.

Evaluation der Behandlung

Von Castillo Morales wurden zahlreiche Fallbeobachtungen mitgeteilt, aber nie eine systematische Evaluationsstudie durchgeführt. Die vorliegenden Studien beschäftigen sich mit der Wirkung auf die Mundmotorik und das Essverhalten oder die Mundmotorik und die Sprachentwicklung; sie sind weder prospektiv noch kontrolliert geplant.

Mundmotorik und Essverhalten

Haberfellner et al. (1977) unternahmen erstmals den Versuch, die Effekte einer längerfristigen Behandlung (6–24 Monate) einschließlich der Anpassung von speziellen Gaumenplatten bei Kindern mit infantiler Zerebralparese zu dokumentieren. Bei allen 10 untersuchten Kindern besserten sich die geprüften Items: Empfindlichkeit der Mundschleimhaut, Kontrolle des Speichels, Nasenatmung, Artikulation. Eine Kontrollgruppe wurde nicht untersucht.

Selley und Boxhall (1986) berichten über die Erfahrungen mit 12 Säuglingen, die aus sehr unterschiedlichen Gründen die orale Ernährung verweigerten (z.B. M. Down, Missbildungssyndrom, Z. n. Pneumonie, psychogene Abwehr). Alle erhielten eine individuell angepasste Gaumenplatte und bei allen besserte sich das Essverhalten innerhalb weniger Tage bis Wochen; sie akzeptierten eine regelmäßige Flaschenernährung über den Sauger.

Limbrock et al. (1991) prüften die Behandlungserfolge einer orofazialen Regulationstherapie verbunden mit der Anpassung von Gaumenplatten bei Kindern mit M. Down. Die Kinder stammten aus der Inanspruchnahmepopulation des Kinderzentrums München. 89 Patienten wurden konsekutiv erfasst und in die Studie einbezogen, 22 brachen die Behandlung aus unterschiedlichen

Gründen ab. Die verbliebenen 67 Kinder (Alter 1 bis 73 Monate) wurden zwischen 7 bis 36 Monaten behandelt, zusätzlich zur krankengymnastischen Behandlung nach Bobath oder Vojta. Es wurden weder eine Kontrollgruppe gebildet noch Kontrollphasen mit und ohne Behandlung eingeplant. Alle Kinder wurden kinderneurologisch und zahnärztlich nach festgelegten Scores zu Beginn und nach Beendigung der Behandlung untersucht. Signifikante Effekte fanden sich hinsichtlich der Zungenposition, der Spannung und Haltung der Lippen, beim Mundschluss und beim Saugen.

Aus der gleichen Arbeitsgruppe stammen zwei mehrjährige Verlaufsstudien über die Wirkung einer Behandlung mit Gaumenplatte bei über 90 Kindern (Alter 0;7 bis 14 Jahre) mit zerebralen Bewegungsstörungen unterschiedlichen Ausmaßes. Die vorliegenden Befunde wurden retrospektiv beurteilt, wobei Behandlungszeiträume von durchschnittlich 6 Monaten ausgewertet wurden. Die Autoren stellten in beiden Kollektiven nicht nur verbesserte orale Atmung und besseren Lippenschluss fest, sondern auch verbesserte Funktionen im Schluckablauf und bei der Zungenbeweglichkeit (Weigert 1992, Weinfurtner 1992). Die Effekte waren bei geringer ausgeprägten Symptomen erwartungsgemäß größer. Eine Verschlechterung der Symptomatik bei einigen Patienten (Speichelflusskontrolle, Saugen und Artikulation) betraf vor allem Kinder mit geistiger Behinderung.

Nach Gisel et al. (1996) ist kritisch anzumerken, dass sich ähnliche Effekte bei verschiedenen sensomotorischen Behandlungsverfahren bei Kindern mit Dysphagie (z.B. bei zerebralen Bewegungsstörungen) bei Evaluationsstudien, die ebenfalls methodisch angreifbar sind, nachweisen ließen. Die Autoren führten eine eigene gut geplante Studie bei 27 Kindern mit CP durch und konnten zeigen, dass sich einige mundmotorische Fertigkeiten signifikant verbesserten, aber das Körpergewicht der Kinder in dem Beobachtungszeitraum von 10 Wochen im untersten Normbereich blieb.

Mundmotorik und Sprachentwicklung

Hohoff et al. (1998) untersuchten die Lautbildung von 10 Kindern mit M. Down (Durchschnittsalter 7 Jahre) im Vergleich zu gleichaltrigen gesunden Kindern in Abhängigkeit von Mundmotorik, Überbiss, Angle Faktor, Hörstörung, logopädischer Behandlung und Mundplattenbehandlung nach Castillo Morales (bei 5 Kindern). Sie setzten hierfür ein semiquantitatives Untersuchungsverfahren ein, die »Sonagraphie« (Aufzeichnung von Frequenz, Amplitude und Zeitdauer) eines Sprechsignals (»Tasse«). Bei den Trisomie-Kindern ergab sich eine höhere Variabilität der Befunde als bei den gesunden, sie artikulierten langsamer und undeutlicher. Es fanden sich aber keine signifikanten Korrelationen zu den geprüften Faktoren, insbesondere nicht zu der logopädischen Behandlung bzw. der früheren Versorgung mit Mundplatten.

Von der gleichen Arbeitsgruppe (Hohoff u. Ehmer 1997) wurde eine retrospektive Fragebogenerhebung über die Sprachentwicklung eine Untersuchung der Mundmotorik von 20 Kindern mit M. Down (Durchschnittsalter 55 Monate) durchgeführt. Nach Angaben der Eltern verlief die Sprachentwicklung der Kinder, die eine Mundplattenbehandlung erhalten hatten, (nicht signifikant) schneller als die der Kontrollgruppe von 20 gleichaltrigen Kindern, bei denen die Behandlung mit Gaumenplatte aus unterschiedlichen Gründen nach einem Monat beendet worden war, obwohl bei den behandelten Kindern die Sprachentwicklung später begann und mehr Risikofaktoren für eine gestörte Sprachentwicklung bestanden. Bei 75% der Kinder hatte sich die Zungen- und Mundhaltung dauerhaft gebessert.

Unerwünschte Wirkungen

Haberstock (1999) weist darauf hin, dass der Mundbereich besonders empfindlich sei und nie mit Druck und Zwang gearbeitet werden dürfe, »da sich sonst ganz andere Beziehungs- und Verhaltensprobleme daraus entwickeln, bis hin zur völligen Nahrungsverweigerung«. In der Tat wird zum Teil mit einer intensiven Behandlung bereits in den ersten Lebensmonaten begonnen, z.B. bei Kindern mit Essstörungen, bei orofazialer Dysregulation oder bei Dysphagie, und selbst wenn keine eindeutigen Effekte auf die Kau- und Schluckmotorik erreicht werden konnten, langfristig weitergeführt. Dadurch kann es zu einer unnötigen Belastung für Kind und Angehörige und zur Verstärkung der Essstörungen kommen.

Zusammenfassende Beurteilung

Die orofaziale Regulationstherapie nach Castillo Morales gibt gute praktische Anleitungen im Umgang mit Kindern mit Störungen des Mundschlusses aufgrund einer generellen Muskelhypotonie oder mit Störungen der Nahrungsaufnahme bei zerebralen Bewegungsstörung. Die theoretischen Vorstellungen über die Wirksamkeit des Konzeptes müssen kritisch beurteilt werden, da sie unter neurophysiologischen Aspekten z.T. wissenschaftlich nicht begründbar sind. Die spezifischen manuellen Behandlungstechniken der sensorischen Stimulation durch Berühren, Streichen, Zug, Druck und Vibration der äusseren Gesichts-, Mund- und Kaumuskulatur können nur unter bestimmten Voraussetzungen eingesetzt werden. Zunächst sind Ausgangsstellungen von Körper- und Kopfhaltung individuell zu schaffen, die auf den Erfahrungen der Physiotherapie nach dem Bobath Konzept beruhen und zu einer verbesserten Muskelspannung und Mobilität von Zunge, Kiefergelenken und Schluckakt führen. Dabei werden auch durch spezielle Techniken die Kopf- und Kieferhaltung kontrolliert.

Es entspricht der allgemeinen Erfahrung, dass insbesondere bei Kindern mit zerebralen Bewegungsstörungen durch Veränderungen der Körperhaltung auch die Kopfkontrolle positiv beeinflusst werden kann und bei einer verbesserten Ausgangssituation in der axialen Kontrolle sich die Mobilität und Zielsicherheit der Greif- und Handfunktionen sowie der Mundfunktionen verbessern. Wenn es gelingt, die Angehörigen adäquat in diesem Bereich anzuleiten und so die Erfahrungen und Effekte aus den Therapiesituationen in den Alltag zu transferieren, ist auch eine nachhaltige Auswirkung auf die Funktionen Lippen- und Mundschluss sowie der damit verbundenen Speichelkontrolle, ebenso wie auf die Akzeptanz von Saug-, Kau- und Schluckfunktionen bei der Fütterung zu erwarten. Inwieweit auch die Artikulationsstörungen beeinflusst werden können, ist ungeklärt. Art und Ausmaß der Effekte wurden allerdings bisher nur in unkontrollierten Verlaufsbeobachtungen oder in Fallberichten dokumentiert. Somit fehlt bisher der wissenschaftlich abgesicherte Nachweis von spezifischen Behandlungseffekten.

Über die Wirksamkeit zusätzlicher Maßnahmen wie der Einsatz einer Gaumenplatte und von anderen Hilfsmitteln zur Stimulation in der Mundhöhle gibt es viele Erfahrungsberichte und Anwendungsbeobachtungen mit positiven Effekten aber ebenfalls keine kontrollierten Studien. Ihr Einsatz erfordert große Erfahrung und sollte spezialisierten Arbeitsgruppen (Neuropädiatrie-Kieferorthopädie) vorbehalten bleiben.

Eine generelle Wirksamkeit konnte für die orofaziale Regulationstherapie bisher nicht nachgewiesen werden. Daher ist eindrücklich vor der Annahme zu warnen, dass eine möglichst frühe und intensive Behandlung besonders effektiv wäre, auch wenn sich Akzeptanz und Mitarbeit des Kindes nur bedingt erreichen lassen oder gar zunehmend Abwehrverhalten auftritt. Die orofaziale Regulationstherapie kann ein Mosaikstein innerhalb eines Gesamtbehandlungskonzeptes bei Kindern mit Störungen der Mundschluss-, Saug-, Kau- und Schluckfunktionen sein, die allerdings nur unter Berücksichtigung anderer Massnahmen indiziert erscheint.

Literatur

1. Barlow SM, Abbs JH (1984) Orofacial fine motor control impairments in congenital spasticity: evidence against hypertonus-related performance deficits. Neurology 34:145-150
2. Bower E, Mitchell D, Burnett M, Campbell MJ, McLellan DL (2001) Randomized controlled trial of physiotherapy in 56 children with cerebral palsy followed for 18 months. Dev Med Child Neurol 43:4–15
3. Butler C, Darrah J (2001) Effects of neurodevelopmental treatment (NDT) for cerebral palsy: AACPDM evidence report. Dev Med Child Neurol 43:778–790
4. Castillo Morales R (1991) Die orofaciale Regulationstherapie. Pflaum, München
5. Castillo Morales R, Molina G, Limbrock GJ (1995) Primäre Zungenbewegungen. Sozialpädiatrie 17:33–35
6. Castillo Morales R (2000) Das Castillo Morales-Konzept: Die motorische Ruhe. Ergotherapie und Rehabilitation 39: 20–24
7. Gisel EG, Applegate-Ferrante T, Benson J, Bosma JF (1996) Oral-motor skills following sensorimotor therapy in two groups of moderately dysphagic children with cerebral palsy: aspiration vs nonaspiration. Dysphagia 11:59–71
8. Haberfellner H, Rossiwall B (1977) Appliances for treatment of oral-sensori-motor disorders.
9. Haberstock B (1999) Castillo-Morales-Konzept. In: Hartmannsgruber R, Wenzel D (Hrsg) Physiotherapie, Band 12, Pädiatrie Neuropädiatrie: 118-139, Thieme Stuttgart
10. Hohoff A, Ehmer U (1997) Die Effekte der Stimulationsplattentherapie nach Castillo-Morales auf die Sprachentwicklung von Kindern mit Trisomie 21. J Orofac Ortop/Fortschritte der Kieferorthopädie 58:330–339
11. Hohoff A, Seifert E, Ehmer U, Lamprecht-Dürssen A (1998) Die Sprachlautbildung von Kindern mit Morbus Down. Eine Pilotstudie. J Orofac Ortop/ Fortschr Kieferorthop 59:220–228
12. Larnert G, Ekberg G (1995) Positioning improves the oral and pharyngeal swallowing function in children with cerebral palsy. Acta Paediatr 64:689–692

13. Limbrock GJ, Hoyer H, Hesse A (1987) Die Mundvorhofspange – eine Ergänzung zur Therapie sensomotorischer Störungen im Mundbereich. der kinderarzt 18: 373–376
14. Limbrock GJ, Fischer-Brandies H, Avalle C (1991) Castillo Morales' orofacial therapy: treatment of 67 children with Down Syndrom. Dev Med Child Neurol 33:296–303
15. Ohrt B (1999) Die Wurzeln des Bobath-Konzepts. Krankengymnastik – Zeitschrift für Physiotherapeuten 3:395–402
16. Orth H, Block R (1987) Die Beeinflussung orofacialer Funktionen durch die Wirbelsäulenhaltung. der kinderarzt 18: 1173–1177
17. Weigert G (1992) Der Einfluss der Gaumenplatte nach Castillo Morales auf die orofazialen Dysfunktionen bei zerebral bewegungsgestörten Patienten. Dissertation, Medizinische Fakultät der LMU München
18. Weinfurtner KB (1992) Gestörte Mundmotorik bei Kindern mit Cerebralparese. Behandlung mit der orofazialen Regulationstherapie nach Castillo Morales. Vergleich der mundmotorischen Befunde mit den Variationen der Gaumenplatten. Dissertation, Medizinische Fakultät LMU München
19. Selley G, Boxhall J (1986) A new way to treat and swalloing difficulties in babies. The Lancet May 24: 1182–1184
20. Von Treuenfels H (1985) Über die Relation von Dysgnathie, Haltungsfehlern und Deformitäten der Wirbelsäule. Dtsch Zschr Biologische Zahn-Medizin

Autoren- und Sachwortverzeichnis

Autorenverzeichnis

Aicardi J.
Hôpital Robert Debré
48, boulevard Sérurier
F-75019 Paris

Assmann B.
Universitäts-Kinderlinik
Im Neuenheimer Feld 150
69120 Heidelberg

Bast Th.
Universitätskinderklinik Heidelberg
Im Neuenheimer Feld 150
69120 Heidelberg

Baumeister F.A.M.
Technische Universität München
Kinderklinik Schwabing
Kölner Platz 1
80804 München

Bäumel C.
Behandlungszentrum Vogtareuth
Abteilung Neuropädiatrie
Krankenhausstraße 20
83569 Vogtareuth

Binder A.C.
Johann Wolfgang-Goethe-Universität
Pädiatrische Neurologie
Theodor-Stern-Kai 7
60596 Frankfurt a.M.

Blankenburg M.
Vestische Kinder-
und Jugendklinik Datteln
Universität Witten/Herdecke
Dr.-Friedrich-Steiner-Straße 5
45711 Datteln

Blaschek A.
Universitätsklinik Heidelberg
Pädiatrische Neurologie
Im Neuenheimer Feld 150
69120 Heidelberg

Boda V.
Johann Wolfgang-Goethe-Universität
Pädiatrische Neurologie
Theodor-Stern-Kai 7
60596 Frankfurt a.M.

Bode H.
Sozialpädiatrisches Zentrum
Schillerstraße 15
89077 Ulm

Boltshauser E.
Kinderspital Zürich
Steinwiesstraße 75
CH-8032 Zürich

Boor R.
Universitätskinderklinik Mainz
Langenbeckstraße 1
55101 Mainz

Borusiak P.
Zentrum für Kinder-
und Jugendmedizin
Klinikum Wuppertal GmbH
Heusnerstraße 40
42283 Wuppertal

Brockhaus A.
Behandlungszentrum Vogtareuth
Abteilung Neuropädiatrie
Krankenhausstraße 20
83569 Vogtareuth

Carmona H.
Universitätsklinikum Freiburg
Neurozentrum
Breisacher Straße 64
79106 Freiburg

Ceballos-Baumann A.O.
Klinikum rechts der Isar
Neurologische Klinik
Möhlstraße 28
81675 München

Dralle D.
Universitätsklinikum Gießen
Feulgenstraße 12
35385 Gießen

Dundurs D.
Westpfalz-Klinikum
Kinderklinik
Hellmut-Hartert-Straße 1
67655 Kaiserslautern

Ebinger F.
Universitätsklinik Heidelberg
Im Neuenheimer Feld 150
69120 Heidelberg

Faist M.
Universitätsklinikum Freiburg
Neurozentrum
Breisacher Straße 64
79106 Freiburg

Feuerstein T.J.
Universitätsklinikum Freiburg
Neurozentrum
Breisacher Straße 64
79106 Freiburg

Forssberg H.
Astrid Lindgren Children's Hospital
SE-17176 Stockholm – Sweden

Forst J.
Friedrich-Alexander-Universität
Orthopädische Klinik
Rathsberger Straße 57
91054 Erlangen

Gold R.
Julius-Maximilians-Universität
Neurologische Klinik
Josef-Schneider-Straße 11
97080 Würzburg

Grohmann K.
Universität Würzburg
Neurologische Klinik
Josef-Schneider-Straße 11
97080 Würzburg

Gruber-Sedlmayr U.
Univ.-Klinik für Kinder-
und Jugendheilkunde Graz
Auenbruggerplatz 30
A-8036 Graz

Härtel C.
Universitätsklinikum Lübeck
Klinik für Kinder- und Jugendmedizin
Ratzeburger Allee 160
23538 Lübeck

Heinen F.
Wedau-Kliniken
Klinik für Kinderheilkunde
und Jugendmedizin
Zu den Rehwiesen 9
47055 Duisburg

Hennig J.
Universitätsklinikum Freiburg
Radiologische Klinik
Hugstetterstraße 55
79106 Freiburg

Homberg V.
Universitätsklinikum Freiburg
Neurozentrum
Breisacher Straße 64
79106 Freiburg

Hoppen Th.
Städt. Klinikum Kemperhof
Klinik für Kinder- und Jugendmedizin
Koblenzer Straße 115–155
56065 Koblenz

Huppertz H.-J.
Universitätsklinikum Freiburg
Neurozentrum
Breisacher Straße 64
79106 Freiburg

Huppke P.
Georg-August-Universität
Zentrum Kinderheilkunde
Robert-Koch-Straße 40
37075 Göttingen

Karch D.
Kinderzentrum Maulbronn gGmbH
Knittlinger Steige 21
75433 Maulbronn

Kehrer M.
Universitätsklinik Tübingen
Abteilung Neonatologie
Hoppe-Seyler-Straße 1
72076 Tübingen

Kessler S.
Universitätsklinikum Kiel
Klinik für Neuropädiatrie
Schwanenweg 20
24105 Kiel

Kieslich M.
Johann Wolfgang-Goethe-Universität
Zentrum der Kinderheilkunde
Theodor-Stern-Kai 7
60596 Frankfurt a.M.

Kirschner J.
Universitätsklinikum Freiburg
Klinik für Neuropädiatrie
und Muskelerkrankungen
Mathildenstraße 1
79106 Freiburg

Klepper J.
Universitätsklinikum Essen
Klinik für Kinderheilkunde
und Jugendmedizin
Hufelandstraße 55
45122 Essen

Klusmann A.
Heinrich-Heine-Universität
Zentrum für Kinderheilkunde
Moorenstraße 5
40225 Düsseldorf

Kölker S.
Universitäts-Kinderklinik Heidelberg
Im Neuenheimer Feld 150
69120 Heidelberg

König St.
Universitäts-Kinderklinik Mannheim
Theodor-Kutzer-Ufer 1–3
68135 Mannheim

Korall H.
Zentrum für Stoffwechseldiagnostik
Reutlingen GmbH
Wörthstraße 47
72764 Reutlingen

Kortmann R.-D.
Universitätsklinikum Tübingen
Abteilung Radioonkologie
Hoppe-Seyler-Straße 3
72076 Tübingen

Krägeloh-Mann I.
Eberhard-Karls-Universität Tübingen
Klinik für Kinderheilkunde
Abteilung III
Hoppe-Seyler-Straße 1
72076 Tübingen

Kühl J.
Universitäts-Kinderklinik Würzburg
Josef-Schneider-Straße 1
97080 Würzburg

Landwehrmeyer G.B.
Neurologische Universitätsklinik Ulm
Steinhövelstraße 9
89075 Ulm

Lidzba K.
Eberhard-Karls-Universität Tübingen
Klinik für Kinderheilkunde
Abteilung III
Hoppe-Seyler-Straße 1
72076 Tübingen

Liebhaber M.
Technische Universität München
Kinderklinik Schwabing
Kölner Platz 1
80804 München

Linder M.
Universitätsklinikum Freiburg
Klinik für Neuropädiatrie
und Muskelerkrankungen
Mathildenstraße 1
79106 Freiburg

Lipinski C.G.
Kinderklinik im Fachkrankenhaus
Neckargemünd
69151 Neckargemünd

Longin E.
Universitäts-Kinderklinik Mannheim
Theodor-Kutzer-Ufer 1–3
68135 Mannheim

Lücke T.
Medizinische Hochschule Hannover
Kinderklinik Abteilung II
Carl-Neuberg-Straße 1
30623 Hannover

Maiwald T.
Universitätsklinik Freiburg
Neurozentrum
Breisacher Straße 64
79106 Freiburg

Mall V.
Universitätsklinikum Freiburg
Klinik für Neuropädiatrie
und Muskelerkrankungen
Mathildenstraße 1
79106 Freiburg

Manzur A.Y.
Hammersmith Hospital
Ducane Road
London W12 OHS – UK

Martin P.
Epilepsiezentrum Kork
Landstraße 1
77694 Kehl-Kork

Merkenschlager A.
Universitätsklinikum Leipzig
Klinik für Kinder- und Jugendliche
Oststraße 21–25
04317 Leipzig

Niederhofer H.
Univ.-Klinik für Psychiatrie
Anichstraße 35
A-6020 Innsbruck

Noser E.
Ostschweizer Kinderspital St. Gallen
Neuropädiatrie
CH-9000 St. Gallen

Ostertag Ch.
Universität Freiburg
Abteilung Stereotaxie
und Neuronuclearmedizin
Breisacher Straße 64
79106 Freiburg

Panteliadis C.
Aristotle University of Thessaloniki
3rd Deparment of Pediatrics
Hippokration Hospital
Konstantinoupoloes 49
54642 Thessaloniki – Griechenland

Philippi H.
Johannes Gutenberg-Universität
Kinderklinik
Langenbeckstraße 1
55101 Mainz

Pohl D.
Georg-August-Universität
Schwerpunkt Neuropädiatrie
Robert-Koch-Straße 40
37075 Göttingen

Preuß N.
Heinrich-Heine-Universität
Zentrum für Kinderheilkunde
Moorenstraße 5
40225 Düsseldorf

Reckert T.
Filderklinik
Im Haberschlai 7
70794 Filderstadt

Reinhold A.
Charité Campus Virchow
Neuropädiatrie
Augustenburger Platz 1
13353 Berlin

Schara U.
Ruhr-Universität Bochum
Klinik für Kinder- und Jugendmedizin
Alexandrinenstraße 5
44791 Bochum

Schilling S.
Medizinische Universität Lübeck
Abteilung für Neuropädiatrie
Ratzeburger Allee 160
23538 Lübeck

Schlack H.G.
Rheinisches Kinderneurologisches
Zentrum
Waldenburger Ring 46
53119 Bonn

Schmitt B.
Kinderspital Zürich
Steinwiesstraße 75
CH-8032 Zürich

Schulze-Bonhage A.
Universitätsklinikum Freiburg
Neurozentrum
Breisacher Straße 64
79106 Freiburg

Schwake C.
Ruhrlandklinik Essen
Tüschener Weg 40
45239 Essen

Schwerin A.
Wedau-Kliniken
Klinik für Kinderheilkunde
und Jugendmedizin
Zu den Rehwiesen 9
47055 Duisburg

Severin T.
Universitätsklinikum Freiburg
Zentrum für Kinderheilkunde
und Jugendmedizin
Mathildenstraße 1
79106 Freiburg

Skirl G.
Klinikum der Friedrich-Schiller-
Universität Jena
Klinik für Kinder- und Jugendmedizin
07740 Jena

Sperner J.
Medizinische Universität Lübeck
Klinik für Kinder- und Jugendmedizin
Ratzeburger Allee 160
23538 Lübeck

Springer S.
Kinderklinik und Kinderpoliklinik
im Dr. von Haunerschen
Kinderspital der LMU
Lindwurmstraße 4
80337 München

Staudt M.
Universitätsklinikum Tübingen
Radiologische Klinik
Hoppe-Seyler-Straße 3
72076 Tübingen

Steinlin M.
Universitätsspital Bern
Medizinische Universitäts-
Kinderklinik
CH-3010 Bern

Straßburg H.M.
Universitäts-Kinderklinik Würzburg
Josef-Schneider-Straße 2
97080 Würzburg

Straub V.
Universitätsklinikum Essen
Zentrum für Kinderheilkunde
Hufelandstraße 55
45122 Essen

Teich M.
Universitäts-Kinderklinik Mannheim
Theodor-Kutzer-Ufer 1–3
68135 Mannheim

Treiss I.
Universitäts-Kinderklinik
Theodor-Kutzer-Ufer 1–3
68167 Mannheim

Utzig N.
Ernst-Moritz-Arndt-Universität
Greifswald
Klinik für Kinder- und Jugendmedizin
Soldtmannstraße15
17487 Greifswald

Vlaho S.
Johann Wolfgang-Goethe-Universität
Pädiatrische Neurologie
Theodor-Stern-Kai 7
60596 Frankfurt a.M.

Vollmer B.
Universitätskinderklinik Tübingen
Hoppe-Seyler-Straße 1
72076 Tübingen

von Maydell B.
Universitäts-Kinderklinik Freiburg
Klinik für Neuropädiatrie
und Muskelerkrankungen
Mathildenstraße 1
79106 Freiburg

Wänninger J.
Behandlungszentrum Vogtareuth
Abteilung Neuropädiatrie
Krankenhausstraße 20
83569 Vogtareuth

Wesendahl M.
Johann Wolfgang-Goethe-Universität
Zentrum für Kinderheilkunde
und Jugendmedizin
Theodor-Stern-Kai 7
60596 Frankfurt a.M.

Wiemer-Kruel A.
Epilepsiezentrum Kork
Landstraße 1
77694 Kehl-Kork

Wilke M.
Technische Universität München
Kinderklinik Schwabing
Kölner Platz 1
80804 München

Willig G.
Zentrum für Kinderheilkunde und
Jugendmedizin
Feulgenstraße 12
35385 Gießen

Wollinsky K.H.
Orthopädische und Neurologische
Klinik der Universität Ulm
Oberer Eselsberg 45
89081 Ulm

Zafeiriou D.I.
1ste Paediatrische Klinik
Aristotle Universitaet
Egnatia St. 106
54642 Thessaloniki – Griechenland

Sachwortverzeichnis